Handbook of

CLINICAL TOXICOLOGY of ANIMAL VENOMS and POISONS

Handbook of
CLINICAL TOXICOLOGY of ANIMAL VENOMS and POISONS

Edited by

JÜRG MEIER
Director
Pentapharm Ltd
Basel, Switzerland

JULIAN WHITE
Director
State Toxinology Services (South Australia)
Women's and Children's Hospital
North Adelaide, Australia

CRC Press
Boca Raton   New York   London   Tokyo

Library of Congress Cataloging-in-Publication Data

Clinical toxicology of animal venoms / editors. Jürg Meier and Julian
  White
    p.   cm.
  Includes bibliographical references and index.
  ISBN 0-8493-4489-1
  1. Venom. I. Meier, J. (Jürg) II. White, Julian, 1952-
  [DNLM: 1. Venoms. 2. Animals, Poisonous. WD 400 C641 1995]
RA1255.C55 1995
615.9′42--dc20

DNLM/DLC
for Library of Congress
                                                      95-17705
                                                          CIP

No claim to original U.S. Government works
International Standard Book Number 0-8493-4489-1
Library of Congress Card Number 95-17705
Printed in the United States of America 1 2 3 4 5 6 7 8 9 0
Printed on acid-free paper

INTRODUCTION

This book realises our long standing desire to produce a form of textbook for the field of clinical toxinology. That the title still refers to "toxicology" represents the reality that as a clinical specialty, toxinology is yet to be fully recognised. We hope that this book will advance toxinology towards specialty recognition within the medical fraternity. However, and more importantly, we hope the information contained herein, brought together for the first time in a single book, will prove useful to all those throughout the world who must diagnose and treat people envenomed or poisoned by animals. We realise that this first attempt at such a book has imperfections, and does not cover every type of venomous and poisonous animal known to man, but nevertheless, the reader will find few significant groups have been omitted. All major groups causing significant morbidity or mortality in humans are mentioned, mostly with detailed chapters, or, as in the case of venomous snakes, a series of chapters. One major problem encountered has been the lack of detailed clinical knowledge on the effects of bites/stings/poisoning by individual species of animal. There are a number of species of snake, and some other animals where such information is available, as detailed in this book. Unfortunately, for many species, including some of probable medical importance, such information is either scarce, incomplete, or simply non-existent. Even case reports may be lacking for some species. A book such as this can only be as good as the information available to those compling it. We therefore urge you, the reader, to write to us with any information from your own experience in medical practice, which may add to the material herein published. Even single case reports can be most useful, if well documented. Case reports of a series of bites/stings by a particular animal species thought to be venomous, all of which had no or trivial effects, are as valuable as those detailing major envenoming, for only through such information can we hope to note those venomous species about which we should have less concern. Equally, if you, the reader, have managed or know of a case of bite/sting/poisoning by an animal, where the clinical details appear to contradict information in this book, then let us know! We do not have a monopoly on knowledge in toxinology. There is undoubtedly a great deal yet for us to learn about the world of venomous and poisonous animals and their interaction with man.

Having discussed the limitations of this book, we wish to express our belief that the book has many strengths, for which we are largely indebted to the chapter authors who have so richly endowed the text, not just through their contributions to the text, but through the many years of work they have given to toxinology, in its various aspects, in the past. Some of the most outstanding contributors to clinical toxinology have written chapters for this book. As the reader will note, there are some large and wonderfully comprehensive chapters which we believe will long stand as essential reviews of their respective topics. To all our chapter authors we say a heartfelt "thank you".

It now remains for you, the reader, to take the information contained in this book, and use it. We hope that many patients will have cause to be thankful for this. Therefore our last thank you is to our readers.

Jürg Meier

Julian White

September 1994

ACKNOWLEDGMENTS

The production of this book has been a long and often problematic process. We (the Editors) wish to thank our respective employers for the generous provision of resources, especially time, so essential to completion of this project. We thank our many colleagues who have assisted, through ideas, comments, provision of illustrations and in other ways. This book has been produced largely by us using personal computers, including "typesetting", but this task has been greatly helped by special cooperation from CRC Press, particularly Jennifer Pate and Carol Messing, to whom we owe a special debt of thanks, and Harvey Kane for supporting this project through numerous delays and missed deadlines.

THE EDITORS

Dr. Jurg Meier, PhD, born in 1954, has studied Natural Sciences, main subject Biology, at the University of Basel, Switzerland. He performed a Ph.D. thesis on the venom of the South American lance adder *Bothrops atrox*, at the Swiss Tropical Institute in Basel under the auspices of Prof. Dr. Thierry A. Freyvogel. He currently is in the position of a Senior Vice President in Pentapharm Ltd., a company, which, beyond other activities, manufactures snake venom components acting on the blood coagulation system. These components are useful tools in basic biomedical research, as well as in the diagnosis and treatment of blood coagulation disorders.

As a member of the executive committee of Pentapharm Ltd., he is also responsible for Pentapharm do Brasil Ltda., the world's largest industrial snake farm, where snakes are bred and kept with the purpose of gaining high quality snake venom in sufficient quantity for the manufacturing process of specific snake venom products. As an associate professor of Zoology, he lectures on venomous and poisonous animals, their venoms and poisons, and supervises Ph.D. students at the University of Basel, Switzerland, who investigate venom-related topics. In 1989, he was elected secretary of the European section of the International Society on Toxinology, a position he currently holds. He is author or co-author of more than 50 publications in the field of toxinology.

Dr. Julian White, M.B., B.S., M.D. (Adel.), F.A.C.T.M., born in 1952, studied medicine at the University of Adelaide. He gained his M.D. in 1988, for work in the field of clinical toxinology. He is Director of State Toxinology Services (South Australia), based at the Women's and Children's Hospital, Adelaide. He is Consultant Toxinologist to most of the Adelaide teaching hospitals, and gives lectures on aspects of toxinology to medical students at the University of Adelaide, health professionals in several institutions, and as part of medical postgraduate training for resident medical staff and trainees in some specialist medical Colleges.

He is a member of the International Society on Toxinology (IST), a Council Member of the Asia Pacific Section of the IST, Vice President, Asia Pacific Association of Clinical Toxicology. He has also been an active member of numerous related professional societies including, the Royal Society of South Australia, the Australian Society of Herpetologists, The Australasian Association of Arachnologists, the Society for the Study of Amphibians and Reptiles, the Herpetologists League, and the Societas Europea Herpetologica.

He has worked on aspects of toxinology internationally through the INTOX Project (IPCS/WHO), for which he has written several Poison Information Monographs, and is an Associate Editor of POISINDEX. He is a Consultant on toxinology to a number of international companies, including some of the major antivenom producers, and to a variety of organisations and institutions outside Australia.

His particular interests in toxinology include snakebite, snake venom research (especially those active on the coagulation system), spiderbite, antivenom, and the development of professional training in clinical toxinology. He is the author or co-author of more than 60 publications in the field of toxinology.

CONTRIBUTORS

Chris Acott
Senior Specialist, Department of
Anaesthesia and Intensive Care, Royal
Adelaide Hospital
North Tce, Adelaide SA 5000 AUSTRALIA

Andre Aeschlimann
Zoological Institute,
University of Neuchatel
2000 Neuchatel
SWITZERLAND

Alejandro C. Alagon
Instituto de Biotecnologia, Universidad
Nacional Autonoma de Mexico
Av. Universidad 2001,
Apartado Postal 510-3,
Cuernavaca, Morelos 62271, MEXICO

Joseph W. Burnett
Professor, Department of Dermatology,
University of Maryland Hospital
405 W. Redwood St., Baltimore, Maryland
21201, U.S.

J. L. C. Cardoso
Hospital Vital Brazil, Instituto Butantan
av. Vital Brazil,
1500, 05503-900 Sao Paulo
BRAZIL

Mireille Chinain
Institut Territorial de Recherches Medicales
Louis Malarde
BP 30 Papeete, Tahiti, FRENCH
POLYNESIA

Lourdes J. Cruz
Marine Science Institute, College of Science,
University of the Philippines
PO Box 1, Diliman, Quezon City 1101,
PHILIPPINES

Richard C. Dart
Rocky Mountain Poison Center
Denver, Colorado 80204
U.S.

Manuel Dehasa-Davila
Instituto de Biotecnologia, Universidad
Nacional Autonoma de Mexico
Av. Universidad 2001,
Apartado Postal 510-3,
Cuernavaca, Morelos 62271, MEXICO

Hui Wen Fan
Hospital Vital Brazil, Instituto Butantan
av. Vital Brazil,
1500, 05503-900 Sao Paulo
BRAZIL

Thierry A. Freyvogel
Swiss Tropical Institute
P.O. Box
4002 Basel
SWITZERLAND

Philippe Glaziou
Institut Territorial de Recherches Medicales
Louis Malarde
BP 30 Papeete, Tahiti, FRENCH
POLYNESIA

Hernan F. Gomez
University of Michigan Medical Center
Dept. of Emergency Medicine
Ann Arbor, Michigan 48109, U.S.

Jose Maria Gutierrez
Instituto Clodomiro Picado, Facultad de
Microbiologia, Universidad de Costa Rica
San Jose, COSTA RICA

Nobuo Kaku
Department of Emergency and Critical Care
Medicine,
Kurume University School of Medicine
Fukuoka, JAPAN

Anne-Marie Legrand
Institut Territorial de Recherches Medicales
Louis Malarde
BP 30 Papeete, Tahiti, FRENCH
POLYNESIA

Slyvia M. Lucas
Hospital Vital Brazil
Department of Biology, Instituto Butantan
PO Box 65, Sao Paulo, BRAZIL

Jurg Meier
Pentapharm Ltd.
P.O. Box
4002 Basel, SWITZERLAND

Dr. Hans Persson
Director, Swedish Poisons Information
Centre, Karolinska Hospital
Box 60500,
10401 Stockholm,
SWEDEN

David Smart
Senoir Specialist in Emergency Medicine,
Royal Hobart Hospital
Hobart Tas 7000 AUSTRALIA

David A. Warrell
Nuffield Dept. of Clinical Medicine,
John Radcliffe Hospital
Headington, OXFORD OX3 9DU,
UNITED KINGDOM

John Williamson
Director of Hyperbaric Medicine,
Department of Anaesthesia and Intensive
Care, Royal Adelaide Hospital
North Tce, Adelaide SA 5000 AUSTRALIA

Dietrich Mebs
Professor, Zentrum der Rechtsmedizin,
University of Frankfurt
Kennedyallee 104, Frankfurt D-6000
GERMANY

Holger Mosbech
Allergy Unit TTA 75 11
National University Hospital
2200 Copenhagen, DENMARK

Lourival D. Possani
Instituto de Biotecnologia, Universidad
Nacional Autonoma de Mexico
Av. Universidad 2001,
Apartado Postal 510-3,
Cuernavaca, Morelos 62271, MEXICO

Kurt Stocker
Pentapharm Ltd.
P.O. Box
4002 Basel, SWITZERLAND

Julian White
Clinical Toxinologist and Director,
State Toxinology Services,
Women's and Children's Hospital
North Adelaide SA 5006 AUSTRALIA

TABLE OF CONTENTS

Chapter 1

VENOMOUS AND POISONOUS ANIMALS - A BIOLOGIST'S VIEW

Jürg Meier

TABLE OF CONTENTS

I. INTRODUCTION

Venomous animals both fascinate and frighten humanity in a way no other living creatures probably do. Personal "polls" evaluated with the contribution of several hundred students attending my lectures on the subject over the last decade revealed that snakes, followed by spiders and scorpions, at least in Europe, seem to be the most feared animals of all. Religious and cultural misconceptions and miseducation as a consequence of poor knowledge on the biology and behaviour of these animals may account for this. However, the most important venomous animals, at least from a medical point-of-view, are doubtless social wasps and bees, since their venoms may lead to life-threatening anaphylactic reactions. In these cases, however, death is not a consequence of the toxic potential of the venoms, but of immunological "nonsense" reactions (anaphylactic shock) taking place in the victim's body. Even in small countries, like Switzerland, two to ten fatalities following bee and wasp stings are reported per year[1].

Venomous animals of medical importance are much better investigated than venomous animals, which have no impact on human activities. This is understandable, although animal

1

venoms have not evolved as tools against human beings. On the contrary, every envenomation of humans by venomous animals is to be seen as either an ultimate emergency reaction in defense or as an unfortunate incident.

As a consequence, it is up to us to prevent painful encounters with venomous animals. There exists a range of simple prophylactic measures to be taken. In following them, accidents may almost completely be prevented. Moreover, should an accident with venomous animals happen, simple first aid measures are applicable to prevent major discomfort in the majority of cases. The most important first aid measure, and this cannot be stressed enough, is to reassure the patient that **he is not going to die just because he has been bitten or stung by a venomous animal**!

Whenever possible, it is advised to see the nearest medical doctor and to be supervised by medical staff for the next couple of hours. Although in the majority of cases, the patient may recover without major signs and symptoms of envenomation, anything from no reaction to death may happen, depending on the animal involved and the circumstances of envenomation.

Most interestingly, people do not consider poisoning following ingestion of animals, when asked about toxic animals. Indeed, poisonous animals are responsible for a high number of intoxications every year. In contrast to venomous animals, where terrestrial organisms are mainly involved, poisonous animals of medical importance are predominantly marine organisms. Here again, prevention is easily performed provided there exists some basic knowledge of the respective organism's biology and distribution.

This book deals exclusively with venomous and poisonous animals of medical importance. Although not covered here and investigated to a much lesser extent, those venomous and poisonous animals which do not harm humans might even be much more fascinating from a biological point-of-view, since venom interactions between different organismic populations in a given ecosystem might reveal a greater understanding of limiting factors and even information flux between different organisms.

II. SOME BASIC DEFINITIONS

When dealing with venomous and poisonous animals, knowledge of the following basic definitions is essential[2,3]:

A. TOXINOLOGY

The term **Toxinology** was introduced in 1962, when the ***International Society on Toxinology*** was founded[4]. This society was established with the aim to accumulate and exchange knowledge on the venoms and poisons derived from animals, plants and microorganisms. Since the word "biotoxin" is often used for toxins derived from these sources, the term "biotoxicology" was taken under consideration for a short time. However, the prefix "bio-" was found to be redundant, because "toxins" are invariably derived from living organisms. Thus, Toxinology was thought to be more appropriate.

Consequently, this field of natural sciences may be defined as follows:

Toxinology *is the science of toxic substances produced by or accumulated in living organisms, their properties and their biological significance for the organisms involved.*

With reference to the animal kingdom, a difference is made between **venoms** and **poisons**.

B. VENOMS

Venoms are produced in specialized tissues or glands (venom glands), which often are connected with application structures (stings, teeth, etc.). The respective animals are referred to as **venomous** and the venoms are of biological significance. **Envenomation** takes place after parenteral application or upon contact.

Upon oral ingestion by mammals, many venoms are destroyed. The animals concerned need their venoms either primarily for self-defense, e.g. the lionfish (Figure 1) or primarily for the aquisition of prey, e.g. snakes and spiders (Figure 2). Venomous animals posses a **venom apparatus** composed of glands, (an) excretory duct(s) and often application devices such as fangs, stings, darts, chelicerae, etc.

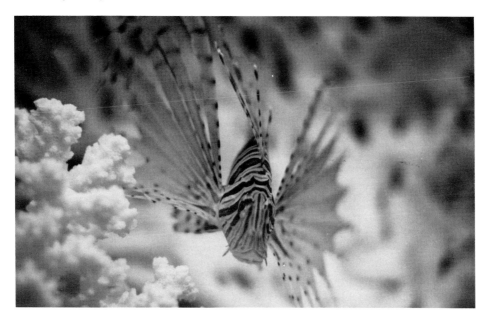

Figure 1. The Lionfish (*Pterois volitans*) is a marine venomous animal, which uses its venom primarily in defense. The venom apparatus is located in the dorsal, pectoral and ventral fins (photo by author).

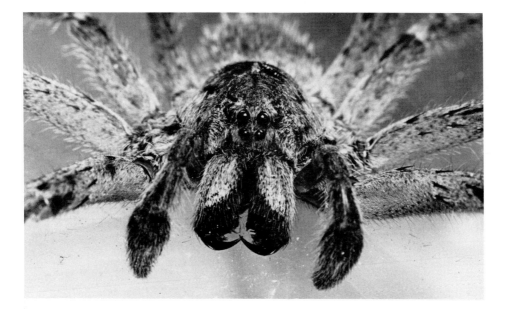

Figure 2. This labidognath spider is a terrestrial venomous animal, which uses its venom primarily for obtaining prey. The venom apparatus is located in the chelicerae seen in the center of the picture below the eyes. With the well visible claws, the animal is able to hold prey animals and to inject its venom (photo courtesy T.A. Freyvogel, Swiss Tropical Institute, Basel).

C. POISONS

Poisons are toxic substances produced in non-specialized glands or tissues (secondary metabolites) or accumulated in an organism after ingestion of prey. The respective organisms are referred to as **poisonous** and the biological significance of poisons is not always known (deterrents, antifeeding agents, etc.). **Poisoning** or **intoxication** takes place after oral ingestion of the respective organism.

Under natural conditions all poisons act upon ingestion, although under artificial conditions, they may act also by a parenteral route.

D. TOXINS

As a rule, neither venoms nor poisons consist of one single chemical substance. On the contrary, they usually are more or less complex mixtures of different chemical substances, which often exert toxic effects by a synergistic action. The toxic substances are referred to as **toxins**.

Toxins are chemically pure toxic substances occurring in venoms and poisons with more or less specific actions on biological systems .

Table 1 gives an overview on the chemical substance groups, to which toxins may be appointed.

E. TOXICITY

Toxinology may not be dealt with without some knowledge of **toxicology**, which is the science of the harmful interactions between chemical substances and biological systems. (For an overview, the reader is referred to J.A.TIMBRELL: "Introduction to Toxicology", 155 pages, London: Taylor & Francis, 1989).

The relationship between the dose of a substance and the response elicited in a biological system is a fundamental concept in toxicology and was probably recognized for the first time by the medieval physician Paracelsus (1493-1541), who stated: "*All substances are poisons; there is none which is not a poison. The right dose differentiates a poison and a remedy*".

Dose *means the amount of a chemical substance (or mixture), which is applied per kilogram (or gram) bodyweight into an organism.*

Thus, if 50 grams (g) of a substance are eaten by an adult of 80 kilograms (kg) bodyweight, he gets a dose of 50 g per 80 kg or 0.000625 g/kg, that means 625 micrograms (μg) per kg bodyweight. If a child of 25 kg bodyweight eats the same amount, he gets a dose of 0.002 g/kg or 2 mg/kg. Thus, the child received a dose, which is 3.2 times higher than that of the adult. Children also usually get higher doses in accidents with venomous or poisonous animals and therefore are more endangered. Even substances used daily like "Salt" (sodium chloride) may become toxic, if they are ingested in very high amounts. For practical reasons, toxicity is therefore defined as follows:

Chemical substances are **toxic***, if they are, due to their physicochemical properties, able, even in very small doses (mg/kg to g/kg), to harm or destroy living organisms.*

Since toxic substances exert their toxic effects by interacting with receptor molecules present in the biological systems affected, only that amount of substance that reaches the receptor(s) is able to exert a toxic effect.

The way in which chemical substances come into contact with biological systems, the route of administration, is therefore of crucial importance for the toxic effect. If a substance is eaten (*peroral* [p.o.] administration), it has to pass the gastrointestinal tract. Thus, before the substance finally enters the body via the small intestine, there are a number of interactions possible. If the toxic substance is e.g. a protein, it will be digested like a steak and there will be no toxic effect at all. If the same substance is administered by a *parenteral* route, e.g. *intravenously* (i.v.) into the venous system, *intramuscularly* (i.m.) into a muscle, *intraperitonealy* (i.p.) into the peritoneum or *intra-* or *subcutaneously* (i.c., s.c.) into or under the skin, other, more or less pronounced interactions are possible. As a rule, the most effective parenteral route is intravenous, followed by intraperitoneal, intramuscular, intra- or subcutaneous injection.

Table 1
Chemical substance groups, to which toxins from venoms and poisons may be appointed

Chemical Substance Group	Example	Present in the Venom or Poison of e.g.
Aliphatic acids	Formic acid	Ants
	Isobutyric acid	Beetles
Polyketides	Okadaic acid	Sponges
	Brevetoxins	Dinoflagellates
Terpenes	Agelasin A	Sponges
	Asperidol A	Corals
Steroids	Bufotoxins	Amphibians
	Cortexon	Beetles
Saponins	Steroidsaponins	Sea stars
	Sapogenins	Sea cucumbers
Derivatives of phenyl propane	Benzoquinone	Beetles
	Hydroquinone	
Indole Alkaloids	Surugatoxin	Mussels
Quinazoline Alkaloids	Ciguatoxin	Fish
	Tetrodotoxin	Amphibians
Pyridine Alkaloids	Nemertillin	Nemertini
	Histrionicotoxin	Amphibians
Purine Alkaloids	Saxitoxins	Flagellates
		Mussels
Steroide Alkaloids	Batrachotoxin	Amphibians
	Samandarin	
Aliphatic Amines	Acetylcholine	Wasps
	Nereistoxin	Annelides
Phenylalkyl Amines	Norepinephrine	Bees
	Leptodactyline	Amphibians
Indole alkyl Amines	5-Hydroxytryptamine	Cnidarians
	Bufotenin	Amphibians
Imidazole Amines	Histamine	Insects
Oligopeptides	Dermorphin	Jellyfish
	Polisteskinin R-1	Wasps
Polypeptides	Noxiustoxin	Scorpions
	Postsynaptic Neurotoxins	Snakes
Proteins	Enzymes	Insects
	Presynaptic Neurotoxins	Snakes

F. FACTORS INFLUENCING TOXICITY

The toxicity of venoms and poisons, respectively, may be influenced to a different extent by the following factors, to name but the most important ones[5-8]:

1. Species

Drastic differences are known between different organisms, since they may react with different sensitivity towards a given venom or poison. Moreover, it has been shown that venomous animals are comparatively resistant to the action of their own venoms.

2. Age and body weight

An organism's sensitivity towards a venom or poison may be altered during age. Variations in sensitivity between adults and youngsters may be due not only to the different body weights, but also to biochemical differences in their metabolism.

3. Sex

At least from experiments with laboratory animals, it is known that variations in sensitivity may depend on the sex. However, a general trend, whether males are more sensitive than females, cannot be drawn.

4. Seasonal variations

Even a seasonal variation in sensitivity towards venoms or poisons sometimes can be detected. However, the mechanisms accounting for this remain unknown to date.

5. Variation of composition

Since venoms and poisons as a rule are complex mixtures of different toxins, individual variations in their composition are well known, both on qualitative and quantitative terms.

6. Geographical variations

Variations between geographically separated populations of the same animal species are also known to be more or less pronounced.

G. THE PROBLEM OF EVALUATING TOXICITY

Most knowledge on animal venoms and poisons has been accumulated by using experimental models and laboratory animals currently used in research institutes. Although these results allow much insight into the pharmacology and toxicology of venoms and poisons, it should be kept in mind, that a conclusive view of the biological significance of animal venoms and poisons is only possible, if their pharmacological action is evaluated in adequate experimental models, e.g. in animals that belong to the natural prey or enemy spectrum of the respective animal species. Due to today´s powerful animal protection movements, however, it is almost impossible to perform such experiments [8].

III. DISTRIBUTION OF VENOMOUS AND POISONOUS ANIMALS

A. DISTRIBUTION ACCORDING TO LIVING SPACE

Table 2 provides an overview on what animals may be expected in marine and terrestrial ecosystems, respectively.

Table 2
Distribution of venomous and poisonous animals according to LIVING SPACE

Marine Ecosystems	Terrestrial Ecosystems
Invertebrates	**Invertebrates**
Protozoans, *Protozoa*	Arachnids, *Arachnida*
Sponges, *Sponigia, Porifera*	- Scorpions, *Scorpiones*
Cnidarians, *Cnidaria*	- Spiders, *Araneae*
Jointed worms, *Annelida*	- Ticks, *Acari*
Horseshoe Crabs, *Xiphosura*	
Crustaceans, *Crustacea*	Centipedes, *Chilopoda*
Molluscs, *Mollusca*	Millipedes, *Diplopoda*
- Conus snails, *Conidae*	
- Mussels, *Bivalvia*	Insects, *Insecta*
- Squids, *Cephalopoda*	- Bees, Ants and Wasps, *Hymenoptera*
Echinoderms, *Echinodermata*	- Beetles, *Coleoptera*
	- Butterflies, *Lepidoptera*
Vertebrates	**Vertebrates**
Lampreys, *Cyclostomata*	Amphibians, *Amphibia*
Fish, *Pisces*	Reptiles, *Reptilia*
Reptiles, *Reptilia*	- Helodermatids, *Helodermatidae*
- Sea snakes, *Hydrophiinae*	- Snakes, *Serpentes*
Mammals, *Mammalia*	Mammals, *Mammalia*

B. DISTRIBUTION IN THE ANIMAL KINGDOM

An overview of the distribution of venomous and poisonous animals in the zoological system is provided in Table 3.

Table 3
Distribution of venomous and poisonous animals in the zoological system

Animal Group, Zoological Name	Venomous Animals Present	Poisonous Animals Present	Animals of Medical Importance
PROTOZOANS, *Protozoa*			
- Flagellates, *Flagellata*	+ +	+ +	*** 1)
- *Rhizopoda*	+ +	+ +	
- Ciliates, *Ciliata*	+ +		
METAZOANS, *Metazoa*			
- Sponges, *Porifera, Spongia*	+	+ +	
- Cnidarians, *Cnidaria*	+ + +	+	***
- Strapworms, *Nemertini*	+	+	
- Jointed worms, *Annelida*	+	+	
- *Arthropoda*			*
-- *Chelicerata*			
--- Scorpions, *Scorpiones*	+ + +		
--- Spiders, *Araneae*	+ +		***
--- Ticks and Mytes, *Acari*	+		***
--- Horseshoe Crabs, *Xiphosuridae*			
-- *Diantennata*		+	***
--- Crustaceans, *Crustaceae*			*** 1)
-- *Antennata*		+	
--- Centipedes, *Chilopoda*			*** 1)
--- Millipedes, *Diplopoda*	+ + +		
--- Insects, *Hexapoda, Insecta*	+ + +	+	*
- Molluscs, *Mollusca*	+ +	+ +	
-- Snails, *Gastropoda*			***
-- Mussels, *Bivalvia*	+	+	
-- Squids, *Cephalopoda*		+ +	***
- Echinoderms, *Echinodermata*	+		*** 1)
- Tunicates, *Tunicata*	+ +	+ +	*
- Chordates, *Chordata*		+ +	***
-- Vertebrates, *Vertebrata*			
--- Lampreys, *Cyclostomata*			
--- Fishes, *Pisces*	+ +	+ +	*** 1)
--- Amphibians, *Amphibia*	+ + +	+ +	
--- Reptiles, *Reptilia*	+ +	+	***
--- Birds, *Aves*			
--- Mammals, *Mammalia*	+	+	*

+   only few animals of the respective group   *   accidents rare
+ +   many animals of the respective group   ***   accidents frequent, fatalities known
+ + +   whole animal group
1) animals often acquire toxicity in connection with food intake of toxic dinoflagellates

IV. THE CONCEPT OF THE BOOK

The book is written in such a way that every chapter dealing with a particular type of envenomation and poisoning, respectively, includes all relevant information on *1)* the animal species responsible, *2)* its venom apparatus, where applicable, *3)* notes on the chemistry and pharmacology of its venom or poison, *4)* epidemiological data, as far as obtainable, *5)* prophylactic measures to be taken to avoid accidents, *6)* simple and accurate first aid treatment, and *7)* information on the clinical management of accidents. Although it is a multi-author volume, each author has been asked to adhere to these principles, when writing their chapters. All clinical information is derived from medical doctors familiar with and experienced in the treatment of respective cases of envenoming and poisoning, respectively.

The book therefore may be used by medical staff facing a given case in their emergency unit, giving them a concise overview about what they have to face and how to manage it. Moreover, the book is also of interest for all those scientists, using animal venoms and poisons as a source for their investigational work or as tools to resolve particular problems in their own research work, providing them all the basic knowledge necessary for the knowledge of the "life behind" the substances used.

V. REFERENCES

1. WÜTHRICH, B. Bienen- und Wespenstichallergie. *LaboLife* Nr. **4/93**: 24-26, 1993.
2. FREYVOGEL, T.A. Poisonous and venomous animals in East Africa. *Acta Tropica* **29**: 401-451, 1972.
3. FREYVOGEL, T.A. AND PERRET, B.A. Notes on toxinology. *Experientia* **29**: 1317 1319, 1973.
4. RUSSELL, F.A. Some historical notes on the naming of the International Society on Toxinology. *Toxicon* **14**: 343-345, 1976.
5. MEIER, J. AND FREYVOGEL, T.A. Comparative studies on the venoms of the Fer-de-Lance (*Bothrops atrox*), carpet viper (*Echis carinatus*) and spitting cobra (*Naja nigricollis*) snakes at different ages. *Toxicon* **18**: 661-662, 1980.
6. MEIER, J. Individual and age-dependent variations in the venom of the Fer-de-lance (Bothrops atrox). *Toxicon* **24**: 41-46, 1986.
7. MEIER, J. AND THEAKSTON, R.D.G. Approximate LD50 determinations of snake venoms using eight to ten experimental animals. *Toxicon* **24**: 395-401, 1986.
8. MEIER, J. AND STOCKER, K. On the significance of animal experiments in toxinology. *Toxicon* **27**: 91-104, 1989.

Chapter 2

POISONOUS AND VENOMOUS ANIMALS - THE PHYSICIAN'S VIEW

Julian White

TABLE OF CONTENTS

I. INTRODUCTION

A. IS THIS BOOK NEEDED?

Emphatically yes! Illness caused by exposure to "natural" toxins, ie. those produced by living organisms, is a significant problem globally. Even within "developed" nations, it is far from insignificant. As an example, calls for advice or help to poisons information centres feature calls about bites and stings prominently. In Australia, the most recent statistics from the largest such centre (in Sydney) show that calls about spiderbite alone are the second most common cause of all calls[1]. Paracetamol is the most common. Calls about bites, stings and poisonous plants or fungi are at least 10% of all calls for most poisons information centres, in some cases exceeding 25%, depending on the country and nature of the service. Furthermore, at least in developed nations, there are a number of "exotic" venomous animals in captivity, in both public and private collections, which may cause bites requiring vigorous treatment and a knowledge of the best management options[2,3].

Even taking the most conservative estimates of morbidity and mortality from venomous or poisonous animals, as will be discussed below, several 100,000 people are affected each year, with deaths exceeding 20,000. These figures are almost certainly a significant underestimate, with snakebites alone accounting for at least 20,000 deaths annually[4]. The economic cost is unknown, but if we consider the lost output of people killed or permanently disabled, plus the cost of alternative support for their dependants, plus the temporary lost output of less severe cases and all the costs of treatment, the figure is likely to be counted in many millions of dollars per year. Indeed, if we put a figure of $10,000 on each case of death or permanent incapacity to work, plus a figure of $1,000 for each less severe case, and rated these at 20% of all cases, with a figure of $100 on all remaining cases, it is possible to guesstimate that the minimum global cost of bites and stings per year is $228,000,000. As it is likely that the figures for morbidity, mortality and cost are all underestimates, the real cost is most probably far higher.

Given the extent of the problem, what is the world doing about it? At least in the medical profession as a whole, the answer is very little. There is no special college or craft group in medicine to accommodate doctors with special expertise in this field, or to encourage or train colleagues in clinical toxinology. Only a few medical schools in the world have specific lectures on clinical toxinology. Currently there are no textbooks dedicated to this medical specialty.

This book is the first to try and address the issue of clinical toxinology of animal venoms and poisons on a global scale. Ironically, while producing this book we became involved with two colleagues in the field of tropical medicine, well aware of the lack of suitable textbooks, who had started to produce a clinical handbook on animal bites and stings for emergency service doctors. This project has proceeded in parallel with our book and we hope the two books will complement each other, as they approach the subject from entirely different perspectives and with different objectives. There are existing texts covering the clinical toxinology of poisonous plants and fungi.

B. THE STRUCTURE OF THE BOOK

We have aimed to make this book a true textbook on clinical toxinology of animal venoms and poisons. In doing so we have sought authors with expertise and clinical experience in all types of illness caused by animal venoms and poisons. In some areas, far more is known about the toxicology and pharmacology of the venoms/poisons than is known about the clinical illness caused by these toxins. We have therefore tried to document what is known, and interpolate it with experience from related areas of clinical toxinology. In some cases this will prove valid. However, this may not always be the case, and all readers of this book are strongly urged to communicate with the editors their own personal clinical experience with particular clinical toxinology cases, if they add to information in this book, and especially if their experience differs from the information given in this book. Clinical toxinology is still a very young medical specialty, and there is undoubtedly much still to learn.

The basic outline of information given in each chapter, and the organisation of the chapters, has been discussed in Chapter 1.

II. CLINICAL TOXINOLOGY

A. WHAT IS CLINICAL TOXINOLOGY?

Toxinology has been defined in Chapter 1. Clinical toxinology is essentially the medical study/specialty of "natural" toxin effects on man, and the medical management of the associated illnesses. Technically it should therefore cover a wide spectrum of problems including injury/illness caused by venomous or poisonous animals, poisonous plants, poisonous fungi, and microbial toxins. Historically illness caused by microbial toxins has been managed by other special areas in medicine, notably microbiologists. For this reason clinical toxinology is not likely to have significant involvement with illness due to microbial toxins, although this area at a research level is now very much part of meetings of toxinologists.

In the past the diagnosis and management of illness due to animal toxins has been managed by the general medical fraternity. In more recent years the emergence of the specialties of emergency medicine and intensive care has seen these groups take a special interest in clinical toxinology, but only as part of a much wider training base. Nevertheless, this has undoubtedly seen some advances in diagnosis and management of bites and stings.

However, it seems to me that most of the major advances in knowledge at the clinical level have arisen as a result of the work of a few doctors who, for a variety of reasons, have made various aspects of clinical toxinology a major focus of their professional life. It would be impossible to list all these people here, but a few names stand out, at least in this author's opinion, as having had a major and positive influence on clinical toxinology of animal toxins in the last 50 years. These include Jack Barnes, Vital Brazil, Wolfgang Bucherl, John Burnett, Charles Campbell, David Chapman, Jean-Phillipe Chippaux, Paul Christensen, Hamilton Fairley, Peter Fenner, Bruce Halstead, Charles Kellaway, Zvonomir Maretic, Dietrich Mebs, Sherman Minton, Hugh Parrish, John Pearn, Alistair Reid, Findlay Russell, Ron Southcott, Struan Sutherland, David Theakston, David Warrell, and John Williamson. There are doubtless others I have omitted, through oversight or ignorance, and to them I apologise.

B. CLINICAL TOXINOLOGY SKILLS

1. An overview

If clinical toxinology is to gain full recognition as a medical specialty, then those who will graduate from training must have a well rounded suit of skills setting them apart from others with involvement in management of clinical toxinology cases[5], particularly colleagues with specialist skills in emergency medicine and intensive care, who can rightly claim to have a significant role in the management of these cases. It is my experience that it is possible for the three groups to work together as a team, to the benefit of patient care, each providing their own particular and vital input into overall management. This is probably the preferred role of the clinical toxinologist; to work as part of a team involved in the optimal diagnosis and management of all cases of significant illness caused by animal toxins. This should be combined with teaching at undergraduate and postgraduate level and advice to health authorities on toxinology matters, such as appropriate policies on antivenom selection, availability and use.

2. Knowing the culprit: biology, taxonomy and distribution

Fundamental to any understanding of clinical toxinology is a clear and detailed knowledge of the animals that produce or deliver the toxins. Biology will encompass the mode of life of each animal species, its place in the micro and macro environment, including how and why it produces or accumulates the venom or other toxin. Behaviour is important as part of this as it points to likely exposure risks, which may be important in diagnosis, in determining which of several possible animal species is likely to be the cause of an illness.

Taxonomy is vital as it defines one animal or animal group from another. Without knowledge of the actual species or group of animal(s) responsible for a specific illness it is very difficult for clinical toxinology to advance, a problem well recognised but infrequently addressed until the recent past. The ability to clearly identify an animal thought to be the cause of an illness is a fundamental skill for a clinical toxinologist. Indeed, there are a number of examples of clinicians with a passion for toxinology who have become important contributors to taxonomy, sometimes even world authorities in a particular area of taxonomy.

Knowledge of the biology and taxonomy/identification of an animal is incomplete without information on distribution. Distribution may be the key to determining which of several similar animals is the probable cause of the illness. As with taxonomy, there are examples of clinicians focussed on toxinology problems who have significantly advanced knowledge of the distribution of some venomous animals, particularly venomous snakes and some marine organisms.

3. Understanding the weapons of attack: toxicology and pharmacology of natural toxins

The reasons for requiring a good knowledge of the toxins, including basic toxicology and pharmacology, are obvious, for it is through this that the clinical effects in man can be understood, explained, and countered by therapies. Ideally the clinical toxinologist will have had experience in basic venom/toxin research, a field which has many potential pitfalls, a comprehension of which will allow better interpretation of the basic research findings published by non-clinical colleagues.

This should be linked to a sound grounding in general principles of toxicology and pharmacology. Related to this is an understanding of immunology, as many toxins interact with the immune system, sometimes with potentially catastrophic results clinically. Indeed, one of the most common and potent specific therapies for venom induced illness is antivenom, reliant for both production and clinical effect on the immune system.

4. Intelligence gathering: diagnosis

It is sometimes assumed by doctors that diagnosis of bites and stings is simple and straightforward. Sometimes this is the case, but often it is not. Cases where there is no clear history to suggest a bite or sting or ingestion of toxin are quite common, especially in children, in which group the presenting symptoms and signs may be misleading. Even where a toxin related illness seems evident, the type of animal and toxin and dose may be in doubt. Correctly looking for and eliciting symptoms and signs relevant to the case is an important practical skill that must be learnt. I have seen a number of patients over the years, who ultimately proved to have significant toxin related illness, in whom quite major signs such as paralysis were missed by experienced and diligent doctors, simply because they had not considered them nor had they seen them frequently. It is quite easy to miss signs of incomplete paralysis, particularly in a child, if concerned about other aspects of their presentation. There is no real substitute for clinical experience in eliciting symptoms and signs, and such experience should be a vital part of any clinical toxinology training.

Increasingly laboratory investigations have a role to play in the diagnosis and management of animal toxin related illness. The development of specific tests for venoms or ingested toxins are the most obvious[6,7], but more widely available and basic tests such as coagulation studies can play a crucial role in determining the extent of envenoming and requirement for therapy[8-10]. All these tests have limitations and a clinical toxinologist should understand both the use of the tests and how they are performed, so that evaluation of results and awareness of causes of possible false results will allow accurate interpretation.

5. The methods of defence: clinical treatment

In some sense, clinical treatment is the core of clinical toxinology, but as in many other areas of medicine, while very important, it is often the correct diagnosis which is crucial to optimal outcome for the patient. Nevertheless, a full understanding of clinical treatment of all types of "natural" toxin related illness is a key component of toxinology training. This should include emergency care skills, use of pharmacologic agents, and very specific and detailed understanding of antidotes, particularly antivenom.

6. Knowing your allies: related medical skills

There are a number of complications of major envenoming that may require the skills of various medical specialties to manage. These include emergency care and resuscitation, intubation and ventilation, intensive care, renal function impairment and dialysis, coagulopathy and its management, myolysis, local tissue damage and management, biochemical abnormalities and their correction. A clinical toxinologist should have knowledge and skills in all these areas, although ideally, working within a team, each particular problem will be handled by the appropriate specialist. Nevertheless, particularly for clinical toxinologists working in some tropical regions, where animal toxin injuries such as snakebite are common, many of the medical specialties will be unavailable; thus basic skills in these areas may literally mean the difference between life and death for the patient.

III. EPIDEMIOLOGY AND CLINICAL TOXINOLOGY

A. PROBLEMS IN EPIDEMIOLOGY OF BITES AND STINGS

As will be clear on reading some of the chapters in this book, detailed epidemiology of animal toxin related illness is unavailable for most animal groups in many and key regions of the world. Where statistics on cases and deaths are available, at least in tropical countries, they may be very incomplete. An example of this is the situation with snakebite in savanna west Africa. The only global survey of this problem, for the World Health Organisation, relied on government statistics, often generated from a very limited number of hospitals. In savanna Nigeria the survey found only 9 snakebite related deaths in 5 years[11]. A subsequent survey investigating at the village level in selected regions of Nigeria found a far higher incidence of snakebite and related deaths, and extrapolated this to the region, estimating as many as 23,000 deaths per year from snakebite, giving a figure over 5 years more than 10,000 times higher than the WHO survey[12]. Both studies had methodological errors[13] and the true figure for this part of Africa lies somewhere between these extremes. A more detailed discussion of this may be found in Chapter 26. However this serves to illustrate one of the problems in assessing the extent of illness caused by animal toxins on a global scale, namely accurate recording of all definite cases. For most rural tropical communities such recording of cases is presently only a dream.

A further problem in recording cases is that the organism responsible is either not known or not reliably recorded. Retrospective diagnosis using tests for residual antibodies is sometimes possible, though there are some technical difficulties with this technique at a laboratory level, let alone in terms of specimen collection and transport[6,12,13]. Furthermore, this takes no account of those cases, possibly numerous, where the cause of the illness is unknown and so may never be listed as possibly due to the effects of an animal toxin. If the patient dies as a result of secondary complications from a primary animal toxin illness, the case may be coded for the complication, not the original illness, again causing under reporting of cases.

B. GLOBAL SIGNIFICANCE OF ENVENOMING: A PERSONAL VIEW

Over the past 12 years, I have had frequent contact with colleagues involved in toxinology throughout the world. Opinions on the likely total global incidence of animal toxin related illness and deaths have varied widely amongst these colleagues. Some have suggested annual mortality rates for their own region far beyond what is currently documented, usually from less developed countries where official reporting is both erratic and inaccurate and likely to significantly underestimate numbers of cases. If these high figures of mortality are accepted then the global annual mortality from snakebite alone is well in excess of 100,000, and for scorpion stings, in excess of 50,000. Given our knowledge of expected mortality rates for snakebite and scorpion sting, based on more reliable evidence than the above mortality rates, then it could be extrapolated that actual cases of snakebites and scorpion stings would number in the millions each year. At the other end of this spectrum there are meticulous researchers who have been conservative in their estimates of case numbers and mortality, yet still suggest an annual mortality for snakebite alone of at least 20,000[4,10,16].

It is my opinion that the annual global mortality related to animal toxins is in the vicinity of 50,000, but possibly considerably higher. The total number of cases, from minor to fatal, is likely to significantly exceed one million, of which at least 10%, or 100,000 will have significant short term or long term effects, incurring costs to the community. If this estimate is correct, and the figures suggested earlier in this chapter are also valid and applied, then the real cost to mankind, each year, of animal toxin related injury, is in the order of $1,000,000,000! Even if this is an overestimate by 50% it yields a very significant monetary cost, let alone cost in human suffering, and amply justifies a substantial international effort to minimise this cost. An important step in such a process would be the establishment of adequate training in clinical toxinology, at all levels of health delivery, with an emphasis on regions at most risk, namely the rural tropics.

IV. FIRST AID

First aid is a key first step in minimising the potential effects of any animal toxin related illness. Because it is essentially applied by non-medical people, either the patient or their companions, it must be safe and easily applied. Unfortunately, partly because it is non-medical treatment, first aid has all too frequently involved the use of unwise or frankly dangerous "treatments", often based on village folk lore, with little relation to our current understanding of envenoming and poisoning.

The key features for first aid are firstly, do no harm to the patient; secondly, use a method that is easy and practical in application; thirdly, use a method which maximises the chance that the patient will reach definitive care safely and in optimal condition, in the circumstances pertaining, and yet minimise the likelihood of ongoing adverse sequelae. To achieve all three of these objectives is not always possible. Some advocate the use of specific techniques focussing on one objective, while forgetting the other two. This is reflected in the wide array of first aid methods advocated or used for snakebite throughout the world. Even within one country, many methods may have been officially approved over the years.

Several years ago, three colleagues (David Theakston, Dietrich Mebs, Ralph Edwards) and I, then working together on a WHO (IPCS) project (INTOX), formulated a general set of guidelines for treating all types of animal toxin illness worldwide, including recommendations on first aid. These were ably reviewed by David Warrell. They are yet to be published by the WHO (IPCS). These guidelines on first aid are given below.

(a) Principles:
The aims of first aid for poisonous and venomous animal bites and stings should be to treat or delay life-threatening effects which may develop before the patient reaches medical care; to hasten the safe transport of the patient to a medical dispensary, clinic or hospital and to avoid harmful measures.

(b) Specific actions:
(i) Patient reassurance - Panic is a common and detrimental response to a bite or sting. This is especially so for snakebites. The patient should be reassured that not all bites or stings result in poisoning/envenoming, even when the animal is dangerous, and many snakes, spiders etc are not dangerous to man, that modern hospital treatment is effective.

(ii) Patient immobility - Movement or exercise of the bitten limb speeds up the spread of venom. Patients should be discouraged, as far as possible, from using the bitten limb; in most cases immobilisation will be beneficial.

(iii) Reduce venom dissipation - Apart from **(ii)** above, specific wound care is not appropriate except as mentioned in special cases in the sections for each animal group.
In particular DO NOT:
Excise the wound
Incise the wound
Apply suction to the wound
Use a tourniquet or constricting band
Use electric shock therapy
Apply or inject chemicals or medicines (e.g. potassium permanganate or condys crystals) to the wound
Apply ice packs
Use any proprietary "snake bite kits".

(iv) Food and drink - In general do not give the patient anything by mouth, including food, alcohol, drugs (especially aspirin, sedatives) or drinks. However, where there is likely to be a considerable delay in receiving medical treatment, consider giving water only by mouth to avoid dehydration.

(v) Identification of the animal hazard - Where possible try to identify the cause of the bite/sting, except where this puts the patient or others at risk. Note descriptive features. If the animal is dead, bring it to hospital with the patient, but handle with extreme care, remembering that even a severed snake's head can bite and inject venom.

(vi) Arrangements should be made to **seek medical advice at the earliest opportunity**, and in most cases the patient should be transferred as quickly and passively as possible to a place where medical attention can be given. Patients can be transferred on a stretcher or trestle, on the crossbar of a bicycle, or a boat, if road transport or conventional ambulances are not available. The worst situation would be if a patient ran for kilometres on a bitten leg.

(vii) Life supportive treatment such as expired air ventilation and external cardiac massage should be used if the patient's condition warrants it. Patients should be laid on their side and the airway kept clear. They may vomit or faint.

(viii) Traditional methods of treatment involving ingestion or application of herbal remedies, tattooing, scarification, incisions, burning, instillation of oily material into the nose etc are very popular in most parts of the rural tropics but should be discouraged as they are, at best, time wasting, and at worst, dangerous or even life-threatening.

Apart from the general principles and methods of first aid listed above, more specific information for each animal group will be found in the relevant chapter of this book. A perusal of these chapters will reveal that unanimity of opinion on this subject, even among experts, has yet to be achieved.

There are, however, several general issues in first aid for animal toxin illness which should be considered. Firstly, there is the use of immobilisation of the bitten limb as a method of retarding venom movement. There appears to be general consensus that immobilisation will, at least in some cases, retard venom movement, particularly if combined with a local bandage to occlude superficial lymphatics (the Australian "pressure immobilisation" technique)[10,14,15,16]. While the use of the bandage may be hazardous in some cases, notably bites causing local tissue damage and oedema, such as some types of snakebite (some cobras, some vipers)[10,16], immobilisation alone appears to have no deleterious effect. Immobilisation in a plaster cast has been shown, experimentally, to retard venom movement (tiger snake, *Notechis scutatus* venom)[17], though the use of a plaster cast is not recommended in the clinical situation. There is also experimental and limited clinical evidence to support the use of immobilisation plus bandaging for Australian snakebite, and by inference, any snakebite where local tissue damage or swelling is not likely[14-19].

Secondly, the use of a true tourniquet as first aid, usually for snakebite, a technique still widely used throughout the world, is not to be recommended. The dangers of this use of a tourniquet are well documented[10,16,20-22]. Given that the vast majority of snakebites will not prove fatal, it is unacceptable to use a first aid technique, such as the tourniquet, which experience has shown will frequently result in significant long term injury to the patient.

Thirdly, another practice, commonly used for snakebite, incising the bite site and sucking out the venom, is not recommended. As with the tourniquet, experience has shown that significant and long term injury can be caused to the patient using the "cut and suck" method[10,16,22]. The recent introduction of special suction/incision devices for treatment of snakebite has reinflamed controversy on this topic[22-26]. In my opinion current evidence does not show sufficient and consistent benefit from these devices, versus their potential hazards, to justify their use. Other methods such as cryotherapy and the local application of either heat or cold have been shown to be at best, ineffective, at worst, hazardous to limb and life[10,16,20,22-24].

V. APPROACH TO DIAGNOSIS

A. GENERAL CONSIDERATIONS

General principles apply to the diagnosis of illness due to envenoming or poisoning, as in any other area of medicine, including the standard approach of history, examination and investigations. The severely envenomed or poisoned patient may require very urgent and abbreviated assessment and institution of remedial measures. Diagnosis may be clear, as in the patient bitten by a "pet" venomous snake, or may be obscure, as in the child presenting unconscious, following a convulsion, with no history of a bite or sting. The latter presentation, at least in my experience, while not common, is certainly far from rare. A clinical toxinologist is likely to see a number of children with severe envenoming, many hours after the bite/sting, the actual cause of their illness not having been discerned by colleagues.

A general approach in collection of useful information from patients with possible envenoming or poisoning by natural toxins is given below. It is not meant to be exhaustive, nor cover all special cases, and clearly some information suggested here may not be relevant for all types of animal toxin associated illness. More detailed and specific information will be found in relevant chapters of this book.

B. HISTORY

1. Details of bite/sting/ingestion

The time that the bite/sting/ingestion occurred is always relevant. Combined with information on first aid, and development of symptoms and signs, if any, it can be used to predict extent of envenoming/poisoning and prognosis, for any particular animal toxin. Similarly, the quantity of toxin introduced is important. Inquire about multiple bites/stings or quantity of the poisonous animal flesh consumed. A description of the offending animal and geographic location at the time of exposure should be obtained, or if unavailable (eg. if the patient is unconscious or is a small child), their location and activity prior to onset of the illness.

2. First aid

Effective first aid applied immediately after the bite/sting will hopefully retard venom movement and so delay envenomation. If first aid has been used details of type, patient's activity prior to and after application, and delay between bite/sting and application should be sought. Use of any "folk medicine" methods, locally or systemically, should be recorded. Ingestion of alcohol prior to or after the bite/sting should be documented, as it may increase the chance of complications from envenoming.

3. General symptoms

General symptoms of envenoming/poisoning are very dependent on the type of animal toxin, as are specific symptoms. Common symptoms applicable include headache, nausea, vomiting, abdominal pain, local bite/sting site pain/swelling/bruising/blistering, collapse, and in children, convulsions. Always note the pattern and timing of onset of symptoms, such as the spread of pain or muscle discomfort.

4. Specific symptoms

Specific symptoms for particular types of toxin action include paralytic symptoms, notably "heavy eyelids" (ptosis), visual disturbance, slurred speech, drooling, difficulty walking and breathing difficulty; myolytic symptoms, including muscle weakness and pain, muscle wasting (late stage) and dark or "blood" stained urine (myoglobinuria); coagulopathic symptoms, including persistent bleeding from the bite/sting site, bleeding gums, haematuria and ecchymosis; and nephrotoxic symptoms, including oliguria or anuria. This list is not exhaustive.

5. Relevant past medical history

Past exposure to horse serum or antivenom, especially if reactions have occurred, is particularly important, although severe acute reactions to antivenom can occur even on first exposure. A history of atopy or asthma may indicate a greater likelihood of reactions to antivenom. Past significant illness, particularly renal impairment or coagulation irregularity, such as warfarin therapy or bleeding diathesis, should always be noted.

C. EXAMINATION
1. Bite/sting site

Examination of the presumed bite/sting site may either cast doubt on the diagnosis, or confirm that a bite/sting is likely to have occurred, and also may indicate that the bite/sting has been multiple (Figure 1), with a consequently increased chance of major envenoming. It is important to realise that even for bites by snakes which cause local tissue injury, bite marks may only be visible at presentation in as few as 50% of cases[27,28], and for many other venomous animals, the bite or sting site is hard to discern in the majority of patients. If the offending organism is available it should be inspected to confirm identity (if possible; Figure 2) and size, or in the case of a suspected ingestion of a poisonous animal, the remaining food items should be kept, for toxin assay, if available. Local effects of the venom may indicate which of several related animals is most likely to be the cause of the bite. Local pain/tenderness, inflammation, oedema, bruising, blistering, ecchymosis (Figure 3), necrosis (Figure 4), bleeding from the wound, and pattern of bite/sting marks may all be useful. Swelling or tenderness of lymph nodes draining the bite/sting area usually indicate that venom has been inoculated and has moved from the bite site, so that systemic envenoming, if not already obvious, is imminent.

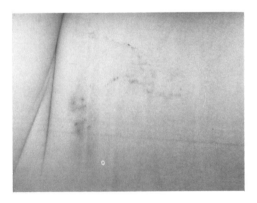
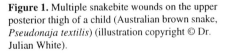
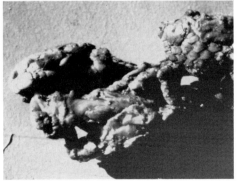

Figure 1. Multiple snakebite wounds on the upper posterior thigh of a child (Australian brown snake, *Pseudonaja textilis*) (illustration copyright © Dr. Julian White).

Figure 2. Dead snake presented with snakebite victim. Such a damaged specimen can prove difficult to identify for the inexperienced (illustration copyright © Dr. Julian White).

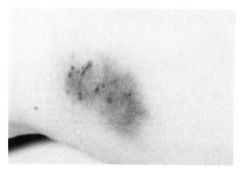
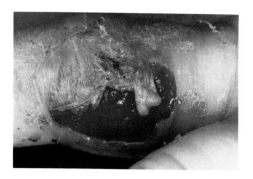

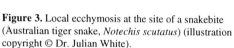

Figure 3. Local ecchymosis at the site of a snakebite (Australian tiger snake, *Notechis scutatus*) (illustration copyright © Dr. Julian White).

Figure 4. Local skin damage following a spiderbite (illustration copyright © Dr. Julian White).

2. General signs

General signs of envenoming/poisoning are widely variable and may not be especially helpful diagnostically. Thus there may be a tachycardia or bradycardia, hypo or hypertension, a low or elevated body temperature, even for the bite of a single species. For some animals however, envenoming/poisoning will cause a typical picture, such as mild hypertension seen with latrodectism (envenoming by widow spiders, *Latrodectus*). In all such cases there will be exceptions.

3. Specific signs

Specific signs of particular toxin induced problems, such as paralysis or coagulopathy, should always be sought. The early signs of paralysis such as ptosis (Figure 5) and mild facial weakness are easily missed, and even moderate to severe paralysis, with respiratory difficulty, can be missed if not systematically examined for. Myolysis is often missed, as it is assumed the apparent weakness is due to paralysis or general debilitation, and the myoglobinuria (Figure 6) is labelled as haematuria. Myolysis can probably mimic many of the signs of paralysis in severe cases, but there should always be biochemical evidence of muscle damage and, usually, at least some degree of muscle movement pain. Untreated it may result in both renal damage and extensive muscle wasting. Signs of coagulopathy, even profound defibrination, may be few and easily missed, yet are highly specific indicators of systemic envenoming[8,9]. Look for persistent bleeding from the bite/sting site and venipuncture sites (Figure 7). If there is an associated haemorrhagin then there may be more obvious signs of bleeding, particularly gingival oozing[10,16].

D. DIFFERENTIAL DIAGNOSIS

In the patient presenting without a history of a bite/sting/ingestion of a toxic animal/flesh, the involvement of an animal toxin in causation of the illness may be easily missed. This is particularly true for children, but may equally apply to adults, especially if obtunded or unconscious on arrival. Include the possibility of envenoming/poisoning in any case of unexplained collapse, convulsions, progressive paralysis (which may present as gait disturbance), local tissue injury, coagulopathy, myolysis, renal impairment, or systemic pain (or even regional pain, such as abdominal or chest pain in latrodectism). While most such presentations will ultimately prove to have a non-animal toxin cause, a case of envenoming missed may result in avoidable morbidity or mortality. Even in some "western" communities, venomous animals are still common in urban environments. In one major Australian capital city, research has shown that of all venomous snakes captured in the metropolitan area each year (amounting to >500 snakes), >10% were actually inside a house! (Geoff Coombe; pers. com.)

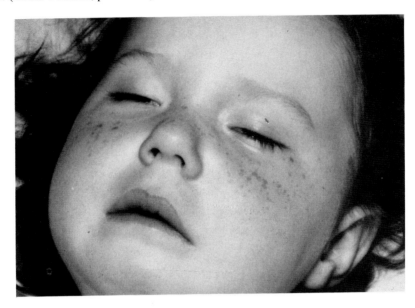

Figure 5. Ptosis in a child as early evidence of neurotoxic paralysis, a sign easily missed (Australian tiger snake bite) (illustration copyright © Dr. Julian White).

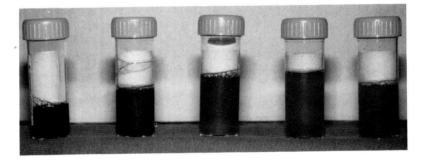

Figure 6. Series of urines taken over 24 hours from a patient with snakebite induced myolysis/myoglobinuria (peak CK >300,000IU; Australian tiger snake bite) (illustration copyright © Dr. Julian White).

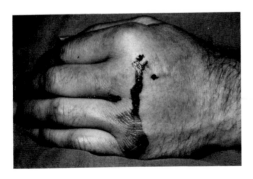

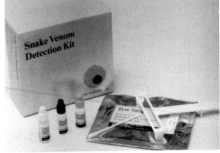

Figure 7. Bleeding from a snakebite wound, often indicating a venom induced coagulopathy (illustration copyright © Dr. Julian White).

Figure 8. Australian Snake Venom Detection Kit (CSL Ltd.) (illustration copyright © Dr. JulianWhite).

E. LABORATORY TESTS

Laboratory tests vary in applicability in animal toxin induced illness. For some quite major types of envenoming, it is possible to manage most cases without the need for laboratory tests. However, where available, laboratory tests may both materially assist in making management decisions, and provide important data on the nature of the envenoming process, of long term value in improving understanding of such processes[8,9,22,29].

1. Venom detection

Venom detection is a technique which, although available for more than 20 years, is nevertheless utilised in only a few places worldwide, despite the important information it can provide the clinician. It has been most widely and successfully used in Australia for snakebite[7,8], where a commercial snake venom identification kit (Figure 8) can demonstrate the presence of venom and type of antivenom needed from minute samples of venom left at the bite site, giving a result within 20 minutes, and not requiring any laboratory equipment or training. There are many other regions of the world where a variety of snake species are known to cause envenoming, requiring different antivenoms, and a kit such as developed for Australia could prove very useful in such areas. Though not currently commercially available, identification of spider venom and even some marine toxins, such as ciguatoxin, might prove useful at a clinical decision making level.

The other important area where such techniques have proved valuable is in epidemiological studies of envenoming, where residual antibodies in individuals may indicate that person's past experience with bites/stings from a wide variety of organisms[6]. These techniques, mostly using a variety of ELISA, have been successfully applied in studies of snakebite and spiderbite. Some technical problems have been encountered, leading to overestimation of past bites[6,13], but it appears these problems can be overcome.

2. Basic blood tests

If no laboratory is available, and the patient may be envenomed by an animal likely to cause coagulopathy, then the simple bedside test for whole blood clotting time can be very useful[10,16]. It requires only a glass test tube and equipment to take venous blood, and may be performed by the clinician or a nurse, taking 20 minutes or less. If there is defibrination, for example, as seen with bites by a variety of snakes in many parts of the world, the blood will either not clot or the clot will be clearly abnormal. This result will usually be available long before even a major hospital laboratory can complete formal laboratory tests of coagulation.

3. Standard laboratory tests

Where available, a combination of one or more of the following tests may prove useful in cases of envenoming/poisoning, depending on the offending animal and the patient's situation:

- Full blood count
- Serum/plasma electrolytes
- Blood glucose
- Renal function (e.g. urea and creatinine)
- Liver enzymes and CK
- Coagulation studies (especially INR, APTT, TCT, Fibrinogen titre and Fibrin(ogen) degradation products)
- Arterial blood gas

VI. CLINICAL MANAGEMENT

A. PRIORITIES

The first priority in managing any patient with an acute condition, be it due to an animal toxin or anything else, is to maintain life, at least until the situation is clear. This may mean urgent attention to the "ABC" of resuscitation, namely airway, breathing and circulation. As obvious as this may seem, it is sometimes overlooked, usually to the tragic detriment of the patient.

Many types of envenoming/poisoning are medical emergencies, requiring priority assessment within the hospital emergency department. A patient presenting with possible snakebite should not be left in the casualty/emergency department waiting room.

Depending on both the nature of presentation, the type of animal toxin involved, and the available facilities, any case where there is significant systemic envenoming/poisoning should usually have an iv line inserted and blood taken at that time for laboratory tests (if applicable). A rapid assessment of major systems should be made, followed up by more detailed assessment as soon as the situation allows. If it is possible that antivenom may be needed, then this should be secured, though not necessarily opened or given. If the hospital does not have appropriate antivenom, then application of good first aid and transfer to an appropriately equipped hospital is often the best course. If in any doubt about the patient's condition and potential for deterioration during transport, then transfer the patient under escort, or use a medical retrieval team.

The patient's welfare is a priority, and any medical attendant inexperienced in or unsure about management of a case of envenoming/poisoning should seek expert advice at the earliest opportunity.

B. GENERAL PRINCIPLES

Priorities have been discussed. For such conditions as snakebite and spiderbite, the patient may initially seem well and show no evidence of envenoming. At this stage they will either be sent to a ward, or be discharged (generally inadvisable if less than 12-18 hours has elapsed since the bite). However, an initially well patient in this situation may develop systemic envenoming several hours later, and unless they are being carefully observed by staff informed about specific problems to watch for, such as paralysis, coagulopathy and renal damage, the onset of envenoming may be missed, and only detected when it is far more advanced, and harder to treat.

C. SPECIFIC TREATMENTS

1. Antivenom

Antivenom is only applicable in the treatment of certain types of envenoming, where it is often the most important single treatment available, substantially reducing morbidity and mortality[7,8,10,16,19,20,22,30]. There are still controversies regarding the use of antivenom, including the use of skin sensitivity testing[10,31] and premedication with adrenaline[7,19,32]. I do not favour either of these practices. The development of newer antivenoms, with a reduced chance of causing immediate type reactions, will largely remove the need for these controversies[33]. The use of antivenom, and its potential problems, is covered in individual chapters dealing with specific animal groups. A complete listing of available antivenoms is provided in Chapter 32.

2. Non-antivenom

A variety of "specific" non-antivenom treatments for envenoming/poisoning are available, ranging from "folk medicine" and plant extracts[34] to agents such as edrophonium or neostigmine in the treatment of classic (post-synaptic neurotoxin) paralysis from snakebite[10,16,35-38]. Details of such treatments, as applicable to specific types of envenoming/poisoning, are discussed in the relevant chapters.

3. Analgesia

Pain is a common feature in many types of envenoming, though certainly not in all. Its causation is quite variable, ranging from mechanical injury at the time of the bite/sting (e.g. sting ray sting) through tissue damage caused by venom (e.g. some jellyfish stings), to direct pain stimulating effects of venom (e.g. latrodectism). Treatment of pain, though not always a medical priority, is usually a priority from the patient's perspective, yet may prove difficult. Narcotic analgesics such as morphine are often inappropriate because of their respiratory depressant effects (e.g. in snakebite), and equally, they may not significantly relieve pain at reasonable doses (e.g. latrodectism). For purely local pain (e.g. some fish stings) the use of local analgesia or even regional nerve blocks may be appropriate, although the "traditional" treatment with hot water should also be tried (see Chapter 12). Antivenom can prove the best "analgesic" in some types of envenoming, indeed may be the only effective treatment (e.g. latrodectism, box jellyfish sting). Oral analgesics are often not very effective and aspirin is contraindicated in some types of envenoming (e.g. snakebite with coagulopathy).

4. Antibiotics

Any bite/sting may act as a site of infection, including tetanus, hence the standard recommendation that all bites receive tetanus immunisation, though tetanus appears to be a rare sequelae of bites and stings[39]. Most bites, particularly if good wound care is observed, will not become infected, and the routine use of prophylactic antibiotics is unwise. Some types of wound are more prone to infection (e.g. sting ray injury) and may justify antibiotics.

D. SPECIFIC PROBLEMS

There are many specific problems relating to particular types of envenoming/poisoning which will be covered in the relevant chapters of this book. A few key problems only are mentioned here. Detailed discussion of these will be found in the relevant chapters.

1. Local wound problems

The local wound following a bite or sting is highly variable, even within injuries caused by a single species of animal. Infection and local pain have been mentioned above. Major tissue injury, with oedema and or tissue damage/necrosis, may occur after some types of bites/stings. Notable examples are some types of snakebite and spiderbite. Particularly for some snakebites, fluid shift into the injured limb may be rapid and massive, threatening both the limb (compartment syndrome)[10,16] and life (hypovolaemic shock)[40,41]. The former may require surgical release of tension, though this is certainly needed far less often than used in the past and should, ideally, be based on objective evidence of raised intra compartmental pressure[10,16,42]. The latter problem, hypovolaemic shock, though not a "local problem", should always be considered and countered in cases of extensive limb oedema. Snakebite patients still die from unrecognised hypovolaemic shock[40,41]. Conversely, problems may occur as a result of incautious use of large volumes of iv fluids, with consequent pulmonary oedema, most likely to occur in children[43].

Necrosis due to venom, as seen in bites by recluse spiders, *Loxosceles* (loxoscelism), may be difficult to treat. Early surgical debridement is usually not helpful, but use of drugs such as dapsone and hyperbaric oxygen therapy have some support (see Chapter 20)[44,45]. Allowing for such treatments, good wound care, including elevation in the early stages, and treatment of secondary infections are important in reducing morbidity.

2. Paralysis

Paralysis due to the effect of neurotoxins is a common feature of the venoms/poisons of many animals. The onset, severity and duration of paralysis is quite variable, both between and within species. For those neurotoxins which take several hours to cause earliest effects of paralysis, and often longer still to cause respiratory paralysis (e.g. some snake venoms), early detection of systemic envenoming and prompt treatment with adequate amounts of appropriate antivenom may either reverse the paralysis (post-synaptic neurotoxins) or at least arrest it before it reaches the critical stage (pre-synaptic neurotoxins). For the latter group, once full paralysis is established, antivenom will not help, and intubation/ventilation is required if the patient is to survive. This may mean the patient is ventilated for days, weeks, occasionally months. For the former group, even if full paralysis has occurred, requiring ventilation, this may only be short term, as either antivenom or possibly anticholinesterase inhibitors may reverse paralysis[10,35-38].

Some neurotoxins act very quickly (e.g. tetrodotoxin), either ingested (fugu poisoning) or inoculated (blue ringed octopus bite), so that major envenoming and complete paralysis may develop in less than an hour. Intubation and ventilation are vital, but may only be required for a few hours.

Incomplete paralysis may also pose a severe risk for the patient, as deglutition may be affected, with the potential for aspiration, long before there is complete respiratory paralysis. This should be remembered and guarded against in all patients where neurotoxic paralysis is a possibility.

3. Coagulopathy and haemorrhage

The management of primary bleeding disorders of envenoming can present a challenge. If there is complete defibrination (e.g. some types of snakebite) this may occur quickly, soon after the bite[29], sometimes without other major evidence of envenoming, and there is no effective clotting function, though platelets may still be effective (but not in all snakebite coagulopathy). Any vessel wall damage can cause significant blood loss. Insertion of subclavian or jugular intravenous/central venous lines in such patients is fraught with danger, and even femoral puncture can result in major haemorrhage, so should be avoided. Specific antivenom, if available, is usually the best treatment of such problems[8,10,16,29,30]. Until all circulating venom is neutralised, additional clotting proteins will only add substrate to the reaction and may deepen the coagulopathy; therefore the use of fresh frozen plasma or cryoprecipitate in such cases is generally inadvisable, unless adequate antivenom therapy has been given[8]. In some types of snakebite (e.g. Malayan pit viper bite) venom at the bite site may act like a depot, with steady or intermittent release into the circulation over many hours, or even days; hence antivenom therapy may need to be repeated[10]. The use of anticoagulants, particularly heparin, advocated in the past, has generally proved unhelpful or worse[10,46,47]. More detailed information may be found in some of the snakebite chapters.

4. Haemolysis

Haemolysis is caused by a variety of venoms, and may vary from mild, without clinical significance (e.g. some snakebites), through to profound, associated with high morbidity and even mortality (e.g. systemic loxoscelism). It is important to neutralise venom using antivenom, if available, and counter any secondary renal damage.

5. Myolysis

Myolysis is usually systemic and may cause several problems, including muscle weakness, potentially severe, muscle wasting, secondary renal damage from high levels of myoglobin, and cardiac arrhythmias secondary to hyperkalaemia.

6. Renal damage

Kidney damage, up to and including severe long term damage (e.g. cortical necrosis in some snakebites), is a common sequelae of envenoming. The role of antivenom in reducing the chance of renal damage is not known. Early and adequate hydration may be helpful. Management of established renal failure is essentially the same as in other causes of kidney damage.

7. Cardiotoxicity

The cardiotoxic effects of venoms are incompletely understood at a clinical level, though a variety of animal venoms cause envenoming with cardiac abnormalities, varying from mild ECG changes through to cardiac arrest. Rapidity of venom absorption and quantity reaching the circulation seem key factors determining the likelihood and severity of cardiac effects. The role of antivenom is uncertain.

VII. REFERENCES

1. **KIRBY, J.** *Annual report of the New South Wales Poison Information Centre, 1993.* Sydney:The Royal Alexandra Hospital for Children, 1994.
2. **WETZEL, W.W., CHRISTY, N.P.** A king cobra bite in New York City. *Toxicon*, **27**:393-395, 1989.
3. **KOPPEL, C., MARTENS, F.** Clinical experience in the therapy of bites from exotic snakes in Berlin. *Hum. Exp. Toxicol.*, **11**:549-552, 1992.
4. **WARRELL, D.A.** Injuries, envenoming, poisoning and allergic reactions caused by animals. In Eds, Weatherall, D.J., Leadingham, J.G.G., Warrell, D.A. *Oxford Textbook of Medicine.* Oxford:Oxford University Press, pps 6.66-6.85, 1987.
5. **WHITE, J.** Clinical toxinology; an Australian perspective. In Eds. Gopalakrishnakone, P., Tan, C.K. *Recent advances in toxinology research; Volume 1.* Singapore:National University of Singapore, 1992.
6. **THEAKSTON, R.D.** Snake venoms in science and clinical medicine; 2. Applied immunology in snake venom research. *Trans. R. Soc. Trop. Med. Hyg.*, **83**:741-744, 1989.
7. **SUTHERLAND, S.K.** Antivenom use in Australia. Premedication, adverse reactions and the use of venom detection kits. *Med. J. Aust.*, **157**:734-739, 1992.
8. **WHITE, J.** Elapid snakes; management of bites. In Eds. Covacevich, J., Davie, P., Pearn, J. *Toxic Plants and Animals: A Guide for Australia*, Brisbane, Queensland Museum, pps 431-457, 1987.
9. **TIBBALLS, J.** Diagnosis and treatment of confirmed and suspected snake bite. Implication from analysis of 46 paediatric cases. *Med. J. Aust.*, **156**:270-274, 1992.
10. **WARRELL, D.A.** Treatment of snake bite in the Asia-Pacific region; a personal view. In Eds.Golalakrishnakone, P., Chou, L.M. *Snakes of Medical Importance (Asia-Pacific Region).* Singapore:National University of Singapore, 1990.
11. **SWAROOP, S., GRAB, B.** Snake bite mortality in the world. *Bul. World Health Org.* **10**:35-76, 1954.
12. **PUGH, R.N.H., THEAKSTON, R.D.G.** Incidence and mortality of snake bite in savanna Nigeria. *Lancet*, 1181-3, 1980.
13. **HO, M., WARRELL, M.J., WARRELL, D.A., BIDWELL, D., VOLLER, A.** A critical re-appraisal of the use of enzyme-linked immunosorbent assays in the study of snake bite. *Toxicon*, **24**:211-221, 1986.
14. **SUTHERLAND, S.K., COULTER, A.R., HARRIS, A.D.** Rationalisation of first aid methods for elapid snakebite. *Lancet*, 183-6, 1979.
15. **SUTHERLAND, S.K., COULTER, A.R., HARRIS, A.D., LOVERING, K.E., ROBERTS, I.D.** A study of the major Australian snake venoms in the monkey (*Macaca fascicularis*); (1) the movement of injected venom; methods which retard this movement, and the response to antivenom. *Pathology*, **13**:13-27, 1981.
16. **WARRELL, D.A.** Venomous bites and stings in the tropical world. *Med. J. Aust.*, **159**:773-779, 1993.
17. **BARNES, J.M., TRUETA, J.** Absorption of bacteria toxins and snake venoms from the tissues; importance of the lymphatic circulation. *Lancet*, 623-6, 1941.
18. **PEARN, J.H., MORRISON, J.J., CHARLES, N., MUIR, V.** First aid for snakebite. *Med. J. Aust.*, **2**:293-4, 1981.
19. **SUTHERLAND, S.K.** Deaths from snakebite in Australia. *Med. J. Aust.*, **157**:740-746, 1992.
20. **RUSSELL, F.E.** *Snake Venom Poisoning* New York:Scholium International, 1983.
21. **TREVETT, A.J., NWOKOLO, N., WATTERS, D.A., LAGANI, W., VINCE, J.D.** Tourniquet injury in a Papuan snakebite victim. *Trop. Geogr. Med.*, **45**:305-307, 1993.
22. **BLACKMAN, J.R., DILLON, S.** Venomous snakebite; past, present and future treatment options. *J. Am. Board Fam. Pract.*, **5**:399-405, 1992.
23. **RUSSELL, F.E.** Snake venom poisoning. *Vet. Hum. Toxicol.* **33**:584-586, 1991.

24. **COHEN, W.R., WETZEL, W., KADISH, A.** Local heat and cold application after eastern cottonmouth moccasin (*Agkistrodon piscivorus*) envenomation in the rat; effect on tissue injury. *Toxicon*, **30:**1383-6, 1992.

25. **REITZ, C.J., GOOSEN, D.J., ODENDAAL, M.W., VISSER, L., MARAIS, T.J.** Evaluation of the Venom Ex apparatus in the treatment of Egyptian cobra envenomation. *Sth. Afr. Med. J.*, **66:**135-138, 1984.

26. **HARDY, D.L.** A review of first aid measures for pitviper bite in North America with an appraisal of extractor suction and stun gun electroshock. In Eds. Campbell, Brodie, *Biology of the Pitvipers*. Texas:Selva Publishing, pp 405-414, 1992.

27. **SILVEIRA, P.V., NISHIOKA, S. DE-A.** South American rattlesnake bite in a Brazilian teaching hospital. Clinical and epidemiological study of 87 cases, with analysis of factors predictive of renal failure. *Trans. R. Soc. Trop. Med. Hyg.*, **86:**562-564, 1992.

28. **NISHIOKA, S. DE-A., SILVEIRA, P.V.** A clinical and epidemiologic study of 292 cases of lance-headed viper bite in a Brazilian teaching hospital. *Am. J. Trop. Med. Hyg.*, **47:**805-810, 1992.

29. **WHITE, J., WILLIAMS, V.** Severe envenomation with convulsion following multiple bites by a common brown snake, *Pseudonaja textilis. Aust. Paediatr. J.*, **25:**109-111, 1989.

30. **MITRAKUL, C., JUZI, U., PONGRUJIKORN, W.** Antivenom therapy in Russell's viper bite. *Am. J. Clin. Pathol.*, **95:**412-417, 1991.

31. **CUPO, P., AZEVEDO-MARQUES, M.M., DE-MENEZES, J.B., HERRING, S.E.** Immediate hypersensitivity reactions after intravenous use of antivenon sera; prognostic value of intradermal sensitivity tests. *Rev. Inst. Med. Trop. Sao. Paulo.*, **33:**115-122, 1991.

32. **TIBBALLS, J.** Premedication for snake antivenom. *Med. J. Aust..*, **160:**4-7, 1994.

33. **SMITH, D.C., REDDI, K.R., LAING, G., THEAKSTON, R.G., LANDON, J.** An affinity purified ovine antivenom for the treatment of *Vipera berus* envenoming. *Toxicon*, **30:**865-871, 1992.

34. **MARTZ, W.** Plants with a reputation against snakebite. *Toxicon*, **30:**1131-42, 1992.

35. **WATT, G., THEAKSTON, R.D.G., HAYES, C.G., YAMBAO, M.L., SANGALANG, R., RANOA, C.P., ALQUIZALAS, E., WARRELL, D.A.** Positive response to edrophonium in patients with neurotoxic envenoming by cobras (*Naja naja philippinensis*). A placebo-controlled study. *N. Eng. J. Med.*, **315:**1444-8, 1986.

36. **WARRELL, D.A., LOOAREESUWAN, S., WHITE, N.J., THEAKSTON, R.D.G., WARRELL, M.J., KOSAKARN, W., REID, H.A.** Severe neurotoxic envenoming by the Malayan krait *Bungarus candidus* (Linnaeus); response to antivenom and anticholinesterase. *Brit. Med. J.*, **286:**678-680, 1983.

37. **CAMPBELL, C.H.** Venomous snakebite in Papua and its treatment with tracheostomy, artificial respiration and antivenene. *Trans. Roy. Soc. Trop. Med.Hyg.*, **58:**263-73, 1964.

38. **WATT, G., MEADE, B.D., THEAKSTON, R.D., PADRE, L.P., TUAZON, M.L., CALUBAQUIB, C., SANTIAGO, E., RANOA, C.P.** Comparison of tensilon and antivenom for the treatment of cobra bite paralysis. *Trans. R. Soc. Trop. Med. Hyg.*, **83:**570-573, 1989.

39. **KERRIGAN, K.R.** Bacteriology of snakebite abcess. *Trop. Doc.*, **22:**158-60, 1992.

40. **KERRIGAN, K.R.** Venomous snakebite in eastern Ecuador. *Am. J. Trop. Med. Hyg.*, **44:**93-99, 1991.

41. **HARDY, D.** Fatal rattlesnake envenomation in Arizona; 1969-1984. *Clin. Toxicol.*, **24:**1-10, 1986.

42. **MARS, M., HADLEY, G.P., AITCHISON, J.M.** Direct intracompartmental pressure measurement in the management of snakebites in children. *Sth. Afr. Med. J.*, **80:**227-228, 1991.

43. **EL-AMIN, E.O., ELIDRISSY, A., HAMID, H.S., SULTAN, O.M., SAFAR, R.A.** Scorpion sting; a management problem. *Ann. Trop. Paediatr.*, **11:**143-148, 1991.

44. **REES, R., ALTENBERN, P., LYNCH, J., KING, L.E.** Brown recluse spider bites; a comparison of early surgical excision versus dapsone and delayed surgical excision. *Ann. Surg.* **202:**659-663, 1985.

45. **JANSEN, J.T., MORGAN, P.N., MCQUEEN, N.N., BENNETT, W.E.** The brown recluse spider bite; controlled evaluation of treatment using the white rabbit as an animal model. *South. Med. J.* **64:**1194, 1983.

46. **WARRELL, D.A., POPE, H.M., PRENTICE, C.R.M.** Disseminated intravascular coagulation caused by the carpet viper (*Echis carinatus*); trial of heparin. *Br. J. Haematol.*, **33:**335-342, 1976.

47. **TIN NA SWE, MYINT LWIN, KHIN EI HAN, TIN TUN, TUN PE.** Heparin therapy in Russell's viper bite victims with disseminated intravascular coagulation; a controlled trial. *Southeast Asian J. Trop. Med. Public Health*, **23:**282-287, 1992.

Chapter 3

BIOLOGY AND DISTRIBUTION OF POISONOUS MARINE ANIMALS

Dietrich Mebs

TABLE OF CONTENTS

I.INTRODUCTION

The sea is a hostile environment for the human intruder. Venomous animals defend themselves or their territory by using stingers or teeth, by venom apparatus as complicated as nematocytes or as simple as spines of fins. Using these tools venom is introduced intradermally or subcutaneously producing local symptoms such as pain, inflammation, necrosis etc. or eventually reaching the circulatory system, whereby the toxins are transported to target organs such as the nervous system, muscle or heart etc. Other animals are poisonous. They produce or accumulate toxins and store them in their body, sometimes in special organs. They are not harmful to man unless they are used as food. Then the toxins, enterally applied, find their way to target organs.

II. SECONDARY METABOLITES IN THE MARINE ENVIRONMENT

Marine organisms produce a huge number of secondary metabolites, perhaps to a larger extent than observed in terrestrial ecosystems[1-3]. These compounds comprise a wide variety of chemical structures ranging from simple molecules such as amines to more complex molecules like alkaloids, terpenes, steroids, peptides or even proteins. Among them some of the most lethal toxins are found: saxitoxin, tetrodotoxin, ciguatoxin, palytoxin, the conotoxins or sea snake toxins. Although considerable progress in marine chemistry led to the discovery of many new compounds with peculiar structures, only a small fraction of marine organisms have been investigated.

These metabolites serve many purposes in the marine ecosystems; they are used for prey capture or for defense, cause antibiosis to prevent microbial infection or overgrowth by competing organisms; they may also have signal functions like pheromones, by deterring and repelling predators or by attracting sexual or symbiotic partners[4]. However, the role these compounds play in the complex interactions of marine organisms is still poorly understood. Until recent years research was mainly motivated by finding new compounds useful for medical purposes or was initiated when these compounds interfered with marine food production and caused serious public health problems.

III. POISONOUS MARINE ANIMALS

In the marine environment poisonous animals are more abundant than commonly anticipated. Their noxious or toxic metabolites act only when ingested, because these animals lack tools or weapons to apply these compounds parenterally. This limits the chances and danger of poisoning, since seafood is a selection of animals, which are normally free of poisons, toxins or harmful substances. Nevertheless these animals are part of the marine food chain and may accumulate noxious compounds from man-made sea pollution (metals, industrial or agricultural chemicals etc.), but may also contain naturally occurring metabolites such as saxitoxin and ciguatoxin.

Many marine animals are known to be poisonous and are avoided and not harvested as sea food; e.g. starfish, sea cucumbers (consumed only after special treatment as trepang or bêche-de-mer), sponges or soft corals. These organisms usually contain considerable amounts of toxic alkaloids, terpenes, steroids or other compounds with a high potential to cause illness or death. Therefore poisoning by marine animals is rarely due to the ingestion of products from the sea which are known to be poisonous. The only exception to this rule is the widespread consumption of puffer fish (fugu) as a delicacy in Japan, where the tetrodotoxin content produces tingling sensations in lips, gums or other symptoms of a slight intoxication depending on the dose. More often poisoning results from the ingestion of sea food such as shellfish, mussels and fish, which became poisonous under certain, hardly predictable circumstances. Thus shellfish poisoning in its various forms; paralytic, diarrhetic, neurotoxic, amnesic, and ciguatera fish poisoning, may easily reach epidemic proportions. In many areas of the world these poisonings are major public health issues and have severe economic impact on shellfish and fishing industries.

IV. RED TIDES

Poisonous sea food like mussels, shellfish or fish are clearly associated with a phenomenon called red tide, the seasonally occurring change of water color due to a bloom of planktonic algae. Dinoflagellates, unicellular algae, are predominantly involved. They produce lethal toxins like gonyautoxins including saxitoxin [5,6]. Plankton feeders such as shellfish filtrate the algae from the water, digest them and accumulate the toxins in various organs where they eventually reach concentrations which do not affect the marine organism, but are lethal for man. Other dinoflagellates do not occcur in the phytoplankton, but are benthic microorganisms, living on the surface of macroalgae and likewise produce toxins such as ciguatoxin [7,8]. These toxins accumulate via the food chain from herbivorous to carnivorous fishes. Planktonic or benthic algae blooms, the red tides, are therefore important to monitor because they easily may lead to the occurrence of toxic compounds in seafood.

Red tides are a natural phenomenon. The factors, which initiate and trigger red tides, are still a matter of speculation. However, human activities leading to the disturbance or destruction of marine ecosystems may well be involved. Massive introduction of nitrogen and phosphorous in coastal waters via sewage or agricultural runoff generally favors a bloom of phytoplankton. Moreover, it seems that algal blooms tend to increase in frequency worldwide. For instance, in 1965 about 40 red tides were observed in the Seto Inland Sea

(Japan) which increased to 300 in 1973. A considerable reduction of pollution by building sewage treatment facilities was followed by a continuous decrease of red tides since 1975[9]. Military activities in the Pacific (nuclear explosions, missile testing etc.) have been linked with increasing ciguatera outbreaks in this area[10].

Toxic algal blooms especially have occurred in alarming proportions in recent years[6]. A red tide which was previously restricted to the Gulf coast of Florida spread northward to North Carolina causing dramatic losses in the shellfish industry in 1987/88. The toxin involved is brevetoxin. An outbreak of a hitherto unknown shellfish poisoning hit Prince Edward Island, Canada, 1987. For the first time domoic acid was found to be involved causing brain damage (amnesic shellfish poisoning). The toxin was traced to a bloom of diatoms, *Nitzschia pungens*, a species, which has a worldwide distribution and which is generally considered to be nontoxic. In 1991 domoic acid was also found on the coast of California killing pelicans which had eaten anchovies. Shellfish and crabs contained high levels of this toxin. Paralytic shellfish poisoning occurred also on the Pacific coast of Guatemala killing 26 people[11].

Whether toxic blooms are on the rise, or the recent observations just reflect more awareness in monitoring such outbreaks more carefully, or are simply due to the fact that people eat more seafood is an open question. Toxic blooms could have occurred without consequences in many areas, when shellfishing was on a smaller scale than nowadays. Since toxins with high lethal potency are involved, which are produced by algae becoming toxin producers unexpectedly, there is an urgent need for research on red tide phenomena and human impact as well as more awareness by public health authorities.

The clinical toxicology of shellfish, ciguatera and fugu poisoning is described in chapters 4,5,6. Other poisonings, which may also cause serious illness and death, are mentioned here such as poisoning by fish, crabs and snails.

V. FISH POISONING OTHER THAN CIGUATERA AND FUGU

Some lesser known forms of fish poisoning (ichthyotoxism) originate from the ingestion of specific fish species or of their organs such as liver, gonads or blood. A few, like scombrotoxism, the second most important fish poisoning after ciguatera, have public health impact; other poisonings are sporadic or even rare[12].

Clupeotoxism may be caused by the ingestion of the flesh of herrings or anchovies (family: Clupeidae; Engraulidae). A sharp metallic taste is usually present; symptoms such as nausea, vomiting, abdominal pain, and diarrhoea follow. Several neurological symptoms like dilated pupils, tingling sensations, muscular cramps, and paralysis followed by coma and death may occur in cases of severe poisoning. Outbreaks of this type of fish poisoning were reported for the Caribbean Sea and the Indo-Pacific. The toxin involved is unknown, perhaps of planktonic origin accumulated via the food chain; treatment of the patient is largely symptomatic.

Gempylotoxic fishes include pelagic mackerels (family: Gempylidae) of the tropical Atlantic and Indo-Pacific oceans. The oil contained in the flesh sometimes provokes diarrhoea similar to that caused by castor oil.

Ichthyotoxism is caused by the ingestion of roe or of the gonads of predominantly freshwater fishes (sturgeons, gars, pikes, carps etc.), but also of some marine species (blennies and sculpins), which appear to become poisonous during the reproductive season. Symptoms include nausea, vomiting, diarrhoea, abdominal pain, weak pulse, cyanosis, cramps. Phospholipids are considered to be the toxic principle involved. Treatment is symptomatic.

Ichthyohaemotoxism is an intoxication observed after drinking the blood of eels (conger, moray eels), a strange and uncommon behaviour. Nausea, vomiting, diarrhoea may occur. The nature of the toxin is unknown.

Reports from Japan indicate that the liver of certain fish species (mackerels) may become seasonally toxic (**ichthyohepatotoxism**). Symptoms of poisoning, including nausea, vomiting, fever, headache and erythema followed by skin desquamation, have been explained by vitamin A overdosage.

Hallucinogenic fish poisoning (**ichthyoallyeinotoxism**) is a strange phenomenon occasionally observed after the ingestion of some coral reef fishes (mullets etc.). Symptoms may develop within minutes including hallucinations, mental depression, dizziness, loss of equilibrium and lack of motor coordination. The toxic principle is unknown. The intoxication is considered to be relatively mild.

Scombrotoxism or **scombroid fish poisoning** is another important sea food intoxication beside ciguatera and shellfish poisoning[13]. However, this is not due to a sea-borne toxin, but to histamine, which is enzymatically produced by bacteria from histidine in the muscle of fish as a result of improper preservation (putrefaction). Fish like mackerel, tuna, bonito (family: Scombridae), but also anchovies, sardines (Engraulidae) and bluefish (Pomatomidae), are predominantly incriminated. Symptoms appear within minutes and are identical to histamine intoxication: headache, dizziness, nausea, vomiting, generalized erythema and urticaria accompanied by extensive pruritus, diarrhoea and in severe cases bronchospasm and respiratory distress; shock may occur and lead to death, if not treated immediately. Antidotes are available; specific treatment by antihistaminics like diphenhydramine, chloropheniramine or cimetidine (H_2-antagonist, in case the patient does not react to diphenhydramine) is most successful. A peppery taste of the fish indicates a high level of histamine. Scombrotoxism is an important public health issue, also involving canned fish[14].

VI. TOXIC CRABS

Various crab species (*Atergatis, Carpilius, Demania, Eriphia, Lophozozymus, Zozymus* etc.) of the Indo-Pacific have been reported to cause severe intoxications when used as a food source, especially as an ingredient of soup[12]. Saxitoxin and its homologues gonyautoxins as well as tetrodotoxin were identified as toxic principles being present in concentrations high enough to cause death[15,16]. These toxins, which are known to be involved in pufferfish and paralytic shellfish poisoning, are obviously produced by bacteria in the crabs (see also chapter 4). Palytoxin, originally found in zoanthid anemones (*Palythoa* sp.), has also been incriminated in fatal cases of crab poisoning[17].

VII. TOXIC SNAILS

Reports from Japan on poisoning by marine snails include various species (*Turbo, Tectus, Charonia* sp.), which are commonly eaten, but may occasionally be poisonous[18]. Saxitoxin, gonyautoxins and also tetrodotoxin have been identified as the causal agents of poisoning. The Japanese ivory shell, *Babylonia japonica*, may also contain glycosides named surugatoxins, which produce atropine-like effects[19].

In cases of crab and snail poisoning reduction of toxin load by emesis and gastric lavage followed by symptomatic treatment is recommended; no specific antidotes are available.

VIII. REFERENCES

1. **KREBS, H.C.** Recent developments in the field of marine natural products with emphasis on biologically compounds. *Prog.Chem.Org.Nat.Prod.* **49**:151-363, 1986.
2. **SCHEUER, P.J.** (ed.) *Marine Natural Products. Chemical and Biological Perspectives.* Vol.**1-5**, New York:Academic Press, 1978-1983.
3. **SCHEUER, P.J.** (ed.) *Bioorganic Marine Chemistry.* Vol.**1-4**, Berlin:Springer Verl.
4. **BAKUS, G.J., TARGETT, N.M. & SCHULTE, B.** (1986) Chemical ecology of marine organisms: an overview. *J.Chem.Ecol.***12**:951-987, 1987-1991.
5. **BADEN, D.G.** Public health problems of red tides. In: Ed. TU, A.T., *Marine Toxins and Venoms.* Handbook of Natural Toxins vol.**3**, New York:M.Dekker, pp. 259-277, 1988.
6. **CULOTTA, E.** Red menace in the world´s oceans. *Science* **257**:1476-1477, 1992.
7. **YASUMOTO, T., NAKAJIMA, I., BAGNIS, R.A. & ADACHI, R.** Finding of a dinoflagellate as a likely culprit of ciguatera. *Bull.Jap.Soc.Sci.Fisheries* **43**:1021-1026, 1977.
8. **WITHERS, N.W.** Ciguatera fish poisoning. In: Ed. TU, A.T., *Marine Toxins and Venoms* . Handbook of Natural Toxins vol.**3**, New York:M.Dekker, pp.31-61, 1988.
9. **CHERFAS, J.** The fringe of the ocean- under siege from land. *Science* **248**:163-165, 1990.
10. **RUFF, T.A.** Ciguatera in the Pacific: a link with military activities. *Lancet,* **Jan.28**:201-205, 1989.
11. **RODRIGUE, D.C., ETZEL, R.A., HALL, S., DE PORRAS, E., VELASZQUEZ, O.H., TAUXE, R.V., KILBOURNE, E.M. & BLAKE, P.A.** Lethal paralytic shellfish poisoning in Guatemala. *Am.J.Trop.Med.Hyg.* **42**, 267-271, 1990.
12. **HALSTEAD, B.W.** *Poisonous and Venomous Marine Animals of the World* (2nd rev.ed.). Princeton:Darwin Press Inc., , 1988
13. **TAYLOR, S.L., STRATTON, J.E. & NORDLEE, J.A.** Histamine poisoning (scombroid fish poisoning): an allergy-like intoxication. *Clin.Toxicol.***27**:225-232, 1989.
14. **MURRAY, C.K., HOBBES, G. & GILBERT, R.J.** (1982) Scombrotoxin and scombrotoxin-like poisoning from canned fish. *J.Hyg.* **88**:215-220, .
15. **YASUMOTO, T., OSHIMA, Y. & KONTA, T.** Analysis of paralytic shellfish toxins of xanthid crabs in Okinawa. *Bull.Jap.Soc.Sci.Fisheries* **47**:957-959, 1981.
16. **NOGUCHI, T., JEON, J:K:, ARAKAWA, O., SUGITA, H., DEGUCHI, Y., SHIDA, Y. & HASHIMOTO, K.** Occurrence of tetrodotoxin and anhydrotetrodotoxin in *Vibrio* sp. isolated from the intestines of a xanthid crab, *Atergatis floridus.* *J.Biochem.* (Tokyo) **99**:311, 1986.
17. **YASUMOTO, T., YASUMURA, D., OHIZUMI, Y., TAKAHASHI, M. & ALCALA, L.C.** Palytoxin in two species of xanthid crab from the Philippines. *Agric.Biol.Chem.,* .**50**:163-167, 1986.
18. **HASHIMOTO, Y.** *Marine Toxins and Other Bioactive Metabolites.* Tokyo:Jap.Soc.of Sciences, 1979, .
19. **KOSUGE, T., ZENDA, H. & OCHIAI, A.** Isolation and structure determination of a new marine toxin, surugatoxin, from the Japanese ivory shell, *Babylonia japonica. Tetrahedron Lett.* **25**:4407-4410, 1972.

Chapter 4

CLINICAL TOXICOLOGY OF SHELLFISH POISONING

David Smart

TABLE OF CONTENTS

I. INTRODUCTION

Shellfish are a significant worldwide source of dietary protein. They are also a vector for a number of food-borne diseases including allergies, infections (viral and bacterial) and toxic poisoning. Bacteria, viruses and toxins accumulate in shellfish because of their technique of filter feeding. Large quantities of seawater are continually filtered by marine shellfish (clams, oysters, mussels and scallops and other molluscs) in order to extract oxygen and nutrients such as particulate food matter and plankton. As a result of this process, heavy metals, toxins and infective micro-organisms are concentrated in the shellfish, causing a health risk when they are ingested by humans. Bacterial and viral diseases are the most common causes of illness resulting from human consumption of shellfish, particularly raw specimens. Table 1 summarises diseases which have been transmitted by shellfish. Exposure to contaminated water is a factor in shellfish transmission of infections[1,2]. Fortunately these infectious diseases are usually self limiting, rarely constituting a threat to life.

Table 1
Diseases commonly associated with shellfish

1.   Infection
     - Bacteria: Salmonella, Vibrio, Staphylococcus
     - Viruses: Norwalk, Hepatitis A
2.   Allergy
3.   Toxic Poisoning
     - Paralytic shellfish poisoning
     - Neurotoxic shellfish poisoning
     - Gastroenteritic shellfish poisoning
     - Amnesic shellfish poisoning
4.   Heavy metal poisoning

Marine intoxications accounted for 13.8% of all food-borne outbreaks of disease in the USA from 1972 - 1982[3,4]. Of the 272 outbreaks due to marine intoxication, 20 outbreaks (7.4%) were toxic shellfish poisoning. Hence, toxic shellfish poisoning is responsible for only 1.1% of all illnesses of food-borne aetiology in the U.S. Four major toxic syndromes have been linked to ingestion of shellfish; paralytic, neurotoxic, diarrhetic, and the recently identified "encephalopathic" or amnesic shellfish poisoning. The general term "toxic shellfish poisoning" applies to all illness caused by toxins in shellfish. Paralytic shellfish poisoning (PSP) is the most common cause of severe illness, producing a similar clinical syndrome to ciguatera and tetrodotoxin intoxication[5], and it has caused a number of fatalities. It is caused by a group of toxins, the saxitoxins, which are produced by unicellular sea algae, the dinoflagellates. Approximately 20 of the 1200 known species of dinoflagellates produce toxins which cause significant illness in man. The dinoflagellates most frequently implicated in outbreaks of severe PSP toxicity are the species *Alexandrium catenella* and *A. tamarense*, *Pyrodinium bahamense* and *P. bahamense* (var compressum). Another dinoflagellate, *Gymnodinium breve* (formerly *Ptychodiscus brevis*) produces toxins which cause a milder clinical syndrome known as neurotoxic shellfish poisoning (NSP). Individuals with NSP do not suffer paralysis and outbreaks of clinical illness mostly occur along the west coast of Florida, U.S.[6] "Diarrhetic" shellfish poisoning (DSP) is a self limiting condition caused by ingestion of shellfish contaminated with the dinoflagellates *Dinophysis* sp. Most cases have been reported in Japan[7]. Amnesic shellfish poisoning (ASP) has recently been described in individuals consuming mussels harvested from water near Prince Edward Island, Canada[8]. A syndrome of gastrointestinal symptoms, headache and memory loss resulted from ingesting mussels contaminated with domoic acid[9]. The source of the domoic acid was the diatom, *Nitzschia pungens* (f. *multiseries*), and four fatalities occurred in the outbreak.

Table 2 summarises the marine plankton linked with toxic shellfish poisoning. The species are predominantly dinoflagellate and the only exception is the diatom *Nitzschia pungens*. All types of shellfish poisoning will be covered in greater detail later; however, several common features are worthy of note. Firstly, the toxins produced by the dinoflagellates and diatoms are heat stable and not destroyed by cooking. When there are large numbers of the organisms in the water during an algal "bloom" their toxins rapidly accumulate in shellfish during filter feeding. The toxins appear to have very little effect on the host shellfish, despite being very toxic to other fish and animals higher in the food chain. Toxic shellfish poisoning occurs when humans ingest affected shellfish. The shellfish are usually bivalved molluscs (i.e. mussels, clams, oysters, scallops and cockles), although other molluscs such as chitons, murex and limpets have caused human illness in addition to sand crabs, horseshoe crabs and reef crabs[10].

Table 2
Organisms linked to toxicity in humans (see Figures 2-6).

Paralytic Shellfish Poisoning (PSP)
  Alexandrium (formerly *Gonyaulax* or *Protogonyaulax*) *tamarense - excavatum*
  Alexandrium catenella
  Pyrodinium bahamense
  Pyrodinium bahamense (var. *compressum*)
  Gymnodinium catenatum
  Cochlodinium catenatum
Neurotoxic Shellfish Poisoning (NSP)
  Gymnodinium breve (formerly *Ptychodiscus brevis*)
Diarrhetic Shellfish Poisoning (DSP)
  Dinophysis fortii
  Dinophysis norvegica
  Dinophysis mitra
  Dinophysis acuminata
  Dinophysis acuta
  Dinophysis rotundata
  Prorocentrum sp.
Amnesic Shellfish Poisoning (ASP)
  Nitzschia pungens f. multiseries

Dinoflagellates are frequently but not always associated with sea discolouration known as "red tides". The association between red tides and seafood toxicity has been known since biblical times[11], and the phenomenon is described in the Bible in Exodus 7:20-21: "And the waters that were in the river turned to blood. And the fish that were in the river died; and the river stank and the Egyptians could not drink the water of the river." Occasionally dinoflagellates may cause bioluminescence. The association of this phenomenon with poisonous mussels was recognised by the North American Indians[12]. Outbreaks of human illness may be linked to dinoflagellate blooms; however, there is often a lead-time between the algal bloom and the onset of clinical illness. This has caused some difficulties for health authorities investigating an outbreak.

II. EPIDEMIOLOGY OF SHELLFISH POISONING

Accurate world-wide data which outline the prevalence of toxic shellfish poisoning in humans are not available. There are a number of problems with data collection. The diagnosis may be missed when clinical symptoms are mild or when small numbers of people are involved and a link with shellfish ingestion is not established. In third world countries, shortages of trained medical and public health personnel may also prevent recognition of the syndrome. Even when the diagnosis is established, cases must be recorded in that country's central database and reported in scientific literature before being available for world-wide epidemiological surveys. Most reports in the scientific literature originate from developed Western nations and they focus on larger outbreaks with more severe illness. In many countries where accurate statistics are collected, public health programmes have reduced the numbers of new cases of toxic shellfish poisoning to low levels. Hence figures from these countries are not representative of the global picture. Researchers can provide at best only rough estimates of the global extent of the problem.

International conferences have provided forums of debate and enabled some estimates to be made of the world-wide prevalence of toxic shellfish poisoning. In 1974 it was estimated that there were 1600 cases of toxic shellfish poisoning world-wide with 300 deaths[13]. Public health data collected in California, U.S. recorded 508 cases between 1927 and 1985 with 32 deaths[14]. Numbers of new cases are declining in the U.S. due to active public health and education programmes, a six month quarantine restricting commercial mussel harvesting every year, and routine monitoring for toxins in commercially produced shellfish[3,15]. Most new cases are sporadic, occurring in individuals who collect "wild" shellfish for private consumption[3].

A. GEOGRAPHIC DISTRIBUTION

Figure 1 depicts areas in the world where outbreaks of toxic shellfish poisoning have been recorded.

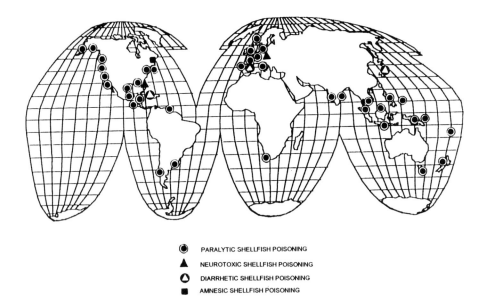

◉ PARALYTIC SHELLFISH POISONING

▲ NEUROTOXIC SHELLFISH POISONING

◖ DIARRHETIC SHELLFISH POISONING

■ AMNESIC SHELLFISH POISONING

Figure 1. World wide distribution of toxic shellfish poisoning. Areas marked indicate geographical regions where toxic shellfish poisoning has occurred, and the type of shellfish poisoning. The map is not quantitative in terms of number of outbreaks or cases

Table 3 summarises outbreaks of human cases of paralytic shellfish poisoning which have been reported between 1968 and 1991 in world literature. The numbers of deaths and case fatality ratios are also tabulated. Even though toxic shellfish poisoning has a world-wide distribution, there are several patterns apparent in its distribution:

(i) There has been a significant global spread of the disease over the last 20 years. It was predominantly a northern hemisphere phenomenon. In recent years outbreaks have occurred in the southern hemisphere, including Chile, New Zealand, Papua New Guinea, Fiji and South Africa[16-20]. This may reflect increasing awareness of the problem in the southern hemisphere or perhaps improved reporting with development of epidemiological data collection systems. It may reflect true spread of disease. A number of toxic dinoflagellate blooms have been recorded in the Indo-Pacific region of the southern hemisphere in recent years, and the prevalence of human illness appears to be increasing[17]. A major outbreak occurred in New Zealand in January and February 1993. This was caused by Gymnodinium breve and 170 cases of human poisoning occurred[18].

(ii) The type of dinoflagellate responsible for human illness via ingested seafood (usually shellfish) varies depending on the geographical area studied. In the southern hemisphere, the organism usually responsible for PSP outbreaks is *Pyrodinium* sp., whereas *Alexandrium* sp., *Gymnodinium* sp. and *Dinophysis* sp. cause PSP, NSP and DSP in the northern hemisphere.

(iii)   Toxic shellfish poisoning has been in the past restricted to temperate regions; however a number of outbreaks have been reported from tropical regions in recent years including Brunei, Sabah, Singapore, Thailand, Venezuela, Guatemala, Papua New Guinea and Fiji[17,19,20,22-26]. Palauan people traditionally have not eaten the cockles *Spondylus* sp and *Lophus cristagalli* because they are "poisonous". These shellfish have been subsequently shown to possess saxitoxin and gonyautoxins I and II, and the dinoflagellate *Pyrodinium* sp. has been identified in the area[27,28].

(iv)   Most outbreaks have been in regions where ocean currents mix with the open coast; however, small outbreaks have been associated with estuarine conditions, for example in Massachusetts U.S.[10]

(v) Although red tides have frequently been linked to outbreaks of human illness from toxic shellfish poisoning, this is not always the case. Maclean in 1984 summarised a number of reports in the Indo-Pacific region including Australia where toxic dinoflagellate blooms occurred resulting in deaths of large numbers of fish[17]. Birds are also victims of the toxicity[29], presumably because the toxin passes up the food chain. A large number of species of dinoflagellates other than those summarised in Table 2 have demonstrated toxicity in field tests; however, they have not been incriminated in human intoxications[10]. These may be responsible for fish and bird mass mortalities. They have been reviewed recently by Hallegraeff[30].

B. SEASONAL INCIDENCE

Outbreaks of paralytic shellfish poisoning have not been detected along the Pacific coast of U.S. and Canada during the colder months of November to January. Most cases have occurred from May to October (late spring to early autumn [fall]). This is the period of closure of commercial shellfish beds in California[14]. European outbreaks have mostly occurred from May to November, and along the Atlantic coast of Canada and U.S. episodes have occurred July to September[10]. The warmer months with greater solar radiation favour proliferation of dinoflagellates. This is supported by observations in the southern hemisphere. In Chile, outbreaks were reported in spring (October and November)[16], and in Tasmania, Australia, highest levels of toxins were recorded in shellfish in the months of January to June (summer and autumn)[31]. The South African outbreak occurred in late autumn[21].

The tropical regions are always warm and outbreaks in Brunei and Sabah occurred in March[17,20,23], and the Papua New Guinea outbreaks occurred in December to February[19].

Table 3
Outbreaks of paralytic shellfish poisoning; 137 deaths in 2334 cases = 5.9%

Year	Country (Ref No.)	Number Affected	Deaths	% Deaths	Shellfish Type	Shellfish Scientific Name	Dinoflagellate	Toxin
1968	United Kingdom[85]	78	0	0	Mussels/Cockles	Mytilus Edulis Cardium sp.	Alexandrium tamarense	? Saxitoxin
1970-72	Chile[16]	Unknown	5		Mussels	Mytilus Chilensis Aulacomya Ater	Mesodinium Ruòrum Dinophysis sp.	Unknown
1972	Papua New Guinea[19]	25	3	12	Cockles	Anadara Maculosa	Pyrodinium Bahamense	Saxitoxin
1976	Palau[27]	NOT STATED			Thorny oyster	Spondylus sp.	Alexandrium sp. Pyrodinium bahamense	Saxitoxin
1976	Brunei[17]	14	0	0	Fish; Chub Mackerel	Rastrelliger sp.	Pyrodinium bahamense	? Saxitoxin
1976	Sabah[23]	201	7 (children)	3.5	Clams/Mussels		Pyrodinium bahamense	
1976	France[86]	17	0	0	Mussels	Mytilus Edulis	Alexandrium tamarense	Gonyautoxins (saxitoxins)
1976	Switzerland[86]	23	0	0	Mussels	Mytilus Edulis	Alexandrium tamarense	Gonyautoxins (saxitoxins)
1976	Germany[86]	19	0	0	Mussels	Mytilus Edulis	Alexandrium tamarense	Saxitoxins
1976	Italy[86]	38	0	0	Mussels	Mytilus Edulis	Alexandrium tamarense	Saxitoxins
1977	Venezuela[26]	171	10 (8 out of 10 children)	5.8	Mussels		Alexandrium tararense. Cochlodinium catenatum. Noctiluca miliaris	? Saxitoxins
1979	South Africa[21]	17	0	0	Mussels	Choromytilus Meridionalis	Alexandrium catenella	Saxitoxins
1927-1980	California, U.S.[14]	508	32	6.3	Mussels, clams, scallops	Mytilus sp., others not stated	Alexandrium catenella	Saxitoxins
1981	India[17]	82	3	3.7	Bivalves ? type	Not stated	Not recorded	

Year	Location				Food	Species	Organism	Toxin
1983	Philippines[17]	250	21	8.4	Mostly fish	Rastrelliger sp. Sardinella sp.	Pyrodinium bahamense (var. compressum)	? Saxitoxins
1983	India[17]	7	1	14	Bivalves ? type	Not stated	Not recorded	
1983	Indonesia[17]	195	4	2	Clupeoid fish	Selaroides sp. Sardinella sp.	?Pyrodinium sp.	
1983 - 84	Sabah[17]	25	11 (children)	44	Shellfish		Uncertain ? P. Bahamense	
1984	Solomon Islands[17]	NOT	STATED		Shellfish	CLINICALLY IDENTIFIED SYNDROME		
1984	Norway[104]	17	2	11.8	Mussels	Mytilus Edulis	Alexandrium sp. Prorocentrum sp.	Saxitoxin
1986	Singapore[22]	10	2	20	Mussels	Perna Viridis	Not identified	Saxitoxin derivatives
1980, 1986	Tasmania, Australia[105]	4	0	0	Shellfish	Not stated	Gymnodinium catenatum	Saxitoxin
1987	Guatemala[24]	187	26	13.9	Clams	Amphichaena Kindermani	Pyrodinium bahamense	Saxitoxin
1981 - 87	Thailand[25]	74	2	2.7	Mussels, Horseshoe crabs	Perna Viridis	Alexandrium sp.	Not identified
1988	Canada[102]	53	0	0	Mussels		Not stated	
1989	El Salvador[106]	106	3	2.8	Clams		Not stated	Saxitoxins
1989	Mexico[106]	99	4	4	Clams		Not stated	
1989	Guatemala[106]	7	0	0	Clams		Not stated	
1976 - 89	Alaska (U.S.)[52]	94	0	0	Butter clams	Saxidomus Giganteus	Not stated	? Saxitoxin
1990	Alaska/ Massachusetts, USA[52]	19	1	5.3	Mussels/Clams	Mytilus sp. Saxidomus Giganteus	Not stated	Saxitoxin

The time of year was not recorded for the Singapore outbreak[22]. Neurotoxic and diarrhetic shellfish poisoning follow a similar seasonal pattern to paralytic shellfish poisoning.

The outbreak of amnesic shellfish poisoning occurred in November and December 1987 (late autumn and winter)[7]. This was due to contamination of shellfish by *Nitzschia pungens*, a diatom. It is likely that factors favouring diatom growth are different to the dinoflagellates.

C. MORTALITY FROM TOXIC SHELLFISH POISONING

Human mortality rates for the paralytic form of toxic shellfish poisoning are falling in Western nations. The death rates for various older series vary from 8.5% to 23.2%[11,15]. The overall mortality rate for the more recent series summarised in Table 3 is 5.9% (137 deaths in 2334 cases). In California, U.S. from 1927 to 1979 there were 30 deaths out of 410 cases of PSP (7.4%). In 1980 there were two deaths in 98 cases (2%). Alaska, U.S. had one death in 107 cases between 1976 and 1990 (0.9%). The availability of advanced life support appears to improve an individual's chances of surviving an episode of PSP. In the U.S. between 1971 and 1977 there were no deaths due to PSP[3]. Six percent of the patients from 1971 - 77 required mechanical ventilation and 32% required hospitalisation. Increased public awareness and early diagnosis also plays a role in preventing deaths from the syndrome.

There appears to be a high mortality in children sustaining toxic shellfish poisoning. All deaths resulting from toxic shellfish poisoning in Sabah Malaysia in 1976 were in children, and eight of 10 deaths reported in Venezuela in 1977 were in children[23,26].

III. DINOFLAGELLATES RESPONSIBLE FOR SHELLFISH POISONING

Dinoflagellates are the second most abundant order of marine organism, outnumbered only by diatoms. Both of these orders of marine phytoplankton have species which produce toxins linked with human illness; however, on a global basis the dinoflagellates are of greatest significance. These organisms form the basis of the marine food chain. Approximately 1200 species of dinoflagellates have been identified and only a small number are toxic to humans (Table 2). Dinoflagellates are unicellular phytoplankton which exhibit properties of both plants and animals. They are motile, possessing a flagellum. Some possess chloroplasts in their cytoplasm for photosynthesis[32]. The chloroplasts are responsible for discolouration of the sea when large numbers are present during dinoflagellate "blooms". A reddish discolouration is often observed; however, many other colours may be noted depending on the species of dinoflagellate which is in bloom[33]. Bioluminescence may also occur during blooms and this has been particularly noticeable with *Alexandrium* species[34].

Dinoflagellates are extremely small, ranging from 20 to 40 micrometres in diameter. They possess subtle differences in their morphology and skilled personnel are required to accurately identify toxic dinoflagellate species. Many structures are only apparent using electron microscopy. The *Alexandrium* species possess an outer shell of polysaccharide plates, and is referred to as an "armoured" dinoflagellate (Figure 2). *Gymnodinium breve* does not possess this polysaccharide shell and has been referred to as a "naked" organism (Figure 3)[32]. Differences in structure are relevant in the toxicity of dinoflagellates towards animals higher in the food chain. *Gymnodinium breve* is particularly toxic to fish because its toxin is absorbed via their gills. More detailed studies of the structure of dinoflagellates has also resulted in changes to their taxonomy over the last two decades[35]. Examples of various dinoflagellate species are depicted in Figures 2 - 6.

41

Table 2 outlines some of the previous terminology used to identify particular dinoflagellates. A detailed account of dinoflagellate classification and taxonomy is beyond the scope of this chapter. It is not necessary to identify the dinoflagellate responsible for an outbreak of toxic shellfish poisoning during initial investigations. Sufficient knowledge is now available after recognising the clinical syndrome to confirm the existence of a toxin, and then precisely identify the toxin. Later investigations may identify the toxic dinoflagellate. Clinical management and preventative measures can be instituted while the above process of identification occurs.

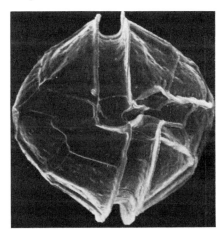

Figure 2. *Alexandrium minutum.* Photo courtesy of Dr G. Hallegraeff PhD.

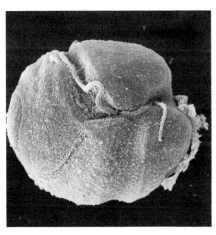

Figure 3. *Gymnodium pulchellum* (very closely related to *Gymnodinium breve*).

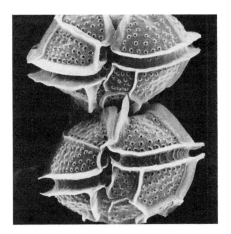

Figure 4. *Pyrodinium bahamense* Photo courtesy of Dr G. Hallegraeff PhD.

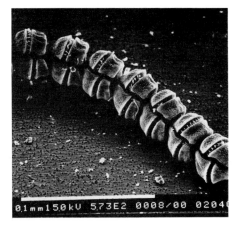

Figure 5. *Gymnodinium catenatum* Photo courtesy of Dr G. Hallegraeff PhD.

A. FACTORS FAVOURING DINOFLAGELLATE BLOOMS

Dinoflagellates spend the colder winter months as benthic resting cysts[36]. Two processes are required to initiate a dinoflagellate bloom. The first is excystment, whereby the "hypnocysts" germinate. This is followed by conversion of the excysted protoplast into a thecate motile cell. Separate factors are involved in each process.

1. Excystment

It has been observed in temperate regions of the world that dinoflagellate blooms and outbreaks of shellfish poisoning occur more frequently in spring and autumn (fall)[10]. Field data and laboratory experiments have demonstrated that excystment of *Alexandrium tamarense* is a temperature dependent process occurring maximally at 16°C[36]. Spring "blooms" of the organism are associated with a rise in water temperature to 16°C and autumn blooms occur as the water temperature falls to 16°C from the summer temperature of 20 - 22°C[37]. Other factors such as available light, salinity and nutrients have not been shown to play a role in the excystment process[38].

Shellfish toxicity can occur without an apparent dinoflagellate bloom. This may be due to ingestion of cysts which are six to ten times as toxic as the swimming cells[38,39]. Factors which disturb marine sediments are thought to increase risk of shellfish toxicity because dinoflagellate cysts become suspended in the water being filtered by the shellfish. These factors include severe storms, tidal mixing, upwellings, currents and dredging operations[36].

Species of dinoflagellates tend to be endemic to specific geographical regions in keeping with resting cysts residing in local ocean sediments. *Alexandrium catenella* is the predominant toxigenic dinoflagellate found along the Pacific coast of North America. *Alexandrium tamarense-excavatum* is the main cause of paralytic shellfish poisoning along the Atlantic coast of North America[10]. *Pyrodinium bahamense* (var. *compressum*) is more frequently found in the Indo-Pacific region, especially South East Asia and nearby Islands[17,19,23,27]. Illness from *Gymnodinium breve* occurs mainly along the coastline of Florida[40,41]. Global spread of dinoflagellates may occur due to human factors. Dinoflagellate cysts have been identified in large numbers in ship ballast water, and may be transported to locations remote from the original "bloom"[38].

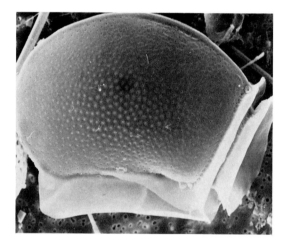

Figure 6. *Dinophysis fortii.* Photo courtesy of Dr G. Hallegraeff PhD.

2. Sustaining factors

After excystment has occurred, many factors contribute to the viability of a dinoflagellate bloom; however, the precise water conditions are not known. "Red tides" are predominantly a coastal phenomenon, and it has been suggested that nutrients and dissolved organic matter from land runoff support the toxic blooms. Conditions of low salinity caused by rainfall or river outflow have been linked to red tide formation[36]. High levels of solar radiation promote dinoflagellate growth. This was a factor producing red tides in Chile in the 1970's[16]. There is evidence that some vertical movement of the biomass of dinoflagellates occurs in the sea in response to variations in ambient light levels during each day[36]. Solar radiation is greatest from late spring to early autumn, consistent with the observed seasonal blooms of dinoflagellates.

Trace metals such as iron may be essential for the growth of dinoflagellates[42,43]. Copper appears to be toxic[44]. Vitamin B12, thiamine and biotin are essential for growth and B12 levels are depleted in seawater surrounding a dinoflagellate bloom.

When large populations of organisms have become established, tides, currents and winds cause their migration along the coast and toxicity may spread to shellfish many kilometres remote from the original dinoflagellate bloom.

B. TOXINS ASSOCIATED WITH TOXIC SHELLFISH POISONING
1. Paralytic shellfish toxins

Much has been learned of these toxins since Sommer and associates proved the association between red tides and shellfish poisoning[45]. The toxins which cause paralytic shellfish poisoning are among the most potent non-protein toxins known. The estimated lethal dose for a human is 0.1 - 1.0 mg[46]. The toxins are a group of heat stable, water soluble tetrahydropurine compounds of which the principal member is saxitoxin (this takes its name from the Alaskan butter clam *Saxidomus giganteus*). The structure of saxitoxin and its derivatives are summarised in Figure 7[45]. Many of the derivatives have been called "gonyautoxins" after the dinoflagellates *Gonyaulax* sp. (now known as *Alexandrium* sp.). A number of dinoflagellates other than *Alexandrium* sp. also produce saxitoxin or its derivatives. These include *Pyrodinium bahamense* (Figure 4) and *Gymnodinium catenatum* (Figure 5)[19,22,28,31]. The toxins have also been identified in bacteria associated with *Alexandrium tamarense*[48].

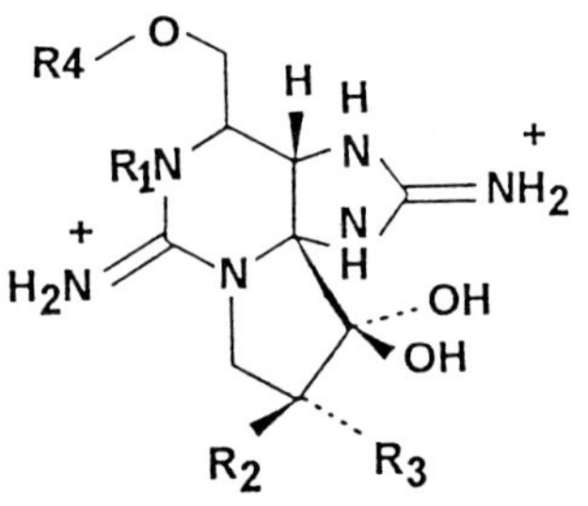

TOXIN	R1	R2	R3	R4
saxitoxin	H	H	H	$CONH_2$
neosaxitoxin	OH	H	H	$CONH_2$
decarbamoyl saxitoxin	H	H	H	H
gonyautoxin I	OH	H	OSO_3	$CONH_2$
gonyautoxin II	H	H	OSO_3	$CONH_2$
gonyautoxin III	H	OSO_3	H	$CONH_2$
gonyautoxin IV	OH	OSO_3	H	$CONH_2$
gonyautoxin V	H	H	H	$CONHSO_3$
gonyautoxin VI	OH	H	H	$CONHSO_3$
gonyautoxin VIII (C1)	H	OSO_3	H	$CONHSO_3$
epi-gonyautoxin VIII (C2)	H	H	OSO_3	$CONHSO_3$
C3	OH	H	OSO_3	$CONHSO_3$
C4	OH	OSO_3	H	$CONHSO_3$

Figure 7. Paralytic shellfish toxins; general structure and variations.

Saxitoxin and its derivatives block the propagation of nerve and muscle action potentials by interfering with membrane sodium ion channels. The usual early increase in permeability to sodium which is associated with an action potential is blocked[49].

Saxitoxin is more effective in blocking nerve and muscle cell membrane sodium channels on a molar and weight basis than all of its derivatives except gonyautoxin III (see Table 4)[50]. The effect of this neural blockade is paralysis. Serial electrophysiological studies (EPS) have revealed that saxitoxin results in prolonged distal latencies, reduced conduction velocities and a moderate reduction of motor and sensory amplitudes in the peripheral nerves of a patient affected by paralytic shellfish poisoning[51]. The effect is similar to tetrodotoxin poisoning and can be distinguished from other acute paralytic illnesses by using EPS.

Table 4
Relative toxicities of the paralytic shellfish toxins (after Genenah and Shimizu, 1981)[50]

Toxin	Specific Toxicity (Mouse Units/mg)	Relative Toxicity
Saxitoxin	5494 +/- 339	100
neo Saxitoxin	2363 +/- 101	43
Gonyautoxin I	3976 +/- 312	72
Gonyautoxin II	2003 +/- 211	36
Gonyautoxin III	5641 +/- 346	103
Gonyautoxin IV	1634 +/- 92	30

Clinically there appears to be a dose-dependent relationship between the severity of illness and the amount of toxin ingested, but this has not been noted in all series[21]. Toxicity of saxitoxin and its derivatives has been measured for many years using a non-specific mouse bioassay method (see later). The method was first described by Sommer and Meyer in 1937[45]. One "mouse unit" corresponds to approximately 0.18 mg of toxin[11]. Toxins from the saxitoxin group can be removed from the shellfish by boiling. Lower concentrations of saxitoxin have been measured in cooked mussels compared with uncooked samples from the same site[52]. High levels have been noted in broth prepared from the *saxidomus* clam[52]. This is consistent with the heat stable, water soluble properties of the toxins. They are not destroyed by boiling; instead the toxins leach out of the shellfish into the supernatant water.

2. Neurotoxic shellfish toxins

Gymnodinium breve produces at least two heat stable toxins known as brevetoxins. These differ from saxitoxin in structure and clinical effect[53-55]. The structures of brevetoxins A and B are depicted in Figure 8. Brevetoxin A is the most potent toxin[55]. Brevetoxins are heat stable, lipid soluble, acid stable and base labile[56,57]. They act by stimulating sodium channels in parasympathetic nerves by keeping "h" gates open and this effect is also noted in adrenergic nerve fibres[58,59]. Bronchospasm occurs when the toxin is inhaled because acetyl choline is released from post ganglionic parasympathetic nerve endings[60,61]. There is some evidence that the toxins inhibit neuromuscular transmission in skeletal muscle[62]; however there is no clinical evidence of paralysis in humans. A mild illness results from ingestion of shellfish contaminated with brevetoxins, and these toxins are unique in that they produce clinical illness when inhaled as an aerosol.

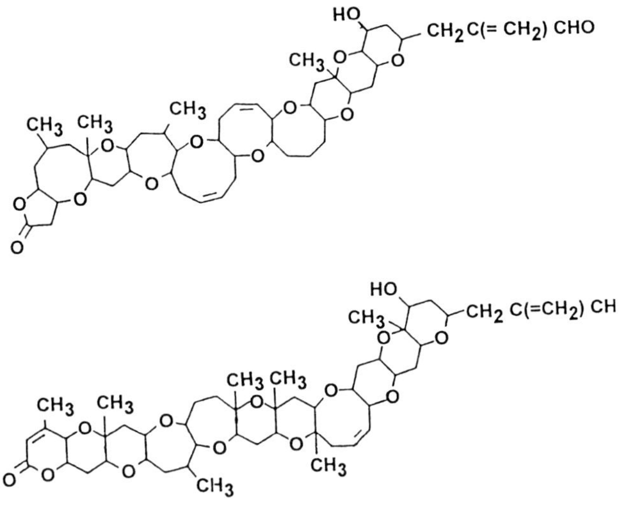

Figure 8. Brevetoxins A (top) & B (bottom).

3. Diarrhetic shellfish toxins

Diarrhetic shellfish poisoning is caused by a group of fat soluble toxins which are distinct from saxitoxins and brevetoxins. These toxins have been isolated in association with outbreaks of gastrointestinal illness in Japan and Europe[63,64]. The toxins have been linked to the dinoflagellates *Dinophysis fortii* (Figure 6), *D. acuminata, D. mitra, D. acuta, D. norvegica,* and *D. rotundata* as well as *Prorocentrum* sp.[18,65,66] The toxins are all derivatives of okadaic acid and their structures and shown in Figure 9.

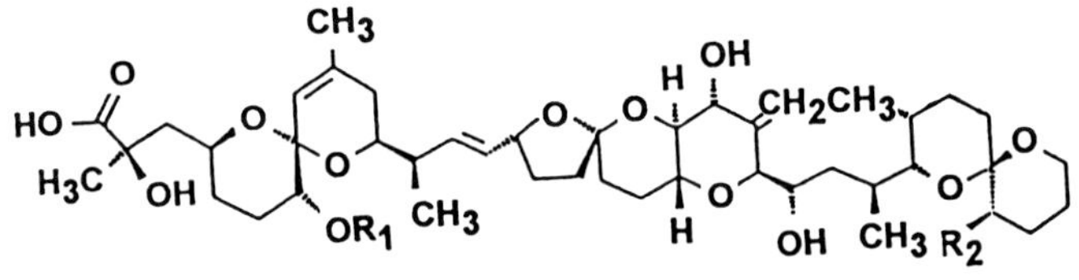

Toxin	R₁	R₂
Okadaic Acid	H	H
Dinophysistoxin-1	H	CH₃
Dinophysistoxin-3	Acyl	CH₃

Figure 9. Okadaic acid and derivatives.

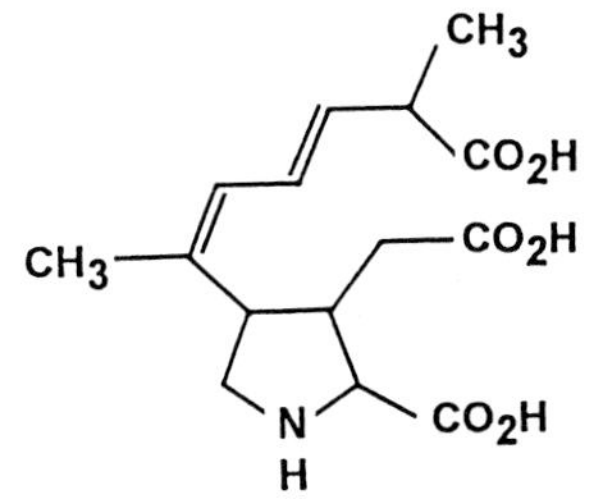

Figure 10. Domoic acid.

4. Amnesic shellfish toxin

Amnesic shellfish poisoning is caused by domoic acid[8]. Domoic acid is produced by the diatom *Nitzschia pungens* (f. *multiseries*) and its structure is depicted in Figure 10. Other diatoms such as *N. pseudodelicatissima* and *N. pseudoseriata* have also been implicated in this form of poisoning[18]. Domoic acid is distinct from the polycyclic toxins produced by the dinoflagellates. It has some structural similarity to glutamic acid, and may function as an excitatory neurotransmitter. Affected individuals experienced a state of "hyper excitation" followed by "chronic loss of function in neural systems susceptible to excitotoxic degeneration"[9]. Severe neuronal necrosis was noted in the hypocampus and amygdaloid nucleus, and dorsal medial nucleus of the thalamus[9]. Domoic acid is a potent depolarising agent of spinal cord ventral root neurons[67]. The effects on the central nervous system correlate with the observed clinical syndrome.

C. DINOFLAGELLATE TOXINS - THE FOOD CHAIN

Dinoflagellate toxins are passed through the food chain to humans via shellfish and, less frequently sea creatures such as crabs and some fish species[68]. The shellfish and other species of marine animals which may harbour dinoflagellate toxins are summarised in Table 5. Crabs and fish become toxic by ingesting dinoflagellates directly or by feeding on affected shellfish. Shellfish accumulate the toxin during the feeding process in which large volumes of seawater are filtered to extract nutrients and oxygen. Toxins dissolved in the seawater and the dinoflagellates themselves form a "soup" which is ingested by the shellfish. Toxins then accumulate in the shellfish without ill effect to this organism. Exposures to 200 - 400 cells per ml of seawater have resulted in poisoned shellfish[10]. Shellfish may also become toxic by ingesting dinoflagellate cysts which reside in marine sediments. The factors which influence dinoflagellate blooms from these cysts have been described in the previous section.

There is considerable variation in the anatomical distribution of the toxin in different species of shellfish[69]. The Alaskan butter clam stores the toxin in its digestive glands, gills and siphon. The toxicity may persist for up to two years after it accumulates in these structures. This may be due to a symbiotic relationship between the toxic dinoflagellate and the body of the clam[70]. Mussels (*Mytilus* spp.) concentrate the toxin in the "hepatopancreas", and the toxin has an elimination half life of 12 days when the shellfish are held in dinoflagellate-free salt water at 15 - 20°C[10]. The adductor muscles of scallops rarely become toxic, even when other parts of the flesh have high concentrations of toxins[10]. The shellfish do not appear to modify toxins once they accumulate[71].

Human illness occurs when affected shellfish, crustaceans or fish are ingested. The toxin is rapidly absorbed from the gastrointestinal tract and the onset of symptoms occurs in less than three hours[9], frequently in less than half an hour. The symptoms and signs are described in a later section. It has been determined that a maximum safe level of toxin is 80 micrograms per 100 grams of flesh[72]. Beyond this level there is significant risk to humans and when detected during the process of routine monitoring of commercial shellfish beds in the U.S., the beds are closed.

IV. PROPHYLAXIS AND FIRST AID MANAGEMENT

Shellfish for human consumption are obtained from two sources:
1. Commercial shellfish farming ventures.
2. Wild shellfish harvested from their natural habitat.
Different strategies are required in order to maintain successful prevention programmes which minimise outbreaks of human illness.

Table 5
Shellfish and other marine animals which have caused human toxicity when ingested[10,107]

Shellfish	Scientific Names
BIVALVED MOLLUSCS	
Mussels	*Mytilus*
	Modiolus
	Aulacomya
	Perna Perna
Clams	*Saxidomus*
	Protothaca
	Spisula
	Mya
	Arctica
	Humilaria
	Mesodesma
	Tapes
	Amphichaena
Scallops	*Pecten*
	Placopecten
	Spondylus
	Hinnites
Oysters	*Crassostrea*
	Ostrea
Cockles	*Cardium*
	Clinocardium
	Spondylus
	Lophus
GASTROPODS	
Atlantic dog winkle	*Thais lapillus*
Moon snail	*Lunatia heros*
Green turban shell	*Turbo marmoratus*
Top shell	*Tectus* sp.
Spider conch	*Lambis lambis*
Rough whelks	*Buccinum undatum*
Ten banded whelk	*Neptuna decemcostata*
OTHER MARINE ORGANISMS	
Chub mackerel	*Rastrelliger* sp.
Scads	*Sellar* sp.
Coral reef crabs	*Atergatis floridus*
	Platypodia granulosa
	Zosimus aeneus
Sand crabs	*Emerita analoga*
Horseshoe crabs	*Carcinoscorpius rotundicauda*
	Tachypleus gigas

A. PREVENTION OF TOXICITY FROM COMMERCIAL SHELLFISH

Commercial ventures are subject to control and surveillance by regulatory authorities in North America and Europe[10]. These authorities monitor shellfish for toxins and have legal power to close the commercial beds if toxin levels exceed established limits. Quarantines are policed by these agencies, for example the annual mussel quarantine in California, U.S.[14] The regulatory authorities are also responsible for investigating outbreaks of toxic shellfish poisoning. The source must be determined, other possible cases traced and action taken to prevent further episodes of human illness. This may involve confiscating affected shellfish and public education programmes. Surveillance by authorities in the U.S. and Canada has been highly effective in reducing the number of deaths from paralytic shellfish poisoning[14,52]. Most cases are now due to consumption of "wild" shellfish[52] or due to previously unrecognised toxins such as domoic acid[8].

The development of the commercial shellfish farming industry has led to greater global awareness of the problem of toxic shellfish poisoning. Outbreaks of toxic shellfish poisoning have significant public health and economic consequences and every effort must be made to prevent their occurrence. Commercial shellfish beds are regularly monitored and tested for toxins. The main method of monitoring toxicity over the last three decades has been the mouse bioassay which was first described by Sommer and Meyer in 1937, and modified by Schantz et al in 1957[45,74]. The basic unit of toxicity is the "mouse unit" (MU). One mouse unit is the amount of toxin which kills a 20 g laboratory white mouse within 15 minutes of an intraperitoneal injection. One MU corresponds to 0.18 micrograms of purified saxitoxin[11]. The mouse bioassay method is sanctioned by the Association of Official Analytical Chemists as an official method[72]. Using conversion charts, toxicity in MU is expressed as microgram equivalents of purified saxitoxin per 100 g of shellfish (µg/100g).

A level of 80 µg saxitoxin per 100 g shellfish was laid down as a quarantine limit for mussel fishery by the Shellfish Sanitation Workshop in the U.S. in 1958[75]. This level was based on epidemiological investigations of Canadian outbreaks in the 1950's[76]. Over the last 30 years, this value has proven a reliable public health guideline. In recent years very few outbreaks have resulted from commercial shellfish beds. With greater awareness of toxic shellfish poisoning, guidelines for other toxins have also been produced. Public health authorities consider that **any** detectable level of brevetoxin per 100 grams of shellfish meat is potentially hazardous for human consumption[76]. Since the discovery of domoic acid as a shellfish toxin in Canada in 1987, mussels are now routinely tested for the presence of domoic acid and no new cases of human illness have been reported. New toxic dinoflagellates are also being discovered when feasibility studies are performed before shellfish farming is introduced to new areas. A recent example is the discovery of toxigenic *Gymnodinium catenatum* (Figure 5)[31,76].

With the discovery of greater numbers of toxic dinoflagellates and toxins produced by other species such as diatoms, considerable research effort has been directed towards developing physical and chemical methods of detecting the toxins. Many methods have been suggested as alternatives to the time-honoured mouse bioassay test. These include high performance liquid chromatography[78], immunoassays[79], house fly bioassay[80], and voltage clamp techniques using animal axons[81]. All of the methods suffer disadvantages including cost and requiring a high degree of technical skill to perform, despite the fact that they are sensitive, reliable tests. There are also problems with determining total toxicity of a mixture of toxins (for example the saxitoxin group) because many of the analogues are interconvertible. Immunological methods are limited by lack of cross reactivity of the antibodies used for the saxitoxin analogues. A tissue culture bioassay has recently been developed and appears to be a valid alternative to the mouse bioassay method[82].

B. PREVENTION OF TOXICITY FROM SHELLFISH HARVESTED FROM THEIR NATURAL HABITAT

Outbreaks of poisoning from naturally harvested shellfish are more difficult to prevent than the commercially produced shellfish, because control is not possible at the "source". Even when public warnings are posted at the shellfish site and closed seasons declared, these may be ignored[83]. The natural environment cannot be controlled; however, monitoring of natural danger signs (red tides, bioluminescence) and toxin levels in high risk areas may enable advanced warning of risk to humans. Quarantines can then be imposed and public education programmes implemented. These programmes and a quarantine on mussel harvesting have been very successful in reducing the number of outbreaks in California, U.S.[14] An additional method of reducing risk of toxicity is to consume "safe" parts of the shellfish - this can be achieved with scallops because the adductor muscle is not toxic.

In endemic areas, public education must be a continuous process to dispel many of the myths concerning toxic shellfish poisoning. For example, a historic "rule of thumb" has been that shellfish should not be consumed in northern hemisphere countries during the months without the letter "r" in their spelling (i.e. May to August)[10]. Toxicity has been recorded in September and October; hence applying the "r" rule will not safeguard against poisoning. This principle is not applicable in the southern hemisphere or tropical countries. Another myth concerns cooking of the shellfish to make them less toxic. Heat does not inactivate the toxin and although there is evidence that toxin levels are reduced by boiling, the shellfish still remain toxic[52]. Research into detoxification of shellfish has been hampered by problems with cost-effectiveness and altered flavour[84]. Prevention and investigation of outbreaks of toxicity from naturally harvested shellfish is best carried out by the same central regulatory authority which monitors commercial shellfish farms. Public education is a major component of this prevention strategy and should include details of the symptoms and signs of toxicity, initial first aid, and where to obtain medical assistance.

C. FIRST AID FOR TOXIC SHELLFISH POISONING

When toxic shellfish poisoning has occurred, the most important issue is to identify the process. The initial symptoms are outlined in Table 6. Many of these symptoms are non-specific and may be attributable to other causes. Establishing a link with recent ingestion of shellfish is very important.

First aid management should include recognition of the syndrome and airway support. If vomiting has not occurred it should not be induced because of the potential for subsequent loss of airway reflexes and respiratory failure, creating a high risk of pulmonary aspiration. Most clinical syndromes progress to maximum severity over 3 - 12 hours, so there is sufficient time to mobilise paramedic services. Only in rare instances is the toxicity fulminant leading to death inside two hours[52]. If respiratory compromise occurs, the affected individual should receive expired-air resuscitation (EAR) and reassurance. Affected individuals will remain completely aware of their surroundings in most instances. If vomiting occurs the patient should be placed on their side in the "coma" position, head lowest. Vomitus should be cleared from the mouth using a finger or suction, then EAR continued. An absent pulse mandates commencement of full cardiopulmonary resuscitation (CPR). Oxygen should be administered when it is available.

When paramedic assistance arrives, support should be continued and the patient transported to the nearest emergency department. All other individuals who ingested the toxic shellfish should also receive medical assessment irrespective of their symptom severity, because they are at risk. Children appear to be particularly at risk of toxicity[17,23,26].

V. CLINICAL SIGNS AND SYMPTOMS OF TOXIC SHELLFISH POISONING

A summary of the clinical features of toxic shellfish poisoning is provided in Table 6. Four main clinical syndromes are apparent: paralytic shellfish poisoning, neurotoxic shellfish poisoning, diarrhetic shellfish poisoning, and amnesic shellfish poisoning which has recently been described as a result of domoic acid toxicity.

A. PARALYTIC SHELLFISH POISONING (PSP)

This is the most common toxic syndrome produced by shellfish, and results in the most severe illness. Its world-wide distribution is summarised in Table 3 and Figure 1.

The onset of symptoms usually occurs within three hours[19,21,22,24,65,85,86], and in many cases may be less than 30 minutes after consumption of affected shellfish[21,41,85]. Earlier onset of symptoms appears to be related to severity of illness[24,65]. Severity of illness has been shown to correlate with the quantity of toxin ingested in some series[86]; however, in other series no relationship has been observed[21]. There is evidence that children may be more susceptible to the toxins; all seven deaths in Sabah, Malaysia in 1976 were children and eight out of 10 deaths from PSP in Venezeula in 1977 were children[23,26]. The case fatality rate of Guatemala in 1987 was 50% for children < 6 years of age, 32% for 7 - 9 year olds and 8% for adults[24].

The initial symptoms of PSP include paraesthesiae of the mouth, lips, tongue and throat followed by feelings of disequilibrium, "floating" or dizziness[19,21,22,24,59,60]. These symptoms may be missed if the patient is sleeping[19]. The paraesthesiae then become more generalised involving the distal upper and lower extremities. Weakness in the upper and lower limbs may then be noted in association with headache, ataxia, nausea and/or vomiting. More severe cases then develop other signs of neurological dysfunction such as dysphagia, dysarthria, diplopia and respiratory difficulty. Death may occur within 12 hours as a result of respiratory failure. In the most fulminant cases death occurs in 2 - 3 hours in the absence of advanced life support[52]. Untreated less severe cases experience symptoms for 2 - 3 days before recovery. The case fatality rate is approximately 5.9% (Table 3) with a range of 0% to 44%. The clinical syndrome is very similar to ciguatera and tetrodotoxin poisoning, prompting some authors to use a general term "pelagic paralysis" to describe the three forms of marine toxicity[9].

Table 6
Clinical features of toxic shellfish poisoning

		Paralytic Shellfish Poisoning PSP	Neurotoxic Shellfish Poisoning NSP	Diarrhetic Shellfish Poisoning DSP	Amnesic Shellfish Poisoning ASP
ONSET		½ - 3 hours, median 1 hour	minutes - 3 hours	½ - 2 hours	¼ - 38 hours, median 5½ hours
INITIAL SYMPTOMS		Paraesthesiae of mouth, lips, throat Disequilibrium, floating feeling	Nausea, abdominal pain, diarrhoea	Diarrhoea, nausea, vomiting, abdominal pain	Nausea, vomiting, abdominal pain
CLINICAL SYNDROME	**MILD TO MODERATE TOXICITY**	Generalised paraesthesia, weakness of arms/legs, headache, ataxia, nausea, vomiting	Circumoral paraesthesia, trunk/limb paraesthesia, ataxia/ incoordination, vertigo, headache	Severe diarrhoea, vomiting, dehydration	Diarrhoea, headache, memory loss, mutism
	SEVERE TOXICITY	Dysphagia Dysarthria Diplopia Limb paralysis Respiratory failure	Bradycardia Convulsions Dilated pupils NO paralysis	Shock in debilitated elderly patients Long term possible risk of gastric cancer	Hemiparesis Ophthalmoplegia Coma Seizures Hypotension Cardiac arrhythmias
DURATION OF ILLNESS		2 - 5 days	2 - 3 days	3 days	24 hours to 12 weeks permanent memory loss
MORTALITY		Up to 44% (average 5.9%)	NIL	NIL	4%

B. NEUROTOXIC SHELLFISH POISONING (NSP)

This produces a milder clinical illness than paralytic shellfish poisoning, is less common and has received less attention in the literature. Cases have been restricted to the West Coast of Florida, although the dinoflagellate has been observed in waters along the coast of Texas and Mexico[87]. It has recently been reported in North Carolina[88] and New Zealand[18]. Clinical illness can result from ingestion of shellfish containing toxins from the organism *Gymnodinium breve*, or from the effects of an aerosol of seawater containing the organism.

Illness from ingestion of affected shellfish has a similar initial presentation to paralytic shellfish poisoning. The onset of symptoms usually occurs in minutes and may be up to three hours after eating the shellfish[7]. Prominent gastrointestinal symptoms are associated with NSP. Affected individuals initially notice nausea, abdominal pains and diarrhoea in association with circumoral paraesthesia which progresses to include the pharynx, trunk and limbs[89]. Ataxia, vertigo and incoordination may occur and rarely convulsions requiring respiratory support[3]. Other symptoms and signs include bradycardia, headache and dilated pupils. Paralysis does not occur, and fatalities have not been recorded[86].

Aerosol exposure to *Gymnodinium breve* results when the organism is destroyed on the coastline by wave action. *Gymnodinium breve* has no protective polysaccharide plates in its cell wall and toxins released into seawater are transported inland as mist in coastal regions[40]. Symptoms include respiratory irritation with cough, dyspnoea, rhinorrhoea and sneezing due to inhalation of the toxins. Bronchospasm may also occur. Eye and skin irritation may also be noted by individuals exposed to the aerosolized toxins. The toxins of *Gymnodinium breve* are more toxic to other species than they are to humans. Deaths of large numbers of fish and sea birds have been associated with blooms of this dinoflagellate[90].

C. DIARRHETIC SHELLFISH POISONING

Symptoms resulting from the toxins produced by the dinoflagellate *Dinophysis* sp. include diarrhoea, nausea, vomiting and abdominal cramps[63]. The onset occurs in 30 minutes to two hours (rarely up to 12 hours) and affected individuals usually recover after 2 - 3 days. In severe cases, the affected individual may suffer dehydration or shock, particularly if they are debilitated and elderly. No fatalities have been recorded from this form of shellfish poisoning; however, okadaic acid and dinophysis toxin-1 may promote gastric tumours[91].

D. AMNESIC SHELLFISH POISONING

This form of shellfish poisoning should be called "excitatory encephalopathic shellfish poisoning" after the syndrome it produces[8]. The onset of symptoms in the first recorded series ranged from 15 minutes to 38 hours after ingestion with a median of 5.5 hours[8]. Initial symptoms affected the gastrointestinal system with nausea, vomiting and abdominal cramps being noted in a majority of patients. Many patients also experienced diarrhoea. Headache (severe) and loss of memory were noted in a significant number of patients. The effect on memory was greatest in older individuals, and many people presented in an acute confusional state. Nineteen of 106 patients required hospitalisation and twelve required treatment in an intensive care unit (ICU). Serious neurological dysfunction was noted in ICU treated patients: coma, seizures, mutism and purposeless facial movements. Seven patients had unstable blood pressure or cardiac arrhythmias, and four patients died from their illness (all were over 70 years of age).

A follow up study of 14 of the most severely affected patients revealed severe anterograde memory deficits despite preservation of other cognitive functions[9]. Eleven of these patients had clinical and electromyographic evidence of motor and sensorimotor neuropathy. Patients who died from the intoxication had focal neural necrosis and loss in the amygdala and hippocampus. Reporting of this syndrome has been limited to the one outbreak in Canada; however, it is of great concern given the number of people affected, the severity of illness, the persistent deficits in memory which occurred in affected individuals[92], and the neuropathology produced by the toxin, domoic acid. This is unlike the effects of dinoflagellate toxins which are reversible provided affected individuals receive advanced life support. Permanent neural pathology is thought to result from the effect of domoic acid on glutamatergic neurones, which impairs glucose metabolism[93].

VI. CLINICAL TREATMENT OF SHELLFISH POISONING

There is no antidote available to treat any of the types of toxic shellfish poisoning. Animal studies examining antisaxitoxin antibodies for the treatment of paralytic shellfish poisoning[94], and kynurenic acid to treat domoic acid toxicity[95], show promise but further research is required before these substances may be used to treat human toxicity. There seems little chance of developing a vaccine because individuals do not become immune to the poisons after they have experienced episodes of toxicity[11]. There are no controlled trials evaluating drug therapy of toxic shellfish poisoning. Documentation in the literature is restricted to anecdotal reports of a small number of drugs which have had little influence on outcome. Atropine and neostigmine have been tried in some series[19] without success. Atropine may even worsen symptoms[96].

Treatment for all forms of toxic shellfish poisoning is supportive and symptomatic. Early active airway management has been associated with a reduction in mortality[21,52,83]. Endotracheal intubation and manual ventilation should be performed if patients suffer respiratory failure from paralysis, or become mentally obtunded with depressed airway reflexes. These patients have a significant risk of pulmonary aspiration, particularly if they are vomiting (a common problem - Table 5). Gastric lavage, administration of activated charcoal and catharsis are recommended; however, there are no clinical trials supporting the efficacy of gastrointestinal decontamination in toxic shellfish poisoning. The recommendation is based on the efficacy of gastrointestinal decontamination in drug over-dose, the subject of a recent review[97].

The treating physician should take into account whether or not the patient has vomited and the degree of poisoning. Patients who have vomited and are still maintaining adequate respiration with intact airway reflexes should receive oral activated charcoal when vomiting has stopped. Patients with mild to moderate toxicity without vomiting should receive careful orogastric lavage prior to activated charcoal, if they present less than six hours after ingestion. Saxitoxin has some anticholinergic activity and may delay gastric emptying[87]. Patients presenting more than six hours after ingestion should receive oral activated charcoal without lavage.

Gastric lavage should be performed in patients only after adhering to the usual precautions concerning airway protection[97]. Alkaline lavage solutions such as isotonic sodium bicarbonate may inactivate the shellfish toxins because they are less stable and have lower toxicity in alkaline media[98,99]. For similar reasons, alkaline diuresis using intravenous sodium bicarbonate has been recommended by some authorities[100]. There is little published clinical data supporting either of these forms of therapy; however, they are worth considering in severe cases.

Individuals with severe toxicity are often critically ill, particularly if they have paralytic shellfish poisoning or domoic acid toxicity[19,24,52]. Management should be in an ICU setting with ventilation and invasive circulatory monitoring if required. Hypotension should be corrected with fluid replacement and inotropes. Continuous electrocardiographic monitoring is required and arrhythmias corrected by conventional means. Full respiratory support should be maintained until the toxin has worn off sufficiently for the patient to maintain their own airway and ventilation. Some investigators have examined other methods of eliminating toxins from affected individuals. Haemodialysis has been tried with probable success in one patient[83]. Charcoal haemoperfusion was successful in animal studies[101].

Supportive therapy has been very successful in recent years leading to a significant reduction in mortality in the U.S. and Canada from paralytic shellfish poisoning[3,4,102]. Provided full support is provided the effects of the toxins are completely reversible over a period of 2 - 5 days. The prognosis is excellent if the patient survives the first 12 hours even if ICU facilities are not available[15].

Unfortunately, supportive therapy was not completely successful in the 1987 outbreak of amnesic shellfish poisoning in Canada[8]. Approximately 15 percent of patients were left with permanent memory deficit despite preservation of intellect. Further investigation of specific antidotes is required in order to prevent significant long term disability from this toxin.

VII. OTHER TOXIC SHELLFISH POISONING SYNDROMES

A. VENERUPIN SHELLFISH POISONING
This is also referred to as asari poisoning. An outbreak of poisoning from short necked clams from Lake Hamana in Japan has been reported[10]. This was associated with a high mortality (114 out of 324 victims) in the absence of paralysis. The incriminated dinoflagellate may have been *Prorocentrum minimum* (var. *mariae-lebouriae*), which produces a heat stable toxin; however, this is controversial[18]. An initial syndrome of headache, gastrointestinal distress and nervousness is followed by liver failure[103]. Clinical management is supportive and symptomatic.

B. CALLISTIN POISONING
Intoxication from the Japanese clam *Callista brevisiphonata* occurs during the months of May to September. A cholinergic group of heat stable toxins builds up in the ovaries during spawning. Symptoms and signs are typical of cholinergic crisis and occur within one hour of ingestion. Affected individuals experience an erythematous urticarial rash, hypersalivation, sweating, nausea, vomiting, diarrhoea, bronchospasm and increased bronchial secretions. Facial numbness and paralysis may be noted in addition to fever, chills and bradycardia. The syndrome is usually self limiting and atropine may be used for profound bradycardia[103].

VIII. CONCLUSIONS

Toxic shellfish poisoning is a world wide problem. With increasing pressure on the marine environment to provide food protein and the development of aquaculture, all nations are at risk of outbreaks of toxicity from this food source. With careful planning, establishment of central regulatory authorities to monitor shellfish toxin levels, and widespread public health programmes, episodes of human illness can be kept to a minimum.

IX. REFERENCES

1.   SALIBA, L. J., Making the Mediterranean safer, *World Health Forum*, **11**, 274, 1990.
2.   MORSE, D. L., GUZEWICH, J. J., HANRAHAN, J. P., et al, Widespread outbreaks of clam and oyster associated gastroenteritis. Role of Norwalk virus, *N Engl J Med*, **314**, 678, 1986.

3.   **HUGHES, J. M.,** Epidemiology of shellfish poisoning in the United States 1971 - 1977, in *Toxic Dinoflagellate Blooms,* Taylor, D. L., Seliger, H. H., editors, New York, Elsevier/North Holland, 1979, 15.

4.   **Centres for disease control,** Food-borne disease outbreaks annual summary 1982, Atlanta. *Centres for Disease Control,* September, 1985, 38.

5.   **MILLS, A. R., PASSMORE, R.,** Pelagic paralysis, *Lancet,* I **(8578),** 161, 1988.

6.   **HEMMERT, W. H.,** The public health implications of Gymnodinium breve red tides, a review of the literature and recent events, in, *Proceedings of the First International Conference on Toxic Dinoflagellate Blooms,* Lo Cicero, V.R., editor, Massachusetts Science and Technology Foundation, Wakefield, Massachusetts, 1975, 489.

7.   **MURATA, M., SCHIMITANI, B., SUGITANI, H., OSHIMA, Y., YASUMOTO, T.,** Isolation and structural elucidation of the causative toxin of diarrhetic shell fish poisoning, *Bull Jpn Soc Sci Fish,* **48,** 549, 1982.

8.   **PERL, T. M., BEDARD, L., KOSATSKY, T., HOCKIN, J. C., TODD, E. C. D., REMIS, R. S.,** An outbreak of toxic encephalopathy caused by eating mussels contaminated with domoic acid, *N Engl J Med,* **322,** 1775, 1990.

9.   **TEITELBAUM, J. S., ZATORRE, R. J., CARPENTER, S., et al,** Neurologic sequelae of domoic acid intoxication due to the ingestion of contaminated mussels, *N Engl J Med,* **322,** 1781, 1990

10   **HALSTEAD, B. W., SCHANTZ, E. J.,** *Paralytic shellfish poisoning,* WHO offset publ., 79, 1, 1984.

11. **MORSE, E. V.,** Paralytic shellfish poisoning: A review. *J Am Vet Med Assoc,* **171,** 1178, 1977.

12. **CARSON, R. L.,** The changing year, in *The Sea Around Us,* Revised edition, Carlson, R. L., editor. New York. Oxford University Press, 28, 1961.

13. **PRAKASH, A.,** An overview, *Proceedings of the First International Conference on Toxic Dinoflagellate Blooms,* LoCicero, V. R., editor, Massachusetts Science and Technology Foundation, Wakefield, Massachusetts, 1, 1975.

14. Leads from the MMWR, Annual Mussel Quarantine - California 1983 *J A M A,* **249,** 3292, 1983.

15. **MEYER, K. F.,** Food Poisoning (concluded), *N Engl J Med,* **249,** 843, 1953.

16. **SERGIO-AVARIA, P.,** Red tides off the coast of Chile, In *Toxic Dinoflagellate Blooms,* Taylor, D. L., Seliger, H. H., editors, New York, Elsevier/North Holland, 1979, 161.

17. **MACLEAN, J. L.,** Indo-Pacific toxic red-tide occurrences 1972 - 1984, in *Toxic Red Tides and Shellfish Toxicity in Southeast Asia: Proceedings of a consultative Meeting held in Singapore, 11 - 14 September 1984,* White, A. W., Anraku, M., Hooi, K-K., editors, Southeast Asian Fisheries Department Centre, 1984, 92.

18. **HALLEGRAEFF, G. M.,** Personal Communication, 5th May 1993.

19. **RHODES, F. A., MILLS, C. G., POPEI, K.,** Paralytic shellfish poisoning in Papua New Guinea, *PNG Medical Journal,* **18,** 197, 1975.

20. **YASUMOTO, T., RAJ, U., BAGNIS, R.,** *Seafood poisonings in tropical regions,* Laboratory of food hygiene, Faculty of Agriculture, Tohoku University, Japan, 1984, 1.

21. **POPKISS, M. E. E., HORSTMAN, D. A., HARPUR, D.,** Paralytic shellfish poisoning, A report of 17 cases in Cape Town, *South Africa Medical Journal,* **55,** 1017, 1979.

22. **TAN, C. T. T., LEE, E. J. D.,** Paralytic shellfish poisoning in Singapore, *Annals Academy of Medicine,* **15,** 77, 1986.

23. **ROY, R. N.,** Red tide and outbreak of paralytic shellfish poisoning in Sabah, *Med J Malaysia,* **31,** 247, 1977.

24. **RODRIGUE, D. C., ETZEL, R. A., HALL, S., et al,** Lethal paralytic shellfish poisoning in Guatemala, *Am J Trop Med Hyg,* **42,** 267, 1990.

25. **SWADDIWUDHIPONG, W., KUNASOL, P., SANGWANLOY, O., SRISOMPORN, D.,** Food borne disease outbreaks of chemical etiology in Thailand, 1981 - 87, *Southeast Asian J Trop Med Pub Hlth,* **20,** 125, 1989.

26. **REYES-VASQUEZ, G., FERRAZ-REYES, E., VASQUEZ, E.,** Toxic dinoflagellate blooms in north eastern Venezuela during 1977. In *Toxic Dinoflagellate Blooms,* Taylor, D. L., Seliger, H. H., editors, New York, Elsevier/North Holland, 1979, 191.

27. **KAMIYA, H., HASHIMOTO, Y.,** Occurrence of saxitoxin and related toxins in Palauan bivalves, *Toxicon,* **16,** 303, 1978.

28. **HARADA, T., OSHIMA, Y., YASUMOTO, T.,** Structures of two paralytic shellfish toxins, Gonyautoxins V and VI isolated from a tropical dinoflagellate, Pyrodinium bahamense var. Compressum, *Agric Biol Chem,* **46,** 1861, 1982.

29. **DE MENDIOLA, B. R.,** Red tide along the Peruvian coast, in *Toxic Dinoflagellate Blooms,* Taylor, D. L., Seliger, H. H., editors, New York, Elsevier/North Holland, 1979, 183.

30. **HALLEGRAEFF, G. M.,** *A review of harmful algal blooms and their apparent global increase,* Phycological reviews 13, Phycologica, March 1993, (in press).

31. **OSHIMA, Y., HASEGAWA, M., YASUMOTO, T., HALLEGRAEFF, G., BLACKBURN, S.,** Dinoflagellate Gymnodinium catenatum as the source of paralytic shellfish toxins in Tasmanian shellfish, *Toxicon,* **25,** 1105, 1987.

32. **STEIDINGER, K. A.**, Collection, enumeration and identification of free living marine dinoflagellates, in *Toxic Dinoflagellate Blooms*, Taylor, D. L., Seliger, H. H., editors, New York, Elsevier/North Holland, 1979, 435.

33. **CLARKE, R. B.**, Biological causes and effects of paralytic shellfish poisoning, *Lancet*, **II, 770**, 1968.

34. **SWIFT, E.**, Bioluminescence, in *Toxic Dinoflagellate Blooms*, Taylor, D. L., Seliger, H. H., editors, New York, Elsevier/North Holland 1979, 459.

35. **TAYLOR, F. J. R.**, The toxic gonyaulacoid dinoflagellates, in *Toxic Dinoflagellate Blooms*, Taylor, D. L., Seliger, H. H. editors, New York/Elsevier/North Holland, 1979, 47.

36. **PROVASOLI, L.**, Recent progress, an overview, in *Toxic Dinoflagellate Blooms*, Taylor, D. L., Seliger, H. H., editors, New York, Elsevier/North Holland, 1979, 1.

37. **ANDERSON, D. M., WALL, D.**, Potential importance of benthic cysts of Gonyaulax tamarensis and G. excavata in initiating toxic dinoflagellate blooms, *J Phycol*, **14**, 224, 1978.

38. **OSHIMA, Y., BOLCH, C. J., HALLEGRAEFF, G. M.**, Toxin composition of resting cysts of Alexandrium tamarense (Dinophyceae), *Toxicon*, **30**, 1539, 1992.

39. **DALE, B., YENTSCH, C. M., HURST, J. W.**, Toxicity in resting cysts of the red-tide dinoflagellate Gonyaulax excavata from deeper water coastal sediments, *Science*, **201**, 1223, 1978.

40. **PIERCE, R. H.**, Red tide (Gymnodinium breve) toxin aerosols: a review, *Toxicon*, **24**, 955, 1986.

41. **HUGHES, J. M., MERSON, M. H.**, Fish and shellfish poisoning, *N Engl J Med*, **295**, 1117, 1976.

42. **GLOVER, H. E.**, Iron in Maine coastal waters: seasonal variation and its apparent correlation with a dinoflagellate bloom, *Limnol Oceanog*, **23**, 534, 1978.

43. **INGLE, R. M., MARTIN, D. F.**, Prediction of the Florida red tide by means of the iron index. Red tide, iron and humic acid levels in streams, *Environ Letters*, **1**, 69, 1971.

44. **ANDERSON, D. M., MOREL F. M. M.**, Copper sensitivity of Gonyaulax tamarensis, *Limnol Oceanog*, **23**, 283, 1978.

45. **SOMMER, H., MEYER, K. F.**, Paralytic shellfish poisoning, *Arch Pathol*, **24**, 560, 1937.

46. **EASTAUGH, J., SHEPHERD, S.**, Infectious and toxic syndromes from fish and shellfish consumption. A review, *Arch Intern Med*, **149**, 1735, 1989.

47. **SCHANTZ, E. J., GHAZAROSSIAN, V. E., SCHNOES, H. K., STRONG, F. M.**, The structure of saxitoxin, *J Amer Chem Soc*, **97**, 1238, 1975.

48. **KODAMA, M., OGATA, T., SAKAMOTO, S., SATO, S., HONDA, T., MIWATANI, T.**, Production of paralytic shellfish toxins by a bacterium Moraxella sp. isolated from Protogonyaulax tamarensis, *Toxicon*, **28**, 707, 1990.

49. **KAO, C. Y.**, Pharmacology of tetrodotoxin and saxitoxin, *Federation Proceedings*, **31**, 1117, 1972.

50. **GENENAH, A. A., SHIMIZU, Y.**, Specific toxicity of paralytic shellfish poisons, *J Agric Food Chem*, **29**, 1289, 1981.

51. **LONG, R. R., SARGENT, J. C., HAMMER, K.**, Paralytic shellfish poisoning, A case report and serial electrophysiological observations, *Neurology*, **40**, 1310, 1990.

52. **Editorial,** Food safety, Paralytic shellfish poisoning USA, Massachusetts and Alaska, June 1990, *Weekly Epidemiological Record*, **25**, 185, 1991.

53. **SPIEGELSTEIN, M. Y., PASTER, Z., ABBOTT, B. C.**, Purification and biological activity of Gymnodinium breve toxins, *Toxicon*, **11**, 85, 1973.

54. **LIN, Y. Y., RISK, M., RAY, S. M., et al,** Isolation and structure of Brevetoxin B from the red tide dinoflagellate Gymnodinium breve (Gymnodinium breve), *J Am Chem Soc*, **103**, 5773, 1981.

55. **SHIMIZU, Y., CHOU, H. N., BANDO, H., VAN DUYNE, G., CLARDY, J. C.**, Structure of brevetoxin A (GB-1 toxin), the most potent toxin in the Florida red tide organism Gymnodinium breve (Gymnodinium breve), *J Am Chem Soc*, **108**, 514, 1986.

56. **DOIG, M. T., MARTIN, D. F.**, Physical chemical stability of ichthyotoxin(s) produced by Gymnodinium breve, *Environ Letters*, **3**, 279, 1972.

57. **BADEN, D. G., MENDE, T. J.**, Toxicity of two toxins from the Florida red tide marine dinoflagellate, Gymnodinium breve, *Toxicon*, **20**, 457, 1982.

58. **ASAI, S., KRZANOWSKI, J. J., LOCKLEY, R. F., et al,** The site of action of Gymnodinium breve toxin within the parasympathetic axonal sodium channel h gate in airway smooth muscle, *J Allergy Clin Immunol*, **73**, 824, 1984.

59. **KRZANOWSKI, J. J., SAKAMOTO, Y., DUNCAN, R., et al,** The mechanism of Gymnodinium breve toxin induced rat vas deferens contraction, *Pharmacologist*, **26**, 175, 1984.

60. **ASAI, S., KRZANOWSKI, J. J., ANDERSON, W. H., et al,** Effects of the toxin of red tide, Gymnodinium breve on canine tracheal smooth muscle: a possible new asthma triggering mechanism, *J Allergy Clin Immunol*, **69**, 418, 1982.

61. **RICHARDS, I. S., KULKARNI, A. P., BROOKS, S. M., PIERCE, R.**, Florida red-tide toxins (brevetoxins) produce depolarization of airway smooth muscle, *Toxicon*, **28**, 1105, 1990.

62. **GALLAGHER, J. P., SHINNICK-GALLAGHER, P.**, Effects of Gymnodinium breve toxin in rat phrenic nerve diaphragm preparation, *Br J Pharmacol*, **69**, 367, 1980.

63. **YASUMOTO, T., OSHIMA, Y., YAMAGUCHI, M.**, Occurrence of a new type of toxic shellfish in Japan and chemical properties of the toxin, In *Toxic Dinoflagellate Blooms*, Taylor, D. L., Seliger, H. H., editors, New York, Elsevier/North Holland, 1979, 395.

64. **KUMAGAI, M., YANAGI, T., MURATA, M., et al**, Okadaic acid as the causative toxin of diarrhetic shellfish poisoning in Europe. *Agric Biol Chem*, **50**, 2853, 1986.

65. **YASUMOTO, T., MURATA, M., OSHIMA, Y., MATSUMOTO, G. L., CLARDY, J.**, Diarrhetic shellfish toxin poisoning, in *Seafood Toxins*, ACS Symp Ser No 262, Ragelis, E. P., editor, American Chemical Society, Washington D.C., 1984, 207.

66. **DICKEY, R. W., BOBZIN, S. C., FAULKNER, D. J., BENCSATH, F. A., ANDRZEJEWSKI, D.**, Identification of okadaic acid from a Caribbean dinoflagellate, Prorocentrum concavum, *Toxicon*, **28**, 371,1990.

67. **BISCO, T. J., EVANS, R. H., HEADLEY, P. M., MARTIN, M. R., WATKINS, J. C.**, Structure-activity relations of excitatory amino acids on frog and rat spinal neurones, *Br J Pharmacol*, **58**, 373, 1976.

68. **OSHIMA, Y., ET AL**, Paralytic shellfish toxins in tropical waters, in *Seafood toxins*, ACS Symp Ser No 262, Ragelis, E. P., editor, American Chemical Society, Washington D.C.,1984.

69. **RAY, S. M.**, Current status of paralytic shellfish poisoning, in *Proceedings of Third International Congress, Food Science and Technology*, 1971, 717.

70. **SHIMIZU, Y.**, Developments in the study of paralytic shellfish toxins, in *Toxic Dinoflagellate Blooms*, in Taylor, D. L., Seliger, H. H., editors, New York, Elsevier/North Holland, 1979, 321.

71. **BOYER, G. L.**, Fix Wichmann, C., Mosser, J., Schantz, E. J., Schnoes, H. K., Toxins isolated from Bay of Fundy scallops, *Toxic Dinoflagellate Blooms*, in Taylor, D. L., Seliger, H. H., editors, New York, Elsevier/North Holland, 1979, 373.

72. **HORWITZ, W.**, editor, *Official methods of analysis of the Association of Official Analytical Chemists*, 13th Edition, Washington DC, Association of official analytical chemists, 298, 1980.

73. **US Department of Health,** Education and Welfare, Public Health Service, *National Shellfish Sanitation Programme Manual of Operations Part 1, Sanitation of shellfish growing areas*, Revised edition, Washington D.C., USDHEW, 1965.

74. **SCHANTZ, E. J., et al**, Paralytic shellfish poisoning VI, A procedure for the isolation and purification of the poison from toxic clam and mussel tissue, *J Am Chem Soc*, **79**, 5230, 1957.

75. *Procedures of the 1958 Shellfish Sanitation Workshop*, Washington D.C., US Department of Health, Education and Welfare, 1958 (Lithographed document).

76. **CLEM, J. D.**, Toxic dinoflagellates, shellfish and public health, in *Toxic Dinoflagellate Blooms*, Taylor, D. L., Seliger, H. H., editors, New York, Elsevier/North Holland, 1979, 33.

77. **ANDERSON, D. M., SULLIVAN, J. J., REGUERA, B.**, Paralytic shellfish poisoning in north west Spain: the toxicity of the dinoflagellate Gymnodinium catenatum, *Toxicon*, **27**, 665, 1989.

78. **SULLIVAN, J. J., WEKELL, M. M.**, Determination of paralytic shellfish poisoning toxins by high pressure liquid chromatography, in *Seafood Toxins*, ACS Symp. Ser. No. 262, Ragelis, E. P., editor, American Chemical Society, Washington D.C., 197, 1984.

79. **CARLSON, R. E., LEVER, M. L., LEE, B. W., GUIRE, P. E.**, Development of immunoassays for paralytic shellfish poisoning, in *Seafood Toxins*, ACS Symp Ser No 262, Ragelis, E. P., editor, American Chemical Society, Washington D.C., 181, 1984.

80. **SIGER, A., ABBOTT, B. C., ROSS, M.**, Response of the house fly to saxitoxins and contaminated shellfish, in *Seafood Toxins*, ACS Symp Ser No 262, Ragelis, E. P., editor, American Chemical Society, Washington D.C., 193, 1984.

81. **DAIGO, K., NOGUCHI, T., KAWAI, N., MIWA, A., HASHIMOTO, K.**, Detection of paralytic shellfish poison by a lobster nerve-muscle preparation, in *Red tides: Biology, Environmental Science and Toxicology*, Okaichi, T., et al, editors, New York, Elsevier, 387, 1989.

82. **JELLETT, J. F., MARKS, L. J., STEWART, J. E., DOREY, M. L., WATSON-WRIGHT, W., LAWRENCE, J. F.**, Paralytic shellfish poison (saxitoxin family) bioassays: automated endpoint determination and standardisation of the in vitro tissue culture bioassay and comparison with the standard mouse bioassay, *Toxicon*, **30**, 1143, 1992.

83. **ACRES, J., GRAY, J.**, Paralytic shellfish poisoning, *Canadian Med Assoc J*, **119**, 1195, 1978.

84. **BOGLOSLASKI, W. J., NEVE, R.**, Detoxification of shellfish in *Dinoflagellate Blooms, Proceedings of the Second International Conference on Toxic Dinoflagellate Blooms*, Key Biscayne, Florida, 1978, 43.

85. **MCCOLLUM, J. P. K., PEARSON, R. C. M., INGHAM, H. R., WOOD, P. C., DEWAR, H. A.**, An epidemic of mussel poisoning in north-east England, *Lancet*, **II, 767**, 1968.

86. **LUTHY, J.**, Epidemic paralytic shellfish poisoning in Western Europe 1976, in *Toxic Dinoflagellate Blooms*, Taylor, D. L., Seliger, H. H., editors, New York, Elsevier/North Holland, 1979, 15.

87. **SAKAMOTO, Y., LOCKEY, R. F., KRZANOWSKI, J. J.**, Shellfish and fish poisoning related to the toxic dinoflagellates, *Southern Medical Journal*, **80**, 866, 1987.

88. **MORRIS, P. D., CAMPBELL, D. S., TAYLOR, T. J., FREEMAN, J. I.**, Clinical and epidemiological features of neurotoxic shellfish poisoning in North Carolina, *Am. J. Public Health*, **81**, 471, 1991.

89. **MCFARREN, E. F., TANABE, H., SILVA, F. J., ET AL**, The occurrence of a ciguatera-like poison in oysters, clams and Gymnodinium breve cultures, *Toxicon*, **3**, 111, 1965.

90. **AHLES, M. D.**, Red tide: a recurrent health hazard, *American J Public Health*, **64**, 807, 1974.

91. **SUGANUMA, M., FUJIKI, H., SUGURI, H., ET AL**, Okadaic acid: an additional non-phorbol-12-tetradecanoate-13-acetate-type tumor promoter, *Proceedings of the National Academy Sciences USA*, 1988, 85, 1768.

92. **ZATORRE, R. J.**, Memory loss following domoic acid intoxication from ingestion of toxic mussels, *Can. Dis. Wkly. Rep.*, **16**, (Suppl. 1E), 101, 1990.

93. **GJEDDE, A., EVANS, A. C.**, PET studies of domoic acid poisoning in humans: excitotoxic destruction of brain glutamatergic pathways, revealed in measurements of glucose metabolism by positron emission tomography, *Can. Dis. Wkly. Rep.*, **16**, (Suppl 1E), 105, 1990.

94. **DAVIS, S. R.**, Neutralisation of saxitoxin by antisaxitoxin rabbit serum, *Toxicon*, **23**, 669, 1985.

95. **BOSE, R., PINSKY, C., GLAVIN, G. B.**, Sensitive murine model and putative antidotes for behavioural toxicosis from contaminated mussel extracts, *Can Dis Wkly Rep*, **16**, (Suppl. 1E), 99, 1990.

96. **SEVEN, M. J.**, Mussel poisoning, *Ann Intern Med*, **48**, 891, 1958.

97. **JAWARY, D., CAMERON, P. A., DZIUKAS, L., MCNEIL, J. J.**, Drug overdose - reducing the load, *Med J Aust*, **156**, 343, 1992.

98. **WILLIS, G., WRIGHT, J.**, Paralytic shellfish poisoning, Vancouver *British Columbia Med J*, **22**, 1980.

99. **PARK, D. L., ADAMS, W. N., GRAHAM, S. L., JACKSON, R. C.**, Variability of mouse bioassay for determination of paralytic shellfish poisoning toxins, *J Assoc. Off. Anal. Chem*, **69**, 547, 1986.

100. Paralytic shellfish, in *Poisindex*, Rumack, B., editor, Denver, Colorado, Micromedex, Inc, 50, 1986.

101. **RAND, P. W., LAWRENCE, F. H., PIRONE, L. A. JR., LAVIGNE, J. R., LACOMBE, E.**, The application of charcoal haemoperfusion to paralytic shellfish poisoning, *J. Maine Med. Assoc*, **68**, 147, 1977.

102. Update, Intoxication following mussel ingestion, *Can Dis Wkly Rep*, **14**, 7, 1988.

103. **AUERBACH, P. S., HALSTEAD, B. W.**, Hazardous aquatic Life, in *Management of Wilderness and Environmental Emergencies*, Second edition, Auerbach, P. S., Geehr, E. C., editors, C. V. Mosby, St Louis, Baltimore, Toronto, 999, 1989.

104. **TANGEN, K.**, Dinoflagellate blooms in Norwegian waters, in *Toxic Dinoflagellate Blooms*, Taylor, D. L., Seliger, H. H., editors, New York, Elsevier/North Holland, 1979, 179.

105. **HALLEGRAEFF, G., SUMNER, C.**, *Toxic plankton blooms affect shellfish farms*, Australian Fisheries December 1986, CSIRO reprint number 158, 1.

106. **Editorial,** Paralytic shellfish poisoning (red tide), *Epidemiol Bull*, **11**, 9, 1990.

107. **TUFTS, N. R.**, Molluscan transvectors of paralytic shellfish poisoning, in *Toxic Dinoflagellate Blooms*, Taylor, D. L., Seliger, H. H., editors, New York, Elsevier/North Holland, 1979, 403.

Chapter 5

CLINICAL TOXICOLOGY OF CIGUATERA POISONING

Philippe Glaziou, Mireille Chinain, and Anne-Marie Legrand

TABLE OF CONTENTS

I. INTRODUCTION

Ciguatera is a human seafood poisoning resulting from the consumption of a large variety of tropical reef fish and possibly of some marine invertebrates. Every year, near to 50,000 people suffer from this typical fish poisoning. The endemic areas are localized within a circumglobal belt which extends approximately from latitudes 35° N to 34° S. The greatest concentrations of ciguatoxic fish are found in the Caribbean and Indo-Pacific regions. According to all available epidemiological information, ciguatera fish poisonings are primarily presenting an insular distribution in the South Pacific Archipelagoes and in the West Indies.

The ecotoxicological phenomenon commonly designated as "ciguatera" is not of recent origin. The poisonous characteristics of certain marine fish were well known to the ancients[1]. Many writings of the navigators referred to the occurrence of fish poisonings in the West Indies and in the Pacific Ocean as well as in the Indian Ocean.

Halstead[1] listed more than 400 fish species implicated. However not all of the fish of the same species caught at the same time in the same place are toxic. Toxic fish specimens contain tiny amounts of polyether compounds highly toxic to humans. Ciguatera toxins can be divided into two classes: the lipid-soluble ciguatoxins and the water-soluble maitotoxins. Their source was demonstrated to be microscopic organisms (dinoflagellates) which appear to spawn and flourish following disturbances and destruction of coral reefs.

II. EPIDEMIOLOGY OF CIGUATERA FISH POISONING

Ciguatera influences the economic and nutritional aspects of tropical island life. Throughout most tropical island countries there is a heavy dependence on the inshore fishery resource to provide reef fish for food. Ciguatera directly impacts on the health of inhabitants, but also has indirect effects on health through avoidance of reef fish which would otherwise provide an important source of protein[2]. This form of poisoning, which seems to be becoming more common, tends to appear in new areas. Since no reliable diagnostic test in humans is available, the diagnosis of ciguatera fish poisoning depends on clinical criteria. No standard case definition is available.

A. GEOGRAPHICAL DISTRIBUTION

Potential risk exists from ingesting fish from tropical and sub-tropical coastal and insular areas of the Pacific and Indian oceans, and the Caribbean. Approximately 400 million people live in areas where ciguatera fish poisoning is present.

Americas: In the United States, most cases occur in Hawaii and southern Florida, or after travel to Caribbean islands. From 1972 to 1977, ciguatera represented 5.8% of the total food-borne diseases reported in the U.S. during this period[3]. In Miami, the estimated annual incidence rate is 50 per 100,000 population[4]. A recent study in Hawaii[5] reported an annual incidence rate of 8.7 per 100,000 from 1984 to 1989, as compared to 2.5 per 100,000 from 1975 through 1981[6]. Cases of human ciguatera fish poisoning in the United States have also been diagnosed in non-endemic states: Texas, Louisiana, Washington D.C., New York, Massachusetts and Maryland[7,8]. Disease in these areas resulted from the consumption of fish caught in other endemic areas and brought into non-endemic areas. In the Caribbean area, sporadic cases and outbreaks have been reported from many islands, including recent reports from the Bahamas, Cayman Islands, Cuba, Martinique, Puerto Rico and the U.S. and British Virgin Islands. Annual incidence in 1983 was 43 per 100,000 in the Cayman Islands, and 41 per 100,000 in Martinique. A household survey in the U.S. Virgin Islands[9] showed an annual incidence rate of 730 per 100,000 population.

Asia and Indian Ocean: Cases have been reported from East Asia, Eastern South Asia, Middle South Asia (particularly from the Maldives) and Western South Asia. Occurrence of ciguatera in Sri Lanka and Indonesia was reported but no reliable information is available. In Japan, 23 ciguatera outbreaks involving 379 patients were recorded during 1949-1980[10].

Oceania and Australia: Ciguatera is prevalent throughout the Pacific Island countries[2]. The South Pacific Commission reported a mean annual incidence of 98 per 100,000 population for the period 1979-1981, and 219 per 100,000 in 1987. Poisoning rates as high as 2% per year have been reported for some islands. Sporadic cases as well as large outbreaks are frequent. The mean annual incidence rate for the period 1986-1990 is between 500 and 1,200 per 100,000 in French Polynesia, Kiribati, Tokelau and Tuvalu; between 100 and 500 per 100,000 in Cook Islands, Fiji, Northern Marianas Islands, Marshall Islands, New Caledonia and Vanuatu, and lower than 100 per 100,000 in all other South Pacific states and territories[11]. In Fiji, ciguatera represents 96.4% of all documented cases of marine food poisoning. In Australia, most cases of ciguatera are not reported to health authorities. From 1976 through 1984, 166 outbreaks have been confirmed, which involved 479 people[12].

Most cases occurred in Queensland. A telephone survey carried out in two towns located in Queensland indicated that 1.8-2.5% of the population had been affected by ciguatera. The annual incidence was estimated at 30 per 100,000[13].

Fish caught in endemic countries can be shipped to any part of the world. Consequently, outbreaks can also be observed in non-endemic countries: 57 of 61 Canadian vacationers in Cuba developed ciguatera fish poisoning[14]. A mass alimentary poisoning occurred in Hungary, also involving travellers[15].

B. AGE AND SEX DISTRIBUTION

Cases aged 1 to 82 years have been observed[16]. Even breast fed infants may be at risk of the disease[17]. An association between illness and age exists; in most studies, the largest age group is that between 30 to 49 years old. Children may be less susceptible to toxic fish[9], but also, eating fish with low levels of toxin over several years could result in a sensitization to the toxin. It seems that men are at a higher risk of poisoning. The sex-ratio (M/F) varies from 1.5:1[16] in French Polynesia, where ciguatera is endemic throughout the year, to 1:1 in Miami[4]. One possible explanation for the difference is that it is not infrequent for a Polynesian fisherman to eat a part of a suspected fish before giving it the next day to the whole family.

C. DISTRIBUTION IN TIME

Very few data are available on trends of ciguatera over time. A notification system has been implemented in the South Pacific area by the South Pacific Commission in 1974[2]. However, the case definition may vary between countries and with time. It seems that ciguatera notification rates are increasing in most areas. This increase could be attributed to at least two factors, or a combination of both: a better effectiveness of reporting systems, or a true increase of incidence rates. This latter factor could be the consequence of changing life styles in islands surrounded with a coral reef. An increased awareness from public health authorities in the area resulted in an increase in the number of notifications[18]. In French Polynesia, where a surveillance system was implemented in 1960, there is no evidence of an increase of notification rates since 1974, but an increase of notifications in August-September and a decrease in March-April have been reported (Unpublished data). Three epidemiologic patterns for ciguatera were described[18]: endemic areas, where cases are observed all the year round; epidemic areas, where only outbreaks are observed; and intermediate areas, where outbreaks exist but cases are also observed between outbreaks. Global climatic changes may also influence the incidence of ciguatera[2]. Over the last 15 years in the Pacific area[2], some countries recorded a decrease in the ciguatera problem (New Caledonia, Marshall Islands), other countries an increase (Kiribati, Tuvalu, French Polynesia), while still other countries recorded an increase followed by a decrease in ciguatera (Tokelau, American Samoa, Western Samoa, Fiji and Vanuatu).

D. INVOLVED FISH SPECIES: BIOLOGY AND DISTRIBUTION

Fish incriminated in ciguatera poisoning are scattered over a wide phylogenetic range having varied biological characteristics. Their habitat, habit, feeding and reproductive processes are very diversified[1]. It appears that under proper circumstances any fish living in a reef area may be a potential vector of ciguatera toxins.

Herewith is a list of the fish families that have been the most frequently incriminated in ciguatera poisonings. The list is arranged phylogenetically by order, but alphabetically inside any order. The short summarizations on the biology of the incriminated families are based on those from Randall[19] and Halstead[1].

Phylum CHORDATA
Class OSTEICHTHYES
Order ANGUILLIFORMES:
Family MURENIDAE
　　Moray eels are a group of savage moderate-sized to large-sized fish. They inhabit a large variety of ecological biotopes in channels, coral ridges, reef flats and lagoon patch reefs. They are carnivorous and predacious, nocturnal in their habits, hiding in holes and under rocks or corals during the day.

Order BELONIFORMES
Family BELONIDAE
　　The needlefish are surface swimmers generally found along coastal areas. Their body is long and slender, prolonged by long jaws and a sharp beak. They are voracious fish feeders.

Order BERYCIFORMES
Family HOLOCENTRIDAE
　　The squirrelfish or soldierfish are brightly coloured species with or without stripes, found near rocky or coral flats. They are predacious, feeding nocturnally on crustaceans, worms and algae.

Order PERCIFORMES
Family ACANTHURIDAE
　　Surgeonfish are a group of small shore fish mostly common in channels and shoal areas. They are predominantly herbivorous, feeding on filamentous algae but they may also ingest small fish and invertebrates.

Family CARANGIDAE
　　Jacks and scads are a large group of oceanic fish living commonly near the coral reefs. Some of the Pacific species are noted for their long distance swimming. They are mostly carnivorous.

Family LABRIDAE
　　Most wrasse species are shore fish inhabiting rocky areas or coral reefs among algae. Some species are herbivorous, but most of them are carnivores.

Family LETHRINIDAE
　　Emperors and scavengers are a group of fish of moderate size. Most of them have a characteristic long muzzle. They are omnivorous, feeding on crustaceans, molluscs and fish as well as biodetritus and corals.

Family LUTJANIDAE
　　Snappers are abundant shore fish common in rocky, coral reef areas. They are voracious carnivores feeding largely on smaller fish.

Family MUGILIDAE
　　Mullet are small to moderate-sized fish, inhabitants of shallow bays and lagoons, swimming in schools near the surface of the water. They have herbivorous feeding habits.

Family MULLIDAE
　　Surmullets or goatfish are small shore fish swimming near coral reefs. They are carnivorous, feeding on various small animals. They have many predators.

Family SCARIDAE

Parrotfish are moderate-sized fish characteristic in that they have their teeth fused into plates. They commonly inhabit shallow water in coral reefs, lagoons and rocky areas. They feed on algae and small animals they ingest along with corals. They contribute to the formation of fine sand.

Family SCOMBRIDAE

Mackerel including the tunas are for the most part swift-swimming pelagic fish running in large schools. They are oceanic fish which come close to the shore during the reproduction period. They feed on a variety of fish and plankton.

Family SERRANIDAE

Seabass or groupers are predacious carnivorous shore fish. They inhabit coral reefs, rocks and sandy areas. Most of them live in shallow water but some species are found in deep water.

Family SPHYRAENIDAE

Barracuda are swift-swimming carnivorous and very voracious fish. Some attain large size. They are common in lagoons, channels and coral reefs.

Order TETRAODONTIFORMES:
Family BALISTIDAE

Triggerfish are a group of small shore fish characterized by their first two dorsal spines modified into a triggerlike device. They are widely distributed. They seem to prefer shallow reef areas, although some are found in deep water. They are omnivorous, ingesting corals, sponges, urchins, algae and various other small organisms. They can travel long distances, following the currents.

The distribution of the most frequently involved fish species is shown in Table 1.

Table 1
Fish species involved in ciguatera fish poisoning in the world (Americas; Western, Central and Eastern Pacific; Asia/India)

Family	Am*	W*	C*	E*	Ind*	Species
MURENIDAE	+			+	+	*Gymnothorax flavimarginatus* (Rüppell)
						G. javanicus (Bleeker)
						G. undulatus (Lacépède)
BELONIDAE	+			+		*Tylosuru scrocodilus* (Peron and Lesueur)
HOLOCENTRIDAE	+			+		*Adiorix spinifer* (Forskål)
						Myripristis murdjan (Forskål)
ACANTHURIDAE	+	+		+	+	*Acanthurus lineatus* (Linné)
						A. triostegus (Linné)
						Ctenochaetus striatus (Quoy and Gaimard)
						C. strigosus (Bennett)
						Naso unicornis (Forskål)
CARANGIDAE	+	+	+	+	+	*Carangoides fulvoguttatus* (Forskål)
						Caranx ignobilis (Forskål)
						C. melampygus (Cuvier and Valenciennes)
						C. sexfasciatus (Q. and G)
LABRIDAE	+	+		+		*Cheilinus undulatus* (Rüppel)
LETHRINIDAE			+	+	+	*Lethrinella conchyliatus* (Smith)
						Lethrinus chrysostomus (Richardson)

The table column headers: Region spanning Am*, Pac* (W*, C*, E*), As/Ind*.

Family	Region					Species
	Am[*]	Pac[*]			As/ Ind[*]	
		W[*]	C[*]	E[*]		
LUTJANIDAE	+	+	+	+	+	*L. harak* (Forskäl)
						L. mashena (Forskäl)
						L. miniatus (Schneider)
						L. xanthocheilus (Klunzinger)
						Aprion virescens (Valenciennes)
						Gymnocranius griseus (Schlegel)
						Lutjanus amabilis (De Vis)
						L. argentimaculatus (Forskäl)
						L. bohar (Forskäl)
						L. fulviflamma (Forskäl)
						L. gibbus (Forskäl)
						L. johni (Bloch)
						L. monostigmus (Cuvier and Valenciennes)
						L. rivulatus (Cuvier and Valenciennes)
						L. sebae (Cuvier)
						Monotaxis grandoculis (Forskäl)
						Plectorhynchus flavomaculatus (Ehrenberg)
						Symphorus nematophorus (Bleeker)
MUGILIDAE				+		*Crenimugil crenilabis* (Forskäl)
						Mugil cephalus (Lacépède)
MULLIDAE				+	+	*Parupeneus porphyreus* (Rüppell)
						Upeneus arge (Jordan and Evermann)
						U. vitattus (Forskäl)
SCARIDAE		+		+	+	*Scarops rubroviolaceus* (Bleeker)
						Scarus ghobban (Forskäl)
						S. gibbus (Rüppell)
						S. harid (Forskäl)
SCOMBRIDAE	+	+	+	+	+	*Acanthocybium solandri* (Cuvier)
						Gymnosarda unicolor (Rüppell)
						Scomberomorus commerson (Lacépède)
SERRANIDAE	+	+	+	+	+	*Anyperodon leucogrammicus* (Valenciennes)
						Cephalopholis argus (Schneider)
						C. leopardus (Lacépède)
						Diagramma pictum (Thunberg)
						Epinephelus aerolatus (Forskäl)
						E. cylindricus (Postel)
						E. microdon (Bleeker)
						E. morrhua (Valenciennes)
						E. tauvina (Forskäl)
						Plectropomus maculatus (Bloch)
						P. melanoleucus (Lacépède)
						P. leopardus (Lacépède)
						Variola louti (Forskäl)
SPHYRAENIDAE	+	+	+	+	+	*Sphyraena barracuda* (Walbaum)
						S. lbleekeri (Williams)
						S. forsteri (Cuvier, Valenciennes)
						S. jello (Cuvier)
BALISTIDAE	+	+		+	+	*Balistoides viridescens* (Bloch, Schneider)
						Pseudobalistes flavomarginatus (Rüppell)
						P. fuscus (Bloch, Schneider)

[*]   Am: Americas
Pac: Pacific (W: Western, C: Central, E: Eastern)
As/Ind: Asia and/or India

E. BIOGENESIS OF CIGUATERA TOXINS; THE FOOD CHAIN ACCUMULATION THEORY

Despite the long history of ciguatera, the process by which ciguatera toxins originate in the body of the fish has been a problem which has given rise to many speculations. Firstly, many theories implicated fish disease or pollution. Later on, field observations and studies of the ciguatera problem suggested that the poison has its origin in the environment of the fish. The first scientific insight on this aspect was given by Randall[19]. The extreme variability of toxicity in any given incriminated fish species, the patchy geographical distribution of ciguatoxic fish in endemic areas and the observation that three types of fish tend to become toxic, the herbivorous reef fish, the detritus-feeding reef fish and large carnivores that feed on these two types of reef fish, lead to the conviction that fish accumulate the ciguatera toxins through their diet from a benthic organism - an alga, a fungus, a protozoan or a bacterium. Discovery of the predicted toxic precursor was possible almost twenty years later when a very important outbreak of ciguatera occurred in the Gambier Islands (French Polynesia). Samples of biodetritus collected on damaged coral surfaces were found to be highly toxic. The high toxicity of these samples was correlated to the great abundance of a microscopic alga which was also found abundant in the gut contents of herbivorous fish[21-23]. Lipid-soluble and water-soluble extracts of the biodetritus fraction containing the microscopic algae yielded two types of toxicity, one closely related to the carnivorous fish toxicity and the other one resembling the toxicity of surgeonfish gut contents described by Yasumoto et al.[21]

F. BIOLOGY OF THE TOXIC PROTOZOANS LEADING TO CIGUATERA POISONING

The primary vector of ciguatera, a benthic microscopic alga, was described by Adachi & Fukuyo[24] as *Gambierdiscus toxicus* (Dinophyceae, Peridiniales, Heteraulacaeae)(see Figure 1a). Some authors have suggested that other species of dinoflagellates, in addition to *G. toxicus*, may be involved in ciguatera fish poisoning[25-27]. These include *Ostreopsis* spp., *Prorocentrum* spp. (see Figure 1b, 1c), *Amphidinium* spp. and *Coolia monotis*, which have been found to produce toxins that may also contribute to the ciguatera syndrome[26-28]. These species are frequently found in association with *G. toxicus*, although their abundance may be inversely correlated to *G. toxicus*[29-33]. Intense competition for space on macroalgal substrates may account for dynamics of these populations[34]. *Ostreopsis* seems to be a more important contributor to the phenomena of ciguatera than is *G. toxicus* in the Caribbean[30,35,36], although toxins extracted from this dinoflagellate seem to differ from ciguatoxins. In contrast, *G. toxicus* appears to be the primary vector of ciguatera in French Polynesia[29,37].

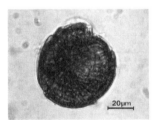 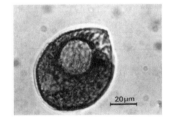 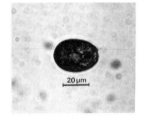

Figure 1. Some potentially ciguatoxic dinoflagellates.
1a. *Gambierdiscus toxicus*;;   **1b.** *Ostreopsis* sp.;   **1c.** *Prorocentrum* sp.

1. Distribution

Populations of ciguatera-causing dinoflagellates are found throughout tropical and subtropical regions of the world: French Polynesia[38,39], the Hawaian islands[40-43], New Caledonia[10,38,44], Vanuatu[38], Guam, Okinawa, Fiji[10], Australia[45] as well as the Atlantic coastal waters of southeastern Florida[31,46-49]. They are also present in the Caribbean sea[26,30,33,35,38,47,50-52] and the Indian Ocean[38,53].

2. Habitats

Ciguateric dinoflagellates are typically associated with coral reef ecosystems but their habitats also include tide pools[47], bays and near docks[31]. Ciguatera outbreaks often follow coral reef disturbances by manmade or natural causes[19,27,54-56]. A time-lag of six months to a year is generally expected between these two events[57]. The resulting dead coral surfaces are then progressively colonized by filamentous or calcareous macroalgae[37,53,58]. Subsequently, toxigenic microorganisms develop on these macroalgal substrates but are also found directly on the surface of dead corals, sand and rocks[21,59]. These cells adhere to their algal substrate by mucus threads or form a mucilaginous matrix over the macrophyte thalli and are often found aggregated within[30]. Colonisation studies on artificial substrates suggest that it may take 8 to 9 months before *G. toxicus* appears on new macrophytic substrates[60]. Ciguatera outbreaks may occur shortly thereafter: the transfer of dinoflagellate toxins to man, via fish consumption, may only require one month[33]. However, coral reef disturbances are not necessarily followed by increases in *G. toxicus* populations and/or ciguatera outbreaks[40,55,61,62]. Others factors, in addition to macroalgal substrate availability, may act as regulating factors of the population densities *in situ*.

G. toxicus is distributed micro-regionally from 0.5 to 30-60 meters, but is generally found in shallow waters (0.5 to 3 m) [33,56,57]. However, cells are usually absent from intertidal substrates, probably because of periodic dilution of this layer by heavy rainfall and/or too high sunlight intensity [57]. Cells may also be occasionally found rafting on the surface of drift algae such as *Turbinaria ornata* or *Sargassum natans*[63], suggesting the existence of a semi-pelagic dispersal mode, explaining the colonisation of new areas.

G. toxicus cells show clear preference for sheltered areas, since highest numbers occur in leeward localities[62], and where land runoff is minimal [27,53,57]. On the other hand, moderate runoff is believed to promote population growth by increasing nutrient input from land [30,53]. Some authors [31,39,53] also report maximum densities of these dinoflagellates at channel sites, suggesting that water motion may play a significant role in regulating the abundance of these populations: water movement may increase exposure to nutrient flow or gases.

3. Substrate preferences and effect of nutrients

In their attempt to determine high risk ciguatera periods, most countries affected by ciguatera have set up monitoring programmes for potentially toxic dinoflagellates. Caution is generally advised if numbers greater than 100 cells of toxic dinoflagellates/g of algae are reported, whereas cell density less than 10 cells/g is unlikely to cause ciguatera[55]. The ciguatera benthic dinoflagellate community is widely dispersed among various macroalgal groups such as Ceramiales (Rhodophyta) [40,48,62,64], Cryptonemiales (Rhodophyta) [27,56,65], Dictyotales (Phaeophyta) [30,33,35,48,51,53], Fucales (Phaeophyta) [27,53], Siphonales and Siphonocladales (Chlorophyta) [33,51,52]. This apparent lack of specificity with regard to the macroalgae substrata is tempered by observations of some specific dinoflagellate/macroalgal associations in the Caribbean [33], which support the hypothesis that the macroalgal hosts supply an important growth factor to their epiphytic dinoflagellate community [34,51,66]. The macroalgae morphology also seems to be a density regulating factor, since *G. toxicus*, *Prorocentrum* spp. and *Ostreopsis* spp. are rarely present on species with broad flat thalli. In contrast, these dinoflagellates demonstrate a very strong preference for the surface of highly branched or tufted macroalgae [57]. The dinoflagellate density also seems to be positively correlated with the macroalgae surface area and negatively correlated with their ash content [34,48].

There is some evidence of the beneficial effect of silicates and oxides (Fe) on *G. toxicus* populations *in natura* [53,60]. Field observations also showed that nitrite, nitrate, ammonia, dissolved phosphate and total dissolved phosphorus present in the "thallisphere" (water directly adjacent to macroalgal thalli) were positively correlated with *G. toxicus* abundance[33].

4. Seasonality

April to October is the period most likely for ciguatera intoxication in the Caribbean[50,67], while an increase of notifications is reported from September to November around St Thomas [68]. There are also reports of seasonal fluctuations of toxic dinoflagellates. Comparison of the optimal *in vitro* growth conditions [48,61,69,70] to the observed seasonality of these dinoflagellates has revealed that temperature and salinity appear to be the main determining factors in the seasonal trends of these species: depending on the localities studied, peak densities are either negatively or positively correlated with temperature. For example, *G. toxicus* and *Prorocentrum* spp. are found most abundantly during the warm water temperature period (t°>26°C) in Tahiti (French Polynesia) [37,65], southwestern Puerto Rico [30] and the Florida Keys [31], and during the cold water temperature period in Mururoa (t°<26°C) [60], in Queensland (Australia) (t°<22°C) [45], and in the Virgin Islands [33]. Likewise, *Ostreopsis* spp. and *P. lima* maximum abundance occur during the cool water season (t°<26°C) in the Florida Keys [31,71] and the Virgin Islands [33]. The abundance of *G. toxicus* is negatively correlated with salinity values [33,60]. These results may help explain the positive correlation between precipitation (thus lower salinity) and abundance of *G. toxicus* [30,33]. However, the degree of rainfall may affect the polarity of response by dinoflagellates, since heavy precipitations often generate high turbidity known to adversely affect the dinoflagellates growth [30,33,53].

The distribution and periodicity of toxic dinoflagellates is the result of a fine balance of multiple factors. The existence of seasonality patterns for most of the incriminated dinoflagellates may allow the determination of high ciguatera risk periods. However, Bomber[31] believes that these dinoflagellates are continually present in coral reef ecosystems and thus continually "pulse ciguatoxins into the food chain". But instances of high toxic dinoflagellate densities without apparent ciguatera have also been reported [55,57,61,64]. The development of *G. toxicus* blooms and the stimulation of toxin production seem to be two separable and distinguishable events [64]. Only under the influence of a "ciguatoxin-inducing factor" is the production of ciguatoxins by a population of *G. toxicus* effective. This inducing factor could be related to *G. toxicus* associated microflora [72], or could be of genetic origin, since only certain strains of *G. toxicus* are capable of producing ciguatoxins[73-75]. Also, Polynesian strains of *G. toxicus* seem to be a more important source of algal ciguatoxins than Caribbean strains.

III. SYMPTOMS AND SIGNS OF CIGUATERA POISONING

A. GENERAL SYMPTOMS

The disease is rarely fatal. From experimentally induced lethality in the fresh water mosquito fish, *Gambusia affinis*, Lewis [76] suggested that, *in natura*, high concentrations of toxin might be lethal to sea fish. Thus, very small quantities of toxins could be present in living fish, resulting in fewer quantities ingested by human individuals. The most extensive studies on clinical features of ciguatera come from French Polynesia [77]. Clinical manifestations appear 2 to 30 hours after eating a toxic fish, and by 24 hours, four groups of symptoms can be identified:

Neurologic manifestations:

The most common presenting complaint of patients is paresthesia, consisting of either numbness or tingling in the extremities, or a painful or hot sensation to the skin when in contact with cold water. Paresthesia is found in 89% of the cases in French Polynesia, 88%

in Fiji [20], 70-76% in Australia [12,78], 70% in Miami[4], 87% in the Caribbean area [79], and 36% of 32 cases in the U.S. Virgin Islands[9]. Pruritus is described in 5% to 89% of the cases (5% in Fiji, 89% in French Polynesia).

Gastro-intestinal tract manifestations:
Diarrhea appears to be common: 32% in Fiji and from 75% to 86% in the other studies. Abdominal pain is also frequently reported.

Cardiac manifestations:
Bradycardia and hypotension are reported in French Polynesia (16%) and Fiji (9%). Cardiovascular disorders have only occasionally been reported in Australia. In Queensland, patients with severe cases of ciguatera have been hospitalized to control the loss of body fluids, the respiratory distress, or the cardio-vascular abnormalities[12]. Cases with tachycardia have also been reported[80].

Other symptoms:
Weakness is the most common symptom in Fiji and in Australia. Many other symptoms have been reported, such as dysuria, chills, sweating, vertigo, neck stiffness, skin rash, ophthalmologic signs[81], generalized pruritic reaction following alcohol ingestion[82], metallic taste in the mouth[83], psychiatric disorders[84], vulvar pruritus[85], polymyositis[86] and polyneuropathy[87].

B. PHYSIOPATHOLOGY
In severe cases, neurologic manifestations have been attributed to an oedema of the adaxonal Schwann cell cytoplasm. These observations have been related to the property of ciguatoxin to increase the permeability of the excitable membrane to sodium[88]. Very few data are available on biological determinations during attacks of ciguatera. Laboratory resources are generally minimal or absent in many of the areas supplying information, and no specific abnormality has been pointed out[16]. Preponderance of paresthesia is related to the fact that paresthesia is considered as the clinical hallmark of ciguatera[16]. In endemic countries, the population has come to recognize it from experience. A recent survey conducted in Noumea, New Caledonia[89] showed that 53% of 500 questioned inhabitants knew the specific symptom of ciguatera, the figure reaching 70% in people having experienced ciguatera. Clinical descriptions of the disease tend to vary from one country to another. In the U.S. Virgin Islands[90], gastrointestinal tract symptoms seem more common: diarrhea was found in 91% of 33 patients and paresthesia in only 54% of patients, as compared with respectively 73% and 89% in French Polynesia. The symptoms of ciguatera tend to disappear in a few days. However, paresthesia, pains, pruritus and weakness may persist several weeks in some cases, with an increase of symptoms following ingestion of proteins of animal origin[18].

A broad range of host responses:
Some patients appear to have mild symptoms after eating a fish known to produce a more severe illness in other persons[16]. The dose relationships and differential distribution of ciguatoxin within a given fish may play a role[91]. A recent study in Tahiti[92] reported differences in the clinical response after fish ingestion related to the nutritional status of the species: diarrhea, ataxia, bradycardia and low blood pressure were found more frequent when the fish were carnivorous. Different symptom profiles with a number of statistically significant differences in the reported frequencies of specific symptoms were reported, supporting the contention that the large variability in symptoms associated with ciguatera poisoning is caused by several closely related but distinct toxins [93,94]. It has been shown that

there are differences in the response depending on whether the patient presented with a first attack or suffered from a second (or subsequent) attack [4,93]: the majority of symptoms listed were significantly more common in those patients experiencing their second or later attack of ciguatera. Factors influencing variability of response to the ingestion of ciguatoxic fish relate both to the fish species and to individual susceptibility.

Differential diagnosis:

Neurotoxic and paralytic shellfish poisoning should be considered for differential diagnosis as these two diseases have a lot of clinical similarities with ciguatera fish poisoning[79]. However, the dinoflagellates responsible for these entities are most common in waters in latitudes above 30° north and below 30° south, whereas the ciguatera organisms are essentially confined to latitudes between 35° north and 35° south[95]. Also, fish poisoning induced by tetrodotoxin or palytoxin should be considered for differential diagnosis in some areas of the South Pacific (New Caledonia).

There is an urgent need for a standard case definition of ciguatera cases. Several difficulties hinder its formulation: no reliable means of detecting ciguatoxins in humans is available, and no specific biologic abnormality in cases has been identified. Even if based on clinical manifestations related to the ingestion of a potentially toxic fish, a standard case definition could allow comparisons between countries as well as the assessment of the trends of incidence rates in a given area.

IV. PROPHYLAXIS

Eradication of the problem associated with ciguatera is highly unlikely unless consumption of reef fish is stopped. Public health measures designed to reduce the morbidity from ciguatera are limited. Many countries prohibit the sale of potentially toxic fish, and provide information to the public. In general, people will not eat a fish that is of a consistently poisonous species, but the decision to eat a fish of a species that is only sporadically toxic will be influenced by the availability of alternative food sources, the perception of seriousness of the consequences, and the presumed ability to predict toxicity. To be effective, ciguatera control measures need a precise identification of risk factors for the disease, the primary factor being the ingestion of toxic fish. Behavioral patterns with individuals who commonly eat potentially toxic fish and are more likely to be poisoned repeatedly need to be assessed, as well as the relationship between the ingested dose and the severity of the disease. A cheap and reliable stick test for the identification of toxic fish is clearly required. Also, the knowledge of environmental parameters and mechanisms that lead to a production of ciguatoxins, hence to ciguatera outbreaks, is needed.

V. CLINICAL MANAGEMENT OF CIGUATERA

Ciguatoxin exerts its effects primarily by altering the membrane properties of excitable cells, thus activating voltage-dependant sodium channels [96,97]. Sodium channels are widely spread in nerve and muscle tissues. Drugs that have been found to be effective experimentally at countering the initial cardiovascular effects of ciguatoxin are atropine, phentolamine, calcium gluconate and lidocaine [98]. To date, the treatment of ciguatera (of the immediate, or of the long term effects) remains symptomatic and supportive, and there is considerable need to find drugs that can treat ciguatera specifically. Such drugs would selectively regulate sodium channel activity with few side-effects[12].

Various drugs have been used for treatment of ciguatera such as folk remedies[99], tocainide[100], amitriptyline and nifedipine[101], antihistamines and steroids[102], and intravenous vitamins B and C associated with calcium and steroids [18]. More recently intravenous mannitol was suggested to be effective [103-105]. However, only one controlled trial has so far been reported, which showed that 250 ml of 20% mannitol given intravenously in one hour was slightly more effective than a combination of vitamins and calcium also given intravenously in one hour [106], for the treatment of mild cases of ciguatera. The possible mechanism of action of mannitol remains obscure. Further pharmacological studies and clinical trials are required before recommending any specific treatment. A recently published experimental study of iv mannitol (1 g/kg) in mice after exposure to ip ciguatoxin did not show any benefit in signs of intoxication or time to death, however the authors urge caution in interpreting this to clinical benefit in man, because of possible species differences in response [107]. The authors point out that there is continued evidence of the clinical effectiveness of iv mannitol in the treatment of humans with ciguatera poisoning [108-110]. They believe that a better animal model for ciguatoxin poisoning is required [108]. For the present, therefore, iv mannitol should be considered in the treatment of significant ciguatoxin poisoning in man.

VI. REFERENCES

1. **HALSTEAD, B.W.** (1967) *Poisonous and venomous marine animals of the world. Vertebrates.* Washington D.C., US Governments Printing Office **2**: 63-330.
2. **LEWIS, R.J.** (1992) Socio-economic impact and management of ciguatera in the Pacific. In: *Proceedings IVth International Conference on Ciguatera Fish Poisoning, Papeete, Tahiti, May 4-7, 1992.*
3. **HUGHES, J.M.** (1979) Epidemiology of shellfish poisoning in United States, 1971-1977. In: *Toxic Dinoflagellate blooms*, Elsevier North-Holland, New York, 23-28.
4. **LAWRENCE, D. N., ENRIQUEZ, M. B. & LUMISH, R. M.** (1980) Ciguatera fish poisoning in Miami. *JAMA* **244**: 254-258.
5. **GOLLOP, J.H. & PON, E.W.** (1992) Ciguatera: A review. *Hawaii Med. J.* 51: 91-99.
6. **ANDERSON, B.S., SIMS, J.K., WIEBENGA, N.H. and SUGI, M.** (1983) The epidemiology of ciguatera fish poisoning in Hawaii, 1975-1981. *Hawaii Med. J.* **42**: 326-334.
7. **CENTERS FOR DISEASE CONTROL** (1980) Ciguatera fish poisoning-Maryland. *MMWR* 29: 610-611.
8. **RUSSEL, F.E.** (1975) Ciguatera fish poisoning: a report of 35 cases. *Toxicon* 13: 383-385.
9. **MORRIS, J.G., LEWIN, P., SMITH, W.C., BLAKE, P.A. & SCHNEIDER, R.** (1982) Ciguatera fish poisoning: epidemiology of the disease on St Thomas, U.S. Virgin Islands. *Am. J. Trop. Med. Hyg.*, **31**: 574-578.
10. **YASUMOTO, T., RAJ, U. & BAGNIS, R.** (1984) Seafood poisonings in tropical regions. In: *Symp. Seafood Toxins in Tropical Regions,* Kagoshima University, Kagoshima, Japan, 74 pp.
11. **DALZELL, P.** (1993) Ciguatera fish poisoning and fisheries development in the South Pacific. In: *Proceedings IVth International Conference on Ciguatera Fish Poisoning, Papeete, Tahiti, May 4-7, 1992.*
12. **GILLESPIE, N.C., LEWIS, R.J., PEARN, J.H., BOURKE, A.T.C., HOLMES, M.J., BOURKE, J.B. & SHIELDS, W.J.** (1986) Ciguatera in Australia. Occurrence, clinical features, pathophysiology and management. *Med. J. Aust.* **145**: 584-590.
13. **CAPRA, M. & CAMERON, J.** (1985) Epidemiological and social surveys of the incidence and of the attitudes towards ciguatera poisoning in two Australian communities. In: GABRIE, C. & SALVAT, B. Eds. *Proceedings of the Fifth International Coral Reef Congress*, Tahiti, 489.
14. **FRENETTE, C., MACLEAN, J.D. & GYORKOS, T.W.** (1988) A large common-source outbreak of ciguatera fish poisoning. *J. Inf. Dis.* **158**: 1128-1131.
15. **DOBI, S., HORVARTH, A., PRINZ, G. & VARNAI, F.** (1990) Imported food poisoning caused by fish toxins. *Orv. Hetil.* **131**: 2201-2203.
16. **BAGNIS, R., KUBERSKI, T. & LAUGIER, S.** (1979) Clinical observations on 3,009 cases of ciguatera (fish poisoning) in the south pacific. *Am. J. Trop. Med. Hyg.* **28**: 1067-73.
17. **BLYTHE, D.G. & De SYLVA, D.P.** (1990) Mother's milk turns toxic following fish feast. Letter. *JAMA* **265**: 2339.
18. **LEGRAND, A.M., BAGNIS, R.** (1991) La ciguatéra : un phénomène d'écotoxicologie des récifs coralliens. *Ann. Inst. Pasteur* **3**: 1-14.
19. **RANDALL, J.E.** (1958) A review of ciguatera, tropical fish poisoning, with a tentative explanation of its cause. *Bull. Mar. Sci. Gulf and Carib.*, **8**: 236-267.
20. **SOROKIN, M.** (1975) Ciguatera poisoning in North-West Viti Levu, Fiji Islands. *Hawaii Med. J.* **34**: 207-210.
21. **YASUMOTO, T., NAKAJIMA, I., BAGNIS, R. & ADACHI, R.** (1977) Finding of a dinoflagellate as a likely culprit of ciguatera. *Bull. Japan. Soc. Sci. Fish.* **43**: 1021-1026.

22. **BAGNIS, R., CHANTEAU, S., YASUMOTO, T.** (1977) Découverte d'un agent étiologique vraisemblable de la ciguatéra. *CR Acad Sci Paris* **28:** 105-108.

23. **CHANTEAU, S.** (1978) Rôle d'un dinoflagellé benthique dans la biogénèse de la ciguatéra. Thèse, Université de Clermont-Ferrand II.

24. **ADACHI, R. & FUKUYO, Y.** (1979) The thecal structure of a marine dinoflagellate *Gambierdiscus toxicus* gen. et sp. nov. collected in a ciguatera-endemic area. *Bull. Jap. Soc. Sci. Fish.* **45:** 67-71.

25. **STEIDINGER, K.A.** (1983) A re-evaluation of toxic dinoflagellate biology and ecology. In: ROUND, F.E. & CHAPMAN, D.J. Eds. *Progress in Phycological Research*, Elsevier Science Publishing Co., pp. 147-188.

26. **TINDALL, D.R., DICKEY, R.W., CARLSON, R.D. & MOREY-GAINES, G.** (1984) Ciguatoxigenic dinoflagellates from the Caribbean Sea. In: RAGELIS, E.P. Ed. *Seafood Toxins*, The American Chemical Society Washington D.C., pp. 225-240.

27. **YASUMOTO, T., INOUE, A., OCHI, T., FUJIMOTO, K., OSHIMA, Y., FUKUYO, Y., ADACHI, R. & BAGNIS, R.** (1980) Environmental studies on a toxic dinoflagellate responsible for ciguatera. *Bull. Jap. Soc. Sci. Fish.* **46:** 1397-1404.

28. **NAKAJIMA, I., OSHIMA, Y. & YASUMOTO, T.** (1981) Toxicity of benthic dinoflagellates in Okinawa. *Bull. Jap. Soc. Sci. Fish.* **47:** 1029-1033.

29. **BAGNIS, R., BENNETT, J., PRIEUR, C., & LEGRAND, A.M.** (1985) The dynamics of three toxic benthic dinoflagellates and the toxicity of ciguateric surgeonfish in French Polynesia. In: ANDERSON, D.M., WHITE, A.W. & BADEN D.G. Eds. *Toxic Dinoflagellates*, Elsevier Science Publishing Co. New York, pp. 177-182.

30. **BALLANTINE, D.L., TOSTESON, T.R. & BARDALES, A.** (1988) Population dynamics and toxicity of natural populations of benthic dinoflagellates in southwestern Puerto Rico. *J. Exp. Mar. Biol. Ecol.* **119:** 201-212.

31. **BOMBER, J.W.** (1985) Ecological studies of benthic dinoflagellates associated with ciguatera from the Florida Keys. Thesis, Florida Institute of Technology, Melbourne, Florida. 104 pp.

32. **CARLSON, R.D.** (1984) Distribution, periodicity and culture of benthic/epiphytic dinoflagellates in a ciguatera-endemic region of the Caribbean. Ph.D. Thesis, Southern Illinois University, Illinois. 308 pp.

33. **CARLSON, R.D. & TINDALL, D.R.** (1985) Distribution and periodicity of toxic dinoflagellates in the Virgin Islands. In: ANDERSON, D.M., WHITE, A.W. & BADEN, D.G. Eds. *Toxic Dinoflagellates*, Elsevier Science Publishing Co. New York, pp. 171-176.

34. **BOMBER, J.W., RUBIO, M.G. & NORRIS, D.R.** (1989) Epiphytism of dinoflagellates associated with the disease ciguatera: substrate specificity and nutrition. *Phycologia* **28:** 360-368.

35. **BALLANTINE, D.L., BARDALES, A.T., TOSTESON, T.R. & DUPONT-DURST, H.** (1985) Seasonal abundance of *Gambierdiscus toxicus* and *Ostreopsis* sp. in costal waters of southwest Puerto Rico. In: *Proceedings Vth International Coral Reef Congress*, **4:** 417-422.

36. **TOSTESON, T.R., BALLANTINE, D.L., TOSTESON, C.G., BARDALES, A.T., DURST, H.D. & HIGERD, T.B.** (1986) Comparative toxicity of *Gambierdiscus toxicus, Ostreopsis cf. lenticularis*, and associated microflora. *Mar. Fish. Rev.* **48:** 57-59.

37. **BAGNIS, R., LEGRAND, A.M. & INOUE, A.** (1990) Follow-up of a bloom of the toxic dinoflagellate *Gambierdiscus toxicus* on a fringing reef of Tahiti. In: GRANELI E., SUNDSTROM B., EDLER, L. & ANDERSON, D.M. Eds. *Toxic Marine Phytoplankton*, Elsevier Science Publishing Co. New York, pp. 98-103.

38. **BAGNIS, R.** (1981) Etude morphologique, biologique, toxicologique et écologique de l'agent causal princeps de la ciguatera, le péridinien *Gambierdiscus toxicus* Adachi & Fukuyo 1979. Thesis, Université de Bordeaux II, France. 180 pp.

39. **YASUMOTO, T., INOUE, A., BAGNIS, R. & GARCON, M.** (1979) Ecological survey on a dinoflagellate possibly responsible for the induction of ciguatera. *Bull. Jap. Soc. Sci. Fish.* **45:** 395-399.

40. **McCAFFREY, E.J., SHIMIZU, M.M.K., SCHEUER, P.J. & MIYAHARA, J.T.** (1990) Seasonal abundance and toxicity of *Gambierdiscus toxicus* Adachi & Fukuyo from O'ahu, Hawaii. In: TOSTESON, T.R. Ed. *Proceedings IIIrd International Conference on Ciguatera*, Polyscience Publications Quebec, pp. 145-153.

41. **SHIMIZU, Y., SHIMIZU, H., SCHEUER, P.J., HOKAMA, Y., OYAMA, M. & MIYAHARA, J.T.** (1982) *Gambierdiscus toxicus*, a ciguatera causing dinoflagellate from Hawaii. *Bull. Jap. Soc. Sci. Fish.* **48:** 811-813.

42. **TAYLOR, F.J.R.** (1979) A description of the benthic dinoflagellate associated with maitotoxin and ciguatoxin, including observations on Hawaiian material. In: TAYLOR, D.L. & SELIGER, H.H. Eds. *Toxic Dinoflagellates*, Elsevier Science Publishing Co. North Holland, pp. 71-76.

43. **WITHERS, N.** (1981) Toxin production, nutrition and distribution of *Gambierdiscus toxicus* (Hawaiian strain). In: *Proceedings IVth International Coral Reef Symposium*, 2, pp. 449-451.

44. **FUKUYO, Y.** (1981) Taxonomical study on benthic dinoflagellates in coral reefs. *Bull. Jap. Soc. Sci. Fish.* **47:** 967-978.

45. **GILLESPIE, N.C., HOLMES, M.J., BURKE, J.B. & DOLEY, J.** (1985) Distribution and periodicity of *Gambierdiscus toxicus* in Queensland, Australia. In: ANDERSON, D.M., WHITE, A.W. & BADEN, D.G. Eds. *Toxic Dinoflagellates*, Elsevier Science Publishing Co. New York, pp. 183-188.

46. **BAGNIS, R., INOUE, A., RONGERAS, S., GALONNIER, M., BENNETT, J., CHANTEAU, S. & PASTUREL J.** (1981) Quelques aspects bioécologiques de *Gambierdiscus toxicus*, péridinien benthique responsable de la ciguatera à Tahiti. *2ème colloque de Microbiologie Marine, Marseille, France, June 24-25.*

47. **BESADA, E.G., LOEBLICH, L.A. & LOEBLICH, A.R.** (1982) Observations on tropical, benthic dinoflagellates from ciguatera-endemic areas: *Coolia, Gambierdiscus* and *Ostreopsis. Bull. Mar. Sci.* **32:** 723-735.

48. **BOMBER, J.W.** (1987) Ecology, genetic variability and physiology of the ciguatera-causing dinoflagellate *Gambierdiscus toxicus* Adachi & Fukuyo. Ph.D. Dissertation, Florida Institute of Technology, Melbourne, Florida. 146 pp.

49. **NORRIS, D.R., BOMBER, J.W. & BALECH, E.** (1985) Benthic dinoflagellates associated with ciguatera from the Florida Keys. I. *Ostreopsis heptagona* sp. nov. In: ANDERSON, D.M., WHITE, A.W. & BADEN, D.G. Eds. *Toxic Dinoflagellates*, Elsevier Science Publishing Co. New York, pp.39-44.

50. **BAGNIS, R.** (1979) Rapport de mission aux Antilles et à l'île de Pâques, *Rapp. Miss. Inst. Rech. Med. Louis Malardé,* 941.

51. **CARLSON, R.D., MOREY-GAINES G., TINDALL, D.R. & DICKEY R.W.** (1984) Ecology of toxic dinoflagellates from the Caribbean sea. Effects of macroalgal extracts on growth in culture. In: RAGELIS, E.P. Ed. *Seafood Toxins*, The American Chemical Society Washington D.C., pp. 271-287.

52. **VALDES MUNOZ, E., POPOWSKY, G., JIMENEZ DOMINGUEZ, C., MARTINEZ, R., BORRERO, N. & BERLAND, B.** (1993) Ciguatera in Cuba: preliminary results. In: *Proceedings IVth International Conference on Ciguatera Fish Poisoning, Papeete, Tahiti, May 4-7, 1992.*

53. **THOMASSIN, B.A., ALI HALIDI, M.E.A., QUOD, J.P., MAGGIORANI, J.M., BERLAND, B., GRZEBYK, D. & COQUEUGNIOT, J.** (1993) Evolution of *Gambierdiscus toxicus* populations in the coral reef complex of Mayotte Island (SW Indian Ocean) during the 1985-1991 period. In: *Proceedings IVth International Conference on Ciguatera Fish Poisoning, Papeete, Tahiti, May 4-7, 1992.*

54. **BAGNIS, R.** (1969) Naissance et développement d'une flambée de ciguatera dans un atoll des Tuamotu. *Revue des Corps de Santé* **10:** 783-795.

55. **BAGNIS, R., JULVEZ, J., ALLAOUI, A., DUBRAY, B., CONAN, H., ALI HALIDI, M.A., MIELI, L. & GALTIER, J.** (1988) Le risque ciguatérique dans l'île de Mayotte (Archipel des Comores). *Rev. Intern. Océanogr. Méd.* 91-92, pp. 43-54.

56. **INOUE, A.** (1987) A contributory dinoflagellate to ciguatera, *Gambierdiscus toxicus*, in French Polynesia. In: INOUE, A. Ed. *Fisheries and Marine Resources in the South Pacific*, Kagoshima University Research Center for the South Pacific, pp. 31-41.

57. **TAYLOR, F.J.R.** (1985) The distribution of the dinoflagellate *Gambierdiscus toxicus* in the Eastern Caribbean. In: *Proceedings Vth International Coral Reef Congress*, 4, pp. 423-428.

58. **CHAINE, M.** (1987) Etude du micro et du meïobenthos algal associés au dinoflagellé *Gambierdiscus toxicus* Adachi & Fukuyo agent causal princeps de la ciguatera par la méthode des substrats neufs artificiels (Atoll de Mururoa, Polynésie Française). Thesis, Université des Sciences et Techniques du Languedoc, Montpellier, France. 149 pp.

59. **BAGNIS, R., CHANTEAU, S., CHUNGUE, E., HURTEL, J.M., YASUMOTO, T. & INOUE, A.** (1980) Origins of ciguatera fish poisoning: a new dinoflagellate, *Gambierdiscus toxicus* Adachi & Fukuyo, definitively involved as a causal agent. *Toxicon* **18:** 199-208.

60. **CAIRE, J.F., RAYMOND, A. & BAGNIS, R.** (1985) Ciguatera: study of the setting up and the evolution of *Gambierdiscus toxicus* population on an artificial substrate introduced in an atoll lagoon with follow up of associated environmental factors. In: *Proceedings Vth International Coral Reef Congress*, 4, pp. 429-436.

61. **BERLAND, B., GRZEBYK, D. & THOMASSIN, B.A.** (1993) Benthic dinoflagellates from the coral reef lagoon of Mayotte Island (SW Indian Ocean); identification, toxicity and preliminary ecophysiological study. In: *Proceedings IVth International Conference on Ciguatera Fish Poisoning, Papeete, Tahiti, May 4-7, 1992.*

62. **TAYLOR, F.J.R. & GUSTAVSON, M.S.** (1985) An underwater survey of the organism chiefly responsible for "ciguatera" fish poisoning in the eastern Caribbean region: the benthic dinoflagellate *Gambierdiscus toxicus*. In: STEFANON, A. & FLEMMING, N.J. Eds. *VIIth Int. Diving Sci. Symp., Italy, 1983.*

63. **BOMBER, J.W., MORTON, S.L., BABINCHAK, J.A., NORRIS, D.R. & MORTON, J.G.** (1988) Epiphytic dinoflagellates of drift algae - another toxigenic community in the ciguatera food chain. *Bull. Mar. Sci.* **43:** 204-214.

64. **GILLESPIE, N.C., LEWIS, R., BURKE, J. & HOLMES M.J.** (1985) The significance of the absence of ciguatoxin in a wild population of *G. toxicus*. In: *Proceedings Vth International Coral Reef Congress*, 4, pp. 437-442.

65. **ASIN, P., CHINAIN, M., MICOUIN, L. & LEGRAND A.M.** (1993) The survey of *G. toxicus* abundance in three points around Tahiti Island. In: *Proceedings IVth International Conference on Ciguatera Fish Poisoning, Papeete, Tahiti, May 4-7, 1992.*

66. **GRZEBYK, D., BERLAND, B. & THOMASSIN, B.A.** (1993) Distribution of ciguateric dinoflagellates in Mayotte Island (SW Indian Ocean). In: *Proceedings International Workshop on Ciguatera Management, Bribie Island, Australia, April 13-16, 1993.*

67. **OLSEN, D.A., NELLIS, D.W. & WOOD, R.S.** (1983) Ciguatera in the eastern Caribbean. *Mar. Fish. Rev.* **1**: 13-18.

68. **McMILLAN, J.P., GRANADE, R.H. & HOFFMAN, P.** (1980) *J. Coll. Vir. Isl.* 6: 84.

69. **DURAND, M.** (1984) Etude biologique , cytologique et toxicologique de *Gambierdiscus toxicus* en culture, dinoflagellé responsable de la ciguatera. Thesis, Université Paris VII, Paris, France. 136 pp.

70. **MORTON, S.L., NORRIS, D.R. & BOMBER, J.W.** (1992) Effect of temperature, salinity and light intensity on the growth and seasonality of toxic dinoflagellates associated with ciguatera. *J. Exp. Mar. Biol. Ecol.* **157**: 79-90.

71. **BOMBER, J.W., NORRIS, D.R. & MITCHELL, L.E.** (1985) Benthic dinoflagellates associated with ciguatera from the Florida Keys. II. Temporal, Spatial and Substrate heterogeneity of *Prorocentrum lima.* In: ANDERSON, D.M., WHITE, A.W. & BADEN, D.G. Eds. *Toxic Dinoflagellates,* Elsevier Science Publishing Co. New York, pp. 45-50.

72. **TOSTESON, T.R., BALLANTINE, D.L., TOSTESON, C.G., HENSLEY, V. & BARDALES, A.T.** (1989) Associated bacterial flora, growth and toxicity of cultured benthic dinoflagellates *Ostreopsis lenticularis* and *Gambierdiscus toxicus. Appl. Envir. Microb.* **55**: 137-141.

73. **HOLMES, M.J., LEWIS, R.J., POLI, M.A. & GILLESPIE, N.C.** (1991) Strain dependent production of ciguatoxin precursors (gambiertoxins) by *Gambierdiscus toxicus* (Dinophyceae) in culture. *Toxicon* **29**: 761-775.

74. **MICOUIN, L., CHINAIN, M., ASIN, P. & LEGRAND, A.M.** (1993) Toxicity of French Polynesian strains of *Gambierdiscus toxicus* in cultures. In: *Proceedings IVth International Conference on Ciguatera Fish Poisoning, Papeete, Tahiti, May 4-7, 1992.*

75. **SATAKE, M., ISHIMARU, T., LEGRAND, A.M. & YASUMOTO, T.** (1993) Isolation of a ciguatoxin analog from cultures of *Gambierdiscus toxicus.* In: SMAYDA, T.J. & SHIMIZU, Y. Eds. *Toxic Phytoplankton Blooms in the Sea,* Elsevier Science Publishing Co. Amsterdam, pp. 575-580.

76. **LEWIS, R.J.** (1992) Ciguatoxins are potent ichthyotoxins. *Toxicon* **30**: 207-211.

77. **BAGNIS, R. & LEGRAND, A.M.** (1987) Clinical features on 12,890 cases of ciguatera (fish poisoning) in French Polynesia. In: Eds. GOPALAKRISHNAKONE, P., TAN C.K. *Progress in venom and toxin research..* National University of Singapore and International Society of Toxinology, Asia-Pacific Section, Singapore, 372-377.

78. **LEWIS, R.J., CHALOUPKA, M.Y., GILLESPIE, N.C. & HOLMES, M.J.** (1988) An analysis of the human response to ciguatera in Australia. In: *Proceedings of the Sixth International Coral Reef Symposium,* Australia, 3: 67-71.

79. **JOHNSON, R. & JONG, E. C.** (1983) Ciguatera: Caribbean and Indo-Pacific Fish Poisoning. *West. J. Med.* **138**: 872-874.

80. **MILLS, A.R. & PASSMORE, R.** (1988) Pelagic paralysis. *The Lancet* **8578**: 161-164.

81. **HAMBURGER, H.A.** (1986) The neuro-ophthalmologic signs of ciguatera poisoning: a case report. *Ann. Ophthalmol.* **18**: 287-288.

82. **CASANOVA, M.F.** (1982) Ciguatera poisoning, medical letter. *Arch. Neurol.* **39**: 387.

83. **PEARCE, R.** (1983) Ciguatera fish poisoning: presentation as a neurologic disorder. *South Med. J.* **76**: 560-561.

84. **LIPKIN, K.M.** (1989) Ciguatera poisoning presenting as psychiatric disorder. *Arch. Gen. Psychiatry* **46**: 248.

85. **DELORD, J.M., MACENO, R. & ARFI, S.** (1984) Prurit vulvaire révélateur d'une ciguatéra. *La Presse Médicale* **13**: 1577.

86. **STOMMEL, E.W., PARSONET, J. & JENKYN, L.R.** (1991) Polymiositis after ciguatera toxin exposure. *Arch. Neurol.* **48**: 874-877.

87. **SOZZI, G., MAROTTA, P., ALDEGHI, D., TREDICI, G. & CALVI, L.** (1988) Polyneuropathy secondary to ciguatoxin poisoning. *Ital. J. Neurol. Sci.* **9**: 491-495.

88. **ALLSOP, J.L., MARTINI, L., LEBRIS, H., POLLARD, J., WALSH, J. & HODGKINSON, S.** (1986) Les manifestations neurologiques de la ciguatéra. *Rev. Neurol.* **142**: 590-597.

89. **LAURENT, D., JOANNOT, P., AMADE, P., MAESSE, P. & COLMET-DAAGE, B.** (1993) Knowledges on ciguatera in Noumea (New Caledonia). In: *Proceedings IVth International Conference on Ciguatera Fish Poisoning, Papeete, Tahiti, May 4-7, 1992.*

90. **MORRIS, J. G. Jr, LEWIN, P., HARGRETT, N. T, SMITH, C. W., BLAKE, P. A. & SCHNEIDER, R.** (1982) Clinical features of Ciguatera Fish Poisoning. A study of the disease in the US Virgin Islands. *Arch. Intern. Med.* **142**: 1090-1092.

91. **BANNER, A. H.** (1976) *Biology and geology of coral reefs.* Acad Press NY.

92. **BAGNIS, R., SPIEGEL, A., N'GUYEN, L. & PLICHART, R.** (1992) Public health, epidemiological and socio-economic patterns of ciguatera in Tahiti. In: *Proceedings of the Third International Conference on*

Ciguatera Fish Poisoning, Porto Rico, TOSTESON, T.R. Ed., Polyscience Publications, Québec, Canada, April 1990. 157-168.

93. **GLAZIOU, P. & MARTIN, P.M.V.** (1993) Study of factors that influence the clinical response to ciguatera fish poisoning. *Toxicon.*

94. **KODAMA, A.M. & HOKAMA, Y.** (1989) Variations in symptomatology of ciguatera fish poisoning. *Toxicon* **27**: 593-595.

95. **HALSTEAD, B. W.** (1978) *Poisonous and Venomous Marine Animals of the World.* Darwin Press; Princeton, NJ, **2**: 325-400.

96. **BENOIT, E., LEGRAND, A.M. & DUBOIS, J.M.** (1986) Effects of ciguatoxin on current and voltage clamped frog myelinated nerve fibre. *Toxicon* **24**: 357-364.

97. **SEINO, A., KOBAYASHI, M., MOMOSE, K., YASUMOTO, T. & OHIZUMI, Y.** (1988) The mode of inotropic action of ciguatoxin on guinea-pig cardiac muscle. *Br. J. Pharmacol.* **95**: 876-882.

98. **LEGRAND, A.M., LOTTE, C. & BAGNIS, R.** (1985) Respiratory and cardiovascular effects of ciguatoxin in cats; antagonistic action of hexamethonium, atropine, propanolol, phentolamine, yohimbine, prazosin, verapamil, calcium and lidocaine. In: GABRIE, C. & SALVAT, B. Eds. *Proceedings of the Fifth International Coral Reef Congress,* Tahiti: 463-466.

99. **BOURDY, G., CABALION, P., AMADE, P. & LAURENT, D.** (1992) Traditional remedies used in the western Pacific for the treatment of ciguatera poisoning. *J. Ethnopharmacol.* **36**: 163-174.

100. **LANGE, W.R., KREIDER, S.D., HATTWICK, M. & HOBBS, J.** (1988) Potential benefit of tocainide in the treatment of ciguatera: report of three cases. *JAMA* **84**: 1087-1088.

101. **CALVERT, G.M., HRYHORCZUK, D.O. & LEIKIN, J.B.** (1987) Treatment of ciguatera fish poisoning with amitriptyline and nifedipine. *Clin. Toxicol.* **25**: 423-428.

102. **WILSON, R.J. & McADAM, J.G.** (1990) Acute cervico-facial oedema and loss of consciousness following ingestion of barracuda fish. *J. R. Army. Corps.* **136**: 163-164.

103. **PALAFOX, N.A., JAIN, L.G., PINANO, A.Z., GULICK, T.M., WILLIAMS, R.K. & SCHATZ, I.J.** (1988) Successful treatment of ciguatera fish poisoning with intravenous mannitol. *JAMA* **259**: 2740-2742.

104. **PEARN, J.H., LEWIS, R.J., RUFF, T., TAIT, M., QUINN, J., MURTHA, W., KING, G., MALLETT, A. & GILLESPIE, N.C.** (1989) Ciguatera and mannitol: experience with a new treatment regimen. *Med. J. Aust.* **151**: 77-79.

105. **WILLIAM, R.K. & PALAFOX, N.A.** (1990) Treatment of pediatric ciguatera fish poisoning. *Am. J. Dis. Child.* **144**: 747-748.

106. **BAGNIS, R., SPIEGEL, A., BOUTIN, J.P., BURUCOA, C., N'GUYEN, L., CARTEL, J.L., CAPDEVIELLE, P., IMBERT, P., PRIGENT, D. & GRAS, C.** (1991) Evaluation de l'efficacité du mannitol dans le traitement de la ciguatéra. In: *Résumé des communications des 2ème journées médicales de Polynésie Française*, Papeete.

107. **LEWIS, R.J., WONG-HOY, A.W., SELLIN, M.** (1993) Ciguatera and mannitol: in vivo and in vitro assessment in mice. *Toxicon* **31**: 1039-1050.

108. **LEWIS, R.J.** (1992) Mannitol: the treatment of choice in the acute phase of ciguatera. In *Ciguatera Information Bulletin.* **2**: 9-10 (LEWIS, R.J., ed.) Noumea: South Pacific Commission.

109. **WILLIAMSON, J.** (1990) Ciguatera and mannitol: a successful treatment. *Med. J. Aust.* **153**: 306-307.

110. **STEWART, M.P.M.** (1991) Ciguatera fish poisoning: treatment with intravenous mannitol. *Trop. Doctor* **21**: 54-55.

Chapter 6

CLINICAL TOXICOLOGY OF FUGU POISONING

Nobuo Kaku, Jürg Meier

TABLE OF CONTENTS

I. BIOLOGY AND DISTRIBUTION OF FISH RESPONSIBLE FOR FUGU (TETRODOTOXIN) POISONING

A number of bony fish of the families Canthigasteridae (sharp-nosed puffer fish), Diodontidae (porcupine fish), Molidae (Ocean sun fish) and Tetraodontidae (puffer fish) of the order Tetraodontiformes (Plectognathi) are known to cause fugu or tetrodotoxin poisoning in humans. Eating of "fugu" (the most commonly used puffer fish in Japan are species from the genus *Fugu*) may be regarded as a national habit in Japan. The respective causative agent is the neurotoxin "tetrodotoxin". These fish do not possess a venom apparatus; the toxin may be found in all organs of the body, although some organs, like the liver and, in females, the ovaries, may contain higher amounts (Table 1).

The body distribution of tetrodotoxin may be different in different fish species and toxin content may vary considerably during the season. Even in individuals of the same species there may be pronounced differences in toxin content. Especially during the reproductive season, the ovaries contain high toxin concentrations. This applies also to freshwater species which may cause tetrodotoxin poisoning, although there, the skin has been shown to contain the highest concentration of tetrodotoxin[2]. The following brief account lists those fish species most often referred to as being poisonous. For more details, see reference 1.

A. Family *Canthigasteridae* (Sharp-nosed puffer fish)

The sharp-nosed puffer (*Canthigaster rivulatus*) is considered to be involved in tetrodotoxin poisoning. The species occurs in the Indo-Pacific Ocean and around Japan.

Table 1

Concentrations (µg TTX/gram fresh tissue) of TTX in different female puffer fish and newts (*Taricha torosus*) (simplified, from[37])

Species	Ovary	Liver	Skin	Intestines	Muscle	Blood
Canthigaster rivulatus	<2	2	40	4	<0.2	
Lagocephalus inermis	0.4	1	<0.2	0.4	0.4	
Sphaeroides alboplumbeus	200	1000	20	40	1	
Sphaeroides basilewskianus	100	40	4	40	< 0.2	
Sphaeroides chrysops	40	40	20	4	< 0.2	<0.2
Sphaeroides niphobles	400	1000	40	400	4	1
Sphaeroides oscellatus	1000	40	20	40	< 0.2	
Sphaeroides pardalis	200	1000	100	40	1	1
Sphaeroides porphyreus	400	200	20	40	1	
Sphaeroides pseudommus	100	10	4	2	<0.2	
Sphaeroides rubripes	100	100	1	2	<0.2	<0.2
Sphaeroides stictonotus	20	<0.2	2	1	<0.2	
Sphaeroides vermicularis	400	200	100	40	4	
Sphaeroides xanthopterus	100	40	1	4	<0.2	
Taricha torosa, female	25	<0.1	25	0.1	2	1
Taricha torosa, male (* testis)	<0.1*	<0.1	80	0.5	8	21

B. Family *Diodontidae* (Porcupine fish)

These spiny marine fish able to inflate themselves when threatened are widely distributed in tropical seas. Species of the genera *Chilomycterus* and *Diodon* are said to contain tetrodotoxin.

C. Family *Molidae* (Ocean sun fish)

The ocean sun fish *Mola mola* , a fish with a diameter of up to 3 meters, lives in tropical and temperate seas, and is considered to be involved in tetrodotoxin poisoning.

D. Family *Tetraodontidae* (Puffer fish)

The puffer fish live in marine, estuarine and fresh water systems, respectively. The genera *Amblyrhynchotes*, *Arothron* (Figure 1), *Chelonodon*, *Fugu*, *Lagocephalus*, *Sphaeroides* and *Tetraodon* of this family are probably the fish most often involved in tetrodotoxin poisoning.

II. OCCURRENCE, ORIGIN, STRUCTURE AND MOLECULAR PHARMACOLOGY OF TETRODOTOXIN

A. OCCURRENCE AND ORIGIN OF TETRODOTOXIN

Tetrodotoxin (TTX) has not only been detected in tissues of fish relevant for fugu poisoning, but also in a number of phylogenetically distinct animal species such as starfishes (*Astropecten* sp.)[3-6], xanthid crabs (*Atergatis floridus, Zosimus aeneus*)[7,8], marine shells and snails (*Charonia saulinae, Babylonia japonica, Tufufa lissostoma*)[9,10], flatworms (*Planocera multitentaculata*)[11], ribbon worms (*Cephalotrix linearis, Lineus fuscoviridis, Tubulanus punctatus*)[12,13], horseshoe crabs (*Carcinoscopus rotundicauda*)[14], in the salivary glands of the Australian blue-ringed octopus (*Hapalochlaena maculosa*)[15], in the skin of frogs (*Atelopus* sp.)[16] and newts (*Taricha* sp.)[17] and even in red calcareous algae (*Jania* sp.)[18]. With the exception of the ribbon worms and the blue-ringed octopus, where it seems to be of importance in the context of prey immobilization, TTX is said to have a protective function in these animals, where it is accumulated in different tissues. Puffer fish, xanthid crabs and ribbon worms are able to secrete appreciable amounts of TTX when disturbed[13,25]. However, its broad occurrence gave evidence for speculation that TTX and its derivatives originate from symbiotic microorganisms. Indeed, in the late eighties, a number of bacterial strains of the genera *Aeromonas* (*A. hydrophila, A. salmonicida*), *Alteromonas* (*A. communis, A. haloplanktis, A. nigrifaciens, A. undina, A. vaga*), *Escherichia coli, Photobacterium phosphoreum, Plesiomonas shigelloides, Pseudomonas* sp. and *Vibrio* (*V. alginolyticus, V. anguillarum, V. costicola, V. cholerae, V. fischeri, V. harveyi, V. marinus, V. parahaemolyticus*) have been shown to produce TTX[19,20]. This hypothesis is further supported by the fact that in newts (*Taricha torosa* and *T. granulosa*, respectively), the skin of which was detoxified by electric stimulation, no *de novo* biosynthesis of TTX occurred[21]. Moreover, puffer fish reared in captivity were shown to lack TTX in their tissues[22]. The trumpet shells (*Charonia* sp.) become toxic by accumulating TTX via the food chain through feeding on TTX containing starfishes (*Astropecten* sp.). It is not yet elucidated why the respective animals are quite resistant to the pharmacologic action of TTX. It has been shown that puffer fish containing TTX are much more resistant against the toxin than those which are essentially free from it[23]. Studies with the blue-ringed octopus revealed that even nerve preparations of this species are not affected by TTX[24]. In conclusion, the biogenesis of tetrodotoxin is still not fully understood.

B. CHEMISTRY OF TETRODOTOXIN

Tetrodotoxin (synonyms TTX, Tarichatoxin, Spheroidine, Maculotoxin, Tetrodotoxine, BJT 1, Babylonia japonica toxin 1, Araregai toxin; 8a(1H)-quinazolineorthoglycolic acid; CA Reg.no. [4368-28-9]; $C_{11}H_{17}N_3O_8$; mol.weight 319.3 D) was known as the causative agent for tetrodotoxin poisoning since the beginning of this century. However, the structure of TTX was only elucidated in 1964 and characterized as an aminoperhydroquinazoline compound with a hemilactal function linking the molecule's two ring systems[26-28]. Meanwhile, three derivatives, tetrodonic acid, 4-*epi* tetrodotoxin and anhydrotetrodotoxin, respectively, have been detected in puffer fish (Figure 2)[29]. TTX is of amphoteric nature, soluble in acidic water, insoluble in organic solvents and stable at ambient temperature[30].

C. TOXICITY OF TETRODOTOXIN

In mice, the LD50 has been determined as 332 µg/kg after oral administration, 10 µg/kg after intraperitoneal and 8 µg/kg after subcutaneous application, respectively[31,32]. Thus, although precise LD50 values should be regarded with caution due the high variability of parameters of the test system, tetrodotoxin is an extremely toxic compound.

D. MOLECULAR PHARMACOLOGY OF TETRODOTOXIN

Tetrodotoxin binds with high affinity (K_D about 10^{-9} M) to the external surface of voltage-gated sodium channels[33]. In so doing, the inward flow of sodium ions through the channel pore is blocked, leading to inhibition of membrane potentials. The cationic (guanidino group) and anionic (acid hydroxyl groups) parts of the molecule seem to be of crucial importance for the biological activity of TTX[34]. Although it is often said that TTX as well as the saxitoxins present in toxic dinoflagellates (see Chapter 4) are channel "blockers" or "occluders", recent data suggest that the structural dependence of TTX action is of a complex nature[35].

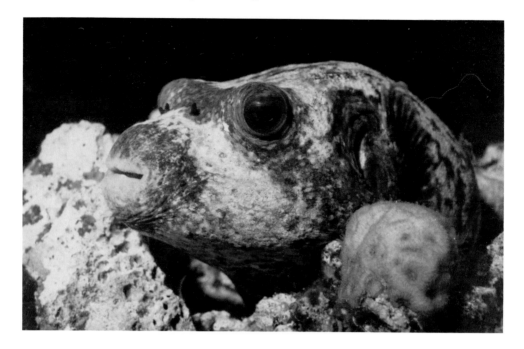

Figure 1. Puffer *Arothron hispidus* (courtesy of Swiss Tropical Institute, Basel, Switzerland).

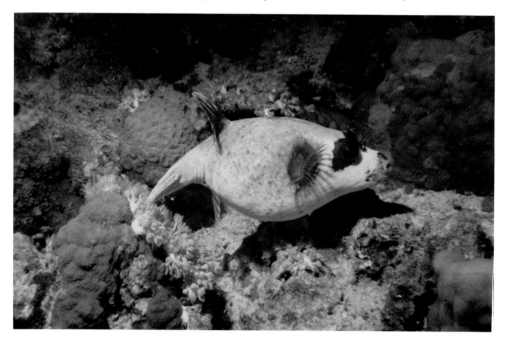

Figure 2. Puffer fish (*Arothron diadematus*) in natural habitat.

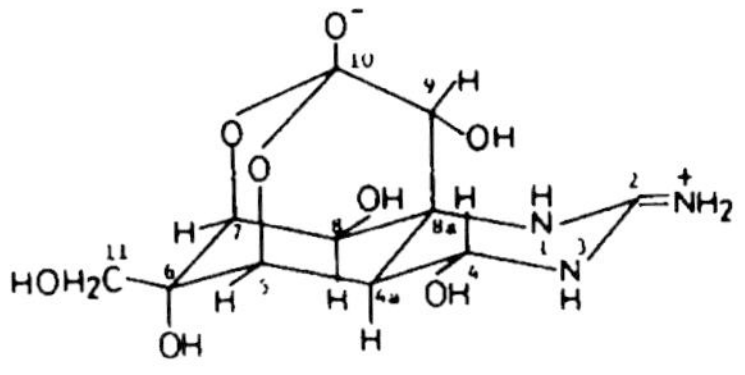

Figure 3. Tetrodotoxin and its derivatives (simplified, from[29]).

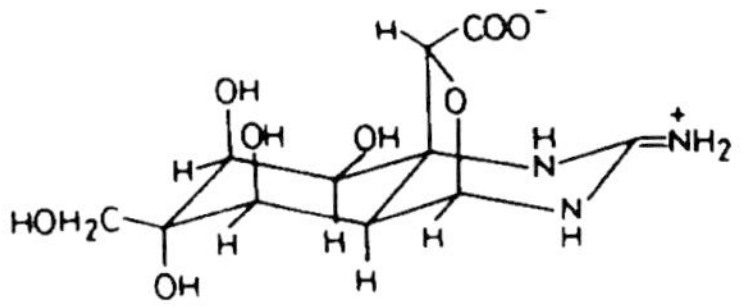

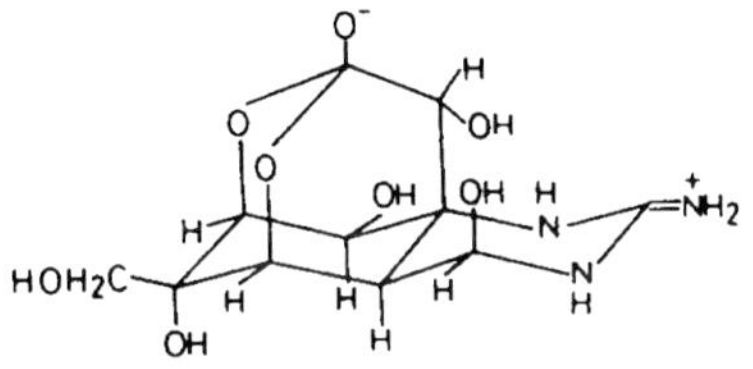

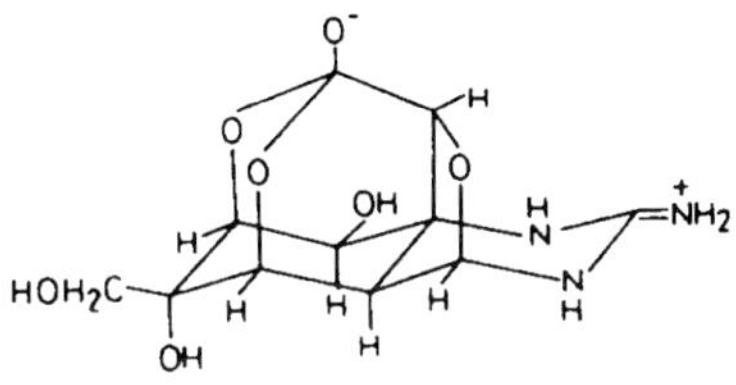

III. EPIDEMIOLOGY OF FUGU (TETRODOTOXIN) POISONING

Tetrodotoxin poisoning may be expected to occur wherever tetrodotoxic fish (see above) are found and eaten. Unfortunately, global statistics regarding tetrodotoxin poisoning are not readily available, with the exception of Japan, where the eating of "fugu" is quite common. Whereas earlier this century more than 100 death cases per year were reported, recent data show an incidence of 45 patients per year and a lethality of about 11 percent (Table 2)[1,36]. The tremendous decline in both incidence and lethality is most probably due to the fact that there are almost no cases of poisoning after fugu consumption in restaurants, since fugu cooks have to pass rigorous examinations before receiving a license. Thus, nowadays, fugu poisoning is most often seen when inexperienced fishermen prepare their own fish.

The puffer fish season in Japan lasts from October until March, the best time being between November and February, since during this period, the flesh is said to have the best flavor. However, human attitude towards fugu meals is controversial: whereas some people describe fugu being just chicken-like in taste, others recommend this fish meat as being a source for exhilaration and euphoria, being accompanied by mild paresthesias of the mouth region, sensations of warmth and flushing skin. To what extent these effects are based on small amounts of TTX present in the meat, or just of autosuggestive origin, remains open.

Table 2
Statistics of fugu poisoning in Japan from 1983 - 1992 (courtesy Ministry of Health and Wellfare, Japan[36])

Year	Number of records	Number of Patients	Number of Deaths
1983	18	34	6
1984	23	39	6
1985	30	41	9
1986	22	38	6
1987	35	52	4
1988	26	46	5
1989	31	45	5
1990	32	52	1
1991	29	45	3
1992	33	57	4
Total	279	449	49
Average	30 records	45 patients	5 deaths

IV. SIGNS AND SYMPTOMS OF FUGU (TETRODOTOXIN) POISONING

The majority of people ingesting TTX containing fish will have only minor poisoning, or no poisoning. Attention should therefore be directed at early detection of those at risk of major poisoning requiring urgent intervention.

The classic symptoms and signs of TTX poisoning are listed in Table 3.

Table 3
Classic symptoms and signs of tetrodotoxin poisoning (after Fukuda and Tani[38]).

STAGE OF POISONING	SYMPTOM/SIGN	ONSET
GRADE 1	Numbness around mouth, perioral parastheseae, with or without gastrointestinal symptoms (nausea).	5-45 mins.
GRADE 2	Numbness of tongue, face, and other areas of skin. Early motor paralysis and incoordination. Slurred speech. Reflexes normal.	10-60 mins.
GRADE 3	Widespread paralysis. Dyspnoea and hypotension. Aphonia. Patient still conscious. Pupils may become fixed, dilated.	15mins to several hours.
GRADE 4	Severe paralysis including severe respiratory muscle paralysis and consequent hypoxia. Hypotension. Cardiac arrhythmias. Bradycardia. Patient may be unconscious. Imminent death due to respiratory failure.	15 mins to 24 hours (death has been recorded 17 mins after ingestion).

Poisoning may be rapid in onset with first symptoms, classically perioral numbness or parastheseae, occurring in 5-15 minutes of ingestion in severe cases. There is at least one report of rapid development of paralysis and respiratory failure resulting in death only 17 minutes after ingestion[1]. The more rapid the onset of symptoms, the more severe the degree of poisoning in most cases. Nausea appears common, but vomiting is not common. The paralysis rapidly advances in severe cases, with associated respiratory problems first manifested as dyspnoea. Even though patients may become progressively and significantly hypoxic, unable to speak or move in response to stimuli, they may remain conscious until a very late stage, aware of comments made about them, though unable to indicate this. This should be remembered by those in professional attendance, and conversation and discussion of the patient's situation guarded appropriately. Cardiovascular manifestations of TTX poisoning include progressive hypotension, bradycardia, depressed AV node conduction, other arrhythmias, and even asystole.

V. CLINICAL TREATMENT OF FUGU (TETRODOTOXIN) POISONING

There is no specific antidote for tetrodotoxin; therefore, treatment is essentially symptomatic and supportive, in addition to detoxification.

The first priority is to ensure vital body functions are maintained; thus, if there is respiratory embarrassment, respiratory support must be given. This may be as simple as oxygen by mask in a mild case, but in any case of significant respiratory problems, the patient may require direct ventilatory support, with formal muscle relaxation, sedation, intubation and mechanical ventilation. The decision to intubate and ventilate will be assisted by objective measures of respiratory function, such as arterial blood gas, peripheral oxygen saturation and direct measurement of respiratory capacity (i.e. vital capacity, FEV1 etc.). However, even prior to respiratory muscle paralysis requiring ventilatory support, paralysis of the oropharyngeal muscles may force intubation and ventilation, as above, to avoid the risk of aspiration and consequent lung damage. While often less clinically important than respiratory problems, hypotension due to TTX does occur and may require vasopressor infusion and iv fluids. Atropine has been suggested, and both iv edrophonium and im neostigmine have been used with success in restoring muscle power[39-42].

The second priority is to remove remaining unabsorbed food from the stomach, to prevent further TTX reaching the circulation. This can be achieved by standard techniques, which, in most hospitals, will include insertion of a naso-gastric tube and aspiration of contents, followed by activated charcoal being given by the tube. Because of the possibility of developing oropharyngeal paralysis, induction of vomiting is not recommended.

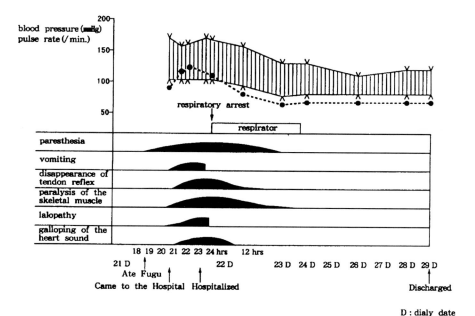

Figure 4. Clinical course of fugu poisoning.

VI. REFERENCES

1. HALSTEAD, B.W., *Poisonous and venomous marine animals of the world,* Princeton, N.J., Darwin Press, 1978 (Rev.Ed.)

2. LAOBHRIPATR, S., LIMPAKARNJANARAT, K., SANGWONLOY, O., SUDHASANEYA, S., ANUCHATVORAKUL, B., LEELASITORN, S. AND SAITANU, K., Food poisoning due to consumption of the freshwater puffer *Tetraodon fangi* in Thailand, *Toxicon* **28**, 1372, 1990.

3. NOGUCHI, T., NARITA, H., MARUYAMA, J. AND HASHIMOTO, K., Tetrodotoxin in the starfish Astropecten polyacanthus, in association with toxification of a trumpet shell, "Boshubora", *Charonia sauliae, Nippon Suisan Gakkaishi* **48**, 1173, 1982.

4. MARUYAMA, J., NOGUCHI, T., JEON, J.K., HARADA, T. AND HASHIMOTO, K., Occurrence of tetrodotoxin in the starfish *Astropecten latespinosus, Experientia* **40**, 1395, 1984.

5. MARUYAMA, J., NOGUCHI, T., NARITA, H., NARA, M., JEON, J.K., OTSUKA, M. AND HASHIMOTO, K., Occurrence of tetrodotoxin in a starfish, *Astropecten scoparius, Agric.Biol.Chem.* **49**, 3069, 1985.

6. MIYAZAWA, K., NOGUCHI, T., MARUYAMA, J., JEON, J.K., OTSUKA, M. AND HASHIMOTO, K., Occurrence of tetrodotoxin in the starfishes *Astropecten polyacanthus* and *A. scoparius* in the Seto Inland Sea, *Marine Biol.* **90**, 61, 1985.

7. NOGUCHI, T., UZU, A., KOYAMA, K., MARUYAMA, J., NAGASHIMA, Y. AND HASHIMOTO, K., Occurrence of tetrodotoxin as major toxin in a xanthid crab *Atergatis floridus, Bull.Jap.Soc.Sci.Fisheries* **49**, 1887, 1983.

8. NOGUCHI, T., DAIGO, K., ARAKAWA, O. AND HASHIMOTO, K., Release of paralytic shellfish poison from the exoskeleton of a xanthid crab *Zosimus aeneus*, in *Toxic Dinoflagellates,* Anderson, D.M. et al., Eds., New York, Elsevier Science Publ., 1985, 293.

9. NARITA, H., NOGUCHI, T., MARUYAMA, J., UEDA, Y., HASHIMOTO, K., WATANABE, Y. AND HIDA, K., Occurrence of tetrodotoxin in a trumpet shell, "Boshubora", *Charonia sauliae, Nippon Suisan Gakkasishi* **47**, 935, 1981.

10. NOGUCHI, T., MARUYAMA, J., UEDA, Y., HASHIMOTO K. AND HARADA, T., Occurrence of tetrodotoxin in the Japanese ivory shell *Babylonia japonica, Nippon Suisan Gakkaishi* **47**, 909, 1981.

11. MIYAZAWA, K., JEON, J.K., MARUYAMA, J., NOGUCHI, T., ITO, K.M. AND HASHIMOTO, K., Occurrence of tetrodotoxin in the flatworm *Planocera multitentaculata, Toxicon* **24**, 645, 1986.

12. MIYAZAWA, K., HIGASHIYAMA, M., ITO, K., NOGUCHI, T., ARAKAWA, O., SHIDA, Y. AND HASHIMOTO, K., Tetrodotoxin in two species of ribbon worm (nemertini), *Lineus fuscoviridis* and *Tubulanus punctatus, Toxicon* **26**, 867, 1988.

13. ALI, A.E., ARAKAWA, O., NOGUCHI, T., MIYAZAWA, K., SHIDA, Y. AND HASHIMOTO, K., Tetrodotoxin and related substances in a ribbon worm *Cephalothrix linearis* (Nemertean), *Toxicon* **28**, 1083, 1990.

14. KUNGSUWAN, A., NAGASHIMA, Y., NOGUCHI, T., SHIDA, Y., SUVAPEEPAN, S., SUWANSAKORNKUL, P. AND HASHIMOTO, K., Tetrodotoxin in the horseshoe crab *Carcinoscopus rotundicauda* inhabiting Thailand, *Nippon Suisan Gakkaishi* **53**, 261, 1987.

15. SHEUMACK, D.D., HOWDEN, M.E., SPENCE, I. AND QUINN, R.J., Maculotoxin: a neurotoxin from the venom glands of the octopus *Hapalochlaena maculosa* identified as tetrodotoxin, *Science* **199**, 188, 1978.

16. KIM, Y.H., BROWN, C.G. AND FUHRMAN, F.A., Tetrodotoxin-occurrence in atelopid frogs of Costa Rica, *Science* **189**, 151, 1975.

17. MOSHER, H.S., FUHRMAN, F.A., BUCHWALD, H.D. AND FISCHER, H.G., Tarichatoxin-tetrodotoxin, a potent neurotoxin, *Science* **199**, 1100, 1964.

18. YASUMOTO, T., NAGAI, H., YASUMURA, D., MICHISHITA, T., ENDO, A., YOTSU, M. AND KOTAKI, Y., in *Tetrodotoxin, Saxitoxin and the Molecular Biology of the sodium channel,* Kao, C.Y. and Levinson, S.R., Eds., New York, Acad.Sciences 1986, 44.

19. YOTSU, M., YAMAZAKI, T., MEGURO, Y., ENDO, A., MURATA, M., NAOKI, H. AND YASUMOTO, T., Production of tetrodotoxin and its derivatives by *Pseudomonas* sp. from the skin of a pufferfish, *Toxicon* **25**, 225, 1987.

20. SIMIDU, U., NOGUCHI, T., HWANG, D.F., SHIDA, Y. AND HASHIMOTO, K., Marine bacteria which produce tetrodotoxin, *Appl. Environ. Microbiology* **53**, 1714, 1987.

21. SHIMIZU, Y. AND KOBAYASHI, M., Apparent lack of tetrodotoxin biosynthesis in captured *Taricha torosa* and *Taricha granulosa, Chem.Pharm.Bull.* **31**, 3625, 1983.

22. SAITO, T., MARUYAMA, J., KANOH, S., JEON, J.K., NOGUCHI, T., HARADA, T., MURATA, T. AND HASHIMOTO, K., Toxicity of the cultured pufferfish *Fugu rubripes rubripes* along with their resistibility against tetrodotoxin. *Bull. Jap.Soc.Sci.Fisheries* **50**, 1573, 1984.

23. SAITO, T., NOGUCHI, T., HARADA, T., MURATA, O., ABE, T. AND HASHIMOTO, K., Resistibility of toxic and nontoxic pufferfish against tetrodotoxin, *Bull. Jap.Soc. Sci.Fisheries* **51**, 1371, 1985.

24. **FLACHSENBERGER, W. AND KERR, D.I.B.,** Lack of effect of tetrodotoxin and of an extract from the posterior salivary gland of the blue-ringed octopus following injection into the octopus and following application to its brachial nerve, *Toxicon* **23,** 997, 1985.
25. **SAITO, T., NOGUCHI, T., HARADA, T., MURATA, O. AND HASHIMOTO, K.,** Tetrodotoxin as a biological defense agent for puffers, *Nippon Suisan Gakkaishi* **51,** 1175, 1985.
26. **TSUDA, K., IKUMA, S., KAWAMURA, M., TACHIKAWA, R., SAKAI, K., TAMURA, C. AND AMAKASU, D.,** Tetrodotoxin. VII. On the structures of tetrodotoxin and its derivatives, *Chem. Pharm. Bull.* **12,** 1357, 1964.
27. **WOODWARD, R.B.,** The structure of tetrodotoxin, *Pure and Appl. Chem.* **9,** 49, 1964.
28. **GOTO, T., KISHI, Y., TAKAHASHI, S. AND HIRATA, Y.,** Tetrodotoxin, *Tetrahedron* **21,** 2059, 1965.
29. **NAKAMURA, M. AND YASUMOTO, T.,** Tetrodotoxin derivatives in puffer fish, *Toxicon* **23,** 271, 1985.
30. **HASHIMOTO, Y.,** *Marine Toxins and Other Bioactive Marine Metabolites*, Tokyo, Jap. Sci. Soc. Press, 1979.
31. **SAKAI, F., SATO, A. AND URAGUCHI, K.,** Über die Atemlähmung durch Tetrodotoxin, *Arch.Exp.Pathol.Pharmakol.* **240,** 313, 1961.
32. **KAO, C.Y. AND FUHRMAN, F.A.,** Pharmacological studies on tarichatoxin, a potent neurotoxin, *J. Pharmacol.Exp.Therap.* **140,** 31, 1963.
33. **KAO, C.Y.,** Tetrodotoxin, saxitoxin and their significance in the study of excitation phenomena, *Pharm.Rev.* **18,** 997, 1966.
34. **HILLE, B.,** The receptor for tetrodotoxin and saxitoxin: a structural hypothesis, *Biophys. J.* **15,** 615, 1975.
35. **STRICHARTZ, G. AND CASTLE, N.,** Pharmacology of marine toxins: Effects on membrane channels, in *Marine Toxins, Origin, Structure and Molecular Pharmacology*, S. Hall and G. Strichartz, Eds., Washington, D.C., ACS Symposia Series, Vol. **418,** 1990, 2.
36. **GOTO, K.,** Japan Poison Information Center, Tokyo, personal communication, 1993.
37. **KAO, C.Y.,** Tetrodotoxin, Saxitoxin and their significance in the study of the excitation phenomena, *Pharmacol. Rev.* **18,** 997, 1966.
38. **FUKUD, A. & TANI, I.,** *Records of Puffer Poisonings*. Report 3, Nippon Igaku oyobi Kenko Hoken (3528), 7-13, 1941.
39. **ELLENHORN, M. & BARCELOUX, D.G.** *Medical Toxicology*, Ney York: Elsevier, 1988.
40. **SIMS, J.K., OSTMAN, D.C.,** Pufferfish poisoning: emergency diagnosis and management of mild human tetrodotoxication. *Ann. Emerg. Med.* **15,** 1094, 1986.
41. **BRADLEY, S.G., KLIKA, L.J.,** A fatal poisoning from the Oregon roughskinned newt (Taricha granulosa). *JAMA*, 1981: **246:**247.
42. **CHEW, S.K., CHEW, L.S., WANG, K.W.,** Anticholinesterase drugs in the treatment of tetrodotoxin poisoning, *Lancet* **2:** 108, 1984.

Chapter 7

BIOLOGY AND DISTRIBUTION OF VENOMOUS MARINE ANIMALS

Dietrich Mebs

TABLE OF CONTENTS

I. GENERAL ASPECTS

The elaboration of toxins is an important strategy for marine organisms surviving in a highly competitive environment (see also Chapter 3). Several methods and procedures are used in the application of venoms and poisons. Venomousness is characterized by the use of a specific apparatus to apply a toxic gland product, a venom. This includes highly effective cell organelles like the nematocysts of the coelenterates, the complicated venom apparatus of the gastropod family Conidae, or the front teeth of sea snakes adapted to inject the secretion of the venom gland. In these organisms venoms are used in an offensive manner, for prey capture and immobilization.

Fish also use some form of puncturing device, dorsal and/or pectoral and/or ventral fin spines (class: Osteichthyes, teleost fish) or caudal stingers like those of the stingrays (class: Chondrichthyes). Venoms applied by these comparatively simple tools are defensive in nature [1]. This type of venomousness is rarely seen among teleost fish and is represented mainly by members of the Scorpaenidae family (lion fish, sculpins, stone fish). Most fish, however, adopt other defensive strategies to avoid predation, such as rapid swimming, schooling or they retreat to holes, reef structures etc.

The clinical toxicology of injuries due to coelenterates, cone shells, sea urchins and sea stars, stingrays, scorpion fish and sea snakes is described in the following chapters. However, a few other venomous marine animals need to be mentioned here such as sponges, cephalopods, weeverfishes, catfishes, toadfishes and rabbitfishes.

II. SOME SPECIAL GROUPS

A. SPONGES

It is dubious to group the sponges under the venomous animals. Although they are known to contain a great variety of secondary metabolites, they are generally considered to be harmless, only a few species causing local reactions upon contact: *Neofibularia nolitangere, N. mordens* (irritating, stinging sponges; Caribbean Sea, coastal waters of Australia), *Microciona prolifera* (red moss; Atlantic coast of North-America), *Haliclona viridis* (green sponge) and *Tedania ignis* (fire sponge; both in the Caribbean Sea). However, these sponges lack a specific venom apparatus. Their secretions have irritating effects on the skin, leading to contact dermatitis including local edema, itching and pain[2]. The toxins involved are unknown. The symptoms usually disappear within days, but may also last several weeks. Treatment, if any, may include corticosteroid or antihistaminic ointment.

A number of sponge species have a skeleton consisting of sharp silica spicules, which remain in the skin after contact and cause a local inflammatory reaction. They may be removed by applying an adhesive tape.

To prevent unexpected skin reactions, sponges should not be touched with unprotected hands.

B. CEPHALOPODS

Although octopuses and squids can be of impressive size possessing long arms equipped with numerous suckers, they are shy and considered to be harmless. Only a small representative of this group, the blue-ringed or banded octopus, *Hapalochlaena maculosa* and *H. lunulata* living in the coastal waters of Australia, New Guinea, the Solomons and of the Philippines, is a really dangerous animal. At low tide, it can be found in tidal pools or under rocks. When excited the animal shows blue rings all over the body and may bite with its jaws, which are shaped like a parrot beak, and introduces a lethal toxin, contained in the saliva, into the wound[3]. This toxin has been identified as tetrodotoxin, which is produced in the salivary glands of the octopus, and which is also well known as the pufferfish toxin [4](see also Chapter 6). It causes essentially the same symptoms as seen in fugu poisoning such as tingling sensations, numbness and progressing paralysis. However, envenoming by the octopus proceeds faster, because of the parenteral application of the toxin. Thus, paralytic symptoms may occur within 15 minutes and fatal cases have been reported[5,6]. Urgent medical intervention is therefore necessary.

The toxin acts on the peripheral nervous system and causes paralysis by blocking the sodium channels of excitable membranes. There exists no specific antidote. Treatment has to be symptomatic including artificial respiration as the patient develops rapidly respiratory deficiency and failure. Complications are mainly due to hypotensive crisis. Although the pressure immobilization technique has been recommended as a first aid measure[3], in most cases this may not be practical, because most bites remain unnoticed until the first symptoms of envenoming occur (e.g. paralysis), by which time venom immobilisation by first aid is of little value, and first aid efforts should be directed towards maintaining respiration and avoiding aspiration of vomitus.

Accidents are always the result of careless handling or playing with an octopus picked up from a tidal pool. It should never be touched with bare hands or placed on unprotected skin.

C. FISH
1. Weeverfish

Echiichthys species (the genus was previously named *Trachinus*), the weeverfish, *E.draco, vipera, araneus, radiatus, lineatus,* are considered to be Europe´s most venomous fish, although envenoming causes mainly local symptoms, and reports of fatal cases are dubious[7]. These fish are found in the coastal waters of the Black, the Mediterranean and North Sea as well as of the Atlantic. They possess four to eight grooved spines in the first dorsal fin and an opercular spine to which glandular tissue is attached, which produces venom. The needle-sharp spines easily penetrate human skin when the fish is handled (removing it from the fishing net or hook) and venom is released by damaging the glandular tissue[8]. It consists of high-molecular protein toxin(s) and produces mainly local pain and edema. Since the toxin is heat labile, treatment with hot water has been recommended, but is not encouraged, because of the danger of scalding[7]. Local injections of anesthetics (lidocaine) have only a short-term effect. General symptoms are uncommon and mainly due to the patient´s overreaction to pain. In contrast to common beliefs, weeverfish envenoming is not life-threatening.

The stargazers (*Uranoscopus* species; worldwide distribution) have two sharp dorsal spines and an opercular spine; however, they do not possess venom glands, and the fish is, therefore, not venomous[8].

2. Catfish

Most catfish species (suborder: Siluroidea) are freshwater species, but a few are found in marine waters like the plotosid catfishes (*Plotosus* sp.). The first spine of the dorsal fin, as well as of the pectoral fin, shows retrorse dentition and is covered by glandular tissue[8]. When the spines penetrate the skin, the venom producing cells are destroyed and venom is released into the wound. It is of proteinaceous nature and causes local pain and edema. The dentation of the surface may cause tissue laceration, but systemic symptoms are uncommon. Treatment is essentially the same as for weeverfish; larger wounds should be cleaned to prevent secondary infections.

3. Toadfish and rabbitfish

Toadfish of the genus *Batrachoides* (Indo-Pacific) and *Thalassophryne* (Caribbean Sea, South-Atlantic) possess hollow opercular and two dorsal spines, which at the base are equipped with a venom gland. The venom is injected by contact and causes local pain and swelling[8].

Rabbitfish, *Siganus* sp., are found in the coral reefs of the Indo-Pacific, but migrated also to the Mediterranean Sea through the Suez Canal. Almost all fins have sharp spines equipped with glandular tissue (venom glands). When penetrating the skin, these glands are damaged and venom is released into the wound causing local pain and edema[8]. Treatment as for weeverfish.

Although surgeonfish (Acanthuridae; worldwide distribution) have a sharp, lancelike, movable spine on each side of the caudal peduncle, which may cause deep and painful wounds, they are not venomous, because no glandular tissue has been detected near or on the spines. The bite of moray eels is not venomous, and the sharp teeth (which may produce severe tissue laceration) are neither grooved nor hollow, and there are no venom glands in the mouth cavity[8].

III. REFERENCES

1. **CAMERON, A.M.** (1976) Toxicity of coral reef fish. In: *Biology and Geology of Coral Reefs* (JONES, O.A. & ENDEAN, R., eds.) pp. 155-176, Academic Press, New York.
2. **FISHER, A.A.** (1978) *Atlas of Aquatic Dermatology.* Grune & Stratton, New York.
3. **SUTHERLAND; S.K.** (1983) *Australian Animal Toxins.* Oxford Univ. Press, Melbourne.
4. **SHEUMACK, D.D., HOWDEN, M.E.H., SPENCE, I. & QUINN, R.J.** (1978) Maculotoxin: a neurotoxin from the venom glands of the octopus *Hapalochlaena maculosa* identified as tetrodotoxin. *Science* **199**, 188-189.
5. **FLECKER, H. & COTTON, B.C.** (1955) Fatal bite from an octopus. *Med.J.Aust.* **2**, 329-331.

6.   **WALKER, D.G.** (1983) Survival after severe envenomation by the blue-ringed octopus (*Hapalochlaena maculosa*). *Med.J.Austr.* **2**, 663-665.

7.   **MARETIC, Z.** (1988) Fish venoms. In: *Handbook of Natural Toxins,* vol.**3**, Marine Toxins and Venoms (TU, A.T., ed.) pp.445-476, M.Dekker, New York.

8.   **HALSTEAD, B.W.** (1988) *Poisonous and Venomous Marine Animals of the World* (2nd rev.ed.), Darwin Press Inc., Princeton.

Chapter 8

CLINICAL TOXICOLOGY OF MARINE COELENTERATE INJURIES

John Williamson and Joseph Burnett

TABLE OF CONTENTS

I. INTRODUCTION

The study of coelenterate envenomation is a relatively new and emerging scientific and medical frontier[1]. This is the direct result of the distinguished work of many pioneers, from medical (e.g. Barnes, Burnett, Cleland, Edmonds, Fenner, Flecker, Halstead, Light, Maretíc, McNeill, Pope, Southcott, Sutherland), biological (e.g. Béress, Cargo, Endean, Haeckel, Hartwick, Kingston, Kramp, Mayer, Ravens, Richet, Totton) and specific scientific (e.g. Baxter, Calton, Crone, Freeman, Keen, Lane, Marr, Russell) disciplines[2,3].

The subject is now gathering scientific momentum, is internationally based[4,5], and an appreciation is dawning of the major and continuous morbidity (with some mortality) associated worldwide with coelenterate injuries. Also emerging among investigators is a more conservation-minded approach to the prevention of injuries from these ancient, intricate and beautiful animals.

A. TAXONOMIC OUTLINE

  Phylum COELENTERATA (CNIDARIA)
    Class CUBOZOA ("Box jellyfish")
      Carybdieds
      Chirodropids

    Class HYDROZOA
      Hydroids
      Physalia species

Limnomedusae
    Gonionemus species

Class SCYPHOZOA (True jellyfish)
    Cyanea
    Catostylus
    Chrysaora species
    Pelagia species
    Rhizostoma species
    Stomolophus species
    Aurelia species

Class ANTHOZOA
    Hard and soft corals
    Anemones

II. GENERAL CONSIDERATIONS

A. INTERNATIONAL EPIDEMIOLOGY[4,5]
1. Mortality

This aspect has always attracted exaggerated emphasis (as it does in most human affairs). Some past records have also been of questionable accuracy. However numerous human deaths have certainly occurred, but the description of venomous coelenterates being "vicious", and "attacking" is nonsense. All such marine envenomations are the direct result of either intentional or accidental interference with the animal by humans. The animals act purely defensively.

Documented human deaths have resulted from envenomation by the following coelenterates:

a. Chirodropids

Chironex fleckeri, the northern Australian box jellyfish [2,6], (Figure 1);
Chiropsalmus quadrigatus in the Philippines and Indo-Pacific;[2,3]
Chiropsalmus quadrumanus in the Gulf of Mexico[7].

Other human fatalities in the Indo-Pacific region from chirodropid envenomations, past and present, are known but firm identification of the animals and accurate records are lacking. Intensive research is current in Australia, the Indo-Pacific and Malaysia, and some documentation is in preparation.

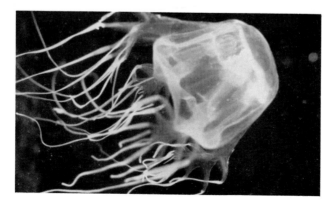

Figure 1. Adult *Chironex* (courtesy Surf Life Saving Queensland, Inc.).

b. Carybdeids

No firm documentation of fatalities exist to date, but are suspected in the Gulf of Oman region (Pratap Chand and Victor, 1992, unpublished observations), and possibly on the west African coast. In northern Australian waters, "Irukandji" envenomation has the potential for a fatal outcome,[8] but none are yet documented.

c. Hydrozoans

The Atlantic *Physalia physalis* ("Portuguese Man-O'War) on the eastern United States coast[9]. Interestingly, there has not been a documented record of a single human Pacific *Physalia utriculus* ("Bluebottle") sting fatality to date, despite thousands of confirmed stingings[4].

d. Scyphozoans

Stomolophus nomurai in the Sea of Japan in northern China[11].

The powerful antigenic properties of many jellyfish venoms are now appreciated,[12] and while a near-death from anaphylaxis from a Mediterranean *Pelagia noctiluca* (Figure 3) sting is known,[13] and the potential for an allergic death in susceptible patients clearly exists, none have yet been recognised.

2. Morbidity

This aspect of coelenterate envenomation is far more significant, numerically speaking. There are uncounted thousands upon thousands of non-fatal coelenterate envenomations worldwide, annually[4,5]. Estimates are only now becoming possible, but accurate international records are still lacking. Their public health significance among maritime populations is only just becoming appreciated[1].

Possibly the commonest known coelenterate injuries are by the familiar and ubiquitous "Bluebottle" jellyfish (e.g. *Physalia utriculus* of the Pacific region), and coral cuts and abrasions[4-6,14]. *Physalia* species non-fatal stings are also very common in South Africa, Portugal, and Pakistan.

3. Geographical distribution of coelenterate injuries

While the extent and variety of coelenterate envenomations is enormous, there is a natural concentration of the animals within tropical oceans. The following data exist:

a. Australia and the Indo-Pacific region

This region contains representatives of every known venomous coelenterate, and accounts for many of the serious stings. The principal animals from the human injury aspect are the cubozoan jellyfish, *Physalia* species, *Rhyzostoma* and *Chrysaora* species, stinging corals, anemones, and the mechanical injuries from coral abrasions and lacerations[6,14]. Of lesser importance are *Cyanea* (hair jelly), *Catostylus* (blubber jellyfish) and (at least in Australia) *Pelagia noctiluca* (the little mauve stinger). *Chrysaora* species stings may be more common in the Malaysian/Thailand region, along with undoubted cubozoan envenomations[2].

b. The Pacific basin

Again, this contains a vast array of venomous coelenterates, with regular and numerous human stingings. Along with the adjoining Indo-Pacific region, these waters contain many stinging corals (e.g. *millepora*), hydroids, hard and soft corals and jellyfish. *Physalia physalis* and perhaps *Catostylus* are among the most plentiful, although the latter's sting is insignificant.

c. The Mediterranean coastlines

The Mediterranean Sea is a rich habitat for coelenterates, and many stings occur there from jellyfish especially. The most frequently encountered stings are from *Pelagia noctiluca* (mauve stinger; Figure 3), *Chrysaora hyoscella*, *Rhyzostoma pulmo* and *Aurelia aurita* (moon jellyfish)[15,16]. Coral abrasions also occur.

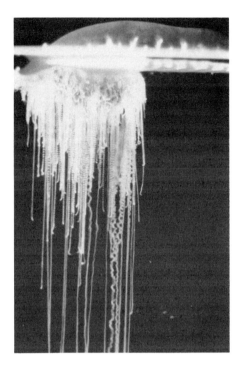

Figure 2. Atlantic *Physalia.*

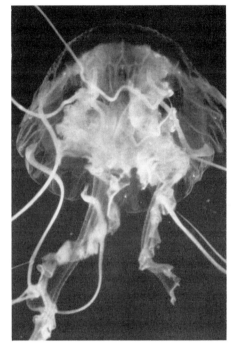

Figure 3. *Pelagia noctiluca.*

d. North America

The North American Sea Nettle, *Chrysaora quinquecirrha*,[17] found in seasonal plague proportions in the Chesapeake Bay estuary, has occupied a key place in the pioneering research into marine venoms by Burnett and colleagues over the past 25 years[12,18,19]. *Physalia* species on both the west (Pacific) and the east (Atlantic) coastlines (see above) are plentiful; the Atlantic *Physalia* is a dangerous sting[9,10,20]. The tropical shores of the Gulf of Mexico and adjoining West Indies, Puerto Rico and Panama regions are the habitat for dangerous chirodropids[7], other cubozoans (e.g. *Carybdea marsupialis, Tamoya haplonema, Tripedalia cystophora*), for *Physalia*, and the ocean-going *Cyanea*.

e. South America

The Atlantic *Physalia* and an *Olindias* species of stinging jellyfish inhabit the tropical east coasts of this continent. Research is in progress.

f. European Atlantic and North Sea shores

Physalia, Pelagia, Chrysaora, Cyanea, Rhyzostoma and *Vallela* species are known. *Physalia, Rhizostoma, Pelagia* and anemone stings, but apparently few deaths, occur on Portugal's beaches[21].

g. Africa

Although little is known about much of this continent's coastline habitats, a large cubozoan is known to inhabit the west coast, and South African *Physalia* occurrence is well documented[22].

h. Northern Indian Ocean shores

This collection of tropical and densely populated coastlines has very numerous coelenterate envenomations yearly. Large cubozoans[23], *Cyanea*, *Pelagia*, *Rhyzostoma*, *Olindias*, *Physalia*, *Chrysaora* and *Aurelia aurita*, as well as unidentified species (Pratap Chand, Victor, Junaid Alam 1993, unpublished observations), are known to occur.

i. China, Japan, and Far Eastern Russia

The range of stinging jellyfish, at least in this region, is impressive, and some of these occur as far north as the cold waters of Vladivostok. *Stomolophus* species (with fatalities),[11] probably *Chiropsalmus* in Okinawa[24] (Tomihara 1992, unpublished observations), *Gonionemus* species in Japan and Vladivostok (Yakovlev and Vaskovsky 1992, unpublished observations), are among the most important stingers.

Overall knowledge of the world distribution of significant coelenterate stingers is meagre at present. Likewise knowledge of the biology and complete life cycles of many medically significant coelenterates remains incomplete.

4. The International Consortium for Jellyfish Stings (ICJS) (Figure 4)

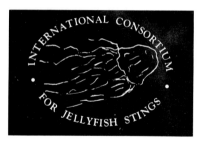

Figure 4. ICJS Logo.

This Consortium began informally with the efforts of a small group of active medical scientists and marine biologists in 1989[4,5,25], in the hope of stimulating interest and communication with involved colleagues around the world. It has now circulated 8 "Newsletters", 4 "Sting Report Summaries"[4] and published a range of international articles[1,8,10,12,14,16,26-29]. Contacts and data bases exist in Baltimore, Maryland, USA, Adelaide, South Australia and Mackay, North Queensland, Australia. The international mailing list now exceeds 130, providing an on-going and accurate source of epidemiological information worldwide[4]. The early data already confirm that marine envenomations are common events, being made even more so by the worldwide increase in recreational diving with self-contained underwater breathing apparatus (SCUBA)[30].

B. THE STINGING APPARATUS OF COELENTERATES

All coelenterates possess one of the most remarkable stinging mechanisms in biology, in the form of the nematocyst. These structures (Figure 5) are present in their thousands on, for example, the tentacles (and often body or bell) of jellyfish, and are used to capture prey. Each microscopic nematocyst contains a micro-dose of sometimes very potent venom, and combines the mechanical functions of a harpoon gun and an injection syringe.

Each nematocyst normally discharges *in situ* in response to a mechanical or chemical stimulation applied to the triggering apparatus (cnidocil) of the investing cell (the nematocyte). Discharge will normally be elicited by items of prey, or accidentally by a human victim, and this sets off an extremely rapid (thousandths of a second!) chain of events (Figure 6)[29]. These events remain imperfectly understood, and are the subject of on-going intensive research[29,31-34]. Currently it is believed that the rapid discharge of the everted thread and polymerized capsular contents of the nematocyst is achieved osmotically by the in-rush of water[29,34]. Penetration by the first-emerging robust spine is efficient, and the largest nematocysts (microbasic mastigophores of *Chironex fleckeri*) can penetrate to a depth in human skin approaching 0.9mm (Figure 7)[35].

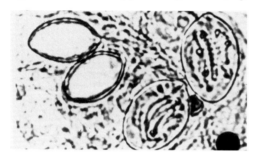

Figure 5. Structure of a nematocyst (courtesy Dr. Robert Hartwick, Townsville).

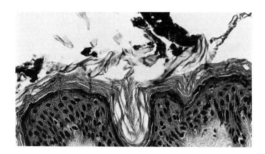

Figure 7. Nematocyst threads in human skin.

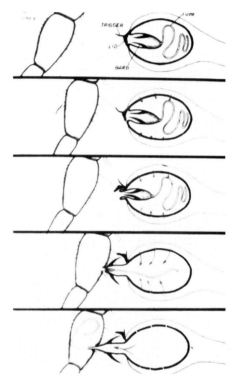

Figure 6. Discharge sequence of a nematocyst (courtesy Dr. Robert Hartwick, Townsville).

It is thus understandable how coelenterate body parts which bear nematocysts (e.g. tentacles) are "sticky" when touched, becoming anchored by the numerous discharged nematocyst threads to the surface of the prey (or human skin). It is estimated that an adult *Chironex fleckeri*, with up to 59 tentacles, may bear some four to five thousand million nematocysts on its tentacles[6]. A hallmark of human envenomation by chirodropids (multi-tentacled box jellyfish) is the presence of densely adherent tentacle material, avulsed from the animal in the water, on the skin of the victim[1,36]. Although visible tentacle material is not seen on the skin following most coelenterate envenomations, discharged and undischarged nematocysts invariably are present, and are of diagnostic and therapeutic importance (see below)[37].

In a classic paper in 1960[37], Barnes documented the fact that the nematocysts from different coelenterate species are morphologically characteristic of the respective species to which they were attached. Thus, like species-specific fingerprints, the examination down a low power microscope of either discharged or undischarged nematocysts scraped from freshly stung skin usually identifies the species of animal which produced the envenomation[2,37]. Dr Robert Hartwick, PhD, of James Cook University, Townsville, North Queensland, Australia, has prepared a diagnostic chart of nematocysts for use in accident and emergency departments of northern Australian coastal hospitals. Another valuable diagnostic feature described by Barnes is the tell-tale imprint that may be left on the relatively hairless human skin by some coelenterate envenomations[36,37]. The architectural arrangements of the nematocyst batteries on tentacles, different in different species, may be reflected in the skin pattern imprinted upon the skin, and rendered visible by the intense acute inflammatory reaction that follows immediately[6,36,37].

1. The envenomation process

Simultaneous discharge of thousands of nematocysts, some bearing a micro-dose of potent venom and each dose deposited into the prey (or human) where it can be rapidly absorbed (e.g. the human dermis), results in a very quickly rising blood level of venom, and the rapid onset of clinical effects[33,36]. In the case of serious human envenomation, massive nematocyst discharge may occur from entanglement in the tentacle material (Figure 8)[36]. Some of the nematocysts in every coelenterate species' cnidom (nematocyst population) are not directly concerned with envenomation, but with grappling of the prey to the tentacle or body of the coelenterate, thus increasing the time and opportunity for the venom-bearing nematocysts to do their work[32,33]. (The systematic morphological classification of nematocysts has been addressed[3].) Chirodropid envenomation is the most rapid envenomation process known; venom absorption may be further enhanced by the struggling of victims rendered incoherent by the immediate and savage pain[26]; such struggling and rubbing of the sting area and any adherent tentacle material will facilitate both further discharge of adherent, unfired nematocysts, and central venom movement from muscle contraction, hence the need in serious envenomations for both restraint of the victim's movements by rescuers and the rapid inactivation of any unfired nematocysts on the skin[1,38].

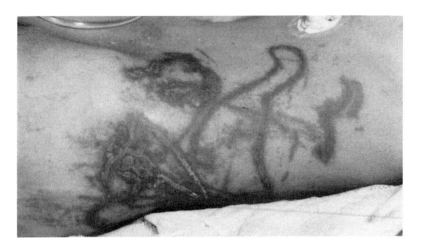

Figure 8. Massive *Chironex* sting (courtesy Surf Life Saving Queensland, Inc.).

In an important conceptual advance, Endean and Rifkin showed that concomitant with the discharge of the nematocyst thread through the vascular skin layers, venom is progressively deposited along the outside of the penetrating thread material, so that transfixion of blood vessels by the thread would deposit venom directly intravascularly[39]. This would explain the almost instantaneous onset of systemic signs and symptoms in seriously envenomated patients.

2. Nematocyst inhibition

While much of the recent data concerning coelenterate envenomation tends to focus upon the more dramatic and potentially life-threatening chirodropid stings, most coelenterate stings are not a threat to life. However nematocyst function, and particularly nematocyst inhibition, is of relevance throughout the phylum, and of general biological and medical importance.

Prior to 1980 it was generally believed that nematocyst inhibition was a relatively straightforward matter. The liberal application of alcohol (e.g. "methylated spirits"[36]) to all fresh box jellyfish (and many other) stings was customary. However even at that time, a large range of different substances was in use for this purpose around the world (including vinegar, paw paw juice, human urine, meat tenderiser, ammonia, local plant extracts and "oily substances"[2]) and commercial interest was attracted[38,40]. Hartwick and colleagues showed the efficacy of 2-10% acetic acid in water as an effective nematocyst inhibitor in chirodropids[38], and subsequent work has verified this - in the form of household vinegar (4-6% acetic acid in water) - as the inhibitor of choice for all cubozoans (box jellyfish)[27,41]. However similar experiments with other coelenterate genera quickly produced confusing and conflicting results, and not a little public confusion[27,42]. It is now appreciated that in the past, and even the present, properly controlled scientific assessment of many substances claimed as effective nematocyst inhibitors is lacking, and that contrary to initial perceptions, nematocyst function is a complex matter; nematocyst inhibition may prove to be partly species-specific[29]. Substance evaluation is profoundly complicated by the placebo effect (many seriously affected envenomation victims are children[7,43]), and by the tendency of lay persons continually to confuse nematocyst inhibition with pain relief (see below). This is an important research frontier.

C. COELENTERATE VENOMS - CHEMISTRY AND PHARMACOLOGY

Halstead has reviewed the toxicology, pharmacology and chemistry of coelenterate venoms to 1988[3]. While an impressive array of biologically active compounds have been isolated from coelenterates, including vasoactive amines (histamine, serotonin and dopamine), prostaglandins and carboxylic acids[3], many of the venoms are labile mixtures of toxic and/or antigenic polypeptides, proteins and enzymes pathogenic to humans[44]. The lability of some venoms to temperature and experimental handling, resulting in molecular fragmentation, aggregation and adhesion to support matrices, has made toxinological study more difficult[45]. It is also now known that the venom content of all nematocysts in a cnidom is not identical[46,47], and that tentacular parenchyma may contain some toxic material that will cause ground tentacle extracts to differ toxinologically from material isolated from nematocysts[46].

Coelenterate venoms exert their effects by either toxicity or allergy. The former is far more common and important. Chemical contents identified have included, along with medium to high molecular weight polypeptides and proteins (14,500 - 600,000)[47,48], elastases, a DNase and histamine (*Physalia physalis*), mouse-lethal acid protease, haemagglutinin, an alkaline protease, a DNase and a collagenase (*Chrysaora quinquecirrha*)[18], proteinase inhibitors (anemones), and a potent group of "palytoxins" which are thought to be non-protein, aliphatic long-chain molecules[3]. Apart from lethal effects in experimental animals which appear to result from cardiotoxicity and/or neurotoxicity[45-47,49], dermatonecrosis, cutaneous vasopermeability, smooth and somatic musculotoxicity, haemolysis, cytotoxicity (mitochondrial inhibition) and cutaneous pain producing substances are documented[18,30].

1. Lethal actions of coelenterate venoms

Again the venom of chirodropids - principally *Chironex fleckeri* - has received most - but not exclusive - attention. The cause of death in humans certainly involves myocardial toxicity[12,18,35,44,47,49]. However both in animals and humans it would appear that certain venom doses possibly lower than those producing actual cardiac arrest can cause respiratory arrest[51,52]. Whether this is a neurotoxic effect[18,53], or is secondary to myocardial and pulmonary insufficiency, or both, is uncertain. Delayed death in humans has followed renal failure (lower nephron nephrosis, perhaps contributed to by haemolysis?)[18]. Potentially fatal envenomation effects have also included anaphylaxis[13], delayed global myocardial dilatation with decompensation[54], and widespread regional (limb) vascular spasm[53]. The pharmacological basis of some of these effects remains unclear. There is circumstantial evidence that the severity of stinging varies seasonally with some coelenterates[3,56], but whether this involves variation in venom composition remains unknown.

2. Jellyfish venom immunology

Along with their toxicity, the antigenicity of particular jellyfish venoms is responsible for the immunological mechanisms that appear in the production of the envenomation reaction. It is the interplay of these toxic and immunological events which determines the clinical course of the patient's sting. Thus immunological mechanisms are of importance for the understanding of envenomation pathogenesis, and offer clues for diagnosis, prophylaxis and treatment. The subject has been recently reviewed by Burnett[57]. It is of historical interest that the first recognition of anaphylaxis in science was using sea anemone venom as antigen[58].

Both humoral and cellular mechanisms are involved. Many moderate coelenterate envenomations lead to a rise in specific immunoglobulin (Ig) titres, particularly IgG after 1 month; but detection of these levels of circulating antibodies requires sensitive tests (e.g. ELISA). In more severely envenomated persons the humoral response is more vigorous, and the cellular immune system is also activated[13,57]. Abnormal cellular immunity reactions, such as exaggerated, prolonged or abberrant T cell responses, may be associated with some protracted or recurrent post-envenomation syndromes. Coelenterate venom-induced immunosuppression has also occurred[57].

As an aid to diagnosis and therapy, hyperimmune or convalescent serum can be used to identify the offending animal[55,59], and even jellyfish parts - information of prophylactic and epidemiological interest. However, significant cross reactivity between various jellyfish venom antigens of both the humoral and cellular immune systems has been observed. Immunoprophylaxis has met with little success to date. However a very successful coelenterate antivenom (*Chironex fleckeri* antivenom) is in regular use in Australia[6,60,61,70].

D. CLINICAL SIGNS, SYMPTOMS AND RECOGNISED SYNDROMES

The clinical effects of coelenterate envenomations are protean in the extreme, from trivial skin itch to virtual immediate cardiac arrest in systole[35,49]. An attempt to organise the effects into "syndromes" has recently been made by Burnett (Table 1)[12].

The skin is usually the first human organ of contact in marine envenomations (hence their interest to dermatologists, who are making important contributions). The exception is "envenomation" (more customarily regarded as "poisoning"[62]) from jellyfish ingestion, in countries (e.g. Japan, Malaysia) where dried jellyfish bell is regarded as a delicacy. Gastrointestinal symptoms and urticaria have been described[12]. Direct eye (corneal) envenomation occurs, usually with spontaneous recovery[63].

An important common skin feature throughout the spectrum of coelenterate envenomations is, however, the production of immediate skin symptoms (usually pain, which can be savage), and signs of an acute inflammatory reaction[59] which can vary from almost nothing visible ("Irukandji" sting, Figure 9) to vesiculation and demarcated, full-thickness skin death (chirodropid sting, Figure 10). Severe pain from certain coelenterate envenomations can render the patient incoherent and irrational, but this does not always correlate with danger to life[6]. Thus pain relief is a major therapeutic need in coelenterate stings, both at first aid and medical levels.

Table 1
Documented clinical response patterns to coelenterate envenomation (modified from Burnett, 1991[12])

Local reactions:

Exaggerated local reaction (angioedema)
Recurrent reactions (up to 4 episodes)
Delayed persistent reactions (several months)
Distant site reactions
Contact dermatitis
Papular urticaria (up to 1 month)
Regional vascular spasm (sea bathers' dermatitis)
Dermatonecrosis
Localised toxic neuropraxia
Superficial thrombophlebitis (Mondor's disease)

Systemic reactions (temporary):

Myocardial dilatation (flabby heart)
Acute pulmonary oedema
"Irukandji"-type (myalgia/panic) syndrome
Disturbed psychic state
Hypertensive crisis
Anaphylaxis
Dysautonomia
Pain-induced prostration
Vaso-vagal reactions

Fatal reactions:

Myocardial systolic standstill
Acute hypoxia with pulmonary oedema
Suspected anaphylaxis
Delayed renal failure
Liver failure

Post-episode dermatitis:

Herpes simplex
Granuloma annulare

Long-term reactions:

Skin:
  keloid formation
  pigmentation
  fat atrophy
  scarring and contractures
  localised gangrene
Ataxia
Blurred vision
Mononeuritis

E. CURRENT MEDICAL MANAGEMENT PRINCIPLES
1. Resuscitation and first aid

As for all human situations where it is indicated, resuscitation takes absolute priority. While the speed of coelenterate envenomation can occasionally defeat resuscitative efforts[6,9,35], this is the exception; more commonly a successful outcome is achieved[6,13,26,36], and pessimism has no place. Every victim of a marine envenomation, no matter how apparently serious, is potentially fully recoverable, provided effective resuscitation is commenced early enough. There is a clinical impression, supported by the known thermolability of most coelenterate venoms[45,51,64], that their acute lethal action in human tissue may be relatively short-lived (e.g. perhaps 40 minutes or less)[51]. This suspicion is strengthened by the fact that few of the 70 or so recorded deaths from *Chironex fleckeri* envenomation appear to have received prompt and sustained resuscitation following the envenomation[6,51], whereas those victims of dangerous stings that are documented, and who did, survived[13,36,51].

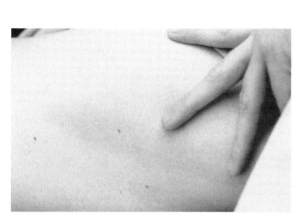

Figure 9. Irukandji sting.

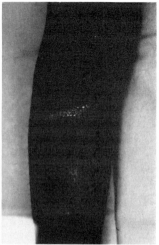

Figure 10. Full thickness skin death.

a. "Bare-handed" resuscitation

The principles of basic or "bare-handed" resuscitation are now widely known and promulgated, and follow the concepts of AIRWAY, BREATHING, CIRCULATION, and DEFINITIVE TREATMENT ("A, B, C, D.")[6,61]. In certain life threatening coelenterate envenomations, the principal practical problem on the beach may be respiratory insufficiency or apnoea alone[51]. In this case prompt expired air resuscitation (EAR) may alone suffice[36,51]. Nothing must be allowed to take priority over resuscitative efforts in a life-threatening coelenterate envenomation.

b. First-aid

With evolving understanding, first-aid techniques for coelenterate injuries have been repeatedly altered during the past 13 years[6,36,38,61], and still present a frontier of intense research[27,29,65,66]. The subject has been bedevilled by two major difficulties, one scientific and one public educational. These are, respectively, the inhibition of nematocyst discharge, and the confusion between nematocyst inhibition and acute analgesia for stings. A third area of current uncertainty concerns venom entrapment techniques[6].

i. First aid and nematocyst inhibition:

This is of first aid importance, to prevent subsequent discharge of unfired adherent nematocysts always present on the victim's skin immediately following a sting; such discharge would increase pain and envenomation. The fresh sting area should never be rubbed with sand, or anything else. Initially alcohol was recommended[36]. Then a benchmark study showed that 2-10% acetic acid in water was an effective nematocyst inhibitor[38]. Subsequently it became apparent that nematocyst inhibition was a complex matter, possibly species specific[27,29,41,42].

Currently, household vinegar (4-6% acetic acid in water) is firmly recommended for nematocyst inhibition of all cubozoan (box jellyfish) stings; this is of most significance for the potentially dangerous chirodropid stings[6,38,61], but could be of importance also for some carybdeid stings[54]. Although a variety of substances for a widely different range of world coelenterates are presently used in an empirical manner, objective tests are lacking. Research continues, and pending further understanding, it is recommended that sea water be used to wash off the adherent tentacles of all jellyfish other than box jellyfish. Fresh water should never be used following natural drying of the sting area in chirodropid stings[56]. Vinegar should not be used for Atlantic *Physalia physalis* (Portuguese Man-o'war) stings[27,42]. Nematocyst inhibition has nothing to do with the relief of pain produced by the venom already injected into the skin.

ii. First aid and venom entrapment:

Sutherland and colleagues made a seminal advance in first aid for envenomation with the development of compressive immobilisation bandaging (Figure 11)[70]. The application of this to serious coelenterate envenomation remains unproven, but is currently suggested for serious chirodropid envenomations[6,62]. The definition of a "serious" such envenomation is any sting:
(i)   involving resuscitation;
(ii)   involving impaired consciousness;
(iii) in which the total sting area is greater than one half of one limb (especially important in children).

To these requirements must be added:
(a) the bandaging must never take priority over, nor distract from, resuscitation;
(b) in chirodropid stings, the bandaging must not precede nematocyst inhibition (vinegar dousing; see above);
(c) application must be within the first minutes of the envenomation, to be most effective[70];
(d) the bandaging must not occlude arterial blood supply; it must never become an arterial torniquet[6,70].

iii. First aid and analgesia (pain relief):

It is natural for lay persons to conclude that any substance recommended for application to a fresh coelenterate sting should be expected to ease the pain. However nematocyst inhibition and analgesia are two distinct and separate phenomena in first aid management. The search for an effective and "universal" analgesic in coelenterate injuries is another research frontier[12]. The best analgesic for Australian chirodropid stings is the specific *Chironex fleckeri* (box jellyfish) Commonwealth Serum Laboratories' antivenom (see below and Figure 12)[6,61,62], but the first aid use of this must obviously be strictly controlled[61]. Ice is an effective and safe topical analgesic for the majority of non-life-threatening coelenterate injuries, and is currently recommended (following vinegar dousing where indicated)[66,67]. The only effective analgesia for the "Irukandji syndrome", and certain other coelenterate stings[55], is systemic narcotics in a medically supervised environment, and is beyond first aid capability[54,68].

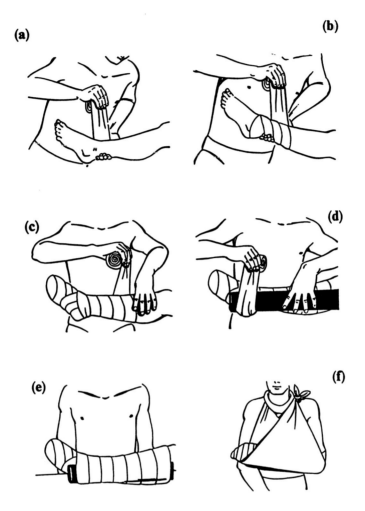

Figure 11. Compressive immobilisation bandaging (courtesy Dr. S.K. Sutherland, Melbourne).

2. Antivenom Usage

Australia, having the largest collection of indigenous venomous marine (as well as terrestrial) animals, is at the forefront of marine coelenterate antivenom development[69]; but this aspect of the subject is still in its infancy[70]. The only coelenterate antivenom presently available and adequately documented is the chirodropid antivenom "Box Jellyfish Antivenom" manufactured by the Commonwealth Serum Laboratories in Melbourne (Figure 12). This is a pungent sheep antiserum, to date remarkably free of serious reactions[69,70], and although its complete efficacy against the cardiotoxic lethal actions of *Chironex fleckeri* venom has been challenged[71], it almost certainly contributes to the preservation of life in dangerous *Chironex fleckeri* stings at least[4,51,70]. It would appear that the antivenom's anti-lethal efficacy may be significantly supplemented by the concomitant injection of verapamil[72], but human trials are lacking. The antivenom's efficacy in pain relief and the minimisation of skin damage is now unquestioned[4,51,60,61,70]. Documented experience with any other coelenterate antivenoms is unknown to the author.

Safe and effective antivenom administration for coelenterate injuries follows the same principles as for any other foreign protein antivenom usage. The antivenom may be given intramuscularly[6,26,61] or intravenously[6,8,35,36]. Premedication is recommended[70] although some controversy exists[73]. A combination of subcutaneous (not intravenous prophylactically) adrenaline and intramuscular hydrocortisone (which significantly reduces the risk of delayed serum sickness[70]), together with intramuscular antihistamines in selected cases, would seem sensible in the in-hospital setting. This is inappropriate for on-beach, urgent box-jellyfish usage for envenomations being managed acutely by paramedical teams[26,61], and as has been mentioned, the track record of safety for this particular antivenom is remarkable to date[70].

3. Training of local ambulance and retrieval facilities

The speed of some of the serious effects of coelenterate envenomations, together with the immediate and sometimes savage pain, conflicts with the remote places where they may occur and the quick availability of skilled medical assistance. An Australian approach has been to train and equip mobile north Queensland ambulance teams, already well skilled in resuscitation and using good communications, to reach remote beaches promptly and carry out appropriate urgent management. This includes provision of antivenom (3 ampoules {60,000 units} of box-jellyfish antivenom) and the skill and equipment to administer it intramuscularly on site for serious stings, when indicated. While this met with some medical opposition initially, the programme is current and successful[26,61]. Extension of this approach to other Australian ambulance services, where the risk exists and distances are great, is being encouraged.

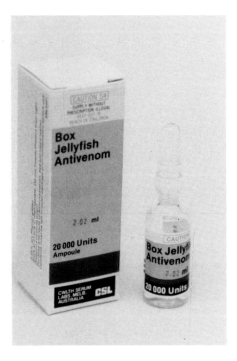

Figure 12. Ampoule of box jellyfish antivenom.

F. PREVENTION

Public education concerning the relatively simple, and very effective, prevention steps to avoid all serious coelenterate envenomation is a never-ending struggle[1]. For it has been said, "People will continue to do, not what they should, but what they want!" Sensationalist and uninformed media reports of "attacks" by various coelenterates are absurdities, and do not help.

Prevention measures can be summarised thus:

KNOW THE RISK SEASONS (e.g. summer)
KNOW THE RISK LOCATIONS (e.g. tropical beaches)
DO NOT HANDLE ANIMALS UNLESS SKILLED
WALK INTO THE WATER, DO NOT RUN OR "DUCK DIVE"
WEAR PROTECTIVE CLOTHING (Figure 13)
SWIM INSIDE SPECIAL ENCLOSURES WHERE AVAILABLE
SWIM AT LOCATIONS WHICH HAVE TRAINED LIFE GUARDS
CARRY 2 LITRES OF VINEGAR IN KNOWN CHIRODROPID AREAS.

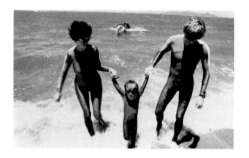

Figure 13. Stinger suits.

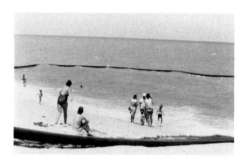

Figure 14. Australian stinger enclosure.

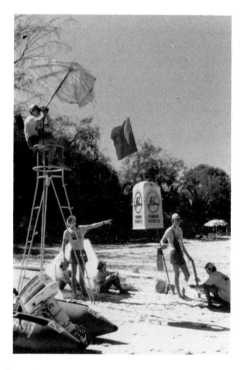

Figure 15. Patrolled north Queensland beach.

III. THE SPECIFIC ANIMALS

A. CLASS CUBOZOA ("BOX JELLYFISH") (WERNER 1975[74])

These are all "box jellyfish", but exist as an *Order* with 4 tentacles only (Carybdeids), and another *Order* with multiple (up to 60) tentacles (Chirodropids). They constitute the most important medical group of coelenterates, and appear (with isolated exceptions[24,75]) to be confined largely to tropical and sub-tropical waters. A classification of the cubozoans is shown (Table 2), but only those of currently known medical significance will be addressed[8]. All stings are potentially identifiable by microscopic examination of fresh skin scrapings[2,37].

Table 2
A classification of cubozoan jellyfish

Order	Genus	Species
Order CARYBDEIDEA	*Tripedalia*	
	Carybdea	*Cb. rastoni*
		Cb. sivickisi
		Cb. alata
	Carukia	*Ca. barnesi*
	Tamoya	
Order CHIRODROPIDEA	*Chironex*	*C. fleckeri*
	Chiropsalmus	*C. quadrigatus HAECKEL, 1880*
		C. quadrigatus BARNES, 1965
		C. quadrumanus MÜLLER, 1859
	Chirodropus	
	Chiropsoides	

1. The Carybdeids

Carukia barnesi and related organisms ("Irukandji syndrome"), *Carybdea rastoni* ("Jimble") and *Tamoya* species ("Fire Jelly", "Morbakka") are medically significant.

a. "Irukandji syndrome"

There is probably more than one animal that produces this syndrome, and it is not clear whether the syndrome is necessarily confined to carybdeid stings[76] (Fenner, P., Williamson, J. and Burnett, J., unpublished data 1993). In the Indo-Pacific the animals are found both in open water and on-shore, sometimes in swarms[4], thus presenting a hazard to both swimmers and divers[76,77].

The animals are predominately tropical, the sting from the tiny carybdeid (Figure 16) is painful, the animal is never seen in the water by the victim, and the mark on the skin may be unremarkable (Figure 9). Some 30-40 minutes later ascending muscle pains begin, becoming total body and prostrating, and presenting the picture of a catecholamine storm[54]. Systemic hypertension can attain dangerous levels. Rarely there may follow a life-threatening cardiac decompensation requiring ventilatory and inotropic support[54,68]. Hospitalisation and narcotic administration are usually essential. The intriguing possibility that compression immobilisation bandaging applied immediately following the sting may ameliorate the subsequent syndrome remains to be adequately tested. The fresh sting should be doused with vinegar[8].

b. "Jimble" (Carybdea rastoni)

This small (4-5cm bell) animal is found in-shore in episodic summertime swarms in South Australia, Western Australia, Japan and Malaysia at least. The sting is painful, leaving an angry but non-dangerous, papular wheal with a red flare. Apply first vinegar for nematocyst inhibition, then ice packs for pain relief[8,67].

c. "Fire Jelly", "Morbakka"[78] (Tamoya species)

This large (bell size up to that of a human head) 4-tentacled animal is found out at sea in the tropics of Australia, the Indo-Pacific, the Gulf of Oman[23] and west Africa at least. It is aptly named, producing an excruciatingly painful sting with its large, ribbon-like tentacles that may leave a cross-hatched pattern on the skin (the only other coelenterates known to do this are chirodropids[6,37]). Isolated accounts of "collapse" occur, but no deaths are known and symptomatic management is appropriate, viz: vinegar dousing, ice packs, and medical referral if necessary.

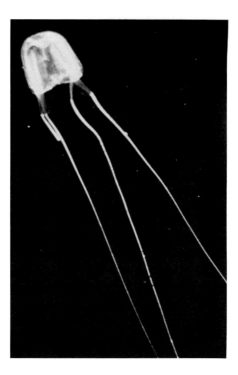

Figure 16. Irukandji jellyfish (courtesy Dr. Robert Hartwick, Townsville).

2. The Chirodropids

These tropical jellyfish are the elite of the marine coelenterate world, and in many respects the Indo-Pacific variety are the most venomous creatures on earth[49]. They have been responsible for at least 60 human deaths to date in Australia, and many more in the Indo-Pacific[2,6,8]. Deaths and serious morbidity continue, especially in the Philippines, and field biological and medical research concerning Malaysian envenomations is proceeding. As described above, much intensive research has already been carried out on the north Australian *Chironex fleckeri*, the most deadly of the chirodropids.

The three known species of greatest medical significance are *Chironex fleckeri*[35], *Chiropsalmus quadrigatus*[8], and *Chiropsalmus quadrumanus*[7]. These animals frequent the shore areas adjacent to mangrove creeks, in which they breed, and from which they swim to feed, in summer[80]. When fishing for their natural prey they favour calm water close to shore, free of snags over clear sandy bottoms, and they extend and trail their curtain of tentacles behind them - thus presenting a major hazard for unwary swimmers. They are large when fully grown (up to 30cm across the bell) (Figure 1), but are virtually invisible under natural conditions, even in clear, sunlit seawater[6]. They are known to occur in the Indo-Pacific[2,36], Okinawa and in the Gulf of Mexico[7].

Massive stings (Figure 8) may be rapidly fatal in the absence of skilled intervention[6,7,35]. However with prompt action on-site, some impressive saves have been documented[26,36,61,79]. Most stings will leave a "cross-hatched" tentacle imprint upon the skin, which, together with multiple wheals of a multi-tentacled animal, are diagnostic of a chirodropid sting. Death is from cardiac standstill in systole or respiratory failure with acute pulmonary oedema (see above)[8,12,35,36,49,51]. As with any envenomation, children are particularly susceptible[43]. Delayed, exzematous-like "allergic" reactions are documented in the absence of further jellyfish contact[6].

a. Management of chirodropid stings

These details have been repeatedly published[6,8,61,69] and can be summarised thus:

1. Retrieve and restrain the victim on the beach[1]; prevent tentacle rubbing and vigorous muscular activity by the victim;
2. Commence and sustain cardio-pulmonary resuscitation (CPR), if indicated[6]; this always takes absolute priority;
3. Douse the sting area liberally with vinegar; do not attempt to remove adherent tentacles prior to this step, unless no vinegar is available, in which case pick off the tentacles carefully using fingers only;
4. For serious stings (see above), apply a compression/immobilisation bandage to stung limbs[69] (see earlier qualification, page 101)
5. Do not leave the patient, but if possible send for informed help;
6. When indicated and if available, administer both oxygen and specific box-jellyfish antivenom (Figure 12) - 3 ampoules (60,000 units) intramuscularly, or if medical skills are at hand, 1 ampoule (20,000 units) intravenously (the latter would require great skill and direct medical supervision on the beach); antivenom should be administered if:
   (i) resuscitation was involved
   (ii) consciousness was or is affected
   (iii) pain relief is unachievable by other means
   (iv) cosmetic damage is anticipated (e.g. facial stings)
   (v) the total sting area is greater than the area equivalent to one half of one limb (especially indicated in children).
7. Transfer all but the most trivial stings to hospital under direct supervision. Do not remove any compression bandages, nor any oxygen administration prior to hospital.
8. In hospital, normal resuscitative and intensive care are maintained, including intravenous access, further antivenom as indicated and appropriate further circulatory and ventilatory support[26].

For less severe stings, neither bandages nor antivenom are necessary, and ice application may suffice for analgesia. Early medical inspection in case of serious local skin damage[6] is wise.

B. *CLASS* HYDROZOA (HYDROIDS)

These include the stinging corals (*millepora*), feather hydroids, the important Portuguese man-o'war or bluebottle, the limnomedusae ("Aquaviva") jellyfish and the intriguing *Gonionemus* species in Eastern Russia. They have a truly world-wide distribution and prevalence.

1. Hydroids

Stinging corals and feather hydroids, armed with nematocyst on their surfaces and arms, sting on contact, producing immediate itching pain, and a series of small red wheals which remain itchy and painful for hours. They are found in tropical and temperate waters everywhere, often attached to submerged wharf piles and wrecks. Some are very beautiful to visualise, and Scuba divers are often stung. They present little danger. Treatment is with sea water washing, and the application of ice. Extensive stings should receive systemic steroids, or less effectively, antihistamines. Heat usually makes the irritation worse, as will sunburn.

2. *Physalia* species (Atlantic "Portuguese man-o'war"; Pacific "Bluebottle")

This "jellyfish" is actually a colony of symbiotic animals with sub-group populations of animals in a single colony specialising in different functions (food capture, reproduction, digestion) (Figure 2)[27]. It is the best known, the widest dispersed and the commonest jellyfish associated with human stinging. Thousands of stingings occur annually in Florida[27],

Queensland[4], Pakistan (Junaid Alam, unpublished data, 1993), South Africa[22], South China (Zhang Mingliang, unpublished data, 1993) and Portugal[21], to name but a few countries. It would appear that the Atlantic species is larger (Figure 2), and more dangerous; several deaths are documented[9,10]. In contrast the smaller Pacific species causes stingings more numerous than can be recorded, but no deaths are known although delayed serious complications have occurred[81]. The animals occur both in-shore and in the open sea in swarms, and are adept sailors by virtue of their left- or right-handed gas filled "sail-floats". Multiple stings on a single person, or involving many persons, occur regularly[4]. (Figure 17).

The sting is a characteric linear collection of elliptical blanched wheals with a surrounding angry red flare. Pain is immediate, intense, but fades over an hour or so to become dull, in most Pacific cases. Recently a larger, more troublesome stinging *Physalia* species has been encountered in Australia, which resembles more the Atlantic species in both morphology and sting syndrome[27]. Also envenomation by the Pakistani *Physalia* may be associated with serious effects (Junaid Alam, unpublished data, 1993)[55]. The situation worldwide is further confused by the fact that nematocyst inhibition in *Physalia* species is in a state of uncertainty, with conflicting experimental results[27,38,43]. Present recommendations are that vinegar dousing should not be used on any *Physalia* sting, worldwide, because this may actually fire undischarged nematocysts on the skin, in stings from the larger *Physalia* animal[27]. Because the taxonomy of the animal, and the clear differentiation between the smaller Pacific (*Physalia utriculus*) and the larger, more dangerous Atlantic (*Physalia physalis*) species remains unclear, the fresh sting should be washed only with sea water, any adherent tentacles picked off, and ice packs applied for pain relief. With more severe effects, medical supervision of systemic pain relief (e.g. morphine) may be required. Needless to say, vigorous resuscitation for the uncommon life-threatening stings is mandatory. No antivenom is available.

3. Limnomedusae

The medical significance of the species *Olindias sambaquiensis* in Brazil, Uruguay and Argentina has been recorded by Dr Hermes Mianzan (Mianzan, unpublished data, 1993), and by Cleland and Southcott in Australia[82,83]. This jellyfish, with its vivid coloured flatish bell, has many tentacles, occurs mainly in summer and its stings can interfere with Brazilian tourist activities. Hundreds of bathers are stung at a time in South America, but no deaths have been reported. The sting can produce burning pain and a red flare. There is no specific treatment, but ammonia solution application is used in Brazil. Results of this treatment are not documented to date. Dermatitis following contact with *Olindias sambaquiensis* in an aquarium has recently been reported[28].

4. *Gonionemus* species

Yakovlev and Vaskovsky (unpublished data, 1993) have recently begun to document the extraordinary effects of the sting of *Gonionemus vertens* in the sea of Vladivostok[67]. This summertime sting results in a 24 hour period of neuropsychiatric derangement in some victims, which abates spontaneously. Nothing is yet known of the toxinology.

C. *CLASS* SCYPHOZOA (TRUE JELLYFISH)

Members of this group are some of the most familiar jellyfish, and include "Hair Jelly" or "Snottie" (*Cyanea* species) and the ubiquitous "Blubber jellyfish" (*Catostylus* species). Members of greater medical significance are the "Sea Nettles" (*Chrysaora* species), "Mauve Stinger" (*Pelagia noctiluca*), *Rhizostoma* species, the "cabbage head jellyfish" (*Stomolophus* species), and the "Moon jellyfish" (*Aurelia* species).

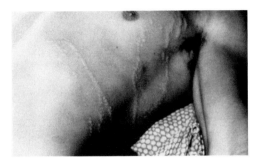
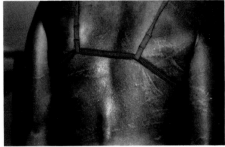

Figure 17. *Physalia* sting (courtesy Surf Life Saving Queensland, Inc.).

Figure 18. *Cyanea* sting.

1. *Cyanea* species

The Hair Jelly can grow to enormous size (feet across the flatish bell) in the open waters of colder oceans, but more commonly is described as "a mop hiding under a dinner plate"! The numerous, hair-like tentacles may extend for metres under the bell, and produce a moderately painful sting and an area of angry looking redness. The pain fades in minutes usually, and although the widespread redness persists, the patient is seldom troubled symptomatically (Figure 18). Vinegar should not be used for this sting[84], but ice packs are appropriate for pain relief.

2. *Catostylus* species

Apart from its familiarity, floating often in large numbers on the surface, and its attractive mosaic pattern on the top of its generous bell, its stumpy tentacles ("a mushroom wearing frilly pants"!), it is of no medical significance. Stinging is scarcely more than a faint prickle. It is of interest that the famous jellyfish lake of Palau contains millions of small, non-stinging *Catostylus* animals.

3. *Chrysaora* species

The Chesapeake Bay animal *Chrysaora quinquecirrha*, the "North American Sea Nettle", occupies an important place in modern toxinological and immunological research into coelenterates venoms. While acknowledging the pioneer work of Freeman[85], Crone[86], Maretic[87,88], and Russell[89], the location of Burnett's team on the Chesapeake Bay, which is regularly infested with summertime sea nettle swarms[90], has significantly accelerated our understanding of coelenterate toxinology[5,10,12,18,45,52] and immunology[12,15,18,19,57].

Different *Chrysaora* species occur plentifully worldwide, including besides the east coast of North America, the Indo-Pacific and Australia[2], Japan and the Indian Ocean[3], and the Mediterranean and Adriatic Seas[15,91].

The animal has long fishing tentacles outside longish mesenteric tentacles, and produces a mild to moderate sting with immediate cutaneous pain, which fades over some hours. It is phylogenetically related to *Pelagia* species. Stings produce elevated IgG and IgE titres in patients' serum which will correlate directly with the severity of the symptoms[92]. The toxin from the fishing tentacle nematocysts is the more potent, showing in animal *in vivo* studies, mouse lethality, haemolysis, dermatonecrosis, vasopermeability, damage to rat liver mitochondria and hepatocytes, and renal necrosis[18,93].

Unlike *Chironex* venom[72], no protection in animals was afforded by verapamil from *Chrysaora* venom[93].

Management of the stings is symptomatic, as no antivenom exists. Partial nematocyst inhibition was previously thought to be achieved by a slurry of sodium bicarbonate[94], but despite a large range of substances (including vinegar) having been applied at various times, a clinically completely effective inhibitor is not yet known[12]. Ice packs must be sustained to be effective analgesia for *Chrysaora quinquecirrha* stings, the pain returning immediately upon removal of the ice[12].

4. *Pelagia* species

The Mauve Stinger is a formidable animal, and a beautiful one (Figure 3). It has existed in plague proportions in the Mediterranean, and is still a frequent cause of stings there[87,88,91]. It has caused the cancellation of surf carnivals in Australia, where it is well known[93]. It phosphoresces at night, hence its name "*Pelagia noctiluca*". It is found in deep water but can approach the shoreline in large colonies. The outer fishing tentacles carry the stinging nematocysts, which also inhabit the outer surface of the bell, making bare-handed handling difficult.

A *Pelagia* species on an Athens beach was responsible for a near-fatal anaphylactic reaction to a sting in a human[13], and its stings generally are accompanied with intense pain, whealing, itching and local swelling, suggesting an allergic propensity for its venom. Post-sting skin pigmentation is documented[16]. There is no antivenom, and treatment is symptomatic, i.e. wash with sea water, apply ice, and seek medical attention for unrelieved pain or systemic symptoms. The apparently high antigenic activity of this venom makes it an attractive target for further immunological research[92].

5. *Rhizostoma* species

The full worldwide distribution of the Rhizostomatidae is uncertain, but they are common in European and Mediterranean waters[3], as well as in South-East Asia and Australia[2]. A typical example is *Rhizostoma pulmo*, which can grow to 65cm across the bell and has a large, dome shaped umbrella covered with minute warts, and 8 oral arms[91]. Handling and contact can produce local urticaria, with sneezing and eye irritation. Some people appear to be sensitized to the animal. Stings from actual contact produce a mild, short-lived burning sensation (Kokelj, F., unpublished data, 1993).

6. *Stomolophus* species ("Cabbagehead Jellyfish")

This animal was considered in the western world as not painful or injurious to man, prior to the work of Dr Zhang Mingliang and colleagues of China[11]. He has recorded both fatality and thousands of stings on a Beidehe Beach, near Beijing. The multiple tentacles produce a cluster of angry wheals, and endotoxaemia can be serious; although preliminary toxinology has occurred[96], little is yet known about the venom. Local skin treatments include "ammonia solutions".

7. *Aurelia* species ("Moon Jellyfish")

The Moon Jellyfish *Aurelia* aurita was considered - and usually is -minimally painful and harmless to man. However Burnett and colleagues recorded a sting from this animal in the Mississippi Sound (Gulf of Mexico) which gave pain, urticaria, ulceration, crusting and regional lymph gland pain which lasted for days[97]. Hyperpigmentation at the sting site was visible 2 weeks later.

D. *CLASS* ANTHOZOA

Included in this Class are the hard and soft corals and the sea anemones.

1. Hard and soft corals

While this group represents a geographically and morphologically diverse international collection all of which sting on contact with their nematocysts, the sting is seldom serious and can be treated symptomatically. However abrasion of skin will also sustain an injury requiring immediate first aid toilet, to avoid secondary bacterial (marine or terrestrial) infection[6,14]. Early (within the first 2-3 hours) scrub with a soft bristle brush, using clean fresh (not sea) water and a mild antiseptic is important. Light bleeding may ensue and is normal. Except in small children, this is not unduly painful or distressing, but removal of the tiny impregnated coral detritus that always contaminates such wounds may prevent months of subsequent morbidity. Appropriate tetanus prophylaxis may be required for deeper wounds.

2. Anemones

These impressive, sessile creatures belong to the taxonomic Order Actiniaria, and include:

Actinodendron pulmosum HADDON 1898
Actinia arboreum QUOY & GAIMARD 1833
Corynactis australia HADDON & DAERDEN 1896 (Corallimorpharia)
Rhodactis howesii SAVILLE-KENT 1893 (Corallimorpharia)
Sagartia elegans
Anemonia sulcata

Very widely dispersed through temperate and tropical waters, they are beautiful in their diversity of colour and fronded, graceful movements; they are among the most photographed of marine animals (Figure 19).

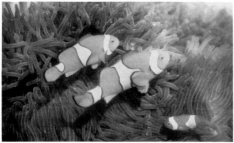
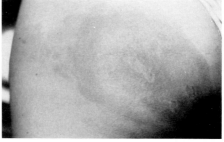

Figure 19. Anemone with pilot fish.

Figure 20. Troublesome Great Barrier Reef *Stoichactis kenti* sting on day 7 (courtesy of Bob and Dinah Halstead, Telita Cruises, Papua New Guinea).

Armed with numerous nematocyst on their waving fronds, they sting on contact, sometimes powerfully and painfully. On Australia's Great barrier Reef one of the most painful is *Actindendron pulmosum* Haddon, whose sting may persist for days. Australian anemone stinging has been well reviewed[2], as have world anemone toxins[98]. The animals contain some potent toxins, but although some stings are not trivial (Figure 20), most do not produce serious morbidity. Divers are particularly susceptible to anemone stings, and wetsuit, facemask (eye protection) and gloves are recommended. It should be noted that Mediterranean "sponge divers disease" or "*maladie des plongeurs*" is in fact due to a sting by an anemone attached to the sponges, at 25 to 45 metres.[3] Treatment is symptomatic; non-infective but unresponsive skin reaction may respond to a short (2 day) course of systemic steroids, under medical supervision.

IV. FUTURE DIRECTIONS

A. RESEARCH

There are many frontiers awaiting the researcher[1]. These include nematocyst inhibition, sting analgesia, clinical management protocols and toxinology and immunology of the venoms. Burnett and colleagues are making significant contributions to these last mentioned fields[27,28,44,45,55,57,72]. The epidemiology of both the animals and the stingings requires a broader international base[4,5]. To this end, the fostering of international collaboration is important, and is one of the main thrusts of the International Consortium for Jellyfish Stings[4,5].

B. MULTI-DISCIPLINARY APPROACH

Crossing boundaries of scientific disciplines releases a multitude of different skills and knowledge. This avoids "re-inventing the wheel", all too frequent in science, and significantly hastens progress. Medical clinicians, marine biologists, biochemists, toxicologists, pure science researchers, photographers, divers, paramedics and lifesaver personnel all have something to contribute[1].

C. PUBLIC EDUCATION

This is on-going and never ending, and has scarcely begun at the co-ordinated international level. It is the key to both prevention and animal conservation. The study of coelenterate injuries brings those involved face to face with the swelling problems of pollution and mindless destruction of the environment. All scientists now have a responsibility to contribute towards correcting this trend.

D. FUNDING

Much of the research carried out on coelenterate injuries over the decades has been by interested enthusiasts, usually in their spare time, and at their own expense. Although much human knowledge will continue to be obtained in this way, governments and populations need now to be persuaded that this subject deserves a higher priority. Research into coelenterate envenomations will contribute not only to environmental preservation, but also to advances in human immunology, pain management, and effective disease therapies - not to mention the reduction in young human death and suffering.

V. REFERENCES

1. **WILLIAMSON, J. A.**, Current challenges in marine envenomation: an overview, J Wilderness Med, 3, 422, 1992.
2. **CLELAND, SIR J. B. AND SOUTHCOTT, R. V.**, *Injuries to Man from Marine Invertebrates in the Australian Region*, National Health and Medical Research Council, Canberra, 1965.
3. **HALSTEAD, B. W.**, *Poisonous and Venomous Marine Animals of the World* (second revised edition), The Darwin Press, Inc., Princeton, New Jersey, 1988, 99.
4. **FENNER, P., WILLIAMSON, J. AND BURNETT, J.**, *Some Australian and international marine envenomation reports, No. 4: Progress summary to March 31, 1992*, International Consortium for Jellyfish Stings, Hyperbaric Medicine Unit, Royal Adelaide Hospital, Adelaide, South Australia. 1992.
5. **BURNETT, J. W.**, *Jellyfish Newsletters, No's 1-8*, International Consortium for Jellyfish Stings, Department of Dermatology, University of Maryland Hospital, Baltimore MD 21201, U.S.A., 1989-1993.
6. **WILLIAMSON, J. A.**, *The Marine Stinger Book*, 3rd edn., Queensland State centre, Inc., Surf Life Saving Australia, Newstead, Queensland, 4006, 1985, 19.
7. **BENGSTON, K., NICHOLS, M. M., SCHNADIG, V. AND ELLIS, M. D.**, Sudden death in a child following jellyfish envenomation by *Chiropsalmus quadrumanus*, JAMA, 266, 1404, 1991.
8. **FENNER, P. J.**, Cubozoan jellyfish envenomation syndromes and their medical treatment in northern Australia, *Hydrobiologia, 216/217, 637, 1991.*

9. STEIN, M. R., MARRACCINI, J. V., ROTHSCHILD, N. E. AND BURNETT, J. W., Fatal Portuguese man-o'-war (*Physalia physalis*) envenomation, *Annals Emerg Med*, 18, 312, 1989.

10. BURNETT, J. W. AND GABLE, W. D., A fatal jellyfish envenomation by the Portuguese man-o'war, *Toxicon*, 27, 823, 1989.

11. ZHANG MINGLIANG, Study on jellyfish *Stomolophus nomurai* stings on Beidehe, *National Med J China*, 9, 499, 1988.

12. BURNETT, J. W., Clinical manifestations of jellyfish envenomation, *Hydrobiologia*, 216/217, 629, 1991.

13. TOGIAS, A. G., BURNETT, J. W., KAGEY-SOBOTKA, A. AND LICHTENSTEIN, L. M., Anaphylaxis after contact with a jellyfish, J Allergy Clin Immunol, 75, 672, 1985.

14. CALLANAN, V., Coral cuts and abrasions, *SPUMS J*, 23, 29, 1993.

15. KOKELJ, F., TUBARO, A. AND DEL NEGRO, P., Effeto dermotossico da *Chrisaora hysoscella* presentazione di un caso, *Giorn It Dermatol*, 124, 297, 1989.

16. KOKELJ, F. AND BURNETT, J.W., Treatment of a pigmented lesion induced by a *Pelagia noctiluca* sting, *Cutis* 1990, 46, 62.

17. BURNETT, J. W., PIERCE, L. H. JR., NAWACHINDA, U. A. B. AND STONE, J. H., Studies on sea nettle stings, *Arch Derm*, 98, 587, 1968.

18. BURNETT, J. W. AND CALTON, G. J., Venomous pelagic coelenterates: chemistry, toxicology, immunology and treatment of their stings, *Toxicon*, 25, 581, 1987.

19. BURNETT, J. W., CALTON, G. J., FENNER, P. J. AND WILLIAMSON, J. A., Serological diagnosis of jellyfish envenomations, *Comp Biochem Physiol*, 91C, 79, 1988.

20. SPIELMAN, F. J., BOWE, E. A., WATSON, C. B. AND KLEIN, E. F., Acute renal failure as a result of *Physalia physalis* sting, *Southern Med J*, 75, 1425, 1982.

21. GONZAGA, R. A. F. Picadas por cnidários, in *Mordedurase e Picadas por Animais da Fauna Portuguesa*, Prémio Bial de Medicina Clínica, Porto, 1984: 157-168.

22. SHANNON, L. V. AND CHAPMAN, P., Incidence of *Physalia* on beaches in the South West Cape Province during January 1983, *South African J Sci*, 79, 454, 1983.

23. COOPER, N. K., Disarming the box jellyfish in Oman, *Medical Corps Internat*, 1, 26, 1991.

24. SHOKITA, S., *Dangerous Animals and Plants of Okinawa*, Okinawa -Shuppan Co., Ltd., Okinawa 901-21 Japan, 18, 1974.

25. BURNETT, J. W., Correspondence to the Editor, *J Wilderness Med*, 1, 135, 1990.

26. BEADNELL, E. C., RIDER, T. A., WILLIAMSON, J. A. AND FENNER, P. J., Management of a major box jellyfish (*Chironex fleckeri*) sting: lessons from the first minutes and hours, *Med J Aust*, 156, 655, 1992.

27. FENNER, P. J., WILLIAMSON, J. A., BURNETT, J. W. AND RIFKIN, J., First aid treatment of jellyfish stings in Australia: response to a newly differentiated species, *Med J Aust*, 158, 498, 1993.

28. KOKELJ, F., MIANZAN, H., AVIAN, M. AND BURNETT, J. W., Dermatitis due to *Olindias sambaquiensis*: a case report, *Cutis*, 51, 339, 1993.

29 RIFKIN, J., WILLIAMSON, J., FENNER, P. AND BURNETT, J., Disarming the box-jellyfish (letter), *Med J Aust*, 158, 647, 1993.

30. WILKS, J., Calculating diver numbers: critical information for scuba safety and marketing programmes, *SPUMS J*, 23, 11, 1993.

31. HULET, W, H., BELLEME, J. L., MUSIL, G. AND LANE, C. E., Ultrastructure of *Physalia* nematocysts, in *Bioactive Compounds from the Sea*, Humm, H. J. and Lane, C. E., Eds., Marcel Dekker, New York, 1974, 99.

32. RIFKIN, J. AND ENDEAN, R., The structure and function of the nematocysts of *Chironex fleckeri* Southcott, 1956, *Cell Tissue Res,* 233, 563, 1983.

33. RIFKIN, J. F. AND ENDEAN, R., Arrangement of accessory cells and nematocytes bearing mastigophores in the tentacles of the Cubozoan *Chironex fleckeri, J Morphol*, 195, 103, 1988.

34. ENDEAN, R., RIFKIN, J. F. AND DADDOW, L. Y. M., Envenomation by the box-jellyfish *Chironex fleckeri*: how nematocysts discharge, *Hydrobiologia*, 216/217, 641, 1991.

35. LUMLEY, J., WILLIAMSON, J. A., FENNER, P. J., ET AL, Fatal envenomation by *Chironex fleckeri*, the north Australian box jellyfish: the continuing search for lethal mechanisms, *Med J Aust*, 148, 527, 1988.

36. WILLIAMSON, J. A., CALLANAN, V. I. AND HARTWICK, R. F., Serious envenomation by the northern Australian box-jellyfish (*Chironex fleckeri*), *Med J Aust*, 1, 13, 1980.

37. BARNES, J. H., Observations on jellyfish stingings in north Queensland, *Med J Aust*, II, 993, 1960.

38. HARTWICK, R., CALLANAN, V. AND WILLIAMSON, J., Disarming the box-jellyfish: nematocyst inhibition in *Chironex fleckeri*, *Med J Aust*, 1, 15, 1980.

39. ENDEAN, R. AND RIFKIN, J., Envenomation involving nematocysts of the box jellyfish *Chironex fleckeri*, *Toxicon*, 3, Suppl., 115, 1983.

40. EASTON, R. G., Disarming the box jellyfish, *Med J Aust*, 1, 335, 1980.

41. FENNER, P. J. AND WILLIAMSON, J. A. H., Experiments with the nematocysts of *Carybdea rastoni*, *Med J Aust*, 147, 258, 1987.

42. EXTON, D. R., Treatment of *Physalia physalis* envenomation (letter), *Med J Aust*, 149, 54, 1988.

43. **VIMPANI, G., DOUDLE, M AND HARRIS, R**. Child accident mortality in the Northern Territory, 1978-1985, *Med J Aust*, 148, 392, 1988.
44. **BURNETT, J. W. AND CALTON, G. J.**, Jellyfish envenomation syndromes updated, *Annals Emerg Med*, 16, 1000, 1987.
45. **OTHMAN, I. AND BURNETT, J. W.**, Techniques applicable for purifying *Chironex fleckeri* (box-jellyfish) venom, *Toxicon*, 28, 821, 1990.
46. **BURNETT, J. W., ORDONEZ, J. V. AND CALTON, G. J.**, Differential toxicity of *Physalia physalis* (Portuguese man-o'war) nematocysts separated by flow cytometry, *Toxicon*, 24, 514, 1986.
47. **ENDEAN, R**. Separation of two myotoxins from nematocysts of the box jellyfish (*Chironex fleckeri*), *Toxicon*, 25, 483, 1987.
48. **NAGUIB, A. M. F., BANSAL, J., CALTON, G. J. AND BURNETT, J. W.**, Purification of *Chironex fleckeri* venom components using *Chironex* immunoaffinity chromatography, *Toxicon*, 26, 387, 1988.
49. **ENDEAN, B.**, Venom of *Chironex*, the world's most venomous animal, in *Venoms & Victims*, Pearn, J. and Covacevich, J., Eds., The Queensland Museum and Amphion Press, South Brisbane, 1988, chap. 3.
50. **AZILA, N. AND OTHMAN, I.** Pharmacological effects of various jellyfishes found in Malaysian waters. International Society of Toxinology meeting, Singapore, November 3, Abstract No. 364, 1991.
51. **WILLIAMSON, J. A., CALLANAN, V. I., UNWIN, M. L. AND HARTWICK, R. F.**, Box-jellyfish venom and humans (letter), *Med J Aust*, 1, 444, 1984.
52. **BURNETT, J. W. AND CALTON, G. J.**, Response of the box-jellyfish (*Chironex fleckeri*) cardiotoxin to intravenous administration of verapamil, *Med J Aust*, 2, 192, 1983.
53. **PRATAP CHAND, R. AND SELLIAH, K.**, Reversible parasympathetic dysautonomia following stinging attributed to the box jelly fish (*Chironex fleckeri*), *Aust NZ J Med*, 14, 673, 1984.
54. **FENNER, P., WILLIAMSON, J., BURNETT, J., et al**, The "Irukandji syndrome" and acute pulmonary oedema, *Med J Aust*, 149, 150, 1988.
55. **WILLIAMSON, J. A., BURNETT, J. W., FENNER, P. J., HACH-WUNDERLE, V., LIM YU HOE AND MADHAV ADIGA, K.**, Acute regional vascular insufficiency after jellyfish envenomation, *Med J Aust*, 149, 698, 1988.
56. **BARNES, J. H.**, Studies on three venomous Cubomedusae, *Symp Zool Soc Lond*, 16, 307, 1966.
57. **BURNETT, J. W.**, Immunological aspects of jellyfish envenomation, International Society of Toxinology Meeting, Singapore, November 3, Abstract No. 118, 1991.
58. **PORTIER, P. AND RICHER, C.**, De l'action anaphylactique de certains venins, *Compt Rend Soc Biol (Paris)*, 54, 170, 1902.
59. **MOATS, W. E.**, Fire coral envenomation, *J Wilderness Med*, 3, 284, 1992.
60. **WILLIAMSON, J. A., LERAY, L. E., WOHLFAHRT, M. AND FENNER, P. J.**, Acute management of serious envenomation by box-jellyfish (*Chironex fleckeri*), *Med J Aust*, 141, 851, 1984.
61. **FENNER, P. J., WILLIAMSON, J. A. AND BLENKIN, J. A.**, Successful use of *Chironex* antivenom by members of the Queensland Ambulance Transport Brigade, *Med J Aust*, 151, 708, 1989.
62. **WILLIAMSON, J.**, venomous and poisonous marine animals, in *Cecil Textbook of Medicine 19th edition*, J. B. Wyngaarden, L. H. Smith and J. C. Bennett, Eds., W. B. Saunders Company, Philadelphia, 1992, 2030.
63. **RAPOZA, P. A., WEST, S. K., NEWLAND, H. S. AND TAYLOR, H. R.**, Ocular jellyfish stings in Chesapeake Bay watermen, *Amer J Ophthal*, 102, 535, 1986.
64. **BARNES, J. H.**, Extraction of cnidarian venom from living tentacle, in *Animal Toxins, a collection of papers presented at the First International Symposium on Animal Toxins, Atlantic City, New Jersey, U.S.A., April 9-11, 1966*, Pergamon Press, Oxford & New York, 1967, 115.
65. **CURRIE, B., HO, S. AND ALDERSLADE, P.** Box-jellyfish, Coca-Cola and old wine, *Med J Aust*, 158, 868, 1993.
66. **EXTON, D. R. P., FENNER, P. J. AND WILLIAMSON, J. A. H.**, Ice packs -an effective first aid treatment for *Physalia* and other painful jellyfish stings. *Med J Aust*, 151, 708, 1989.
67. **WARRELL, D. A. AND FENNER, P. J.**, Venomous bites and stings, *Brit Med Bull*, 49, 423, 1993.
68. **MARTIN, J. C. AND AUDLEY, I.**, Cardiac failure following Irukandji envenomation, *Med J Aust*, 153, 164, 1990.
69. **SUTHERLAND, S. K.**, *Australian Animal Toxins: The creatures, their toxins and care of the poisoned patient*, Oxford University Press, Melbourne, 1983, chap. 3.
70. **SUTHERLAND, S. K.**, Antivenom use in Australia: premedication, adverse reactions and the use of venom detection kits, *Med J Aust*, 157, 734, 1992.
71. **ENDEAN, R. AND SIZEMORE D. J.**, The effectiveness of antivenom in countering the actions of box-jellyfish (*Chironex fleckeri*) nematocyst toxins in mice, *Toxicon*, 26, 425, 1988.
72. **BURNETT, J. W., OTHMAN, I. B., ENDEAN, R., FENNER, P.J., CALLANAN, V.I. AND WILLIAMSON, J. A.**, Verapamil potentiation of *Chironex* (box-jellyfish) antivenom, *Toxicon*, 28, 242, 1990.
73. **FATOVICH, D. M., TURNER, V. F. AND HIRSCH, R. L.**, Premedication before antivenom therapy, *Med J Aust*, 156, 510, 1992.

74. **WERNER, B.**, Bau und Lebensgeschichte des Polypen von *Tripedalia cystophora* (Cubozoa, class. nov., Carybdeidae) und seine Bedeutung für die Evolution der Cnidaria, *Helgoländer wiss. Meeresunters*, 27, 461, 1975.

75. **HOVERD, W. A.**, Occurrence of the order Cubomedusae (Cnidaria: Scyphozoa) in New Zealand: collection and laboratory observations on *Carybdea sivickisi*, *New Zealand J Zool*, 12, 107, 1985.

76. **KIZER, K. W.**, Decompression sickness or Portuguese Man-Of-War envenomation?, *Wilderness Med*, 1, 7, 1984.

77. **WILLIAMSON, J.**, "Irukandji" syndrome or decompression sickness or cerebral arterial gas embolism? A differential diagnostic trap for practitioners of diving medicine in North Queensland, *SPUMS J*, 15, 38, 1985.

78. **SOUTHCOTT, R. V.**, The "Morbakka", *Med J Aust*, 143, 324, 1985.

79. **MAGUIRE, E. J.**, *Chironex fleckeri* (sea wasp) sting, *Med J Aust*, 2, 1137, 1968.

80. **HARTWICK, R. F.**, Distributional ecology and behaviour of the early life stages of the box-jellyfish *Chironex fleckeri*, *Hydrobiologia*, 216/217, 181, 1991.

81. **HALSTEAD, B. W.**, *Poisonous and Venomous Marine Animals of the World* (second revised edition), The Darwin Press, Inc., Princeton, New Jersey, 1988, chap IV, plate 9.

82. **CLELAND, SIR J. B. AND SOUTHCOTT, R. V.**, *Injuries to Man from Marine Invertebrates in the Australian Region*, National Health and Medical Research Council, Canberra, 1965, 26.

83. **MIANZAN, H.**, Distribución de *Olindias sambiquiensis* Muller, 1861 (Hydrozoa, Limnomedusae) en al Atlántico Sudoccidental. *IHERINGA, ser Zool*, 69, 155, 1989.

84. **FENNER, P. J. AND FITZPATRICK, P. F.**, Experiments with the nematocysts of *Cyanea capillata*, *Med J Aust*, 145, 174, 1986.

85. **FREEMAN, S. E.**, Actions of *Chironex fleckeri* toxins on cardiac transmembrane potentials, *Toxicon*, 12, 395, 1974.

86. **CRONE, H. D.**, Chemical modification of the haemolytic activity of extracts from the box jellyfish *Chironex fleckeri* (cnidarian), *Toxicon*, 14, 97, 1976.

87. **MARETIC, Z., RUSSELL, F. E. AND LADAVAC, J.**, Epidemic of stings by the jellyfish *Pelagia noctiluca* in the Adriatic, *Toxicon*, 17(Suppl.1), 115, 1979.

88. **MARETIC, Z.**, The blooms of jellyfish *Pelagia noctiluca* along the coast of Pula and Istria in 1977-1983 with special reference to epidemiology, clinics and treatment. Workshop on jelly-fish blooms in the Mediterranean, Athens, 31 October - 4 November 1983, United Nations Environment Programme, 1983, 83.

89. **RUSSELL, F. E., GONZALEZ, H., DOBSON, S. B. AND COATS, J. A.**, *Bibliography of Venomous and Poisonous Marine Animals and their Toxins*, Office of the United States Naval Research, Arlington, Virginia,1984, 86.

90. **BURNETT, J. W., PIERCE, JR., L. H., URIWAN NAWACHINDA AND STONE, J. H.**, Studies on sea nettle stings, *Arch Derm*, 98, 587, 1968.

91. **AXIAK, V.**, Long-term programme for pollution monitoring and research in the Mediterranean, Workshop on jelly-fish blooms in the Mediterranean, Athens, 31 October - 4 November 1983, United Nations Environment Programme, 1983, 23.

92. **RUSSO, A. J., CALTON, G. J. AND BURNETT, J. W.**, The relationship of the possible allergic response to jellyfish envenomation and serum antibody titres, *Toxicon,* 21, 475, 1983.

93. **MUHVICH, K. H., SENGOTTUVELU, S., MANSON, P. N., MYERS, R. M., BURNETT, J. W. AND MARZELLA, L.**, Pathophysiology of sea nettle (*Chrysaora quinquecirrha*), envenomation in a rat model and the effects of hyperbaric oxygen and verapamil treatment, *Toxicon*, 29, 837, 1991.

94. **BURNETT, J. W., RUBINSTEIN, H. AND CALTON, G. J.**, First aid for jellyfish envenomation, *Southern Med J*, 76, 870, 1983.

95. **CLELAND, SIR J. B. AND SOUTHCOTT, R. V.**, *Injuries to Man from Marine Invertebrates in the Australian Region*, National Health and Medical Research Council, Canberra, 1965, 156.

96. **BURNETT, J. W. AND CALTON, G. J.**, The chemistry and toxinology of some venomous pelagic coelenterates, *Toxicon*, 15, 177, 1977.

97. **BURNETT, J. W., CALTON, G. J. AND LARSEN, J. B.**, Significant envenomation by *Aurelia aurita*, the moon jellyfish, *Toxicon*, 26, 215, 1988.

98. **MEBS, D. AND GEBAUER, E.**, Isolation of proteinase inhibitory, toxic and hemolytic polypeptide from a sea anemone, *Stoichatus* sp. *Toxicon*, 18, 97, 1980.

Chapter 9

CLINICAL TOXICOLOGY OF *Conus* SNAIL STINGS

Lourdes J. Cruz and Julian White

TABLE OF CONTENTS

I. INTRODUCTION

Conus snails are some of the most successful predators in marine communities. Paleontological evidence suggests that the >300 recognized *Conus* species evolved from an older stem group of gastropods, the worm-hunting turrids or slit shells around the Caenozoic period[1]. The cones, which belong to the superfamily Toxoglossa ("poison tongue"), family Conidae, have radiated since then into three feeding types[2]: worm-hunters, mollusc-hunters and fish-hunters. Their success as predators depends on their use of an efficient venom apparatus that can inject a cocktail of very potent peptides to quickly overpower the prey. Most dangerous to man are the fish-hunting species, particularly the geography cone, *Conus geographus* (see Figure 1) because many of their venom components are very active not only on fish but also on other vertebrates including humans.

II. EPIDEMIOLOGY

A. DISTRIBUTION OF *Conus* SPECIES

The *Conus* species are most abundant in the warmer areas of the Indo-Pacific region[3,4]. Of the >300 species listed by Walls[3], 91% are represented in the Pacific, 69% in the Indian Ocean and only 15% are found in the Atlantic Ocean. Very few species are found in the temperate regions such as the southern coast of South Africa and the southern coast of Australia including Tasmania[3]. In the western Pacific region, cones are found only as far north as southern Japan and in the eastern Pacific region as far north as San Francisco and as far south as the coast of Peru. In the western Atlantic area, cones are found along the coast from Georgia to northern Brazil. Many species are widely distributed from the western Indian Ocean to the eastern Pacific region whereas others have extremely restricted localities[3].

Cones have a variety of habitats ranging from shallow waters of the intertidal zone to very deep waters (600 meters), from muddy or sandy bottoms and coral rubble to reef platforms, from barren substrates to sea grass areas of algal turfs[2,5,6]. They are mainly nocturnal, preferring to stay buried under the substrate or hidden in crevices during the day.

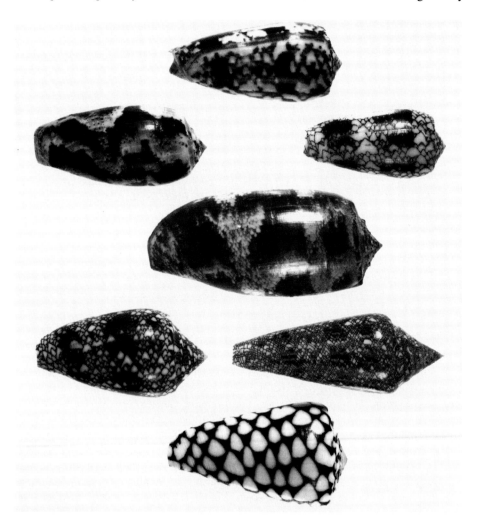

Figure 1. *Conus* species reputedly responsible for severe and deadly envenomations. Center; *C. geographus* Clockwise from top; *C. striatus, C. omaria, C. gloriamaris, C. marmoreus, C. textile, C. tulipa.* The most dangerous species is *C. geographus.* The single story of a human fatality due to *C. gloriamaris* has not been verified.

Four *Conus* species have been reported[7-12] to produce very severe envenomations in humans: *C. geographus, C. textile* (cloth-of-gold cone)*, C. omaria* (pearled cone)*,* and *C. marmoreus* (marble cone) (see Figure 1). These cones are relatively common in shallow water and widespread in the Indo-Pacific region. During the day, *C. geographus* hides in sandy pockets, under rocks or in reef crevices. The three other species usually burrow in sandy substrates and coral rubble or under rocks and corals.

B. THE VENOM

The toxicity of the venom varies between species, and each species produces its own unique set of biologically active peptides[13-17]. In tests using laboratory animals, the most toxic venoms are from the fish eaters followed by venoms from the mollusc- and worm-hunting species[18-20]. Venoms from mollusc hunters have no obvious effects when injected intraperitoneally in mice. However, human lethalities have been reported not only for fish hunters but also for mollusc-hunting species such as *C. textile* [8,21] and *C. marmoreus*[21].

The major components of the venom of *C. geographus* are small peptides which synergistically block the neuromuscular junction to rapidly paralyze prey[13-15]: the ω-conotoxins block calcium channels at the presynaptic terminal, α-conotoxins inhibit the acetylcholine receptors at the postsynaptic end, and μ-conotoxins block the muscle sodium channels. The venom contains many other peptides (see Table 1) that can affect various receptors and ion channels in the central nervous system[16,17]. However, it is believed that the ω-, α- and μ-conotoxins are mainly responsible for the characteristic reaction of the prey to the deadly *C. geographus* sting. In mice, ω-conotoxins produce an effect only when injected intracranially[22]. Perhaps in humans also, ω-conotoxins are not active on the peripheral nervous system and do not contribute to the overall paralysis observed in *C. geographus* envenomation.

Table 1
Classes of peptides found in *Conus geographus* venom

Class	Mode of Action	Number Isolated	Number of Amino Acids in Peptide
α-Conotoxin	Inhibits acetylcholine receptors	3	13 - 15
μ-Conotoxin	Blocks muscle sodium channel	7	22
ω-Conotoxin	Blocks neuronal calcium channel	5	27 - 30
Conantokin	Inhibits glutamate receptors of the NMDA subtype	1	17
Conopressin	Agonist of vasopressin receptor	1	9
Miscellaneous[a]	Unknown	4	16 - 34

[a] Many other peptides have been detected but not yet isolated from the venom.

All the α-conotoxins so far isolated from the venom of *C. geographus* and *C. magus* are active on mammalian systems but two of three α-conotoxins obtained from *C. striatus* are much less active in mice than in fish[23,24]. This is probably one of the reasons why there are more human fatalities from *C. geographus* than from *C. striatus* in spite of their similar size.

In comparing the venom of different *Conus* species, it has become clear that the cones utilize many variations of the overall strategy of synergistically acting toxins. For example, the venom of *C. magus* and *C. striatus* have been found to contain α- and ω-conotoxins but μ-conotoxins have not yet been isolated from their venoms. Instead, both species appear to contain peptides which cause repetitive firing in neuromuscular preparations[25].

In addition to the neuroactive peptides, *Conus* venoms contain other components such as hydrolytic enzymes[26,30] and toxic proteins[31-38]. Low molecular weight non-peptide biologically active components have been found in venom from some species: 5-

hydroxytryptamine [39] and a cholinomimetic compound suspected to be an alkaloid [40, 41] in *C. californicus*, arachidonic acid in *C. textile* [42], quaternary ammonium compounds such as homomarine, g-butyrobetaine and N-methyl-pyridinium in 5 species [20], and serotonin from *C. imperialis* (the imperial cone) [43].

The venom apparatus (see Figure 2) consists of a long convoluted venom duct which starts from the muscular venom bulb to the anterior portion of the oesophagus. The venom is synthesized by cells lining the lumen of the duct and it is injected into the prey through the hollow disposable radula tooth positioned at the end of the extensible proboscis. Cytological data suggest that final processing of the venom might take place as the venom goes through the proboscis [44]. The venom extracted directly from the venom duct is usually milky whereas injected venom is usually clear; recent evidence indicates a difference in the composition of the extracted and injected venom [45]. This may explain the discrepancy between the reported human lethalities due to the stings of mollusc-hunting species and the observed ineffectiveness of the extracted venom when injected intraperitoneally in mice [44].

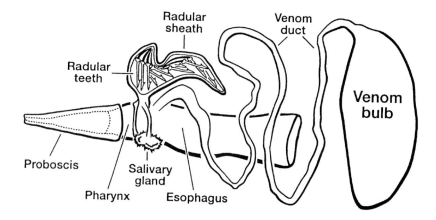

Figure 2. Diagram of the venom apparatus of *Conus* species. The venom is synthesized in the duct. When the cone is ready to sting, one of the disposable harpoons from the radular sac is positioned at the tip of the proboscis. Contraction of the venom bulb pushes the venom from the duct through the proboscis and hollow harpoon to the victim.

C. ENVENOMATIONS

Man's encounters with marine cones are mostly in connection with gathering them for food, shell craft and shell collections. On account of the varied colors and patterns on their beautiful shells, the *Conus* species are a favorite among collectors, and the rarer ones like *Conus gloriamaris* (the glory-of-the-sea cone) and *Conus cedonulli* (the matchless cone) have commanded high prices. The more common ones, especially those found in the intertidal region, are eaten by people living in fishing villages in many islands of the Indo-Pacific region. A combination of man's appreciation for beautiful shells and his relative ignorance of the venomous nature of *Conus* species has led to careless handling of these snails. Table 2 gives a list of species which have reportedly stung humans. Since the first case of stinging was recorded in the literature, more than 70 cases including ~26 human fatalities have been reported [7-12, 21, 46,47].

Most stinging cases have occurred in the western and central Pacific areas. Even though the statistics are not impressive and cone snails do not present a public health problem, a sting can be very severe, even deadly. In the 1984 report of Yoshiba[12], he estimated a worldwide fatality rate of 38% for all reported *Conus* stings and a 66.7% fatality rate for *C.*

geographus sting cases. However, as with most envenomations, mild cases are generally not reported and the actual rate is probably substantially lower.

Compared to envenomation by other venomous animals, *Conus* sting cases are quite rare. Cone snails are generally shy animals and tend to retract into their shells when disturbed. Their venom apparatus is used mainly for catching prey but under certain circumstances, they can be provoked to sting defensively. Reports of stinging of humans by cones have occurred under the following circumstances: the shell was scraped with a knife to remove the periostracum and examine its pattern[9,48], the cone was held for a long time or kept in a pocket or basket touching the body [21,49], the animal was handled after the shell was broken[7], the cone was disturbed in its natural habitat and picked up or unknowingly touched while picking up some other organisms [26,50]. High risk situations include prolonged handling, destruction of the shell, and disturbance of the cone in its natural habitat.

Table 2
Conus species reported to have stung humans

Type	Species	Prey Preference	Shell Length mm
Species responsible for confirmed fatalities	*C. geographus*	Fish	70-153
	C. textile	Mollusc	40-129
	C. marmoreus	Mollusc	50-150
Species suspected of causing fatalities	*C. striatus*	Fish	60-130
	C. gloriamaris	Mollusc	75-147
Species responsible for severe envenomations	*C. omaria*	Mollusc	35-85
	C. tulipa	Fish	30-84
Species responsible for other sting cases	*C. aulicus*	Mollusc	70-162
	C. catus	Fish	25-50
	C. ermineus	Fish	30-70
	C. imperialis	Marine worm	40-105
	C. leopardus	Marine worm	75-222
	C. litteratus	Marine worm	75-150
	C. lividus	Marine worm	30-81
	C. magus	Fish	40-75
	C. nanus/ sponsalis	Marine worm	15-32
	C. obscurus	Fish	20-41
	C. pennaceus	Mollusc	30-85
	C. pulicarius	Marine worm	30-75
	C. quercinus	Marine worm	50-144

The list is based on stinging cases reported in the literature[7-12] and on unpublished reports[47] from the Philippines. The shell lengths of adult specimens were obtained from Walls[3].

III. SYMPTOMS AND SIGNS

A. INITIAL SENSATION OF STING

The sting of cones is generally felt with a sharp intense pain as reported for *C. geographus* [7,9,51], *C. ermineus* [53], and *C. striatus* (striated cone)[50]; it has been described as "not unlike the sting of a wasp" for *C. tulipa* (tulip cone)[7-9] and similar to that "produced by the burning of phosphorus under the skin" for *C. aulicus* (the court cone)[7-9]. This is immediately followed by numbness of the stung portion of the body, usually a hand or finger. There are a couple of cases where immediate numbness and no sharp pain were reported[7-9,48] and in one report, the victim was not aware of being stung[49].

B. SYMPTOMS PRODUCED BY STINGS OF FISH-HUNTING *Conus* SPECIES

In *C. geographus* stings, the development of symptoms is relatively rapid [27-29, 48]. The immediate numbness around the site of stinging spreads rapidly upwards to the rest of the extremity then to the shoulder, throat and lips; within 30 min partial paralysis and difficulty in speaking may develop. The victim feels faint and numbness spreads thoughout the body. In very severe cases, this is followed by a progression of symptoms - from inability to speak, blurring of vision with diplopia, paralysis of most voluntary muscles, cyanosis then unconsciousness within an hour. In less severe cases, there is general muscle weakness, ataxia, diminished reflexes, slurred speech, difficulty in swallowing and breathing. Depending on the severity of the case, coma followed by death may occur in 40 min to 5 hr. Respiratory failure due to paralysis of the diaphragm muscle is believed to be the cause of death [19, 49].

The very rapid onset of signs of paralysis in victims of *Conus geographus* envenomation compared to that in Elapidae snakebite victims (2 to 3 hours after the bite[53]) is probably due mainly to the difference in size of their neurotoxins. Conotoxins generally consist of 13 to 30 amino acids whereas snake neurotoxins have about 60 to 70 amino acids (post-synaptic) or substantially larger, sometimes with subunits (pre-synaptic). Conotoxins are also more tightly folded with an average of one disulfide bridge for every 6 to 10 amino acids compared to one disulfide bridge per about 15 amino acids in snake postsynaptic neurotoxins[16,54]. The small and tightly folded structure of conotoxins can therefore be more rapidly transported from the site of injection to the toxin target site. In addition, *Conus* venom contains many other peptides some of which like conopressin-S and conopressin-G have been suggested[55] to act as accessory peptides in facilitating dispersal of the major toxins.

In those who survive a *C. geographus* sting, general numbness and muscular weakness may persist for a few days and numbness at the sting site may persist much longer. In isolated cases, nausea, vomiting, dizziness and fever were also observed[7-9].

Very few detailed reports on stings by other fish-hunting *Conus* species are available. *C. striatus* was listed by Caras[10] as one of the species responsible for human fatality but no details were given. The only other account of a sting by this species involves a woman from Fiji who experienced slight swelling and intense pain in the stung finger[50]. She felt very faint. A serous blister, which later became a blood blister, developed at the site of sting. In about 2 hours, the stung finger tip was still painful when pressed, but numb otherwise. The finger was still numb after a week and remained numb for "a long time".

The single available report on *C. tulipa* [8], which is closely related to *C. geographus*, indicated immediate numbness of the hand. When examined by a doctor at 25 min, the patient appeared drowsy, pale and clammy. There was excessive salivation, weak movements of the left wrist and fingers with complete numbness of the left hand and distal left forearm. The victim complained of chest constriction which disappeared on injection of antihistamine and adrenaline but the other symptoms remained unchanged in 4 hours. The patient gradually recovered with movement returning to two fingers in two days but the remaining fingers remained numb for 2 weeks. Complete recovery took 3 months.

In the report on a sting by *C. ermineus* (turtle cone), a fish-hunting species from the Atlantic[52], "discrete paresthesia in the left hand, from fingers along arm to the shoulder" and "discrete thermohypoesthesia in the anterior-external side of left forearm" were felt in 5 to 30 min. The case was relatively mild and the symptoms regressed after 45 min but localized pain at the site of puncture lasted for 24 hours.

The symptoms produced by the smaller fish-hunters are comparatively mild. *Conus magus* produced numbness and swelling of the stung extremity whereas the tiny *C. obscurus* (obscure cone) produced redness, soreness and swelling[8,9].

C. SYMPTOMS PRODUCED BY STINGS OF MOLLUSC-HUNTING *Conus* SPECIES

Among the mollusc-hunters, *C. textile* has reputedly caused several human fatalities. Two of the 6 reported lethal cases turned out to be due to *C. geographus* and two are from undocumented reports but two lethalities appear to be certainly due to *C. textile*[7-9, 21]. The first case was that reported by Rumphius in 1705[8] and the second one is a recent unpublished report from Tawi-Tawi, Philippines[21]. The progression of symptoms was much slower than for *C. geographus* and, with medical attention, the fatal outcome probably could have been avoided in the Tawi-Tawi case. The symptoms reported include numbness of the hand in 25 min and its paralysis in 9 hours. The victim became very weak and had little appetite. He died after a couple of days without receiving any medical treatment. In this case, the snail was initially referred to by the victim's relative as *C. gloriamaris* but later identified as *C. textile*. A case of a fatal *C. gloriamaris* sting in Cebu, Philippines has come to our attention but this has not yet been verified.

In the milder cases of *C. textile* stings, numbness and swelling of the stung extremity were generally observed[7-9, 47]. In the one case reported from Hawaii[56], the symptoms included immediate shortness of breath, severe headache in 15 min, severe stomach cramps in 9 hours and extreme nausea up to 12 hours. The victim recovered on the following day except for localized pain at the site of puncture.

Two lethalities from *C. marmoreus* stings in the Philippines have come to our attention but only one has been documented [21, 47]. The progression of symptoms was also much slower than that for *C. geographus* with numbness and paralysis of the leg developing after 7 hours. The victim felt very weak and had little appetite. He developed a fever and died after 3 days. The sting case occurred in one of the remote islands of Tawi-Tawi where no medical service was available.

A relatively severe case of *C. omaria* envenomation in an 8-year old girl was reported from Hawaii [56, 57]. The following symptoms developed during the first 2 hours: slurred speech, shallow breathing, absence of reflexes in lower legs, arms and neck, and increased heart rate. Eventually there was complete paralysis of the respiratory muscles. With artificial respiration, the victim recovered and regained consciousness after 2 hours; she completely recovered after about 20 hours.

D. SYMPTOMS PRODUCED BY OTHER *Conus* SPECIES
No lethality has ever been reported from a sting by a worm-hunting species[7,8]. Symptoms described are mild and generally include severe and sharp pain which disappears in about two hours.

E. FACTORS AFFECTING THE SEVERITY OF ENVENOMATION
The severity of envenomation produced by a particular *Conus* species is influenced by a number of factors such as potency of its venom, size of the animal, size of its venom duct and size of the radula. *C. geographus,* the species responsible for most human fatalities, is the largest fish-hunting *Conus* species. *C. magus*, another fish-hunter, has an equally toxic venom but stings by this species have produced only mild symptoms. Since it is a smaller species (see Table 2) and its venom duct is comparatively short and thin for its shell size, it is not capable of injecting enough venom to produce severe effects in man. On the other hand, *C. geographus* has a large venom apparatus, and a relatively long radula (~1.2 cm for a 10 cm shell, a 1:8 ratio[8]), which can penetrate deeper and inject more venom into the victim. *C. textile,* a mollusc-hunting species responsible for a couple of deaths, is also a relatively large species with a large venom duct and long radula (1:8 ratio of radula length to shell length[8]). The other two species reputed to have caused fatalities are the fish-hunting *C. striatus* and the mollusc-hunting *C. marmoreus*; both species can be about as large as *C. geographus*. As for the worm-hunters, although some species can be very big, their venom ducts are generally quite small and their toxins are not very effective on mammals.

For the victim, age and physical condition can greatly influence the severity of resulting symptoms. As in the case of the *C. omaria* stinging an 8-year-old girl, the symptoms were very severe despite *C. omaria* being a relatively small mollusc-hunting species.

IV. PROPHYLAXIS

A. PREVENTION OF *Conus* STINGS
Conus stings can be avoided by proper handling of the animal. To avoid stings, the animal must first be disturbed with a long tool to make it retract into its shell. It should always be picked up from the broad or posterior end of the shell since the proboscis and harpoon come out of the aperture from its anterior end. The proboscis is very extensible and may reach within striking distance of the hand holding the shell. When handling the animal, it should be released as soon as the proboscis comes out of the rostrum. Cones should never be placed on the palm of the hand and never held longer than necessary. They should not be stored in pockets or in bags and baskets touching the body. A cone found partially buried under the sand or hidden in a crevice should be completely exposed by digging it out and disturbed with a long tool until the animal retracts into its shell before it is picked up.

B. PUBLIC EDUCATION
Since reported cases of stings are quite rare, many people are unaware of the danger of handling *Conus* species. Information about the cones should be included in leaflets regarding poisonous and venomous marine animals for distribution to the general public in seaside resorts and fishing villages.

V. FIRST AID TREATMENT OF *Conus* STINGS

In devising a first aid treatment for *Conus* envenomation, the primary consideration should be the prevention of toxin transport from the injection site, particularly since conotoxins act very rapidly. The stung extremity should immediately be cooled and kept lower than the heart to prevent further spreading of the toxin to other parts of the body and the patient should be kept still until medical help becomes available. The "pressure immobilization bandage" suggested for snakebites[53] will probably be effective also for *Conus* sting cases, and is our recommendation for first aid (see chapter on Australian snakebite for further discussion and method). In published reports, measures such as forcing the tiny puncture to bleed[50] and application of torniquet have been used[7-9, 56], but are not recommended. Since tissue necrosis does not seem to be a problem in *Conus* stings, a properly applied tourniquet might theoretically be helpful. However, experience with snakebite has shown that tourniquets used as first aid by non-medical personel can and do result in significant iatrogenic injury; hence, they cannot be recommended as routine first aid in envenoming. As with any poisoning potentially causing respiratory failure, maintenance of vital functions will always take precedence in first aid management. Expired air (mouth to mouth) ventilation of the patient may well be lifesaving. The other paralytic problem of oropharyngeal muscle paresis leading to the risk of aspiration of vomitus must be remembered and the airway secured with the patient nursed on their side.

VI. CLINICAL MANAGEMENT

Conus envenomation, particularly if the responsible species is *Conus geographus* or an unidentified species, should be treated as a life threatening emergency. Due to the usual intense pain associated with the sting, the patients are generally aware of what has happened. However, there was a report in which the patient was unaware of being stung[49];

in such an instance, a description of the patient's activities immediately before the symptoms appear would be helpful. The puncture mark is very tiny and may be difficult to discern on presentation of the patient at the hospital. Immediate numbness of the stung extremity appears to be a common symptom[7-9, 46, 49-52, 56].

The onset of paralysis is very rapid and the greatest danger is from respiratory failure due to respiratory muscle paralysis or aspiration secondary to oropharyngeal muscle paresis. Oxygen should be given as soon as the victim shows the initial signs of paralysis and artificial respiration administered with the first signs of respiratory difficulty, preferably by intubation and ventilation. As this may require both formal paralysis and sedation, it is important that the extent of venom induced paralysis and depression of CNS function be fully documented prior to such intervention. Assisted ventilation may only be needed for a short period, up to several hours, rarely longer. There is no specific antidote or antivenom. The role of anticholinesterases is uncertain, though edrophonium has been recommended, based on limited experience with tetrodotoxin poisoning. The patient could be given the Tensilon test, and if responsive, edrophonium or neostigmine could be tried. Analgesics, glucocorticoids and antihistamines have been given to victims to alleviate local pain and possible allergic reactions; however, their role is uncertain [77-79, 46, 49-52, 56]. Antibiotics have been administered also in a few cases to prevent infection at the sting site[50]. As with any penetrating wound, tetanus prophylaxis should be ensured. As there is penetration of the radula there is potential for a portion to be embedded in the wound, causing a foreign body reaction and acting as a focus for infection; therefore, all cone shell wounds, irrespective of systemic envenoming, should be inspected carefully for remaining portions of the radula tooth, which should be removed promptly if found.

Acknowledgement: Support for the *Conus* project in the Philippines was provided by the National Research Council of the Philippines, the Marine Science Institute, University of the Philippines, Diliman, and the International Foundation for Science, Stockholm, Sweden.

VII. REFERENCES

1. **KOHN, A. J.**, Tempo and mode of evolution of Conidae, *Malacologia*, 32, 55, 1990.
2. **KOHN, A. J.**, The ecology of *Conus* in Hawaii, *Ecol. Monogr.*, 29,47, 1959.
3. **WALLS, J. G.**, *Cone shells*, T. F. H. Publications Inc. Ltd., HongKong/Singapore, 1979, 1011.
4. **SPRINGSTEEN, F. J. AND LEOBRERA, F.** M., *Shells of the Philippines*, Carfel Shell Museum, Manila, Philippines, 1986, 219.
5. **KOHN, A. J.**, Microhabitat factors affecting abundance and diversity of *Conus* on coral reefs, *Oecologia (Berlin)*, 60, 293, 1983.
6. **KOHN, A. J. AND NYBAKKEN, J.** W., Ecology of *Conus* on Eastern Indian Ocean fringing reefs: Diversity of species and resource utilization, *Int. J. on Life in Oceans and Coastal Waters*, 29, 211, 1975.
7. **CLENCH, W. J. AND KONDO, Y.**, The poison cone shell, *Amer. J. Trop. Med.*, 23, 105, 1943.
8. **KOHN, A. J.**, Venomous marine snails of the genus *Conus*, in *Venomous and Poisonous Animals and Noxious Plants in the Pacific Region*, H. C. Keegan and W. V. McFarlane, Eds., Pergamon Press, Oxford, 1963, 83.
9. **MCMICHAEL, D. F.**, Mollusks - classification, distribution, venom apparatus and venoms, symptomatology of stings, in*Venomous Animals and Their Venoms.*Vol. III, W. Bucherl and E. E. Buckley, Eds., Academic Press, London, 1971, Chap. 3.
10. **CARAS, R.**, *Venomous Animals of the World*, Prentice Hall, Inc., New Jersey, 1974, 29.
11. **OLIVERA, B. M.**, Interview of E. Zambo, *Carfel Philippine Shell News*, Jul-Aug, 6, 1979.
12. **YOSHIBA, S.**, An estimation of the most dangerous species of cone shell *Conus geographus* venoms lethal dose in humans. *Jap. J. Hygiene*, 39, 565, 1984.
13. **CRUZ, L. J., GRAY. W. R. AND OLIVERA, B. M.**, *Conus* venoms: a rich source of neuroactive peptides, *J. Toxicology-Toxin Reviews*, 4, 107, 1985.
14. **GRAY, W. R., OLIVERA, B. M. AND CRUZ, L. J.**, Peptide toxins from venomous *Conus* snails, *Annu. Rev. Biochem.*, 57, 665, 1988.
15. **OLIVERA, B. M., GRAY, W. R., ZEIKUS, R., MCINTOSH, J. M., VARGA, J., RIVIER, J., DE SANTOS, V. AND CRUZ, L. J.**, Peptide neurotoxins from fish-hunting cone snails, *Science*, 230, 1338, 1985.

16. **OLIVERA, B. M., RIVIER, J., CLARK, C., RAMILO, C. A., CORPUZ, G. P., ABOGADIE, F. C., MENA, E. E., WOODWARD, S. R., HILLYARD, D. R., AND CRUZ, L. J.,** Diversity of *Conus* neuropeptides, *Science*, 249, 257, 1990.

17. **OLIVERA , B. M., RIVIER, J., SCOTT, J. K., HILLYARD, D. R., AND CRUZ, L. J.,** Conotoxins, *J. Biol. Chem.*, 266, 22067, 1991.

18. **WHYTE, J. M. AND ENDEAN, R.,** Pharmacological investigation of the venoms of the marine snail *Conus textile* and *Conus geographus, Toxicon*, 1, 25, 1962.

19. **ENDEAN, R. AND RUDKIN, C.,** Studies of some venom of Conidae, *Toxicon*, 1, 49, 1963.

20. **KOHN, A. J., SAUNDERS, P. R. AND WIENER, S.,** Preliminary studies on the venom of the marine snail *Conus, Ann. N.Y. Acad. Sci.*, 90, 706, 1960.

21. **SABAL, R. AND ROMERO, J.,** unpublished report, 1992.

22. **OLIVERA, B. M., MCINTOSH, J. M., CRUZ, L. J., LUQUE, F. A. AND GRAY, W. R.,** Purification and sequence of a presynaptic peptide toxin from *Conus geographus* venom, *Biochemistry,* 23, 5087, 1984.

23. **ZAFARALLA, G. C., RAMILO, C., GRAY, W. R., KARLSTROM, R., OLIVERA, B. M., AND CRUZ, L. J.,** Phylogenetic specificity of cholinergic ligands: a-conotoxin SI, *Biochemistry*, 27, 7102, 1988.

24. **RAMILO, C. A., ZAFARALLA, G. C., NADASDI, L., HAMMERLAND, L. G., YOSHIKAMI, D., GRAY, W. R., KRISTAPATI, R., RAMACHANDRAN, J., MILJANICH, G., OLIVERA, B. M., AND CRUZ, L. J.,** Novel a- and w-conotoxins from *Conus striatus* venom, *Biochemistry*, 31, 9919, 1992.

25. **YOSHIKAMI, D.,** unpublished data, 1990.

26. **MARSH, H.,** The radular apparatus of *Conus, J. Moll. Stud.*, 43, 1, 1977.

27. **PALI, E. S., TANGCO, O. M. AND CRUZ, L. J.,** The venom duct of *Conus geographus*: Some biochemical and histologic studies, *Bull. Phil. Biochem. Soc.*, 2, 30, 1979.

28. **JIMENEZ, E. C., OLIVERA, B. M. AND CRUZ, L. J,** Localization of enzymes and possible toxin precursors in granules form *Conus striatus* venom, *Toxicon supplement*, 3, 199, 1983.

29. **BALBIN-ROMERO, B. J. AND CRUZ, L. J.,** Acetylcholinesterase of *Conus geographus* venom: partial purification and characterization, *Acta Medica Philipp.*, 23, 79, 1987.

30. **MIRANDA, R .R.,** *Partial purification and characterization of* Conus textile *venom phosphodiesterase I*, M.S. Thesis (Biochemistry), College of Medicine, Univ. of the Philippines, Manila, 1982.

31. **CLARK, C., OLIVERA, B. M. AND CRUZ, L. J.,** A toxin from *Conus geographus* venom which acts on the vertebrate central nervous system, *Toxicon* , 19, 691, 1981.

32. **KOBAYASHI, J., NAKAMURA, H., HIRATA, Y. AND OHIZUMI, Y.,** Isolation of a cardiotonic glycoprotein, striatoxin, from the venom of the marine snail *Conus striatus, Biochem. Biophys. Res. Commun.*, 105, 1389, 1982.3

33. **KOBAYASHI, J., NAKAMURA, H. AND OHIZUMI, Y.,** Tessulatoxin, the vasoactive protein from the venom of the marine snail *Conus tessulatus, Comp. Biochem. Physiol.*, 74B, 381, 1983.

34. **SCHEITZ, H., RENAUD, J. F., RANDIMBIVOLOLOA, N., PREAU, C., SCHMID, A., ROMEY, G., RAKOTOVAO, L. AND LAZDUNSKI, M.,** Purification, subunit structure and pharmacological effects on cardiac and smooth muscle cells of a polypeptide toxin isolated from the marine snail *Conus tessulatus, Eur. J. Biochem.*, 161, 787, 1986.

35. **KOBAYASHI, J., NAKAMURA, H, HIRATA, Y. AND OHIZUMI, Y.,** Isolation of eburnetoxin, a vasoactive substance from the *Conus eburneus* venom, *Life Sci.*, 31, 1085, 1982.

36. **KOBAYASHI, J., NAKAMURA, H. AND OHIZUMI, Y.,** Potent excitatory effects of a cardiotonic protein from the venom of the marine snail *Conus magus* on the guinea-pig left atria, vas deferens and ileum, *Toxicon*, 23, 783, 1985.

37. **WHYSNER, J.A. AND SAUNDERS, P. R.,** Studies on the venom of the marine snail *Conus californicus, Toxicon,* 1, 113, 1963.

38. **WHYSNER, J. Z. AND SAUNDERS, P. R.,** Purification of the lethal fraction of the venom of the marine snail *Conus californicus, Toxicon*, 4, 177, 1965.

39. **COTTRELL, G. A. AND TWAROG, B. M.,** Active factors in the venom duct of *Conus californicus, Br. J. Pharmac.*, 44, 365P, 1972.

40. **ELLIOTT, E. J.,** Cholinergic response in the heart of the clam *Mercenaria mercenaria*: Activation by *Conus californicus* venom component, *J. Comp. Physiol.*, 129, 61, 1979.

41. **ELLIOTT, E. J. AND KEHOE, J.,** Cholinergic receptor in aplysia neurons: Activation by a venom component from the marine snail *Conus californicus, Brain Res.*, 156, 387, 1978.

42. **NAKAMURA, H., KOBAYASHI, J., OHIZUMI, Y. AND HIRATA, Y.,** The occurrence of arachidonic acid in the venom duct of the marine snail *Conus textile, Experientia*, 38, 897, 1982.

43. **MCINTOSH, J. M., FODERARO, T. A., LI, W., IRELAND, C. M., AND OLIVERA, B. M.,** Presence of serotonin in the venom of *Conus imperialis, Toxicon*, (in press).

44. **OLIVERA, B. M., HILLYARD, D. R., RIVIER, J., WOODWARD, S., GRAY, W. R., CORPUZ, G. P., AND CRUZ, L. J.,** Conotoxins: targeted peptide ligands from snail venoms, in *Marine Toxins - Origin, Structure, and Molecular Pharmacology*, S. Hall, G. Strichartz, Eds., ACS Symposium Series 418, 1990, Chap. 20.

45. **HOPKINS, C., ZAFARALLA, G. C., AND OLIVERA, B. M.,** unpublished data, 1989.

46. **ALCALA, A. C.**, Recent cases of crab, cone shell, and fish intoxication on southern Negros Island, Philippines, *Toxicon,* Suppl. 3, 1, 1983.

47. **CORPUZ, G. P., AND CRUZ, L. J.**, unpublished report, 1988.

48. **LYMAN, F.**, Charlie Garbutt meets tragic death, *Shell Notes*, 2, 78, 1948.

49. **RICE, R. D. AND HALSTEAD, B. W.**, Report of fatal cone shell sting by *Conus geographus* Linnaeus, *Toxicon*, 5, 223, 1968.

50. **TSURIEL, P. S.**, A *Conus striatus* sting in Fiji, *Levantina,* 15, 168, 1978.

51. **TSURIEL, P. S.**, First record of a *Conus* sting from Elat, *Levantina*, 14, 150, 1978.

52. **TSURIEL, P. S.**, A case of *Conus ermineus* sting in West Africa, *Levantina*, 18, 204, 1979.

53. **WHITE, J.**, Clinical Toxicology of snakebite in Australia and New Guinea, In Eds., J. White and J. Meier, *Clinical Toxicology of Animal Venoms and Poisons,* CRC Handbook of Toxicology Series, CRC Press, Boca Raton, Chap. 28.

54. **KARLSSON, E.**, Chemistry of protein toxins in snake venoms, in *Snake Venoms*, C.-Y., Lee, Ed., Handbook Exp. Pharmacol., 1979, vol. 52, 159.

55. **CRUZ, L. J., CORPUZ, G. P., RAMILO, C. A., ZAFARALLA, G., JOHNSON, B., LEITNER, T., YOSHIKAMI, D., AND OLIVERA, B. M.**, The biological role and pharmacological uses of conotoxins, in *Proc. 7th Asian Symposium on Medicinal, Plants, Spices and Other Natural Products*, L. J. Cruz, G. P. Concepcion, M. A. Mendigo, and B. Q. Guevara, Eds., ASOMPS VII Nat. Org. Com., Marine Sci. Inst., Univ. Philippines 1992, 90.

56. **KOHN, A. J.**, Cone shell stings, *Hawaii Medical J.*, 17, 528 (1958).

57. **PETRAUSKAS, L. E.**, A case of cone shell poisoning by "bite" in Manus Island, *Papua & New Guinea Med. J.*, 1953, 1, 67.

Chapter 10

CLINICAL TOXICOLOGY OF SEA URCHIN AND STARFISH INJURIES

Dietrich Mebs

TABLE OF CONTENTS

I. INTRODUCTION

Sea urchins (class: Echinoidea) and starfishes (Asteroidea) belong to the animal phylum Echinodermata which also include brittle stars (Ophiuroidea) and the sea cucumbers (Holothuroidea). These marine animals are characterized by their radial symmetry and by the calcareous skeleton and plates which form the thick body wall. Spines, spicules or pedicellariae are used for defense or, as in the latter case, also for prey capture.

Although most echinoderms are poisonous, containing a variety of toxic substances in their body such as steroid glycosides or terpenes[1], only a few are able to cause injuries or envenoming symptoms in humans; namely one starfish, the crown-of-thorns starfish *Acanthaster planci* and various sea urchin species[2].

II. EPIDEMIOLOGY OF INJURIES AND ENVENOMING

Generally echinoderms are slow moving, non-aggressive animals. Beach walkers, swimmers, snorklers and divers are at risk of injury by spines of sea urchins or the crown-of-thorns starfish by stepping on them or by careless handling of these animals. Although accidents occur very often along tropical and subtropical beaches, serious consequences or envenoming are rather rare[2]. In most cases patients ask the physician to remove broken spines which penetrated the skin. Injuries by echinoderms are not a public health problem.

III. MEDICALLY IMPORTANT ECHINODERMS

A. BIOLOGY AND DISTRIBUTION

The crown-of-thorns starfish, *Acanthaster planci,* is of relatively large size (up to 40 cm diameter) and possesses 7 to 23 arms. Its aboral (dorsal) surface is covered by series of sharp spines. The starfish inhabits the coral reefs of the Indo-Pacific, usually in a low population density (2 to 3 specimen per km^2). However, because of still unknown reasons it may occur in mass-population, as happened twice in the Great-Barrier-Reef of Australia during the last 25 years. As it feeds on the living corals, such events often lead to severe damage of the affected reef[3].

Sea urchins have a mainly globular, sometimes flattened body shape. Numerous short or long spines articulate on the calcareous plates which form the body shell. Pedicellariae are situated between the spines. These organs are used in defense or to procure food. Sea urchins are common in all oceans and live in shallow waters as well as in the deep sea.

Most of these echinoderms have a nocturnal activity cycle; however, they are also found during the day.

B. VENOM APPARATUS

The sharp calcareous spines of *Acanthaster planci* are covered by integument which contains numerous venom-producing glandular cells[2]. When penetrating the skin either the epidermis is removed or the spines break off and both remain embedded in the wound.

Sea urchins possess two types of venom apparatus: spines and pedicellariae[2]. Although most spines are solid and do not constitute a venom organ, others such as those of *Diadema* urchins are long (up to 30 cm), sharp, hollow and have a rough surface (Figure 1). They easily break off in the wound and release a bluish liquid, which is believed to be venomous. The short spines of the leather urchins (*Asthenosoma, Areosoma, Phormosoma* species) possess a venom organ at the tip which is composed of muscular and connective tissue enclosing a venom sac (Figure 2). Epithelial cells appear to secrete a venom which is stored in the sac and released when squeezing the sac[2].

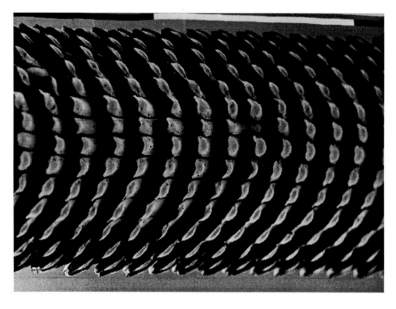

Figure 1. Spine of *Diadema* sea urchin (SEM picture; white bar represents 1mm) (courtesy of Dr. J. Meier, Basel).

Pedicellariae are small delicate organs which consist of two parts, a thin stalk with a terminal head (Figure 2). Two to four (but most often three) pincer-like calcareous valves or jaws are covered by venom-producing glandular tissue. Venom ducts empty near the fang-like tip of the valves. Muscles move the valves which act as pincers seizing prey when touching the pedicellariae. Venom is injected and the prey is paralyzed. Pedicellariae of most sea urchins are not able to penetrate the human skin; however, those of some species (*Toxopneustes* sp.) are extraordinarily large and able to inject venom even through human skin[2].

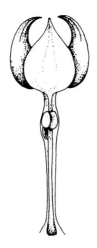 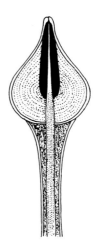

Figure 2. Sea urchin pedicellaria (left), globiferous type, showing the head, which consists of three calcareous valves attached to the supporting stalk. Diagrammatic presentation of the tip of an aboral spine (right) of a leather sea urchin (*Asthenosoma*). The venom sac (black) is completely encased with a sheath of muscle and connective tissue (modified from [2]).

C. VENOM: CHEMISTRY AND PHARMACOLOGY

The mucous secretion from the glandular epithelium of the spines of *Acanthaster planci* is venomous and of protein nature. It causes edema and local necrosis; myotoxicity seen in experimental animals is due to phospholipase A_2 activity of the venom[4,5]. A toxin lethal to mice was isolated and characterized as a glycoprotein of 25 kDa [6]. The steroid glycosides (thornasterosid) present in high concentration in the starfish body are obviously not involved in envenoming.

Data on sea urchin venoms are scarce. The aqueous blue content of *Diadema* spines causes an increase of blood pressure in experimental animals. The presence of noradrenaline has been suggested[7]. The chemical nature of the very painful venom of leather urchins is unknown. Basic proteins lethal to mice, of 20 and 25 kDa molecular weight respectively, have been isolated from pedicellariae of *Toxopneustes pileolus* and of *Tripneustes gratilla* [8,9].

IV. CLINICAL SIGNS AND SYMPTOMS

Contact with the spines of *Acanthaster planci* which deeply penetrate skin and muscle layers (several centimeters) cause severe pain lasting one or two hours. A slight edema develops around the site of injury and nausea and vomiting may also occur[2,10]. In some cases circulatory problems have been reported. The spines easily break off and remain embedded in the skin where they initiate inflammation and granuloma tissue formation if they are not removed.

Injuries by the long spines of *Diadema* urchins also produce burning pain[2]. The fragments of the broken spines which are not absorbed may cause discomfort for weeks. They are difficult to remove from the skin because of their rough surface. Immediate pain which can be excruciating is the result of even slight contact with leather sea urchins. However, the pain disappears within 20 to 30 minutes followed by numbness of the body part affected.

The pincing pedicellariae of *Toxopneustes* sea urchins still hang on the skin even when the sea urchin has been removed, and venom is continuously injected. This causes severe pain which decreases in intensity gradually after 15 minutes, but paralytic symptoms may also develop involving facial muscles, tongue and eyelids[2]. Although pain usually disappears after one hour, facial paralysis may continue for several hours. Death of a female pearl diver has been reported who became unconscious after an accidental contact with the urchin and drowned[11].

V. PROPHYLAXIS

Most injuries caused by the crown-of-thorns starfish and by sea urchins occur by stepping on them. Wading in bare feet in turbid waters, especially at night, should be avoided. Sneakers provide some protection; however, even the sole may be penetrated by the sharp spines. Do not handle the crown-of-thorns starfish with unprotected hands, use thick gloves; this also applies to most sea urchin species, especially *Toxopneustes pileolus*.

VI. FIRST AID TREATMENT

Leaving the water immediately and removal of the broken spines or of the pedicellariae still hanging on the skin by forceps are the main first aid treatment recommended. Bathing the wound area in hot water is not effective and not recommended. Do not press or pound the wound area to crush the spine into smaller fragments.

VII. CLINICAL MANAGEMENT

Most injuries caused by echinoderms do not need medical attention except when broken spines have to be removed from wounds. Probing the spine puncture or even X-raying gives an idea whether or not spine fragments remain. If those embedded fragments are not removable by forceps, a small incision may be necessary for surgical exploration, especially if spines have penetrated joint capsules. Otherwise the spine fragments cause inflammation, are encapsulated and granuloma tissue will develop during the wound healing process.

The wound area should be cleaned. Infections are rare. Pain, which is mostly of short duration and tolerable, may be treated by local anesthetics (lidocaine) or oral or parenteral analgesia. Corticosteroids are of no value. General symptoms are rarely due to envenoming, but are either caused by systemic reaction to pain or anxiety reactions and should be treated accordingly. Sedation of the patient e.g. by benzodiazepines may be useful. Tetanus prophylaxis, if indicated.

VIII. REFERENCES

1. **KREBS, H.C.** Recent development in the field of marine natural products with emphasis on biologically active compounds. *Prog.Chem.Organic Natural Prod.* **49**:151-363, 1986.
2. **HALSTEAD, B.W.** *Poisonous and Venomous Marine Animals of the World* (2nd rev.ed.). Princeton, Darwin Press Inc., 1988.
3. **MORAN, P.J.** *Acanthaster planci* (L.): biogeographical data. *Coral Reefs* **9**:95-96, 1990.

4. **SHIOMI, K., ITOH, K., YAMANAKA, H. & KIKUCHI, T.** Biological activity of crude venom from the crown-of-thorns starfish *Acanthaster planci*. *Bull.Jap.Soc.Sci.Fisheries* **51**:1151-1154, 1985.

5. **MEBS, D.** A myotoxic phospholipase A_2 from the crown of thorns starfish *Acanthaster planci*. *Toxicon* **29**:289, 1991.

6. **SHIOMI, K., YAMAMOTO, S., YAMANAKA, H. & KIKUCHI, T.** Purification and characterization of a lethal factor in venom of the crown-of-thorns starfish (*Acanthaster planci*). *Toxicon* **26**:1077- 1083, 1988.

7. **ALENDER, C.B.** A biologically active substance from spines of two diadematid sea urchins. In: *Animal Toxins* (F.E.Russell & P.R.Saunders, eds.) p.145-155, Oxford:Pergamon Press, 1967.

8. **NAKAGAWA, H. & KIMURA, A.** Partial purification of a toxic substance from pedicellariae of the sea urchin *Toxopneustes pileolus*. *Jap.J.Pharmac.* **32**, 966-968, 1982.

9. **MEBS, D.** A toxin from the sea urchin *Tripneustes gratilla*. *Toxicon* **22**:306-307, 1984.

10. **SUTHERLAND, S.K.** *Australian Animal Toxins*. Melbourne:Oxford Univ.Press, 1983.

11. **HASHIMOTO, Y.** *Marine toxins and their bioactive marine metabolites*. Tokyo:Jap.Sci.Societies Press, 1979.

Chapter 11

CLINICAL TOXICOLOGY OF VENOMOUS STINGRAY INJURIES

Chris Acott and Jürg Meier

TABLE OF CONTENTS

I. EPIDEMIOLOGY

Rays do not attack man. Accidents usually occur when bathers are wading through shallow water and accidentally step on a ray hidden in the sand or mud. The ray then quickly raises its tail like an arch as a defensive reflex exposing the spine beneath. This spine is responsible for any injury by the ray. Other accidents occur when anglers or fishermen find rays on their fishing lines or in their net. The excited animal strikes out in a defensive manner with its tail and spine.

II. BIOLOGY OF STINGRAYS

Among rays, only the stingrays can be considered dangerous to man. They are characterised by one or several stings on the back of the tail which is spread out when moving. Stingrays may be subdivided into six families, one found in fresh water (Potamotrygonidae) and five marine ones: Dasyatidae (stingrays), such as the European species *Dasyatis pastinaca* and *D. violacea*, encountered in the Atlantic, occasionally in the North and in the Mediterranean Sea; Gymnuridae, worldwide in tropical seas; Myliobatidae, world-wide, often encountered in shoals; Rhinopteridae, world-wide, also in the Mediterranean Sea; and Urolophidae, world-wide. Table 1 gives a systematic overview, and Figure 1 shows the characteristic outline of the different body forms. The smallest stingrays have a body diameter of 30 cm, often even less, while giant stingrays (some *Dasyatis* species) reach a diameter of more than 2 m and often weigh more than 300 kg.[1-3] Stingrays are present in all tropical waters and have been found at depths of 150 m. They are also found in brackish water lagoons and estuaries. Fresh water species can be found in the Amazon, Parana, Rio Magdalena and Orinoco rivers of South America, the Niger and Benoue Rivers of Africa and in the Mekong River of Laos and Vietnam.[1]

They are bottom dwellers and are usually found buried in the sand with their eyes protruding. They feed on worms, molluscs and crustaceans. When disturbed they immediately try to escape.

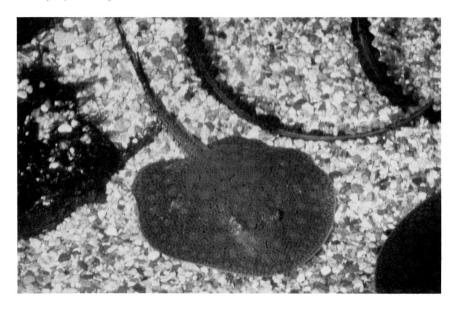

Figure 1. Freshwater stingray, *Potamotrygon* sp. (courtesy of Dr. A. Moser, Swiss Tropical Institute, Basel).

Table 1
Systematics of Venomous Stingrays (simplified according to Castex, 1967[1])

Family	Genus	Number of Species
DASYATIDAE	*Dasyatis*	30
(Sting or Whip Rays)	*Himantura*	13
	Taeniura	4
	Urogymnus	-> not venomous, lack of tail spine
GYMNURIDAE	*Gymnura*	11
(Butterfly Rays)		
MYLIOBATIDAE	*Aetobatus*	3
(Eagle Rays)	*Aetomylaeus*	4
	Myliobatis	11
	Pteromylaeus	3
POTAMOTRYGONIDAE	*Disceus*	1
(Fresh water Stingrays)	*Potamotrygon*	19
RHINOPTERIDAE	*Rhinoptera*	4
(Cow nosed Rays)		
UROLOPHIDAE	*Trygonoptera*	3
(Small Stingrays)	*Urotrygon*	8
	Urolophus	

III. VENOM APPARATUS

The stingray's venom apparatus is a striking organ (spine) on the dorsal surface of the tail. It consists of one (in some species several), serrated spine on the back part of the tail (Figure 2). These spines vary in size and development as well as in their position on the tail. Thus, in Gymnuridae for example, the spine is under developed, small and close to the root of the tail, while in the Myliobatidae, the sting is situated near the root of the tail, but is greater and more developed. The most effective are the spines of Dasyatidae and Urolophidae which are located towards the end of the tail. The ray's tail has a wide range of movement and so can cause a deep lacerated wound. The spines of big rays can reach 30 cm in length.[2,3] The two last cited ray families are the most dangerous to man.

The flat, pointed spines consist of a bone-like material (vasodentin) the edges of which are lined with recurved short barbs. On the underside of the spine are two grooves which are filled with sponge-like glandular tissue which produces the venom. These run along the length of the spine. Bone and glandular tissue are enveloped by the epidermis (Figure 3). Venom is injected into the wound by the tearing off of the glandular tissue which may also remain in the wound. Very often the spine breaks off and will also remain in the wound either entirely or in parts. Broken spines are regenerated.

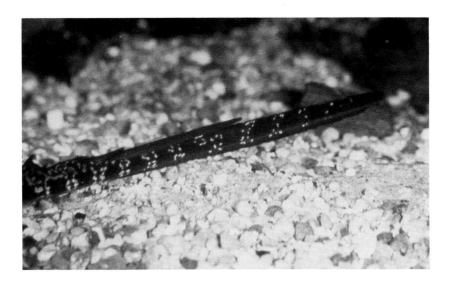

Figure 2. Detail of the tail with stinger *Potamotrygon* sp. (courtesy of Dr. A. Moser, Swiss Tropical Institute, Basel).

IV. VENOM COMPOSITION

Stingrays do not possess distinct venom glands and so extraction of the venom is difficult. This has hindered research into the effects of the venom. The venom appears to be a mixture of proteins which are heat sensitive (both to elevated and low temperatures). A great part of the venom's toxicity is lost by freeze drying. Venom extracts of *Urolophus halleri* were enzymatically active (5`-nucleotidase, phosphodiesterase, but no proteolytic activity) and showed an LD_{50} of about 28mg/kg. The venom does not block neuromuscular transmission. It may disturb cardiac and circulatory functions, probably by a direct effect on the myocardium.[4-6]

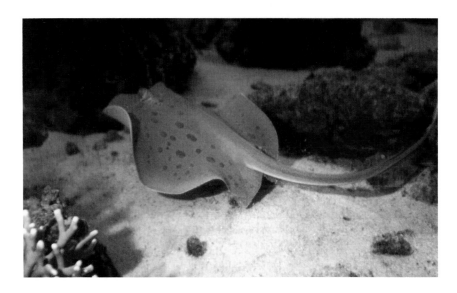

Figure 3. Blue spotted stingray (*Taeniura lymma*) in its natural habitat, the Red Sea.

V. PROPHYLAXIS

When wading in water shuffle. This will avoid treading on the stingray and it will also encourage the stingray to move out of the way. Do not run into the water or jump out of a boat into shallow water unless there is a clear view of the bottom. Beware rays concealed under sand on the bottom.

If swimming watch where your hands and feet are placed. Divers should avoid swimming close to the sea bed.

Other precautionary methods that have been used include prodding the sea bed with a stick before walking on it.

Never deliberately provoke or scare the ray; all attacks are defensive. Given adequate time and space the ray will always move out of the way.

VI. ENVENOMING AND CLINICAL SYMPTOMS AND SIGNS

Most stingray injuries are to the lower limbs. The spine may cause a deep laceration (up to 18cm long) or a penetrating puncture wound. Two deaths have been recorded in Australia due to the spine penetrating the thoracic cavity[12], and a similar accident has occurred in New Zealand.[13] Other recorded deaths and serious injury have been associated with complications of the wound (i.e. septicaemia and tetanus) due to poor wound management.[10,11] Laceration of major vessels has occurred and exsanguination is reported. Similarly there may be major injury to important structures, including vessels, nerves, tendons and muscle, or internal organs if the wound is on the trunk.

Usually at the time of injury the pain is not severe; however, over the next 30-90 minutes the pain becomes intense and can cause the victim considerable distress.[14,15] At first the wound bleeds profusely (some clinicians have wondered if there is some anticoagulant properties for the venom), but this slowly decreases and the wound becomes a bluish-grey colour.[12,14,15]

Oedema may develop in the affected limb, but this is a variable sign.

General symptoms include nausea, vomiting, syncope, salivation, muscle cramps, diarrhoea, convulsions and circulatory collapse. These symptoms are associated with severe envenoming, while severe distress due to local pain is the most common problem in all stingray injuries.[14,15]

VII. FIRST AID

Remove the victim from the water and danger. Attention to the ABC of first aid is essential. Wash the wound with sea water to remove the venom and any gland tissue present. If there is major bleeding suggesting damage to a large vessel, staunch bleeding with local pressure. Bathe the affected part in warm water (fresh if available). The stingray's venom is presumed to be heat labile, and so the aim of bathing in warm to hot water is to inactivate any venom present [2,6,14,15]. The water should be 45° - 50^OC so as not to scald the victim,[14,15] but to be hot enough to inactivate the venom. Place the contralateral limb in the water first to ensure the temperature is bearable without injury, then immerse the affected limb. Often when the water cools, or the affected limb is removed from the water, the pain returns. Reimmerse again in hot water. This process may need to be repeated several times, but after 2 hours of intermittent immersion, it is of doubtful value and should be discontinued.

Do not apply a tourniquet or use the pressure immobilisation technique.[14] Do not incise the wound or rub anything on it.[14] Do not inject any local anaesthesia into the wound, because this may spread wound contamination deeper.

VIII. CLINICAL TREATMENT

In cases where the pain is severe, hot water may only afford temporary relief, and so regional anaesthesia may be needed. Local anaesthetic (without adrenalin) can be injected around the wound edges.[15] However, in severe situations the regional techniques incorporating blocking the nerve supply to the limb may be needed [14,15] (i.e. brachial plexus block). These regional techniques not only give good analgesia, but will enable surgical exploration of the wound.

Significant wounds should be surgically explored and debrided. There may be underlying damage to major structures, including vessels, nerves, tendons or muscle, requiring appropriate immediate or delayed repair. All wounds should be considered as being potentially contaminated, and may also contain some glandular and integumentary sheath material along with necrotic tissue. Part of the spine may have also been left in the wound. Remnants of the spine may not be radio-opaque; thus X-rays may not help in localisation. Ultrasound may be useful in localising spine fragments.

Tetanus prophylaxis is an important part of the management of **any** stingray wound, minor to severe.[12,14,15]

After debridement the wound should be left open, and closed later. The patient should be reviewed over the following week to detect early evidence of developing wound infection.

Any wound that continues to be infected needs surgical exploration to remove all dead tissue and any foreign body that may have been left behind (i.e. spine). Infection equals poor wound care and debridement, with a probable retained foreign body.

IX. REFERENCES

1. **CASTEX, M.N.**, Fresh water venomous rays. In *Animal Toxins*, Russell, F.E. and Saunders, P.R., Eds., Oxford, Pergamon Press, 1967, 167.

2. **HALSTEAD, B.W.**, Venomous Fishes, In *Venomous animals and their venoms*, Vol. 2, Bucherl, W. and Buckley, E.E., Eds., New York, Academic Press, 1971, 588.

3. **HALSTEAD, B.W.**, *Poisonous and venomous animals in the world*, 2nd revised Ed., Princeton, Darwin Press, 1988.

4. **RUSSELL, F.E., AND VAN HARREFELD, A.**, Cardiovascular effects of the venom of the round stingray, *Urobatis halleri*, *Arch. Int. Physiol.*, 62, 232, 1954.

5. **RUSSELL, F.E., BARRIT, W.C., AND FAIRCHIELD, M.D.**, Electrocardiographic patterns evoked by venom of the stingray, *Proc. Soc. Exp. Biol. Med.*, 96, 634, 1957.

6. **RUSSELL, F.E., FAIRCHIELD, M.D., AND MICHAELSON, J.**, Some properties of the venom of the stingray, *Med. Arts Sci.*, 12, 78, 1958.

7. **CROSS, T.B.**, An unusual stingray injury - the skindiver at risk, *Med.J.Aust.*, 2, 947, 1976.

8. **RUSSELL, F.E.**, Injuries by venomous animals in the United States, *J.Amer.Med. Assoc.*, 177, 903, 1961.

9. **RUSSELL, F.E.**, Marine toxins and venomous and poisonous marine animals, *Adv. Mar. Biol.*, 3, 255, 1965.

10. **MARINKELLE, C.J.**, Accidents by venomous stingrays in Colombia, *Ind. Med. Surg.*, 77, 988, 1966.

11. **RUSSELL, F.E., PANOS, C.T., KANG, L.W., WARNER, W.M., AND COLKET, T.C.**, Studies on mechanisms of death from stingray venom. A report of two fatal cases, *Am. J. Med. Sci.*, 235, 566, 1958.

12. **FENNER, P.J., WILLIAMSON, J.A., AND SKINNER, R.A.**, Fatal and non-fatal stingray envenomation, *Med. J. Aust.*, 151, 621, 1989.

13. **WILLIAMSON, J.A.**, Personal communication.

14. **SUTHERLAND S.**, *Australian Animal Toxins.*, 1st Edition, Oxford University Press, 1983.

15. **EDMONDS, C.**, *Dangerous marine creatures*, Reed Books, 1989.

Chapter 12

CLINICAL TOXICOLOGY OF VENOMOUS SCORPAENIDAE AND OTHER SELECTED FISH STINGS

John Williamson

TABLE OF CONTENTS

I. INTRODUCTION

Venomous fish are characterised by the possession of glandular tissue which elaborates a poison, together with a defensive apparatus (e.g. spines) for the traumatic delivery of the poison into the tissues of an attacking predator (Figure 1).

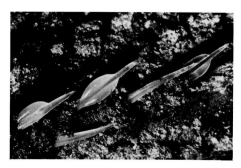 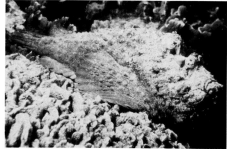

Figure 1. Spines of stonefish (courtesy Surf Life Saving Queensland, Inc.).

Figure 2. Stonefish (courtesy Surf Life Saving Queensland, Inc.).

Members of the Family Scorpaenidae (Phylum CHORDATA; Class OSTEICHTHYES (formerly TELEOSTOMI); Order PERCIFORMES), together with other Families in this Order (vertebrate fishes), suffer taxonomically somewhat from a confusing array of "common names"[1]. This tends to hinder their accurate field identification, and hence the medical study of their envenomations. Precise medical understanding remains relatively meagre. There exists present uncertainty regarding the degree of threat to human life by some members of this group of fishes, particularly the stonefishes (Order PERCIFORMES)[2-4].

A. THE PRINCIPAL VENOMOUS FISH OF MEDICAL SIGNIFICANCE
(Stingrays are discussed in Chapter 11)

The monumental work of Halstead[1] remains a leading source of international information, supplemented by various other writings[3,5-10]. The Family "Scorpaenidae" may in fact include two Families, "Scorpaenidae" (scorpionfishes) and "Synanceiidae" (stonefishes)[1].

1. Family Scorpaenidae

(Family Synanceiidae: Stonefishes (Figure 2))

Stonefish, devil fish, warty-ghoul.

Synanceia horrida;
Synanceia trachynis;
Synanceia verrucosa.

Lionfish, scorpionfish, zebra fish, butterfly cod, bullrout, cobbler, rascasse, stingfish (Figure 3).

Apistus carinatus;
Brachirus species;
Centropogon species;
Gymnapistes marmoratus;
Helicolenus dactylopterus;
Inimicus species;
Minous adamsi;
Notesthes robusta;
Pterois species;
Scorpaena species;
Sebastodes species.

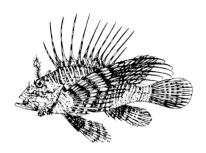 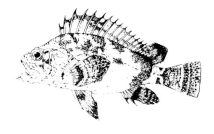

Figure 3a. Butterfly cod (courtesy of Dr. R.V. Southcott and Mr. I. Munro).

Figure 3b. Bullrout (courtesy of Dr. R.V. Southcott and Mr. I. Munro).

2. Family Trachinidae: Weeverfishes

Trachinus species (Figure 4)

3. Order Siluriformes, Suborder Siluroidei: Catfishes

Includes   Family Ariidae   (forked-tailed catfish Figure 5);
               Family Plotosidae (eel-tailed catfish);
               Family Siluridae

4. Other venomous fishes

Order Perciformes:
          Jacks (Family Carangidae);
          Rabbitfishes (Family Siganidae);

Scats (Family Scatophagidae);
Stargazers (Family Uranoscopidae);
Surgeonfishes (Family Acanthuridae);
Order Batrachoidiformes (Haplodoci):
Venomous toadfishes (Family Batrachoididae).

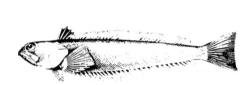

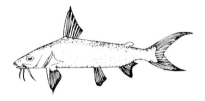

Figure 4. Weeverfish (courtesy of Dr. B.W. Halstead).   **Figure 5.** Fork-tailed catfish (courtesy of Dr. R.V. Southcott and Mr. I. Munro).

II. DISTRIBUTION AND EPIDEMIOLOGY

Venomous fish of medical significance are found world wide (including in the Mediterranean Sea and in the Arctic regions). However tropical seas contain a majority of the species, and are the locations for many documented human stings. The temperate to warm seas and shores of the Indo-Pacific, India, South Africa, Australasia, Philippines, China, Japan and the U.S. feature prominently. All human envenomations are the result of a defensive response of the animals to either intentional or accidental interference by humans; none of these animals "attack" human beings, despite lurid media reports to the contrary. A common accidental encounter is by fisherman, aquarists or other fish handlers[11]. Most envenomations occur on feet (wading) or hands (handling)[6]. The increasing forays of tourists (including recreational scuba divers) into the world's seas are resulting in a general increase in the risk of human envenomations; no longer are such envenomations confined to marine occupational workers.

A. FATALITIES

Documentation exists regarding human deaths from the following fish envenomations. The number of references discovered is quoted for each animal, but the geographical locations of each were not determined.

Zebrafish[1,12] (6 references), including in the Philippines;

Weeverfish[13] in Europe (7 references);

Catfish[10,14] in the tropics (2 references);

Stonefish[3,13] (4 references), including in Africa.

No conclusive evidence of an Australian death from stonefish envenomation[2,3,5,6] (where such events are common[5] (Figure 8)) has yet been found.

Precise interpretation of some fatality documentation is made difficult by the frequent use of "common names" for the accused animals, combined with the age and language of publication of some of the references.

III. VENOM APPARATUS: GENERAL FEATURES

Venomous fish spines may be located in a variety of anatomical sites on different animals[1], including dorsal (the most common), pectoral, opercular, shoulder, pelvic, anal and caudal. Studies of the evolution of the venom apparatus in fish[15] have shown a trend from the simplest unicellular gland, elaborating poison into the integumentary sheath of the epidermal spine (as in an *Arius* species of catfish), to the elegant "grooved-spine-encapsulated-venom-gland" apparatus of the stonefish (Figure 1; see below). Such apparatus, irrespective of its sophistication, is capable of erection, efficient penetration of human flesh, and the deposition in the wound of the associated poison (Figures 1 & 7).

IV. SPECIFIC ANIMALS AND GROUPS

A. FAMILY SCORPAENIDAE (SYNANCEIIDAE)
1. Stonefishes (Figure 2)
Common names: Stonefish, devil fish, warty-ghoul.
Species names:　*Synanceia horrida* (Indian Stonefish);
　　　　　　Synanceia trachynis (Estuarine Stonefish);
　　　　　　Synanceia verrucosa (Reef Stonefish).
　　　　　　Conflict of opinion remains concerning a distinction between *Synanceia horrida* and *Synanceia trachynis*.[1,5]
Stonefish are medically the most important of the venomous fish.

a. Distribution and incidence
Throughout the tropical and warmer temperate oceans, from the central Pacific west through the Indo-Pacific to the east African coastline. Their habitat can extend northwards to the Gulf of Oman and southern Japan, and southwards to beyond New Zealand. They are typically found in shallow waters, but have been photographed at depths of 30 metres[6]. Their true incidence tends to be underestimated because of their superb camouflage[4]; they are now known to be more common on the Australian east coast than previously appreciated - at least by the white man![5] They are stationary bottom-dwellers, but as true fish possess powerful pectoral fins and are capable of sudden short bursts of speed and/or lightning jaw movement to capture passing prey.

b. Appearance (Figure 2)
Stonefish are the complete masters of camouflage. They become covered with slime and mud, and, with their craggy, scaleless, tubercle-covered, rock-like exterior, are absolutely indistinguishable from their surroundings when still (Figure 6). Many human envenomations result from a fossiker or snorkeller standing on, or picking up, "a rock"! The deeper specimens can show spots of colour[6]. They average about 20cm in length but may attain 40cm or more[5].

c. The venom apparatus (Figures 1 and 7)
This is displayed in immense detail by Halstead[1] and Endean[16]. Stonefish possess the most evolved venom apparatus of all the venomous fishes, and it is purely defensive. The paired venom glands associated with each of the 13 dorsal spines are partially (proximally) and completely (distally) enclosed in each of the two laterally placed grooves in each spine. The glands themselves are full of granular, proteinaceous venom and completely invested by a tough connective tissue layer; their ducts are sealed by fibrous tissue, thus preventing accidental venom discharge[5].

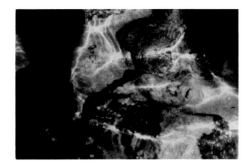

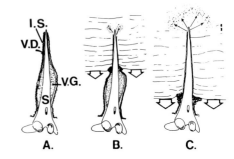

Figure 6. Stonefish camouflaged.

Figure 7. Sting mechanism, (From Sutherland, 1983).

A foot or a hand pressing down on the fish produces immediate erection of the spines, the front 3 or 4 becoming vertical to the dorsum of the animal. Each spine tip protrudes from the connective tissue sheath and pierces the "offending" overlying structures; the penetration of the spine forcibly unblocks the duct, compresses the venom-packed gland inside its non-elastic connective tissue sheath, and expels venom "violently"[15] from the gland out the spine tip into the depths of the wound. Granular venom mixed with gland cells are injected, and venom regeneration time is uncertain,[9] but may take 3 weeks[16]. A venom yield from *Synanceia trachynis* of some 6mg per spine, and 49-88mg per fish is recorded[17].

d. Venom composition and pharmacology

Synanceia venom was the first of the scorpaenid venom to be studied[18,19], and Australian workers have since sustained a distinguished place in this research[16,17,20,21]. Various studies have been made of the venom from all 3 species of *Synanceia*.[21-23] The venom contains heat-labile and antigenic protein toxins[17] with molecular weights up to 158,000, and which exhibit myotoxic, neurotoxic, vascular-leakage and myocardial effects in experimental animals, but no effects on blood coagulation[5,17,21,23]. The much studied haemolytic effects are of no clinical significance[5]. The haemolytic, lethal and vascular permeability-increasing effects are probably produced by the same molecule, which may be more accurately described as "cell membrane damaging", or cytolytic[23]. Venom in the venom glands retains its toxicity for at least several days after the fish has died[19].

The intra-peritoneal LD_{50} in mice is 1.3-2.0mg/kg[17,23]. Intravenous (IV) injections into mice were fatal within 30 minutes, but animals surviving beyond this time did so indefinitely[24]. In 250 g body weight guinea pig a subcutaneous injection of 4mg causes muscular weakness, coma and then death within 3 hours[17]. IV injections of either *Synanceia verrucosa* or *Synanceia horrida* venom into rabbits produced systemic hypotension, respiratory arrest, atrio-ventricular block and ventricular fibrillation[24]. (These 2 venoms are now considered to be identical[1].) Life was not extended in these animals by ventilatory support. Hypotension and respiratory failure occur with IV injections of *Synanceia horrida* venom into the dog and the chicken[17]. The venoms probably possess myotoxic properties in animals which seriously affect diaphragmatic musculature ahead of myocardium[25]. Structural studies of the venom molecules are presently lacking.

e. The sting: clinical features

A stonefish sting is a dreadful experience[3,6] repeatedly attested to by patients as the most painful experience of their life, far eclipsing that of natural childbirth or of ureteric colic. An eloquent and unadorned description by an Australian aboriginal is quoted by Sutherland[5] from *"Confessions of a Beachcomber"*[26]:

"Suppose that fella nail go along your foot, you sing out all a same bullocky all night. Leg belonga you swell up and jump about(?) Bingie (belly) *belonga you, sore fella. Might you die."*

While Australian fatalities have apparently yet to occur[2,6] the evil reputation of the stonefish sting is justified. Upon spine(s) penetration (usually a human hand or foot) the pain is immediate, savage and increasing, and comes to involve the whole of the affected limb[11]. Victims in documented stonefish envenomations in Australia rapidly become incoherent from the pain, not from any other central effects of the venom. However this deranged state may lead to the victim placing himself at risk of further injury. Various systemic effects such as diaphoresis, nausea, hypotension and syncope[2,17] may conceivably result from the savage pain; however direct systemic toxic effects should not be overlooked. (The possibility exists of a rare anaphylactic reaction to the antigenic venom.[5,27]) The envenomated part cannot be touched, swells rapidly, and usually quite massively, with a classical blue discolouration of the tissues around the visible puncture site (Figure 8).

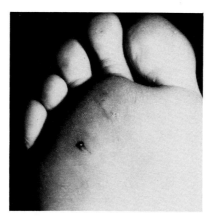

Figure 8. Stonefish sting wound.

Smith's description of human fatalities in the Seychelles and Mozambique included agonising pain following envenomation in the foot (both cases), followed by rapid "collapse", central cyanosis, pulmonary oedema ("frothing at the mouth"), unconsciousness, and death "well within the hour"[28]. Direct intravascular deposition of the venom was postulated by Smith in the Mozambique case, as the victim's foot showed no local reaction. One may also wonder if the venom of the animals in Smith's report may differ (qualitatively and/or quantitatively) from the Australian species? Records of deaths days or months following envenomation[1] must raise suspicions of non-specific complications such as infection. Secondary tetanus infection is certainly a theoretical possibility from a stonefish wound[5,6].

Despite the massive local oedema, which can spread to involve an entire distal limb, and the unhealthy local tissue discolouration, extensive tissue necrosis in stonefish envenomation seems conspicuous by its absence (this is in contrast to stingray envenomation - see Chapter 11).

Neither is local circulatory insufficiency, muscle paralysis or haemorrhage a feature. Local capillary refill is normally retained.

f. First aid

Necessary resuscitation measures for any effects on consciousness or breathing must always take priority[6]. However first aid relief of the conscious patient's agony is of the greatest importance and should also be treated as a matter of urgency.

The first aid principles apply equally well to any venomous fish sting, and are summarised thus:

1. Resuscitation as required;

2. Plunge the envenomated part into comfortably hot (not boiling!) water. Do not ask the patient to gauge the temperature of the water. He/she will be too distraught. Rescuers should do this themselves first. This measure will usually reduce (not eliminate) the pain, but will be thankfully received by the suffering patient. Maintenance of immersion, and of the water temperature is necessary to prevent full return of the pain.

3. If the skills and facilities are available on site, local infiltration of the envenomated area with **no more than 2mg/kg body weight of plain** lignocaine or bupivicaine will also ease the pain. (Care must be taken not to administer an accidental intravascular injection.)

4. Seek medical aid. All venomous fish stings warrant early medical contact.

5. *Further Comments*:

- **never apply an arterial torniquet to a venomous fish sting**.
- do not apply compression/immobilisation bandaging[29] to wounds from any venomous fish stings[5,6]. Retardation of venom at the site will only increase local pain and tissue damage.
- elevation of the envenomated limb may not be possible if hot water immersion is in use. Immersion takes priority.
- with the exception of stingray injuries (Chapter 11), and catfish spines[10] (see below), it is relatively unusual for a wound from a venomous fish to have a visible foreign body (e.g. broken off piece of spine) retained. However such can be present, hidden in the depths of the wound, and will only be revealed by a competent medical examination (see below).
- do not incise the puncture wound, unless informed medical opinion has been sought. Amateur incision is seldom of benefit and carries risks.
- do not inject potassium permanganate, or other irritant solutions into the wound[5]. Although previously recommended[30], their availability is unlikely, their efficacy is unclear, and they may produce further tissue damage. Although emetine hydrochloride is on record as providing impressive pain relief in stonefish stings,[30] it is now safer to use local anaesthetics.

g. Clinical management

Again, the principles of clinical management described, allowing for specific minor variations, apply equally well to any venomous fish sting.

1. Adequate pain relief is an urgent requirement. This is most adequately achieved by a regional anaesthetic block (e.g. ankle block, wrist block), and can be dramatically effective.

2. If the identity of the offending animal can be confirmed with certainty (often difficult or impossible[2,6]) as a stonefish, and the patient has significant pain and/or local effects, specific stonefish antivenom[1,5,20] should be administered (see below). This will also produce effective analgesia[5].

3. Contrast radiography is advised to detect or exclude any retained foreign body[5,6].

4. The decision to incise and explore the wound will vary according to the features of each individual case. Skilled surgical exploration under appropriate anaesthesia, performed early, with removal of any foreign material and the successful washout of deposited venom may improve outcome. However in the majority, this measure is not necessary, and is contraindicated for the unskilled.

5. Tetanus prophylaxis and wound toilet is advisable.

6. The management of delayed, severely contaminated or infected wounds requires surgical wound debridement and toilet, culture of infected material, careful tetanus prophylaxis, appropriate antibiotic therapy and follow-up care. Awareness of the special requirements for marine pathogens is important[8].

7. Bed rest and immobilisation of the injured part is helpful.

8. *Further Comments*:

- attempts to control the acute pain of stonefish (and some other venomous fish) stings by the administration of systemic narcotic analgesics alone are a strictly medical matter, may be ineffective[30] and may produce respiratory depression and impaired consciousness.
- suspect a retained foreign body or a marine pathogen[8] in any non-healing venomous fish wound being actively treated.
- venomous fish wounds not given early medical treatment may remain painful and disabling for months[2,5].

h. Antivenom therapy [5,20]

Australia's Commonwealth Serum Laboratories (CSL) in Melbourne produce a specific stonefish antivenom[1,5], which is a hyperimmunised horse antiserum prepared against the venom from the dorsal spines of *Synanceia trachynis*[20]. The antivenom has been shown to destroy the venom's *in vitro* lethal, vascular permeability-increasing and haemolytic properties[23]. One ampoule of 2.0ml will neutralise *in vitro* 20mg of venom[5]. Its clinical efficacy for both analgesia and diminution of venom-induced tissue damage is now well established[5,31].

At present levels of understanding, this antivenom should not be routinely administered to other than stings from *Synanceia* species. However there is circumstantial evidence that it may be effective for serious, or non-responding, stings from other scorpionfish[1,32].

CSL stonefish antivenom is recommended only for intramuscular (IMI) use. Premedication is recommended[31]. The choice of specific premedicant drugs is controversial[31], but might include an IMI antihistamine, and subcutaneous adrenalin 0.25mg. Prophylactic corticosteroids may prevent later serum sickness[31]. Patients with an allergy history require especially careful premedication. Facilities for resuscitation and the management of anaphylaxis must be immediately to hand.

The recommended antivenom doses are[5]:

- 1 - 2 puncture wounds, give 1 ampoule IMI (2000 units)
- 3 - 4 puncture wounds, give 2 ampoules IMI (4000 units)
- more than 4 puncture wounds, give 3 ampoules IMI (6000 units).

There is evidence, especially following the use of a large volume of antivenom, that a short course of prophylactic steroids (e.g. 100mg hydrocortisone or equivalent, daily for 4 days), commencing with the antivenom administration, may reduce the risk of delayed serum sickness[31].

I. Prophylaxis

The principles of prevention of stonefish envenomation apply to any venomous fish sting.

1. Be aware that a stonefish will not be seen until a sting occurs, and even then maybe not! Their camouflage is total.

2. Always wear thick-soled shoes, for wading or fossiking on littoral reefs or shores. The spines can penetrate thin shoes.

3. Never reach for a submerged "rock" with bare hands or feet. Touch only what you or your guide identify as safe.

4. Do not search by hand into hidden crevices in the sea.

5. Do not "tease" marine life, or handle animals unnecessarily.

6. Do not jump bare-foot from a boat into the shallows, unless the bottom is clearly visible and free of marine life.

7. Wear a bracelet alerting your companions, if you have a serious allergic condition, and/or are on powerful medications.

2. Other Scorpaenidae

Common Names: Lionfish, scorpionfish, zebra fish, butterfly cod, bullrout, cobbler, rascasse, stingfish.

Such is the bewildering array of species among the Scorpaenidae, and so many of their features are shared that apply to their venomous potential that Halstead selects three species, (1) *Pterois volitans* (Linnaeus; lionfish, zebrafish - slender spines), (2) *Scorpaena guttata* (Girard; the Californian scorpionfish - shorter, thicker, less slender spines), (3) *Synanceia horrida* (Linnaeus; stonefish - stout, powerful spines), as representatives of the spectrum of features of the Scorpaenidae[1].

Two species, the butterfly cod (genus *Pterois*), and the Australian bullrout (genus *Notesthes*), are selected here for comparison with the stonefish (genus *Synanceia*), discussed above. Together these three species also illustrate the essential medical elements of all known venomous scorpionfish, with the knowledge presently available.

a. Pterois *species*

Along with the genus *Dendrochirus*, these fish are among the most photographed (Figure 3). They grow to some 35cm in length and are very widely distributed throughout the Indo-Pacific, Australia, Japan, China, Indian Ocean and the Red Sea. They are gaily adorned with striped and coloured appendages; hence one of their common names, "zebrafish". These they display while floating still or moving very slowly among coral reefs, to photographers' delight. These same features make them popular aquaria fish; not surprisingly aquarists are among the most commonly envenomated[11]. When an enemy approaches, they can rapidly rotate their body to present a suitable array of defensive spines. They possess 12 to 13 elongated and slender dorsal spines, and very large pectoral fins with the upper rays often produced beyond the membrane of the fin as filaments[7]. *Pterois* also has anal and pelvic spines; all spines have associated venom glands and enveloping integumentary sheaths. The grooved spines contain the venom-producing glandular epithelium, but only a poorly developed venom duct.

Human envenomation invariably results from interference with the animal, and produces immediate and severe pain at the puncture site of the spine(s). Hot water will relieve the pain somewhat (see above). Deaths are claimed from "zebrafish" envenomations[1,12].

Only limited study of *Pterois* venoms has occurred, but in general they are believed, along with *Urolophus* (stingray), *Trachinus* (weeverfish) and *Scorpaena* venoms, to be similar to stonefish venoms[32]. Envenomations should be managed accordingly (see above).

A polyvalent(?) horse serum antivenom for scorpion fish stings (also used for weeverfish, see below), for IV use, was available from the Institute of Immunology, Rockerfellerova 2, Zagreb, Yugoslavia. (Theakston, R. D. G. and Warrell, D. A., WHO Collaborative Centre for Control of Antivenoms, Liverpool School of Tropical Medicine, Liverpool, England, 1991.) However no further details are known.

b. Notesthes *species*

The typical example, *Notesthes robusta* (Gunther), has an Australian distribution and is associated with human stings in brackish or freshwater rivers; thus it presents a non-marine hazard. Some uncertainty exists whether it has a freshwater or marine life cycle[33]. All 15 of the strong dorsal spines, the 3 anal spines and the single pair of pelvic spines bear venom sacs. There are also venomous, long, stout upper jaw and operculum spines. The venom is believed to be protein and regenerates at least partially, within 6 days[34]. Bullrouts are sedentary, cryptic and solitary[33]. They love beds of ribbongrass or other water plants for habitats, and are very difficult to see. Human stings may involve multiple spine penetration, and as with stonefish, the pain is immediate and excruciating. However pain will usually ease a little after 4 hours or so. Again like stonefish stings, the tissues around the puncture site may become bluish. Hot water will relieve the pain significantly (see above).

Management of bullrout stings should be conducted as for stonefish stings (see above). Although no firm data exist, the administration of the Australian stonefish antivenom would seem logical for non-responding bullrout stings.

B. FAMILY TRACHINIDAE: WEEVERFISHES

Common names: Weever, dragonfish.

Known venomous species: Genus *Trachinus* (Figure 4).

> *Trachinus draco* ("Greater weeverfish" - the largest);
> *Trachinus araneus* ("Araneus weeverfish");
> *Trachinus radiatus* ("Vive à tête rayonnée");
> *Trachinus vipera* ("Lesser weeverfish").

1. Distribution

Weevers are small venomous marine fishes found along Mediterranean and eastern Atlantic coastlines, as far north as Denmark[35]. Species of weeverfish are also present in the Australian and Indo-Pacific area, but the former at least are not related and have no spines, and the latter have apparently not been examined to date for the presence of spines (Dr J Rifkin, PhD, personal communication). Their presence in Chile is disputed[36]. Of no real commercial value, they favour flat, muddy or sandy inlets. The smaller weevers tend to be found in shallower waters, but spawning in the shallows during early summer months occurs with all species.

2. Appearance (Figure 4)

Weevers range in size according to species, but the largest, *Trachinus draco*, has attained 45cm in length. A more standard length is 21cm. These fishes bury themselves in soft bay mud or sand with eyes, head, and opercular and dorsal stings exposed. Thus effectively camouflaged, they dart out with impressive speed and skill, to spine their prey. They possess 5 readily visible dorsal spines (another one or two not so easily seen), and a "dagger-like" opercular spine on each side of the head, all venomous and enveloped by integumentary sheaths. Touching their body produces a lightning-fast, defensive and accurate opercular spine response!

3. The venom apparatus

The 2 opercular and 6 or 7 dorsal spines are grooved and have spongy venom glands attached, which extend to the tips in undamaged spines. There appear to be no excretory ducts[1]. The dorsal spines are relatively solid and stout with sharp tips. They are contained in the dorsal fin which is instantly erected in defense. The opercular spines are held in adduction against the head at rest. They are instantly abducted by powerful "cheek" muscles when needed, and are applied with accuracy, speed and precision to prey, or against any threat. Penetration of a spine simultaneously deposits clear, grey, fresh venom into the wound.

4. Venom composition and pharmacology

Following major European contributions during the early decades of the 20th century, considerable toxicological, pharmacological and chemical research into *Trachinus* venom, using experimental animals, has occurred[13,37-39]. (This is a natural consequence with a venomous animal prevalent among European civilisations.)

The venom is a protein mixture, not all components of which are toxic in animals[38]. It is antigenic, labile with storage and handling, can produce intense local tissue destruction, and has no effect on neuro-muscular transmission[37]. The venom produces respiratory depression, hypotension and cardiac ischaemic changes with arrhythmias in cats[38]. *Trachinus vipera* venom appears to contain 5-hydroxytryptamine[39], and weeverfish venom has been observed to produce peripheral vascular disorders[40]. Russell considers the systemic toxic effects of stingray, scorpionfish, weeverfish and stonefish to be similar[32].

5. The sting: clinical features

Swimming and wading along sandy sea bottoms invites weeverfish envenomation. The pain is instantaneous, burning, comes to involve the entire affected limb or part, and within 30 minutes or so increases to reduce the patient to writhing and sometimes screaming incoherence. The similarity to stonefish sting is close (see above). Local erythema and swelling quickly follow, but unlike stonefish stings, significant local tissue damage, proceding to gangrene, may occur[1]. Secondary bacterial infection is particularly likely following neglected weeverfish stings.

Deaths are documented[13,37,38] but at least 3 of those in the literature were from delayed secondary septicaemia[32]. As with many marine envenomations, early neglect of weever stings may produce protracted morbidity. Serious allergic reactions are not documented, but are possible[27].

6. First aid

This is identical to that for *Synanceia* stings and stingray envenomations (see above, and Chapter 11). Again, hot water immersion should be employed, but compression/ immobilisation bandaging[29], or amateur wound incision, should not.

7. Clinical management

This is identical with that for stingray stings (see Chapter 11), and closely similar to that for stonefish stings. Unlike the latter, selected cases of weeverfish envenomation may require local excision of necrotic tissue. Certainly analgesia is of the highest priority, and regional anaesthetic block is an effective method[40]. The use of IV calcium gluconate for this purpose has been advocated[41], but is not without cardiac risk and cannot be supported in preference to regional anaesthetic block. (The role of calcium blockade for a different purpose is of current interest in serious chirodropid jellyfish stings[42].)

8. Antivenom therapy

There is report of a horse antiserum for intravenous use against weeverfish envenomation, prepared at the Institute of Immunology, Rockerfellerova 2, Zagreb, Yugoslavia (see scorpionfish, above). No further details are known.

9. Prophylaxis

General principles are enumerated above for stonefish and scorpionfish stings. Of particular note is the ability of weeverfish to retain life and stinging ability long after removal from the sea. Handling of a "dead" weeverfish requires caution. Snorkellers, swimmers and divers should be warned of the dangers of travelling close to sandy bottoms in the sea.

C. ORDER SILURIFORMES, SUBORDER SILUROIDEI (NEMATOGNATHI): CATFISHES

Includes:Family Ariidae (forked-tailed catfish Figure 5);

Family Plotosidae (eel-tailed catfish);

Family Siluridae

Common names include: sea catfish, saltwater catfish, freshwater catfish, estuary catfish, armoured catfish, cobbler, catfish eel, striped catfish, stonecat.

1. Distribution

Including up to 1000 different species in some 9 Families, venomous catfishes are worldwide, predominately tropical, and inhabit both freshwater streams and the sea. The majority are freshwater species. Certain Families are restricted to one or other continent (e.g. Family Dorididae in South American fresh waters). Their habitats coincide with that of edible fish, for the commonest human envenomation occurs on the hand in fish handlers with catfish on a fishing line, or in a net, or handling a discarded and apparently dead catfish. Waders in streams, estuaries and sea shallows may be envenomated on the feet[10,43]. Marine catfish (e.g. *Plotosus lineatus* [Oriental catfish], *Arius thalassinus* [Arabian Gulf catfish]) may live among seaweed and cluster in schools.

2. Appearance

Catfish species vary widely in their shapes and sizes. They may be stumpy or elongate and "eel-like", have forked or pointed tails, have small, short heads or elongated, large heads, and can vary from less than finger length (the Amazonian *Urinophilus* species) to huge (*Silurus glanis*, length 4 metres, weight 275 kg!)[43]. However catfish in the length range 6-40cm are more usual. They have no true scales, and commonly have thick, slimy skin. Some have bony plates. Their camouflage in their natural surroundings can be impressive.

Typically a group of paired sensory "barbels", or fleshy whiskers, protrude from the chin, mouth and nostril parts; these are harmless appendages (Figure 5).

The spine weaponry of catfish is typically a single, stout, serrated dorsal fin spine, sharply tipped, and a pair (right and left) of serrated pectoral fin spines. Each spine is covered by a skin-like enveloping sheath, and, when the fish becomes agitated, is capable of being locked firmly into the erected or extended position by a complex and efficient bony articular apparatus located at each spine base[43,44].

3. The venom apparatus

This consists of the three erectile spines, sheath venom glands, and a pair of axillary venom glands. Most venomous catfishes have the spines enveloped in an integumentary sheath which also contains venom glands distinct from the axillary glands. The process of penetration by the extended, sharp spines is accompanied by the disruption of this sheath, and the deposition of venom from the sheath glands into the wound. While the role of the axillary glands of the catfishes (and their venomous secretions) remains unknown, it has been suggested that the pore from each axillary gland supplies further venom to the outside of the ipsilateral pectoral spines, which would be carried into the wound[45]. However Cameron and Endean consider that the axillary gland secretions play no defensive role[46]. The powerful, locked and serrated spines can lacerate, and not infrequently can snap off and remain in the wound[10]. Recently it has been suggested that additional toxic epidermal secretions elaborated over the entire body of some catfish species (proteinaceous crinotoxins) also play a part in the spinous envenomation process. This has been described for *Plotosus lineatus*[47] and *Arius thalassinus*[48].

4. Venom composition and pharmacology

The toxicology of catfish venom upon laboratory animals received early attention in 1918 and 1944[43]. The pharmacology and chemistry of two of the more dangerous species has since been studied further[47,48]. In animals, the venom from *Plotosus lineatus* (plototoxin) produced muscular spasm, respiratory distress, neurotoxic, leucopaenic, haemolytic, and lethal effects; it produced local tissue destruction with necrosis. The venom exhibited some immunological activity, was labile to storage, but could be preserved by freezing[49]. The crinotoxin of *Plotosus lineatus* contains oedema-forming and haemolytic factors, and that of *Arius thalassinus* acetyl-choline-like and prostaglandid-releasing components. Both animals' crinotoxic effects in experimental animals, and *in vitro*, can be significantly attenuated by pretreatment with indomethacin[47,48]. Edmonds describes catfish venom as being a water-soluble, vasoconstrictor protein, which is heat labile and to which an immunity can develop[50]. No source details are provided. Recently the chemistry, pharmacology and apparent wound-healing properties of "fright-induced" epidermal secretions of another Arabian Gulf saltwater catfish (*Arius bilineatus* Valenciennes) have received some attention in Kuwait University[51]. The precise role of such secretions in actual human envenomations requires further study.

5. The sting: Clinical Features

In common with many venomous fish stings, catfish envenomation is accompanied by immediate "hot-pin like" pain, which may radiate up the affected limb. Accompanying spotted skin rashes in the envenomated skin area are described[10]. The hand is by far the most common sting site in humans[10], (see above), but stings on the feet occur[43]. Unlike stonefish venom, catfish venom produces painful muscular spasms and intense local pallor of surrounding tissues, with subsequent local ischaemia and necrosis. Surrounding local redness and swelling quickly follow the actual envenomation. The wound commonly contains pieces of spine, and secondary infection is common, especially in neglected wounds, and potentially dangerous in immuno-compromised victims[52]. Such a sequence has resulted in a septicaemic death[10]. Other deaths are claimed[43]. The powerful and serrated catfish spines may produce a combination of trauma and envenomation (c.f. stingrays), with damage to tendons and nerves[10]. Regional lymphadenopathy is not uncommon. There is no practical distinction between the clinical effects of freshwater and saltwater catfish stings.

Note: Considering the more exotic catfish, one species, the Amazonian pygidid catfish, *Urinophilus*, can actually penetrate the urethral orifice in immersed mammals, including man. It is one of the few known parasitic vertebrates. Yet another, an Egyptian species (*Malapterus*), gives an electric shock when touched![43]

6. First aid

This is identical to that for stingray injuries (see Chapter 11). Hot water immersion (see above) is recommended.

7. Clinical management

As for stingrays (Chapter 11).

8. Antivenom therapy

No antivenom is known, although research would seem justified.

9. Prophylaxis

As for any other venomous fish (see above).

D. OTHER VENOMOUS FISHES

Order Perciformes: Jacks (Family Carangidae);
         Rabbitfishes (Family Siganidae);
         Scats (Family Scatophagidae);
         Stargazers (Family Uranoscopidae);
         Surgeonfishes (Family Acanthuridae)
Order Batrachoidiformes (Haplodoci): Venomous toadfishes (Family Batrachoididae).

While the miscellaneous remainder of known venomous fishes and the injuries they produce are covered by the principles already discussed above, some special features are worthy of mention.

1. Jacks (family Carangidae)

This is a Family of oceanic and coastal fishes adapted for rapid swimming. They are characterised by the possession of two separate anal spines, anterior to the anal fins, in addition to the seven or so dorsal spines. The spines can be held depressed against the body or erected. The anal stings seem to be especially venomous and can be locked into the erected state.

The sting is instantly painful, "bee-like", and the pain persists for 30 minutes. Hawaiian fishermen are often stung. Hot water immersion of the affected part should be used for analgesia (see above).

2. Rabbitfishes (family Siganidae)

These fishes have an impressive array of spines (13 dorsal, 7 anal, 4 pelvic). Their particular distinguishing feature is the first and last rays of the ventral fins, which are spinous. They are throughout the central and western Pacific and in the Red Sea[53]. The sting is similar to, and should be treated as, a scorpionfish sting (see above).

3. Scats (family Scatophagidae)[53]

A small Family of perch-like fishes in the Indo-Pacific region. They typically have 11-12 dorsal, 2 anal and 2 ventral spines, plus venom glands and integumentary spine sheaths. Pain from a sting is instant, severe, and "electric-shock like"[54]. Management is the same as for scorpionfish stings (see above).

4. Stargazers (family Uranoscopidae)

Small, carnivorous, bottom-dwelling fish, with an unattractive, square-shaped head and a mouth and eyes that face vertically upwards. They have no fin spines, but two shoulder spines with sheaths and venom glands. They are tropical and Mediterranean in distribution.

Vague reference to Mediterranean fatalities is made by Halstead[53]. Treat as for scorpionfish stings.

5. Surgeonfishes (family Acanthuridae)

Common names: Doctorfish, tang, spinetail.

These fish are predominately tropical dwellers, but also occur in Japanese waters. The wound is inflicted by an erectile paired caudal spine. The pain is intense, can be protracted, and seems to include an envenomation.[53] Manage as for scorpionfish stings.

6. Venomous toadfishes (family Batrachoididae)

These unattractive bottom-dwellers have two short (about 1cm) dorsal spines, and a pair of opercular spines, one on each side of the head. The spines are well enveloped in a covering sheath which has venom glands. The spines are needle-like with a hollow lumen and a distal opening[55]. The fish are widely distributed in tropical oceans, including South America. They lie buried in the sand or bottom mud, and envenomation is usually from being stepped on. Intense pain, local swelling, and secondary infections are all described. Treat as for a scorpionfish sting (see above).

Footnote: Close-up, sharply focussed photos of fresh wounds produced by any venomous fish are of great value, especially if accompanied by clinical details, and, if possible, a reliable identification of the responsible animal. Such photos would be gratefully received by the International Consortium for Jellyfish Stings, and would be with full acknowledgement if and when published. The address of the author will suffice for forwarding photos and details, which should include the precise geographical locality of the sting or envenomation.

VII. REFERENCES

1. **HALSTEAD, B. W.,** *Poisonous and Venomous Marine Animals of the World*, 2nd revised edn., The Darwin Press, Princeton, NJ, 1988, chap. XXI.
2. **FLECKER, H.,** Injuries from stonefish, *Med J Aus,t* 2, 371, 1956.
3. **CAMERON, A.,** Stonefishes, in *Venoms & Victims*, Pearn, J. and Covacevich, J., Eds., The Queensland Museum, South Brisbane, 1988, chap. 7.
4. **WILLIAMSON, J. A.,** Current challenges in marine envenomation: an overview. *J Wilderness Med*, 3, 422, 1992.
5. **SUTHERLAND, S. K.,** *Australian Animal Toxins: The Creatures, Their Toxins, and Care of the Poisoned Patient*, Oxford University Press, Melbourne, 1983, chaps. 28 & 29.
6. **WILLIAMSON, J. A.,** *The Marine Stinger Book*, 3rd edn., Queensland State Centre, Inc., Surf Life Saving Australia, 1985, 54.
7. **MACKAY, R. J.,** A guide to common venomous fishes, in *Toxic Plants & Animals: a Guide for Australia*, Covacevich, J., Davie, P. and Pearn, J. Eds., Queensland Museum, South Brisbane, 1987, 147.
8. **AUERBACH, P. S. AND HALSTEAD, B. W.,** Hazardous aquatic life, in *Management of Wilderness and Environmental Emergencies*, 2nd edn., Auerbach, P. S., Geehr, E. C., Eds., Mosby-Year Book, Inc., St. Louis, 1988, chap. 34.
9. **EDMONDS, C.,** *Dangerous Marine Creatures*, Reed Books Pty. Ltd., French's Forest, NSW, 1989, 52.
10. **MCKINSTRY, D.M.,** Catfish stings in the United States: Case report and review, *J Wilderness Medicine*, **293:** 1993
11. **KIZER, K. W., MCKINNEY, H. E., AND AUERBACH, P. S.,** Scorpaenidae envenomation: A five-year poison center experience, *JAMA*, 253, 807, 1985.
12. **HERRE, A. W.,** A review of the scorpaenoid fishes of the Philippines and adjacent seas, *Philippine J Sci*, 80, 381, 1952.
13. **MARETIC, Z.,** Fish venoms, in *Handbook of Natural Toxins: Vol. III; Marine Toxins and Venoms*, Tu, A.T., Ed., Marcel Dekker, Inc., New York. 1988:445-478.
14. **HALSTEAD, B. W.,** *Poisonous and Venomous Marine Animals of the World*, 2nd revised edn., The Darwin Press, Princeton, NJ, 1988, 802.

15. **CAMERON, A. M. AND ENDEAN, R.,** Epidermal secretions and the evolution of venom glands in fishes, *Toxicon*, 11, 401, 1972.
16. **ENDEAN, R.,** A study of the distribution, habitat, behaviour, venom apparatus, and venom of the Stonefish, *Aust J Marine Freshw Res*, 12, 177, 1961.
17. **WIENER, S.,** Observations on the venom of the stone fish (*Synanceja trachynis*), *Med J Aust*, 1, 620, 1959.
18. **BOTTARD, A.,** L'appareil à venin des poissons, *Compt. Rend. Acad. Sci.*, 108, 534, 1889.
19. **DUHIG, J. V. AND JONES, G.,** Haemotoxin of the venom of *Synanceja horrida*, *Aust J Exp Biol Med Sci*, 5, 173, 1928.
20. **WIENER, S.,** The production and assay of stone-fish antivenene, *Med J Aust*, 2, 715, 1959.
21. **AUSTIN, L., GILLIS, R. G. AND YOUATT, G.,** Stonefish venom: Some biochemical and chemical observations, *Aust J Exp Biol Med Sci*, 43, 79, 1965.
22. **DEAKINS, D. E. AND SAUNDERS, P. R.,** Purification of the lethal fraction of the Stonefish *Synanceja horrida* (Linnaeus), *Toxicon*, 4, 257, 1967.
23. **KREGER, A. S.,** Detection of a cytolytic toxin in the venom of the stonefish (*Synanceia trachynis*), *Toxicon*, 29, 733, 1991.
24. **SAUNDERS, P. R.,** Venom of the Stonefish *Synanceja verrucosa*, *Science*, 129, 272, 1959.
25. **AUSTIN, L., CAIRNCROSS, K. D. AND MCCALLUM, I. A. N.,** Some pharmacological actions of the venom of the Stonefish, *Synanceja horrida*, *Arch Int Pharmacodyn Ther*, 131, 339, 1961.
26. **BANFIELD, E. J.,** *Confessions of a Beachcomber*, Angus and Robertson, Sydney, 1977.
27. **TOGIAS, A. G., BURNETT, J. W., KAGEY-SOBOTKA, A. AND LICHTENSTEIN, L. M.,** Anaphylaxis after contact with a jellyfish, *J Allergy Clin Immunol*, 75, 672, 1985.
28. **SMITH, J. L. B.,** Two rapid fatalities from stonefish stabs, *Copeia*, 3, 249, 1957.
29. **SUTHERLAND, S. K.,** *Australian Animal Toxins: The Creatures, Their Toxins, and Care of the Poisoned Patient*, Oxford University Press, Melbourne, 1983, chap. 3.
30. **WIENER, S.,** Stone-fish sting and its treatment, *Med J Aust*, 2, 219, 1958.
31. **SUTHERLAND, S. K.,** Antivenom use in Australia, *Med J Aust*, 157, 734, 1992.
32. **RUSSELL, F. E.,** Marine toxins and venomous and poisonous marine animals, *Adv Marine Biol*, 3, 255, 1965.
33. **HARRIS, J. AND PERAN, J.,** Bullrout stings, in *Toxic Plants & Animals: a Guide for Australia*, Covacevich, J., Davie, P. and Pearn, J. Eds., Queensland Museum, South Brisbane, 1987, 155.
34. **CAMERON, A. M. AND ENDEAN, R.,** The venom and apparatus of the scorpionfish *Notesthes robusta*. *Toxicon*, 4, 111, 1966..
35. **HALSTEAD, B. W.,** Weever stings and their medical managements, *U.S. Armed Forces Med J*, 8, 1441, 1957.
36. **BERG, L. S.,** Classification of fishes both recent and fossil {In English and Russian}, J. W. Edwards, Ann Arbor, Mich., 1947.
37. **RUSSELL, F. E. AND EMERY, J. A.,** Venom of the weevers *Trachinus draco* and *Trachinus vipera*, *Ann N Y Acad Sci*, 90, 805, 1960.
38. **SKEIE, E.,** Toxin of the weeverfish (*Trachinus draco*): Experimental studies on animals, *Acta Pharmacol Toxicol*, 19, 107, 1962.
39. **CARLISLE, D. B.,** On the venom of the lesser weeverfish *Trachinus vipera*, *J Marine Biol Assoc U.K.*, 42, 155, 1962.
40. **LINARES DEL RIO, F., MONICHE GARCIA PUMARINO, M. AND HERRUEZO PEREZ, A.,** Therapeutic application of anaesthetic blocks in weever-fish stings. *Rev Esp Anestesiol Reanim*, 36, 57, 1989.
41. **MARETI, Z.,** Erfahrungen mit Stichen von Giftfischen. *Acta Tropica*, 14, 157, 1957.
42. **BURNETT, J. W., OTHMAN, I. B., ENDEAN, R., FENNER, P.J., CALLANAN, V. I. AND WILLIAMSON, J. A.,** Verapamil potentiation of *Chironex* (box-jellyfish) antivenom, *Toxicon*, 28, 242, 1990.
43. **HALSTEAD, B. W.,** *Poisonous and Venomous Marine Animals of the World*, 2nd revised edn., The Darwin Press, Princeton, NJ, 1988, chap. XIX.
44. **MANN, J. W. AND WERNTZ, J. R.,** Catfish stings to the hand, *J Hand Surg*, 16A, 318, 1991.
45. **TANGE, Y.,** Beitrag zur Kenntnis der Morphologie des Giftapparates bei den japanischen Fischen, XV, bei *Plotosus anguillaris* (Lacépède), *Yokohama Med Bull*, 6, 255, 1955.
46. **CAMERON, A. M. AND ENDEAN, R.,** The axillary gland of the plotosid Catfish *Cnidoglanis macrocephalus*, *Toxicon*, 9, 345, 1971.
47. **SHIOMI, K., TAKAMIYA, M., YAMANAKA, H., KIKUCHI, T. AND SUZUKI, Y.,** Toxins in the skin secretion of the oriental catfish (*Plotosus lineatus*): immunological properties and immunocytochemical identification of producing cells, *Toxicon*, 26, 353, 1988.
48. **AL-HASSAN, J. M., THOMSON, M., ALI, M., FAYAD, S., ELKHAWAD, A., THULESIUS, O. AND CRIDDLE, R. S.,** Vasoconstrictor components in the Arabian Gulf catfish (*Arius thalassinus*) proteinaceous skin secretion, *Toxicon*, 24, 1009, 1986.
49. **TOYOSHIMA, T.,** Serological study of the toxin of the fish *Plotosus anguillaris*, Lacépède (in Japanese), *J Japan Protoz Soc* 6, 45, 1918.

50. **EDMONDS, C.,** *Dangerous Marine Creatures*, Reed Books Pty. Ltd., French's Forest, NSW, 1989, 69.
51. **AL-HASSAN, J. M., DYSON, M., YOUNG, S.R., THOMSON, M. AND CRIDDLE, R.S.,** Acceleration of wound healing responses induced by preparations from the epidermal secretions of the Arabian Gulf catfish (*Arius bilineatus* Valenciennes), *J Wilderness Med* 2, 153, 1991.
52. **MURPHEY, D. K., SEPTIMUS, E. J. AND WAAGNER, D. C.,** Catfish-related injury and infection: report of two cases and review of the literature. *Clin Inf Dis* 14, 689, 1992.
53. **HALSTEAD, B. W.,** *Poisonous and Venomous Marine Animals of the World*, 2nd revised edn. The Darwin Press, Princeton, NJ, 1988, chap. XXIII.
54. **CAMERON, A. M. AND ENDEAN, R.,** Venom glands in scatophagid fish, *Toxicon,* 8, 171, 1970.
55. **HALSTEAD, B. W.,** *Poisonous and Venomous Marine Animals of the World*, 2nd revised edn. The Darwin Press, Princeton, NJ, 1988, chap. XXII.

Chapter 13

CLINICAL TOXICOLOGY OF SEA SNAKEBITES

Julian White

TABLE OF CONTENTS

I. INTRODUCTION

Sea snakes are a diverse group of marine or aquatic front fanged venomous snakes, widely distributed from the East coast of Africa to the West coast of the Americas. They generally have potent venom exerting effects in man at the systemic level, and a number of species can cause human fatalities.

II. EPIDEMIOLOGY OF SEA SNAKEBITE

A. THE SEA SNAKES: DISTRIBUTION, VENOMS, CHARACTERISTICS

The sea snakes are proteroglyphous venomous reptiles, principally inhabiting the marine environment, though a few species are found in estuaries or even in fresh water lakes, the latter thought to have had previous connections to the sea. With the exception of the pelagic species, the yellow bellied sea snake, *Pelamis platurus*, all sea snakes are found either close to shore or around coral reefs, in continental shelf waters rather than in deep ocean waters. They feed principally on fish (mostly elongate fish, including eels) and are bottom feeders, except for *Pelamis*, which is a surface feeder. Most bear fully formed live young (viviparous) and never need come ashore, while some, the Laticaudids, come to shore to lay eggs (oviparous). All sea snakes are contained within one Family, Hydrophiidae, subdivided into 2 subfamilies, Hydrophiinae and Laticaudinae. There is a clear relationship to the Elapid (cobra) venomous snakes and some authors have speculated that either the sea snakes have evolved from the Indo-Australian elapids or vice versa.

The distribution of the sea snakes as a family is shown in Figure 1. It should be noted that the distribution map encompasses large tracts of open ocean, where the only sea snake present would be *Pelamis platurus*. There has been some suggestion recently that sea snakes have succeeded in colonising the Carribean via the Panama Canal. The author has not personally confirmed this range extension however; therefore, it is not shown on Figure 1.

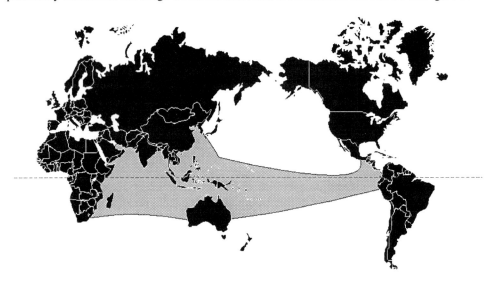

Figure 1. Distribution of Family Hydrophiidae, sea snakes.

A listing of all sea snakes, with salient details, is given in Table 1. For some species available information is incomplete as reflected in the Table.

B. SEA SNAKEBITE EPIDEMIOLOGY

Until the 1950's there was little literature on the epidemiology of sea snakebite, suggesting a very small number of cases. However, as with other types of snakebite, it appears that few records do not equate to few cases. This was clearly demonstrated by Reid, whose papers on sea snakebite remain the most comprehensive on this topic[1-9].
He noted 31 cases of sea snakebite recorded worldwide from 1825 to 1942, yet 30 cases were admitted to hospital in one year from one village in Malaya, once the local population were convinced to seek medical treatment for sea snakebites.

While underuse of medical treatment for sea snakebite may be lessening in some regions, particularly Malaysia, it is possible that in many parts of the Indo-Pacific rim where such bites are probably common amongst fishermen that few cases are reported still. It is therefore not possible to give figures of persons bitten and numbers dying from sea snakebite worldwide. Reid[9] estimated that in the late 1950's there were 150 cases of sea snakebite annually in the Malayan fishing villages surveyed, representing about 10% of all such villages in the country, giving an annual figure of about 1,500 cases for Malaya alone. It might be extrapolated that for all fishing communities within the Indo-Pacific region, this figure for Malaya could be multiplied by between 10 and 50, giving a total worldwide annual rate of bites between 15,000 and 75,000. In one of Reid's[9] series there was an overall fatality rate of 8%, covering a variety of species. However, virtually all fatalities were following bites by *Enhydrina schistosa*. As the series were of hospital cases, it seems likely that the overall fatality rate for all bites is well below 8% and should have fallen further with the availability of specific sea snake antivenom. If we suppose a current fatality rate of between 1% and 5%, then annual fatalities worldwide from sea snakebite would be between 150 and 3750. As pointed out by Reid[9], the chance of dying from sea snakebite within these coastal communities is relatively low, only 10% or less of the number dying from accidental drowning.

The main risk group for sea snakebite is the fishing community, particularly those using traditional methods. The majority of bites occur in men engaged in fishing, particularly using drag nets and gape nets, and also hook line methods, while drive-in nets, palisade traps, lift nets and falling nets seem less likely to entrap sea snakes. A single fisherman might encounter up to 100 sea snakes in a day's work. Overall, from Reid's[9] series, handling nets, sorting fish, and treading on the snake while fishing were the main causes of bites. However, there were significant numbers of cases of people, especially children, bitten while swimming or bathing, most commonly treading on the snake, either in coastal waters or in rivers, up to 5km inland.

Although northern Australian waters are populated by a wide variety of sea snakes, including some of the most dangerous species, there are few reports of sea snakebite, and no fatalities. In the case of remote aboriginal communities this may merely reflect lack of adequate reporting. Significant bites have been reported in recreational beach users from Queensland waters[10,11] and as far south as Sydney's Bondi Beach[12]. Bites have also occurred in fisherman, including modern commercial fishing boats, which may catch large numbers of sea snakes in nets.

III. SYMPTOMS AND SIGNS

A. GENERAL CONCEPTS OF ENVENOMING

As with other snakebites, sea snakes may bite and leave bite marks, yet fail to inject enough venom to cause any significant effects in the human victim. This incidence of "dry bites" will vary from species to species, but overall it appears that about 80% of all sea snakebites will result in either no envenoming or only trivial envenoming.[9] Of the remaining 20% of cases, about 40% were fatal in Reid's[9] series (on very small numbers) and, with antivenom therapy, this number should fall to almost zero. Nevertheless, severe, life threatening envenoming can and does occur following sea snakebites, and is often more severe in children, both in the Malayan and Australian experience.

Table 1
Details of each species of sea snake[9,13-17]

Scientific Name	Common Name	Distribution	Length	Scalation	Venom Quantity	Toxicity	Lethality
HYDROPHIINAE							
Acalyptophis peronii		Aus,SEA	1.0m	23-31/140-210/d/	0.33mg	0.079 sc	
Aipysurus apraefrontalis		Aus	0.5m	17/140-155/d/18-25s			
Aipysurus duboisii		Aus	0.7m	19/150-165/d/23-35s	0.43mg	0.044 sc	
Aipysurus eydouxii		Aus, SEA	1.0m	17/124-150/d/23-35s	0.60	>4 iv	
Aipysurus foliosquama		Aus	0.6m	19/135-155/d/20-30s			
Aipysurus fuscus		Aus	0.6m	19/155-180/d/20-40s			
Aipysurus laevis	Olive brown sea snake	Aus	1.2m	21-25/135-155/d/25-35s	6.6mg	0.13 im	
Aipysurus tenuis		Aus	1.02m	19/185-195/d/35-40s			
Astrotia stokesii	Stoke's sea snake	Aus, SEA, Ind	1.2m	45-63/226-286/d/	31.3	0.32 iv	
Disteira kingii		Aus	1.5m	37-39/324-342/d/			
Disteira major		Aus	1.3m	37-43/230-266/d/	22.8	0.21 iv	
Disteira nigrocincta		Ind					
Emdocephalus annulatus		Aus	0.75m	15-17/125-145/s/20-40s	0.15	>25 iv	
Emydocephalus ijimae		Jap					
Enhydrina schistosa	Beaked sea snake	Aus, SEA, Ind	1.2m	49-66/239-322/d/	8.5 (79)	0.04 ip	sev *
Ephalophis greyi		Aus	0.5m	19-21/159-169/d/28-33s			
Ephalophis mertoni		Aus	0.5m	36-39/158-160/d/29-35s			
Hydrelaps darwinensis		Aus	0.5m	25-29/163-172/d/27-39sd			
Hydrophis belcheri		Aus, SEA					
Hydrophis bituberculatus		Ind					
Hydrophis brookii		Aus, SEA, Ind			1.1		
Hydrophis caerulescens		Aus, SEA, Ind	0.6m	37-39/266-287/			
Hydrophis cantoris		Ind					
Hydrophis cyanocinctus	Annulated sea snake	SEA, Ind	1.7m	37-49/345-432/	8.2 (80)	0.24 ip / 0.12 im	mild *
Hydrophis elegans		Aus	1.0m	35-49/323-514/	5.5		
Hydrophis fasciatus	Banded small headed sea snake	Aus, SEA, Ind	1.0m	30-36/220-287/		0.18 iv	mild *
Hydrophis gracilis	Graceful small headed sea snake	Aus, SEA, Ind	0.7m	35-48/195-293/			
Hydrophis inornatus		Aus, SEA	0.7m				
Hydrophis klossi		Ind			1.0	0.2 ip	
Hydrophis lapemoides		Ind					
Hydrophis mamillaris		Ind					
Hydrophis melanocephalus		Aus, SEA	1.0m	29-34/289-358/	0.13	0.11 sc	
Hydrophis melanosoma		SEA, Aus	1.0m	37-43/266-368/			

Scientific Name	Common Name	Distribution	Length	Scalation	Venom Quantity	Toxicity	Lethality
Hydrophis obscurus		Aus, Ind	0.5m	29-35/331-345/		0.16 im	mild *
Hydrophis ornatus	Reef sea snake	Aus, SEA, Ind	1.0m	39-59/246-336/	8.5		
Hydrophis parviceps		SEA					
Hydrophis semperi		Lake Taal					
Hydrophis spiralis	Yellow sea snake	SEA, Ind			2.1	0.25 ip	mild *
Hydrophis stricticollis		Ind					
Hydrophis torquatus		Ind, SEA					
Kerilia jerdoni		Ind, SEA			2.8	0.53 ip	mild
Kolpophis annandalei		SEA					
Lapemis curtus		Ind					
Lapemis hardwickii	Hardwicke's sea snake	Aus, SEA, Ind	1.0m	23-45/114-235/	1.9 (15)	0.26 ip	mild *
Pelamis platurus	Yellow bellied pelagic sea snake	Pelagic	0.7m	49-67/264-406/	0.25	0.09 iv	mild *
Praescutata viperina		SEA, Ind					
Thalassophis anomalus		SEA					
LATICAUDINAE							
Laticauda colubrina	Yellow lipped sea krait	Aus, SEA, Ind	1.0m	21-25/210-250/d/29-47d		0.42 iv	?mild
Laticauda crockeri		Lake Tegano					
Laticauda laticaudata		Aus, SEA, Ind	1.0m	19/225-245/d/30-47d		0.3 im	
Laticauda semifasciata		SEA				0.34 sc	
Laticauda schistorhynchus		SEA					

KEY: Scientific Name= commonly accepted taxonomic designation, may vary in some publications. **Common Name**= commonly accepted vernacular name, other names may be more common in some parts of distribution. **Distribution**= very general distribution; Aus= Australian/PNG and adjacent waters; SEA= Asian/Pacific waters; Ind= Indian Ocean continental waters. **Length**= total length in metres. **Scalation**= mid body scale count/total ventral scale count/anal divided(d)or single(s)/subcaudal scale count, single(s) or divided(d). **Venom quantity**= dry wt. in mgs. **Toxicity**= LD_{50} in mg/kg mouse with route, subcutaneous(sc), intramuscular(im), intraperitoneal(ip), intravenous(iv). **Lethality**=expected clinical severity of majority of bites; mild, mod(erate), sev(ere), *=fatalities recorded or suspected.

B. THE ONSET AND DEVELOPMENT OF ENVENOMING

Sea snakebite is usually painless, without local swelling, and fang marks may not be easy to distinguish. There may be one or two fang marks, but occasionally there may be numerous teeth marks from other (non-fang) teeth in the upper, or even lower jaw. Scratch marks rather than fang punctures may be seen in some cases. In Reid's[9] series, all patients complained of early "coldness", irrespective of whether actual envenoming occurred later. Symptoms due to anxiety were common, early, and included peripheral shut down with cold, clammy skin, feeble pulse, rapid shallow breathing, and even collapse. The onset of these anxiety symptoms were not related to envenoming, and Reid[9] found a placebo injection often resolved the situation.

For those minority of cases where envenoming did occur, onset of symptoms of poisoning varied from 30mins. to 3½hrs., but in cases developing severe envenoming, the latent period never exceeded 2hrs.

In most cases, the first symptom of envenoming is associated with myolysis, namely muscle aches and pains. Occasionally these are preceded by dizziness, dry throat, nausea and vomiting, and generalised non-specific weakness. The muscle pain may involve the neck, trunk, face, and limbs, and initially may manifest as stiffness, becoming more severe over 30mins., with development of pain on muscle movement. This progresses rapidly to passive muscle movement pain, the pain of movement causing an apparent weakness, previously interpreted as evidence of true neurotoxic paralysis. Neurological examination may be normal at this stage. The myolysis may become more severe, the patient remaining as motionless as possible to alleviate muscle movement pain. Damage to the jaw muscles may result in a "pseudo-trismus". There may be headache, sweating, nausea, vomiting, and thickness or swelling of the tongue. Reid[9] notes that a few patients may deny any muscle pain, noting only weakness, but passive movement of muscles may elicit pain. Myoglobinuria becomes evident about 3-6hrs. after envenoming.

After some hours the patient may develop a "true paresis", characterised by a flaccid paralysis, with ptosis, ophthalmoplegia, no tongue protrusion, dysarthria, inability to sit up, and depressed or absent tendon reflexes. Limb movement may be preserved. This may progress to more severe paralysis, and eventually to complete respiratory paralysis. This stage may be reached in a few hours, up to 60hrs. In this late stage there may be hypertension and sweating. At an earlier stage of paralysis, when glossopharyngeal function is impaired, there is a risk of vomiting with aspiration, which may precipitate a much earlier respiratory failure.

In addition to the myoglobinuria, there will be an associated rise in plasma/serum CK, and liver enzymes (notably SGOT), often with rising urea, creatinine, a hyperkalaemia (possibly with ECG changes), and a moderate leukocytosis is "invariable". There is no evidence of coagulopathy or thrombocytopenia or significant haemolysis.

C. GENERAL SYMPTOMS AND SIGNS OF ENVENOMING

These have essentially been covered above. It is important to remember that anxiety is a common early sequelae of sea snakebite, producing typical symptomatology, which is independent of envenoming, and will occur in many cases where no envenoming has occurred. In addition, some typical general symptoms of envenoming may occur in the 20% or less of bite victims who are actually significantly envenomed. These include headache, nausea, vomiting, and collapse.

D. SPECIFIC TOXIN EFFECTS AND COMPLICATIONS

The specific effects of sea snake toxins are those of myolysis and neurotoxic paralysis. Most current clinical evidence suggests that the latter is not of major importance clinically, most of the "paralysis" type symptoms and signs being ascribed to the effect of myotoxins on skeletal muscle throughout the body. A case of *Astrotia stokesii* bite with severe paralysis and only minor myolysis casts some doubt on this[10].

The myotoxins in sea snake venom have been studied clinically[9]. In effect they appear to act in a similar manner to the phospholipase A_2 myotoxins demonstrated from a number of Elapid and Viper venoms. Histological samples from muscles of sea snakebite patients with myolysis, taken either as biopsies or at autopsy, showed widespread hyaline necrosis of skeletal muscle only. Individual fibres are affected, sometimes with normal intact fibres adjacent to necrotic fibres. In some muscles, less than 20% of fibres might be affected, while in other muscles in the same patient, all fibres would be necrotic. The necrotic material becomes an amorphous mass, with contraction beneath the intact sarcolemma. Regeneration and repair of damaged muscle commences about 1-2 weeks after the bite, with regeneration from surviving muscle nuclei, allowing rebuilding within the original sarcolemmal sheath. Biopsy at 6 months shows only a little fine scarring.

Secondary renal damage may occur as a result of the extensive myolysis. Distal tubular necrosis was found in fatal cases dying more than 48hrs. after the bite.

The neurotoxins in sea snake venom have been extensively studied[15,18,19]. With the exception of a few postsynaptically active phospholipase A_2 toxins from *Laticauda semifasciata*, all are classic snake venom postsynaptic neurotoxins, low molecular weight basic proteins, mostly of the short chain variety. Classic short chain neurotoxins have 60-62 amino acids, cross linked with 4 disulphide bonds. Some neurotoxins from sea snakes are slightly larger; 69 aa from *Laticauda colubrina* and 66 aa from *Laticauda semifasciata*. All have a very similar structure and mode of action. They have a central core, with three projecting "fingers" or loops; near the tip of the central one of these loops is the active site. The toxins bind to the acetylcholine receptor on the muscle endplate of the skeletal muscle neuromuscular junction. It has been proposed that this is effected, in part, by penetration of a receptor tryptophan residue deep into the "hydrophobic tryptophan cleft" of the toxin. Binding may be slow, but release is far slower, so that binding is often characterised as "irreversible". The sea snake toxins are similar in both structure and action to other snake venom postsynaptic neurotoxins and related toxins, such as cobra cardiotoxin. A number of the sea snake neurotoxins have been sequenced: the erabutoxins (*L. semifasciata*), the laticotoxins (*L. laticaudata*), and toxins from *Enhydrina schistosa*, *Lapemis hardwickii*, and *Hydrophis cyanocinctus*.

E. PROGNOSTIC INDICATORS

Patients who develop myoglobinuria following sea snakebite are, by definition, envenomed. Those that have clinical evidence of muscle damage, notably muscle movement pain, within 2-3hrs. of the bite, are likely to develop moderate to severe envenoming. Conversely, those patients who have no objective evidence of envenoming or myoglobinuria at 4 or more hours after the bite, in the absence of effective first aid, are unlikely to develop significant envenoming. As with other guidelines on prognosis for snakebite, there will be exceptions to the above, so that it would be prudent to carefully observe all sea snakebite patients for a period well in excess of 4 hours.

IV. PROPHYLAXIS

A. AVOIDANCE OF BITES

The main risk group for sea snakebite, fishermen, especially those using drag nets or similar techniques, should be aware of the risk of sea snakebite. Careful handling of nets and the use of tools to remove snakes, rather than use of bare hands, might reduce the incidence of bites. Many bites occur when the fisherman (or other) accidentally stands on a submerged sea snake. Apart from due care, and avoidance of situations where such accidents might happen, not easy to achieve for many traditional fishermen, specific methods to avoid such incidents are not obvious. Bathing in estuaries and adjacent sections of rivers entering the sea, in sea snake prone regions, is another cause of sea snakebites, and thus caution should be exercised in such locations. This knowledge might influence the siting of tourist complexes. However, the real risk of sea snakebite to casual or recreational bathers remains small. It was estimated by Reid[9] at one bite per 270,000 man bathing hours on Penang Island.

B. PUBLIC EDUCATION ON SNAKEBITE

In areas where sea snakes are common, public education on high risk areas and activities might reduce the risk of bites. More importantly, correct first aid (see below) should be emphasised, as this should reduce the number of patients presenting with advanced envenoming. The at-risk populations should be encouraged to apply correct first aid immediately following a bite, and then seek urgent medical attention. This educational advice must be accompanied by complementary education of health professionals in the diagnosis and management of sea snakebite, coupled with provision of appropriate treatment facilities, including ready availability of specific sea snake antivenom.

V. FIRST AID TREATMENT

A. PRINCIPLES AND THEORY OF FIRST AID

Some sea snake venom components are low molecular weight toxins which might be readily absorbed into the capillaries at the bite site, thus precluding effective first aid. However, experience with Elapid venoms in Australia has demonstrated that a significant proportion of venom is absorbed and transported in the lymphatic system. It has been shown clinically and experimentally that Australian Elapid venoms can be immobilised at the bite site for prolonged periods using a combination of a local mild compressive bandage and immobilisation of the limb with a splint[16]. Details of this method may be found in Chapter 28.

B. RECOMMENDED FIRST AID

The recommended first aid for sea snakebite worldwide is the application of the Australian type snakebite compression/immobilisation bandage and splint, as detailed in Chapter 28. It is not clear from clinical reports whether this method will effectively retard sea snake venom movement. However, the method, when correctly applied, is both safe and relatively easy to achieve. It is unlikely to do harm, and may prove beneficial.

Older methods of snakebite first aid, such as the tourniquet, local wound incision, suction, or excision, or use of locally applied chemicals, are all now considered inappropriate and should never be used for sea snakebite.

VI. CLINICAL MANAGEMENT

A. GENERAL CONSIDERATIONS

As mentioned earlier, the majority of sea snakebites will not result in envenoming. This should always be borne in mind by the treating physician, together with the fact that of the 20% or less who are envenomed, up to 40% or more will develop severe, even life threatening envenoming. It should also be remembered that if optimum treatment facilities are available, particularly specific sea snake antivenom, then virtually no patient should die as a result of sea snakebite.

All sea snakebites seen within 4 to 6 hours of the bite, even if initially symptom free, should be treated as a medical emergency requiring urgent assessment.

B. DIAGNOSIS
1. Approach to diagnosis

The diagnosis of sea snakebite may be straightforward, if the victim can clearly give a history of being bitten by a sea snake, and the clinical features fit; namely the bite caused little or no local pain or reaction. If the patient presents unwell following a bite sustained while in an area frequented by sea snakes, then the presence of small or indistinct bite marks without significant local pain or reaction makes a diagnosis of sea snakebite likely. This would be more so if the bite was to a lower limb after treading on a moving object in water. A bite with marked local pain or reaction is much more likely to have been caused by something other than a sea snake (e.g. spiny fish, sting ray, jellyfish, echinoderm etc). Other marine organisms can envenom without causing much local pain or reaction. Notable amongst these is the blue ringed octopus, *Hapalochlaena* spp., and a few of the cone shells, *Conus* spp. However, clinical reports suggest that for both these organisms, bites are unlikely to occur through brief contact. Indeed, most severe cases have followed the victim actually picking up and holding the organism, in which case a clear history should differentiate from sea snakebite. Sea snakebites are not infrequently prolonged, the snake continuing to bite and hang on to the victim, requiring it to either be shaken off, or otherwise detached. This is far less common with land snakebites. Some species of sea snake regularly come ashore, but bites from sea snakes on land appear rare.

2. Role of venom detection

Venom detection for sea snake venom is technically possible using a variety of techniques, but is not used clinically at present. There is a report of testing for snake venom in a case of suspected sea snakebite in Australia, where cross reactivity with King Brown snake antivenom was noted, the significance of which is uncertain[12].

In most cases the diagnosis of sea snakebite will be reasonably evident after careful history taking and examination. The decision on whether to use antivenom will depend on clinical criteria and evidence of myolysis. As only a single sea snake antivenom is available, there is no requirement to determine the species of sea snake involved for antivenom therapy; therefore, venom detection has no useful role in determining such therapy.

3. Role of Laboratory Investigations

The principal effects of sea snake systemic envenoming are those of myolysis and its complications. The key diagnostic laboratory tests are therefore related to the detection of myolysis; myoglobin in the urine and raised enzymes such as CK and SGOT in the plasma/serum. Renal function may be impaired secondary to myolysis; so urea, creatinine and electrolytes should be measured. If there is significant myolysis then there may be hyperkalaemia, which should be checked for. ECG monitoring may also be helpful in detecting hyperkalaemia. A non-specific leukocytosis is a very common feature of systemic envenoming. Coagulation studies are not helpful.

4. Assessing extent of envenoming

Once the diagnosis of definite or possible sea snakebite has been made, it is necessary to determine if there is systemic envenoming and its extent. As discussed earlier, if systemic envenoming is going to develop, it will usually manifest within 4 hours of the bite, and if severe, usually within 2 hours of the bite. There will be exceptions to this. Firstly the physician must differentiate between anxiety symptoms and true envenoming. Muscle weakness and movement pain are the classic indicators of systemic sea snake envenoming. Once present, their extent and rate of progression, if any, towards severe envenoming with generalised weakness and respiratory distress will determine the severity of envenoming. A patient who has had correct effective first aid applied immediately following the bite and who has remained still thereafter may be symptom free until the first aid is removed, and timing of onset should then be taken from that time, not the time of the bite. A patient who is initially symptom free should be frequently reassessed. Urine output should be constantly measured and urine checked for myoglobin (by urine dipstick testing for "haemoglobin").

C. TREATMENT
1. General approach to treatment
All definite or possible sea snakebites seen within the first 4-6hrs. after the bite, and all those showing symptoms of envenoming should be treated as a medical emergency requiring urgent assessment. Adequate hydration should be ensured, where possible using an intravenous line and restriction of oral intake to clear fluids. Renal output should be established early, by catheterisation if necessary, and urine frequently sampled for myoglobin (see above). A full assessment of the patient should be made, with particular note of symptoms and signs of myolysis and associated paresis. Frequent clinical reassessment should be made.

2. Antivenom therapy and its complications
If the patient has significant systemic envenoming, as evidenced by symptoms and signs of myolysis or paresis, or laboratory evidence of myolysis, then antivenom therapy is indicated. This should be commenced as soon as it is clear there is significant systemic envenoming. The most appropriate antivenom is CSL Sea Snake Antivenom (CSL, Parkville, Melbourne, Australia). The minimum dose is 1 ampoule. Multiple ampoules may be required in some severe cases, where the snake has injected an abnormally large quantity of antivenom. The antivenom is made by hyperimmunising horses with *Enhydrina schistosa* venom. This has been shown effective in neutralising the effects of many other sea snake venoms, as listed in Table 2[16,20]. CSL Tiger Snake Antivenom has also been shown to have some neutralising effect against sea snake venoms, and may be used as an alternative if specific sea snake antivenom is unavailable. However, several ampoules of Tiger Snake Antivenom may be needed to reach equivalence with Sea Snake Antivenom.

Sea Snake Antivenom, as with other current snake antivenoms, should be given intravenously. It is preferable to do so through the side arm of an established IV line. Depending on the size of the patient and the volume to be given, it is preferable to dilute antivenom about 1:10 with saline/hartmans/dextrose or other carrier IV solution. Prior to commencing infusion of antivenom, have an appropriate dose of adrenaline drawn up ready to give, should anaphylaxis to the antivenom occur. Consider prophylactic measures prior to antivenom if there is a history of allergy or asthma. Commence the infusion of antivenom slowly, while carefully observing the patient and monitoring for hypotension or bronchospasm. Increase the rate if no reaction occurs, aiming to give the whole initial dose over about 15mins.

As with most antivenoms, in addition to early reactions, delayed reactions may occur, notably serum sickness. This should be explained to the patient prior to discharge. A course of prophylactic oral steroids may be warranted to prevent serum sickness, especially if a large volume of antivenom has been given.

3. Neurotoxicity and its treatment
The role of true neurotoxicity in sea snake envenoming is uncertain. Earlier literature suggested that neurotoxicity was the main feature of envenoming, however Reid[5,9] determined that myotoxicity was the main clinical problem and that its effects could explain the apparent neurotoxicity in these cases. However, a case of severe envenoming of a child by *Astrotia stokesii* in Australia, in which there was rapid development of classic paralysis

without evidence of major myolysis, may indicate that in some circumstances the neurotoxins in many sea snake venoms may play a dominant role[10].

The treatment of neurotoxicity, should it be a part of sea snake envenoming, is essentially the same as for other snakebites with paralysis. Specific antivenom should be given as soon as there is early evidence of developing paralysis, in the hope of preventing progression to full paralysis. Should the latter occur, or as soon as there is either significant respiratory impairment or poor glossopharyngeal function (i.e. risk of aspiration of vomitus), then the patient should be intubated and ventilated, with sedation and formal paralysis as necessary.

Table 2
Venoms neutralised by CSL Sea Snake Antivenom[16,20]

Species of Sea Snake	Venom Quantity*	Quantity Neutralised**
Enhydrina schistosa	8.5 (79)	10
Aipysurus laevis	6.6	13
Astrotia stokesii	31.3	18
Disteira major	22.8	11
Hydrophis cyanocinctus	8.2 (80)	59
Hydrophis elegans	5.5	57
Hydrophis spiralis	2.1	130
Hydrophis stricticollis		11
Lapemis hardwickii	1.9 (15)	102
Laticauda semifasciata		17

* Average venom quantity milked from snake, where known, in dry weight, mg.
** Quantity of venom in dry weight, mg., neutralised by one ampoule of CSL Sea Snake Antivenom.

4. Myotoxicity and its treatment

The role of antivenom in reducing the extent of myolysis is uncertain. It seems possible that venom, once having reached the systemic circulation, may rapidly leave the circulation and reach target organs, notably the neuromuscular junction. Here the myotoxins may rapidly fix to the muscle and commence the process of membrane and intracellular damage. It is not known if antivenom can slow or reverse this process, once started; therefore, the best hope for antivenom response would be early administration before any damage had occurred. In many cases, this would not be possible, due to time between the bite and reaching treatment. Furthermore, it would mean that antivenom should be given prior to the development of symptoms of envenoming. This would necessitate essentially all sea snakebite victims receiving antivenom, a costly and potentially hazardous regimen. In practical terms, antivenom is only given once there is already evidence of myolysis. Nevertheless, there is some clinical experience to suggest that it is effective despite the onset of paralysis, and therefore antivenom therapy remains the treatment of choice for systemic sea snake envenoming.

Other measures should also be adopted to manage myolysis. Good hydration should be ensured with adequate IV therapy. Urine output should be maintained and monitored. The level of myolysis should be monitored with CK levels and qualitative measurement of urine myoglobin (quantitative measurement of urine myoglobin is, in most labs, very expensive). Potassium level should be monitored, and hyperkalaemia looked for, using regular or continuous ECG. Some authors believe alkalinisation of the urine is useful if there is significant myoglobinuria. While physiotherapy may not be either helpful, or tolerated, in the early stages of myolysis, in the recovery period, an exercise program is worthwhile to assist full muscle recovery. Where myolysis is so severe that there is either respiratory distress or glossopharyngeal dysfunction, then intubation and ventilation should be considered, as discussed above for neurotoxicity.

5. Other Issues in treatment

Sea snakebites rarely result in significant local problems, and local infection does not appear to be a clinical problem. Hence prophylactic antibiotics are not required. Tetanus immunisation should be ensured. Renal failure, if it occurs, should be treated along standard lines.

VII. REFERENCES

1. **REID, H.A.** Sea snake bite research. *Trans. Roy. Soc. Trop. Med. Hyg.* **50:**517-542, 1956.
2. **REID, H.A.** Sea snake bites. *B.M.J.* **2:**73-78, 1956.
3. **REID, H.A.** Antivenene reaction following accidental sea snake bite. *B.M.J.* **2:**26-29, 1957.
4. **REID, H.A.** Sea snake bite and poisoning. *The Practitioner* **183:**530 534, 1959.
5. **REID, H.A.** Myoglobinuria and sea snake poisoning. *B.M.J.* **1:**1284-1289, 1961.
6. **MARSDEN, A.T.H., REID, H.A.** Pathology of sea snake poisoning. *B.M.J.* **1:**1290-1293, 1961.
7. **REID, H.A.** Diagnosis, prognosis and treatment of sea snake bite. *Lancet* **2:**399-402, 1961.
8. **REID, H.A.** Sea snake antivenene; successful trial. *B.M.J.* **2:**576-579, 1962.
9. **REID, H.A.** (1975) Epidemiology and clinical aspects of sea snake bites. In Ed. DUNSON, W.A. *The Biology of Sea Snakes.* University Park Press, Baltimore. pps. 417-462, 1975.
10. **MERCER, H.P., McGILL, J.J., IBRAHIM, R.A.** Envenomation by sea snake in Queensland. *Med. J. Aust.* **1:**130-132, 1981.
11. **ACOTT, C.J.** Sea snake envenomation. *Med. J. Aust.* **144:**448, 1986.
12. **FULDE, G.W.O., SMITH, F.** Sea snake envenomation at Bondi. *Med. J. Aust.* **141:**44-45, 1984.
13. **MINTON, S.A.**. Geographic distribution of sea snakes. In Ed. DUNSON, W.A. *The Biology of Sea Snakes.* University Park Press, Baltimore. pps. 21-32, 1975.
14. **COGGER, H.G.**. Sea snakes of Australia and New Guinea. In Ed. DUNSON, W.A. *The Biology of Sea Snakes.* University Park Press, Baltimore. pps. 59-140, 1975.
15. **TAMIYA, N.** Sea snake venoms and toxins. In Ed. DUNSON, W.A. *The Biology of Sea Snakes.* University Park Press, Baltimore. pps. 385-416, 1975.
16. **SUTHERLAND, S.K.** *Australian Animal Toxins.* Oxford University Press, Melbourne. pps. 159-184, 1983.
17. **LIMPUS, C.** Sea snakes. In Eds. COVACEVICH, J., DAVIE, P., PEARN, J. *Toxic Plants and Animals: A Guide For Australia.* Queensland Museum, Brisbane. pps. 195-204, 1987.
18. **TU, A.T., FULDE, G.** Sea snake bites. *Clinics in Dermatology* **5:**118-126, 1987.
19. **MEBS, D., HUCHO, F.** Toxins acting on ion channels and synapses. In Eds. SHIER, W.T., MEBS, D. *Handbook of Toxinology.* Marcel Dekker, New York. pps. 493-600, 1990.
20. **BAXTER, E.H., GALLICHIO, H.A.** Cross neutralisation by tiger snake (*Notechis scutatus*) antivenene and sea snake (*Enhydrina schistosa*) antivenene against several sea snake venoms. *Toxicon* **12:**273-278, 1974.

Chapter 14

CLINICAL TOXICOLOGY OF BLUE RINGED OCTOPUS BITES

Julian White

TABLE OF CONTENTS

I. INTRODUCTION

The only octopuses clearly capable of causing severe toxin induced morbidity or mortality in man are small species of the genus *Hapalochlaena*, found in the Indo-Pacific region, predominantly in the coastal waters around Australia. While many bites do not result in envenoming, severe paralysis due to the neurotoxin, tetrodotoxin, can occur.

II. EPIDEMIOLOGY

The precise range of this genus of octopuses is uncertain. Two species are common in Australian coastal waters; *H. maculosa* in southern waters, and *H. lunulata* in northern waters. A recent fatality in Singapore due to *Hapalochlaena* sp. extends the range into South East Asian waters[1]. The genus is also found in coastal New Zealand waters[2]. The Singapore case may indicate that genus is represented in waters around parts of Indonesia and New Guinea, although this is not substantiated by case material at this time.

With the exception of the recent Singapore case, all significant cases of morbidity and all fatalities are limited to Australian waters. Sutherland[3] has summarised these cases in a review of blue ringed octopus bites. This data is summarised in Table 1.

Personal experience with suspected and confirmed bites by *H. maculosa* in South Australia is that the majority of bites do not result in envenoming of any significance, at a ratio of at least 5:1. The bite is either not felt or causes a minor sting, but there is often blood at the bite site. All cases have involved placing an octopus, removed from the water, on an exposed area of skin. The single case with symptomatology involved an adult female tourist who placed an octopus in the cleavage of her bikini, where she was bitten, with subsequent perioral parasthesiae and minimal muscular weakness, without significant respiratory involvement.

It appears clear that with the exception of a single case of unconfirmed envenoming[3], all bites have occurred after the octopus has been removed from the water and placed in contact with the victim. The majority of cases occur in the warmer months, possibly reflecting the increased recreation in coastal areas at that time, rather than differences in abundance of the octopus.

Despite the apparent commonness of these octopuses in areas frequented by humans, recorded bites are very few, and deaths rare.

Table 1
Recorded bites from Australian blue ringed octopuses
(afterSutherland[3])

Age & Sex	Date & Place	Species	Incident, Symptoms, Outcome
M, adult	May 1950, Wollongong, NSW	*H. maculosa*	Picked up octopus but felt no bite, then vomiting at 10mins, leg weakness, visual problems. Recovery after several days. ?no respiratory symptoms.
M, 21yrs	October 1954, near Darwin, NT	*H. lunulata*	Picked up octopus & placed on shoulder, no bite felt, but bleeding wound. Within mins. developed dry mouth & dyspnoea, then nausea, vomiting. Developed complete respiratory failure, failed to respond to ventilation, and died about 2hrs after the bite.
M, child	April 1961, Swansea, NSW	*H. maculosa*	Bitten on hand and rapidly developed dyspnoea & vomited. Spasmodic jerking of limbs for several hrs, improved by 8hrs, eventual recovery.
M, 21yrs	December 1961, Cowes, VIC	*H. maculosa*	Picked up octopus and placed on arm. Within mins. developed paralysis including respiratory, requiring assisted ventilation for 3hrs, with eventual recovery.
M, 33yrs	December 1962, Beaumaris, VIC	*H. maculosa*	Bitten on hand with almost complete paralysis within 15mins. Required 1hr of assisted ventilation.
M, 23yrs	June 1967, Camp Cove, NSW	*H. maculosa*	Octopus placed on back of hand, no bite felt, but after 10mins, felt dizzy. Within mins could not swallow, dyspnoea, and shortly after, respiratory failure, then respiratory arrest, and death despite attempts at expired air resuscitation. Time to death less than 90mins.
F, adult	December 1968, Shell Harbour, NSW	*H. maculosa*	Carrying shells inside wet suit. Felt faint during dive and at 10mins, exhaustion. Did not feel bite but found octopus against skin (from shell?). Became nauseous, then jerking spasms of whole body, lasting 6hrs. At 12hrs developed a pruritic urticarial truncal rash, followed by joint effusions over the next few days.
M, 28yrs	November 1977, Geraldton, WA	?	?stood on octopus which fell out of lobster pot and felt bite on foot. No symptoms.
M, 11yrs	March 1979, Gosford, NSW	*H. maculosa*	Handling octopus, no bite felt, but within mins developed parasthesiae of hand and periorally, and nausea. Rapidly developed slurred speech ataxic gait and cerebellar signs, but no respiratory failure. Recovery within 24hrs.
M, 41yrs	April 1979, Adelaide, SA	*H. maculosa*	Bitten on finger?, developed slight weakness around shoulders, rapidly recovered. Some bite site swelling.
M, 43yrs	September 1981, South Stradbroke Island, QLD	?	Bite on hand after picking up octopus. Collapsed (?cardio-pulmonary arrest) in transit to hospital and in full arrest with fixed dilated pupils on arrival. He responded to ECM, with return of cardiac function, but with fixed dilated pupils still. He was ventilated and after 6hrs pupils became reactive, with returning neuromuscular function. Over the next few days he recovered except for memory loss/dysfunction.
M, 16yrs	December 1980, Sydney, NSW	?	Walked through a rock pool, felt something brush against foot, and later developed weakness, parasthesiae, numbness of hands and face, chest tightness, dyspnoea. He rapidly collapsed, with respiratory failure and aspiration of vomitus. He was ventilated and remained so for ?several days. He was asthmatic and it appears at least some of his respiratory problems were related to this[3].

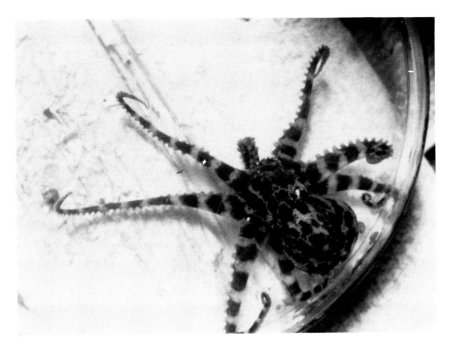

Figure 1. Southern blue ringed octopus, *Hapalochlaena maculosa* (illustration © Dr. J. White).

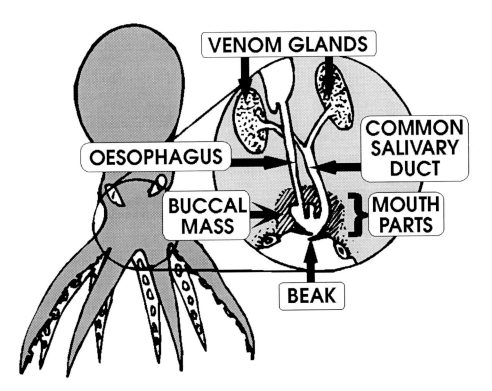

Figure 2. Diagrammatic representation of the venom apparatus of *H. maculosa* (illustration © Dr. J. White).

III. VENOM AND VENOM APPARATUS

The venom of the blue ringed octopus is produced in the paired posterior salivary glands (Figure 2). The venom leaves the glands via ducts, which combine into a common salivary duct, opening in the mouth region, adjacent to the "beak"[3,4]. The venom is inoculated into the victim during the process of biting. There are no fangs or sting. It appears that the act of biting affords the octopus the chance to inoculate venom under pressure, in experimental animals apparently reaching a depth of up to 5mm into the dermis[4].

The principle toxic component of the venom is tetrodotoxin (TTX)[5]. Details on the pharmacology of TTX may be found in Chapter 6 (Fugu poisoning). It is a presynaptic neurotoxin, blocking sodium channels on axons, has a MW of 319D and an LD_{50} of 9mg/kg (mice, iv & sc.).

IV. SYMPTOMS AND SIGNS

The symptoms and signs of envenoming by the blue ringed octopus are those of TTX poisoning. It appears that a significant number of bites by the octopus do not result in clinically detectable envenoming. The ratio of such "dry" bites to effective bites is not known, but is probably greater than 1:1. The octopus must be in contact with the skin to bite the victim and cause envenoming. This almost invariably occurs when the octopus is taken out of the water and placed on the victim's skin, most often the hand or forearm. When distressed the octopus produces warning colouration, particularly small blue rings all over the body and arms, giving rise to the common name. The bite may be felt, but often is not felt, although difficulty in removing the octopus probably reflects the act of biting. Frequently there are a few small marks left on the skin surface with associated bleeding. Local pain is not common.

The principal symptoms and signs are systemic, reflecting the systemic action of TTX, and may occur within a few minutes of the bite. Because the bite is trivial, often the first realisation the victim may have, that a bite has occurred, is the onset of systemic symptoms. This has obvious implications for the likely effectiveness of first aid. The symptoms of TTX poisoning are essentially similar to those seen with TTX ingestion. There is numbness or parasthesiae involving the lips, then face and tongue, with rapid development of generalised muscle weakness and dyspnoea. Speech is often quickly affected, and oropharyngeal paralysis may precipitate respiratory difficulty prior to full paralysis of respiratory muscles. Possibly within 15 minutes of the bite, in extreme cases, respiratory paralysis is so severe that respiratory, then cardiac arrest may occur, unless first aid measures are instituted. Nausea seems to be an inconstant feature, vomiting is not common, and cardiovascular manifestations of TTX poisoning do not receive prominence in case reports.

Death may be rapid and is due to respiratory failure.

V. PROPHYLAXIS

As bites only occur when the octopus is molested, and almost invariably, only after it has been removed from the water and placed on the victim's skin, all bites are preventable. To ensure public awareness of the potential danger of handling the blue ringed octopus, repeated public education campaigns are needed. Education of school children should include information on the octopus. Areas where the octopus is common and frequently encountered should be signposted with appropriate warnings.

VI. FIRST AID TREATMENT

Due to the rapidity of onset of life threatening sequelae of envenoming by the blue ringed octopus, prompt and appropriate first aid will often be crucial in securing a favourable outcome for the patient. If the patient is still in the water, quickly move them to dry land. If the patient is aware of a bite having occurred prior to the onset of symptoms, then application of the Australian snakebite technique of first aid is appropriate (pressure immobilisation bandage and splint [6]; see Chapter 27). More often, the first indication of problems will be onset of systemic envenoming. Providing the patient is not in respiratory distress, application of the bandage, as above, should be a priority. However, if there is developing respiratory distress, expired air breathing takes priority and is potentially life saving. As aspiration of vomitus is a real risk, nurse the patient on their side, and pay careful attention to airway patency, which may be compromised by oropharyngeal paresis and vomitus. Providing there is adequate maintenance of respiration, cardiac arrhythmias or arrest are not likely, so ECM will only rarely be needed. If there has been significant delay between respiratory arrest and commencement of resuscitation, then full cardiopulmonary arrest is much more likely.

VII. CLINICAL MANAGEMENT

All patients with definite or suspected blue ringed octopus bite seen within 6 hours of the bite should be admitted for observation. In practice, however, if significant envenoming has occurred, systemic envenoming will be manifest well before 6 hours, often within minutes of the bite, and by time of arrival at a hospital, the patient will often have established respiratory failure, if this is going to occur. In this situation, rapid establishment of the respiratory and cardiovascular status is imperative, accompanied by measures to maintain vital functions. Thus clearing the airway, intubation and ventilation, establishment of an iv line, and ECM (if indicated) will be priorities. The completely paralysed patient may only need ventilation for a few hours. If on arrival the patient has early symptoms of systemic envenoming without dyspnoea, establish an iv line, hydration, document muscle power, and establish respiratory status with arterial blood gasses and vital capacity. Monitor closely until at least 6 hours post bite. Institute respiratory support when indicated.

Any patient presenting more than 6 hours after a suspected blue ringed octopus bite, without symptoms of envenoming, is most unlikely to have been envenomed. After a brief period of observation, they can be discharged.

VIII. REFERENCES

1. **WILLIAMSON, J.A.H.** The blue ringed octopus bite and envenomation syndrome. *Clinics in Dermatol.* 5: 127-133, 1987.
2. **SUTHERLAND, S.K.** Australian Venomous Animals and Their Venoms. Melbourne: Oxford University Press. 1983.
3. **WALKER, D.G.** Survival after severe envenomation by the blue ringed octopus (*Hapalochlaena maculosa*). *Med.J. Aust.* 2: 663-665, 1983.
4. **SUTHERLAND, S.K., LANE, W.R.** Toxins and mode of envenomation of common ringed or blue banded octopus. *Med. J. Aust.* 1: 893-898. 1969.
5. **SHEUMACK, D.D., HOWDEN, M.E.H., SPENCE, I.,** Maculotoxin: a neurotoxin from the glands of the octopus *Hapalochlaena maculosa* identified as a tetrodotoxin. *Science* 199: 188-189. 1978.
6. **SUTHERLAND, S.K., DUNCAN, A.W.** New first aid measures for envenomation: with special reference to bites by the Sydney funnel web spider *Atrax robustus. Med. J. Aust.* 1: 378-379, 1980.

Chapter 15

BIOLOGY AND DISTRIBUTION OF TICKS OF MEDICAL IMPORTANCE

André Aeschlimann and Thierry A. Freyvogel

TABLE OF CONTENTS

I. INTRODUCTION

Ticks are haematophagous ectoparasites, and thus belong to parasitology. However, the saliva of several species of ticks has a neurotoxic action, and can cause paralysis in their hosts. Looked at from this angle, ticks might be considered to belong in the province of the toxinologist. What, one might ask, is the decisive criterion for ascribing a group of animals to the fields of either parasitology or toxinology? The answer seems to be that parasitic animals whose saliva has toxic properties, but where these are facultative, are primarily to be considered as parasites. On the other hand, animals whose toxicity is obligatory - that is, essential for their survival - clearly belong to the field of toxinology. Such distinctions may sound rather academic; they are indeed man-made and somehow artificial. Yet they remind us how complex Nature is, and that there are limits to its meaningful compartmentalization by the human mind. It also brings to our attention the fact that ticks are endowed with manifold fascinating capacities, which are well worth scientific investigation in themselves. However, ticks have an importance which goes beyond the bounds of pure science - in most parts of the world ticks are important pests, causing damage and disease, and they are often the vectors of dreaded pathogens.

This chapter is meant to introduce ticks in general, emphasizing their mode of life and interrelations with their hosts. A clinical perspective is given in Chapter 16. For more exhaustive information on the geographic distribution of ticks, their biology and on the human and animal pathogens transmitted by some of them, a wide literature is available. The short reference list at the end of this chapter is far from complete; it should, however, suffice to facilitate access to the more relevant existing publications, especially the two volumes on the biology of ticks published recently by Sonnenshine[1]. Incidentally, both tables and all figures have been produced at the Institute of Zoology of the University of Neuchâtel.

II. THE TICKS

A. TAXONOMY

Ticks belong to the *Arthropoda*. They have an ovoid body which appears homogeneous, all traces of external segmentation having been lost in the course of embryonic evolution. The fore-part of the body bears a capitulum which includes the mouthparts with which blood is taken up. There are four pairs of legs. There are neither antennae nor wings. Ticks thus appear to be more closely related to spiders than to insects.

In fact, they belong to the *Chelicerata* (Table 1, Figure 1). The capitulum comprises paired dorsal chelicerae, a pair of lateral pedipalps and one ventral hypostome. Chelicerae and hypostome surround the buccal orifice and together form the piercing device, the rostrum. The hypostome bears hooks which attach the tick firmly to the skin of its host (Figure 2 a and b).

Within the *Chelicerata*, ticks and mites form the order of the *Acarina*. Most acarines are tiny animals, less than 1 mm in body length, but adult ticks can be between 3 and 23 mm long. The ticks belong to the suborder *Metastigmata* (or *Ixodida*), characterised by paired lateral respiratory openings, the stigmata, which are located on either side of the body, about half-way between its anterior and posterior ends.

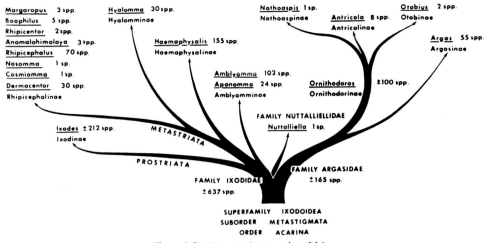

Figure 1. Phylogeny and systematics of ticks.

Table 1
The systematics of ticks (Ixodida)

Phylum	ARTHROPODA
Sub-Phylum	CHELICERATA
Class	ARACHNIDA
Order	ACARINA
Sub-Order	METASTIGMATA (= IXODIDA, ticks)
	(3 families; 11 sub-families; 19 genera; approx. 800 species known today)

Family	Sub-Family	Genus
IXODIDAE	**PROSTRIATA**	
	Ixodinae	*Ixodes*
	METASTRIATA	
	Amblyomminae	*Amblyomma*
		Aponomma
	Haemaphysalinae	*Haemaphysalis*
	Hyalomminae	*Hyalomma*
	Rhipicephalinae	*Margaropus*
		Boophilus
		Rhipicentor
		Anomalohimalaya
		Rhipicephalus
		Nosomma
		Cosmiomma
		Dermacentor
NUTTALLIELLIDAE	Nuttalliellinae	*Nuttalliella*
ARGASIDAE	Argasinae	*Argas*
	Ornithorinae	*Ornithodoros*
	Otobinae	*Otobius*
	Antricollinae	*Antricola*
	Nothoaspinae	*Nothoaspis*

The *Metastigmata* comprise three distinct families[2]. The most extensive (in terms both of genera and of species), is that of the *Ixodidae* (Figure 3 a), which are also called the "hard ticks" because they have a sclerotized dorsal shield or scutum. This covers about one third of the dorsal surface in (unfed) female ticks, all other areas of the integument posterior to the scutum remaining flexible (alloscutum); in males the scutum (sometimes called conscutum) covers virtually the entire dorsal surface. The second family is that of the *Argasidae* or "soft ticks" (Figure 3 b), which have an integument which is tough and "leathery" all over. The third (or second ?) family, that of the *Nuttallielidae*, is thought to be represented by but one single species, *Nuttalliella namaqua*, known from southern Africa[3]; it will not be further discussed in this paper.

In all, some 800 species of ticks are known to exist, of which 640 are ixodids and 160 argasids. Compared with the numbers of species which make up certain insect families, the figures for ticks are rather modest. Nevertheless, only about 20 tick species have been studied in detail, and then most often in conjunction with the transmission of pathogens. What follows in this chapter on the morphology, anatomy, life cycle, host specificity and ecology of ticks will be based on the results obtained from studies undertaken on these comparatively few tick species.

B. MORPHOLOGY AND ANATOMY
In the following comments ixodid and argasid ticks will be compared.

1. Morphology
Ticks are flattened dorsoventrally. As was mentioned above, the body is ovoid in shape and homogeneous. In *Ixodidae*, the capitulum is visible from above; it projects forwards beyond

the anterior outline of the body. In*Argasidae*, the capitulum is not visible from above, since it is situated ventrally, in a depression called the camerostoma.

In ixodid females the scutum can be easily seen, because it contrasts with the rest of the dorsal integument. In ixodid males, the conscutum covers the entire dorsal surface, and thus does not contrast with the rest of the integument. The scutum permits easy distinction between females and males.

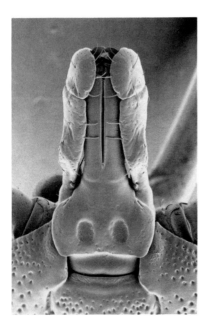
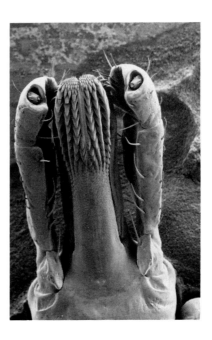

Figure 2. Rostrum of an*Amblyomma variegatum* female.
2a. Dorsal view: to right and left the pedipalps, in between the paired cheliceres, all affixed onto the basis capituli, 54x.

2b. Ventral view: note the rows of hooks on the hypostome; on either side the pedipalps, 98x.

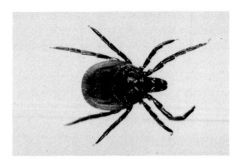
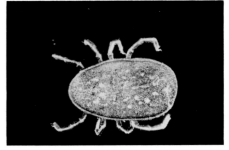

Figure 3a. *Ixodes ricinus* female (unfed), dorsal view: note the comparatively long rostrum, the sclerotized shield and the flexible alloscutum.

Figure 3b. *Argas* sp. female (unfed): note the "leathery" appearance of the integument; the rostrum remains hidden because of its small size and ventral position.

In argasid ticks there is no scutum. The sexes differ in size, the females being larger. The genital orifices, too, are shaped differently; crescent-shaped in the females and quadrangular in the males.

In ixodid and argasid ticks of both sexes, "Haller's organ" can be observed on the dorsal part of the tarsus of the first pair of legs (Figure 4). This organ consists of an accumulation of sensory hairs, separated in two groups. The first one is located at the bottom of a posterior capsule, most often covered by a thin membrane (except for some Ixodes species), with a slit which allows contact with the outside world. The second one is found in an anterior pit, a tiny integumentory depression surrounded by a heavily sclerotized rim. Additional sensory hairs are arranged either singly or in smaller groups, in front and behind these two most characteristic amassings. All these sensory hairs function as either chemo-, thermo-, hygro- or mechano-receptors. They are linked with the underlying peripheral nervous system. The Haller's organ enables the ticks to locate themselves in their surroundings, to find their hosts and an adequate spot to bite.

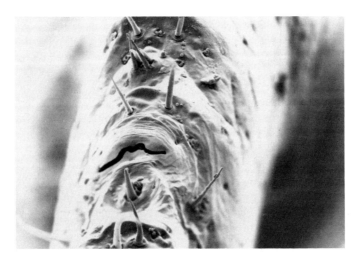

Figure 4. Haller's organ (*Amblyomma variegatum* female): note the slit of the undulated membrane covering the posterior capsule (centre of picture) and (below it, i.e. distally) the anterior pit.

2. Anatomy

Only those inner organs which are directly involved in the transmission of pathogens by ticks will be mentioned here.

The midgut shows numerous diverticula, the ramifications of which extend into all the body cavities of the tick, and which enable it to take up large quantities of blood. A precondition for the spectacular engorgement of tick females, of course, is the flexibility of the outer integument, in particular the alloscutum. Pathogens that are taken in by the tick with its blood meal therefore find themselves at first in the lumen of that vast "stomach". All its diverticula are in close contact with the other organs in the body cavity once the tick is engorged.

The paired salivary glands are equally important in pathogen transmission, for it is most often there that the infectious forms assemble, waiting for the opportunity to be injected into their vertebrate host when the tick takes its next blood meal. As has been indicated in the introduction, the salivary glands are relevant also in conjunction with toxicoses such as tick paralysis and sweating sickness, which will be dealt with in Chapter 16. The salivary glands, incidentally, assume various other functions, most important for the ticks' biology and physiology. In some instances they produce a kind of cement with which the tick attaches itself more firmly to its host. They also produce anticoagulant substances, which prevent the clotting of the blood while it is being sucked in. They do produce enzymes and other substances, including hygroscopic and immuno-suppressive compounds. In ixodids, moreover, during the meal they control the tick's water metabolism, in that they excrete surplus water and ions from the ingested serum back into the host. Thus, ixodids rid themselves of unwanted liquid and concentrate the solid parts of the blood in the lumen of the intestine. With regard to the numerous vital functions the salivary glands fulfill, it is not surprising to find their histology and cytology highly sophisticated[4,5,6]. In Argasidae, the function of controlling the water-balance is assumed by the coxal organs, which are a unique feature of this family. These are specialized paired glands, situated between the first and second pair of legs, which expel the surplus water onto the skin of the host.

The reproductive organs can also play an important role in relation to pathogen transmission. Eggs may be invaded by pathogens in the ovaries - a process which means that young larvae may be infective already after hatching and even before they have taken their first blood meal. In fact, in some parasitic diseases transovarian transmission has been found to represent a major epidemiological factor. Mating-bound transmission, from male spermatophores to female egg-cells, could also take place in theory, but its occurrence has not (yet) been established with certainty.

C. LIFE CYCLE

The life of an individual tick is characterized by a succession of ectoparasitic and free-living phases. All ticks' life cycles consist of four succeeding stages: the egg, the larva, the nymph(s) and the adult (Table 2).

In the *Ixodidae*, out of the egg hatches a hexapod larva, which takes a first blood meal and moults to an octopod nymph. After a second blood meal, the nymph moults again, and becomes an adult, either female or male. As a rule, mating takes place on the skin of the host, during a blood meal. In the genus Ixodes, mating may take place during a free-living phase, prior to the third blood meal. This poses the question of how the sexes meet; the answer is, presumably, that pheromones are produced. Once engorged, the female drops to the ground, lays her eggs (between 2,000 and 20,000, depending on the species) and dies. No development towards a succeeding life stage is possible without a previous blood meal. Each blood meal, irrespective of the developmental stage, lasts for several days; ixodid ticks are considered "long feeders".

The life-cycle of *Argasidae* is basically the same as that of the *Ixodidae*. However, there are several nymphal stages, the number being species-specific. Each stage needs a blood meal and is followed by a moult. The females may oviposit repeatedly. They do not necessarily die after oviposition; they may take another bloodmeal and oviposit again. A single copulation may be sufficient for several batches of viable eggs (less than 200 at a time). Also, in some species of argasid ticks, the larvae do not feed at all, their vitelline reserve enabling them to moult into the first nymphal stage without any intake of blood. Among the *Ixodidae* the number of blood meals in each individual's life is constant, but among the argasid ticks the number of blood meals an individual takes during its lifetime may vary, and will usually be higher. Finally, each single blood meal lasts only between fifteen minutes and an hour. Argasids are "short feeders".

III. MEDICAL AND VETERINARY IMPORTANCE OF TICKS

As ectoparasites, ticks may trouble their hosts in various ways and cause a variety of symptoms collectively known as "tick worries" - not to be confused with diseases indirectly caused by ticks as a result of the transmission of pathogens.

A. TICK WORRIES

Besides being a nuisance ticks may cause lesions, anaemia or toxicoses as well as various other sequelae, including immunosuppression and allergies[7,8].

1. Lesions

When the tick feeds, a skin lesion is produced at the site of penetration. The more powerful the rostrum, the more extensive will the lesions become. Ticks may occur in very large numbers on a single host animal, and the bites may become sources of secondary infection; so, damage may be extensive. In animals whose hide is used for the making of leather, one result can be that the skin loses all its commercial value (Figure 5).

Table 2
The life cycles of Ixodid and Argasid ticks

	IXODIDAE (hard ticks)			ARGASIDAE (soft ticks)
	monophasic	diphasic	triphasic	polyphasic
Egg ↓ **Larva** ↓ **Nymph** ↓ **Adult** ♀ x ♂ **Egg laying**	N M N M N El	N M N M N El	N M N M N El	N M N M N M N M N etc. N El/El/El...
	♀: dies after a single egg laying of several thousand eggs			♀: can lay 50 to 200 eggs on successive occasions

⌐ = on the host   ♀ x ♂ = copulation

N = Nutrition   M = Molting   El = Egg laying

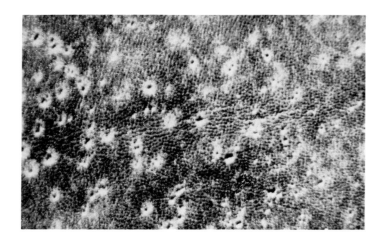

Figure 5. Cow leather, badly damaged due to numerous tick bites.

2. Anaemia

Female ixoxid ticks take up comparatively large quantitites of blood, up to 20 times their own body weight. Since they often occur in large numbers and may reinfest their hosts repeatedly over long periods of time, they can cause increasing anaemia in their hosts, followed by loss of weight, diminution of milk production and general weakness.

3. Toxicoses

As mentioned in the Introduction, several tick species may cause "tick paralysis". This will be dealt with in Chapter 16.

4. Miscellaneous

Besides substances causing paralysis, other toxins may also be injected into the host when a tick takes a blood meal. Some of these toxins have been found to lead to immunosuppression, which may be followed by the re-appearance of latent infections. Others were found to act as allergens, i.e. to cause allergic reactions.

To sum up: owing to their sheer numbers, to the quantity of blood taken up, and to the properties of their saliva, ticks represent a considerable hazard to animal husbandry and even to man (in particular with reference to tick paralysis), quite apart from their role as vectors of pathogenic organisms.

B. TRANSMISSION OF PATHOGENS

A surprisingly wide variety of pathogens are transmitted by ticks. They include microorganisms, protozoans and metazoans[9]. Ticks might be the most versatile vectors among the arthropods; they are capable of transmitting the highest number of different pathogen species. This applies to tick species as well as to single specimens. *Ixodes ricinus*, e.g., may harbour simultaneously TBE virus, *Borrelia burgdorferi* and *Rickettsia helvetica*. Among the microorganisms there are obligatory intracellular organisms (e.g. tick-borne encephalitis viruses and rickettsiae of the spotted fever group), and other bacteria, including various spirochaetes like *Borrelia burgdorferi*, the agent of Lyme disease, or *B.duttoni*, the agent of African relapsing fever. It is even suspected that *Yersinia tularensis* may be transmitted by ticks. The tick borne protozoans include several species of *Babesia* and of *Theileria*. Among the metazoans transmitted by ticks one finds filarial helminths such as *Acanthocheilonema* (*Dipetalonema*) and *Macdonaldius*.

1. Transmission routes

There are several routes - the salivarial, coxal, stercoral, regurgitation, effraction and ingestion route - of transmission of pathogens by ticks, depending on host behaviour, on the biology of the ticks concerned, on their chance of picking up one pathogen or another, and on the possibilities of transstadial (larva - nymph, nymph - adult) and transovarian (adult female - egg/larva) transmission.

Unicellular parasites, including microorganisms, are transmitted by and large via the salivary glands. Spirochaetes transmitted by *Argasidae* may also use the route of the coxal glands. *Borrelia burgdorferi* may possibly be regurgitated. *Coxiella burnetti*, a rikettsia-like bacterium, is excreted with the tick's faeces and later inhaled into the lungs; this is an example of what is known as the stercoral route. As for filariae, their stage 3 larvae leave the tick actively, breaking through the integument and invading the final host by penetrating through the skin at the site of the lesion made by the tick rostrum.

Several tick species contribute to the survival of pathogen populations in susceptible hosts by combining transstadial with transovarian transmission (Figure 6). Transovarian transmission is not possible for all pathogens; no transovarian transmission has been observed with either *Theileria* or *Acanthocheilonema*. Where it does occur, it may may take place through several consecutive tick generations. In this case the tick population simultaneously assumes the role of both vector and reservoir. How effective this is depends on the pathogens concerned. Transmission of rickettsiae is 100% transovarian, and of *B. duttoni* 40%. For *B. burgdorferi*, however, this route accounts for only 3 - 6% of transmission, and for encephalitis viruses only for 0.1%. Such figures provide some indication as to how relevant transovarian transmission may be under given epidemiological circumstances.

2. Natural transmission foci

A natural transmission focus has been defined as the smallest area which permits sustaining the complete life cycle of a pathogen over longer periods of time. Thus, a natural focus must accomodate ticks, capable of pathogen transmission, the ticks' blood donor hosts and the reservoir of the pathogens concerned. Since ticks barely migrate and since many reservoir animals are rather sedentary, natural foci frequently are much localized and may function as autonomous entities over prolonged periods of time. The creation of new foci largely depends on particularly favourable conditions, such as the emigration of young animals, or the dissemination of ticks by either birds or mammals, whether migrants or passers-by[10].

3. Interrelations of natural foci and tick life cycles

In order to understand how natural foci work, adequate knowledge of the interrelations between ticks and their hosts is indispensable. Details of the life cycles of the various tick species may be essential (Table 2). With reference to their life cycles, *Ixodidae* are either *tri-, di-* or *monophasic*; with reference to their hosts, they are either (tri-), *di-* or *monoxenous*. To take a first example: a triphasic tick is one which will search for an appropriate host three times in its life, two moults occurring in between, during free living phases. To take a second example: a dixenous tick is one which is likely to feed on a first kind of host, predominantly of smaller size, as a larva and as a nymph, while it uses to feed on a comparatively large host animal as an adult tick. [There are virtually no trixenous ticks. *Ixodes ricinus*, most common in Switzerland, though, shows a tendency to trixeny in that its larvae feed on lizards, birds and rodents, its nymphs on birds, rodents and other small mammals, and its adults exclusively on large animals, either wild or domestic (Figure 7).] With diphasic/dixenous ticks, larvae and nymphs stay on the same host for two consecutive blood meals and the intermittent moult. The second moult, the one from nymph to adult, takes place off the host, mostly in the soil, during a free living phase. Once adult, the tick has to search for another host to feed on. As to monophasic and, consequently also monoxenous ticks, they feed on a single host throughout their lives, as larva, nymph and adult. The vast majority of species concerned belong to the genus *Boophilus*. They may act as vectors of pathogens only when they get infected by transovarian route.

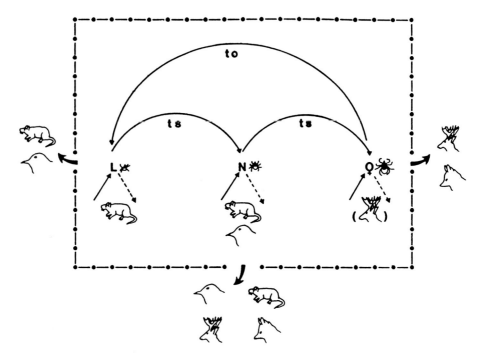

Figure 6. Transmission of pathogens by *Ixodes ricinus* in a natural transmission focus: a tick may get infected at the larval stage (L), pass on the infection to the nymph (N) transstadially (ts) and onwards to the adult tick (female shown). The female can further transmit trans-ovarially (to) onto the next tick generation. The interrupted arrows point out the infectiveness of the ticks for wild animals (or man). The straight, full arrows indicate an infection of the ticks. As *I. ricinus* barely migrate, they stay in a natural transmission focus. Their dissemination becomes possible by phoresis, when the ticks are attached to migrating host animals. This way (fat, bent arrows) new natural foci may ensue.

The *Argasidae* are all polyphasic since they go through several nymphal stages. Thus, they have to search for new hosts repeatedly. Their search for a host may, however, be rendered less strenuous by the fact that they are (facultatively) monoxenous, i.e. that they may feed on only one host species. Monoxeny, in fact, may be seen as an evolutionary simplification. As a consequence, argasid ticks will live in rather restricted habitats, in permanent, close vicinity with their hosts. Monoxenous ticks, thus, often are *endophilous*; they are to be found in burrows, nests or other shelters, where, by the way, variations of temperature and humidity are low. Other tick species, particularly among the *Ixodidae*, are *exophilous*. They climb upon vegetation, to await their hosts. Thanks to the Haller's organ they are capable of locating a host animal approaching and, once on it, to make out an adequate bite site.

Thus, three categories of behavioural phenomena determine the ticks' interrelations with their environment and, with them, also their role as vectors of pathogens: the tri-, di-, mono- or polyphasy; the (tri-), di- or monoxeny - and with it the host-specificity; and the endo- and exophily, in the sense of the most intimate interchange with the environment.

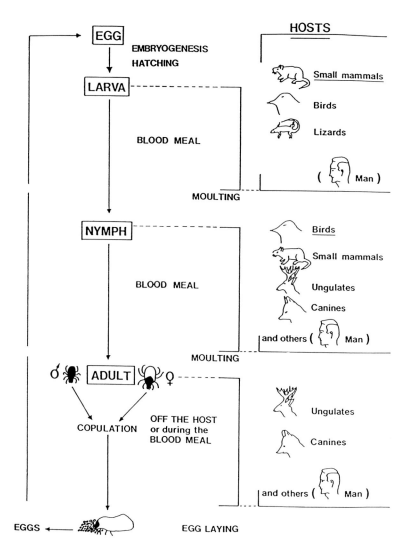

Figure 7. Life cycle of the triphasic, trixenous and exophilous tick *Ixodes ricinus*; note that man can be its host at each of its developmental stages.

IV. HANDLING TICKS

A. COLLECTION OF TICKS
1. From a host

Collecting ticks from a freshly captured host animal presents no difficulties. Also, an essential bit of information is obtained with the identification of the host. One has to keep in mind, though, that host animals may migrate or move from one place to another. It is further recommended to note the exact location of the ticks collected on their host, e.g. around the ears, in the underarm, inguinal or peri-anal region, or in between fingers and toes, for there is a certain habitat specificity. On the other hand, the identification of semi- or fully engorged ticks may prove tricky, for species specific characteristics pertaining to the integument become blurred due to its extension during blood intake.

Thus, either trapping rodents or other small mammals (e.g. carnivores), or netting birds, under circumstances are not to be avoided; thereby, well established, "classical" methods may be used. Capture/release methods permit an estimation of the re-infestation rates of hosts, provided these were marked prior to release. In countries like Switzerland, trapping mammals and netting birds, in fact, contribute much to the existing collections, mainly with regard to subadult specimens and endophilous tick species. As to collecting ticks from domestic or game animals, neither are there any particular difficulties encountered. One has to be aware, though, that ticks use to leave host animals rather soon once these are dead.

2. Free living phases

Most successfull is the "flag method". It consists in dragging along a piece of clear coloured material over the vegetation of the site selected for collecting ticks. *Exophilous* ticks will get trapped in the mesh of the cloth used. This method provides accurate results with reference to the site where ticks were awaiting for their hosts and to their number (in relation to the size of the "flag").

An other method is to lay out frozen carbondioxide cubes on the soil of the site selected and to cover them with a blanket. The emanating carbondioxide gas will stimulate the Haller's organ and attract ticks under the blanket. The personal experience gained by one of us (A.A.) with this method were, however, not very encouraging.

As to *endophilous* ticks, a careful search of burrows, nests and all kinds of refuges and resting sites is recommended. The personal experience made by the other author (T.A.F.) with the argasid *Ornithodoros moubata* in the East African savannah was that by entering a warthogs' burrow, he acted as a bait and attracted numerous adults and subadults on his clothing, in particular his cap[11]. The same soft tick species was also found in the soil of human habitations; the specimens were undug by scratching the soil, near the base of the mudwalls, with little sticks.

B. PRESERVATION OF TICKS
1. Live ticks

Except for a few species originating from dry areas, ticks are rather susceptible to low humidity and desiccation. They thus ought to be kept in tubes wherein the air is saturated with moisture. The bottom of the tubes may be covered with a layer of moist gypsum; in addition, a piece of humidified folded filter paper does help to keep the atmosphere in the tubes damp. In case of need some fresh blades of grass may provide the humidity wanted. In any way, the sooner the ticks collected are transferred into climatized laboratory conditions, the higher will be their chances of survival. Some species, e.g. *I. ricinus*, easily withstand temperatures as low as 5°C; pathogens present in such ticks, too, will remain viable for several days after collection of the ticks.

2. Dead ticks

They are best preserved in 80% ethanol. The morphological characteristics remain intact. The colours of enamelled scutum and conscutum may fade away, but can be revived by the addition of a drop of chloroform to the alcohol in the tube.

C. PREVENTION OF TICK BITES

By far not all ticks are infective, nor do all their bites cause worries as described earlier in this paper. Yet, they are resented as a nuisance. The following rules may help to prevent tick bites; they apply mainly to *I. ricinus*, the most common tick in Switzerland:
- Avoid, whenever possible, forests with dense undergrowth. Ticks of all stages may be awaiting for blood donors on vegetation.
- Stay within a road or path; avoid repeated contact with vegetation alongside it.
- Wear long trousers and shirts with long sleeves.

- Wear boots and introduce the trouser legs into your socks. Ticks are so prevented to enter into direct contact with your skin.
- Wear bright colours. Ticks are more easily detected when moving around.
- Search body, head and vestments carefully when returning from an outing; search yourself and your dog. Ticks often move around in their search for an appropriate bite site on their host. (In theory, at this stage, they still could move over from dog to man or vice versa.)
- Use an anti-tick collar for your dog, or possibly apply an acaricidal spray.

D. REMOVAL OF TICKS ATTACHED

The removal of ticks attached onto a host is not necessarily easy. This applies in particular to adults of species with a long rostrum, deeply embedded in the host's skin.

Slight anaesthesia[8], with either ether or ethanol, or the onset of asphyxia with oil or ointment, may facilitate extraction of the capitulum in that they cause the tick to loosen its grip and to partially retract cheliceres and hypostome. After some 10 to 20 minutes a firm hold is kept on the rostrum, at the level of the skin, with fine forceps or tweezers, and the tick removed with a straight, firm and steady movement, along the tick's longitudinal axis. No rotating movement is needed; care should be taken not to break the rostrum.

Removing a tick with fingers alone is to be avoided. Usually, several attempts are necessary if one does not want to crush the tick. In addition, the ongoing handling of the tick may cause it to either regurgitate or to salivate, whereby the transmission of pathogens may be the consequence.

V. REFERENCES

1. **SONNENSHINE, D.E.**, Biology of Ticks, Oxford University Press, vol.1 1991, vol. 2 1993.
2. **HOOGSTRAAL, H., AND AESCHLIMANN, A.**, Tick-Host Specificity, Mitteil. Schweiz. Entomol. Ges., 55, 5, 1982.
3. **HOOGSTRAAL, H.**, Argasid and Nuttalliellid ticks as parasites and vectors, *Adv. Parasitol.*, 24, 135, 1985.
4. **FAWCETT, D. W., DOXSEY, S. AND BUSCHER, G.**, Salivary gland of the tick vector (*R. appendiculatus*) of East Coast Fever. I. Ultrastructure of the type III acinus, *Tissue and Cell*, 13, 209, 1981.
5. **FAWCETT, D.W., DOXSEY, S. AND BUSCHER, G.**, Salivary gland of the tick vector (*R. appendiculatus*) of East Coast Fever. II. Cellular basis for fluid secretion in the type III acinus, *Tissue and Cell*, 13, 231, 1981.
6. **FAWCETT, D. W., BINNINGTON, K. AND VOIGT, W. P.**, The cell biology of the tick salivary gland, in *Morphology, Physiology and Behavioral Biology of Ticks*, Sauer, J. R. and Hair, J. A., Ellis Horwood, Chichester, 1986, 22.
7. **HOOGSTRAAL, H.**, *African Ixodoidea. 1. Ticks of the Sudan*, Bureau of Medicine and Surgery, U.S. Navy, 1956.
8. **MOREL, P.**, *Maladies à tiques du bétail en Afrique*, in *Précis de parasitologie vétérinaire tropicale*, Institut d'Elevage et de Médecine vétérinaires des Pays tropicaux, Ministère de la Coopération et du Développement, République française, 1981.
9. **PETERS, W.**, A Colour Atlas of *Arthropods in Clinical Medicine*, Wolfe Publishing Ltd, London, 1992.
10. **AESCHLIMANN, A.**, *Ticks and disease: susceptible hosts, reservoir hosts, and vectors*, in *Parasite-Host Associations. Coexistence or Conflict ?*, Toft, C. A., Aeschlimann, A., Bolis, L., Oxford University Press, 1991.
11. **GEIGY, R. UND MOSER, H.**, Untersuchungen zur Epidemiologie des afrikanischen Rückfallfiebers in Tanganyika, *Acta Trop.*, 12, 327, 1955.

Chapter 16

CLINICAL TOXICOLOGY OF TICK BITES

Julian White

TABLE OF CONTENTS

I. INTRODUCTION

The extent of true tick envenoming worldwide is not known. The envenoming syndrome of major clinical significance following tick bites is tick paralysis, induced by neurotoxins in the tick saliva. However, only a few species of tick have the capacity to cause such effects in man. Globally, ticks are of far more importance medically as vectors for disease, a subject not covered in this chapter, as this is not a form of envenoming. The same applies to veterinary aspects of tick bite; however, there appear to be several other tick toxin induced diseases in domestic animals[1].

II. EPIDEMIOLOGY OF TICK BITE

A. THE TICKS

Ticks are invertebrates, members of the class Arachnida, subclass Acari, order Meostigmata. They have 4 pairs of walking legs and no antennae, a feeding device (hypostoma) and are all ectoparasites of terrestrial vertebrates, particularly mammals. Ticks of medical importance are found in two distinct families; Ixodidae (hard ticks) and Argasidae (soft ticks). The Ixodid ticks are in the majority (at least 644 species[2]). They have a hard body plate, or cuticle, unlike the Argasid ticks (at least 149 species[2]), the cuticle of which is not rigid, and "leathery". Argasid ticks feed, then drop off the host, the feeding process often taking only 5 to 25 mins. In contrast, Ixodid ticks in the adult phase (females) may remain attached to the host, feeding, for a considerably longer period of time, up to 11 days, possibly more. In general, it appears that the longer the period of attachment, the more likely is paralysis. Tick paralysis is a phenomenon associated with Ixodid ticks, and the following description of feeding biology relates to this group.

Ixodid ticks appear to feed at the end of each of the three phases of their life cycle: larval, nymphal and adult. Depending on the species of tick, there may be separate hosts for each phase of the life cycle, or a single host for all phases. In general, the first phase (larval) commences with hatching of eggs, then the 6 legged minute larvae crawl up vegetation to attach to passing host animals. After a variable period of feeding, they fall off and undergo a moult to the 8 legged nymph phase. Again the nymph climbs vegetation to attach to a passing host for further feeding. This feeding may last several days (7 days for *Ixodes holocyclus*[3]), after which the nymph falls off and undergoes a further moult into an adult, male or female, tick. After attaching again to a host the female will feed, usually until mating, after which she will fall off and, over a period of time, lay eggs, then die. At least for *I. holocyclus*, the male tick feeds not on the host, but on the female tick, while copulating[3]. The tick feeds by first gaining access to the skin by cutting a hole through the epidermis with the mouthparts (chelicerae and hypostoma), a process which may take 3-5 minutes[4], sometimes anchoring to the host with "cement" (though not in *I. holocyclus*), then exuding saliva and commencing sucking of blood, the tick's food. The saliva contains anticoagulants, other antigenic substances, and, in the case of species causing tick paralysis, a neurotoxin.

Most work on the tick neurotoxins has been on the Australian paralysis tick, *Ixodes holocyclus*. The toxins are difficult to collect in sufficient quantity to characterise. In reviewing this research, Stone[1] notes that for this species, the toxin is a pronase resistant protein, produced in the salivary gland (Cell "b" of the granular acinus II), with a MW of about 50 kD, and named Holocyclotoxin. It functions as a presynaptic neurotoxin at the neuromuscular junction. Experimentally, peak production appears to be at about day 5 of the female tick feeding cycle. Studies on the toxin from the North American tick, *Dermacentor andersoni*, have shown a similar presynaptic neurotoxic action at the NMJ[1,2]. A list of ticks reported as causing paralysis (in animals) is given in Table 1.

B. TICK PARALYSIS IN AUSTRALIA

The current extent of tick paralysis in Australia is unknown. Sutherland[3], in an excellent review of this subject, listed all known tick bite fatalities. Earliest reports of tick bite fatality in Australia date to the early part of the 20th century, since which time some 20 fatalities are recorded. Significantly, this means tick paralysis has killed more Australians than either latrodectism or funnel web spider bite, both generally considered more clinically important.

A listing of these fatalities is given in Table 2. However, there are no recorded fatalities since 1945. As tick paralysis may present as progressive ataxia and paralysis of unknown origin, the true cause may only be discerned on discovery of the tick, and if this were not thought of or looked for, it is entirely possible that the diagnosis of tick paralysis might be missed. While this is unlikely to have occurred often, if at all, since the publicity generated by the paper of Taylor and Murray in 1946[7], prior to that time it seems likely that some fatal cases would have been missed. More importantly in some respects, paralysis appears to be the less common outcome of humans parasitised by *I. holocyclus*.

Table 1
Global distribution of tick associated paralysis in animals, after Stone[1]

Family	Species	Country
Ixodid (hard) ticks	*Amblyomma maculatum*	Uruguay
	Amblyomma variegatum	Nigeria
	Dermacentor andersoni	Canada, U.S.
	Dermacentor auratus	India
	Dermacentor occidentalis	U.S.
	Dermacentor variabilis	U.S.
	Haemaphysalis punctata	Crete, Macedonia
	Hyalomma truncatum	South Africa
	Ixodes cornuatus	Australia
	Ixodes crenulatus	Moldavia, Transcarpathia, Ukraine
	Ixodes hirsti	Australia
	Ixodes holocyclus	Australia
	Ixodes ricinus	Crete, "U.S.S.R.", Turkey, Yugoslavia
	Ixodes rubicundus	South Africa
	Ixodes scapularis	U.S.
	Rhipicentor nuttalli	South Africa
	Rhipicephalus evertsi	South Africa
	Rhipicephalus sanguineus	U.S.
Argasid (soft) ticks	*Argas africolumbae*	Upper Volta
	Argas miniatus	Brazil
	Argas persicus	South Africa, India, Upper Volta, U.S.
	Argas radiatus	U.S.
	Argas sanchezi	U.S.
	Argas walkerae	South Africa
	Ornithodoros lahorensis	U.S.S.R.

It has been suggested that in tropical Australia, many, possibly most, residents have been bitten by ticks on one or more occasions[10]. The bite is usually of "nuisance value only, some local itching remaining for one or two days after removal of the embedded hypostome"[10]. Other problems associated with tick bite in Australia include anaphylaxis, local allergic reactions, bite site infection, granuloma due to retained mouth parts, and tick-borne diseases (such as North Queensland tick typhus)[1,3,10-12].

While no recent reports document the incidence of tick paralysis, the report of Pearn gives some insight into possible occurrence of this condition. Six children with tick paralysis were admitted to the major Queensland children's hospital over a 5 year period (1971-1975)[10,13]. However, all these cases occurred over a 17 month period within the 5 year time span. As with the fatal cases listed in Table 2, the precise identification of the tick is often not accomplished, so that the above figures relate to tick paralysis, not necessarily paralysis only by *I. holocyclus*, but also possibly by related species. Details of the 6 paediatric cases above are given in Table 3. Overall, it is clear that those at most risk of tick paralysis are children, particularly those under 5 years, and perhaps the elderly or infirm. The high risk area for bites is around the head, particularly the scalp, and in and behind the ears. Peak incidence of cases is in the spring and summer, though cases can occur at any time of year.

Table 2
Reported fatalities due to tick paralysis in Australia, after Sutherland[3].

Year	Age	Sex	Site of tick	Interval*	Reference
1904	13yrs	F	ear drum	18hrs	5
1909	13mths	F	behind ear	1 day	6
1910	3yrs	M	forehead	-	5
1913	3yrs	F	chest near axilla	7hrs	5
1916	2yrs	M	-	-	5
1921	10mths	M	side of neck	-	5
1921	3yrs	M	-	several days	5
1923	16mths	M	scalp	30mins	5
1927	39yrs	M	behind ear	-	7
1927	6yrs	F	scalp	several hours	8
1929	3½yrs	F	scalp	2 days	9
1935	1½yrs	F	-	-	7
1935	2yrs	F	-	-	7
1936	75yrs	M	-	-	7
1936	30yrs	F	-	-	7
1937	27mths	F	scalp	-	7
1939	2mths	F	breast	1 day	8
1941	23mths	F	back of shoulder	-	7
1942	3yrs	M	behind right ear	-	7
1945	27mths	-	occipital region	6 days	7

*Interval = time between removal of tick and death of victim.

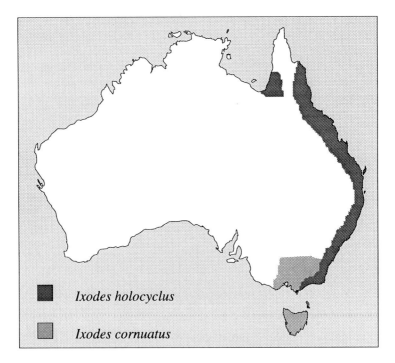

Figure 1. Approximate distribution of the two principal species of paralysis tick in Australia.

On current evidence, tick bite paralysis is almost completely limited to the eastern coastal regions of Australia, consistent with the known range of *I. holocyclus* (Figure 1). However, given current mobility of human populations, it would be possible for a tick to be aquired while in this range, yet envenoming occurring only after the victim had moved elsewhere. Theoretically, at least, cases of tick envenoming might present for medical care anywhere in Australia; thus, tick envenoming should be considered in any case of unexplained paralysis or disturbance of gait, and the recent travel history of the victim should be ascertained.

There is a single case report of severe paralysis following confirmed bite by another species of tick, *I. cornuatus*[14]. The patient was a 3 year old boy, the tick was behind the left ear, and presentation history was of lethargy, slurred speech, ataxia, bulbar muscle paresis, generalised hypotonia and left seventh nerve palsy, all developing over the preceding 12 hours. Complete paralysis followed, requiring ventilation for nearly 5 days.

Table 3

Details of 6 non-fatal paediatric cases of Australian tick paralysis, after Pearn[10,13].

Age	Sex	Site of Bite	Presenting features	Clinical Course After Removal of Tick	Peripheral Muscle Paralysis	Reflexes (DTR)	Ptosis	Facial Weak-ness
3yr 11mth	F	Behind ear	Ataxia	Fever, paralysis, able to walk at 3days, full recovery after 5days	Total paralysis of lower limbs, partial paralysis of upper limbs	Hypo-reflexic or absent	Present	Present; no ophthal-moplegia
2yr 7mth	F	Scalp	Dysarthria	Paralysis, unable to walk until day 6	Almost total paralysis 1 day after removal of tick	Areflexic; recovery at 4 days	Present	Present
3yr	F	Scalp	Weak repetitive cough & stridor	Severe flacid paralysis, unable to walk until day 8	Ascending flacid paralysis, worsening after removal of tick	Areflexic; recovery at 11 days	Present	Present
5yr	F	Behind ear, over VIIth CN	Left Bell's palsy	VIIth CN palsy only improved after 3 days, full recovery by day 5	No generalised paralysis	Normal	Left only	Left Bell's palsy
3yr 11mth	M	Scalp	Ataxia	Initial progression of paralysis, then resolution over several days	Moderate paralysis lower limbs, but able to stand	Normal	Absent	Absent
3yr 2mth	F	Scalp	Ataxia	Progressed to almost complete paralysis by day 4, rapid resolution after antivenom	Ascending flacid paralysis, with respiratory distress 3 days after tick removed	Areflexic	Present	Present

C. TICK PARALYSIS IN NORTH AMERICA

As with Australia, the current extent of tick envenoming in North America is unclear, although one review in 1988 suggested that there had been no change in incidence in recent years, in contrast to a tick-borne disease, Lyme Disease, which had shown a steady increase in the preceeding decade[15]. The subject has been reviewed by Murnaghan and O'Rourke, whose work forms the basis of this review[2]. The first recorded instances of tick paralysis were in 1912, from British Columbia, Oregon and Idaho. The ticks implicated were Ixodid ticks, *Dermacentor andersoni* and *D. variabilis*. There is also a single fatality attributed to *Haemaphysalis cinnabarina*. *D. andersoni* is found in north west North America, where it appears to be essentially the sole species likely to cause tick paralysis. Within Canada, most reports of cases are from British Columbia, virtually all from the valleys of the Frazer, North Thompson, Okanagan, Columbia and Kootenay rivers, with a few cases from Alberta, and Sasketchewan. For British Columbia, 305 confirmed cases occurred between 1900 and 1968, 127 of which occurred prior to 1928. In this series, the incidence of fatality was 10%.

D. andersoni is found in the western states of the U.S. as well, including Washington, Montana, Oregon, Idaho, Wyoming, Nevada, Utah, Colorado, Arizona, New Mexico, and California (only in the northern parts of the last three states). However, reports of tick paralysis cover a more limited distribution, essentially confined to the Northwestern Rocky Mountain states; Washington (14), Montana (52), Oregon (15), Idaho (23), Wyoming (4), Colorado (6), totalling 114 cases in all (by 1978). It is apparent that tick paralysis does not coincide with tick distribution fully, so that some areas with evident tick populations, and almost certainly tick bites to man, do not have ticks causing paralysis. The reasons for this variability in ability to cause tick paralysis is uncertain. It is also interesting to note that the incidence of tick paralysis does not correlate well with incidence of tick-borne disease. In particular, while there are more recorded cases of tick paralysis from British Columbia than all of the north western U.S. there are only 2 recorded cases of tick-borne spotted fever (to 1978). *D. andersoni* tick paralysis occurs principally in April, May and June (when ticks are more prevalent, and perhaps humans more active in tick areas). As in Australia, children are more likely to be affected, with most deaths from this group (total cases 139/166 in children under 16 yrs age; mostly under 7 yrs; all deaths were in children, 12%).

D. variabilis is found in central and eastern states in the U.S., and the southern portion of Canadian states, from Saskatchewan to Nova Scotia. As with *D. andersoni*, cases of tick paralysis have a more limited range, essentially from the eastern and southern states of the U.S. (New York, Pennsylvania, Virginia, North Carolina, South Carolina, Georgia, Kentucky, Tennessee, Missouri, Alabama, Florida), and not at all from Canada. At least 40 cases of tick paralysis due to *D. variabilis* have been reported from the above states, but also a few cases due to *Amblyomma maculatum* and *A. americanum*. Most cases of *D. variabilis* tick paralysis occur in June and July.

D. TICK PARALYSIS IN OTHER CONTINENTS

Tick paralysis has also been recorded from other regions of the world[1,2]. Non-fatal cases have been reported from South Africa, due to *Rhipicephalus simus*, *Hyalomma transiens*, *H. truncatum*, and *Ixodes rubicundus*. Only in the case of the first species was the paralysis apparently typical (i.e. generalised). Tick paralysis has also been reported from Algeria and Somalia. Europe is also not immune, as there are scattered case reports of tick paralysis from the U.K., France, Spain, and Greece. There are isolated reports from Israel, Mexico, and Russia.

E. TICK TOXICOSES OTHER THAN PARALYSIS, IN ANIMALS

Stone[1] has reviewed this subject. He noted 4 types of non-paralysing tick toxicoses in domestic animals. The relationship of these with human disease is unclear.

Type 1: Fever, profuse moist eczema, anorexia and debilitation, found in cattle, sheep and pigs, in central, eastern and southern Africa, in southern India and Sri Lanka. Associated with the small bontpoot tick, *Hyalomma truncatum*.

Type 2: Rapidly lethal condition affecting young calves and sheep, from the Kalahari and Namibia, caused by the sand tampan (tick), *Ornithodoros savignyi*.

Type 3: Pyrexia, anaemia, wasting and necrosis of lymph nodes, affecting cattle from southern Africa, and associated with massive infestations by the brown ear tick, *Rhipicephalus appendiculatus*.

Type 4: Pyrexia, anorexia, possible liver dysfunction, affecting cattle, from Australia, due to the cattle tick, *Boophilus microplus*. There is some contention that Type 4 is not a true tick toxicosis.

In relating these animal tick toxicoses to human disease, it is of value to note that the species causing most cases of tick paralysis in domestic animals are essentially those causing the disease in man: *I. holocyclus, I. rubicundus, D. andersoni, D. variabilis* and also, in animals, *Rhipicephalus evertsi, Argas walkerae, A. radiatus*.

F. OTHER TICK INDUCED INJURIES, EXCLUDING TICK-BORNE DISEASES.

While it seems likely that many ticks, both Ixodid and Argasid, may bite man and cause some reaction, in most cases these reactions are relatively minor, so they go unreported in the medical literature. There are occasional reports indicating the frequence of tick bites in some populations, such as a study from Australia which showed up to 39% of soldiers on exercise were infested by ticks, all of whom had a local reaction (see next section)[16]. Southcott[17], in his review of arthropod injuries in man, notes a variety of ticks that have been reported to bite man (Table 4).

Table 4
Ticks reported to bite man, in Australia

Tick Species	Paralysis	Other effects
Ixodid (hard) ticks		
Ixodes confusus	not reported	
Ixodes kohlsi	not reported	
Ixodes holocyclus	severe	
Ixodes tasmani	not reported	
Ixodes fecialis	not reported	
Ixodes cornuatus	can occur	
Haemaphysalis bancrofti	not reported	
Haemaphysalis longicornis	not reported	
Haemaphysalis humerosa	not reported	
Amblyomma loculosum	not reported	
Amblyomma moreliae	not reported	
Amblyomma postoculatum	not reported	
Amblyomma triguttatum	not reported	
Argasid (soft) ticks		
Ornithodoros gurneyi	not reported	prolonged local itching and swelling, occasional systemic reaction
Argas persicus	not reported	unconfirmed bites in man, local effects

III. SYMPTOMS AND SIGNS

A. TYPES OF TICK ENVENOMING

The principal type of tick envenoming of clinical importance in man is tick paralysis. This will be the major focus of the rest of this clinical discussion. However, the reader should note that tick paralysis is undoubtedly much in the minority as a manifestation of tick bite in man. Far more common is the local irritation caused by the bite[3,10], without attendant systemic symptoms, in addition to which there may also be an allergic reaction, either local, or occasionally generalised[3,10-12]. Secondary infection is always possible, with consequent symptomatology, but is apparently not common.

As an example of the frequency of both tick bites, and reactions, a study of soldiers on field exercises in Western Australia showed 26% and 39% of all soldiers at each of two camps, were infested by one or more ticks, from lymphal to adult stage[16]. All soldiers infested showed some reaction locally, often not initially, but over a period of 24-48 hours post removal of ticks, local papular or papulopustular lesions occurred, taking several days to subside. In none of these cases was there any evidence of systemic toxicosis. In this series, the tick was *Amblyomma triguttatum*. A similar study on troops in a camp in Arkansas, U.S. found significant frequency of tick bites (*Amblyomma americanum*), with greater than 50% of all troops being bitten, and 40% reporting greater than 10 ticks found attached[18]. This study did not report any cases of paralysis.

Tick bite is also associated with local granuloma formation, presumably due to retention of mouth parts, rather than reaction to tick saliva (venom). The incidence of granuloma is unknown, but appears uncommon.

Mild systemic illness may follow bites by some ticks, such as the Australian kangaroo tick, *Ornithodoros gurneyi* (Argasid), which is reported to cause local itching and swelling at the bite site which may last days to weeks, or if allowed to complete feeding (up to 20 mins), lasting up to several months[17]. The nature of the systemic illness is ill defined, varying from mild malaise and headaches, through to a single case where early collapse occurred (possibly of allergic aetiology).

Allergic reactions do occur following some tick bites, varying from mild local swelling and pruritis, through regional swelling, to true "anaphylactic" reactions. These are well documented for the Australian paralysis tick[3,10-12].

Scrub itch due to multiple bites by larval *I. holocyclus* has been described from Australia, particularly in the warmer months[3,19-21]. Symptoms vary from an itchy rash to allergic dermatitis.

Several tick toxicoses, other than paralysis, have been noted in animals at least (see previous section)[1]. As case reports of these conditions occurring in man are not available, it is uncertain if similar toxicoses affect humans. Diligent reporting of all cases of toxicoses in man, due to tick bite, may, in the future, allow clarification of the above.

B. THE ONSET AND DEVELOPMENT OF ENVENOMING

From a clinical standpoint, tick envenoming is essentially synonymous with tick paralysis. Hereafter, discussion of tick envenoming will therefore relate to tick paralysis only. The initial tick bite and infestation may be noticed as minor local irritation or pruritis, even swelling, or may go completely unnoticed. The systemic illness, usually confined to the development of progressive and widespread skeletal muscle paralysis, is unlikely to develop immediately after commencement of feeding by the tick. In most reported cases of tick paralysis, this has commenced only after the tick has been feeding for several days[1-3,10,13,22-25]. A unique feature of tick paralysis in Australia is the common finding that paralysis may worsen after removal of the tick, occasionally with a delay of up to 4 days before maximal paralysis is evident[3,10]. At least for North American tick paralysis in children, the child is usually irritable for 12 to 24 hrs prior to the onset of paralytic symptoms, which often commence in the lower limbs, with weakness and unsteady gait[2,22-25]. Both ascending flacid paralysis and acute ataxia may be the presenting sign[24-26]. Similarly in Australia the lower limbs are usually affected first and worst, unsteady gait being a common presenting symptom[3,10,13]. If untreated the paralysis may deepen and spread to involve the upper limbs, the neck and face and cranial nerves, and finally, muscles of respiration. While ptosis is a common feature, at least in Australian tick paralysis, it is either not noticed early, or develops after the lower limb weakness and ataxia[10,13]. This is quite distinct from snakebite paralysis, where ptosis is nearly always the first, or one of the first, sign of developing paralysis. Death due to tick paralysis may only occur some hours to days after onset of paralysis, and is the result of either respiratory failure due to complete respiratory paralysis, or aspiration pneumonia due to bulbar paralysis, which may therefore present a hazard well before paralysis is otherwise complete. Apart from the flacid paralysis, examination will usually reveal hyporeflexia or areflexia. The pupils may be dilated and unresponsive to light.

There is at least one report of Australian tick paralysis associated with cardiac failure, ascribed to acute myocarditis[27], and a second possible case[8]. In the prime case, the child developed acute cardiac failure 18hrs after removal of the tick, which responded after 24hrs of "conservative" therapy. ECG changes noted were prolonged Q-T interval, depressed S-T segments, low voltage P and T waves.

There is a single case report from Australia, associating tick bite with subsequent myolysis about a week later, the peak CK being 2100 IU/l[3]. The child was investigated for other causes of myolysis, all proved negative; thus, a presumptive diagnosis of myolysis due to the tick bites was made. Myolysis has also been reported following North American tick bite, due to *Dermacentor andersoni*, but in this case the degree of myolysis was less impressive (108 IU/l) and occurred within the first 24 hours[28].

C. GENERAL SYMPTOMS AND SIGNS OF ENVENOMING

Apart from the irritability seen in children prior to the onset of paralysis, general symptoms and signs of envenoming appear absent or few, and not specific. Pain, dizziness, vertigo, photophobia, nausea and vomiting and urinary retention have been reported but are clearly rare.

D. PROGNOSTIC INDICATORS

Tick paralysis and fatality due to tick paralysis is more likely in children, particularly those under 5 years. It is also more likely if the tick has been attached for several days. The more extensive the paralysis at time of first diagnosis, the more likely is progression to even more severe paralysis. In Australia, such progression is not uncommon after removal of the tick[10,13]. Clearly, severe paralysis, including bulbar paralysis, puts the patient at more risk, including the possibility of aspiration pneumonia. For tick paralysis in North America, removal of the tick is usually associated with progressive recovery, taking from 3 days to greater than a week[2,24-26].

IV. PROPHYLAXIS

A. AVOIDANCE OF BITES

Apart from avoiding areas of the world where ticks are found, not practical for most people at risk, avoidance of tick bite is difficult. As the ticks usually initially gain access to their host by attaching as the host brushes against vegetation, care in selecting clothing and ways of moving through vegetated areas might help. Long boots have been suggested as providing a degree of protection. If active in areas where tick infestation is likely, it is advisable to regularly check for ticks, including cryptic areas such as the scalp, behind the ears, and in the external auditory canal. The value of insect repellants in discouraging ticks is unproven[18].

B. PUBLIC EDUCATION ON TICK BITE

Given the prevalence of ticks and tick bite in areas where tick paralysis occurs, it seems likely that most people will be aware of ticks. Public education campaigns to inform about ticks, tick bite, and tick paralysis might prevent the establishment of ticks in many cases, and in those where paralysis does start to develop, earlier presentation for treatment through greater awareness of the possible diagnosis might reduce the number of patients progressing to severe paralysis. However, given the small number of severe cases, even in areas where tick bite is common, such as Queensland, Australia, the cost-benefit ratio would probably not favour extensive and expensive campaigns.

V. FIRST AID TREATMENT

The primary purpose of first aid in envenoming is to prevent the systemic spread of venom from the site of inoculation, and limit any deleterious local effects of envenoming. In tick paralysis, neither of these two objectives is likely to be met by first aid, as by the time there is clinical evidence of envenoming the salivary venom has already attained widespread body distribution and the local effects are, in comparison, minor. Hence prevention of envenoming by avoidance of bites, and regular body searches while at risk, to expeditiously remove ticks, are of more value than first aid. In the case of a person, usually a child, developing the early symptoms and signs of paralysis, first aid should be directed towards getting the child to medical care quickly, and maintenance of vital functions, if imperilled. Particularly watch for developing bulbar and respiratory paralysis, keep the patient fasted, and nurse on the side to avoid the chance of aspiration of vomitus.

VI. CLINICAL MANAGEMENT

A. GENERAL CONSIDERATIONS

The single most important aspect of tick paralysis is to recognise it as such, a subject covered below under Diagnosis. Apart from this, it should be remembered that tick bite is common, but tick paralysis is not. A particular species of tick may cause tick paralysis (but uncommonly) in one part of its range, but fail to do so entirely in another part of its range. This undoubtedly has to do with variability in salivary content, only some ticks from certain areas actually producing the appropriate toxin in significant amounts.

It should also be realised that when a case of tick paralysis presents, it is potentially a medical emergency, requiring priority assessment and management. Though rapid death after onset, common in some other forms of envenoming, is unlikely with tick paralysis, it can occur, and the more rapidly the correct diagnosis is made the greater the probability of avoiding serious consequences for the patient, at least in most cases.

B. DIAGNOSIS
1. Approach to diagnosis

The first rule of diagnosis of any envenoming is to actually think of envenoming as a cause of the patient's symptoms and signs. This certainly applies to tick paralysis. Include tick paralysis in the differential diagnosis of anyone presenting with acute onset of ataxia, lower limb weakness, or more generalised paralysis, and in cases presenting in extremis following a convulsion, in whom a history of respiratory or speech difficulties or generalised weakness preceded the convulsion. This is particularly true for children. In seeking the diagnosis, do not lose sight of the immediate needs of the patient, and attend to these, particularly in regard to securing adequate respiratory function, if imperilled, and avoiding the possibility of aspiration of vomitus.

Seek a history of possible exposure to tick bite, including recent trips to tick infested areas. Enquire about the progression of symptoms, i.e. the time interval from exposure to ticks, to onset of symptoms, and the timing of progression of symptoms thereafter. Enquire about past exposure to ticks and general health. In children, in particular, ascertain if there was a period of irritability prior to onset of weakness. Ataxia being a common early feature in children, specifically ask about unsteady walking or reduced mobility in the very young. Examine the patient thoroughly, checking for ticks, particularly in cryptic areas such as the scalp, behind the ears, in the external auditory canal, under skin folds such as under breasts, and in the groin and perineal/genital areas. Check for evidence of paralysis in lower limbs, upper limbs, and cranial nerves, looking for symmetric weakness. Check for hypotonic or absent deep tendon reflexes. Check for adequacy of the gag reflex. Look for evidence of secondary problems such as allergic reactions to the saliva and local infection. While considering tick paralysis within the differential diagnosis of progressive weakness, as mentioned above, also consider other diagnoses if tick paralysis is initially the diagnosis considered.

Differential diagnosis of tick paralysis encompasses a variety of envenomings, infections and other conditions. Essentially any disease which can cause paralysis of non-traumatic onset should be considered, and vice versa, tick paralysis should be in the differential diagnosis of patients presenting with non-traumatic paralysis. A variety of venomous snakes may cause neurotoxic paralysis similar to that seen in tick paralysis. In Australia such snakes are common in areas where *I. holocyclus* is found, e.g. taipans (*Oxyuranus scutellatus*), tiger snakes (*Notechis scutatus*), rough scaled snakes (*Tropidechis carinatus*), death adders (*Acanthophis antarcticus*) and brown snakes (*Pseudonaja textilis*). In North America, however, the only snakes likely to cause paralysis (e.g. *Crotalus scutellatus* and *Micrurus* spp.) are not found in areas where tick paralysis is recorded. In Europe, similarly, there is no co-occurrence of tick paralysis and snakes able to cause paralysis. In Africa, some species of cobra which cause paralysis may occur in areas where tick paralysis has been reported, but as cases of the latter are very scarce in this region, and the snake bites show other symptoms and signs suggesting the causal agent, confusion here seems unlikely. Amongst other diseases to be considered are poliomyelitis, Guillaine-Barre syndrome, diphtheria, myasthenia, and acute toxic and inflammatory neuropathies and myopathies. In most, but not all cases, a careful search of the victim will reveal an attached tick. It is important to remember that for the Australian tick, *I. holocyclus*, maximal paralytic features may occur 1 to 4 days after removal of the tick.

2. Role of venom detection

Clinically relevant venom detection for tick salivary toxins is not presently available, and does not appear likely in the foreseeable future.

3. Role of laboratory investigations

Laboratory investigations in tick paralysis are, in general, not helpful in establishing the diagnosis[10]. Their main role is assisting the assessment of the extent of envenoming, and in particular, if there is respiratory difficulty due to severe paralysis, arterial blood gas analysis may be helpful in assessing the current and ongoing respiratory function.

4. Assessing extent of envenoming

The extent of envenoming at the time of first diagnosis may not indicate the maximum extent of envenoming, at least in Australia. A child presenting with mild ataxia, on whom a tick is found and removed, may actually progress to more severe neurological involvement over the next 1 to 4 days. Therefore all patients presenting with infestation by a species of paralysis tick should be admitted and observed for at least 24 hours after removal of the tick, or if in Australia, then for at least 4 days.

C. TREATMENT
1. General approach to treatment

The paramount objective in tick infestation is to remove all ticks, mandating a thorough search of all parts of the patient's body, including cryptic areas such as the scalp, behind the ears, in the external auditory canal, in flexures, and the groin and perineal areas. If the patient already has major paralysis with either bulbar paresis or respiratory distress, then management of these problems will take precedence, and may require intubation and ventilation.

Removal of the tick must be performed carefully. The body should not be gripped. Rather, the tick should be levered off the skin, by placing the jaws of fine forceps on either side of the hypostome and pulling away from the skin. The use of irritants beforehand, such as alcohol, to induce tick disengagement is commonly recommended, though not really of proven value. One recent study using North American ticks, *Dermacentor variabilis* and *Amblyomma americanum*; did not show any value in the use of irritants (petroleum jelly, fingernail polish, alcohol, lighted match)[29]. The same study showed careful mechanical removal was effective and did not leave embedded mouth parts. The wound should be carefully inspected for remains of tick mouthparts. After removal of one tick, always check carefully for the presence of other ticks.

General measures include establishment of an iv line, hydration, and nursing the patient on their side.

2. Antivenom therapy and its complications

For Australian paralysis tick bite an antivenom is available and does appear to confer some benefit in treatment, but may not reverse established paralysis[3,10,13,14]. It should only be used if there is significant systemic envenoming including involvement of respiratory muscles or those of the oropharynx. Like other antivenoms, reactions may occur, though appear to be infrequent. The initial dose should be 1 ampoule (CSL specific tick antitoxin, 20ml/ampoule, canine origin). Sutherland[3] suggests an initial dose of 2 ampoules if there is severe paralysis. Occasionally further doses may be needed. It is given iv, preferably diluted, with infusion commenced slowly. Appropriate medications should be drawn up prior to commencing antivenom therapy. Serum sickness is not likely to be common following tick antivenom and prophylactic steroids are therefore not generally recommended.

3. Neurotoxicity and its treatment

The three elements of treatment of tick paralysis are (i) secure adequate respiratory function, (ii) remove all ticks from the patient, (iii) administer tick antivenom (Australia only). The role of the latter, though still recommended, is not entirely clear. Some cases have shown dramatic reversal of paralysis following antivenom therapy[10,13], while others have shown little benefit[14]. Antivenom does appear effective in treating domestic animals with tick paralysis, especially if given early.

4. Other issues in treatment

Like any bite or sting, secondary infection can occur. While tetanus following tick bite in man does not appear to have been reported, tetanus prophylaxis is advisable. Human cases of tick envenoming do not appear to be common enough to warrant immunisation programmes, but in domestic animals, at least in Australia, this may be a consideration, with an estimate of at least 20,00 affected animals per year, with in excess of 10,000 deaths (from a limited area of NSW alone)[1].

VII. REFERENCES

1. **STONE, B.F.** (1986) Toxicoses induced by ticks and reptiles in domestic animals. In Ed. Harris, J.B. *Natural Toxins. Animal, Plant and Microbial*, Oxford, Clarendon Press.
2. **MURNAGHAN, M.F., O'ROURKE, F.J.** (1978) Tick paralysis. In Ed. Bettini, S. *Handbook of Experimental Pharmacology; Vol. 48; Arthropod Venoms,* Berlin, Springer Verlag. pps 417-464.
3. **SUTHERLAND, S.K.** (1983) *Australian Animal Toxins,* Melbourne, Oxford University Press.
4. **BALASHOV, Y.S.** (1968) Blood sucking ticks (Ixodoidea): vectors of diseases to man and animals. *Mix. Pub. Ent. Soc. Amer.* 8:161-376.
5. **FERGUSON, E.W.** (1924) Deaths from tick paralysis in human beings. *Med. J. Aust.* 2:346-348.
6. **CLELAND** (1912) Injuries and diseases of man in Australia attributable to animals (except insects), *Aust. Med. Gaz.,* 32 (12):295-299.
7. **TAYLOR, F.H., MURRAY, R.E.** (1946) *Spiders, ticks and mites.* Service Publication Number 6. Sydney: School of Public Health and Tropical Medicine, University of Sydney.
8. **HAMILTON, D.G.** (1940) Tick paralysis: a dangerous disease of children. *Med. J. Aust.* 1: 759-765.
9. **SINCLAIR, C.W.** (1930) A fatal tick bite. *Med. J. Aust.* 1: 554.
10. **PEARN, J.** (1977) The clinical features of tick bite. *Med. J. Aust.* 2:313-318.
11. **GAUCI, M., LOH, R.K.S., STONE, B.F., THONG, Y.H.** (1989) Allergic reactions to the Australian paralysis tick, *Ixodes holocyclus*: diagnostic evaluation by skin test and radioimmunoassay. *Clin. Exper. Allergy* 19: 279-283.
12. **STONE, B.F., BINNINGTON, K.C., GAUCI, M., AYLWARD, J.H.** (1989) Tick/host interactions for *Ixodes holocyclus*: role, effects, biosynthesis and nature of its toxic and allergenic oral secretions. *Exper. Applied Acarology* 7: 59-69.
13. **PEARN, J.** (1977) Neuromuscular paralysis caused by tick envenomation. *J. Neurol. Sci.* 34:37-42.
14. **TIBBALLS, J., COOPER, S.J.** (1986) Paralysis with *Ixodes cornuatus* envenomation. *Med. J. Aust.* 145:37-38.
15. **GODDARD, J.** (1988) The changing status of tickborne disease in the U.S. *Military Medicine* 153: 513-519.
16. **PEARCE, R.L., GROVE, D.I.** (1987) Tick infestation in soldiers who were bivouacked in the Perth region. *Med. J. Aust.* 146:238-240.
17. **SOUTHCOTT, R.V.** (1976) Arachnadism and allied syndromes in the Australian region. *Rec. Adelaide Child. Hosp.* 1:97-186.
18. **GODDARD, J., MCHUGH, C.P.** (1990) Impact of a severe tick infestation at little rock AFB, Arkansas on Volant Scorpion military training. *Military Medicine* 155: 277-280.
19. **SUTHERST, R.W., MOORHOUSE, D.E.** (1971) *Ixodes holocyclus* larvae and scrub itch in south east Queensland. *Southeast Asian J. Trop. Med. Public Health* 2: 82-83.
20. **LEE, D.J.** (1975) *Arthropod bites and stings and other injurious effects.* Sydney: School of Public Health and Tropical Medicine, University of Sydney.
21. **MOOREHOUSE, D.E.** (1981) Ticks and their medical importance. In Ed. Pearn, J.H. *Animal Toxins and Man,* Brisbane: Queensland Department of Health.
22. **ROSE, I.** (1954) A review of tick paralysis. *Can. Med. Assoc. J.* 70: 175-176.
23. **COSTA, J.A.** (1952) Tick paralysis on the Atlantic seaboard. *Amer. J. Dis. Child.* 83: 336-347.
24. **HALLER, J.S., FABARA, J.A.** (1972) Tick paralysis: case report with emphasis on neurological toxicity. *Amer. J. Dis. Child.* 124: 915-917.
25. **ABBOTT, K.H.** Tick borne diseases. *Dis. Nerv. Syst.* 5: 19-21.
26. **CHERINGTON, M., SNYDER, R.D.** (1968) Tick paralysis: neurophysiological studies. *New Eng. J. Med.* 278: 95-97.
27. **PEARN, J.H.** (1966) A case of tick paralysis with myocarditis. *Med. J. Aust.* 1: 629-630.
28. **BOFFEY, G.C., PATERSON, D.C.** (1973) Creatine phosphokinase elevation in a case of tick paralysis. *Can. Med. Assoc. J.* 108: 866-868.
29. **NEEDHAM, G.R.** (1985) Evaluation of five popular methods for tick removal. *Paediatrics* 75: 997-1002.

Chapter 17

BIOLOGY AND DISTRIBUTION OF SCORPIONS OF MEDICAL IMPORTANCE

Sylvia M. Lucas and Jürg Meier

TABLE OF CONTENTS

I. INTRODUCTION

Scorpions are very ancient animals, and several fossil species are described. The oldest is *Dolichophonus loudonensis* from the Middle Silurian rocks of Scotland, described by Laurie[1]. Stormer[2] discovered a giant fossil, *Gigantoscorpio willsi*, from the Lower Carboniferous of Scotland, with a length of about 300- 350 mm. The aspect of these fossils is very similar to scorpions actually living today.

There are about 1,400 species described but only a few are medically important. The World Health Organization[3] listed species from the genera: *Centruroides*, *Tityus*, *Androctonus*, *Buthus*, *Buthotus*, *Leiurus* and *Parabuthus*, all belonging to the family of BUTHIDAE, as capable of causing clinically significant envenoming. The distribution of these genera of medical importance is shown in Figures 3,8,11,12,15,16,17.

II. SYSTEMATIC POSITION

Scorpions are Arthropoda of the class Arachnida and constitute the order of Scorpiones, with nine living families: Bothriuridae, Buthidae, Chactidae, Chaerilidae, Diplocentridae, Ischnuridae, Iuridae, Scorpionidae and Vaejovidae. This classification is based on morphological characters, although some researchers use techniques involving DNA sequencing, to identify species, subspecies and races.

III. MORPHOLOGY

The body consists of a cephalothorax (prosoma) and an abdomen (opisthosoma). The cephalothorax is dorsally covered by the carapace which has median and lateral eyes. In the front of the cephalothorax are situated the chelicerae with pincer-like claws used for feeding, to produce sound and as a taste organ. Also on the cephalothorax are the pedipalps, used for prey detection and immobilization, in courtship and mating and for self-defense; and the four pairs of legs. Ventrally the cephalothorax is protected by the sternum and the coxae of the legs.

The abdomen is divided into a wide anterior mesosoma (preabdomen) and a long and slender posterior metasoma (postabdomen). The mesosoma consists of seven segments. On the ventral side, the first segment bears paired genital opercula, the second comprises the pectines, a pair of comb-like structures, which, according to Foelix and Müller Vorholt[4], are mechanoreceptors and chemoreceptors. The next four segments present the spiracles or stigmata, the openings of the respiratory organs. The metasoma consists of five segments and the telson, which ends in a sting or aculeus and contains the two poison glands. Each gland is invested dorsally and mesally with a muscle layer. The glands are separated by a median vertical septum. Each gland has an exit duct which opens near the tip of the sting. The glands are enclosed in a basement membrane, within which is a layer of connective tissue. Between this tissue and the lumen is a single layer of secretory epithelium. According to Bücherl[5,6], two kinds of epithelial cells exist: very small subcoidal cells attached to the basement membrane, with small elliptic nuclei, and the functional epithelial cells. These cells produce venom as long as their nuclear and cytoplasmatic substances remain vital. Then the cells will degenerate and are replaced by a basal cuboidal cell. The scorpion ejects the venom by the voluntary contraction of the muscle layer of the glands.

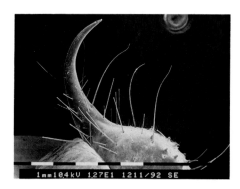

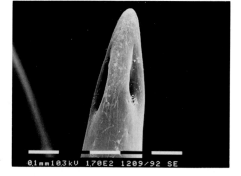

Figure 1. Telson, lateral view, (courtesy Dr. J. Meier; Basel)

Figure 2. Tip of stinger with the two venom orifices, (courtesy Dr. J. Meier; Basel)

IV. BIOLOGY

Scorpions occur in tropical and temperate regions of the world, within 50 degrees North and South of the Equator. They live in forests, savannas, deserts, and some species are even found in the mountains over 5,000 m of altitude. All scorpions are nocturnal, hiding during the day under stones, under wood, under tree bark, in termite hills, and other protected places. Some species seem to be attracted by human habitation and live around the human dwellings and even inside of them.

The main food of scorpions are insects and arachnids. In some species (*Bothriurus* sp.) cannibalism was observed. Scorpions do not hunt for food but wait for their prey, which is detected by sensory hairs, called trichobothria, localized mainly on the pedipalps. The prey is seized in little portions and predigested chemically in the preoral cavity. Scorpions can live for several months without food and sometimes even without water.

Reproduction: the courtship dance of scorpions has been observed by several researchers. The male grasps the pedipalps or chelicerae of the female and then the pair begins to move forward and backward to find a proper place for mating. The male ejects a capsule of sperma, the spermathophore, which is fixed to the soil. The male tries to pull the female over the spermathophore so that her genital openings are directly in contact with the spermathophore and the sperm can be absorbed. This fertilization mechanism is similar to that found in pseudoscorpions and was observed for the first time in scorpions by two different investigators, working independently[7,8]. Parthenogenesis was observed in two species: *Tityus serrulatus* and *Tityus uruguayensis*[9,10].

The young are born alive and immediately after birth try to mount on the tergites of the female, where they remain until the first moult. Then the venom glands become functional and the little scorpions can survive alone. Polis and Sissom[11] presented a comparison of the post-birth life history of scorpions of seven families. The age to reach maturity is variable, for example, in the species *Tityus serrulatus* from 17 to 25 months[9], in *Pandinus gambiensis* 39 to 83 months[12]. The longevity is also quite variable, from only several months to several years; for *Pandinus gambiensis* a maximum longevity of 96 months has been reported[12].

V. LIST OF GENERA AND SPECIES OF MEDICAL IMPORTANCE

The species responsible for serious human accidents belong to the family Buthidae. According to Sissom[13], this family contains 48 genera and over 500 species.

A. GENUS *Tityus* C. L. KOCH, 1836

The genus presents the following characters: tergites I-IV with a distinct median longitudinal keel, immobile finger of chelicerae with one tooth, inner side of the movable finger of the pedipalps generally with 11-22 oblique rows of granules, without secondary granular rows.

Distribution: Central and South America and The West Indies.

The number of described species is over 100.

Several species responsible for human accidents occur in human dwellings and their vicinity. Bücherl[5] cited that often whole cities may be "invaded", like Ouro Preto and Belo Horizonte in Brazil, where a great number of these specimens can be found inside houses, hiding during the day behind furniture, in shoes and in clothes. The Instituto Butantan, Sao Paulo, Brazil received over 25,000 scorpions captured during one week in a small town of the State of Minas Gerais.

1. *Tityus serrulatus* Lutz and Mello, 1922
Total length: 60-70 mm

The cephalothorax and the first six tergites are yellowish brown, the last tergite, the segments of the tail, legs, pedipalps and chelicerae are pale yellow, the ventral side of the fifth caudal segment is blackish. The dorsal paramedian keel of the caudal segments II-IV presents bigger posterior granules which are very distinct, especially on the fourth segment.

Distribution: the most common species in the State of Minas Gerais, also frequent in the State of São Paulo, Brazil.

Habitat: under stones, rocks, loose bark of trees, in the "termites house".
Venom quantities: obtained by electrical stimulation in the Arthropod Laboratory, Instituto Butantan, São Paulo, Brazil during 1992: 0.43 mg. (average of 1,500 extractions).

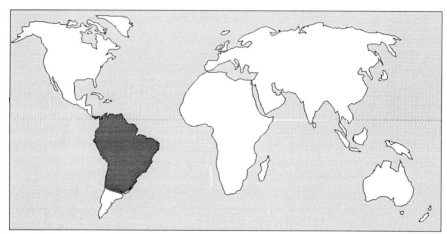

Figure 3. Approximate global distribution of scorpions of the genus *Tityus.*

2. *Tityus bahiensis* (Perty, 1830)
Total length: 60-70 mm
    The cephalothorax and tergites are uniformrly brown-reddish, the legs with black spots, also a dark spot on the tibia of the pedipalps.
Distribution: species described from Salvador, State of Bahia; and in the State of São Paulo (Brazil) where it is the most common scorpion. The species also occurs in the Brazilian States of Santa Catarina and Mato Grosso do Sul, as well as in Argentina (Misiones, Province of Buenos Aires)[5].
Habitat: in fields, under stones, rocks, preferably in places where the sun shines during the morning period; they also dig and live in holes between 20 to 30 cm deep.
Venom quantities: obtained by electrical stimulation in the Arthropod Laboratory, Instituto Butantan, São Paulo, Brazil during 1992; 0.33 mg. (average of 1,500 extractions).

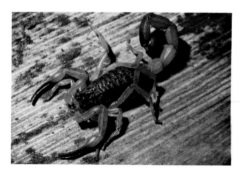

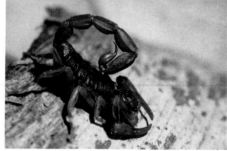

Figure 4. *Tityus baliiensis,* (courtesy Dr. J. Meier; Basel).

Figure 5. *Tityus cambridge,* (courtesy Dr. J. Meier; Basel).

3. *Tityus stigmurus* (Thorerr, 1877)
Total length: 60 mm
    Truncus pale yellow to brownish-yellow. The cephalothorax presents a triangular black spot in front of the median eyes and the tergites present a longitudinal median, black band.

209

Distribution: States of the north-east of Brazil: Bahia, Sergipe, Alagoas, Pernambuco, Paraiba.
Habitat: under loose barks of trees, under stones, in crevices of ravines.
Venom quantities: obtained by electrical stimulation in the Arthropod Laboratory, Instituto Butantan, São Paulo, Brazil during 1992; 0.25 mg. (average of 1,500 extractions).

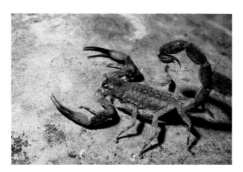 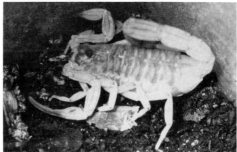

Figure 6. *Tityus stigmurus,* (courtesy Dr. J. Meier; Basel).   **Figure 7.** *Tityus serrulatus,* (photo © Dr. J. White).

4. *Tityus trinitatis* Pocock, 1897
Total length: 60 to 75 mm
   Truncus in females dark-brown to almost black, males dark reddish brown with the last three segments of the tail black, legs dark brown, pedipalps brown, more light-colored.
Distribution: Trinidad and Venezuela. The scorpions are very frequent in the sugar cane plantations of southern Trinidad from Couvaa to Siparia and in the coconut plantations of the north-eastern region[14].
   Other species cited in literature as producing a venom with neurotoxic activity: *T. cambridgei, T. clathratus*[16]*, T. trivittatus dorsomaculatus*[6]*, T. discrepans*[16].

B. GENUS *Centruroides* MARX, 1889

   Tergites I to IV with a distinct median longitudinal keel; tail, chiefly in males, not posteriorly dilated, but segments distinctly elongated, tail longer in males than in females; 7 to 9 oblique rows of granules on the movable finger of pedipalps, not overlapping at the apices and flanked, externally and internally by large, dentate, lateral granules; between the lateral granules are one to four much smaller granules. Diaz Najera[17] presented an identification key for the medically important species of the genus occurring in Mexico. Stahnke and Calos[18] presented an identification key for 37 different species. The genus comprises 40 species and occurs from southern United States to northern South America and in the West Indies.

1. *Centruroides noxius* Hoffmann, 1932
Total length: 40 to 50 mm
   The truncus is uniformly brownish-reddish to blackish, with a narrow, light colored, lateral band on each side, without longitudinal stripes. Cephalothorax and abdomen uniformly dark. Vesicle with a strong, subaculear tubercle.
Distribution: Nayarit, south region of Sinaloa, Mexico.

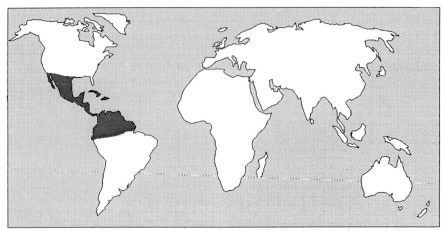

Figure 8. Approximate global distribution of scorpions of the genus *Centruroides.*

2. *Centruroides suffusus* Pocock, 1902
Total length: 50 to 80 mm.
Color: tergites with two broad, dark, longitudinal bands; carapace light colored laterally, sometimes in area of post-median furrow, otherwise entire median posterior part of carapace darker. Tail of the male at least 8.25 times longer than the carapace.
Distribution: central region of the State of Durango, north of Zacatecas, Mexico.

3. *Centruroides infamatus* (C. L. Koch, 1845)
Adults 60-70 mm in length. A slender scorpion with a thin tail.
Color: Usually straw coloured and similar to *C. suffusus.* Has lines on the cephalothorax replaced by broad stain and two longitudinal stripes on the preabdomen. The tail of the males shorter, not over 7.51 times longer than the carapace.
Distribution: Michoacan, Jalisco, Zacatecas, Durango and Vera Cruz, Mexico.

4. *Centruroides elegans* (Thorell, 1876)
Adults 85 mm long.
Color: tergites with two broad, longitudinal bands, posterior margin of tergites I to VI yellowish to light brown and pretergites with an intense, black point, four dark lines on the cephalothorax.
Distribution: Jalisco, Guerrero, Nayarit and Tres Marias Islands, Mexico.

5. *Centruroides limpidus* (Karsch, 1879)
Two subspecies are described: *C. l. limpidus* (Karsch,1879) and *C. l. tecomanus* Hoffmann, 1932.
Adults about 70 mm (*C. l. limpidus*) to 75 mm (*C. l. tecomanus*) in length.
Color: tergites I to VI with an intense black spot on pretergites, and another larger, but more diffuse, spot on posterior border; the two dorsal, longitudinal black bands begin as a transverse black line on the posterior border of carapace. The subaculear tooth is weakly developed.

Centruroides limpidus limpidus: The adult is light to dark yellow in color. The cephalothorax has four well defined lines, the preabdomen two well-marked longitudinal stripes and the subaculear spine reduced to a small tubercle.
Centruroides limpidus tecomanus: The color and other distinguishing features are the same as *C. limpidus limpidus*, but the subaculear spine is well developed.

211

Distribution: central Guerrero, Morelos, southern Puebla and along the western coast of Mexico.

6. *Centruroides sculpturatus* Ewing, 1928

Adult length about 65 mm.

Color: tergites without two dark, longitudinal bands, uniformly colored or bicolored, fifth caudal segment of a darker color than the other caudal segments. The subaculear tubercle is obsolete or small and spinoid.

Distribution: Arizona, eastern California (U.S.) and western and northern Mexico.

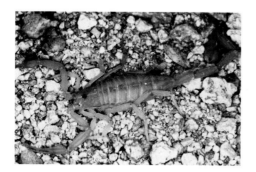 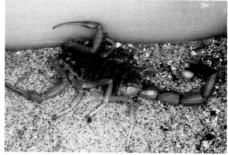

Figure 9. *Centruroides sculpturatus,* (photo © Dr. J. White).

Figure 10. *Leiurus quinquestriatus,* (photo © Dr. J. White).

C. GENUS *Leiurus* (HEMPRICH AND EHRENBERG, 1829) VACHON, 1949

The genus is characterized by the presence of five crests on the first two tergites and by the presence of at least three crests on the posterior tergites. Vachon[19] gave a redescription of the genus and of the species *L. quinquestriatus quinquestriatus*. Levi, Amitai and Shulov[20] gave a redescription of the other subspecies *L. quinquestriatus hebraeus*, and summarized the differences between the two subspecies. The authors cited a third subspecies: *L. quinquestriatus brachycentrus* from Gedda, Arabia

Distribution: northeastern Africa through the Middle East.

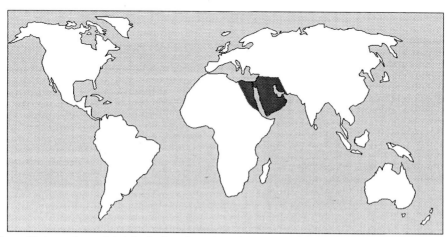

Figure 11. Approximate global distribution of scorpions of the genus *Leiurus*.

1. *Leiurus quinquestriatus hebraeus* (Birula, 1908)

Total length: females from 64 to 95 mm, males from 53 to 77 mm. Great variations exist among animals of the same locality as well as among specimens from different areas[20].

Color: yellowish to light orange-brown, last segment of the tail sometimes slightly darker than the other segments. Area between prosomal median-posterior crests granulated and often with a pair of granulated crescents; fifth mesosomal tergite on sides heavily granulated, but granules usually not arranged in rows; mesosoma, ventrally without conspicuous crests, and only toward the back do they gradually become somewhat distinct; granules of ventral crests of 2nd and 3nd metasomal segments gradually become bigger and coarser toward the back, and are different from crests of neighbouring segments; aculeus shorter than vesicle and only in a few cases rarely approaches the same length.

Distribution: Israel, Jordan, Syria and Lebanon.

2. *Leiurus quinquestriatus quinquestriatus* (Hemprich and Ehrebberg, 1829)

Total length: female 80 mm, male 70 mm

Area between prosomal median-posterior crests smooth or scarcely graduated; fifth mesosomal tergite on sides, often with short crestlike rows of granules; mesosoma, usually with distinct and elevated crests on four posterior sternites ventrally; ventral crests of 2nd and 3rd metasomal segments are regularly granulated even in females; aculeus usually distinctly longer than vesicle.

Distribution: North Africa, mainly Egypt.

D. GENUS *Buthus* LEACH, 1815

Central, lateral and posterior median keels of the carapace forming an " H " or " lyre-like " design; the immobile finger of the chelicerae with two ventral teeth; movable finger of pedipalps with three granules; tibial spurs present on legs III and IV.

Three species are described.

Distribution: Egypt, Ethiopia, Libya, Israel, Jordan, southern Spain and south of France.

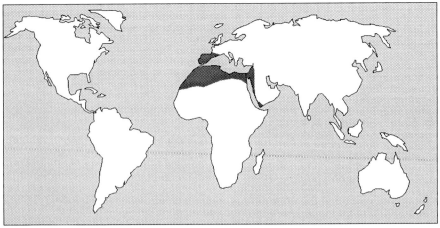

Figure 12. Approximate global distribution of scorpions of the genus *Buthus.*

1. *Buthus atlantis* (Pocock, 1889)

Total length: up to 9 cm

Yellow to brownish

Subspecies: *B. atlantis atlantis* (Pocock, 1889), *B. atlantis parroti* (Vachon, 1949)

Distribution: Atlantic coast of Morocco

2. *Buthus maroccanus* (Birula, 1903)
Total length: 5 to 6 cm
Uniformly black body
Distribution: Area of Rabat, Morocco

3. *Buthus martensi* (Karsch, 1879)
Total length: up to 6 cm
Brown to yellowish body
Distribution: Korea, Mongolia and China

4. *Buthus occitanus* (Amoreux, 1789)
Total length: 4 to 7.5 cm
Yellowish body
Subspecies: *B. occitanus occitanus* (Amoreux, 1789), *B. occitanus tunetanus* (Herbst, 1800), *B. occitanus mardochei* (E. Simon, 1878), *B. occitanus malhommei* (Vachon, 1949), *B. occitanus paris* (Koch, 1839)
Distribution: throughout the Mediterranean coasts and some Mediterranean islands

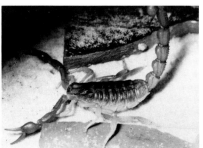

Figure 13. *Buthus occitanus,* (photo © Dr. J. White).   Figure 14. *Androctonus australis,* (photo © Dr. J. White).

E. GENUS *Androctonus* HEMPRICH AND EHRENBERG, 1829
    The central, lateral and median posterior keels of the carapace do not form an " H " or " lyre-like " design as in the genus *Buthus*; the fourth caudal segment with a strongly developed dorsal keel, caudal segments increasing in width and depth posteriorly.
Eight species are described.
Distribution: North Africa, Middle East and Asia.

1. *Androctonus aeneas* (Koch, 1839)
Total length: up to 8 cm
Uniform dark body with black-olive to chocolate-brown extremities.
Subspecies: *A. aeneas aeneas* (Koch, 1839), *A. aeneas liouvielli* (Pallary, 1924)
Distribution: From Tunisia to Morocco, high lands

2. *Androctonus crassicauda* (Olivier, 1807)
Total length: up to 8.5 cm
Dark, black-brown body with clearer extremities
Subspecies: *A. crassicauda gonneti* (Vachon, 1948)
Distribution: North Africa

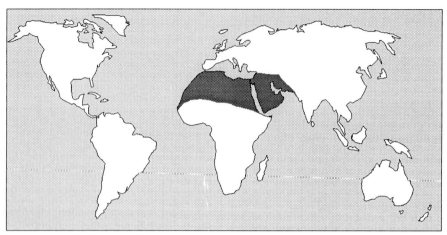

Figure 15. Approximate global distribution of scorpions of the genus *Androctonus*.

3. *Androctonus mauretanicus* (Pocock, 1902)
Total length: up to 9 cm
Uniform, dark-brown to black body
Subspecies: *A. mauretanicus mauretanicus* (Pocock, 1902), *A. mauretanicus bourdoni* (Vachon, 1948)
Distribution: Morocco

4. *Androctonus sergenti* (Vachon, 1948)
Total length: up to 7.5 cm
black-brown body, extremities and belly slightly clearer
Distribution: Morocco, restricted area (Anti-Atlas)

5. *Androctonus hoggarensis* (Pallary, 1929)
Total length: up to 7 cm
Dark green to brownish body, extremities clearer
Distribution: Highlands of Algeria and Morocco

6. *Androctonus australis* (L., 1758)
Total length: up to 10 cm
brown-yellowish body
Subspecies: *A. australis hector* (Koch, 1839)
Distribution: Algeria and Tunisia to Libya and Egypt

7. *Androctonus amoreuxi* (Audouin and Savigny, 1812 and 1827)
Total length: up to 12 cm
Brown-yellowish species (very similar to *A. australis*)
Distribution: from Egypt to Senegal

F. GENUS *BUTHOTUS* (VACHON, 1949)
   Only one out of about twenty different species of this genus is known to be medically significant.

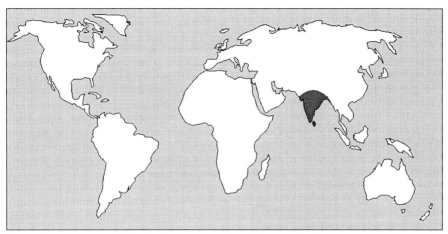

Figure 16. Approximate global distribution of scorpions of the genus *Buthotus*.

1. *Buthotus tamulus* (Fabricius, 1828)
Total length: up to 10 cm
Yellow to brownish to black
Distribution: Indian subcontinent

G. GENUS *Parabuthus* (POCOCK, 1890)
From about thirty different species recognized in this genus the following species are known to be medically significant.

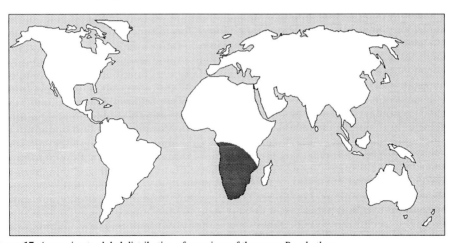

Figure 17. Approximate global distribution of scorpions of the genus *Parabuthus*.

1. *Parabuthus transvaalensis* (Mason, 1965)
Total length: up to 14 cm
brownish
Distribution: South Africa

2. *Parabuthus triradulatus* (Mason, 1965)
Total length: up to 10 cm
brownish
Distribution: South Africa

3. *Parabuthus villosus* (Mason, 1965)
Total length: up to 14 cm
brownish
Distribution: South Africa

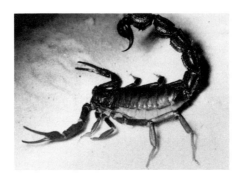

Figure 18. *Parabuthus transvaalensis,* (photo © Dr. J. White).

VI. PROPHYLAXIS AND FIRST AID TREATMENT

The majority of accidents occur inside human dwellings or in their vicinity.
As preventive measures the following are advisable:

- avoid the spread of domestic garbage in the vicinity of the house, in order to control domestic insects, like cockroaches, the main food for scorpions;
- avoid the accumulation of wood, building material like bricks and tiles, near the house; use gloves for protection during work, because these animals like to hide under such materials;
- periodically clean vacant lots around the house;
- care has to be taken when putting on shoes and clothes;
- keep furniture, mainly the bed, away from the wall;
- do not walk barefooted in the darkness as scorpions are active at night.

Scorpions in heavily infested areas can be trapped using a simple method: "just dampen a burlap sack or other rather heavy piece of cloth and spread it over the ground in the evening. During the night, scorpions will crawl under it and then can be readily killed the following morning" [21,22]. The floor level of the house must be at least 20 cm above the ground and the steps at the entrance should be separated at least 6 cm from the wall of the house[23]. Placing a layer of tiles around the house to prevent scorpions from climbing the walls has also been recommended[23]. Russell[24] used ultra-violet light for collecting scorpions, because the cuticle of these animals has the ability to fluoresce.

The main natural enemies of scorpions are birds (chicken, ducks, owls), monkeys and bats. These animals could be used for biological control of scorpions. Chemical control has some problems: scorpions have the ability to hide for several months. The use of residual insecticides in a kerosene solvent (DDT, Chlordane, Lindane) is recommended[21,22,25].

First aid for scorpion sting varies with the region and type of scorpion. Application of a pressure immobilisation bandage, as used for some snakebites (see Chapter 28), may delay venom absorption, but also may intensify local pain. The use of tourniquets, cutting or local suction is potentially hazardous and is not recommended.

Antivenom therapy is most often used in children, depending on the seriousness of symptoms.

VII. ANTIVENOMS

A list of hyperimmune sera currently available for the treatment of scorpions bites and other forms of envenoming has recently been published[26]. This is summarised in Table 1.

Table 1
List of available antivenoms for the treatment of scorpion envenoming[26]

Antidote	Source	Specific Name
01- Scorpion antivenom (Ar, F, E)	Institute Pasteur, Rue de Docteur Laveran Algiers, ALGERIA Phone: 2132653497	*Androctonus hector* (North African scorpion)
02- Scorpion antivenom (Ar, F, E)	Institute Pasteur, Place Charles-Nicole, Casablanca, MARROCOS Phone: 2122275778 212227520	*A. mauretanicus* (North African scorpion)
03-Anti- scorpionic (Ar, F, E)	Institute Pasteur, 13 Place Pasteur, Tunis, TUNISIA Phone: 283022-4 Telex: 14391 PASTU	*A. australis* (North African scorpion) [10,000] , *Buthus occitanus* (North African scorpion) [100,000] [southern and central Tunisia]
04- Scorpion antivenom (E, A)	The South African Institute for Medical Research, P.O. BOX 1038, Johannesburg 2000, SOUTH AFRICA Phone: 725-0511 Telex: 4-22211 Gram: BACTERIA	*Parabuthus transvaalicus* Scorpion (South Africa) North Transvaal [50 - 100]
05-Antivenin Centruroides (S)	Laboratorios " MYN " S.A., Av. Coyoacan 1707, Mexico City 12 D.F. MEXICO	*Centruroides spp.* Scorpion (Central America)
06-alacras polyvalent (S)	Anti-³ Laboratorio Zapata, Mexico City D.F., MEXICO Phone: 592-87-70/ 561-12-11/ 592-88-93	*C. suffusus C. noxius* Scorpions
07- Alacramyn antiscorpion serum lyophilized (E)	Grupo Pharma, S.A. de C.V., Zapata Labs., Mexico City, MEXICO Phone: 592-87-70/ 561-12-11/ 592-88-93	*C. noxius C. s. suffusus C. l. limpidus* Scorpions [50 - 100] [Durango, Nayarit, Michoacan, Colima, Guanajuato, Sinaloa Guerrero, Morelos, Jalisco, Zacatecas, Puebla, San Luis Potosi states]
08- Soro Anti-escorpionico genus Tityus (P)	Instituto Butantan, Av.Vital Brazil 1500, Caixa Postal 65, São Paulo - SP BRAZIL Phone: (011) 813-7222 FAX: (011) 815-1505 Telex: 11-83325-BUTA BR	*Tityus serrulatus T. bahiensis* Scorpions (Brazil)
09- Antivenin (scorpion)	Refik Saydan Central Institute of Hygiene, Ankara, TURKEY	*Androctonus crassicauda* (Israeli scorpion) *Leiurus quinquestriatus* (yellow scorpion)
10- Scorpion antivenom Twyford (North Africa) (E, Ar, G)	Twyford Pharmaceuticals GmbH, Postfach 21 08 05, D-6706 Ludwigshafen am Rhein, GERMANY Phone: (0621) 589-2688 FAX: (0621) 589-2896 Telex: 464823	*A. australi,s B. occitanus, L. quinquestriatus* (North African scorpions) [> 100 of each species]

Antidote	Source	Specific Name
11- Polyvalent scorpion antivenom (E, Pe)	Institut d'Etat des Serums et Vaccins, Razi Hessarek, B.P. 656, Teheran, IRAN Phone: 02221-2005	*A. crassicauda* (Israeli scorpion) *Buthotus salcyi* , *Mesobuthus eupeus, Odontobuthus riae, Scorpio maurus* Scorpions [> 10,000] [Iran]
12- Monovalent scorpion venom anti-serum (Hi, E)	Central Research Institute, Kasauli, (Simla Hills) (H.P.) INDIA Phone: C.R.I. 22	*B. tamalus* (Indian red scorpion) [> 100] [Parel, Bombay]
13- Scorpion antivenom (E)	Lister Institute of Preventive Medicine, Elstree, Herts, U.K. Phone: 081-954 6297	*A. australis, B. occitanus* (North African scorpions), *L. quinquestriatus* , (Yellow scorpion), *A. crassicauda* (Israeli scorpion)

Language on label : (A) Afrikaans ; (Ar) Arabic ; (E) English ; (F) French ; (G) German ; (Hi) Hindi ; (P) Portuguese ; (Pe) Persian ; (S) Spanish.

VIII. REFERENCES

1. **LAURIE, M.**, On a silurian scorpion and some additional eurypteride remains from the Pentland Hills, *Royal Soc. Edinburgh Trans*, **39,** 575, 1899.
2. **STORMER, L.**, *Gigantoscorpio willsi* a new scorpion from the lower Carboniferous of Scotland and its associate preying microorganisms, Skrifter utgitt av Det Norske *Videnskaps-Akademi 1 Oslo, I. Mat.-Naturv. Klasse. Ny Serie No.* **8,** 4, 1963.
3. **WORLD HEALTH ORGANIZATION**, Progress in the characterization of venoms and standardization of antivenoms, *WHO Offset Publication*, **58,** 6, 1981.
4. **FOELIX, R. F. AND MÜLLER-VORHOLT, M.**, The fine structure of scorpion sensory organs. II. Pecten sensilla, *Bul. British Archnol. Soc.*, **6,** 2, 68, 1983.
5. **BÜCHERL, W.**, Classification and Biology of Scorpions, in *Venomous Animals and their Venoms*, III *Venomous Invertebrates*, Bücherl, W. and Buckley, E. E., Eds., Academic Press, New York London, 1971, chapt. 55.
6. **BÜCHERL, W.**, Venoms of Tityinae, in *Handbuch der experimentellen Pharmakologie, Arthropod Venoms*, Bettin, S., Ed., Springer Verlag, Berlin Heidelberg New York, 1978, chapt. 14.
7. **ALEXANDER, A. J.**, The courtship and mating of the scorpion *Opisthophtalmus latimanus, Proc. Zool. Soc. London*, **128 (4),** 529, 1957.
8. **ANGERMANN, H.**, Indirekte Spermatophorenübertragung bei *Euscorpius italicus* Hbst. Scorpiones, (Chactidae), *Naturwissenschaften*, **42,** 323, 1955.
9. **MATTHIESEN, F. A.**, Parthenogenesis in scorpions, *Evolution*, **16,** 255, 1962.
10. **COVELO DE ZOLESSI, L.**, La partenogenesis en el escorpion amarillo *Tityus uruguayensis* Borelli,1901, *Rev. Fac. Hum. Cien., ser. cienc. biol.*, **1 (3),** 25, 1985.
11. **POLIS, G., A. AND SISSOM, W. D.**, Life history, in *The Biology of Scorpions*, Polis, G. A., Ed., Stanford University Press, Stanford, California, 1990, chapt. 4.
12. **VACHON, M., ROY, R. AND CONDAMIN, M.**, Le developpement post-embryonnaire du Scorpion *Pandinus gambiensis* Pocock, *Bulletin de l'Institut Français d'Afrique Noire, Ser. A*, **32,**412, 1970
13. **SISSOM, W. D.**, Systematics, Biogeography and Paleontology , in *The Biology of Scorpions*, Polis, G. A., Ed., Stanford University Press, Stanford, California, 1990, chapt. 3.
14. **WATERMAN, J. A.**, Some notes on scorpion poisoning in Trinidad, *Caribbean Med. J.*, **19 (1-2),** 113, 1957.
15. **FLETCHER, P. L., FLETCHER, M. D., VON EICKSTEDT, V. R., LUCAS, S., POSSANI, L. D. AND MARTIN, B. M.**, Comparative analysis of venoms from American scorpions, Abstracts of the *2nd. Symposium of Brazilian Society of Toxinology*, Campinas, São Paulo, Brazil, July 1992.
16. **BORGES, A., ARANTES, E. C. AND GIGLIO, J. R.**, Isolation and characterization of toxic proteins from the venom of the Venezuelan scorpion *Tityus discrepans* (Karsch), *Toxicon*, **28 (9),** 1011, 1990.
17. **DIAZ-NAJERA, A.**, Alacranes de la Republica Mexicana, *Rev. Invest. Salud. Publ. (Mex)*, **26 (2),** 109, 1966.
18. **STAHNKE, H. L. AND CALOS, M.**, A key to the species of the genus *Centruroides* Marx (Scorpionioda, Buthidae), *Ent. News*, **88 (5 & 6),** 111, 1977.
19. **VACHON, M.**, Etudes sur les scorpions, *Archs. Inst. Pasteur Alger*, **27,** 66, 1949.

20. **LEVI, G., AMITAI, P. AND SHULOV, A.,** *Leiurus quinquestriatus hebraeus* (Birula, 1908) (Scorpiones, Buthidae) and its systematic position, *Israel J. Zool.*, **19 (4),** 231, 1970.

21. **STAHNKE, H. L.**, Scorpions, Poisonous Animals Research Lab., Arizona State College, Tempe, Arizona, 1956.

22. **BÜCHERL, W.**, EscorpiÆes e escorpionismo no Brasil. IV. ConsideraçÆes em torno de substancias escorpionicidas e outras medidas de combate aos escorpiÆes, *Mem. Inst. Butantan*, **27,** 107, 1955/1956.

23. **MAZZOTTI, L. AND BRAVO-BECHERELLE, M. A.**,Scorpionism in the Mexican Republic, in Keegan H. L. and McFarland, W. W., Eds., *Venomous and poisonous animals and noxious plants of the Pacific Area*, Pergamon Press, New York, 119, 1963.

24. **RUSSELL, F. E.**, Scorpion collecting, *Toxicon*, **6,** 307, 1966.

25. **STAHNKE, H. L.**, The Genus *Centruroides* (Buthidae) and its Venoms, in *Handbuch der Experimentellen Pharmakologie, Arthropod Venoms*, Bettini S., Ed., Springer Verlag, Berlin Heidelberg New York, 1978, chapt. 12.

26. **THEAKSTON, R. D. G. AND WARRELL, D. A.**, Antivenoms: a list of hyperimune sera currently available for the treatment of envenoming by bites and stings, *Toxicon*, **29 (12),** 1419, 1991.

Chapter 18

CLINICAL TOXICOLOGY OF SCORPION STINGS

Manuel Dehesa-Davila, Alejandro C. Alagon and Lourival D. Possani

TABLE OF CONTENTS

I. INTRODUCTION

This chapter encompasses the clinical toxicology of scorpion stings, using as a model the scorpions from the genus *Centruroides* of Mexico. Statistical estimates indicate that in Mexico about a quarter of a million sting accidents occur in humans every year. Also, due to the diversity of climates, about 136 different species and sub-species of scorpions are endemic in Mexico[1]. Fortunately only eight species and sub-species are clinically important for man[1,2].

Scorpions are arachnids well distributed geographically, in tropical and sub-tropical areas of the world, and possess a venom apparatus composed of a pair of glands and a sting. The species important for human health contain in their venoms small molecular weight peptides capable of causing impairment of cell function by interfering with ion channel permeability of the membranes of excitable cells.

In this chapter we will present and discuss some of the general aspects of the venom, symptoms and signs of envenomation, prophylaxis and clinical management, based on the author's own experience, especially in the treatment of persons stung by scorpions. More than ten thousand cases were treated by our group in different clinical facilities. Some references are also included concerning scorpions in other parts of the world.

II. EPIDEMIOLOGY OF SCORPION STINGS IN MEXICO

A. THE SCORPIONS: DISTRIBUTION AND CHARACTERISTICS

Worldwide, there are more than 1,000 scorpion species distributed in six families: Buthidae, Scorpionidae, Diplocentridae, Chactidae, Vejovidae and Bothriuridae[3]. Although all scorpions are venomous, less than 50 species (belonging to the Buthidae family) can be considered dangerous to humans[3].

In Mexico, the only species of scorpions of medical importance are from the genus *Centruroides*, which belongs to the Buthidae family. There are at least 30 different species and subspecies from this genera described by Hoffmann[1,2].

The scorpions are arthropods that belong to the class Arachnida and to the order Scorpionida. They have two main body divisions: the prosoma or cephalothorax and the opisthosoma or abdomen. The abdomen is further subdivided into an anterior mesosoma (preabdomen) and a posterior metasoma (postabdomen or "tail"). Both of these regions are segmented. The tail-like metasoma terminates in a bulbous segment called the telson. This structure possesses a sharp, curved stinger or aculeus. A scorpion is equipped with a pair of pedipalps that look like claws; the small chelicerae between the bases of the pedipalps; four pairs of legs, all on the prosoma; and a pair of pectines, which are ventrally located, have comb-like structure and are sensorial organs[3]. For additional information on the morphology of scorpion, please refer to Chapter 17.

Centruroides scorpions belong to a New World genus with its center of distribution in Mexico (Figure 1). These scorpions are also found in the southern states of the United States, Central America, the West Indies and in several countries of South America. Specifically, the species of medical importance occur in Western New Mexico, Arizona, areas along the basin of the Colorado river in California, and in Mexico, in the Pacific States from the North of Sonora down to the West-side of Oaxaca and in some regions of some Central States such as Durango, Aguascalientes, Zacatecas, Guanajuato and Morelos[4]. Figure 2 illustrates representative species of Mexican scorpions.

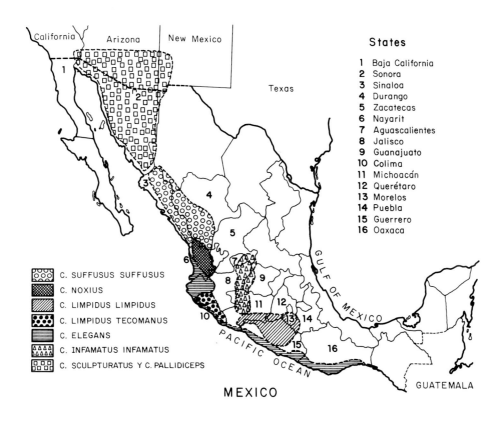

Figure 1. Geographical distribution of Mexican scorpions dangerous to humans. The Mexican States are indicated by numbers, while the scorpion species by various graphic representations (see legend)[5].

Scientific name: *Centruroides*

Species (States in Mexico, or U.S.)

Centruroides bertholdi (Jalisco)

**Centruroides elegans* (Nayarit, Jalisco, Michoacán, Colima, Guerrero)

Centruroides exilicauda (Sonora, Baja California Norte, California in U.S.)

Centruroides flavopictus (Veracruz)

Centruroides fulvipes (Guerrero)

**Centruroides infamatus infamatus* (Zacatecas, Aguascalientes, Guanajuato, Michoacan)

**Centruroides limpidus limpidus* (Colima, Guerrero, Morelos)

**Centruroides limpidus tecomanus* (Colima)

Centruroides margaritatus (Oaxaca)

Centruroides nigrescens (Oaxaca)

Centruroides nigrovariatus (Oaxaca)

**Centruroides noxius* (Nayarit)

**Centruroides pallidiceps* (Sonora, Sinaloa, Arizona in U.S.)

**Centruroides sculpturatus* (Sonora; Arizona and New Mexico in U.S.)

**Centruroides suffusus suffusus* (Durango)

The most dangerous species are highlighted with an asterisk (*). See also the map of geographical distribution in Figure 1. In Mexico the dangerous species are distributed along the Pacific coast, comprising 16 states of the country, while in the U.S. the dangerous species occur mainly in Arizona and New Mexico. The morphological characteristics of *Centuroides* sp., including the most dangerous species, are listed in Chapter 17.

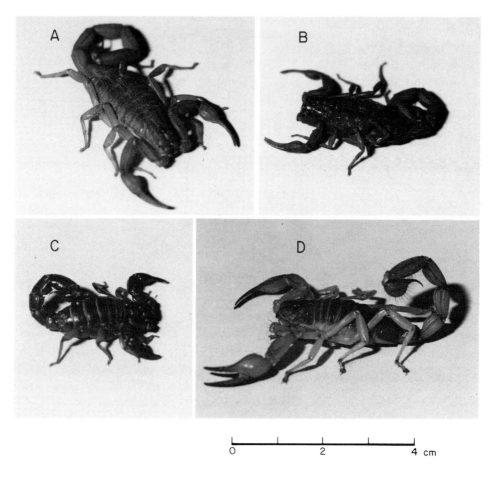

Figure 2. Representative photos of Mexican scorpions. In A: adult female of the species *Centruroides limpidus limpidus*; B: adult female of *Centruroides noxius*; C: adult *Vejovis mexicanus*; D: young *Hadrurus concolorous*. The two latter species are non-dangerous to man.

B. SCORPION STINGS IN MEXICO

Scorpionism is a public health problem in many states of Mexico. Unfortunately, the epidemiological data are incomplete and the exact number of accidents is unknown. Original estimates on the number of cases were published by Mazzotti and Bravo-Becherelle[6] and reported by Monroy-Velazco[7]. Numbers as high as 100,000 cases of accidents per year were reported for the 60's and 70's. Lopez-Acuña & Alagon have compiled data (presented in the technical session of the Sociedad Mexicana de Salud Publica) in 1976 suggesting numbers close to 200,000 per year, with 700 to 800 fatalities. Dehesa-Davila[8] and Possani et al.[9] confirm estimates higher than 250,000 stings per year in Mexico. Table 1 summarises unpublished data from statistics collected by the authors in the city of Leon, Guanajuato. Also included are partial data from the states of Nayarit and Morelos. There have been about 69,000 accidents in 9 years of observation. The city of Leon alone had approximately 7,540 stings per year (data recorded only from the Red Cross Hospital and one of the Social Security Clinics of the city), during this period. Yet, the city of Leon is not the most important in Mexico in terms of scorpionism[8]. The mortality rate is 0.01%.

Table 1
Partial statistical data of scorpion stings in mexico

Year	Guanajuato	Morelos	Nayarit	Mortality
1981	6649	n.c.	n.c.	0
1982	8044	n.c.	n.c.	1
1983	7342	n.c.	1759	17
1984	7928	1564	1068	25
1985	7289	2641	1063	8
1986	7989	3042	1206	7
1987	n.c.	3775	1510	1
1988	n.c.	3661	1109	6
1989	n.c.	n.c.	1814	0
TOTAL	45,241	14,683	9,529	65
GLOBAL	69,453			

* Only Red Cross Hospital and one clinic of IMSS (Mexican Institute of Social Security) in Leon, Guanajuato. n.c.= not compiled.

III. VENOM COMPOSITION AND PHARMACOLOGY

A. STRUCTURE AND MODE OF ACTION OF SCORPION TOXINS

In humans and experimental animals toxic polypeptides of scorpion venom are responsible for the symptoms of intoxication. There are two groups of similar peptides in the venoms of *Centruroides*: one is composed of long-chain peptides that affect sodium channels, and the second consists of short-chain peptides which block potassium channels of excitable membranes (mainly nervous and muscular tissues). The binding of these toxins to the cation channels (Na^+ and K^+) causes most of the toxicological symptoms of the venom. The binding is reversible, but different toxins have different affinities[10-15]. Recently, another class of peptides was described in the venom of the scorpion *Buthotus hottentota*, which affects the Ryanodine-sensitive Ca^{2+}-channel[16], and similar peptides were found in the venom of the genus *Hadrurus* from Mexico[17]. The literature of the last five years reflects the importance of the structure and function relationship of toxins from scorpions collected in many different parts of the world[18-23]. Figure 3 is an example of the primary structure of toxins isolated from scorpions of the genus *Centruroides*. In this figure both classes of scorpion toxins are represented: long-chain (Na^+-channel blockers) and short-chain (K^+-channel blockers).

B. HUMAN DATA

It is only possible to obtain a rough estimate concerning the amounts of venom that result in envenomation in humans. This approximation is based on the amount of venom extracted by electrical stimulation from the telson of anaesthetized scorpions. The average amount of venom that can be obtained from a single animal varies from 100 μg in small species (i.e. *Centruroides noxius*) to 600 μg in the large species (i.e. *Centruroides elegans*). These experimental values set the range of variation on the amount of venom toxic to humans. It is unlikely that a scorpion in a normal situation will inject more venom than is extracted under extreme stress (electrical stimulation). Scorpions usually inject venom subcutaneously, from where it is distributed all over the body by the circulatory system.

The human lethal dose is probably less than 100 to 600 µg of venom. This is the maximum amount of venom that a single scorpion has in the glands (telson) at any one time. Ismail[24] demonstrated that the venom is distributed very rapidly into the tissues by the intravenous route ranging between 4 - 7 minutes and overall elimination half-lives of 4.2 to 13.4 hr.

Toxin Amino acid sequence of Na⁺-channel blockers[13]

	1	10	20	30	40	50	60	66
Cn2	KEGYLVDKNTGCKYECLKLGDNDYCLRECKQQGYKGAGGYCYAFACWCTHLYEQAIVWPLPNKRCS							
CssII	KEGYLVSKSTGCKYECLKLGDNDYCLRECKQQYGKSSGGYCYAFACWCTHLYEQAVVWPLPNKTCN							
Clt1	KEGYLVNHSTGCKYECFKLGDNDYCLRECRQQYGKGAGGYCYAFGCWCTHLYEQAVVWPLPNKTCS							
Cn3	KEGYLVELGTGCKYECFKLGDNDYCLRECKARYGKGAGGYCYAFGCWCTQLYEQAVVWPLKNKTCR							
CsE1	KEGYLVKKSDGCKYDCFWLGKNEHNTCECKAKNQGGSYGYCYAFACWCEGLPESTPTYPLPNK-CS							
CsE2	KEGYLVNKSTGCKYGCLKLGENEGNKCECKAKNQGGSYGYCYAFACWCEGLPESTPTYPLPNK-CSS							
CsE3	KEGYLVKKSDGCKYGCLKLGENEGCDTECKAKNQGGSYGYCYAFACWCEGLPESTPTYPLPNKSC-							
CsEI	KDGYLVEK-TGCKKTCYKLGENDFCNRECKWKHIGGSYGYCYGFGCYCEGLPDSTQTWPLPNK-CT							
Cn1	KDGYLVDA-KGCKKNCYKLGKNDYCNRECRMKHRGGSYGYCYGFGCYCEGLSDSTPTWPLTNKTC-							

Toxin Amino acid sequence of K⁺-channel blockers[14]

	1	10	20	30	39
Cn NTX	TIINVKCTSPKQCSKPCKELYGSSAGAKCMNGKCKCYNN				
Cn II-10.2	TFIDVKCGSSKECXP...				
CII II-10.11.4	TVINVKCTSPKQCLLPCKQI...				

Figure 3. Primary structure of scorpion toxins. These amino acid sequences were taken from the indicated references (13-14), where the abbreviations correspond to: Cn, *C. noxius*; Css, *C. suffusus suffusus*; Clt, *C. limpidus tecomanus*; CsE, *C. sculpturatus*; Cll, *C. limpidus limpidus*, and NTX to noxiustoxin.

C. ANIMAL DATA

LD_{50} values determined in experimental animals vary according to the species and strain of animal used. For example the LD_{50} estimated for *Centruroides limpidus limpidus* venom in seven different strains of mice averaged (intraperitoneal injection) at 2 mg/kg mouse with the extremes of variation being 0.61 mg/kg for the SSA strain and 3.31 mg/kg for the BALB/k strain[25]. The LD_{50} of *Centruroides infamatus infamatus* venom injected intraperitoneally into mice was 1.27 mg/kg, but was only 0.166 mg/kg in Wistar strain rats using the same route. *Centruroides noxius* seems to be the most toxic venom, with an LD_{50} of 0.26 mg/kg mouse intraperitoneally[26]. *Centruroides limpidus tecomanus* has an LD_{50} of 0.65 mg/kg, while that of *Centruroides sculpturatus* is 1.12 mg/kg in mice injected intraperitoneally[27].

1. *In vitro* data

Most of the data on the mechanism of action of the toxins from the scorpion venoms were obtained by *in vitro* experiments using excitable tissues such as squid axons, several types of heart cells, dorsal root ganglion cells, synaptosomes from brain tissues, and others. Whole-cell clamp and patch-clamp techniques, or single channels incorporated into artificial bilayer membranes, were used to identify the channels affected by toxins purified from the venom of *Centruroides* scorpions[12,28-31].

2. Elimination by route of exposure

Elimination of venom occurs mainly through urinary excretion, although bile secretion may play an important role[32]. People stung by *Centruroides* scorpions may have clinical symptoms for as long as one week, especially near or at the site of the sting (unpublished observations).

IV. SYMPTOMS AND SIGNS

A. GENERAL COMMENTS

Centruroides scorpions have a tendency to hide above the ground; therefore, they are frequently found under loose bark on trees, crevices in dead trees, logs and walls or at the base in dry leaves of palms and corn plants. They may also thrive in lumber piles, bricks, stones and other debris or in soil cracks. Poorly built houses offer scorpions many niches to live. Indeed, they are often associated with human habitations because they enter homes and hide during daylight hours in places offering darkness and close contact (shoes, folded blankets, heaped clothing, hanging pictures, etc). Scorpions are almost exclusively nocturnal. *Centruroides* scorpions are not aggressive; accidents occur when they are inadvertently touched in their hiding places or when they are wandering in search of food. In Mexico, there is an increase in the morbidity and mortality rate that in some places coincides with the rainy season and in others with the beginning of spring. The most dangerous *Centruroides* species dislike damp places preferring dry indoor locations[33].

All species belonging to the *Centruroides* genus or other genera; dangerous or harmless are called "scorpions" in English speaking countries, and "escorpiones" or "alacranes" in Spanish speaking countries.

1. Risk factors

Envenomation and prognosis will depend on a number of factors, some of them attributable to the arthropod and some to the victim. For the arthropod these are: (i) species, (ii) condition of the telson at the moment of the sting, (iii) number of stings and quantity of venom injected. For the victim: (i) age, weight and health of the victim, (ii) concomitant disease (i.e. diabetes, hypertension, heart disease, etc.) and (iii) effectiveness of the treatment. From the onset of the first signs and symptoms of envenomation to the development of severe envenoming may take a very short time; in most cases this progression can take only 5 to 30 minutes. Prognosis: serious systemic complications such as heart failure, pulmonary oedema, convulsions and coma worsen the prognosis. Respiratory failure is usually the cause of death, but other severe complications, like cardiocirculatory shock, may lead to death[8,34].

B. ONSET, EVOLUTION AND CLINICAL PICTURE

Local evidence of the sting in the skin of the victim is often minimal or absent. Patients report intense pain or a burning sensation with intense pruritus and hyperesthesia. Some redness and inflammation with local oedema can be observed at the sting site. The pain occurs instantaneously after the sting and can last for several days; paresthesia can be present for several weeks and is usually the last symptom to disappear.

1. Local symptoms and signs

Immediately after the sting there is burning pain, which is followed by pruritus and hyperaesthesia. Mild inflammation sometimes occurs.

2. General symptoms and signs

General symptoms are not always observed and do not have an apparent sequence. They include some or all of the following: hyperexcitability, restlessness, hyperthermia, tachypnoea, dyspnoea, tachycardia or bradycardia, profuse sweating, nausea, vomiting, gastric hyperdistention, diarrhoea, lachrymation, nystagmus, mydriasis, photophobia, excessive salivation, nasal secretion, dysphagia with a sensation of hair in the throat, dysphonia, cough, bronchorrhea, pulmonary oedema, arterial hypertension or hypotensive heart failure, circulatory shock, convulsions, ataxia, fasciculations and coma.

In evaluating envenomation it is important to consider that it is more serious in children and people of advanced age or with debilitating diseases[35-38].

C. SPECIFIC TOXIN EFFECTS AND COMPLICATIONS

Lachrymation, mydriasis, photophobia, nystagmus, nasal secretion, a characteristic sensation of hair in the throat with dysphonia, cough and dysphagia are some of the most consistent symptoms observed following envenomation.

1. Cardiovascular

There is ample experimental and clinical evidence that venoms from different scorpion species release catecholamines from the sympathetic nervous system and stimulate the cardiac adrenergic endings[39-45].

Usually, there is an initial period of hypertension that can be followed by hypotension. Likewise, tachycardia predominates although bradycardia may also be observed. These contradictory effects may depend on the system preferentially affected by the toxins, either cholinergic or adrenergic[46,47].

The evolution of these phenomena plus the direct action on the conducting system of the heart can lead to cardiac arrhythmia and heart failure and secondarily may cause pulmonary oedema.

Gonzalez-Romero[48] treated 722 patients stung by *Centruroides suffusus*: 38% had electrocardiographic abnormalities, from which 12.8% corresponded to bundle branch block, 10.2% first-degree atrioventricular block and 15% alterations in the ventricular repolarization (in the majority of cases reversible), and the remaining 62% of patients had other abnormalities.

The profuse loss of fluids (sweating, vomiting, diarrhoea) may also contribute to circulatory collapse. Continuous electrocardiogram (ECG) monitoring will permit the early diagnosis and treatment of cardiac arrhythmia and commencement of ventilatory support through oxygen therapy or positive pressure respiration.

2. Respiratory

Tachypnoea is often present. Dyspnoea is a common finding in severe cases. Respiratory failure, the usual cause of death, reflects paralysis of the respiratory muscles, particularly the diaphragm, due to a reflex stimulation of vagal afferent fibers. Bronchial hypersecretion and pulmonary oedema may also be contributing factors[34,47,49,50]. Catecholamines in very large doses may cause brief periods of apnea. Thus, it seems that the pathogenesis of respiratory failure is multifactorial[50]. Respiratory arrest has been occasionally observed following *Centruroides sculpturatus* sting[38]. Most of the available pathological data are based on experimental envenomation. These studies emphasized the presence of different degrees of pulmonary oedema with diffuse parenchymal hemorrhages[50].

3. Neurologic

Central nervous system

There is currently no experimental evidence that scorpion neurotoxins can cross the blood-brain barrier. However, some effects may indicate a direct action on the central nervous system, such as the hyper-excitability and the restlessness, very often observed even in mild cases[51]. The high levels of catecholamines released by the venom may also provide some explanation for these symptoms. Coma can be present in severe envenomation, mostly in children.

Peripheral nervous system

The peripheral nervous system is the main target of scorpion neurotoxins. Most of the time, their clinical effects reflect the action of neurotransmitters, like acetylcholine and catecholamines that are released by the action of the toxins[51,52].

Autonomic nervous system

The autonomic nervous system includes parasympathetic and sympathetic pathways. Both are stimulated by scorpion venom. The most common parasympathetic manifestations are: salivation, lachrymation, gastric hyperdistention, diarrhoea, bradycardia and hypotension. The main sympathetic effects are mydriasis, tachypnea, tachycardia and hypertension. In the course of the envenomation one effect can be predominant, but mixed effects are also observed. This is the reason for finding variable symptomatology as discussed by Freire-Maia[46].

Skeletal and smooth muscle

Spasms, muscle contraction and twitches are due to stimulation of skeletal muscle by the venom[53]. These effects reflect the action of the toxins at a presynaptic level[54]. The most notorious effects on smooth muscle are abdominal pain and diarrhoea. The contraction and or relaxation of smooth muscle of the intestine induced by the venom are due to the release of chemical mediators, such as acetylcholine and catecholamines; but other mediators such as substance P could also be released[46].

4. Gastrointestinal

Excessive salivation, nausea and vomiting are characteristic features of scorpion envenomation. Also, an increase in motility of the intestine with diarrhoea is common. Gastric hyperdistention is frequently observed. These effects are basically explained by the peripheral action of the toxins on cholinergic nerve fibers (vagus nerve) which would act through muscarinic and H2 receptors[55-58]. Experimental data show a dramatic increase in volume, acid and pepsin output of gastric juice and a significant decrease in its pH. From a clinical point of view it is necessary to be very cautious with patients that suffer peptic ulcers. Acute pancreatitis was reported in humans stung by the scorpion *Tityus trinitatis* and by *Leiurus quinquestriatus*[59-62]. It was suggested that this could be explained in part by the release of acetylcholine from pancreatic nerve endings[63]. Fletcher *et al*[64] proposed a mechanism that involves ion channels (Na^+, Ca^{2+} and K^+) in the case of *Tityus serrulatus* venom.

5. Miscellaneous

Skin contact: No effect on intact skin.

Hepatic: The liberated chemical mediators such as catecholamines may provoke increase of liver glycogenolysis, with a consequent hyperglycemic effect in blood[32,65].

Urinary tract: In severe envenomation urinary incontinence may be observed or urinary retention[35].

Kidney: *Tityus serrulatus* decreased renal plasma flow, urine and sodium excretion in dogs[66]. These effects could be due to the release of catecholamines from renal nerve endings.

Endocrine and reproductive system: No known effects.

Hematologic: Longnecker reported that the venom of *C.sculpturatus* caused a sustained platelet aggregation in dogs[67]. One possible explanation is that the release of catecholamines induces platelet aggregation and this contributes to a defibrination syndrome. However, the venom of *C. limpidus limpidus* does not seem to affect platelet aggregation in human blood (author's unpublished observations).

Immunologic: In very rare cases of repetitive exposure, allergic reactions have been reported (author's unpublished observations)[68].

Metabolic: A hyperglycemic effect has been documented in *Centruroides* envenomation. The release of catecholamines is expected to increase hepatic glycogenolysis (as mentioned above) and at the same time inhibit insulin release[69,70].

Acid base disturbances: Blood acidosis associated with hypercapnia occurs in patients with severe respiratory failure, or shock[50].

Fluid and electrolyte disturbances: Dehydration due to vomiting, profuse sweating and diarrhea must be carefully monitored.

Pregnancy: A case of a pregnant woman (first trimester) who aborted was reported following a sting of *Leiurus quinquestriatus*[71]. There is no information on *Centruroides* species in this respect, nor is there any information on possible foetal damage. However, the toxins can potentiate the action of agonists such as acetylcholine, serotonin and bradykinin enhancing the autorhythmic activity of the uterus[51].

V. PROPHYLAXIS

A. CIRCUMSTANCES OF STINGS AND HEALTH EDUCATION

In areas endemic for dangerous scorpions it is suggested that shoes and clothes be shaken out before dressing. Since scorpions are nocturnal animals, before going to sleep it is recommended to look between covers, around the bed, walls and ceilings. There are some architectural features of housing that are recommended in order to avoid the entrance of scorpions into houses. The scorpions can not climb smooth and well-polished surfaces. Mazzotti[6] recommends the use of screens on windows and a row of glazed tiles around the outside walls of the house (including stairs) in order to protect against scorpion invasion. The children's bed can be protected by a gauge-cloth envelope.

Accidents occur with both dangerous and non-dangerous scorpions, either in rural or in urban areas. Many accidents take place in houses, buildings or schools. Some species of *Centruroides* invade human dwellings, where they can get into shoes, clothing or inside furniture. They crawl on walls and ceilings, from where they can fall and sting people. Frequently people are stung while picking up domestic objects containing the hidden scorpions[33].

In endemic areas, particularly in the dark, it is recommended not to touch unseen objects, but use artificial light.

Additionally, it should be noted that most venomous species of *Centruroides* are resistant to commonly used home-insecticides[72].

B. PERSPECTIVES ON PRODUCTION OF A VACCINE

In the past, some attempts have been made to prepare a possible immunogen for vaccination of experimental animals[73]. A toxic fraction of the venom from *Centruroides noxius* was detoxified with glutaraldehyde and was shown to produce neutralizing antibodies in rabbits. Purified antibodies protected mice against the lethal effect of the toxic fraction (number II from Sephadex G-50 gel filtration)[73]. Detoxification of scorpion toxins by acetylation was also reported for pure toxins of *Androctonus australis* and *Buthus occitanus tunetanus* by Delori et al[74]. These authors conclude that the use of fraction II from Sephadex G-50 is the most suitable substrate for obtaining a potent acetylated anatoxin that is capable of producing neutralizing antibodies against several venoms of African scorpions. A more recent review on this subject is also available[75]. Heneine et al[76]. showed that iodination of fraction T2 from the venom of *Tityus serrulatus* abolishes its lethal capacity, without changing its immunological properties.

More recently, several synthetic peptides were prepared with amino acid sequences corresponding to the primary structure of whole toxins and/or segments of the primary structure of toxins of the scorpion *Centruroides noxius* for immunization purposes[77]. Some peptides are immunogenic and produce neutralizing antibodies against the native toxin, when injected in passive immunization protocols. Unfortunately, other peptides cause hypersensitivity of preimmunized animals, when challenged directly with native toxin. These experiments are in progress, and it is difficult to foresee, at this moment, the possibility of a vaccine against scorpion venom[78].

Several questions should be addressed before a real vaccine can be obtained and applied in humans. The first question, only partially answered by the publications mentioned above[78], is the selection of an adequate antigen, i.e. homogeneous, non-toxic, which can be obtained in sufficient amounts with an acceptable grade of quality for human use. The second question is the route of administration and the adjuvant needed, if any. The next important question is to determine the levels of neutralizing-circulating antibodies and the duration of such levels after immunization. A scorpion sting is an acute event. The envenomed organism needs a prompt and efficient response. Further problems could be presented by the need to prepare different antigens, according to different geographical areas of the world, or different species of scorpions living in the same area. Finally, an outbred strain, like humans, is bound to present a wide variety of different responses to the same antigens.

Newer approaches, using cloned toxin-genes[79-82] and recombinant DNA techniques might present an alternative strategy for studying the problem of vaccine preparation against scorpion stings. While these questions are awaiting answers the prospective development of a vaccine is no more than a dream, and serotherapy continues to be the only choice for treatment of scorpionism.

VI. FIRST AID TREATMENT

A. PRINCIPLES AND RECOMMENDATIONS

Scorpion accidents constitute a significant problem, mainly in children under five years old, and elderly and emaciated or malnourished adults. If not adequately treated, often lethal consequences can result.

Unfortunately, there is no simple way for a medical doctor and the public to distinguish between a dangerous and a harmless species. Several different species can live in the same location.

The following steps can be used in cases of scorpion sting:
- Immobilize the patient and the affected part;

- Avoid incisions;
- A constriction bandage could be placed close to the site of sting, but the application of tourniquets should be avoided;
- The use of local suction is recommended by some, but remains controversial. It is a technique widely accepted in Mexico, where it appears effective, based on anecdotal evidence. Suction is applied at the site of the sting (oral suction is very effective if immediately applied, and providing there is no damage to the oral mucosa; the venom must be spat out immediately);
- Apply cold packs or immerse the stung area in ice water for the first two hours (intermittently) to help slow absorption;
- Obtain medical attention or transport to hospital;
- If the offending scorpion has been killed, take it with the victim to hospital for identification.

The victim must be kept calm and warm, and given reassurance. Immobilize the affected part in a functional position. Watch for any untoward reaction, and transport the victim to the nearest medical facility as quickly as possible. On admission, local antisepsis must be performed: give analgesics if pain is severe. Keep the patient under observation for at least 4 hours. Tetanus prophylaxis is recommended although not mandatory.

Avoid incisions. The local extraction of venom by suction with the mouth through the orifice made by the stinger is often recommended, but its efficacy is not proved. As little as one microgram of purified toxin is potent enough to cause local anaesthesia in humans with impairment of movements (unpublished personal experience). A few tenths of micrograms of purified material are probably lethal to humans.

VII. CLINICAL MANAGEMENT

A. DIAGNOSIS

A patient describing a well documented history of scorpion sting presents no problem in diagnosis. However, the possibility that the victim could have been stung by a non-dangerous scorpion should be taken into consideration. Thus clinical observations are of utmost importance in confirming envenoming. With children under the age of four years old it is common to hear them crying loudly, and it is also very common to miss the offending scorpion. In this case if there is sneezing and nasal pruritus one can suspect a scorpion sting and consequent envenomation.

B. TREATMENT
1. Antivenom production

A recent review by Theakston and Warrell[83] compiled addresses and names of most institutions around the world that produce scorpion antivenoms, which has been updated for this chapter (see also Table 1, Chapter 17 and Chapter 32). The following countries are reported to be currently producing antivenom against scorpions: Algeria, Brazil, England, Germany, India, Iran, Mexico, Morocco, South Africa, Tunisia, Turkey, U.S. and Venezuela[83].

In Mexico, *Centruroides* polyvalent antivenom is produced in horses by injecting with a mixture of venom from the most important species (*C. noxius*, *C. l. limpidus*, *C. l. tecomanus*, and *C. suffusus suffusus*). It is enzymatically digested and lyophilized. The antivenom cross-reacts with other *Centruroides* spp. venoms, and protects against all venomous species in Mexico. There are two producers of antivenom against *Centruroides* species:

1. Gerencia General de Biologicos y Reactivos. Health Ministry. M. Escobedo 20, C.P. 11400 Mexico D.F., Mexico. Suero Antialacran - ampoule with lyophilized immunoglobulins. One ampoule neutralizes 150 LD_{50} in mice tested intraperitoneally.

2. Laboratorios BIOCLON (before MYN, Zapata, and Grupo Pharma). Calzada de Tlalpan 4687, C.P. 14050 Mexico D.F., Mexico. Suero Antialacran (Alacramyn)[*] - ampoule with lyophilized immunoglobulins. One ampoule neutralizes 150 LD_{50} in mice tested intraperitoneally. [*]Registered Trademark of Bioclon, Mexico.

A third producer of antivenom is located in the U.S. The antivenom from Arizona is prepared in goats following immunization with venom of *C. sculpturatus*[84]. The lyophilized product is distributed free throughout the state of Arizona. The mailing address is: Antivenom Production Laboratory, Arizona State University, Tempe, Arizona 85281, U.S.

Other producers of antivenom for scorpion stings in Latin America are:

- Instituto Ezequiel Dias, Belo Horizonte - Minas Gerais, Brazil
- Centro de Biotecnologia, Facultad de Farmacia Universidad Central, Caracas, Venezuela, The Centro de Biotecnologia in Venezuela prepares an antivenom against *Tityus discrepans* (personal communication Dr. Jeanette Scannone).

2. Antivenom therapy

In Mexico specific treatment consists of the administration of *Centruroides* polyvalent antiserum. Its application will depend on the presence of two or more general symptoms listed previously (section IV.B).

The quantity of antivenom to be used is determined by the clinical symptoms and their evolution over time. The lyophilized immunoglobulins contained in the ampoules are dissolved in 5 ml of water for injection. There is always uncertainty in the progression of the envenomation and it is almost impossible to predict the evolution of the symptomatology. Thus, in earlier stages of envenomation, one or two vials are enough to control the symptoms. However, when the patient comes to the hospital in later stages of envenomation it might be necessary to use up to four vials of antivenom. This is valid for both children and adults. In Mexico it is considered advisable to administer an antihistamine (i.e., chlorpheniramine) together with antivenom. Faster neutralizing effects are obtained if the intravenous route of injection is used. Intramuscular injection of the antivenom is also effective. The use of the antivenom is not recommended in the absence of systemic symptoms of envenomation.

Currently there are no uniform criteria for treatment of scorpion sting envenomation. Several reports are available in the literature[7-9,37,41,44,57,58,85,86].

In Mexico, from a total of 38,068 cases of envenomation by *Centruroides* scorpions, the application of antivenom (mixed with an antihistamine) was reported in 20,293 cases[8]. Skin tests, or other procedures, were not performed to determine possible hypersensitivities. None of the patients developed immediate allergic reactions. No deaths were recorded. Cases of late development of serum sickness, although possible, were not documented, mainly because the patients did not return to the hospital. The conclusion of this work is that there is no doubt that the administration of antivenom is the most important therapeutic measure in neutralizing the circulating venom.

In Brazil, the group of Freire-Maia *et al*[44] has reported treatment of 3,860 patients stung by *Tityus serrulatus* with a very high rate of success due to the prompt use of antivenom. The mortality rate was 0.28%. All deaths were in children, principally because of late admission to the hospital (3 or more hours after the accident). The serotherapy consisted of intravenous injection of 20 - 40 ml of antivenom from Butantan Institute, Sao Paulo, Brazil[57,58].

In Tunisia, specific antivenom is considered the main therapeutic measure for severe cases of envenomation by the scorpions *Androctonus australis* and *Androctonus aeneas*[85].

In Israel, Gueron and Ovsyshcher[41] reported that antivenom therapy is of great value in cases of severe envenomation by *Leiurus quinquestriatus* or by *Buthotus judaicus* when it is used in early stages of envenomation. Similarly, Hershkovich *et al*[86], used antivenom in 96% of 53 cases in which it was indicated. The offending scorpion was identified as *Leiurus quinquestriatus*. Allergic reactions occurred in 4 cases, 2 of which developed symptoms of anaphylaxis. Fortunately, none of these cases were fatal.

3. Role of laboratory investigations

Detection of venom in biological fluids of the patient is very difficult, and is not a common practice. Radiolabeled antibodies or immunoenzymatic assays are being prepared by some laboratories for such purposes, and might find future application in toxicological analysis. In the initial steps of evaluating envenomation, standard blood tests are of very little value, however in complicated cases arterial blood gas, serum glucose, red blood cells and amylase levels can be helpful for clinical treatment, if known.

4. Examples of clinical treatment

The clinical cases reported here were taken from the records of the Red Cross in Leon, Guanajuato, Mexico.

Case 1

Male, 4 months of age. The baby was in his bed and suddenly began to cry. The mother picked him up and discovered a scorpion behind his head. Ten minutes later he was crying very loudly and had excessive salivation, dyspnea, hyperexcitability, nystagmus, bronchial secretions, tachycardia, respiratory failure, abdominal distension, meteorism, ataxic movements and profuse sweating. He was assessed medically 30 minutes after the sting. The pulse rate was 170, respiration 34, white cells 7.5×10^9/l with 5% eosinophils, glucose 142 (normal 60 - 100 mg/dl) (his last feed was 4 hours before). Treated with intravenous fluids and antivenom (only one vial) plus chlorpheniramine intravenously, symptoms disappeared after 3 hours.

Case 2

Female, 48 years. Patient stung twice on her hand. Within five minutes she felt intense pain, local hyperesthesia, stammer, photophobia, excessive salivation and sensation of hair in the throat. At the hospital her arterial pressure was 160/110, pulse rate 102, respiration 28, and there was ocular redness. Laboratory tests: Glucose 212 mg/dl (normal 60 - 100 mg/dl) with glucosuria. Antivenom was given by intravenous route 30 minutes after the sting. Recovery completed within two hours. The patient was sent to a diabetic clinic to investigate possible diabetes mellitus (later analysis indicated that she was not diabetic).

Case 3

Female, 8 years. Patient stung in her hand 45 minutes earlier. On admission to the hospital she had intense pain at the site of the sting, hyperaesthesia, pruritus, nasal pruritus, nasal secretion, salivary secretion, sensation of hair in the throat, cough, bronchorrhea, nausea and vomiting, abdominal pain, tachycardia and hyperexcitability. Treated with one vial of antivenom intravenously plus chlorpheniramine. Recovery was complete within three hours.

In all the above cases, the offending scorpion was positively identified as *Centruroides infamatus infamatus*.

5. Other issues in treatment

Other medical measurements are:

- Fluid and electrolyte monitoring (appropriate administration of intravenous fluid, when required);
- Support of cardiorespiratory functions by control of blood pressure, monitoring vital signs, resting in Fowler position;
- Aspiration of nasopharyngeal secretions;
- Correction of acid - base balance disturbances;
- Tetanus prophylaxis;
- Treatment of pain with non-central nervous system depressing analgesics, such as acetaminophen;
- Precautions, in order to avoid bronchial aspiration by the patient when vomiting.

Atropine, neostigmine and steroids have been used in the past for treatment of scorpion envenomation, but they have not been proved to be of important clinical value in *Centruroides* and *Tityus* cases. Experimental data showed that atropine might potentiate the hypertensive effect and increase the severity of the pulmonary oedema induced by scorpion toxin in the rat[43]. However, if there is severe bradycardia (secondary to sinus arrest or any kind of atrioventricular block), atropine should be given (0.05 - 0.1 mg/kg). Application of drugs such as barbiturates or narcotics might increase central respiratory depression in scorpion envenomation.

Acknowledgements: This work was supported in part by Howard Hughes Medical Institute (grant No.75191-527104), Universidad Nacional Autonoma de Mexico (DGAPA No. IN202689 and IN300991), and Consejo Nacional de Ciencia y Tecnologia (CONACyT grant No.0018-N9105) to L.D. Possani. The scholarship received by M. Dehesa-Davila from CONACyT is greatly acknowledged. Suggestions and reading this manuscript by Dr. Paul Fletcher Jr was appreciated.

VIII. REFERENCES

1. **HOFFMANN, C. C.,** Distribucion geografica de los alacranes peligrosos en la Republica Mexicana. *Bol. Inst. Higiene* (Mex) **2:**321-330, 1936.
2. **HOFFMANN, C. C., NIETO, D. R.,** Segunda contribucion al conocimiento de los alacranes mexicanos. *Anales Inst. Biologia,* **10:**83-92, 1939.
3. **KEEGAN, H.L.,** *Scorpions of medical importance.* University Press of Mississipi, Jackson, MI, , 1980, 140 pp.
4. **DIAZ NAJERA, A.,** Contribucion al conocimiento de los alacranes en Mexico. *Rev. Invest. Salud Publ. (Mex),* **30:**111-122, 1970.
5. **DIAZ NAJERA, A.,** Alacranes de Mexico. Identification de alacranes colectados en 235 lugares. *Rev. Inst. Salubr. Enferm. Trop.,* (Mex) **XXVI:**15-30, 1964.
6. **MAZZOTI, L., and BRAVO-BECHERELLE, M. A.,** Scorpionism in the Mexican Republic. In: *Venomous and Poisonous Animals and Noxious Plants of the Pacific Area,* Keegan, H.L. and McFarlane, W. V., Eds., Pergamon Press, London, 1963, 119.
7. **MONROY-VELASCO, J.,** Alacranes venenosos de Mexico. *Rev. Mex. Cien. Med. Biol.,* (Mex) **1:**1., 1961.
8. **DEHESA-DAVILA, M.,** Epidemiological characteristics of scorpion sting in Leon, Guanajuato, Mexico. *Toxicon,* **27:**281-286, 1989.
9. **POSSANI, L. D., CALDERON, E. S., OLAMENDI, T. P., DEHESA- DAVILA, M. and GURROLA, G. B.,** Proteccion contra el alacranismo. In: *Vacunas, Ciencia y Salud.* Escobar G. A., Valdespino G. J. L., Sepulveda A. J., Eds., Secretaria de Salud, Mexico D. F., 1992, chap 44.
10. **POSSANI, L.D.,** Structure of scorpion toxins. In: *Handbook of Natural Toxins.* Anthony T.Tu., Ed., Marcel Dekker, New York, 1984, 513-550.
11. **CARBONE, E., WANKE, E., PRESTIPINO, G., POSSANI, L.D. and MAELICKE A.,** Selective blockage of voltage dependent K^+ channels by a novel scorpion toxin. *Nature,* **296:**90-91, 1982.
12. **SITGES, M., POSSANI, L.D. and BAYON, A.,** Characterization of the actions of toxins II-9.2.2. and II-10 from the venom of the scorpion *Centruroides noxius* on transmitter release from mouse brain synaptosomes. *J. Neurochem.* **48:**1745-1752, 1987.

13. **ZAMUDIO, F., SAAVEDRA, R., MARTIN B. M., GURROLA-BRIONES, G., HERION, P. and POSSANI, L. D.,** Amino acid sequence and immunological characterization with monoclonal antibodies of two toxins from the venom of the scorpion *Centruroides noxius* Hoffmann. *Eur. J. Biochem.,* **204:**281-292, 1992.

14. **POSSANI, L.D., VALDIVIA, H. H., RAMIREZ, N. A., GURROLA B. G. and MARTIN M.B.,** K$^+$ channel blocking peptides isolated from the venom of scorpions. In: *Recent Advances in Toxinology Research* Eds. Gopalakrishnakone, P., Tan, C.K., Singapore Vol. 1 p. 39-58, 1992.

15. **RAMIREZ A. N., GURROLA G. B., VALDIVIA H. H. and POSSANI L. D.,** Binding affinities of Mexican scorpion toxins to brain synaptosomal membranes. *Proceedings 10th World Congress on Animal Plant and Microbial Toxins.* Abstract No. 301 pp 355, 1992.

16. **VALDIVIA H. H., FUENTES O., EL-HAYEK R., MORRISSETTE J., and CORONADO, R.,** Activation of the Ryanodine receptor Ca2+ release channel of sarcoplasmic reticulum by a novel scorpion venom. *J Biol. Chem.,* **266:**19135-19138, 1991.

17. **COSSIO, R., MARTIN, B.M., CORONAS, F.V., VALDIVIA, H., ALAGON, A.C. and POSSANI L.D.,** Isolation and characteristics of a phospholipase from the venom of the Mexican scorpion *Hadrurus concolorous. XIX Congress of the Mexican Biochemical Society, Sociedad Española de Bioquímica. VII PAABS Congress.* p. 82, 1992.

18. **MEVES, H., RUBLY, N. and WATT, D.D.,** Effect of toxins isolated from the venom of the scorpion *Centruroides sculpturatus* on the Na$^+$ currents of the node of Ranvier. *Pflügers Arch.,* **393:**59-62, 1982.

19. **MEVES, H., SIMARD, J.M. and WATT D.D.,** Biochemical and electrophysiological characteristics of toxins isolated from the venom of the scorpion *Centruroides sculpturatus. J. Physiol. (Paris),* **79:**185-191, 1984.

20. **MEVES H., SIMARD J.M., and WATT D.D.,** Interactions of scorpion toxins with the sodium channel. In: *Tetrodotoxin, saxitoxin and the molecular biology of the sodium channel.* Kao, C. Y. and Levinson, S.R., Eds., Annals New York Academy of Sciences Vol. 479 New York, 1986 pp 113-132.

21. **GIMENEZ-GALLEGO, G., NAVIA M.A., REUBEN J.P., KATZ G.M., KACZOROWSKI, G.J. and GARCIA M.L.,** Purification, sequence and model structure of charabdotoxin, a potent selective inhibitor of calcium-activated potassium channel. *Proceedings of the National Academy of Science* USA **85:**4814-21, 1988.

22. **MENEZ, A., BONTEMS, F., ROUMESTAND, C., GILQUIN, B. and TOMA, F.,** Structural basis for functional diversity of animal toxins. *Proceedings of the Royal Society of Edinburgh,* **99B (1/2):**83- 103, 1992.

23. **ZLOTKIN, E. F., MIRANDA, F. and ROCHAT, H.,** Chemistry and pharmacology of Buthinae scorpion venoms. In: *Arthropod Venoms,* Bettini, S., Ed., Springer-Verlag, Berlin, pp. 317-369, 1978.

24. **ISMAIL, M., and ABD-ELSALAM, A.,** Are the toxicological effects of scorpion envenomation related to tissue venom concentration?. *Toxicon,* **26:**233-256, 1988.

25. **ALAGON, A.C., GUZMAN, H.S., MARTIN, B.M., RAMIREZ, A. N., CARBONE, E. and POSSANI,, L.D.,** Isolation and characterization of two toxins from the Mexican scorpion *Centruroides limpidus limpidus* Karsh. *Comp. Biochem. Physiol.,* **89B:**153-161, 1988.

26. **DENT, M. A. R., POSSANI, L. D., RAMIREZ, G. A. and FLETCHER, P. L. Jr.,** Purification of two mammalian toxins from the venom of the Mexican scorpion *Centruroides noxius* Hoffmann. *Toxicon,* **18:**343-350, 1980.

27. **POSSANI, L. D., FLETCHER, P. L. JR., ALAGON, A. B. C., ALAGON, A. C. and JULIA, J.Z.,** Purification and characterization of a mammalian toxin from venom of the Mexican scorpion *Centruroides limpidus tecomanus* Hoffmann. *Toxicon,* **18:**175-183, 1980.

28. **CARBONE, E., PRESTIPINO, G., SPADAVECCHIA, L., FRANCIOLINI, F., and POSSANI L.D.,** Blocking of the squid axon K+ channel by noxiustoxin: a toxin from the venom of the scorpion *Centruroides noxius. Pflügers Arch.,* **408:**423-431, 1987.

29. **PRESTIPINO, G., VALDIVIA, H.H., LIEVANO, A., DARSZON, A., RAMIREZ A.N. and POSSANI, L.D.,** Purification and reconstitution of potassium channel proteins from squid axon membranes. *FEBS Letters* **250:**570-574, 1989.

30. **YATANI, A., KIRSH, G. E., POSSANI, L. D. and BROWN, A. M.,** Effects of two new world scorpion toxins on single channel and whole cell cardiac sodium channel. *Amer. J. Physiol.,* 254 (*Heart Circ. Physiol.*), **23:**H443-H451, 1988.

31. **KIRSH, G. E., SKATTEBOL, A., POSSANI, L. D. and BROWN, A. M.,** Modification of Na$^+$ Channel Gating by a scorpion toxin from *Tityus serrulatus. J. Gen. Physiol.,* **93:**67-83, 1989.

32. **EL-ASMAR, M. F., SOLIMAN, S. F., ISMAIL, M., OSMAN O.H.,** Glycemic effect of venom from the scorpion *Buthus minax* (L. Koch) *Toxicon,* **12:**249-251. 1974.

33. **MAZZOTTI, L. and BRAVO-BECHERELLE, M.A.,** Escorpionismo en la Republica Mexicana. *Rev. Inst. Salubr. Enfer. Trop. (Mex.),* **21:**3-19, 1961.

34. **DEL POZO, E.C., & GONZALEZ, J.Q.,** Efecto del veneno de alacran en el sistema respiratorio. *Rev. Inst. Salubr. Enfer. Trop. (Mex.),* **6:**77-84, 1945.

35. **FLORES-PEREZ, R.,** Sintomatologia y tratamiento de la picadura de alacran. *Rev. Inst. Enferm. Trop. (Mex.)*, **23:**175-179, 1963.
36. **LAGUNAS-FLORES, A. and ROJAS-MOLINA, N.,** Experiencia clinica en 147 niños con picadura de alacran en Acapulco, Guerrero, Mexico. *Rev. Med. IMSS* (Mex.) **21:**270-275, 1983.
37. **DEHESA-DAVILA, M.,** Avances en el tratamiento farmacologico de la picadura de alacran. *Rev. Salud Publica de Mexico* (Mex.) **28:**83-91, 1986.
38. **STAHNKE, H.L.,** The genus *Centruroides* (Buthidae) and its venom. In: *Arthropod Venoms*. Handbook of Experimental Pharmacology, Bettini S., Ed., Vol.48, Berlin, Springer-Verlag 277-307, 1978.
39. **GUERON, M., ADOLPH, R., GRUPP, I., GRUPP, O., GABEL, M. and FOWLER, N.O.,** Hemodynamic and myocardial consequences of scorpion venom. *Am. J. Cardiol.*, **45:**979-983, 1980.
40. **GUERON, M. and YAROM, R.,** Cardiovascular manifestations of severe scorpion sting. *Chest*, **57:**156-158, 1970.
41. **GUERON, M. and OVSYSHCHER I.,** Cardiovascular effects of scorpion venoms. In: *Handbook of Natural Toxins*, Ed. Tu, A., Vol. 2 New York, Marcel Dekker, pp 639-657, 1984.
42. **MOSS, J., KAZIC, T., HENRY, D. P. and KOPIN, I. J.,** Scorpion venom-induced discharge of catecholamines accompanied by hypertension. *Brain Research* **54:**381-385, 1973.
43. **FREIRE-MAIA, L., PINTO, G. I. and FRANCO, I.,** Mechanism of the cardiovascular effects produced by purified scorpion toxin in the rat. *J. Pharmac. Exp. Ther.*, **188:**207-213, 1974.
44. **FREIRE-MAIA, L. and CAMPOS, J.A.,** Pathophysiology and treatment of scorpion poisoning. In: *Natural Toxins*. Characterization, Pharmacology and Therapeutics. Pergamon Press. pp 139-159, 1989.
45. **DEL POZO, E.C., ANGUIANO, G.L. and GONZALEZ, J.Q.,** Efectos del veneno de alacran en el sistema vasomotor. *Rev. Inst. Enferm. Trop.*, (Mex.) **5:**227-239, 1944.
46. **FREIRE-MAIA, L., AZEVEDO, A. D., and LIMA, E. G.,** Pharmacological blockade of the cardiovascular and respiratory effects produced by Tityustoxin in the rat. In: *Animal, Plant and Microbial Toxins*. Ohsaka, A., Hayashi, K., and Sawai, Y., Eds., Vol.2, Plenum Press, New York, pp. 287-298, 1976.
47. **CANTOR, A., WANDERMAN, K. L., OVSYSHCHER, I. and GUERON, M.,** Parasympathomimetic action of scorpion venom on the cardiovascular system. *Israel J. Med. Sci.* **13:**908-912, 1977.
48. **GONZALEZ-ROMERO, S., GONZALEZ, H. J. A., GONZALEZ, R. A., FLORES, M. E. and MIJANGOS, V. G.,** Alteraciones electrocardiograficas en sujetos picados por alacran. *Arch. Inst. Cardiol. (Mex)*, **61:**15-20, 1991.
49. **DEL POZO, E.C.,** Farmacologia del veneno de *Centruroides* en Mexico. *Rev. Invest. Salud Publica, (Mex)* **28:**51-66, 1968.
50. **SOFER, S. and GUERON, M.,** Respiratory failure in children following envenomation by the scorpion *Leiurus quinquestriatus*: hemodynamic and neurological aspects. *Toxicon,* **26:**931-939, 1988.
51. **WATT, D.D. and SIMARD, J.M.,** Neurotoxic proteins in scorpion venom. *J. Toxicol.*, 3 **(2 and 3):**181-221, 1984.
52. **DINIZ, C. R., PIMENTA, A. F., COUTINHO-NETTO, S., POMPOLO, M. V., GOMEZ and BOHM.,** Effect of scorpion venom from *Tityus serrulatus* (Tityustoxin) on the acetylcholine release and fine structure of the nerve terminals. *Experientia (Basel),* **30:**1304- 1305, 1974.
53. **DEL POZO, E.C. and ANGUIANO, L.G.,** Efecto del veneno de alacran en musculo estriado. *Rev. Inst. Salubr. Enferm. Trop. (Mex.)*, **8:**231-237, 1947.
54. **VITAL BRAZIL, O., NEDER, A. C. and CORRADO, A. P.,** Effects of mechanism of action of *Tityus serrulatus* venom on skeletal muscle. *Pharmacol. Res. Comm.*, **5:**137-150, 1973.
55. **GONZAGA, H. M. S., ALZAMORA, J.R., CUNHA-MELO, J.R. and FREIRE-MAIA, L.,** Gastric secretion induced by scorpion toxin. *Toxicon*, **17:**316-318, 1979.
56. **CUNHA-MELO, J.R., GONZAGA, H. M. S. ALZAMORA, F. and FREIRE- MAIA, L.,** Effects of purified scorpion toxin (tityustoxin) on gastric secretion in the rat. *Toxicon*, **21:**843-848, 1983.
57. **CAMPOS, J. A., SILVA, O. A., LOPEZ, M. and FREIRE-MAIA, L.,** Signs, symptoms and treatment of severe scorpion sting in children. *Toxicon*, **17:** (suppl. 1), 19, 1979.
58. **CAMPOS, J. A., SILVA, O. S, LOPEZ, M. and FREIRE-MAIA, L.** Signs, symptoms and treatment of severe scorpion poisoning in children. In: *Natural Toxins*, Eaker, D. and Wadstrom, T. Eds. Oxford, Pergamon Press, p. 61, 1980.
59. **BARTHOLOMEW, C.,** Acute scorpion pancreatitis in Trinidad. *Br. Med. J.* March; 666-668, 1970.
60. **BARTHOLOMEW, C., McGEENY, K. F., MURPHY, J.J., FITZGERALD, O. and SANKARAN, H.,** Experimental studies on the aetiology of acute scorpion pancreatitis. *Br. J. Surg.*, **63:**807-810, 1976.
61. **SOFER, S., SHALEV, H., WEIZMAN, Z., SHAHAK, E., GUERON, M.** Acute pancreatitis in children following envenomation by the yellow scorpion *Leiurus quinquestriatus*. *Toxicon*, **29:**125-128, 1991.
62. **POSSANI, L.D., MARTIN, B. M., FLETCHER, M. D. and FLETCHER, P. L.,** Discharge effect on pancreatic exocrine secretion produced by toxins purified from *Tityus serrulatus* scorpion venom. *J. Biol. Chem.*, **266:**3178-3185, 1991.
63. **GALLAGHER, S., SANKARAN, H. and WILLIAMS, J. A.,** Mechanism of scorpion toxin-induced enzyme secretion in rat pancreas. *Gastroenterology,* **80:**970-974, 1981.

64. **FLETCHER, P. L. Jr., FLETCHER, M. D. and POSSANI, L. D.,** Characteristics of pancreatic exocrine secretion produced by venom from the Brazilian scorpion, *Tityus serrulatus. Eur. J. Cell Biology,* **58:**259-270, 1992.

65. **ANGUIANO, G., BEYER, C. and ALCARAZ, M.,** Mecanismo fisiologico de la hiperglicemia causada por veneno de alacran. *Bol. Inst.Est. Med. Biol. (Mex.),* 14:93-101, 1956.

66. **XAVIER, M. S., CARDINI, J. F., MACHADO, R. P. and ALZAMORA, F.,** Effect of phentolamine on the renal action of norepinephrine and scorpion venom. *Brazilian J. Med. Biol. Res.,* **19:**536A, 1986.

67. **LONGNECKER, G.L. and LONGNECKER, Jr. H.E.,** *Centruroides sculpturatus* venom and platelet reactivity: Possible role in scorpion venom-induced defibrination syndrome. *Toxicon* **19:**153-157, 1981.

68. **VELASCO-CASTREJON, O.,** Choque anafilactico por picadura de alacran. *Rev. Med. Univ. Aut. Guadal. (Mex.),* 5:74-77, 1971.

69. **JOHNSON, D. G., HENRY, D. P., MOSS, J. and WILLIAMS, R. H.,** Inhibition of insulin release by scorpion toxin in rat pancreatic islets. *Diabetes,* 25:645-649, 1976.

70. **JOHNSON, D. G. and ENSINCK, J.,** Stimulation of glucagon secretion by scorpion toxin in the perfused rat pancreas. *Diabetes,* 25:654-649, 1976.

71. **MAREI, Z.A. and S.A. IBRAHIM.,** Stimulation of rat uterus by venom from the scorpion *L. quinquestriatus. Toxicon,* **17:** 251- 258, 1979.

72. **MAZZOTI, L., MARTINEZ PALACIOS, A. and RAMIREZ J.,** Ensayo experimental sobre la accion del dieldrin en la especie *Centruroides limpidus. Rev. Inst. Salubr. Enf. Trop. (Mex),* 22:179-182, 1962.

73. **POSSANI, L.D., FERNANDEZ DE CASTRO, J. and JULIA, J.Z.,** Detoxification with glutaraldehyde of purified scorpion (*Centruroides noxius* Hoffmann) venom. *Toxicon,* **19:**323-329, 1981.

74. **DELORI, P., VAN RIETSCHOTEN, J. and ROCHAT H.,** Scorpion venoms and neurotoxins: An inmunological study. *Toxicon,* **19:**393-407, 1981.

75. **EL-AYEB, M. and DELORI, P.,** Immunology and Immunochemistry of scorpion neurotoxins. In: *Insect poisons, allergens and other invertebrate venoms.* Handbook of Natural Toxins. Ed. Tu, A., chap 18 pp 607-638, 1984.

76. **HENEINE, L.G.D., CARDOSO, U.N., DANIEL, S.P. and HENEINE I.F.,** Detoxification of the T2 fraction from a scorpion (*Tityus serrulatus,* Lutz and Mello) venom by iodination and some immunogenic properties of the derivatives. *Toxicon,* 24:855-894, 1986.

77. **POSSANI, L. D., GURROLA, G. B., PORTUGAL T. O., ZAMUDIO F. Z., VACA, L. D., CALDERON E. S. A., and KIRSCH, G.E.** Scorpion toxins: A model for peptide synthesis of new drugs. In: *Proceedings of the first Brazilian Congress on proteins.* Ed. Benedito Oliveira & Valdemiro Sgarbieri. Unicamp pp 352-367, 1990.

78. **CALDERON-ARANDA, E. S., HOZBOR, D. and POSSANI, L. D.** Neutralizing capacity of murine sera induced by different antigens of scorpion venom. *Toxicon,* 1993.

79. **BOUGIS P.E., ROCHET H. and SMITH L.A.,** Precursors of *Androctunus australis* scorpion neurotoxins. *J. Biol. Chem.,* **264:**19259- 19265, 1989.

80. **GUREVITZ M., URBACH D., ZLOTIKIN E., AND ZILOBERBERG N.,** Nucleotide sequence and structure analysis of a cDNA encoding an alpha insect toxin from the scorpion *Leiurus quinquestriatus* hebraeus. *Toxicon* 29:1270-1272, 1991.

81. **ZLOTKIN, E.F., EITAN M., BINDOKAS V.P., ADAMS M.E., MOYER M., BURKHART W. and FOWLER E.,** Functional duality and structural uniqueness of depressant insect-selective neurotoxins. *Biochemistry* 30:4824-21, 1991.

82. **BECERRIL B., VAZQUEZ A., GARCIA C., CORONA M., BOLIVAR F. and POSSANI L.D.,** Cloning and characterization of cDNAs that code for Na^+ channel blocking toxins of the scorpion *Centruroides noxius* Hoffmann. *Gene* 1993.

83. **THEAKSTON R. D. G. and WARRELL D.A.,** Antivenoms: A list of hyperimmune sera currently available for the treatment of envenomation by bites and sting. *Toxicon* 29:1419-1470, 1991.

84. **GATEAU T., BLOOM, M. and CLARCK, R.,** Action of specific *Centruroides sculpturatus* antivenom in the treatment of scorpion sting. A clinical review of 151 cases. In: *Recent Advances in Toxinology Research.* Eds. Gopalakrishnakone, P. and Tan, C.K., University of Singapore Press, Vol. 2, 12-24., 1992,

85. **GOYFFON, M., VACHON, M. and BROGLIO N.,** Epidemiological and clinical characteristics of the scorpion envenomation in Tunisia. *Toxicon,* **20:**337-344, 1982.

86. **HERSHKOVICH, Y., ELITSUR, Y., MARGOLIS, C. Z., BARAK, N., SOFER, S. and MOSES, S. W.,** Criteria map audit of scorpion envenomation in the Negev, Israel. *Toxicon,* **23:**845-854, 1985.

Chapter 19

BIOLOGY AND DISTRIBUTION OF SPIDERS OF MEDICAL IMPORTANCE

Sylvia M. Lucas and Jürg Meier

TABLE OF CONTENTS

I. INTRODUCTION

The number of described species of spiders is very high, over 30,000, and in principle, with the exception of a few groups (Uloboridae and Holoarchaeidae) which have no venom glands, all spiders must be considered as venomous. However, the World Health Organization[1] listed only four genera as responsible for severe human poisoning: *Latrodectus, Loxosceles* and *Phoneutria* (infraorder Araneomorphae) and *Atrax* (infraorder Mygalomorphae). A number of cases of spiderbites are described in the literature, involving different species. Maretic and Lebez[2] discussed the problem of the bites of *Lycosa tarentula*, considered for a long time to cause a necrosis of human skin. Levi and Spielman[3] related five probable cases of poisoning by *Chiracanthium mildei*, a spider living inside houses in the vicinity of Boston, U.S.

Maretic[4] believed that a number of spider species, apart from the major genera noted above, can present a real danger to human beings. Ori[5] related 10 spider accidents in Japan between 1954 -1974, only one caused by the dangerous species *Latrodectus hasselti*, the other cases involving genera such as *Chiracanthium* and *Theridion*, which in general are not considered of medical importance.

Russell and Gertsch[6], based on their own experience, cited that from approximately 600 suspected spider bites in the United States, 80% have been caused by arthropods other than spiders or by other diseases.

Schmidt[7] gave a historical review of spiderbites in the world since ancient times and concluded that only 0.1% of the described species are dangerous for human beings. Wong et al.[8] listed between 50 to 60 species in the United States which have been implicated in medically significant accidents in human beings, covering 24 genera, 4 of them not native but "imported " into the country accidentally.

Ori[9], following the classification of Yaginuma, listed more than 100 species including notorious spiders and species of medical importance, but also some dubiously venomous spiders such as *Grammostola mollicoma* and other *Mygalomorph* spiders.

Maretic[10] noted that a spider may not necessarily be venomous for human beings for a variety of reasons:

- the venom does not contain toxic fractions which affect humans;
- the quantity of venom which the spider injects is insufficient to cause envenoming in humans;
- the chelicerae are not strong enough to penetrate human skin;
- the likelihood of contact with humans, resulting in bites, is very low.

Ribeiro et al.[11] investigated 515 cases involving wolf spider bites (*Scaptocosa raptoria*, Lycosidae) registered at the Hospital Vital Brazil, São Paulo, Brazil, and demonstrated that this spider does not present an active venom for human beings.

In this chapter we will only discuss the notoriously dangerous species of the genera *Latrodectus, Loxosceles, Phoneutria* (infraorder Araneomorphae) and *Atrax/Hadronyche* (infraorder Mygalomorphae) which are responsible for severe envenoming in humans, often requiring antivenom treatment.

II. SYSTEMATIC POSITION

Spiders are Arthropoda of the class Arachnida and constitute the order Araneae or Araneida.

Several classifications of this order are proposed:

- According to the vertical or horizontal position of the chelicerae:
  Order Araneae (Araneida)
  suborder Mesothelae
  suborder Labidognatha (Araneae Verae)
  suborder Orthognatha (Mygalomorphae)

- According to the position of the spinnerets:
  Order Araneae (Araneida)
  suborder Mesothelae
  suborder Opisthothelae
      infraorder Mygalomorphae (tarantulas)
      infraorder Araneomorphae (true spiders)

III. MORPHOLOGY

The body of the spider consists of a prosoma (cephalothorax) and an opisthosoma (abdomen); they are connected together by a narrow stalk, the petiolus or pedicel. The cephalothorax is protected dorsally by a hard plate, the carapace, and ventrally by the sternum, labium and coxae of the legs. The eyes are situated on the cephalothorax, sometimes grouped upon a tubercle or disposed in rows. The cephalothorax can also present a thoraxic groove and radial furrows; sometimes it is possible to distinguish a cephalic and a thoracic region. The chelicerae are situated in front of the cephalothorax or below.

The two venom glands are situated partly in the cephalothorax and partly in the chelicerae, with the exception of the Mygalomorph spiders where they are contained wholly in the chelicerae. The glands consist of three principal parts: a muscular coat, a secreting layer and the duct of the gland. Suomalainen[12] studied the structure of the venom gland in several species of 16 different spider families and concluded that the structure is fairly uniform in all species. The greatest differences are found in the secretory part of the gland: a syncytium consisting of star-shaped cells with very long branches. Secretion takes place from the branches into the spaces between the cells. Järlsfors et al.[13] studied the innervation of the venom-secreting cells in the black-widow spider (*L. mactans*), and observed that the glandular epithelium is also innervated and probably this nervous supply stimulates or regulates the synthesis of the venom.

All the limbs articulate on the cephalothorax; the first pair are the chelicerae, with a basal segment and a claw. Near the end of these is the opening of the venom duct; the second pair are the pedipalps, with six segments, which in adult males are the copulatory organs; the other four limbs are the legs, each with seven segments.

The abdomen is commonly sac-like, non-segmented, with the exception of the spiders of the infraorder Mesothelae. On the ventral side of the abdomen are found the epigastric furrow, with the opening of the reproductive organs, and also the openings of the lungs. The spinnerets, normally six, responsible for the emission of silk, are situated at the end of the abdomen and just behind them is the anus.

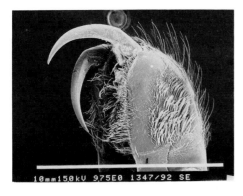

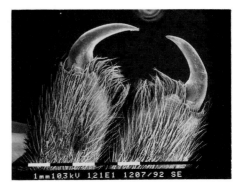

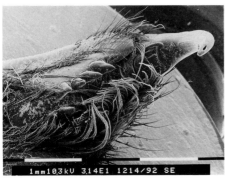

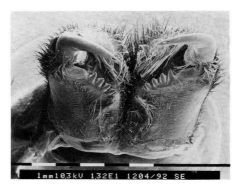

Figure 1a. Fangs and chelicerae of a mygalomorph spider.

Figure 1b. Fangs and chelicerae of an aranaeomorph spider

IV. ARANEOMORPH SPIDERS

A. THE SPIDERS OF THE GENUS *Phoneutria* (PERTY, 1833) (CTENIDAE)

Although the genus *Phoneutria* was described by Perty in 1833[14], the species were included for many years in the genus *Ctenus* Walckenaer, 1837, and only in 1936 Mello Leitåo[15] reestablished the former designation.

The genus is characterized by: (i) the disposition of the eyes in three rows: the first nearer to the edge of the chelicerae with two eyes, the second with four, and the third with two; (ii) by the presence of a dense scopulae on the inner side of the palpal segments and (iii) by the presence of five pairs of spines on the ventral side of the first and second tibia.

The spiders are known by the popular name: "banana spiders".

Measurements: adults reach a total body length of 3.5 cm and have a leg span up to 15 cm.

1. Coloration and general aspect

The description of the color is based on the species *P. nigriventer* (Keyserling, 1891). The body is covered with short, adherent hairs, grayish to brownish gray, and the chelicerae are covered with red hair on the basal segment. The dorsal side of the abdomen shows a bright design of paired spots, forming a longitudinal band and oblique lateral rows, also of smaller spots, but more or less discernible. The ventral side of the abdomen is black in females and orange in males. The legs show numerous spines and white spots.

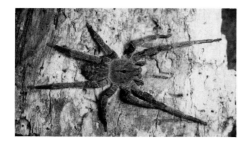 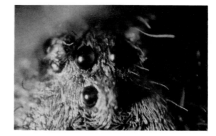

Figure 2a. Banana spider, *Phoneutria nigriventer.*   **Figure 2b**. Eye structure of Banana spider, *Phoneutria nigriventer.*

2. Habitat

The habitat of *P. nigriventer* and *P. keyserlingi*, occurring mostly in the State of Sǎo Paulo, Brazil, is well known. The specimens are frequently found near human dwellings, where they find shelter and abundant food (insects such as cockroaches and crickets). They live beneath fallen trees, within crevices of ravines, in heaped up wood, under building refuse, in banana plants and fruits, in palm trees and bromeliads. They display nocturnal and erratic habits, hunting actively, dominating their prey with the effectiveness of their venom and they do not make webs. They "invade" houses and nearby buildings, mainly during the mating season: the months of March and April in the southeast of Brazil. During daytime they hide in dark places such as shoes, clothes, etc.

3. Biology

Bücherl[16] and Tretzel[17] described the biology of *P. nigriventer* and *P. keyserlingi*, and Simo and Bardler[18] the postembryonic development of *P. keyserlingi*. From hatching to adulthood takes about three years. After mating, the female makes one to four egg-sacs, producing up to 3,000 eggs. The young molt 8 to 10 times in the first year, 4 to 7 times in the second and 2 to 3 times in the third year. After mating they can continue to live for several months. The sex ratio between females and males may be, according to Bücherl[19], from 1 to 5. Tretzel mentioned a longevity for males of one and a half years, for females of two and a half years. Bücherl cited four to five years for females. In the laboratory, specimens used for venom extraction in the Instituto Butantan, Sǎo Paulo, Brazil, survive only several months.

Very little is known about the species *P. reidyi* and *P. fera*, of the Amazonas region, collected by the technical staff of the Instituto Butantan in the region of Tucurui and Balbina (Para and Amazonas, Brazil), before the closing of the floodgates of the hydroelectric power stations. During faunal rescue a great quantity of these spiders was found between dry leaves of coconut palms, semi-submerged, where the yellowish color mingled with the substratum, thus causing unexpected accidents.

4. Venom quantities

Bücherl[20] noted that the dried venom, obtained from a single spider (*P. fera*), varies widely and cited: during winter a maximum of 0.8 to 1.8 mg and a minimum of 0 to 0.08 mg was collected; at warm temperatures a maximum of 0.5 to 2.5 and a minimum of 0 to 0.6 mg. In the Arthropod Laboratory at the Instituto Butantan using electrical stimulation between 0.5 to 0.9 mg is obtained from *P. nigriventer*.

5. Venom activities

Kaiser[21] described the presence of a proteolytic enzyme in the venom of *P. nigriventer*. This was later confirmed by Kaiser and Raab[22]. From the venom of the same species Diniz[23] isolated two peptides which elicit the contraction of the guinea-pig ileum. The same author detected the presence of L-histamine and 5-hydroxy-tryptamine. Fisher and Bohm[24] demonstrated that the venom also contains free glutamic acid, aspartic acid and lysine. Schenberg and Pereira Lima[25] investigated the physiological aspects such as local pain, sneezing, lacrimation, hypersalivation, erection, hypotensive response, on various vertebrates (dogs, rats, guinea pigs, rabbits). Entwistle et al.[26] submitted the venom to gel filtration and separated 11 fractions which were tested for their neurophysiological activity in invertebrates (locust); from one of these fractions they isolated a pure polypeptide with a molecular weight between 5500 and 5900 and determined its amino acid composition. Cicarelli et al.[27] studied the toxicity of the venom and its LD_{50} in mice. Fontana and Vital Brazil[28] investigated its mode of action on muscle contraction in rats and found that it activates the sodium channel in muscle and nerve cell membranes. Rezende et al.[29] isolated three neurotoxic fractions, lethal for mice. These toxins have molecular weights between 5000 and 9000. They also described the presence of a non-neurotoxic peptide, active on the smooth muscle.

6. List and distribution of species

The papers of Bücherl[30,31], Schmidt[32], Schiapelli and Gerschman de Pikelin[33] and von Eickstedt[34,35] contributed to the elucidation of the systematics as well as to the better knowledge of the geographical distribution of the species.

P. fera Perty, 1833
distribution: Amazonas, Ecuador, Peru and Guyanas

P. keyserlingi (Pickard Cambridge, 1897)
distribution: Espirito Santo, Rio de Janeiro, São Paulo, Parana, Santa Catarina and Rio Grande do Sul, Brazil

P. nigriventer (Keyserling, 1891)
distribution: São Paulo, Minas Gerais, Mato Grosso do Sul, Rio de Janeiro, Parana, Santa Catarina and Rio Grande do Sul, Brazil

P. reidyi (Pickard Cambridge, 1897)
distribution: Amapa, Amazonas, Distrito Federal, Mato Grosso, Roraima and Rondonia, Brazil

P. colombiana Schmidt, 1956
distribution: Colombia

P. boliviensis (Cambridge, 1897)
distribution: Costa Rica to Bolivia

7. Epidemiology

The spiders are aggressive, trying to bite, assuming a characteristic position. The accidents involving spiders of the genus *Phoneutria* occur mainly in Central and South America. Some accidents are related in other regions, involving spiders which are transported in loads. The Brazilian Health Ministry presented the first data about spiderbites in Brazil in 1991[36]. From January 1988 to December 1989 a total of 4,836 spiderbites were reported in the country. The species from the genus *Phoneutria* was responsible for 1,857 accidents, occurring in the southeast and south. Trejos et al.[37] described some accidents involving spiders of the genus *Phoneutria* in Costa Rica. Valerio[38] confirmed the presence of *P. boliviensis* in several localities of Costa Rica. Schmidt[39] gave some data about spiderbites in Germany due to the presence of spiders of the genus *Phoneutria* in bananas imported from Guatemala, Ecuador, Colombia and Brazil. Similar accidents are reported in Argentina and Uruguay. Personal communication from Penaranda, in 1992, gives notice of accidents caused by *Phoneutria* in La Paz, Bolivia.

B. THE SPIDERS OF THE GENUS *Latrodectus* WALCKENAER 1805 (THERIDIIDAE)

The genus is characterized by: (i) the disposition of the eyes in two rows, the lateral separated from each other; (ii) tarsus IV with a comb of bristles on the ventral side; (iii) the first leg is usually longer than the fourth; (iv) the abdomen of the female is globe like, showing on the ventral side usually an hourglass design; (v) males are much smaller than females.

The different species are known as black-widow spiders, and also by various local names: Karakurt in the Russian Steppes, Malmignatto in Italy, Red back spider in Australia, Katypo in New Zealand, Arana del Lino, del Trigo in Argentina and Uruguay, Pallu or Guina in Chile, Casampulga in Guatemala, Arana Capulina in Mexico and Central America, Button Spider in South Africa, Menavodi in Madagascar.

Measurements: females: total length between 8-13 mm; males: total length 3 mm.

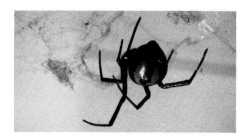
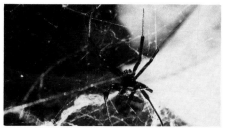

Figure 3a. South American widow spider, *Latrodectus curacavensis.*

Figure 3b. South American widow spider in web structure.

1. Coloration and general aspect

L. geometricus varies from pale yellow white to almost jet black[40]. Lamoral[41] confirmed this statement and observed that most of the specimens he studied in South Africa were found to match the ground coloration of their body to that of their habitat. Spiders cannot alter the ground coloration of their body once they have reached maturity. Shulov[42] described the young spiderlings of *L. tredecimguttatus* from Israel as black with light spots which gradually change in color from brownish-yellow to red. *L. pallidus* in adult females present a uniform pearly-white, or light brown-yellow dorsal surface, with six small brownish-black punctuations. The other species, *L. revivensis* with regard to coloration resembles in certain aspects *L. tredecimguttatus* and sometimes resembles *L. pallidus*, with regards to the coloration.

McCrone and Levi[43] described the female of *L. curacaviensis* with a black abdomen with white marks, but the authors examined preserved specimens, and probably the marks are red.

L. mactans is generally described as black with red spots and a red hourglass design on the ventral surface of the abdomen, sometimes more distinct and sometimes less. Even totally black specimens are described.

2. Habitat

The species present a high diversity of habitats; some are very common near the human dwellings. They make an irregular web of very tough silk in protected places as under stones, in stumps, building materials. In Israel *L. tredecimguttatus* make their web on the ground, *L. revivensis* at the height of 35 to 40 cm above the soil and *L. pallidus* at a height of 40 to 60 cm[42]. *L. curacaviensis* at the coast of Rio de Janeiro (Brazil) make their webs of about 2 square meters in the branches of the *Ipomoea* arbusts[44]. At a beach, within an extension of 3 km., Bucherl collected 1,400 spiders and observed that the specimens are more common in the month of May and June[44]. Probably, they are carried by the wind. He also found specimens near the houses, inside old shoes, tin cans, old cameras, and among fallen leaves of *Ficus* trees. Mowsznicz[45] found in Uruguay three or four adult females within one square meter and the spiders make their webs in agricultural areas and rocky fields. He observed that in some years the spider population was very high. Lamoral[41] observed the nest and web structure of *L. geometricus* and *L. mactans* in South Africa and noted differences between the two. He discussed the general belief that all Theridiidae webs are disorganized and structureless. MacKay[46] observed that two different species in South Africa, *L. geometricus* and *L. rhodensiensis*, are found in the same habitat, often living at a distance of a meter from each other. Several investigators observed that in some years the population of spiders of the genus *Latrodectus* increase, probably due to climatic conditions and because of the decrease of parasites and predators and other factors, giving origin to an epidemic Latrodectism.

3. Biology

Several researchers studied the biology of the different species of black-widow[41,47-51]. McCrone and Levi[43] described the courtship and copulatory behavior of *L. bishopi* in laboratory and gave some data about the development of this species and *L. mactans*, both from the *L. curacaviensis* group. *L. mactans* females required from 5 to 8 molts for maturity and *L. variolus* females 7 to 8. In both species the sex ratio is 1:1. Abalos and Baez[52] used about 170,000 specimens of *Latrodectus* for the production of antivenom. They collected these specimens in the nature, in different localities of Argentine. They belong to the species *L. geometricus* and to the *L. curacaviensis* of the *L. mactans* group. They reared also spiders in laboratory and observed that the males of the *L. curacaviensis* group undergo four ecdyses until the adult stage, females eight. The first egg-sac develops seven days after copulation. In captivity they observed up to eight egg-sacs in 120 days and the number of eggs ranged between 83 to 326. The mother spider looks after the egg-sacs and watches over them constantly, but neglects completely the emerged spiderlings. The data observed for the spiders of the group *L. mactans* are very similar, but in this case the mother shows maternal habits toward her brood and the spiderlings are fed with prey captured by her. Kaston[53] made a comparative study of the biology of the American black widow spider: *L. mactans*, *L. variolus* and *L. hesperus*. He observed that even under uniform environmental conditions, there was a considerable variation with respect to the number of molts, the interval between molts, and the length of time it took for the spider to mature. *L. hesperus* and *L. variolus* live longer than *L. mactans*, and it was observed that *L. mactans* have a maximum longevity of 127 and 849 days, respectively, males and females; *L.hesperus* 196 and 952 and *L. variolus* 155 and 822 days.

4. Venom quantities

Bücherl[19] cited an average of 0.60 mg of dried venom obtained by electrical stimulation for the species: *L. curacaviensis* and *L. mactans*.

5. Venom activities

Probably due to the seriousness of the human accidents and the worldwide occurrence of the spiders of the genus *Latrodectus*, the venoms, mainly from the species *L. tredecimguttatus* of the Mediterranean Region and *L. mactans* from North America, have been studied by several investigators. Grasso[54] studied the extract of the venom apparatus of *L. tredecimguttatus* and isolated and purified a neurotoxin with an amino acid composition consisting of 1219 residues per 130,000 molecular weight molecule. Frontali et al.[55] working with the venom of the same species isolated a pure fraction called B 5. Tzeng and Siekevitz[56] first called this fraction B 5 α-latrotoxin. This toxin is an active neurotoxin which affects the transmitter release from nerve endings of the vertebrates. Fedorova and Magazanik[57] isolated from the α-latrotoxin a homogeneous protein of mol. wt. 120 KDa , labelled α-latroinsectotoxin which acts on presynaptic nerve endings of insects preparations. Akhunov et al.[58] succeeded in showing that the venom of *L. tredecimguttatus* contains peptides possessing bradykinin potentiating activity. Grishin[59] purified seven high mol. wt neurotoxins from the venom of *L. tredecimguttatus*. These protein neurotoxins induce a massive release of the neurotransmitter from affected nerve endings, being specific either for the insect (latroinsectotoxin), or for the vertebrate (α-latrotoxin), or for the crustacean (α latrocrustatoxin). Kiyatkin et al.[60] presented the structure of a low molecular weight protein copurified from the α latrotoxin.

6. List and distribution of species

The genus has a worldwide distribution and several different species occur between the latitudes of 50^0 North and 45^0 South. After the last revision of Levi[61] based mainly on morphological characters, like the structure of the male palpal organs, female genitalia and color, the number of species was reduced to six. This was contested by several investigators who used biological, immunological and other characters for the species identification. As Martindale and Newlands[62] concluded, the *Latrodectus* taxonomy will require a detailed field and laboratory study of each species. Levi[63] also concluded that the taxonomy of the genus is far more complex than was previously thought and that it is time for a new revision using new characters and more sophisticated methods.

Rower[64] listed 29 species and subspecies reduced by Levi[61] to six; Brignoli[65] and Platnick[66] listed 15 species:

L. antheratus (Badcock, 1932)
Paraguay, Argentina

L. corallinus Abalos, 1980
Argentina

L. curacaviensis (Muller, 1776)
Curaçao

L. dahli Levi, 1959
Socotra, Israel and former U.S.S.R.

L. diaguitia Carcavallo, 1959
Argentina

L. geometricus C. L. Koch, 1841
Cosmopolitan

L. hesperus Chamberlin and Ivie, 1935
North America, Israel

L. mactans (Fabricius, 1775)
North America

L. mirabilis (Holmberg, 1876)
Argentina

L. pallidus Cambridge, 1872
Libya to former U.S.S.R.

L. quartus Abalos, 1980
Argentina

L. revivensis Shulov, 1948
Israel

L. rhodesiensis Mackay, 1972
South Africa

L. tredecimguttatus (Rossi, 1790)
Mediterranean Region

L. variegatus Nicolet, 1849
Chile, Argentina

7. Epidemiology

According to the geographical distribution of the genus with species occurring in warm zones of the different continents, a high number of accidents are related. Jelinek et al.[67] stated that in Fremantle, Western Australia, between 1982 and 1987, 150 patients were admitted to their hospital with definite red-back spiderbite (*Latrodectus*), of whom 32 (21%) received antivenom. Also these authors estimated that the annual number of *Latrodectus* spiderbites in Australia lies between 830 and 1,950 cases. Maretic and Gonzales-Lorenzo[68] reported 180 cases of Latrodectism proceeding from the rural environment in Spain and Yugoslavia. They discussed the increase of spiderbites as a direct consequence of the increase of spiders, influenced by ecological factors, in some years.

Maretic and Habermehl[69] made a distinction between the " urban Latrodectism ", in the United States, for example, and the " rural Latrodectism " in rural zones of Europe. In urban areas accidents happen occasionally, but in the rural areas the number of accidents is so high that it assumes epidemic characteristics. Schenone and Correa[70] studied the Latrodectism in Chile. *L. mactans* is found in rural areas in thirteen regions in Chile. Most of the accidents occur during day time, particularly during agricultural work. The sex distribution of the cases is 84.4% and 15.6% for male and female, respectively. Grisolia et al.[71] related their experience with 281 *Latrodectus* spiderbites in Buenos Aires, Argentina over a period of two years (1979 - 1980) and related that 80% of the bitten persons are workers from the rural zones. An increase of accidents was noted from December to March. Penaranda (peronal. communication) related that in Bolivia, Department of Tarija, the accidents with *L. mactans* are frequent and some deaths occurred. In South Africa, Zumpt[72] made some references to spiderbites, involving two different *Latrodectus* species. Newlands[73] mentioned *L. mactans* and *L. geometricus* as medically important species in South Africa. In Brazil accidents with spiders of the genus *Latrodectus* are mentioned by Schwab Rodrigues et al.[74] in the State of Bahia, and by Machado[75] in the State of Rio de Janeiro.

C. THE SPIDERS OF THE GENUS *Loxosceles* HEINECKEN AND LOWE, 1835 (LOXOSCELIDAE)

The genus is characterized by the presence of six pearly-white eyes disposed in three diads, the chelicerae are fused together at their base, the labium is fused with the sternum, the cephalothorax is somewhat depressed with a conspicuous longitudinal thoracic furrow and the legs are slender and long. The different species are known by regional names as: violin spiders or brown spiders (U.S.), Arana de los rincones (Chile), arana homicida (Argentine) and aranha marrom (Brazil).

Measurements: females: 8 to 15 mm; males slightly smaller.

1. Coloration and general aspect

The species are brown, some are very dark, others pale-yellowish; several present a yellowish to orange design on the carapace. Gertsch[76,77] gave a detailed description of the coloration, measurements and general aspect of the different species described for North, Central and South America, and West Indies.

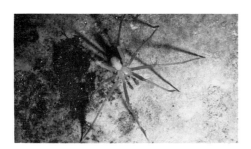

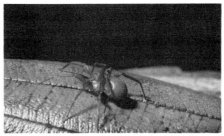

Figure 4a. Male South American recluse spider, *Loxosceles gaucho.*

Figure 4b. Female South American recluse spider, *Loxosceles gaucho.*

2. Habitat

The species are of nocturnal activity; they make irregular white webs forming a sheet over surfaces, under stones, in holes in the ground, under the bark of trees, and also inside human dwellings or in the vicinity. Because of their sedentary habits and because they avoid light, they are seldom seen, but they can be found in almost any undisturbed place. The flattened body permits squeezing into narrow cracks. As cited by Gertsch[77] human beings provide ideal habitats for the spiders of this genus in and around the buildings. They move into facilities like barns, chicken coops, garages, storage sheds and into human houses, where they hide in crevices of the walls, behind furniture and other places. These specimens were sometimes "transported" inattentively by man. Bücherl[78] related that he collected over 8,000 specimens every year for venom extraction and antivenom production. He found those specimens in the city of São Paulo, Brazil, in places like old factories and inside human dwellings and the vicinity. Lowrie[79] observed *L. laeta* in the laboratory and concluded that this species has the ability to withstand long periods without water or food, and probably this fact can explain the wide dispersal of this species. Huhta[80] found *L. laeta* in the buildings of the University of Helsinki, and mainly during the winter months of 1970-1971 the spider became more numerous. A systematic search revealed that the whole ground floor of the bulding was infested. In 1964, Levi and Spielman[81] related an identical case: the spider had produced a dense population inside the Cambridge Museum. Along the coast region of Peru, Delgado[82] made some ecological observations involving the species *L. rufipes*. He found these spiders mainly under big stones, in precolombianic ruins, where they always chose dry places. The enemies of the spiders are wasps and ants, but also the human being by destroying their natural habitat.

3. Biology

Hite et al.[83] studied the biology of *L. reclusa* in the laboratory. From the collected spiders they obtained 146 egg sacs. Five females produced a maximum of five egg-sacs; 43 produced more than one. The time from oviposition to the emergence of the spiderlings was 25 to 39 days. A maximum of 300 eggs was laid by one female and the maximum number of spiders was 158. The number of eight instars was observed. Males lived 301 to 796 days with an average of 543 days, and females 356 to 894 days with an average of 628 days. Elzinga[84] observed the same species in the laboratory and cited a higher longevity, i.e. a maximum of 1,755 days for one female. Twenty-five of the observed females survived more than 1,000 days; for males a maximum of 897 days was recorded. Galiano[85,86] studied the biology of *L. laeta*. She observed that the number of instars is variable: 8.57 % of the males and 41.89 % of the females reached the maturity with 9 moults; and 82.85 % of the males and 44.59 % of the females with 10 moults, and other males and females need one more moult. Concerning longevity, there are significant differences between sexes and between mated and unmated individuals of both sexes; for mated males she cited a longevity of 696 days and for mated females 1,536 days; unmated males and females have a higher longevity.

4. Venom quantities

Bücherl[78] gave the average of 0.10 mg of venom obtained by electrical stimulation, probably for the species *L. gaucho*. In the Instituto Butantan an average between 0.05 to 0.07 mg of dry venom is obtained from the same species, also by electrical stimulation.

5. Venom activities

Geren et al.[87] using standard techniques for the fractionation of proteins, obtained from the venom of *L. reclusa* two major components: a high molecular fraction, lethal to mice, and another of low molecular weight which proved to be non-toxic. Their molecular weight is in the range of 24,000. The high-molecular fraction was further separated into three peaks by Sephadex G 100; the latest eluting fraction was lethal to mice and caused necrotic lesions in rabbits. Suarez et al.[88] obtained from the venom of the species *L. laeta* a highly purified fraction of molecular weight approximately 20,000. Cicarelli et al.[27] studied the electrophoretic and immunochemistry behavior of *L. gaucho* venom. They used polyacrylamide electrophoresis techniques to determine the presence of 11 fractions and used immunodiffusion and immunoelectrophoresis in agar gel techniques for the determination of the number of specific and non-specific immunogenic components of the venom. Barbaro et al,[89] using a technique of Gel filtration on Sephadex G 100, obtained from the venom of the species *L. gaucho* three fractions: fraction A containing the higher mol. wt components (approximately 35,000), fraction B containing lower mol. wt.

components (approximately 15,000) and fraction C containing very low mol. wt components (probably small peptides). The dermonecrotic and lethal activities were detected exclusively in fraction A.

6. List and distribution of the medically most important species

The spiders of this genus have a wide distribution in the temperated and tropical regions. According to Gertsch[77] and Gertsch and Ennik[90] native species are known only from two principal centers: Africa and the Americas. In their opinion the species range from temperate South Africa northward through the tropics of that continent into the Mediterranean region and southern Europe. Only two of these species live in the warmer parts of Europe. The genus is strongly represented in the Americas, with species known from temperated and tropical North and South America. Gertsch[77] listed 30 species from South America, and Gertsch and Ennik[90] listed 54 species for North and Central America and The West Indies. Two of these species, related to the *laeta* group of South America, are endemics in Central America; two species that can be called "cosmopolitan ": *L. laeta* and *L. rufescens,* have been brought into North America by commercial vehicles. In Africa about 20 species are described.

L. gaucho Gertsch, 1967
Brazil, also register of occurrence in Tunisia

L. laeta (Nicolet, 1849)
America, also register of occurrence in Australia and
Finland

L. reclusa Gertsch and Mulaik, 1940
U.S.

L. rufescens (Dufour, 1820)
Cosmopolitan

L. rufipes (Lucas, 1834)
Guatemala, Panama and Colombia

L. parrami Newlands, 1981
South Africa

7. Epidemiology

The spiders of this genus normally do not bite. They only do so when pressed against the body within clothes, bed clothes and bath towels, thus not permitting them to escape. Sometimes the spider is not found and the accident is identified only through the symptoms. The accidents occur mostly inside the houses during summer time when the spiders are more active. Several cases of loxoscelism are cited in the literature in the United States[91-93], in South Africa[94,95], in Israel[96], and in Australia[97]. In some countries the population of the dangerous species *L. laeta* has been found, but loxoscelism is only a serious problem of public health in South America, mainly in Chile and Peru.

Macchiavello[98] in Chile was the first who associated the necrotic skin lesions with the bite of the common house-spider *Loxosceles laeta*. In Brazil the species responsible for accidents are: *L. gaucho, L. intermedia* and *L. laeta*. The accidents occur mainly in the southern region of the country (41.44 %).

V. MYGALOMORPH SPIDERS

A. THE SPIDERS OF THE GENUS *Atrax* CAMBRIDGE, 1877 (HEXATHELIDAE)

The genus is characterized by a glabrous and shiny carapace with an arched caput, the eye tubercle is low, the labium is almost square with numerous cuspules, the fangs groove with an inner and outer row of large teeth , four spinnerets, the large pair may be relatively long or short, and the terminal segment is digitiform, always longer than it is wide. The species are known as funnel-web spiders.

Measurements: large spiders have a body length of 1.5 to 4.5 cm; males are much smaller than females; in several species the males present on the second leg a tibial aphophysis.

1. Coloration and general aspect

The spiders are dark brown; sometimes the abdomen may be quite pale in color. The cephalothorax is smooth and shiny.

2. Habitat

The spiders make their tube-like web in or under rocks, and on the base of stumps. Being ground or log dwellers, some species live in trees, but they always give preference to moist places with a few exceptions. Around the entrance of the spider's house, some support lines surrounding rocks and sticks can be observed. Some species live near human dwellings, making their webs around house foundations. After maturity the males assume an errant way of life and, according to Sutherland[99], they often enter the houses particularly in the summer months after a heavy rain.

3. Biology

Kaire[100] maintained for several years a colony of several hundred *A. robustus* in the laboratory. The average survival time of spiders in captivity was 4 months; spiders surviving 6 months also were observed. Males have a significantly shorter lifespan than females. Egg-sacs were made and laid from the last days of July to the end of October. Gray and Sutherland[101] observed a mating activity from October to April. The mother takes care of the egg-sac and after approximately three weeks the spiderlings hatch and dig themselves into the soil, making a small web around the hole. The spiders, according to Sutherland[99], take several years to reach maturity, and it is believed that the females may live for perhaps eight years or longer; males probably have only one season of reproductive activity, living a short period only.

4. Venom quantities

Kaire[102] obtained by electrical stimulation an average of 0.31 mg for females and 0.28 mg for males; frequently he obtained much higher averages, for example: two males produced together, on their first milking, 1.6 mg of dry venom.

5. Venom activities

Sutherland[103,104] studied the venom of the species *A. robustus*. The venom contains high concentrations of hyaluronidase which is responsible for the rapid spread in tissues. Also some other components were isolated as a gamma-aminobutyric acid and a spermine complex associated with indole lactic acid. The whole venom, called Atraxotoxin, experimentally acts upon neuromuscular endings, releasing acetylcholine, adrenalin and noradrenalin from the autonomic nervous system. The venom of the male spider is five-times more toxic than that of females. Men and monkeys appear to have a special susceptibility to the venom. Brown et al.[105] studied the venom of the species *A.versutus* and cited the amino acid sequence of lethal neurotoxin which they called Versutoxin. The venom of both, males and females, contained this polypeptide toxin having similar chromatographic and electrophoretic properties to Robustoxin, a lethal neurotoxin isolated from the venom of the males of *A. robustus*.

6. List and distribution of species

According to Gray and Sutherland[101] the genus is primarily confined to southeastern Australia. Their main geographic range extends from southern Queensland to N.S.W., Victoria and Tasmania and west to the Mount Lofty and Flinders Ranges regions of South Australia. Outside Australia, *Atrax* has been recorded from Papua New Guinea and the Solomon Islands. Gray[106] includes only *A. robustus* and two other species in this genus (see relevant sections of Chapter 20).

7. Epidemiology

Sutherland[99] cited that cases of human envenomation are quite common, with at least 230 cases every year in Australia. Most accidents occur in summer and males are bitten twice as much than females. In general the bites occur in the extremities. Some fatal cases are registered, the majority of them involving children. The species *A. robustus*, which is limited to an area radiating out for some 160 kilometers from the centre of the city of Sydney, is considered a dangerous species to human beings. Maretic[10] cited that until 1980, 14 fatalities were due to *A. robustus* male bites. The other species, *Hadronyche formidablis*, is a tree dwelling funnel-web spider living near the northern coast of New South Wales and in southern Queensland.

VI. PROPHYLAXIS AND FIRST AID TREATMENT

Spiders often are attracted by civilization where they find a favourable habitat and plenty of food. In general they are not aggressive with an exception of the species of the genera *Atrax* and *Phoneutria*. They only try to bite when it is impossible to escape. Many spiders have nocturnal habits, hiding during the day in shoes, clothes, behind curtains and furniture.

The natural enemies of spiders are birds, insectivorous mammals, lizards, frogs, and several different parasites.

As preventive measures the following are advisable:

- avoid the spreading of domestic garbage in the vicinity of houses; under no circumstances should garbage and building debris be thrown on vacant lots;
- lawns have to be mown and shrubs with large leaves should not be planted near the houses;
- periodically clean vacant lots around the house or, if too big, at least a 1 to 2 m strip near the back yard; garden has to be cleaned;
- avoid storage of debris and building material near the house;
- mainly in rural areas, care has to be taken when putting on shoes and clothes;
- seal doorsills and windowslits to avoid the entrance of spiders into the house, mainly at the beginning of the night, when these animals become more active;
- do not walk bare-footed inside the house, mainly in the darkness;
- periodically clean the house, (air clothes and bedding when kept a long time without use), move aside furniture, clean the walls behind pictures and curtains;
- avoid accumulation of superfluous materials such as paper and cardboard boxes;

- remove, using a broom, spiders webs and egg-sacs on the walls, inside houses or around them;
- use thick leather gloves and shoes to avoid accidents when working in the garden, in the field, or when removing garbage;
- control domestic insects, like cockroaches, which are the main food of the spiders.

Mc Crone[107] recommended 5 to 10% DDT or 2% Lindane for spider control; BHC used in closed areas at the rate of 1/6 oz of the product per 130 cu. yds is the most effective insecticide; the application must be repeated after 30 days to destroy any broods which may have emerged. Levi and Spielman[81] used Lindane for controlling a brown spider (*L. laeta*) infestation in a large building of the Harvard University. It was made up in a 1.0% formulation, with 1.0% Chlordane, in deodorized kerosene and was applied in a coarse spray to the floors of the infested areas . Each of the rooms was then closed and a 1.0% Lindane solution applied as a space-spray with an aerosol dispenser. Another application of Lindane and Chlordane was applied to the floors one month later. Gorham[108] mentioned that, probably, in the case of *Loxosceles* spider infestation; every contact or fumigant insecticide can be used. Lindane, Chlordane, Malathion, Dichlorvos and Paradichlorobenzene have been recommended. On the other hand, the author agrees that although insecticides have their place in spider control, a good housekeeping is essential.

When an accident occurs it is important to try to collect the spider for identification and to facilitate the diagnosis. According to the seriousness of the symptoms, an antivenom therapy is necessary.

A list of currently available antivenoms was published by Theakston and Warrell[109].

VII. ANTIVENOMS

A list of currently available antivenoms was published by Theakston and Warrell[109]. Table 1 summarises their data for spider antivenoms. A further updated list is to be found in Chapter 32.

Table 1
List of available spider antivenoms (after Theakston and Warrell[109])

Antidote	Source	Specific Name
01- Spider antivenom (E, A)	South African Institute for Medical Research, P.O. BOX 1038, Johannesburg 2000, SOUTH AFRICA Phone: 725-0511 Telex: 4-22211 Gram: BACTERIA	*Latrodectus mactans indistinctus* (Black Widow spider) [Cape Peninsula, Cape Town] [1000]
02- Antivenim (*Latrodectus mactans*) MSD (E)	Merck, Sharp and Dohme Int., P.O. BOX 2000, Rahway, NJ 07065, U.S. Phone: 215-661-5477 FAX: 215-661-5319	*L. mactans* (Black Widow spider) [approx 600]
03- Soro anti-aracnidico polivalente (P)	Instituto Butantan, Av. Vital Brazil, 1500 Caixa Postal 65, São Paulo - SP - BRAZIL Phone: (011) 813-7222 FAX: (011) 815-1505 Telex: 11-83325 BUTA BR	*Phoneutria* spp. (Banana spider) *Loxosceles* spp. (Brown recluse spider) *Tityus serrulatus* (Scorpion) *T. bahiensis* (Scorpion)

Antidote	Source	Specific Name
04- Soro anti-loxoscelico (P)	As above	*L. reclusa* (Brown recluse spider)
05- Soro anti-loxoscelico (S)	Institutos Nacionales de Salud, Departamento de Animales Venenosos, Calle Capac Yupanqui no. 1400, Apartado no. 451, Lima - PERU Phone: 5114678212	*Loxosceles* spp. (Brown recluse spider)
06- Anti-*Latrodectus mactans tredecimguttatus* serum (E and other on request)	Institute of Immunology Rockerfellerova 2, Zagreb, YUGOSLAVIA Phone: 430-333 FAX: (041) 277-278 Telex: 21864 VACC YU	*L. mactans tredecimguttatus*(European widow spider) [3,000] [Yugoslavia]
07- Red-backed spider antivenom (E)	Commonwealth Serum Laboratories, 45 Poplar Road, Parkville, Victoria 3052, AUSTRALIA Phone: (03) 389 1911 FAX: (03) 389 1434 Telex: AA 32789	*L. hasselti hasselti* (Red-backed spider) (female) [> 100] [Australia, Central Victoria]
08- Funnel-web spider antivenom (E)	As above	*Atrax robustus* (Sydney funnel-web spider) (male) [> 100] [Australia, Gosford area of NSW]

Language on label: (A) Afrikaans; **(E)** English; **(P)** Portuguese; **(S)** Spanish.

VIII. REFERENCES

1. **WORLD HEALTH ORGANISATION,** Progress in the characterization of venoms and standardization of antivenoms. *WHO Offset Publication*, **58**:6, 1981.
2. **MARETIC, Z. AND LEBEZ, D.,** *Lycosa tarentula* in fact and fiction, *Bulletin du Museum National D''Histoire Naturelle*, 2 serie, 41 (1), 1969 (1970).
3. **SPIELMAN, A. AND LEVI, H. W.,** Probable envenomation by *Chiracanthium mildei* a spider found in houses, *Amer. J. trop. dises.*, **19, 4,** 729, 1970.
4. **MARETIC, Z.,** Arachnologorum Congressus Internationales V. Brno 1971, Toxicity of "non-venomous spiders".
5. **ORI, M..** Ten human cases of spider bites, *Eisei Dobutsu*, **26 2/3,** 83, 1975.
6. **RUSSELL, F. E. AND GERTSCH, W. J,** Last word on Araneism, *Am. Arachnol.*, **25,** 7, 1982.
7. **SCHMIDT, G. E.,** Wie gefährlich sind Spinnenbissvergiftungen ?, *Natur und Museum*, **117 (7),** 197, 1987.
8. **WONG, R. C, HUGHES, S. E. AND VOORHEES, J. J.,** Spider Bites, *Arch. Dermatol.*, 123, 1987.
9. **ORI. M.,** Biology of and poisonings by spiders, in *Handbook of Natural Toxins*, 2, Tu, A., Ed., Marcel Dekker Inc. New York and Basel, 1984
10. **MARETIC, Z.,** III Spider Venom and their effect, in *Ecophysiology of Spiders*, Nentwig, W., Ed., Springer Verlag, Berlin Heidelberg, 1987, 142.
11. **RIBEIRO, L. A., TANUS JORGE. M., PIESCO, V. R. AND NISHIOKA, S. A.,** Wolf spider bites in São Paulo, Brazil : a clinical and epidemiological study of 515 cases, *Toxicon*, **28,** 715, 1990
12. **SUOMALAINEN, K. U.,** Histological studies on the poison glands of Araneids, *Ann. Zool. Fenn.*, **1,** 89, 1964.
13. **JÄRLSFORS, U., SMITH, D. S. AND RUSSELL, F. E.,** Innervation of the venom-secreting cells in the Black Widow Spider (*Latrodectus mactans*), in *Toxins of Plant and Animal Origin*, 1, De Vries, A. and Kochva, E., Eds., London, 1971, 159.
14. **PERTY, M.,** Arachnides Brasiliensis, in *Delectus Animalium articolatorum, quae in itinere per Brasiliam ann. 1817-1820 colligerunt*, Spix, J. B. and Martius, F. P., Eds., Monachii, Hamburg, 1833, 191.
15. **MELLO LEITÅO, C. F.,** Contribution à l'étude des Ctenides du Brésil, *Festschr. Strand*, **1,** 1, 1936.
16. **BÜCHERL, W.,** Estudos sobre a biologia e a sistematica do genero *Grammostola*, *Monogr. Inst. Butantan*, 1, 1951.

17. **TRETZTEL, E.,** Haltung, Zucht und Entwicklung von *Phoneutria fera* (Perty) und anderen Spinnen, *Der Zoologische Garten* (NF) **23, 1/3,** 74, 1957.
18. **SIMO, M. AND BARDIER, G.,** Desarrollo postembrionario de *Phoneutria keyserlingi* (Pickard Cambridge, 1897) (ARANEAE, CTENIDAE), *Bol. Soc. Zool. Uruguay,* **5,** 15, 1989.
19. **BÜCHERL, W.,** Spiders, in *Venomous Animals and Their Venoms,* III, Bücherl, W. and Buckley, E. E., Eds., Academic Press, New York, 1971, chap. 51.
20. **BÜCHERL, W.,** Studies on Dried Venom of *Phoneutria fera, Amer. Ass. Advancement of Science,* **44,** 95, 1956.
21. **KAISER, E.,** Fermentchemische Untersuchungen an Spinnengiften, *Monatshefte für Chemie,* **84 (3),** 482, 1953.
22. **KAISER, E. AND RAAB, W.,** Collagenolytic activity of snake and spider venom, *Toxicon,* **4,** 251, 1967.
23. **DINIZ, C. R.,** Separation of proteins and characterization of active substances in the venom of Brazilian spiders, *Anais Acad. Bras. Cienc.,* **35,** 283, 1963.
24. **FISCHER, F. G. AND BOHN, H.,** Animal Toxins VIII. The venoms of the Brazilian Tarantula, *Lycosa erythrognatha* and the spider, *Phoneutria fera, Hoppe-Seyler's Z. Physiol. Chem.,* **306,** 265, 1957.
25. **SCHENBERG, S. AND PEREIRA LIMA, F. A.,** *Phoneutria nigriventer* venom. Pharmacology and biochemistry of its components, in *Venomous Animals and Their Venoms,* III, Bucherl, W. and Buckley, E. E., Eds., Academic Press, New York, 1971, chap. 52.
26. **ENTWISTLE, I. D., JOHNSTONE, R. W. A. , MEDZIHRADSZKY, D. AND MAY, E. T.,** Isolation of a pure toxic polypeptide from the venom of the spider *Phoneutria nigriventer* and its neurophysiological activity on an insect femur preparation, *Toxicon,* **20, 6,** 1059, 1982.
27. **CICARELLI, R. M. B., VILLARROEL, M. S. AND ROLIM ROSA, R.,** Evaluation of the toxic activity of *Phoneutria nigriventer* venom in terms of LD_{50} and titration of the antivenom in mice, *Mem. Inst. Butantan,* **47/ 48,** 27, 1983/1984.
28. **FONTANA, M. D. AND VITAL BRAZIL, O.,** Mode of action of *Phoneutria nigriventer* spider venom at the isolated phrenic nerve-diaphragm of the rat, *Brazilian J. Med. Biol. Res.,* **18,** 557, 1985.
29. **REZENDE, L. J., CORDEIRO, M. N., OLIVEIRA, S. B., AND DINIZ, C. R,** Isolation of neurotoxic peptides from the venom of the " armed spider " *Phoneutria nigriventer, Toxicon,* **29 ,** 10, 1225, 1991.
30. **BÜCHERL, W.,** Biology and venoms of the most important South American spiders of the genera *Phoneutria, Loxosceles and Latrodectus, Am. Zool.,* **9,** 157, 1969.
31. **BÜCHERL, W., LUCAS, S. AND VON EICKSTEDT, V. R.,** Spiders of the family CTENIDAE, subfamily PHONEUTRIINAE. VI Bibliographia Phoneutriarum, *Mem. Inst. Butantan,* **34,** 47, 1969.
32. **SCHMIDT, G.,** Zur Herkunftsbestimmung von Bananenimporten nach dem Besatz an Spinnen, *Z. Angew. Ent.,* **36,** 400, 1954.
33. **SCHIAPELLI, R. D. AND GERSCHMAN DE PIKELIN, B.,** Diagnosis de *Phoneutria reidyi* (F.O.Pickard Cambridge, 1897) and *Phoneutria boliviensis* (F.O. Pickard Cambridge, 1897) ((ARANEAE,CTENIDAE), *Rev. Soc. Ent. Arg.,* **34 (1/2),** 31, 1972.
34. **VON EICKSTEDT, V. R. D.,** Estudo sistematico de *Phoneutria nigriventer* (Keyserling, 1891) e *Phoneutria keyserlingi* (Pickard Cambridge, 1897) (ARANEAE, CTENIDAE), *Mem. Inst. Butantan,* **42/43,** 95, 1978/1979
35. **VON EICKSTEDT, V. R. D. ,** ConsideraçÆes sobre a sistematica das especies amazonicas de *Phoneutria* (ARANEAE,CTENIDAE), *Revta. bras. Zool. Sào Paulo* **1 (3),** 183, 1983.
36. **MINISTERIO DA SAUDE,** Araneismo: analise epidemiologica, Brasilia, D.F., 1991.
37. **TREJOS, A., TREJOS, R. AND ZELEDON,** Aracnidismo por *Phoneutria* en Costa Rica (ARANEAE,CTENIDAE), *Rev. Biol. Trop.,* **19 (1,2),** 241, 1979.
38. **VALERIO, C. E.,** Sobre la presencia de *Phoneutria boliviensis* (Cambridge) (ARANEAE, CTENIDAE) en Costa Rica, *J. Arachnol.,* **11,** 101, 1982.
39. **SCHMIDT, G.,** Die Spinnenfauna der importierten Bananen, *Deutsches Ärzteblatt-Ärztliche Mitteilungen,* **67,** 42, 3106,1970
40. **SMITHER, R. H. N.,** Contribution to our knowledge of the genus *Latrodectus* in South Africa, *Ann. S. Afr. Mus.,* **36 (3),** 263, 1944.
41. **LAMORAL, B. H.,** On the nest and web structure of *Latrodectus* in South Africa, and some observations on body colouration of *L. geometricus* (ARANEAE : THERIDIIDAE), *Ann. Natal Mus.,* **20 (1),** 1, 1968.
42. **SHULOV, A. AND WEISSMAN, A.,** Notes on the life habits and potency of the venom of three *Latrodectus* spider species of Israel, *Ecology,* **40 (3),** 515, 1959.
44. **BÜCHERL, W.,** *Latrodectus* e latrodectismo na America do Sul. II. Bio-ecologia de *Latrodectus* do grupo "curacaviensis" nas praias dos Estados do Rio de janeiro e Guanabara, *Rev. Bras. Pesq. Med. Biol.,* **1 (2),** 83, 1968.
45. **MOWSZWICZ, B. H.,** La Arana del Lino, *Bol. Informativo,* Publicacion Extra, Mus. Nac. Hist. Nat., 1968.
46. **MACKAY, I. R.,** A New Species of Widow Spider (Genus *Latrodectus*) from Southern Africa (ARANEAE: THERIDIIDAE), *Psyche,* **79 (3),** 236, 1972.

47. **BAERG, W. J.,** The black-widow and five other venomous spiders in the United States, *Univ. Arkansas Agr. Exp. Sta. Bull.*, **608,** 43, 1959.

48. **BLAIR, A. W.,** The life history of *Latrodectus mactans, Arch. Intern. Med.*, **54,** 844, 1934.

49. **DEEVEY, G. B. AND DEEVEY, E. S.,** A life table for the black widow, *Trans. Connecticut Acad. Sci.*, **36,** 115, 1945.

50. **SHULOV, A.,** On the biology of two *Latrodectus* spiders in Palestine, *Proc. Linn. Soc. London*, **152,** 309, 1940.

51. **JENNINGS, D. T. AND MC DANIEL, I. N.,** *Latrodectus hesperus* (ARANEAE, THERIDIIDAE) in Maine, *Ent. News*, **99 (1)** 37, 1988.

52. **ABALOS, J. W. AND BAEZ, E. C.,** The spider genus *Latrodectus* in Santiago del Estero, Argentina, in *Animal Toxins*, First International Symposium on Animal Toxins (Atlantic City, New Jersey, U.S.A., April 9-11, 1966), Pergamon Press, Oxford, New York, 1967, 59.

53. **KASTON, B. J.,** Comparative biology of American black widow spider, *San Diego Soc. Nat. Hist. Trans.*, **16 (3),** 33, 1970.

54. **GRASSO, A.,** Preparation and properties of a neurotoxin purified from the venom of the black-widow spider (*Latrodectus mactans tredecimguttatus*), *Bioch. Biophys. Acta*, **439,** 409, 1976.

55. **FRONTALI, N., CECCARELI, B., GORIO, A., MAURTO, A.,SIEKEVITZ, P. TZENG, M. C. AND HURLBUT, W. P.,** Purification from black-widow spider venom of a protein factor causing the depletion of synaptic vesicles at neuromuscular junctions, *J. Cell. Biol.*, **68,** 462, 1976.

56. **TZENG M. C. AND SIEKEVITZ, P.,** The effect of purified major protein factor (alfa-latrotoxin) of black-widow spider venom on the release of acetylcholine and norepinephrine from mouse cerebral cortex slices, *Brain. Res.*, **139,** 190, 1978.

57. **FEDOROVA, I. M. AND MAGAZANIK, L. G.,** The effects of alfa-latroinsectotoxin of black-widow spider venom on the transmitter release from insect nerve endings, *Ninth European Symposium on Animal, Plant and Microbial Toxins*, Lohusalu, Estonia, 23-26 Sept. 1990 (Abstracts of the Symposium in: *Toxicon*, **29, 3,** 283, 1992.)

58. **AKHUNOV** 1991 Abstract *Toxicon:*

59. **GRISHIN, E. V.,** Neurotoxin from spider venoms, Third International Symposium, *Neurotoxins in Neurobiology*, Piriapolis, Uruguay, 16-20 March 1991 (Abstract: *Toxicon*, **29, 10,** 1165, 1991).

60. **KYIATKINK** 1992 Abstract *Toxicon*

61. **LEVI, H. W.,** The spider genus *Latrodectus* (Araneae, Theridiidae), *Trans. Amer. Micr. Soc.*, **78, 1,** 7, 1959.

62. **MARTINDALE, C. B. AND NEWLANDS, G.,** The widow spider: a complex of species, *South African Journal of Science*, **78,** 78, 1982.

63. **LEVI, H. L.,** On the Value of Genitalic Structures and Coloration in Separating Species of Widow Spiders (*Latrodectus sp.*) (ARACHNIDA, ARANEIDA, THERIDIIDAE), *Ver. Naturwiss. Ver. Hamburg (NF)*, **26,** 195, 1983.

64. **ROEWER, C. FR.,** *Katalog der Araneae*, Bremen, Bruxelles, 424, 1942.

65. **BRIGNOLI, P. M.,** *A Catalogue of the Araneae*, Merrett, Ed., Manchester University Press, Manchester, 1983, 408.

66. **PLATNICK, N. I.,** *Advances in Spider Taxonomy*, Merrett, Ed., Manchester University Press, Manchester, 1981, 197.

67. **JELINEK, G. A., BANHAM, N. D. G. AND DUNJEY, S. J.,** Red-back spiderbites at Fremantle Hospital, 1982 - 1987, *Med. J. Australia*, **150,** 693, 1989.

68. **MARETIC, Z. AND GONZALEZ-LORENZO, D.,** Caracter profesional del latrodectismo en paises mediterraneos, con especial referencia a experiencias en Yugoslavia y Espana, *Rev. Clin. Espanola*, **160 (4),** 225, 1981.

69. **MARETIC, Z. AND HABERMEHL, G.,** Latrodektismus bei Menschen und Tieren sowie grosse Tierseuchen des vorigen Jahrhunderts hervorgerufen durch Latrodektus, *Dtsch. Tierarzt. Wschr.*, **92,** 245, 1985.

70. **SCHENONE, H. AND CORREA L. E.,** Algunos conocimientos practicos sobre la biologia de la arana *Latrodectus mactans* y el sindrome del latrodectismo en Chile, *Bol. Chil. Parasit.*, **40,** 18, 1985.

71. **GRISOLIA, C. S., PELUSO, F. O. STANCHI, N. O. AND FRANCINI, F.,** Epidemiologia del latrodectismo en la Provincia de Buenos Aires, Argentina, *Rev. Saude Publ. S.Paulo*, **26 (1),** 1, 1992.

72. **ZUMPT, F.,** Latrodectism in South Africa, *South Afric. Med. J.*, 385, 1968.

73. **NEWLANDS, G.,** Review of the Medically Important Spiders in Southern Africa, *South Afric. Med. J.*, **49, 10,** 823, 1975.

74. **SCHWAB RODRIGUES, D. AND BRAZIL NUNES, T.,** Latrodectismo na Bahia, *Rev. Baiana Saude Publ.*, **12 (1/3),** 38, 1985.

75. **MACHADO, O.,** *Latrodectus mactans*, sua ocorrencia no Brasil, *Bol. Inst. Vital Brazil*, **V (4),** 153, 1948.

76. **GERTSCH, W. J.,** The Spider Genus *Loxosceles* in North America, Central America and the West Indies, *Amer. Mus. Novitates*, **1907,** 1, 1958.

77. **GERTSCH, W. J.,** The Spider Genus *Loxosceles* in South America, *Bull. Amer. Mus. Nat. Hist.*, **136 (3),** 121, 1967.
78. **BÜCHERL, W.,** Biologia de Artropodes Peçonhentos, *Mem. Inst. Butantan*, **31,** 85, 1964.
79. **LOWRIE, D. C.,** Starvation longevity of *Loxosceles laeta* (Nicolet) (ARANEAE), *Ent. News.*, **91 (4),** 130, 1980.
80. **HUHTA, V.,** *Loxosceles laeta* (Nicolet) (ARANEAE, LOXOSCELINAE), a venomous spider established in a building in Helsinki, Finland, and notes on some other synanthropic spiders, *Ann. Ent. Fennici*, **38 (3),** 152, 1972.
81. **LEVI, H. W. AND SPIELMANN, A.,** The biology and control of the South American brown spider, *Loxosceles laeta* (Nicolet), in a North American Focus, *Amer. J. Trop. Med. Hyg.*, **13, 1,** 132, 1964.
82. **DELGADO, A.,** Investigacion ecologica sobre *Loxosceles rufipes* (Lucas), 1834, en la region costera del Peru, *Mem. Inst. Butantan*, **33 (3),** 683, 1966.
83. **HITE, J. M., GLADNEY, W. J. LANCASTER JR., J. L. AND WHITCOMB, W. H.,** Biology of the Brown Recluse Spider, Arkansas Experiment Station, *Bulletin* **711,** 1, 1966.
84. **ELZINGA, J.,** Observations on the Longevity of the Brown Recluse Spider, *Loxosceles reclusa* Gertsch & Mulaik, *J. Kansas Ent. Soc.*, **50 (1),** 187, 1977.
85. **GALIANO, M. E.,** Ciclo biologico y desarrollo de *Loxosceles laeta* (Nicolet) (ARANEAE), *Acta Zool. Lilloana*, **23,** 431, 1967.
86. **GALIANO, M. E. AND HALL, M.,** Datos adicionales sobre el ciclo vital de *Loxosceles laeta* (Nicolet) (ARANEAE), *Physis*, **32 (85),** 277, 1973.
87. **GEREN, C. R., CHAN, T. K., HOWEL, D. E. AND ODELL, G. V.,** Isolation and characterization of toxins from brown recluse spider venom (*Loxosceles reclusa*), *Arch. Biochem. Biophys.*, **174,** 90, 1976.
88. **SUAREZ, G., SCHENONE, H. AND SOCIAS, T.,** *Loxosceles laeta* venom, partial purification, *Toxicon*, **17,** 291, 1971.
89. **BARBARO, K. C., CARDOSO, J. L. C., EICKSTEDT, V. R. D. AND MOTA, I.,** Dermonecrotic and lethal components of *Loxosceles gaucho* spider venom, *Toxicon*, **30, 3,** 331, 1992.
90. **GERTSCH, W. J. AND ENNIK, F.,** The Spider Genus *Loxosceles* in North America, Central America and the West Indies, *Amer. Mus. Novitates*, **175 (3),** 265, 1983.
91. **SCHMAUS, L. F.,** Case of arachnidism (spiderbite), *J. Amer. Med. Assn.*, **92,** 1265, 1929.
92. **GOTTEN, H. B. AND MACGOWAN, J. J.,** Blackwater fever (hemoglobinuria) caused by a spider bite, *J. Amer. Med. Assn.*, **115,** 1457, 1940.
93. **ATKINS, J. A., WINGO, C. W. AND SODEMAN, W. A.,** Probable cause of necrotic spiderbite in the Midwest, *Science,* **126,** 3263, 1957.
94. **NEWLANDS, G., ISAACSON, C. AND MARTINDALE, C.,** Loxoscelism in the Transvaal, South Africa, *Transac. Royal Soc. Trop. Med. Hyg.*, **76 (5),** 610, 1982
95. **NEWLANDS, G.,** Review of southern African spiders of medical importance, with notes on the signs and symptoms of envenomation, *South Afric. Med. J.*, **73,** 235, 1988.
96. **EFRATI, P.,** Bites by *Loxosceles* Spiders in Israel, *Toxicon*, **6,** 239, 1969.
97. **SOUTHCOTT, R. V.,** Spiders of the genus *Loxosceles* in Australia, *Med. J. Aust.*, **1,** 406, 1976.
98. **MACHIAVELLO, A.,** Cutaneous Arachnoidism, or gangrenous spot of Chile, *Puerto Rico J. Publ. Health Trop. Med.*, **22, 4,** 425, 1947.
99. **SUTHERLAND, S. K.,** Treatment of arachnid poisoning in Australia, *Aust. Family Physician*, 395, 1977.
100. **KAIRE, G. H.,** The Sydney funnel-web spider (*Atrax robustus*) in captivity, *Vic. Nat.*, **81,** 38, 1964.
101. **GRAY, M., R. AND SUTHERLAND, S. K.,** Venoms of DIPLURIDAE, in *Handbuch der experimentellen Pharmakologie, Arthropod Venoms*, 48, Bettini, S., Ed., Springer Verlag, Berlin Heidelberg, 1978, 121.
102. **KAIRE, G. H.,** Observations on some funnel-web spiders (*Atrax* species) and their venoms, with particular reference to *Atrax robustus*, *Med. J. Aust.*, **2,** 307, 1963.
103. **SUTHERLAND, S. K.,** The Sydney funnel-web spider (*Atrax robustus*), fractionation of the female venom into five distinct components, *Med. J. Aust.*, **2,** 593, 1972.
104. **SUTHERLAND, S. K.,** Isolation, mode of action and properties of the major toxin (Atraxotoxin) in the venom of the Sydney funnel-web spider (*Atrax robustus*), *Proc. Aust. Soc. Med. Res.*, **3,** 172, 1973.
105. **BROWN, M. R., SCHEUMACK, D. D., TYLER, M. I. AND HOWDEN, M. E. H.,** Amino acid sequence of versutoxin, a lethal neurotoxin from the venom of the funnel-web spider *Atrax versutus, Biochem. J.*, **250,** 401, 1988.
106. **GRAY, M. R.,** Distribution of funnel-web spider, in *Toxic Plant and Animals: A Guide for Australia*, Covacevich, J., Davie, P. and Pearn, J., Eds., Queensland Museum, 504 pp, 1987. Brisbane, 312, 1987.
107. **MC CRONE, J. D. AND STONE, K. J.,** The widow spiders of Florida, Florida Department of Agriculture, 2, 1965.
108. **GORHAM, J. R.,** The Brown Recluse Spider *Loxosceles reclusa* and Necrotic Spiderbite, A New Public Health Problem in the United States, *J. Envir. Health* **31,** 138, 1968.
109. **THEAKSTON, R. D. G. AND WARRELL, D. A.,** Antivenoms: a list of hyperimmune sera currently available for the treatment of envenomings by bites and sting, *Toxicon,* **29, 12,** 1419, 1991.

Chapter 20

CLINICAL TOXICOLOGY OF SPIDER BITES

Julian White, J.L. Cardoso, Hui Wen Fan

TABLE OF CONTENTS

I. INTRODUCTION

Spiders are ubiquitous animals, found in virtually every habitat occupied or used by man. They are common in urban environments as well as rural areas and are found in most houses. Estimates of density of spiders in rural environments have been as high as 2,000,000 per acre (4.9×10^6 per hectare)[1], but comparable figures for urban environments are not available. All spiders are predators, feeding on a variety of other animals, but for most species the dominant food items are insects. Spiders are therefore overall great allies of man, without which mankind would now find much difficulty in surviving. It is against this background that the problems caused by spiderbite in clinical medicine should be assessed.

This Chapter will first cover some general information about spiders and spiderbite, then will detail information on each medically important group of spiders.

II. A MEDICAL OUTLINE OF SPIDER TAXONOMY

The large number of described species of spiders, and the numerous species as yet undescribed, the small size of most, the superficial similarity of all spiders, the lack of useful taxonomic texts for identification, the lack of skilled spider taxonomists and the lack of distribution data for many species combine to make the task of identifying the spider culprit quite difficult for the treating clinician. Nevertheless, it is possible in many cases to at least partially identify the spider, and every attempt should be made to do so, as there is a paucity of data linking most species of spider with the effects of their bite on man.

A. AN APPROACH TO IDENTIFYING SPIDERS

The bulk of all spiders, and certainly virtually all causing injury to man, belong to one of two subclasses, the "primitive" spiders, Mygalomorphae (=Orthognathae) or the "modern" or "true" spiders, Araneomorphae (=Labidognathae). Distinguishing between these two groups is usually easy. Key features are shown in Figures 1,2,3. The fang position, chelicerae disposition and book lungs are particularly useful diagnostic characters. It is also often easy to distinguish between mature male and female spiders, on the basis of the external secondary sexual organs, namely the pedipalps, which are swollen or bulbous in the male, as shown in Figures 4,5,6,7,8.

B. MYGALOMORPHAE

The major taxonomic divisions within Mygalomorphae are listed in Table 1. This is not a complete list of all families, many genera are omitted, and it may not conform with all existing taxonomic outlines. Mygalomorph spiders are generally medium to large spiders, with robust body and legs, prominent forward facing chelicerae, large paraxial fangs, two pairs of book lungs and small eyes set in a "binacle" on the anterior cephalothorax. They are principally terrestrial in habit, often utilising a burrow structure as retreat, in which they spend most of their lives. Males leave their burrow to locate females and are generally less robust in build than females, though not necessarily smaller in overall dimensions. The venom glands are situated in the chelicerae.

C. ARANAEOMORPHAE

Araneomorph spiders are considerably more diverse in size, shape, habit and habitat than the Mygalomorphs. Some major taxonomic groups are listed in Table 2. This list of families is far from exhaustive, and only a few of the very many genera are listed here. As with Mygalomorphs, Araneomorph spider taxonomy remains in a state of flux and the family listings herein may not conform to some taxonomic outlines.

III. EPIDEMIOLOGY OF SPIDERBITE GLOBALLY

Detailed figures on the extent of spiderbite to humans, and even the far narrower subset of clinically significant spiderbite are not available. Limited studies, usually covering a single species or genus of spiders are published. A better guide may be the records of poisons information centres (PICs). Those which take calls from all sections of the community may give the most useful guide to the significance of spiderbite. In Australia, PICs take calls from the general public. The category of "bites and stings" is consistently about 10% of all calls, and within this group, spiderbite is often the largest component, though occasionally edged out by calls about bee and wasp stings[2]. For Australia's largest PIC, in Sydney, which takes calls from throughout Australia "after hours", spiderbite is the second most common cause of calls (paracetamol is the most common)[3]. American PICs deal with a smaller percentage of calls about bites and stings (3.6%) and within that group, spiderbite is less important (17%)[2,4]. In North America in the 1950's Parrish found spiderbite caused 6 to 7 fatalities per year, but non-fatal cases (very much more common) were not recorded[5]. Russell has noted a wide variety of spider species which are implicated in significant bites in humans[6]. In Europe information is less available, but reports of latrodectism alone indicate that spiderbite certainly occurs[7]. In South America a variety of spiders cause clinically significant spiderbite[8-11], and latrodectism and necrotic arachnidism are recorded from Africa[12-14]. The situation in Asia is unclear, though latrodectism certainly occurs in eastern regions of the former Soviet Union[7,8]. Since most spiderbites are not fatal, it is likely that in most regions cases are not recorded. This is particularly so for the rural tropics where spiderbite must occur, probably very frequently, and possibly with significant morbidity.

Because spider bite is poorly documented it is not possible to state how many people are bitten by spiders globally each year, nor even how many of these bites cause significant medical problems. The number of fatal cases is not known, though has recently been estimated at less than 200 annually for the whole world[15], suggesting that spiderbite is a minor problem, especially compared to snakebite. Assuming the above figure is aproximately correct, this hides the extent of spiderbite morbidity, ranging from severe local pain lasting less than 24 hours through to extensive skin necrosis causing long term, even permanent, morbidity. While the annual number of cases within this spectrum of morbidity is uncertain, it is likely to be measured in tens of thousands, quite possibly far higher. The economic cost is therefore likely to be considerable when considered globally.

Table 1
Some major taxonomic divisions within the Mygalomorph spiders

Family	Genus	Common Name	Distribution
BARYCHELIDAE	*Idiomata*	Brush foot spiders	Australia
THERAPHOSIDAE	*Aphonopelma, Selenocosmia, Theraphosa, Lasiodora, Grammostola, Brachypelma*	Tarantulas, hairy spiders, aranas de caballo, matacaballos, bird eating spiders	Worldwide
ACTINOPIDAE	*Misulena*	Mouse spiders	Australia
CTENIZIDAE	*Aganippe, Anidiops, Arabantis, Blakistonia, Conothele, Misgolas, Bothriocyrtum, Ummidia, Hebestatis, Actinoxia, Eucteniza, Aptostichus, Myrmekiaphila, Cyclocosmia*	Trapdoor spiders	Worldwide
HEXATHELIDAE	*Hexathele, Hadronyche, Atrax*	Australian funnel web spiders, sheet web tarantulas	Australia, North America
DIPLURIDAE	*Brachythele, Euagrus, Microhexura, Calisoga, Cethegus, Aname, Chenistonia, Kwonkan, Stanwellia, Teyloides*	Sheet web tarantulas	Worldwide
ATYPIDAE	*Atypus, Calommata*	Atypical tarantulas, purse web spiders	Americas, Europe, Japan, Africa, parts of Asia
MECICOBOTHIIDAE	*Hexura, Megahexura, Hexurella*	Sheet web atypical tarantulas	Western U.S. and parts of Argentina
ANTRODIAETIDAE	*Atypoides, Antrodiatus, Aliatypus*	Atypical tarantulas	North America, Japan

MYGALOMORPH   *ARANEOMORPHS*

VENTRAL SURFACE (Underside)

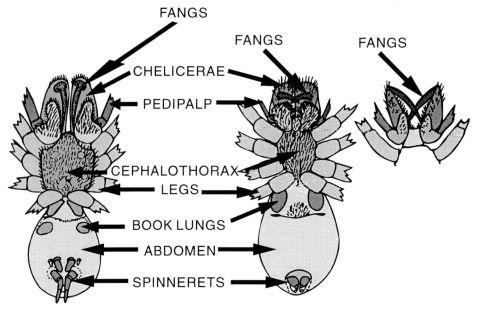

DORSAL SURFACE (Topside)

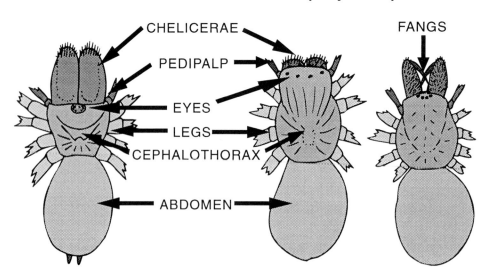

Figure 1. Diagramatic representation of principle distinguishing features of spiders of Suborders Mygalomorphae and Aranaeomorphae (illustration © Dr. J. White).

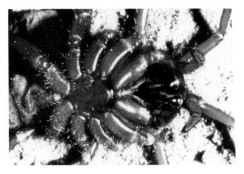

Figure 2. Underside of Mygalomorph spider, showing parallel (paraxial) fangs (photo © Dr. J. White).

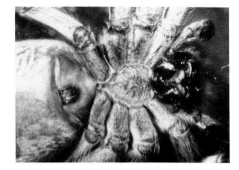

Figure 3. Underside of Araneomorph spider showing crossed (diaxial) fangs (photo © Dr. J. White).

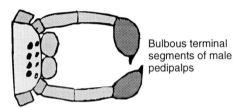

Bulbous terminal segments of male pedipalps

Figure 4a. Diagramatic representation of the male spider pedipalp, with characteristic bulbous end containing secondary sexual organ.

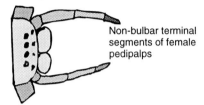

Non-bulbar terminal segments of female pedipalps

Figure 4b. Diagrammatic representation of the female spider pedipalp, lacking the bulbous end seen in male spiders.

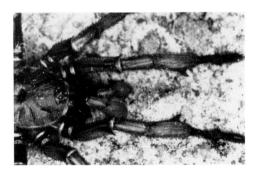

Figure 5. Close up of male spider pedipalp, with bulbous end (Trapdoor spider, *Aganippe subtristis*) (photo © Dr. J. White).

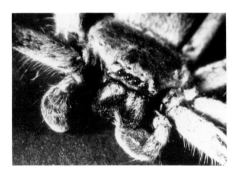

Figure 6. Close up of male spider pedipalp, with bulbous end (Huntsman spider, *Heteropoda* sp.) (photo © Dr. J. White).

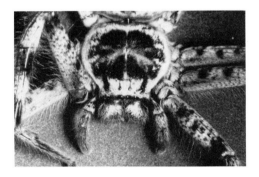

Figure 7. Close up of female spider pedipalp, without bulbous end (Huntsman spider *Pediana* sp.) (photo © Dr. J. White).

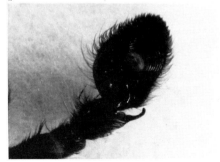

Figure 8. Close up of terminal segment of male pedipalp, showing bulbous end, for semen transfer (photo © Dr. J. White).

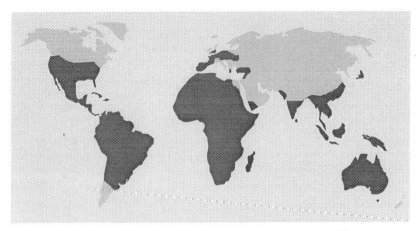

Figure 9. Approximate worldwide distribution of Mygalomorph spiders.

Table 2
Some major taxonomic divisions within the Araneomorph spiders

Taxonomic Group	Genus	Common Name
FILISTATIDAE	*Filistata*	
DYSDERIDAE	*Disdera crocata*	
SEGESTRIIDAE	*Ariadna, Segestria*	
LOXOSCELIDAE	*Loxosceles*	Recluse and fiddleback spiders
OONOPIDAE	*Gamasomorpha*	
PHOLCIDAE	*Pholcus*	Daddy long legs spiders
SCYTODIDAE	*Scytodes*	Spitting spiders
OECOBIIDAE	*Oecobius*	Hackled band spinners
DICTYNIDAE	*Badumna, Amaurobius*	Black house spider
STIPHIDIIDAE	*Corasoides*	Sheet web spiders
AGELENIDAE	*Tegenaria*	
HAHNIIDAE	*Hahnia*	
CTENIDAE	*Phoneutria*	Banana spiders
ZORIDAE	*Argoctenus*	
CYCLOCTENIDAE	*Cyclotenus*	
MITURGIDAE	*Miturga*	Miturgid spiders
ANYPHAENIDAE	*Amaurobioides*	
DOLOMEDIDAE	*Dolomedes*	Water spiders
CLUBIONIDAE	*Chiracanthium, Clubiona, Supunna*	Clubionid spiders
GNAPHOSIDAE	*Lampona, Hemicloea*	White tailed spiders, rock spiders
SELENOPIDAE	*Selenops*	
SALTICIDAE	*Phidippus, Breda, Servea*	Jumping spiders
HETEROPODIDAE	*Delena, Heteropoda, Isopoda, Olios*	Huntsman spiders
THOMISIDAE	*Sidymella, Diaea*	Crab spiders
PHILODROMIDAE	*Philodromus*	Crab spiders
LYCOSIDAE	*Lycosa*	Wolf spiders
OXYOPIDAE	*Oxyopes, Peucetia*	Lynx spiders
ZODARIDAE	*Storena*	
ULOBORIDAE	*Philoponella*	
DEINOPIDAE	*Deinopus*	Net casting spiders
NICODAMIDAE	*Nicodamus*	
ARANEIDAE	*Araneus, Arachnura, Argiope, Eriophora, Gasteracantha, Nephila, Phonognatha, Cyrtophora*	"Typical" spiders, orb weaving spiders
LINYPHIIDAE	*Linyphia*	Sheet web spiders
THERIDIIDAE	*Achaearanea, Argyrodes, Latrodectus, Steatoda, Theridion*	Therids, widow spiders, Australian red back spider, house spiders
MIMETIDAE	*Arcys*	
TETRAGNATHIDAE	*Tetragnatha*	Four jawed spiders
MICROPHOLCOMMATIDAE	*Micropholcomma*	

Table 3
Species of spiders reported to cause effects after biting humans[6,8,9,11,12,15,44,58,76,79,86,93,96]

Family	Scientific Name	Common Name	Distribution
MYGALOMORPHS			
Ctenizidae	*Aganippe*	Trap door spiders	Australia
	Arabantis spp.	Trap door spiders	Australia, East Indies
	Bothricyrtum spp.	Trap door spider	California
	Dyarcyops	Trap door spider	Australia, New Zealand
	Ummidia spp.	Trap door spider	North and Central America
Hexathelidae	*Atrax* spp. & *Hadronyche* spp.	Funnel web spiders	Australia
Theraphosidae	*Harpactirella*	Trap door spider	South Africa
	Pamphobetus spp.	Tarantula	South America
	Aphonopelma spp.	Tarantula	North America
	Dugesiella spp.	Tarantula	North America
	Selenocosmia	Tarantula	East Indies, India, Australia
Dipluridae	*Trechona* spp.	Funnel web spider	Central and South America
Actinopodidae	*Missulena* spp.	Mouse spider	Australia
ARANEOMORPHS			
Agelenidae	*Tegenaria agrestris*		Europe, North America
Araneidae	*Araneus* spp.	Orb weaver	Worldwide
	Argiope spp.	Orb weaver	Worldwide
	Neoscona spp.	Orb weaver	Worldwide
Clubionidae	*Chiracanthium* spp.	Sac spider	Worldwide
	Liocranoides	Running spider	Appalachia and California
	Trachelas spp.	Sac spider	North America
Ctenidae	*Cupiennius* spp.	Banana spider	Central and South America, West Indies
	Elassoctenus harpax	Hunting spider	Australia
	Phoneutria spp.	Banana spider	Central and South America
Desidae (Amaurobiidae)	*Ixeuticus (Badumna)* spp.	House spider	New Zealand, Southern California
Dysderidae	*Dysdera* spp.	Dysderid	Worldwide
Filistatidae	*Filistata* spp.	Hackled band spider	Worldwide
Gnaphosidae	*Drassodes* spp.	Running spider	Worldwide
	Lampona spp.	White tailed spider	Australia, New Zealand
	Herpyllus spp.	Parson spider	North America
Loxoscelidae	*Loxosceles* spp.	Recluse spiders	Worldwide
Lycosidae	*Lycosa* spp.	Wolf spiders	Worldwide
Miturgidae	*Miturga* spp.	Miturgid spiders	Australia, New Zealand
Oxyopidae	*Peucetia* spp.	Lynx spider	Worldwide
Salticidae	*Phidippus* spp.	Jumping spider	Worldwide
	Holoplatys sp.	Jumping spider	Australia
	Mopsus spp.	Jumping spider	Australia
	Thiodina spp.	Jumping spider	Americas
Siariidae	*Sicarius* spp.	Six eyed crab spider	Africa
Sparassidae	*Heteropoda* spp.	Huntsman spiders	Worldwide
	Isopoda spp.	Huntsman spiders	Australia, New Guinea, East Indies
	Olios spp.	Huntsman spiders	Americas, Australia
Theridiidae	*Latrodectus* spp.	Widow spiders	Worldwide
	Achaeranea tepidariorum	Grey house spider	Worldwide
	Steatoda spp.	False black widow	Worldwide
Thomisidae	*Misumenoides* spp.	Crab spider	Americas
Zoridae	*Diallomus* spp.	Zorid spider	Australia

A wide range of spiders have been "reported" as causing injury to man, the validity of which is uncertain in some cases, while in others, the toxicity of these spiders is beyond question. Russell suggested that at least 200 species of spiders had been implicated as medically significant[6]. His list, updated, is shown in Table 3.

IV. GENERAL CONCEPTS, SYMPTOMS AND SIGNS FOR SPIDERBITE

A. GENERAL CONCEPTS OF SPIDERBITE

Spiderbite may result in a wide variety of symptoms and signs in the human victim, depending on both assailant and victim factors. Some of these are listed in Tables 4 and 5.

Table 4
Factors affecting symptomatology of spiderbite related to the spider

• The species of spider.	Most species of spider are harmless to humans.
• The sex of the spider.	For several species known to be toxic to man, a specific sex is more toxic, e.g. for widow spiders only the female is clinically toxic to humans, while for Australian funnel web spiders, both sexes are toxic, but only the male has caused fatalities.
• The maturity of the spider.	Usually only adult spiders are clinically toxic to humans
• The individual spider.	As with most other venomous animals there is likely to be variation in venom components and toxicity, both between individuals of the same species and even for a given individual spider over time, dependent on maturity, when venom was last expelled and season.
• The quantity of venom injected.	This will vary greatly.
• Attack position.	For any given species of spider, fang length will be within a narrow range depending on the size of the spider and angle of attack when biting a human victim will determine how effectively the fangs may penetrate skin and inject venom.
• Gut secretions.	For many species of spider, the fang tips at rest are quite close to the mouth parts and it is possible that digestive secretions from the mouth may enter the wound caused by the act of biting a human with the fangs, with consequent effects being due to these digestive secretions as well as the venom. This may be important in causation of some clinically significant local effects of spiderbite.
• Bacterial flora on the fangs, mouth parts and adjacent structures.	The act of biting a human with a fang has the potential to contaminate the wound with any bacteria on adjacent areas of the spider, with the consequence that clinically significant local effects of the bite may be due, at least in part, to secondary infection introduced by the act of biting. The bacterial flora on relevant areas of spiders is not known.
• The number of times the spider bites the human victim.	Multiple bites are, in general, more likely to result in clinically significant effects.
• The length of time the spider takes to make each bite.	A brief glancing strike is, in general, less likely to result in clinically significant effects than will occur if the spider "hangs on", taking some time to bite. However, this is only relative, as the toxicity of the spider concerned is clearly of greater importance.

Table 5
Factors affecting symptomatology of spiderbite related to the human victim

• The age of the human victim.	In general a child or an elderly adult is more likely to suffer clinically significant consequences of a spiderbite than a normal healthy adult. Interestingly this principle is not universal. In the authors experience in Australia with latrodectism (envenoming by widow spiders) it is often large, muscular adult men who seem worst affected by the bite and require the most antivenom to reverse envenoming.
• The size of the victim.	In general the larger the human, the more body mass to dilute any venom and its effects, thus small children are usually at greater risk (but not caveat for latrodectism noted above).
• The position of the bite.	Clearly there are some areas of the body where it will be more difficult for a spider to successfully penetrate the skin and inject venom, such as where the skin is thicker or calloused. For bites causing local tissue injury, bites on peripheral or dependent areas, such as the feet and lower legs, are more likely to result in problems.
• Pre-existing health of the human.	Pre-existing disease may make the results of any spiderbite worse than might be expected in healthy people. Of concern are diseases either decreasing natural immunity to infection or reducing the capacity of local tissue at the bite site to withstand venom effects (e.g. peripheral vascular disease).
• Allergic reactions.	Individual inappropriate immune responses to venom may result in a far more clinically significant bite than would otherwise occur. This may be an "anaphylactic" type reaction, which appears rare with spiderbite, or a more localised reaction which may result in significant and continuing tissue damage. A classic example of atypical local reaction to a bite is the development of pyoderma gangrenosum, which has been associated with loxoscelism.

From these spider and victim associated factors it will be clear that in assessing the most common or likely effect of a bite by a given species of spider, it is important to consider all these factors in each reported case. Unfortunately there is a considerable amount of published material on spiderbite, both scientific and popular, in which assessments of the effect of spiderbite are made without adequate regard to confounding factors. This has resulted in various spider species being linked with particular effects without sufficient substantiating evidence, and sometimes erroneously being accused of causing effects such as skin necrosis. To clearly identify a particular species of spider with a particular syndrome of envenoming with local or systemic effects, it is necessary to have a series of case reports which meet certain criteria. These are:

- The spider must have been caught in the act of biting the human victim.
- The spider must have been kept and identified by a person skilled in identifying spiders.
- The effects of the bite must have been carefully documented and clearly shown to be due to the effects of the bite/venom by exclusion of other factors, where applicable, such as local infection introduced by the bite, specific allergy type reactions to the bite/venom, pre-existing local or systemic disease which might influence outcome (such as peripheral vascular disease, immunologic deficiency etc.).

If the above criteria are met then the case reports have validity. There are some partial exceptions to the above. Most important of these is distinctive symptomatology for the bite of a particular species, notably the widow spiders (latrodectism). These spiders have been well documented as causing a particular set of symptoms and signs which are distinctive and do not appear to be caused by other types of spiders. For epidemiological purposes it seems reasonable to accept series of cases which meet the clinical criteria for latrodectism, even if all the above criteria are not met by each case in the series. Similarly for loxoscelism, case series are often accepted where the criteria for entry are clinical symptoms and signs, without necessarily having a clearly identified spider culprit in every case. For loxoscelism this may not be entirely valid, as it is now accepted that some other sympatric species of spiders have the potential to cause similar skin damage in humans.

Details of symptomatology for selected species of spiders are given in sections of this chapter dealing with major spider groups of clinical importance.

V. GENERAL PRINCIPLES OF PROPHYLAXIS FOR SPIDERBITE

A. AVOIDANCE OF BITES

Spiders are ubiquitous in areas inhabited by humans. They cannot be avoided even in urban environments of "developed" nations. It is fortunate that most species are either reluctant to bite, unlikely to interact with humans in a way that bites may occur, or are not toxic to humans. Some specific measures can be taken to avoid bites by clinically significant species, and these are listed in sections of this chapter dealing with these species.

In more general terms, keeping dwellings clean and free of insect prey which may attract spiders may reduce the likelihood of bites. Avoidance of placing parts of the body in unseen areas where spiders may live will also reduce the chance of bites. This may mean using gloves for gardening in some areas, making sure clothing and footwear is not left in areas where spiders may enter and placing furniture away from walls (notably beds and chairs).

B. PUBLIC EDUCATION ON BITES

In some regions, where spiderbite is a clinically significant problem, public education about avoiding bites may prove useful, either through targetted campaigns or use of more general published information. It is the author's experience that it is far easier to scare a population with misinformation about spiderbite than it is to educate them about the facts on spiderbite.

C. IMMUNIZATION AGAINST SPIDERBITE

Unlike some hymenopteran stings, spiderbite rarely causes severe immediate ("anaphylactic") type reactions and so specific desensitisation is not necessary or practical in affected individuals. Mass immunisation against bites by a particular species of spider causing clinically significant problems has not been reported. As with snakebite, there are some theoretical problems which make such an approach problematic. For species that cause severe life threatening reactions, such as the Australian funnel web spiders, it is unlikely that normally circulating levels of specific antibody induced by immunisation would be adequately protective, and they would not reach protective levels rapidly enough to be useful. For those spiders causing local necrosis the situation is less clear. It may be that even low levels of circulating specific antibody would reduce or even prevent significant local tissue injury, but in general, administration of large amounts of antivenom (i.e. specific antibody) has not proved very helpful in reducing the extent of local venom injury following bites by a variety of animals, such as snakebite.

VI. GENERAL PRINCIPLES OF FIRST AID FOR SPIDERBITE

First aid for spiderbite varies considerably depending on the type of spider involved. Some details are given in the later sections of this chapter. As with any first aid for bites and stings, the first principle must be to do the patient no harm. For most spiderbites there is no need to use any first aid. Methods causing imperilled circulation to the bitten area are generally inadvisable, and tourniquets should not be used. An exception to this is the Australian funnel web spiders, where the Australian snakebite type first aid is considered appropriate (pressure immobilisation bandage). For latrodectism most first aid only worsens local pain.

VII. GENERAL PRINCIPLES OF CLINICAL MANAGEMENT OF SPIDERBITE

A. GENERAL APPROACH TO THE MANAGEMENT OF SPIDERBITE
1. General Approach to the Patient

With the exception of Australian funnel web spiderbite, most spiderbites are not immediately life threatening. They should be attended to promptly however, as in some cases, early treatment may reduce long term effects.

2. Diagnosis
a. Clinical

Establish the circumstances of the definite or suspected bite. Was a spider seen or felt biting? Was it caught (encourage patients to catch the spider and bring it with them) and is it available for identification? Any spiders brought in should be kept, preserved in alcohol (not formalin which alters colouration significantly), and later identified by an expert, if available. What were the immediate and subsequent effects of the bite, both locally and systemically, if any? Determine the patient's general health and pre-existing disease and medications, if any. Has the patient had clinically significant spiderbite previously and is this relevant to the current presentation? Examine the bite area, looking for evidence of fang marks, though these are often hard to see, mutiple bites, local erythema, oedema, bruising, blistering, and necrosis. Are the draining lymph nodes involved? Are there any systemic signs such as sweating, tachycardia, hypertension (or hypotension), excessive lachrymation, piloerection, muscle spasm, priapism, respiratory difficulty or pulmonary oedema?

b. Venom detection

Venom detection is not presently available commercially to determine which type of spider caused a particular bite, but has been used experimentally, particularly for loxoscelism in Brazil, where it has been possible to detect antibodies to *Loxosceles gaucho* venom[16]. The future role of venom detection is uncertain for spiderbite, unlike snakebite, as there are a large range of species of spiders which might need to be included in test systems, and obtaining sufficient venom for development and ongoing manufacture of test systems is both difficult and generally expensive. It is to be hoped that this situation will change, as the ready availability of venom detection for spiderbite would greatly increase our knowledge and ultimately assist development of more precisely targetted treatment.

c. Laboratory investigations

There are generally no specific markers notable for spiderbite amongst the array of routine laboratory tests available. For loxoscelism there are some specific tests which, if positive, strongly suggest the diagnosis, but these are not widely available[17-20]. Unlike snakebite, markers of systemic envenoming such as coagulopathy and myolysis are not seen with spiderbite. Where cases have been reported with either coagulopathy or myolysis, this is generally a secondary phenomenon, not directly related to specific venom effects.

3. Treatment
a. General

If there is systemic envenoming of significance, particularly if it potentially imperils life, then this should take precedence, notably establishment of airway and maintenance of adequate respiratory and cardiovascular function. In some bites, particularly some cases of Australian funnel web spider bite, where rapid development of severe pulmonary oedema may occur, respiratory problems may initially dominate, and may require intubation and other measures. However, for the vast majority of spiderbites such problems are unlikely. Treatment will then include careful wound care, symptomatic treatment and specific treatment (where applicable and available). Tetanus prophylaxis is usually recommended, though cases of tetanus following spiderbite are very rare, if they occur at all.

b. Antivenom

The specific treatment of spiderbite is the use of antivenom in most cases where any specific treatment is available. Antivenom for spiderbite is apparently not as widely used and accepted as for snakebite. There are antivenoms available for latrodectism, Australian funnel web spider bite, loxoscelism and *Phoneutria* bites[21]. For the former two, antivenom, used correctly, is both effective and definitive treatment. The role of antivenom in loxoscelism is less clear, but it is useful in *Phoneutria* bites. Details are given in the relevant sections below.

c. Local necrosis

The treatment of local necrosis after spiderbite is controversial. Antivenom appears to have only a limited value, if any[22,23]. Experience suggests that early surgery to debride the wound is generally unhelpful or worse[24-28]. Late (>2 weeks) debridement may be necessary and justified in a few cases. Steroids do not appear useful, at least in most cases[26,29-31]. Conservative treatment is often the best treatment, or, as stated by one author, "The 'benign neglect' approach nearly always results in an excellent outcome"[32]. This may overstate the final result in severe cases, where long term scarring may occur despite all therapy, or lack thereof. Antibiotic therapy is clearly needed if local infection occurs, but is less certain as prophylactic therapy[25,32]. The choice of antibiotic is unclear but should probably cover staphylococcal and streptococcal bacteria[25]. In Australia flucloxacillin is usually tried first, though this is not necessarily a recommendation. The use of more radical treatments such as dapsone or hyperbaric oxygen is still the subject of debate, but if available, both may have some value in treating significant local tissue destruction, at least for loxoscelism (see below)[23,25,27,32-40].

VIII. THE AUSTRALIAN FUNNEL WEB SPIDERS: *Atrax* AND *Hadronyche*

(This section and others in this chapter dealing with the genera Atrax and Hadronyche are based on a monograph on funnel web spider bite, prepared for the IPCS INTOX Project by Dr. White, but assisted by Dr. M. Grey, Australian Museum, Sydney, and Dr. M. Fisher, Royal North Shore Hospital, Sydney. The author is most grateful to these two colleagues for their input into the monograph, and hence their contribution to this section of the chapter.)

The funnel web spiders, Family Hexathelidae, Subfamily Macrothelinae (Atracinae), are found in Australia, in two genera, *Atrax* and *Hadronyche*, comprising about 35 species, many, possibly all, being potentially dangerous to man[41,42]. At least 13 fatalities are known following funnel web spider bites, all ascribed to the male Sydney Funnel Web, *Atrax robustus* (Figure 10). The known distribution for each genus is shown in Figures 11 & 12[41,42].

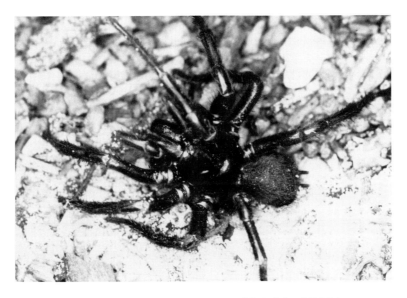

Figure 10. Male Sydney funnel web spider, *Atrax robustus* (photo© Dr. J. White).

A. BIOLOGY AND DISTRIBUTION
1. Biology

They are mostly terrestrial spiders, which build typical silk-lined tubular burrow retreats, with a collapsed "tunnel" or open "funnel" entrance from which irregular silk triplines radiate out over the ground. These distinctive surface triplines, whose function is to alert the spider to the movement of prey animals in the vicinity, provide a reliable means of identifying the retreats of funnel web spiders. Exceptions, which lack triplines but may have trapdoors, are those *Hadronyche* from South Australia, viz. *Hadronyche adelaidensis, Hadronyche eyrei, Hadronyche flindersi.*

The silk entrance tube may be split into 2 openings, in a Y or T form. In the case of *Hadronyche formidabilis* the burrow may be in the hollow of a tree trunk or limb, many metres above ground level.

Significant numbers of these spiders may aggregate their burrows within a small area, forming colonies. The spiders usually forage at the burrow entrance, seizing prey that walks over the triplines. Adult male spiders leave the burrow permanently to seek a mate. Such wandering male spiders may enter houses, sometimes even find their way into clothing, and thus account for many bites.

Most funnel web spiders are ground or log dwellers but at least two are tree dwellers (*Hadronyche formidabilis* and *Hadronyche cerberea* the Northern and Southern tree funnel web spiders respectively). They are moist adapted animals largely restricted to temperate to sub-tropical regions of south east Australia in both sclerophyll and closed (rain-forest) forest habitats. At the western edges of distribution some species occupy dryer woodland habitats where they dig deep burrows in sheltered microhabitats (shaded ground in leaf litter, under rocks or logs etc.). Typically funnel web spiders prefer sheltered microhabitats and in many urban areas these are plentiful, e.g. garden rockeries, dense shrubberies, wooden sleeper or stone paths and retaining walls and any long-term ground detritus such as old building materials. In areas such as the damp garden suburbs of Sydney, urbanisation may actually have increased funnel web abundance.

2. Taxonomy

In addition to the general features of Mygalomorph spiders, funnel web spiders also have the following distinguishing characteristics[41,42]:

(a) They are large to very large spiders, body length 15 - 45 mm (excluding the jaws or chelicerae), dark brown to black in colour overall, the abdomen often dark plum coloured. The carapace covering the front part of the body is almost hairless and so appears smooth and glossy. The body lacks any obvious patterning.

(b) Spinnerets obvious, four in number, the apical segments of the large posterior spinnerets always longer than wide.

(c) Eyes closely spaced.

(d) The labium, a small ventral plate found on the ventral cephalothorax in the midline, immediately in front of the sternum, and between the two maxillae, is studded with many short peg-like spines (cuspules).

(e) The fang grooves, into which the fangs fold at rest, have a row of strong teeth along both margins (marginal teeth), and a variable number of smaller teeth within the groove itself.

(f) Carapace foveal groove concave forwards.

(g) The tarsal segments of the legs are spined and lack thick scopulae or claw tufts.

(h) The second leg of male spiders may have a spur (spined apophysis) of variable shape, on the ventral tibia. However, males of many *Hadronyche* species lack obvious apophyses.

Distinguishing features for each genus are:

Atrax: Carapace weakly raised and obviously longer than wide. Central fang groove teeth confined to basal half of groove. Male second leg with a large, conical tibial apophysis. Posterior lateral spinnerets with a long cylindrical apical. The principal species is the Sydney funnel web spider, *Atrax robustus*, but there are two other species yet to be fully described.

Hadronyche: Carapace moderately to strongly raised, often almost as wide as long. Central teeth typically occupy full length of fang groove in one or several rows, but occasionally restricted to basal region. Male second leg with a variably developed rounded tibial apophysis or apophysis absent. Apical segment of posterior lateral spinnerets of variable length but often rather short. There are at least 32 species of *Hadronyche*, many of which are yet to be fully described. Principle species include *H. adelaidensis*, *H. cerberea*, *H. eyrei*, *H. flindersi*, *H. formidabilis*, *H. infensa*, *H. meridiana*, *H. modesta*, *H. pulvinator*, *H. valida*, *H. venenata*, and *H. versuta*.

3. Distribution

Funnel web spiders (Australian) are restricted to south-eastern Australia.

Atrax is confined to south-eastern coastal Australia and adjacent highlands (Figure 11). *Atrax robustus*, the Sydney funnel web spider, has a distribution centering on Sydney, extending north to the Hunter River and south to the Shoalhaven River, and narrowing westwards as far as Lithgow[41,42].

Hadronyche has a considerably wider distribution (Figure 12). Many species distributions can be related to local topography. Overall, the distribution of *Hadronyche* is correlated with the coastal trend of the eastern highlands from Tasmania to south east Queensland, where the western trend of the main range into dryer inland regions approximates the northern limits of the genus[41,42].

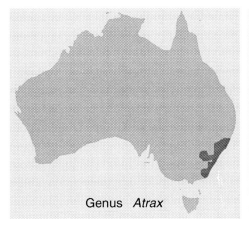 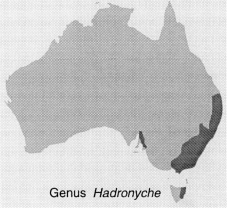

Figure 11. Australian distribution of funnel web spiders of the genus *Atrax*.

Figure 12. Australian distribution of funnel web spiders of the genus *Hadronyche*.

B. VENOM

Paired flask-shaped venom glands in the chelicerae connect via 4 mm venom ducts to openings at the base of the paired paraxial fangs, approximately 6 mm long in *Atrax robustus*. At rest the fangs are folded into the fang grooves on the ventral surface of the chelicerae, but for attack the front of the body is elevated above the prey and the fangs open downwards on widely separated chelicerae preparatory to the downward thrust of attack[43,44].

The venom exits the fang near its tip, and is apparently under some degree of voluntary control, as venom initially exuded on the fang tip when the spider is threatened can then be withdrawn back into the fang. Venom yield has been reported for *Atrax robustus* as 0.28 mg for females and 0.175 mg for males, on milking, and 0.25 mg (F) and 0.81 mg (M) on dissection of spiders. An average figure was 140 µg dry weight. Yields are apparently higher in summer than winter months[44,45].

While the venoms of most species of *Hadronyche* and the two unnamed *Atrax* have not been studied, those known to cause significant clinical effects in man, particularly *Atrax robustus*, have been examined in detail. Consensus of these studies is that lethal activity (for man) is contained in just one component of these multicomponent venoms. In *Atrax robustus* male venom toxicity is consistently several times (4-6) higher than female venom.

1. Venom Composition

a. Robustoxin (from male Atrax robustus *venom)*

(Note: A component with similar or identical properties to robustoxin has been described by other authors, and named atraxotoxin (and possibly atraxin). As the most complete studies are for robustoxin, this name is adopted as the "type" even though, historically, atraxotoxin has precedent[44,46-50].)

Robustoxin is a unique presynaptic neurotoxin, lethal in man, other primates, and newborn mice, but non-lethal in many other laboratory animals (or lethal only at very high doses)[51-53].

It is a protein, MW 4854 (calculated from amino acid sequence), with 42 amino acid residues, with a high proportion of basic residues, 8 cysteine residues with 4 disulphide bridges and has a pI >9 and an LD_{50} (SC newborn mice) of 0.16 mg/kg. Robustoxin alone causes a typical syndrome of envenomation in primates and man of whole male *Atrax robustus* venom[51-53].

b. Versutoxin (from male and female Hadronyche versuta *venom)*

Structurally very close to robustoxin, a protein neurotoxin, MW 4852, 42 residues, highly basic, pI >9, 4 disulphide bridges. 8 residues are different to robustoxin, and these are considered conservative changes. LD_{50} (SC newborn mice) is 0.22 mg/kg. Versutoxin alone causes a syndrome of envenomation in primates and man almost typical of whole male *Atrax robustus* venom, the difference being the sustained hypotension typical of robustoxin, which is not seen with either versutoxin or whole *Hadronyche versuta* venom. There is strong antigenic cross-reaction between robustoxin and versutoxin[52].

c. Venoms of important related species

Hadronyche formidabilis - Venom is reported as approximately equal in toxicity (both male and female) to male *Atrax robustus* venom, and has caused similar cases of envenomation in man (no definite fatalities), and therefore probably contains a robustoxin-like component[44].

Hadronyche infensa - Venom reported as approximately equal or greater in toxicity (females and males) to male *Atrax robustus* venom, and therefore may contain a robustoxin-like component[44].

d. Other physico-chemical characteristics

Several other components or properties of male *Atrax robustus* venom have been reported. These include: GABA; Spermine Complex; Lactic acid; Trimethylsilyl or pentafluoropropionate derivatives; Citric acid; Glycerol; Urea; Glucose; Glycine; Spermidine; Tyramine; Octopamine[44,46-48].

2. Pathophysiology of Envenoming

The venom, when injected experimentally in monkeys, rapidly causes systemic problems, these being immediate (if given IV) and delayed about 2 minutes (if given SC), suggesting that the venom may be rapidly transported from the bite site systemically. The role of lymphatics in venom transport is uncertain, but in view of the rapid envenomation often seen, lymphatic transport of most venom seems unlikely. However, the compression-immobilisation technique of first aid is effective[54].

Having reached the systemic circulation the main toxin (to man) in the venom is rapidly distributed to target organs, principally nerve cells, and particularly synaptic junctions where the toxin is apparently bound presynaptically (autonomic and motor neurons).

There is no published information on the half-life of the venom or its components. Human fatalities have occurred from 15 minutes to 6 days after bites. Cases with survival following severe systemic envenomation have an average hospital stay of 14 days (if **no** antivenom treatment)[44].

Studies on the mode of action of both whole venom and robustoxin have been hampered by low availability of venom and relative resistance to venom in many common laboratory animals, contrasting with the exquisite sensitivity to venom toxins in primates, including man (50 - 100 times more sensitive in some preparations)[44].

The clinical effects of funnel web spider envenoming in man (and monkeys) appear directly attributable to one venom component, robustoxin. This appears to act as a presynaptic neurotoxin. On the autonomic system the venom causes both inhibition of neurally mediated release of transmitters (e.g. noradrenaline, acetylcholine) and an increase in spontaneous transmitter release. A similar action on the skeletal muscle neuromuscular junction has been postulated[44,54-56].

Given the current paucity of relevant *in vitro* studies of the mode of action of the venom, the detailed *in vivo* studies in primates (*Macaca fascicularis*) are most relevant. In summary, the effects recorded after experimental envenomation (IV or SC) with whole venom from male *Atrax robustus* were:

(a) Cardiovascular - initial fall in blood pressure (BP), then rise to hypertensive level, lasting several hours, followed by return to normal or progressive hypotension (lethal). Tachycardia, ventricular ectopic beats, bigemeny and transient second degree atrio-ventricular blocks were seen, though not in all monkeys.

(b) Pulmonary oedema - seen in 3 of 9 monkeys.

(c) Acid-base disturbances - all developed acute metabolic acidosis about 1 hour post envenomation, resolving spontaneously by 4 hours. Most developed a respiratory acidosis.

(d) Intracranial hypertension - seen in all monkeys.

(e) Temperature - all developed hyperthermia.

(f) Catecholamine excretion - marked increase in urinary catecholamines, peaking at about 2 hours after envenomation.

(g) Fluid shifts - all showed haemoconcentration.

(h) Creatine kinase - all showed massive rises in CK.

(i) Pharmacological denervation - both pre and post-envenomation administration of atropine + phenoxybenzamine + propranolol abolished the major features of envenomation and allowed survival of "massive" doses of venom.

The lethal dose for adult humans is not known, but a single bite from an adult male *A. robustus* is potentially lethal and the average venom yield is 176 μg. The recommended initial dose of antivenom is sufficient to neutralise *in vitro* about 8 times this amount of venom. Children, especially those under 12 years of age, are more susceptible to severe or lethal envenoming, presumably due to a lower body mass, hence higher concentrations of venom.

Most experimental animals, being relatively resistant to the venom, are not equatable to human toxicity. For experimental purposes two groups of animals appear useful, having susceptibility to the venom of male *A. robustus*, sufficient for comparative clinical studies (monkeys) or for toxicity assay (newborn mice)[44,45,57].

- Monkeys (*Macaca fascicularis*)
    lethal dose 0.2 mg/kg
- Newborn mice (up to 2 days old, 2 g weight)
    lethal dose 1.5 μg/kg

While not demonstrated in clinical cases, theoretically adrenaline might have adverse effects in an envenomed patient (and is therefore not recommended as pre-medication for antivenom therapy), because catecholamine levels may already be elevated as a result of envenomation[44].

Both experimentally and clinically, atropine and diazepam may ameliorate the toxic effects of venom.

Experimentally the effects of venom (on isolated nerve-muscle preparations) are suppressed by gallamine, suxamethonium, lignocaine and tetrodotoxin; are enhanced by physostigmine; and are unaffected by neostigmine, choline or acetylcholine.

C. EPIDEMIOLOGY

Funnel web spiderbite is restricted to the range of these spiders in parts of eastern and southern Australia. The number of bites occurring yearly is not known, but there is some evidence to suggest that only a minority of bites results in significant envenoming. Indeed, possibly as few as one in ten cases require antivenom. Since the introduction of specific antivenom in 1980, there have been over 40 cases treated; thus if the ratio of 1:10 is correct, there is an average of about 30 to 40 cases per year.

Highest risk is in areas where dangerous species occur, especially *Atrax robustus*, but also *Hadronyche infensa, Hadronyche formidabilis, Hadronyche versuta, Hadronyche cerberea,* and *Hadronyche sp.7,* such as the Sydney-Newcastle-Illawarra region, but even those species not yet confirmed as dangerous should be treated with caution; therefore the true risk area should be considered as the entire range of the two genera, involving parts of Queensland, New South Wales, Victoria, Tasmania and South Australia. It is possible for vagrant male spiders to be accidentally transported well beyond the natural distribution; thus cases of envenoming might occur anywhere connected to the natural range by transport systems. It is unlikely that the spider would survive extended sea or air travel, so cases outside of Australia are unlikely to occur, except from deliberately imported specimens.

Some potentially high risk activities in areas where known lethal species occur include:

- Walking barefoot, especially at night, outside places of abode.
- Dressing in items of apparel left on or near the floor where wandering male spiders might easily enter, including footwear.
- Working in areas likely to have high concentrations of spiders, e.g. gardens and other disturbed sheltered urban habitats in some parts of the Sydney region.
- Activities associated with camping.
- Activities associated with handling spiders such as in laboratories milking venom, or field researchers. NOTE: No bites in such circumstances are recorded.

High risk times for funnel web spiderbite are particularly during the mating period, when male wandering activity and abundance is highest. The summer-autumn period (December-June) is the time of greatest activity for males of many species. While most bites occur during this period funnel web spiders can be encountered throughout the year. In addition pesticide spraying to kill spiders stimulates wandering activity and excitability in much of the target funnel web population and is not recommended. Increased activity after heavy rainfall also occurs because of burrow flooding.

D. SYMPTOMS AND SIGNS
1. General

In the majority of cases of funnel-web spider bite, systemic envenomation does not occur, and any symptoms are confined to the local effects of the bite. The outcome cannot be predicted at the outset however, and all bites should be assumed to be potentially lethal.

2. Local

One or two large fangs enter the victim with some force. The bite is very painful for about 30 minutes or more, with local erythema, and occasionally local piloerection, sweating, and muscle fasciculation. Local necrosis does not occur.

3. Systemic

Onset of systemic envenomation may occur from 10 minutes up to an hour or more after the bite (with further delay if appropriate first aid used).

Earliest systemic symptoms are usually perioral tingling around the mouth which often occurs within 15 mins of the bite, tongue spasms, followed by nausea and vomiting, abdominal pain, profuse sweating, brisk salivation, lachrymation, and severe dyspnoea.

The level of consciousness may rapidly deteriorate, with confusion or coma. Hypertension is usually noted at this time. Severe pulmonary oedema may develop quite early, and is a potential cause of fatality, particularly in children. The pulmonary oedema is mixed in origin, similar to neurogenic pulmonary oedema, with catecholamine release, high filling pressures, and membrane leak.

While classic neurotoxic paralysis does not occur, local and generalised muscle fasciculation is commonly seen, including spasms of muscle groups such as jaw musculature. In severe cases coma has been reported, and some authors believe it may be due to raised intracranial pressure (not relieved by adequate control of oxygenation or BP), although this has not been proven in man. However clinical experience suggests coma is not common, and is probably a dubious sign of envenomation, most envenomed patients being anxious and alert until anaesthetized. Patients treated with antivenom do not develop coma on current experience.

After several hours the above symptomatology may subside, with decreased secretions, although generalised muscle activity and coma may continue. There may be a gradual resolution or an insidious and intractable hypotension may develop, sometimes preceded by a brief period of semi-normality. The hypotension may end in death due to irreversible cardiac arrest, a possible mode of death in fatal cases in adults, sometimes many hours after the bite.

The venom does not cause primary coagulopathy or renal failure, though these may occur as complications.

Funnel web spider envenomation is a complex multisystem disease.

4. Course, prognosis, cause of death

The likelihood of systemic envenomation is not presently predictable from the appearance of the bite site or local symptoms.

The only recorded fatalities have followed bites by male *Atrax robustus*[44,58-76]. Severe envenomation not ending fatally has occurred following bites by *Hadronyche formidabilis* (male specimens, but females also considered dangerous), and *H. infensa* (one possible fatal case), and more recently, *H. versuta, H. cerberea,* and *Hadronyche sp.7*[44,76,77]. *H. versuta* in any case should be considered as potentially dangerous since its venom contains a robustoxin-like substance, Versutoxin[78]. Bites from virtually all other funnel web spiders are unknown. A single bite from *H. adelaidensis* did not result in envenomation[79].

Sutherland[44] has noted that children usually die in the asphyxial stage (important role of pulmonary oedema) early, often within 1 - 2 hours of the bite (shortest time 15 minutes, longest 3 days), while adults die later, often due to intractable hypotension or secondary complications, mean 11 hours (excludes one case dying at 6 days with complications including coagulopathy, renal failure and brain damage). This picture is clearly modified by the growing experience with patients treated by specific antivenom therapy, which has proved most efficacious in modifying symptomatology, and preventing a fatal outcome.

5. Systematic description of clinical effects
a. Cardiovascular

Initial fall in BP and development of tachycardia, followed by hypertension lasting several hours, and cardiac arrhythmias, followed by apparent resolution which in severe cases heralds the onset of intractable hypotension, and ultimate cardiac arrest in fatal cases. Peripheral circulatory failure with peripheral cyanosis has been recorded (mostly based on monkey studies)[80-82].

b. Respiratory

There may be early development of severe pulmonary oedema. While some clinicians have described this as akin to the adult respiratory distress syndrome, with increased pulmonary capillary membrane permeability[72], it appears more likely it is akin to neurogenic pulmonary oedema, which is mixed in origin, with catecholamine release, high filling pressures, and membrane leak.

c. Neurologic
i. CNS

Early development of impaired consciousness or coma in severe cases has been noted, either directly due to venom effects, or secondarily due to causes such as hypoxia (pulmonary oedema)[70,72]; however, it is general clinical experience that patients do not present with or develop early coma, but rather are anxious and alert. Raised intracranial pressure may develop and may be lethal (experimentally in monkeys, not shown in man).

ii. Peripheral nervous system

There are widespread effects of the neurotoxic action of robustoxin and analogues with spontaneous transmitter release, and failure of response to stimuli, manifest as muscle fasciculations, tremors, spasms, and patchy weakness (which is usually a late manifestation).

iii. Autonomic

There are widespread effects of the neurotoxic action of robustoxin or analogues on synapses in the sympathetic and parasympathetic systems, with spontaneous release of transmitters, manifest as alterations in vascular tone, and excessive secretions, especially salivation and lachrymation, and piloerection.

d. Other effects
i. Gastrointestinal

Specific effects of toxin not generally noted, although nausea and vomiting are common, and gastric distension is noted.

ii. Metabolic

Patients may develop acute metabolic acidosis early followed by respiratory acidosis. Fluid shift out of circulation (cf. pulmonary oedema) may occur. Hyperthermia is reported. Massive rises in serum creatine phosphokinase may occur and marked catecholamine excretion in urine (studies in monkeys).

E. PROPHYLAXIS

Prevention of bites depends on the at risk populations being aware of the habits of the funnel web spiders, particularly the males, whose wanderings are most likely to bring them into contact with humans, including entering dwellings. High risk activities and circumstances, as listed under epidemiology (above), should be minimised or avoided.

F. FIRST AID

Sutherland's work on first aid methods is now widely accepted as the standard, although tourniquets are still used as first aid in a disturbingly high number of cases[44,54,55,75]. Of more importance is the finding that in many cases no first aid has been used, a situation which is most disturbing considering the rapidity of onset of life threatening problems in severe cases and the effectiveness of correct first aid in delaying such problems. Possibly even more vigorous public education would help.

First aid for funnel web spiderbite is the same as for Australian snakebite (see chapter 27), namely the use of a pressure immobilisation bandage[44,54,55]. Severe, even life threatening envenoming can develop very quickly, and deaths within the first hour are reported, so correct and urgent application of first aid and transport to hospital is crucial[44]. Respiratory or cardiovascular collapse require priority first aid management, if they occur. The spider should be removed from the victim carefully, if still attached, ensuring no further bites occur, then placed in a container and brought to the hospital with the victim. A broad bandage, such as crepe (but even torn strips of clothing or pantyhose may be used), should be applied over the bite area as quickly as possible, while keeping the victim still and calm. The bandage is applied at firm pressure, as for a sprained ankle, not so tight that it impairs circulation to the distal limb significantly. Further bandage is then used to bind the rest of the bitten limb, at the same pressure as above. The limb is then immobilised using a splint. If applied correctly this first aid can safely be left in place until the patient reaches a hospital where definitive treatment (i.e. antivenom) is available.

G. TREATMENT
1. General principles

All cases of suspected bite by funnel web spiders occurring in areas inhabited by *Atrax robustus*, *Hadronyche formidabilis*, *H. infensa* and *H. versuta* should be treated as potentially life threatening emergencies[44,76,84-88]. This is especially true of bites to children from male *A. robustus*.

If appropriate first aid has not been applied and it is within 2 hours of bite or symptoms of systemic envenomation are present, then it should be applied prior to assessment at a funnel web spider treatment centre. If first aid has been applied it should be left in place until the patient is at a treatment centre (exception: arterial tourniquet where viability of the limb is at stake, but beware rapid massive envenomation on removal).

Main principles of medical management are:
(a) Maintain life through general measures including life support systems if indicated.
(b) Neutralise venom with specific antivenom (funnel web spider antivenom, CSL, Melbourne) if systemic envenomation is present.
(c) Strive to avoid secondary complications, e.g. hypoxia and hypoxic damage, brain damage, renal failure, coagulopathy.

2. Laboratory Tests

There are no specific assays for funnel web spider venoms. While the development of a venom assay, akin to those developed for Australian snake venoms, might allow further clinical and experimental study of venom actions, because of the nature of funnel web spider envenomation compared to snakebite, it would not be likely to have the same clinical impact as the snake Venom Detection Kit (CSL Melbourne), and from both a clinical management and economic viewpoint is of quite dubious value.

All tests are to determine the extent of effects of venom systemically, e.g.
- Arterial blood gases - extent of hypoxia and response to treatment.
- Serum/plasma electrolytes, acid base, renal function - extent of metabolic acidosis, secondary renal impairment.
- Serum creatine kinase - secondary elevation.
- Complete blood picture - early evidence of secondary coagulopathy, haemo-concentration.
- Coagulation studies - required if suspicion of secondary coagulopathy (rarely present, not usually seen acutely in the first 8 hours after bite).
- Urinary catecholamines - may be significantly elevated.

3. Life supportive procedures and symptomatic treatment

Severe funnel web spider envenomation is a complex multi-system disease, best managed in an ICU setting, preferably in a treatment centre with previous experience in handling such cases. Good IV line access should be urgently established at the place of first medical contact, prior to transfer to a treatment centre (i.e. a hospital stocked with CSL funnel web Antivenom).

a. Respiratory

Severe pulmonary oedema causing hypoxia and respiratory failure demands urgent ICU management which classically includes intubation and mechanical ventilation (intermittent positive pressure ventilation, IPPV; positive end expiratory pressure, PEEP), oxygen, possibly high dose steroids (now believed contraindicated), and later, possibly diuretics (role uncertain)[44,70,72]. CVP line, arterial line, and Swan-Ganz catheter have proved valuable for monitoring.

b. Circulatory

This is usually managed in conjunction with respiratory problems. Isoprenaline, and volume replacement with SPPS or albumin, may be required. Dopamine is probably contraindicated.

In the early stages where hypertension and tachycardia are a problem, sympathetic blockade has been suggested[44]. While alpha blockade has been used, it requires massive doses, and beta blockade might well prove lethal in this situation and is not advocated for funnel web envenomation[45].

c. Pharmacologic

Atropine has proved valuable, e.g. for para-sympathetic blockade. Diazepam has also been suggested, but only when ventilation is supported.

There is some suggestion that prolonged immobilisation of venom at the bite site using recommended first aid may allow local destruction of venom.

4. Antivenom

The availability since 1981 of specific funnel web spider antivenom (CSL, Melbourne) has dramatically changed the pattern of funnel web spiderbite envenomation sequelae. In all cases where envenomation has occurred it is the definitive and preferred treatment[44,71,74,76,90,91].

Sutherland has defined the following as clinical indicators of systemic envenomation by male *A. robustus*[44]. The presence of any of the following is an indication of envenomation for which antivenom is required:

- Muscle fasciculation in the limb involved or remote from the bite, usually first seen in tongue or lips when systemic spread of venom has occurred.
- Marked salivation or lachrymation.
- Piloerection.
- Significant tachycardia.
- Hypertension in a previously normotensive patient.
- Dyspnoea.
- Disorientation, confusion, or a depressed level of consciousness.

In most cases of bites by funnel web spiders, no symptomatology will develop, other than local pain of limited duration due to the mechanical trauma of the bite. These patients do not require antivenom.

Funnel web spider antivenom is prepared by hyperimmunising rabbits with male *A. robustus* venom, and is therefore a rabbit immunoglobulin. The average quantity per ampoule is 100 mg of purified rabbit IgG, which is enough to neutralise *in vitro* the average venom yield from at least 4 adult male *A. robustus*.

Sutherland recommends prophylactic pre-treatment with antihistamine and a steroid, about 15 minutes prior to antivenom[44]. Pre-medication with adrenaline is not recommended[44]. Subcutaneous testing for allergy is not recommended[44]. The antivenom should be given intravenously, initially very slowly. The initial dose is a minimum of 2 ampoules, or 4 ampoules for a severe case, and repeated in 15 minutes if no improvement. As with all antivenoms, everything should be prepared to treat anaphylaxis should it occur; however, anaphylaxis has not been reported in these cases, and theoretically it is unlikely it could occur in severe cases due to the neuroendocrine response. The dosage is the same for children and adults. Serum sickness has not occurred following therapy with funnel-web spider antivenom. In the unlikely event of occurrence, steroid therapy may be worth consideration. The antivenom prepared against *A. robustus* venom has now been shown potent against bites by other species[76].

- Adult dosage: Minimum 2 ampoules, most cases will require 4 or more ampoules. Up to 8 ampoules are sometimes required in severe cases and in one case of double bite by *A. robustus*, 18 ampoules were required to fully reverse all symptoms (Dr. I. Whyte, personal communication, 1995).
- Child dosage: As for adults.

While systemic envenomation by male *A. robustus* and some other funnel web spiders is a severe, potentially fatal complex multi-system illness, the advent of specific antivenom has significantly modified the likely outcome and problems encountered. Its development and dissemination by Sutherland and colleagues at CSL Melbourne has been the crucial step in ameliorating this envenomation syndrome and dramatically reducing the likelihood of fatalities. As a result, much of the pre-antivenom controversy about management practices and medication is now largely redundant. The important work of Fisher and others had established valuable precedents in the successful treatment of severe envenomation in an ICU setting, prior to antivenom availability[70,72].

IX. OTHER MYGALOMORPHS

Numerous other Mygalomorph spiders are known to have or are likely to have bitten humans, but for most species, these bites are minor. For some species, irritation of the skin from fine abdominal hairs is far more significant clinically than the effects of a bite, as is the case with the large Mexican orange kneed tarantula, *Brachypelma emelia*, which is sometimes kept as a pet (Figure 13)[92,93]. The Arizona Tarantula, *Aphonopelma chalcodes*, though large, does not seem to cause clinically significant bites, or only short lived local symptoms including oedema, pain and lymphadenitis (Figure 14)[11,94,95]. The Australian trapdoor spiders, notably *Aganippe subtristis*, though aggressive when dug up from their burrow home (Figure 15, 16), do not appear to cause any significant injury if they bite[79,96]. The male mouse spiders, *Missulena* spp. (Figure 17, 18), also Australian, are reported to have very toxic venom, but human bite cases substantiating this are virtually non-existent (a single case from Queensland)[44]. The Australian Theraphosid, *Selenocosmia stirlingi* (Figure 19, 20), has been reported to cause a systemic illness following a bite, but not life threatening[11,63]. Several South American mygalomorphs are reported to be possibly or definitely toxic to man, causing neurotoxic symptoms, but details are scant (*Sericopelma* sp., *Phormictopus* sp. *Acanthoscurria* sp.)[11]. The South African spider, *Harpactirella* sp., can apparently cause local pain and even collapse[11].

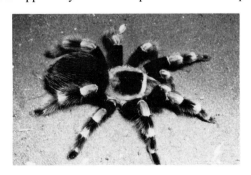

Figure 13. Mexican orange kneed tarantula, *Brachypelma emelia* (photo © Dr. J. White).

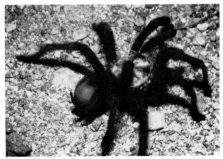

Figure 14. Arizona tarantula, *Aphonopelma chalcodes* (photo © Dr. J. White).

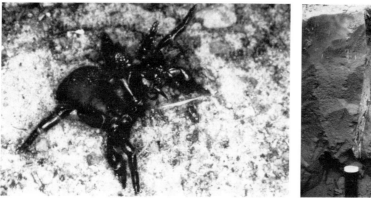

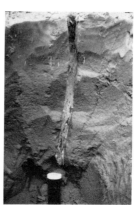

Figure 15. Australian trapdoor spider, *Aganippe subtristis* (photo © Dr. J. White).

Figure 16. Excavated burrow structure of trapdoor spider.

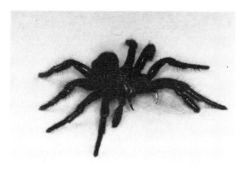

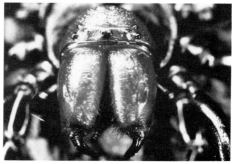

Figure 17. Australian mouse spider (male), *Missulena* sp. (photo © Dr. J. White).

Figure 18. Close up of face of mouse spider (photo © Dr. J. White).

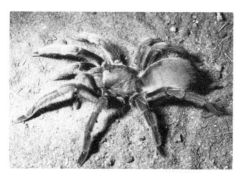

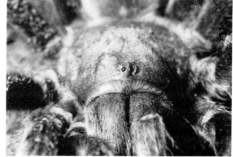

Figure 19. Australian "bird eating" spider, *Selenocosmia stirlingi* (photo © Dr. J. White).

Figure 20. Close up of face of bird eating spider (photo © Dr. J. White).

X. THE WIDOW SPIDERS: LATRODECTISM

(This section and other sections of this chapter dealing with *Latrodectus* are based on a monograph on widow spiderbite, prepared for the IPCS INTOX Project by Dr. White, but assisted by Dr. Robert Raven, Queensland Museum, Brisbane. The author is most grateful to Dr. Raven for his input into the monograph, and hence his contribution to these sections of the chapter.)

The single most medically important group of spiders worldwide is the Widow spider group, genus *Latrodectus*, the bite of which may result in a characteristic set of symptoms and signs, known as latrodectism. These spiders are members of Family Theridiidae, which contains a wide variety of species, several others of which may be harmful to man. They are typically small to medium sized spiders, usually with a globular abdomen, relatively small cephalothorax, and long thin legs. They utilise a web structure for prey aquisition. In the case of the Widow spiders, this includes the use of sticky drop lines. They are cosmopolitan, well able to survive, even thrive, in urban environments, and are thus likely to come in contact with man. Typical species are shown in Figures 21,22,23,24. The worldwide distribution of Widow spiders is shown in Figure 25. The taxonomy of *Latrodectus* is contentious and is currently being reviewed. It is likely that significant changes will be made in the forseeable future.

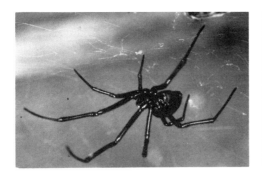

Figure 21. Female widow spider, *Latrodectus mactans*, from Arizona, U.S. (photo © Dr. J. White).

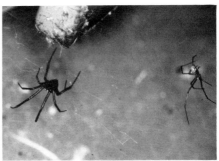

Figure 22. Female and male widow spider together in web (photo © Dr. J. White).

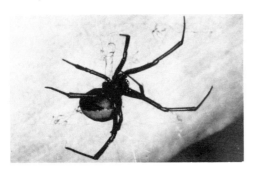

Figure 23. Female Australian red back spider, *Latrodectus hasseltu* (photo © Dr. J. White).

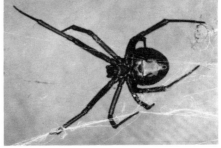

Figure 24. Underside of female red back spider (photo © Dr. J. White).

A. BIOLOGY AND DISTRIBUTION
1. Biology

Widow spiders are found in many diverse habitats throughout the world, their anthropochorus nature derived from the rich variety of suitable habitats provided by human urban environments and transport vehicles. In nature they seem to prefer drier habitats, seemingly most content in desert or near desert conditions.

2. Taxonomy

The taxonomy of the genus *Latrodectus* has been one of the most highly disputed and least resolved problems facing arachnologists. An indication of the intensity of the argument is given by the unusually hostile exchange between Dahl[97] and Cambridge[98] at the turn of the century (see Levi for summary[99]). Cambridge[100] listed 43 species and he recognized only 6 as distinct.

The situation remained unresolved for many years. In 1959, noted theridiid taxonomist Herbert W. Levi revised the genus *Latrodectus* and again only 6 species were recognized[99]. Many groups had almost identical genitalia. However, traditionally, differences in genetalic structure had always been the indicator *par excellence* of species differences. The problem then lay in establishing the significance of the abdominal pattern of the various "races" or "subspecies" in the face of almost identical genitalia. In Argentina, Abalos[101] noted correlations between habitat or microhabitat and abdominal pattern. To these differences he assigned species significance and those have not been contested. Levi later revised all of his previous conclusions about species differences in *Latrodectus*[102]. Many studies were done in the U.S. and elsewhere in which the species used was listed as *L. mactans*, the black widow. Clearly, a number of species were included within that catch-all name. At best, in some cases, data can be recovered where only one or two species are known from the country in which the study specimens were taken. This has clear implications in interpreting both toxinologic and clinical data from the literature which must be considered by the reader in using the information in this chapter.

Widow spiders are large comb-footed spiders. The lateral eyes on each side are separated from each other. The legs are of medium length; first usually longer than the last. The abdomen is usually subglobular. Males are much smaller than females. The ventral surface of the abdomen usually has a red hourglass mark or vestiges of this. The web is strong, usually with a tubular retreat of tough silk[99].

3. Distribution

The genus *Latrodectus* is found worldwide (see Figure 25) as far north as central Europe (50°N) in the U.S.S.R., but not extending much north of France in western Europe[7,106,108,109]. They are not known from the United Kingdom yet (but there are some recent unconfirmed reports of imported *L. hasseltii*). They are found north to about latitude 40°N in North America[106]. In the Southern Hemisphere they reach the southern tips of Africa and Australia and southern Argentina[7,12,44,86,93,106,107].

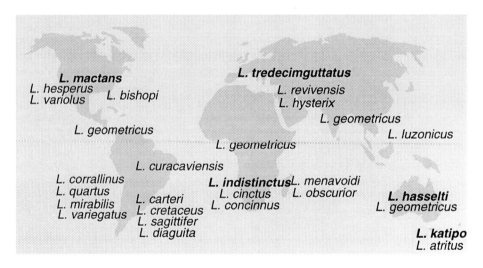

Figure 25. Worldwide distribution of widow spiders, genus *Latrodectus*.

Table 6
Species of *Latrodectus*[103] and some common names

Genus	Species	Common Name
Latrodectus	(whole group)	Araignee a cul rouge; Arana capulina (Mexico and Central America); Arana naranja (Antilles); Arana venenosa de Chile; Black spider (Jamaica); Black widow (North America); Casampulga (Guatemala); Menavoudi (Malagassy); Pallu or Guina (Chile); Lucacha (Peru); Atocatl (Mexico); La Coya; Poto Colorado (Chile); Cojo (Columbia); Mico mico (Bolivia); Veuve noire (France); Viuda negra (Spain); Laualaua (Philippines)
"	*ancorifer*	
"	*antheratus*	
"	*aruensis*	
"	*atritus*	
"	*bishopi*	
"	*carteri*	
"	*cinctus*	
"	*concinnus*	
"	*corallinus*	
"	*cretaceus*	
"	*curacaviensis*	Araignee orange de Curaco
"	*dahli*	
"	*diaguita*	
"	*elegans*	
"	*geometricus*	Brown widow
"	*hahli*	
"	*hasseltii*	Redback spider, jockey spider, murra-ngura, kapara, kana-jeri[104]
"	*hesperus*	
"	*hystrix*	
"	*indicus*	
"	*indistinctus*	Button spider, black widow, knoppie-spinnekop[12]
"	*insularis*	
"	*katipo*	Katipo
"	*limacidus*	
"	*luzonicus*	
"	*mactans*	Black widow
"	*menavodi*	
"	*mirabilis*	
"	*obscurior*	
"	*pallidus*	
"	*quartus*	
"	*renivulvatus*	
"	*revivensis*	
"	*rhodesiensis*	
"	*sagittifer*	
"	*schuchi*	
"	*stuhlmanni*	
"	*tredecimguttatus*	Ragno velenoso, palangium, tarantula, malmignatto, ragno venefico, ragno rosso, malmignatte, latrodecte di volterra, karakurt
"	*variegatus*	
"	*variolus*	

B. VENOM
1. Venom Composition

Venom is produced in venom glands situated in the cephalothorax. The glands contain holocrine secretory epithelium covered by a layer of intrinsic musculature resting on a basal membrane or extracellular gland sheath. There appear to be several populations of secretory cells. Droplets of secretion are released when contraction of the intrinsic musculature causes compression of the extracellular gland sheath, resulting in expulsion of venom[44].

Expelled venom travels through paired ducts traversing the cephalothorax, then chelicerae, exiting at the base of each of the paired fangs located at the basal end of the chelicerae. It then travels through the hollow fangs exiting near the tip.

During the act of biting the spiders cephalothoracic musculature contracts also adding compressive pressure to the glands.

The venom of *Latrodectus* spp. is multicomponent, but the major toxic fractions are variations of a protein, latrotoxin, with most varieties being non toxic to man. However, one common component, alpha latrotoxin, with a MW of 130,000 D, is active against man[44].

Only the actions of alpha latrotoxin, which is the neurotoxin active against mammalian tissues, are of relevance in human envenomation, although some of the other venom fractions are of relevance in non-clinical research. Alpha latrotoxin is a potent stimulator of release of transmitter substances from neurons throughout the nervous system. Thus it causes depletion of synaptic vesicles and an initial increase in mepps coresponding to releases of the transmitter acetyl choline at the vertebrate neuromuscular junction, equating to a variable presynaptic blockade and consequent patchy paralysis of voluntary muscle[44,110-113]. Similarly it has been shown to cause depletion of the transmitter catecholamines at adrenergic nerve endings in the autonomic nervous system[113,114], and stimulation of release of the transmitters acetylcholine, norepinephrine, and gamma amino butyric acid from brain synaptosomes[116,117]. It also appears to have similar actions at sensory nerve terminals[118]. Alpha latrotoxin has been shown to increase the permeability of lipid bilayer membranes by forming ionic channels[119], and it has been suggested that it stimulates transmitter release by both increasing nerve ending permeability to cations and directly stimulating release by a process of redistribution of membrane components, possibly also inhibiting vesicle recycling[120]. The membrane effects of the venom appear specific to neuronal tissue, suggesting either a differential toxic binding by specific cell types or differential responses of cells to uniformly bound toxin[110,119], although the apparent concentration of the toxin in neural tissue may suggest the former[121].

No detailed information is available on toxic doses of venom in man. However from clinical data it is clear that untreated latrodectism is potentially lethal, with deaths reported throughout the worldwide range of *Latrodectus* spp., specifically from Italy, Australia, Argentina, Chile, Madagascar, South Africa, and the U.S.A.[107]. In the U.S. a fatality rate of 6% has been reported[122], although this may well be an overestimate due to case selection[107]. More recently, a mortality rate of 5-10% has been reported for latrodectism in the Middle East[123], though this figure is probably again an overestimate. In a 10 year period (1950-1959) 65 people died as a result of spider bite in the U.S., all but 2 being attributed to latrodectism[5]. A series of 463 cases of *L. tredecimguttatus* bite in Uzbekistan did not result in any fatalities[109].

Extensive animal data on both whole venom and fractions toxicity are available. For whole venom there is a wide range of susceptibility depending on the target species, an effect repeated for the fractions. The data for *L. mactans tridecimguttatus* whole venom toxicity for various species are summarised in Table 7[110].

Table 7

Toxicity of *Latrodectus* venom in experimental animals[110]

Test Animal	LD$_{50}$ (mg./kg.)*
Frog	145 +/- 32
Canary	4.7 +/- 1.7
Blackbird	5.9 +/- 2.7
Pigeon	0.36 +/- 0.07
Chick	2.1 +/- 0.57
Cockroach	2.7
Housefly	0.6
Guinea pig	0.075
Mouse	0.90

2. Pathophysiology of Envenoming

There is little substantiative data on rate and mode of absorption of widow spider venom in man, but it is well established on clinical grounds that venom travels principally via the lymphatic system until reaching the blood stream and it appears that a significant proportion of the venom remains at or near the bite site where it is presumably eventually metabolized[110,121].

Again, there is little data on the distribution of the venom in man, but clinical evidence suggests that latrodectism principally involves the nervous system, and by inference venom is widely and effectively distributed throughout the nervous system. Animal experiments indicate this is the case, with peak concentrations in the central nervous system and peripheral nerves in guinea pigs, but venom was also detected in the lungs, heart, liver, spleen, and a large amount remained locally around the bite site[121,124].

Data on the metabolism and half life of venom in man is essentially clinical, indicating that venom may directly or indirectly cause envenoming effects which without specific (antivenom) treatment can cause symptomatology for several days or even weeks, but that the most severe effects usually start to dissipate after about 24 to 36 hours. However experience with the late use of specific antivenom where such therapy has dramatically and rapidly effected a resolution of symptomatology even five days after the bite suggests that there was a significant quantity of active venom still present and at effector sites at the time of therapy; thus the active venom components may have a long half life in man.

C. EPIDEMIOLOGY

Of those spiders clearly identified with a particular syndrome of envenoming, the widow spiders, *Latrodectus* spp., causing latrodectism, are the most significant. Their global distribution, commonness in many areas, moderate to high likelihood of contact with man within their habitat and potent venom ensure that they cause numerous bites. Fortunately only the minority of bites result in significant envenoming, and fewer still require antivenom therapy.

Risk factors for widow spider bite include working in areas infested with widow spiders, particularly if working with bare hands. It is typically considered an occupational hazard, especially for farmers in some regions such as Argentina[124] and Yugoslavia[106,125]. High risk farming activities have included harvesting and threshing of cereal and other crops, harvesting of grapes, and work in some rural buildings. In Australia in the past a high percentage of bites were to the genitalia while using stand-alone toilets (outback dunny), e.g. 64%[61], 80%[58,126]. However these toilets are now much less common, so that this mechanism of bites appears to be reducing in frequency. In Australia the red-back spider *L.hasselti* is common along fence lines, in sheds, and around gardens and rubbish, and most bites now occur when humans are working in or near these environments. In urban areas introduced populations of widow spiders may reach plague proportions putting large metropolitan populations at risk, especially while gardening or working in hot metal sheds or along metal fence lines.

Bites are more common in the warmer months in subtropical and temperate areas, but may occur at any time of year. In tropical areas bites occur at all times of the year.

Epidemics of latrodectism are well documented and have been recently reviewed[106,127]. These epidemics appear directly related to an abnormal increase in spider population density. In one epidemic in Yugoslavia spider densities for *L.mactans tridecimguttatus* reached several specimens per square meter[128]. Such massive increases of spider numbers are usually temporary, and related to ecological change or climatic aberration. A second important component in epidemics of latrodectism is an increase in man-spider contact. This has particularly related to large scale movements of people into an area where spiders are common, and historically is most often associated with troop movements. Since 866 A.D. epidemics have been recorded from the following places (number of reports in brackets, from Maretic[106]): Italy (5), Sardinia (2), France (1), Corsica (3), Spain (2), Bulgaria (1), Yugoslavia (6), Russia (6), Morocco (1), Uruguay (1), New Zealand (1). Recently epidemic loxoscelism has been reported from Uzbekistan[109].

The highest risk areas are those where widow spiders are known to inflict a potentially lethal bite. The most venomous species appear to be *L. hasseltii* from Australia, and *L. indistinctus* from southern Africa, based on clinical reports.

a. North America

L. mactans is the most important species in this group in North America, though several other species can cause bites, notably *L. hesperus* and *L. geometricus*. Of all deaths from poisonous and venomous creatures in the U.S. between 1950 and 1959, only 65 (14.1%) were due to spiders, 63 of these attributed to *Latrodectus* spp.[5]. In comparison, in the same series, there were 138 deaths due to snakebite and 229 deaths due to insect stings, most or all of the latter presumably due to anaphylactic type reactions to bee or wasp stings. Most bites and deaths occurred in the southern and eastern states (Figure 26; Table 8). Where the time interval between bite and death was noted (n=54) only 17 (32%) occurred in the first 24 hours. Given the nature of latrodectism it might be inferred that many of the deaths were due to secondary problems such as pneumonia. Of those deaths, 20 were in children under 10 years of age (31%), yet this age group accounts for less than 25% of all widow spider bites. The other major group noted was people over 50 years age, who accounted for 52% of all deaths, though well under 50% of all bites. In a more recent series of 163 cases of latrodectism there was one death attributed to bronchospasm[129].

Table 8
Deaths from spider bite in the U.S., 1950 to 1959

Region	Number of Deaths
New England States	0
Middle Atlantic States	1
East North Central States	3
West North Central States	10
South Atlantic States	14
East South Central States	11
West South Central States	21
Mountain States	4
Pacific States	1

b. South America

Latrodectism occurs throughout the Americas, from Canada to Patagonia including central America, and the islands of the Caribbean. Latrodectism in South America is less well documented than for North America, and appears to be less common, representing only a small proportion of spiderbite cases seeking medical attention, at least in eastern regions such as Brazil. However, latrodectism is apparently infrequent in Colombia and Brazil where it is largely limited to the south. A recent study from Brazil showed only 0.22 % of cases of spiderbite seen at hospitals were definitely due to *Latrodectus* spp. (see Table 12). Cases have been reported from Argentina[130,131]; Colombia[132]; Brazil[132,133] and Uruguay (unpublished data). Severe envenoming is reported from Chile[135]. At least in Brazil, latrodectism appears to be less severe than seen in North America, Australia and some other regions.

c. Europe

Latrodectism exists throughout much of Europe, especially the more southern regions, including Spain, Italy and the Balkans. It has been reported occurring in France, Corsica, Portugal, Spain, Italy, Sardinia, Yugoslavia, Greece, Greek Islands, Bulgaria, Hungary, Rumania, Poland, and Russia[7,106].

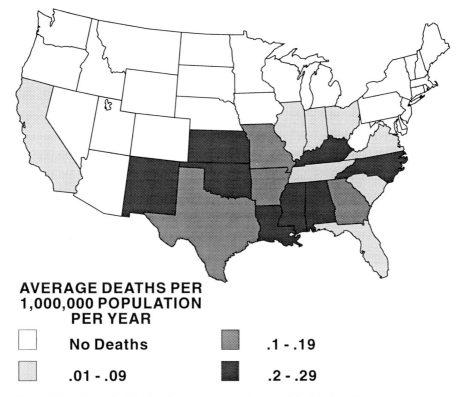

**AVERAGE DEATHS PER
1,000,000 POPULATION
PER YEAR**

☐   **No Deaths**   ▨   **.1 - .19**

▨   **.01 - .09**   ■   **.2 - .29**

Figure 26. Incidence of spiderbites (Latrodectism) deaths in the U.S., After Parrish.

d. Africa

Most information on latrodectism in Africa originates from southern Africa, where *L. indistinctus* is the most important species[12,14]. However reports suggest that it occurs throughout Africa, encompassing all of north Africa including Egypt, Lybia, Tunisia, Algeria, Morocco, the Atlantic islands of Madeira, Canary Islands, Porto Santo, St. Helena, and the Gold Coast, Senegal, Congo, Cameroun, Togo, Sudan, Ethiopia (Abysinia), Kenya, Zimbabwe, South Africa, and Madagascar[12,14,7,106,107-109].

e. Asia

Latrodectism is less well reported for most of Asia, although isolated reports and unsubstantiated information given to the author suggests that it may be quite common in central Asia. It has been reported from Asiatic Russia, Mongolia, Turkey, Syria, Lebanon, Israel, Saudi Arabia, Yemen, Aden, India, Nepal, Sri Lanka, Maldives, Loyalty Islands, Myanmar, Indonesia, Borneo, New Guinea, Vanuatu, Marianas, Malaysia, Polynesia, Bismark Archipelago, Philippines, Hawaii, islands of the western Pacific, south of Okinawa, and on Ryukyu and Ishigaki[7,106,109].

f. Australia

Latrodectism is the most common form of medically significant spiderbite in Australia[44,86,96,136,137]. One report listed 2144 cases of bite by the local species, *L. hasselti*, nearly all of which required antivenom therapy[137]. However, as this series was generated from returns to the antivenom producer, this is hardly surprising, and other reports from Western Australia[136] and the author's experience in South Australia suggest that most cases of bites by the red back spider do not result in significant envenoming, which is likely to occur in only 20% or less of cases. Latrodectism also occurs in New Zealand and New Caledonia[106].

D. SYMPTOMS AND SIGNS

All known cases of human envenomation by *Latrodectus* spp. are due to bites by female widow spiders.

Bites may occur on any part of the body where the spider may gain access, including inside clothing. The area most frequently bitten varies with location and historical era; thus for farmers harvesting in Yugoslavia most bites are to the hand or arm[106], while in Australia in the past when the "outback toilet" was common most bites were to the exposed genitalia occasioned while using the toilet, 64% of cases[61], and even as high as 80%[126], while more recent surveys in Australia have shown a steady decline in this method of bites, 22%[138], and most recently 9.7%[137]. Currently in Australia most bites occur on the extremities, 74%[137].

Severity of symptomatology and rates of envenomation is variable both within species and between different geographic populations of each species, and between species. A significant proportion of all *Latrodectus* bites will not result in envenomation or symptomatology. Despite earlier reviews which suggested most bites were significant, a more comprehensive review of latrodectism in Australia showed that only 21% had symptoms sufficiently severe to require antivenom therapy[136].

The syndrome of envenomation by *Latrodectus* spp., latrodectism, has consistent syndromic features that often are distinctive enough to make the diagnosis likely even if the spider was not identified. However a wide range of less frequently seen symptoms and signs may occur which may make diagnosis difficult, and cause other conditions to be considered initially, the classic example being acute abdomen.

1. Local effects

Even if a significant bite has occurred it may cause little or no local pain initially, or just a sensation of a mild sting. In one series from Yugoslavia 58% of patients did not experience local pain at the time of the bite[139]. Similarly patients bitten while asleep may not be woken by the initial bite, thus obscuring the identity of the culprit[106]. After a variable period, usually between 5 to 60 minutes after the bite, symptomatology occurs. This is usually manifest as local pain of increasing severity, either at the bite site and spreading to involve most of the bitten limb and eventually the regional lymph nodes, a sequence that may take 30 mins. to several hours and is typical of Australian latrodectism (*L. hasselti*)[44,86]; or in the regional lymph nodes only, as noted from Yugoslavia (*L. mactans tridecimguttatus*)[106]; or local pain only which is mild to moderate and may be of brief duration, subsiding prior to development of more generalized symptoms, as noted in North America (*L. mactans, L. mactans hesperus*)[93]. The local wound may be invisible, or present as one or two puncture marks, or associated with local erythema, or with central blanching surrounded by erythema, sometimes with red lines extending towards draining lymph nodes. There may be local sweating, and occasionally local swelling, heat, or pruritis. However the dominant local feature of latrodectism is pain.

2. General

Only the minority of cases will develop generalized symptomatology from latrodectism, but these are distinctive from all regions where latrodectism occurs[7,12,15,44,86,93,106,127,136-156]. When such problems do develop they may do so after about one hour, but more usually will gradually develop over many hours, and onset may be delayed for 12 hours or more. Systemic latrodectism is more severe in the young, the elderly, and the infirm. Systemic spread of venom is frequently heralded by swollen or tender regional lymph nodes. The dominant systemic manifestation of latrodectism is pain. The pain may be generalized, or localized to parts of the body nearer the bite site; thus upper limb bites may cause predominant pain in the face, neck or chest (the latter occasionally being mistaken for cardiac pain), while bites to the lower limb frequently result in predominant abdominal pain, which may mimic acute abdomen. Bites to any part of the body may cause abdominal pain. Muscle cramps and spasms are common and may result in board-like rigidity of some muscle groups, notably those of the abdomen (less common for Australian latrodectism). There may be profuse sweating which may be localized to an area quite distant to the bite site, or may be generalized (more common in Australian latrodectism). The patient will usually have a marked malaise, feel generally weak, and may have difficulty in performing simple tasks. There may be a generalized muscle weakness, but true paralysis is rare. Other symptoms noted include nausea, vomiting, parasthesiae, pyrexia, insomnia, dizziness, headache, generalized rash, hypertension, diarrhoea, haemoptysis, dyspnoea, dysuria, severe trismus, anorexia, periorbital oedema, generalized arthralgias, generalized tremors, restlessness, photophobia, lachrymation, psychosis, bradycardia or tachycardia and apparent anuria secondary to sphincter spasm. Of note in latrodectism from North America and Europe is *Facies Latrodectismica*, a flushed and sweating face contorted in a painful grimace with swollen eyelids, a strong blepharoconjunctivitis, lachrymation, and often chelitis, rhinitis, trismus of masseters, photophobia, and often early miosis followed by later midriasis, increased fundal filling of veins, and occasionally tinnitus[106,140] .

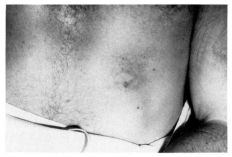
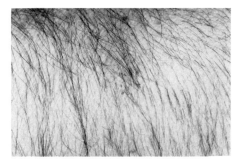

Figure 27. Local erythema and peticheae following a bite by an Australian widow (red back) spider (photo © Dr. J. White).

Figure 28. Central blanching with surrounding erythema following a bite by an Australian widow (red back) spider (photo © Dr. J. White).

Infants may present differently, typically screaming with pain, which may come in spasms with calm periods interspersed, and with more rapid onset of symptomatology, often more severe, and abdominal pain and rigidity appears more common. The spider may be found in the bedding or clothes if searched for. The sudden onset of severe pain, regional skin changes (erythema), and a marked tachycardia in an apyrexic infant is suspicious of latrodectism[44,157].

3. Course

There are essentially three major outcomes of a *Latrodectus* bite:

1) A trivial bite with minimal local symptoms and no general symptoms. This is a common outcome of bites. No sequelae.

2) A locally painful bite which may cause moderate to severe local pain for up to several hours, but which does not progress to generalized latrodectism. Moderately common. No sequelae, but note some cases may initially present this way, and may progress to generalized latrodectism only many hours later, possibly after local symptoms have resolved.

3) Development of generalized (systemic) latrodectism. This occurs only in the minority of cases, despite some publications which suggest it is the usual outcome. In Australia it has been reported as present in only 22% of cases despite the apparent high frequency of cases of widow spider bite in that continent[136].

The progression of symptomatology in systemic latrodectism is of very variable rate, from a matter of a few hours to several days, but in most cases the peak is at about 24 hours. However if untreated there may be residual symptoms lasting several days up to a week or more, and the patient may feel debilitated for a much longer period. In the recovery phase there may be an intense burning sensation in the soles of the feet[153]. Antivenom dramatically curtails the natural progression, and most patients achieve a complete termination of symptomatology[44,86,93,106,127].

4. Prognosis

Most patients will develop only minimal or mild envenomation. Of those who develop generalized latrodectism most will recover substantially within one week even without treatment. Death is a rare outcome and is most likely in the young, the elderly, or the infirm. In North America a death rate of 6.7% has been reported[122], but this is most likely an overestimate due to selection of cases and in untreated cases the actual death rate is almost certainly considerably lower than this[106]. In most regions there have been no deaths in patients treated with antivenom. In Australia there have been no deaths reported from latrodectism since the introduction of specific antivenom in 1956[44,137,141]. In Australian fatal cases time to die varied from 6 hours to 30 days, with only one case dying in under 24 hours, an infant of only 3 months age dying at 6 hours[61].

5. Cause of Death

Information on the cause of death in cases of latrodectism is scant. In a 15 year old male there was severe pulmonary oedema, marked hyperaemia of pia and the brain, oedema of medullary pia, and hyperaemia of the liver, kidneys, cortex of the adrenal glands and other organs at autopsy[106,154]. In a fatal case from Australia the only finding at autopsy was intense lymph gland enlargement along the spinal column[60,158]. Some of the complications of latrodectism such as severe hypertension, cardiac disturbances, and renal damage may lead to fatal outcomes (e.g. cerebral haemorrhage, heart failure, myocardial ischaemia, renal failure, secondary infections etc.)[106]. Respiratory paralysis does not appear to be a significant cause of death in latrodectism.

6. Systematic description of clinical effects
a. Cardiovascular

Both bradycardia and tachycardia have been reported, but the usual sequence appears to be an initial tachycardia followed by later bradycardia which in untreated cases may become severe[106]. Other problems reported include arrythmias[106,144,159-162], ECG abnormalities[93], cardiac insufficiency[163], extrasystoles[162], systolic murmurs[122,161] and palpitations[122].

ECG changes reported include high P_2 and P_3 waves, slurring of the QRS complex, depression of the ST segment and T waves, and prolongation of the QT interval[106].

Atrial fibrillation 72 hrs. after the bite and 24 hrs. after resolution of symptoms has been reported in a bedouin man[165]. Urinary VMA was increased in this patient.

Hypertension is a common finding in latrodectism, usually seen once systemic envenomation is established, as there may be an initial hypotension after the bite[106]. Severe hypertension occurs occasionally, and pressures as high as 250 systolic, 170 diastolic may be seen, at least in Australian cases of latrodectism, although this is an unusual complication, at about 3% of cases with systemic involvement[137,141]. It has been speculated that the hypertension is due to a direct effect of the venom on the vasomotor centres of the

CNS, with secondary release of adrenaline from the adrenal glands, and noradrenaline from the sympathetic system[106,124,166,167].

The venom causes marked vasoconstriction, except the vessels in the skin of the head where marked vasodilatation may occur[106]. This may have implications for those patients with myocardial function or perfusion defects prior to the bite.

b. Respiratory

True respiratory paralysis due to latrodectism is a doubtful entity, for which there are few case reports. A series from Australia noted 10 cases (in a series of over 2000 cases) which required assisted ventilation[137], while an earlier series reported "paralysis" without details[141], but a major review of latrodectism worldwide did not note respiratory paralysis[106]. However patients with pre-existing respiratory problems, notably asthma, may be at increased risk of respiratory problems due to latrodectism, as the venom increases bronchial secretion and bronchoconstriction[106]. Pulmonary oedema is reported[168].

c. Neurologic
i. CNS

The venom has direct CNS activity, mediating a variety of effects via the central effects, including effects on the motor, sensory, and autonomic systems. There is direct excitatory activity, with EEG changes experimentally[124,128]. The toxin breaches the blood brain barrier[169]. Psychic disturbances may occur including acute psychoses[128,150,170], deep torpor[150], prolonged amnesia[149], confusional states[147], insomnia[137,141,147,150,152,162,171,172], visual disturbances, hallucinations and deleria[122,147,153,173].

ii. Peripheral nervous system

The pain which is the hallmark of latrodectism is at least partly mediated through a direct effect of the venom on the sensory system as well as a central.
iii. Autonomic nervous system

There is an increase in all secretions, particularly profuse sweating, but also increased salivation, lachrymation, rhinitis, and increased secretions in the gastrointestinal tract, urethra, and bronchi may occur[106]. Midriasis, miosis, priapism, and ejaculation may all occur.

d. Skeletal and smooth muscle

There is a generalized muscular hypertonia due to direct venom effects on the neuromuscular transmission system, and this may manifest as boardlike abdominal rigidity, or there may be clonic contractions, a fine tremor, or fibrillations[106,128,137,141,161].

e. Gastrointestinal

Through effects on the nervous system there may be gastrointestinal symptoms. Nausea and vomiting may occur, in up to 50% of cases in some series[128], but usually less (20%, 24% in Australia)[137,141]. There may also be heartburn type indigestion, stomach dilatation, and hypersalivation[106].
i. Differentiation from acute abdomen

Latrodectism may mimic acute abdomen and in children particularly where a history of spiderbite may not be available latrodectism should be considered in the differential diagnosis of acute abdominal pain[106,124,142]. Table 9 lists key differentiating points between latrodectism induced abdominal pain and a true intra-abdominal pathology[106,174].

Table 9
Differentiation between latrodectism and acute abdomen as a cause of acute abdominal pain

Symptom or sign	Latrodectism	Acute Abdomen
Report of spiderbite, or local evidence of a bite	may be positive	negative
history of gastric problems or symptoms	negative except by coincidence	mostly positive
collapse or shock	not frequent	frequent
blood pressure	increased	low or normal
facies	facies latrodectismica	sometimes facies abdominalis
localization of pains in the abdomen	usually absent	present
radiographic evidence of intra abdominal air	negative	may be positive
rigidity of musculature	positive	negative
pains in thighs and feet	positive	negative
motoric restlessness, anxiety	positive	negative

ii. Hepatic

No reports of significant hepatic involvement in clinical cases, apart from one report of enlargement of the liver[175], but experimentally in rats latrodectism has caused parenchymetous degeneration and necrotic zones in the liver[176].

f. Urinary

In patients with systemic latrodectism the majority may show oliguria or even anuria during the first 12 hours, most likely due to urinary retention secondary to venom effects on the sphincter, or decreased urinary output secondary to dehydration, itself secondary to profuse sweating, vomiting, salivation, or initial shock[106].

i. Renal

Though rare, renal injury has been described[124], including nephritis[155]. Experimentally in rats renal oedema and degeneration or necrosis of the tubular epithelium has been seen[176].

ii. Other urinary problems

The urine may be of high specific gravity, and albuminuria and sediment with leukocytes, erythrocytes, and rough granular casts may occur[122,124,141,156,172,177]. Priapism and even ejaculation may occur[122,144,153,173,178]. Dysuria may occur[137,141].

g. Dermatologic

Apart from the local effects of the venom at the bite site a rash may occur, usually several days later (in untreated cases). Typically the rash occurs on the fourth day, and may be scarlatiniform, morbilliform, or papulous, localized around the bite site, or generalized, and it may be pruritic[106]. In Australia this rash is often described as "prickly heat" and may occur in 4% of envenomed cases[137].

The local appearance of the bite site typically may result in a small area of local erythema, which may be associated with local sweating or piloerection. There may be an area of central blanching, which may be sharply demarcated by a reddish-blueish border (usually seen several hours later[169]), and local oedema may occur. There may be ray like beams of erythema corresponding to lymphatic drainage, and local anaesthesia, hypoaesthesia, or hyperaesthesia may occur[106,127,128,137,141]. Local necrosis is not usually seen, though may occur following *L. mactans tridecimguttatus* bites in Yugoslavia[128]. This may be the result of local treatment however[179].

h. Eye, ear, nose, throat; local effects

Generally not affected, but periorbital oedema, conjunctivitis, and tinnitus have been reported following envenoming by *L. hasselti* in Australia[137,141].

i. Haematological

Non-specific effects include leukocytosis, with neutrophilia, lymphopenia, eosinophilia, haemoconcentration, and monocytosis[106,122,141,172]. ESR is said to be normal[106] although there is a report of raised ESR from Australia[141], and a coagulopathy is not seen, at least as a primary effect of the venom[172]. However haemoptysis has been reported[137].

j. Immunologic

No specific effects on the immune system have been noted, other than initial transport of the venom via the lymphatic pathways and subsequent concentration in lymph nodes seen clinically as swelling or tenderness of regional nodes. Lymphopenia has been noted[106]. A bite from *Latrodectus* does not appear to result in immunity for subsequent bites, and Wiener[141] found no neutralizing antibodies in the sera of 8 patients who had had latrodectism (not treated with antivenom) 2 to 7 months previously.

k. Metabolic

Acid base disturbances have not been noted. However, a slight hyponatraemia, hypochloraemia, and hyperkalaemia, hyperphosphataemia, has been described[128]. Disturbances of fluid and electrolytes would be expected if there is dehydration, a not uncommon finding in severe latrodectism[106]. A transitory hyperglycaemia may occur and there may be a rise in blood urea[106,127]. A rise in urinary VMA in association with atrial fibrillation is reported[165].

l. Allergic reactions

Though details are not given anaphylactic shock to the venom has been reported[137]. An apparent death due to anaphylactic reaction to the venom has occurred in Australia[44].

m. Pregnancy

There are few case reports of latrodectism in pregnant women. A bite by *L. mactans hesperus* in the U.S. to a 20 week pregnant woman resulted in both local and abdominal pain and cramps, relieved by antivenom therapy, with delivery of a normal baby 18 weeks later[180]. Similarly bites by *L. mactans tridecimguttatus* did not cause abortion in women bitten during the 2nd., 4th., and 8th. months of pregnancy[128]. Latrodectism treated with antivenom in pregnant women has not caused abortion or deleterious effects to the foetus in Australia[44].

n. Myolysis

Myolysis does not appear to be a problem with latrodectism, but there is a single case report from Australia suggesting a rise in CK associated with envenoming by the Australian red back spider[181].

E. PROPHYLAXIS

There are no specific measures available to avoid bites from widow spiders, other than the more general principles of prophylaxis outlined earlier in this chapter.

F. FIRST AID

There is no agreed definitive first aid measure for latrodectism, and the use of tourniquets, compressive bandages and similar methods of delaying venom movement are not useful, and are not recommended. Indeed they may make the pain worse for the patient. Similarly local scarification, incision, or excision is not recommended and is potentially harmful. Local application of heat can make the pain worse[147]. It is sometimes suggested that application of a local ice pack may relieve the local pain in the early stages, although there is no trial to prove this. Transport the patient to a medical facility for assessment and treatment. Respiratory and heart failure are very rare in latrodectism and only exceptionally will patients require respiratory support while being transported to medical care. Therefore in nearly all cases the patient may be safely transported in private transport. If the patient is unconscious nurse on side and keep airway clear. Do not give the patient alcohol.

G. TREATMENT
1. General Principles
Latrodectism is rarely, if ever, immediately life threatening, even in small children, though it is symptomatically very distressing in severe cases. Correct treatment will both give the patient good symptomatic relief and greatly foreshorten the period of significant envenoming and (for adults) lost productivity. If there is a suspicion of a *Latrodectus* spp. bite observe the patient closely for at least 3 hours after the bite (some centres routinely observe these patients for at least 6 hours even if asymptomatic). Establish past medical history, including allergic tendencies and past exposure to horse serum or antivenom, and any associated reactions to such therapy. Determine if the patient is dehydrated, and treat accordingly including intravenous therapy if indicated. If the patient has evidence of envenomation with symptomatology then consider specific treatment measures rather than control of significant pain using analgesics alone.

2. Diagnosis
Before treatment can be commenced a definite or probable diagnosis of latrodectism or bite by a *Latrodectus* spp. spider must be established. This may be obvious, i.e. the patient saw the spider bite and brought it in for identification, or it may be obscure, i.e. a small child brought in for assessment of abdominal pain or just screaming due to cause unspecified, or the presentation may be between these two extremes. As there is no laboratory test diagnostic of latrodectism, diagnosis must usually be on purely clinical grounds.

a. Clinical
Latrodectism is likely if the patient has severe generalized pain without other pathologic cause, particularly abdominal pain associated with a non-tender but rigid abdomen, and the diagnosis is more certain if there is a history of preceding bite or pain in a localized area, or if there is profuse sweating without fever, or if there is associated hypertension. The range of symptoms in latrodectism is great (see above). Be aware that a significant number of people bitten by *Latrodectus* spp. will not develop envenomation (up to 80%), and that envenomation may develop late, after 6 to 24 hours, or may present with atypical symptomatology. Maintain a high index of suspicion for the diagnosis, especially in young children who may give a misleading history and present as an apparent abdominal emergency.

b. Laboratory tests
There is no specific test for latrodectism. Other laboratory tests should be performed only as indicated on general clinical grounds, i.e. serum electrolytes if there is dehydration, tests for renal function if there is a suspicion of renal problems, chest X-ray if there is pulmonary oedema, a white cell count if there is a suspicion of infection or other intra-abdominal pathology, and such other tests as may be indicated.

3. Life supportive procedures and symptomatic treatment
Life is rarely threatened by latrodectism, although the patient may feel very ill subjectively and may even think they are dying. Those at most risk of a fatal outcome are

children under 16 years age, adults over 60 years. age, and those with other medical problems, notably myocardial instability or ischaemia where envenomation may precipitate infarction. All those with severe envenomation should be considered at risk.

Life supportive treatment is therefore not usually required and if needed should be directed to control of specific problems that arise. If there is significant respiratory distress then consider respiratory support, commencing with oxygen therapy and proceeding to intubation and ventilation only if required (very rarely needed). Similarly support cardiac function as indicated clinically.

As discussed above, the principle symptom in most patients with symptomatic envenomation is severe pain. It is general experience that oral analgesics will not be helpful in pain relief for most patients, and even narcotic analgesics such as morphine and pethidine may often prove ineffective. Simple measures, notably immersing the patient in a bath of hot water, apparently did give temporary relief of pain in some cases[147], but if more definitive treatments are available such older remedies are not recommended. The best relief of all symptomatology, especially pain, is specific antivenom therapy. As an alternative to antivenom, calcium gluconate iv has been widely reported, as has the use of antispasmodic and muscle relaxent drugs; however, there is ample evidence these are not as effective as antivenom.

4. Antivenom

The principle decision in treating a case of latrodectism is whether or not to use specific antivenom therapy. The alacrity with which it is used is dependent not just on availability but local medical custom and artificial restraints imposed by national legal systems (e.g. in North America). Alternative therapies to antivenom are also discussed later.

The definitive treatment of systemic envenomation by *Latrodectus* spp. is neutralization of venom by antivenom. However the indications for antivenom therapy differ from region to region despite the relative uniformity of latrodectism worldwide. A variety of antivenom manufacturers produce specific anti-*Latrodectus* antivenom each based on venom milked from local species, but given the apparent homogeneity of the principle venom component responsible for human symptomatology across the range of species and geographic boundaries, it would appear that all such antivenoms would have significant and useful neutralizing capacity for any case of latrodectism. Thus countries which do not produce their own antivenom should be able to use the antivenom produced by their nearest regional producer.

For most regions of the world it is accepted that the antivenom should be used if the patient has significant systemic envenomation, that is if the patient has generalized pain or regional pain distant to the bite site (e.g. abdominal pain), or other symptoms or signs of systemic envenomation such as muscle cramps or fasciculation, profuse sweating, hypertension etc. as discussed earlier. Antivenom should be given as soon as possible once indicated on clinical grounds, but a long delay between development of symptoms and availability of antivenom should not preclude its use if the patient is still symptomatic, as antivenom has proved very efficacious even several days after the onset of envenomation[142].

Route of administration of antivenom is variously recommended as iv or im, depending on the country and severity of envenomation. Excluding North America the most usual recommendation is that im is the preferred route as it gives a good therapeutic response within 60 mins. (often within 20 mins.), and is less likely to result in significant adverse reactions than iv. However if the patient has life threatening or very severe envenomation mandating a rapid response then the iv route is indicated. In either case the incidence of anaphylaxis to such antivenoms is very low, estimated at well under 1%. In a large series from Australia where latrodectism and its treatment with antivenom is common, only 11 of 2062 patients receiving antivenom developed anaphylaxis (0.54%), and in no case was this fatal, and 5 of these 11 received undiluted antivenom iv, a practice best avoided[137]. If antivenom is to be given iv it is preferable to dilute it about 1 in 10 with sterile normal saline solution. Any patient receiving antivenom is at risk of anaphylactic type reactions which may occur immediately or after 5 to 60 mins., rarely longer, and therefore it is essential that prior to giving antivenom by any route full provision is made to treat acute reactions including the immediate availability of adrenaline in appropriate dosage drawn up ready in a syringe, and resuscitation equipment.

Premedication prior to antivenom therapy is controversial, but particularly in view of the low rate of reactions to anti-*Latrodectus* antivenom premedication with subcutaneous adrenaline, or im/iv antihistamine or hydrocortisone is not recommended as a routine practice. It may be considered if the patient is known to be allergic to the antivenom or horse serum, or if the facilities for treatment of anaphylaxis are not ideal (e.g. in some rural hospitals etc.).

Pretesting for allergy to antivenom using a small subcutaneous test dose of antivenom is not a useful procedure and is not recommended. It is still advocated by the North American producer of antivenom and by some physicians in the U.S. where failure to perform such testing may have legal implications should a reaction to the antivenom occur. Those practitioners using antivenom in the U.S. would have to consider this in deciding on what course to follow; however, it is the opinion of the authors of this monograph that such pretesting for antivenom sensitivity is not a medically valid practice.

For those treating latrodectism in the U.S. the guidelines for use of antivenom published within that country are different to those recommended in this chapter. In general the current recommendations in the U.S. are that antivenom should be reserved for patients with severe or life threatening envenomation, and then only used after the challenge with subcutaneous antivenom is negative. If the patients meet these criteria the antivenom is given iv rather than im. Premedication is not recommended.

The argument against antivenom except in severe cases in North America is related to the relative chances of dying from latrodectism versus dying from anaphylaxis to antivenom. This is summarised by[151] estimating the natural death rate from latrodectism at less than 1%, but even in individuals who skin test negative for antivenom reaction there is an (alleged) 9% chance of anaphylaxis (80% in those who skin test positive) and 36% incidence of serum sickness. On this basis it is argued that the antivenom carries a higher risk of both death and long term reactions than does latrodectism. This may reflect the relative quality of the commercial North American antivenom compared to that produced in some other regions, or it may reflect some problem in generation of information on the adverse effects of antivenom in North America. These levels of problems with anti-*Latrodectus* antivenom are not reported in other parts of the world where such antivenoms are commonly used. In particular in Australia where latrodectism is common, with probably thousands of cases per year[136], there are large series of cases published showing a very low incidence of any adverse reactions to antivenom therapy, and no deaths[137,138]. It is clear that patients with latrodectism not treated with antivenom will have an acute illness lasting 2 to 3 days, and may be debilitated for a considerably longer period. This has a major cost both in terms of patient suffering, and in economic cost. If such patients are treated with antivenom the illness is usually completely aborted, and they may not even require hospitalization. This is a clear saving in both suffering and economic cost and would appear to amply justify the risks of antivenom therapy.

In view of the lower use of antivenom for latrodectism in the U.S. there are other recommended treatments for the majority of patients.

In parts of South America, such as Argentina, where antivenom is available, its use is restricted to patients with severe systemic involvement[145].

It is the opinion of the principle author of this chapter that antivenom is the recommended therapy of latrodectism and that its use should not be restricted to severe cases, but should extend to all cases with significant symptomatology, an opinion based on extensive experience treating latrodectism in Australia.

- Adult dosage: The initial dosage of antivenom will depend on the product being used and the manufacturer's recommendations. The volume depends on the degree of refinement of antivenom. In most instances the contents of one ampoule is the appropriate dose, and only if the response is incomplete and the patient still has significant symptomatology should a second ampoule be considered. Only in unusual circumstances would further antivenom be needed. In excess of 5 ampoules of CSL Ltd Red Back Spider Antivenom have been used occasionally in Australia.
- Child dosage: The dosage of antivenom is the same in children as in adults.

5. Alternatives to antivenom therapy

A wide variety of therapies for latrodectism have been advocated, but most are unproven or ineffective. However the use of iv calcium gluconate has been well accepted in many areas and is now the recommended treatment for most cases in North America in the opinion of many authors[12,151,182-187]; however, in children it may have only transitory benefit[151,188], and at least one dissenting view, recommending antivenom in preference to other therapies, is published[143]. The mode of action of calcium gluconate is not clear, but repeated anecdotal reports and at least one small prospective trial have shown it to have limited efficacy[183]. At least for latrodectism in North America it has been shown as effective therapy for patients presenting with symptomatology 3 or more hours after the bite, which probably equates to mild to moderate cases[183]. It was not effective in relieving the symptoms, notably failing to relieve pain, in cases presenting in less than 3 hours after the bite, equating to moderate to severe cases. Repeated doses were sometimes needed. The recommended regimen is 10% calcium gluconate solution, given iv with the patient under cardiac monitoring; for an adult start with 2-3 ml. as a slow iv push, and increase dose in 2 ml. increments until there is relief of symptoms, repeating as necessary to control symptoms[151].

a. Calcium Gluconate

Apart from its use in North America as an alternative to antivenom therapy, it has gained a wider acceptance in many regions as an adjunct to antivenom. First proposed in 1935[189], its value has largely been reported on the basis of anecdotal experience, with the exception of one small series from North America[183] which did show benefits in mild to moderate cases of latrodectism. It is generally recommended as an early adjunct therapy to relieve pain prior to definitive antivenom therapy, but its effect is generally brief, about 15 to 30 mins[12]. Interestingly it has not gained acceptance as therapy in Australia where many cases of latrodectism occur. It is potentially hazardous and should only be given with the patient being cardiac monitored[151].

b. Muscle relaxents

A number of authors have proposed muscle relaxant drugs as therapy for latrodectism based on the predominance of pain due to muscle spasm as the principle symptom of envenomation. A small trial of calcium gluconate versus muscle relaxant (methocarbamol) did not show any value in muscle relaxant drug therapy[183]. Despite this muscle relaxants are still advocated by some North American authors, methocarbamol and diazepam being the 2 most often recommended drugs[148,185-187]. Suggested doses are; methocarbamol 5-10 mg. iv in adults, repeated 3-4 hourly for about 24 hrs., or diazepam 0.1 mg. /kg. iv 4-5 hourly for 1-2 days (in children)[148].

c. Other drug therapies

Bell and Boone reported the use of neostigmine methylsulphate (2 ml. of 1:2000, im) and atropine (0.4 mg., im) with good response including relief of pain in a case of severe latrodectism in a 16 year old boy who had failed to respond to iv calcium gluconate, pentobarbital, codeine, or aspirin[161]. Relief was temporary requiring repeat doses every 4 hrs. for a total of 4 doses. Artaza et al. proposed the use of neostigmine in order to abbreviate the symptoms due to acetylcholine depletion[135].

Weitzman et al. reported a case of atrial fibrillation occurring 72 hrs. after a bite, and after the symptoms of latrodectism had abated (no antivenom therapy), which failed to respond to propanolol or digoxin, but which stabilized and reverted with iv oxprenolol[165].

Analgesics frequently fail to provide effective relief of pain in latrodectism and are not recommended except as adjunctive treatment[106].

Antihistamines have not been accepted as useful in managing latrodectism[106].

Corticosteroids have shown limited effect in alleviating symptoms in latrodectism but this effect is minor compared with the effect of specific antivenom therapy, and even in comparison to iv calcium gluconate[106].

Magnesium sulphate iv has a similar effect in latrodectism as calcium therapy but the effect is short-lived and not as easily or safely repeated as calcium and it has not proved a useful therapy[106].

d. Non-drug treatments

Apart from a variety of "traditional" remedies including dancing ('Tarantism"[106,180]), it does appear that immersing the patient in a bath of water as hot as they can bear will relieve the symptoms at least partially, but the effect is only temporary and may require repeated immersions[106,147].

6. Complications of latrodectism

Major complications of latrodectism are rare.

Mild hypertension is a common finding in latrodectism, but severe hypertension, though less common (3%[137]), should be excluded. It is best treated by antivenom therapy but adjunctive drug therapy may also be required.

Pulmonary oedema has been reported and responded rapidly to specific antivenom therapy[168].

Envenomation may result in myocardial infarction in patients with pre-existing cardiac ischaemic problems[106].

Cerebral haemorrhage is reported to have occurred[106].

Renal failure may occur[106].

DIC has occurred but is rare[106].

Though rare, psychosis due to latrodectism is a documented problem[106].

Wound infection: Local wound infection at the bite site is only rarely seen in latrodectism. As the fangs are potentially contaminated tetanus prophylaxis should be considered.

XI. THE RECLUSE SPIDERS: LOXOSCELISM

Family Loxoscelidae contains the second most medically important group of spiders worldwide, the recluse spiders, genus *Loxosceles*. At least some of these spiders have venom capable of causing skin necrosis in man, and less commonly a systemic illness which is sometimes fatal.

A. BIOLOGY AND DISTRIBUTION

1. Biology

Recluse spiders are, as the common name suggests, reclusive, using irregular web structures. They are found in urban environments, including within dwellings, but, because of their small size and habit, are often overlooked. The only evidence of their presence in a case of suspected loxoscelism may be the finding of exoskeletal casts.

2. Taxonomy

The recluse spiders are cosmopolitan, found either as natives or exotics in many inhabited regions of the globe. Like the other spiders discussed herein, their taxonomy is still in a state of flux. Some of the more important species are shown, with distribution, in Figure 33 .

They are small to medium sized spiders, with a distinctive pattern on the dorsal cephalothorax in some species, the so called "violin" or "fiddle" shape that is represented in some common names for these spiders (see Figure 32). They have 6 eyes. Their eye structure is distinctive (Figure 29) and they have long very thin legs and a comparatively diminutive cephalothorax and abdomen (Figures 30,31,32). They are widely distributed (Figure 33).

3. Distribution

Loxosceles spp. occur naturally in North America in the southern states (principally *L. reclusa*)[8,23-2638,190,191], Central America (principally *L. rufipes*)[191], South America (principally *L. laeata, L. gaucho*)[116,191-196], Europe (principally *L. rufescens*)[191,197], Africa (principally *L. rufescens, L. parrami*)[12-14,191], and parts of Asia. They have been accidentally introduced to other regions, such as parts of Australia (*L. rufescens*, Adelaide; *L. leata*, Sydney)[96]. An approximate distribution for some major species is shown in Figure 32. The total number of species is in excess of 50, only a few of which have been implicated in loxoscelism.

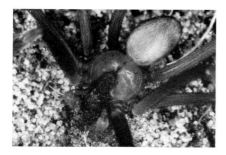

Figure 29. Close up of face of *Loxosceles* to show distinctive eye structure (photo © Dr. J. White).

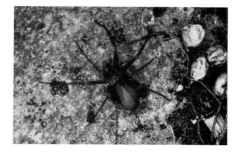

Figure 30. *Loxosceles reclusa* (photo © Dr. J. White).

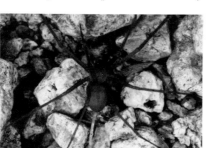

Figure 31. *Loxosceles arizonica* (photo © Dr. J. White).

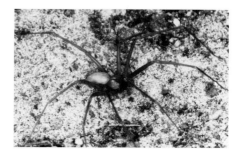

Figure 32. *Loxosceles rufescens* (photo © Dr. J. White).

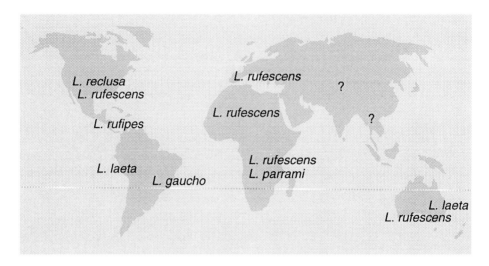

Figure 33. Distribution of some key species of *Loxosceles.*

B. VENOM

1. Venom composition

There have been a variety of studies of *Loxosceles* venom, but the exact mechanisms causing the local necrosis and systemic illness in man are still controversial. Given that the pathophysiology is poorly understood, several aspects have to be considered in understanding the mechanisms of action:

1. Sphingomyelinase D is clearly an important component of *Loxosceles* venom, responsible, at least in part, for local skin necrosis, intravascular haemolysis and platelet aggregration[23]. A dermonecrotic fraction has been isolated from *L. gaucho* venom, a common cause of loxoscelism in Brazil[198].

2. The role of polymorphonuclear leucocytes seems to be important in the development of local vasculitis, the putative cause of necrotic lesions. This led to new therapeutic approachs in loxoscelism[36,199], using inhibitors of chemotaxis, which have proven beneficial clinically.

3. The hemolytic activity may be related to G6PD deficiency[200]. Complement activation and other factors are apparently not involved.

2. Pathophysiology of envenoming

As discussed above, the precise mechanisms involved in loxoscelism are still the subject of debate, but the consensus view appears to be that the pathophysiology is multifactorial, involving both primary tissue damage by the venom, and inducing secondary damage, both by vascular injury (± local vascular occlusion by thrombosis) and release of tissue destructive enzymes from polymorphs. A recent report suggests that the naturally occurring glycoprotein, serum amyloid P, may be essential in mediating the destructive effects of sphingomyelinase D in the spider venom[201]. This venom component induces platelet aggregation and serotonin secretion, the former action requiring serum amyloid P and calcium ions. It may be that sphingomyelinase D induced binding of serum amyloid P to damaged platelet membranes mirrors a more general interaction, involving a wide variety of cell types. Serum amyloid P is known to bind to amyloid fibrils and is part of the process of amyloidosis. This may therefore provide an explanation for the slow healing seen with loxoscelism, and the occasional development of pyoderma gangrenosum type lesions.

C. EPIDEMIOLOGY

Loxoscelism occurs in many parts of the world. In some areas not usually associated with loxoscelism, necrotic arachnidism occurs and some of these cases may be loxoscelism, possibly due to introduction of *Loxosceles* spp. as accidental exotics. This has occurred in Australia at least[96].

1. North America

Loxoscelism is well known in parts of North America, particularly the southern and western regions, though the range of these spiders is thought to be limited (Figure 34)[8,23-26,38,190,191,202]. The range is not generally thought to extend to Canada, though "loxoscelism" has been reported from parts of western Canada (north west region and Okanagan Valley, British Columbia) and Ontario, based on clinical appearance rather than finding the spider in association with the bite[203-207]. It appears that many cases of local tissue damage caused by events other than loxoscelism are nevertheless blamed on loxoscelism by less well informed members of the medical profession, and this is likely to have skewed the literature on the epidemiology of loxoscelism in North America. Rates of cases are not well documented. In South Carolina at least 478 cases were recorded in 1990, possibly less than half of all cases seen medically as only 43% of doctors surveyed responded with data[190]. In comparison, in the same study there were only 143 cases of black widow spider bite. *Loxosceles reclusa* is the most important species clinically.

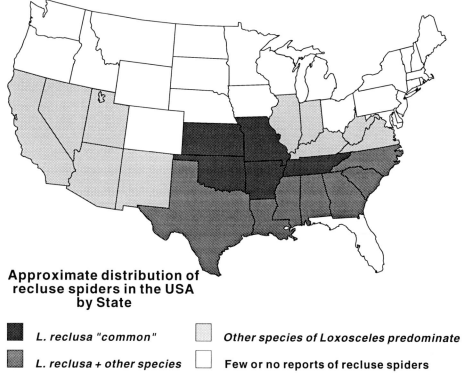

Approximate distribution of recluse spiders in the USA by State

■ *L. reclusa "common"*   ▨ *Other species of Loxosceles predominate*
▨ *L. reclusa + other species*   □ Few or no reports of recluse spiders

Figure 34 . Approximate distribution of *Loxosceles* in North America.

2. South America

Loxoscelism is the most severe form of araneism in South America. Cases are reported in Brazil[208]; Chile[191-193]; Argentina[209]; Peru[195] and Uruguay (Iseglio & Galasso; pers. com.). Principle species appear to be *L. laeta* and *L. gaucho*. In Chile 216 cases were recorded in

Santiago from 1955 to 1988[193]. 73.6% occurred in the "hot" season, 86.6% occurred in houses, especially bedrooms, while sleeping or dressing and the spider was seen in 60% of cases. 67.6% of bites were to the limbs.

At Hospital Vital Brazil most of the cases are included in the cutaneous form, as shown in Table 10 .

Table 10
Comparative data from South America

Reference	Number of Cases with Cutaneous Form	Number of Cases with Viscero-cutaneous Form	Fatal Cases
GAJARDO-TOBAR, R.(1966)[194]	178 (89.0%)	22 (11.0%)	7 (03.5%)
ROSENFELD, G (1972)[208]	114 (85.7%)	19 (14.3%)	5 (03.8%)
SCHENONE, H.(1975)[192]	- (00.0%)	- (00.0%)	4 (00.9%)
SCHENONE, H. (1989)[193]	(84.3%)	(15.7%)	(3.7%)
HVB (1972-76)	236 (96.7%)	8 (03.3%)	1 (00.4%)
CARDOSO, J.L.C.(1988)[196]	236 (97.5%)	6 (02.5%)	- (00.0%)

3. Europe

Loxoscelism probably does occur sporadically in Europe, both due to endemic species, notably *L. rufescens*, and exotics from the Americas, but the extent is not well documented and is probably quite minor.

4. Africa

Loxoscelism, though not common, does occur, at least in southern Africa south of 17^0S. The principal species appear to be *L parrami* (Witwatersrand)*, L. spiniceps* (Natal, Transvaal, Botswana, Zimbabwe)*, L. pillosa* (South West Africa, Namibia, north-western Cape) and *L. bergeri* (South West Africa, Namibia)[12]. They frequently invade dwellings and therefore bites to humans might be considered quite likely, but analysis of the literature suggests that loxoscelism is at most, uncommon, in southern Africa, where several other spiders are thought to be a more common cause of skin necrosis (e.g. *Chiracanthium lawrencei*, ?*Sicarius* sp.)[12,13]

5. Asia

There is a lack of information on loxoscelism in Asia, and if it does occur, it is apparently uncommon to rare. The exception is the Middle East, where loxoscelism does occur in Israel[22], and probably in some other countries in the region. In Israel the principle species is *L. rufescens*. A recent retrospective study noted that bites were more common in warmer months (summer, 43%; spring, 31.5%; autumn, 20%; winter, 6%)[22].

6. Australia

There are no reports of loxoscelism from Australia, but quite a few reports suggesting necrotic arachnidism is widespread in urban areas, though frequency is not known[44,79,86,210-225]. Attention has focussed on local species, without good evidence in support. *L. rufescens* and *L. laeta* have both been reported as exotics established in Adelaide and Sydney respectively[96]. The author has treated numerous cases of "necrotic arachnidism" in the last 10 years, in none of which was a spider seen to bite, but in at least some of the cases, the local effects were consistent with cutaneous loxoscelism[79,86]. A recent case in a young healthy adult male, on the upper thigh, with extensive skin necrosis in the absence of infection almost certainly represents loxoscelism, as a specimen of *L. rufescens* was found in the bedclothes adjacent to the bite area on awakening from sleep, at the time of initial discovery of the thigh lesion. Discomfort, possibly due to a bite was felt in bed the previous evening. *Loxosceles* casts were found in the bedroom and under the floorboards. The author considers it likely that many, possibly most, of the cases of true venom induced skin necrosis seen in Australia will ultimately prove to be loxoscelism.

D. SYMPTOMS AND SIGNS

The diagnosis is often based on the clinical picture since the spider is not identified in most of cases (Table 11). Preliminary studies applying immunoassay (ELISA) have been developed in order to detect *Loxosceles* venom in necrotic skin lesions[16] and specific IgG antibodies in patients[197].

Table 11
Positive identification of *Loxosceles* spider in cases of suspected loxoscelism

Source	Number of Cases	Spider Identified as *Loxosceles* (%)
GAJARDO-TOBAR, R. (1966)[194]	200	36 (18.0%)
SCHENONE, H. (1975)[192]	133	15 (11.2%)
SCHENONE, H. (1989)[193]	216	(10.6%)
ROSENFELD, G. (1972)[208]	453	41 (9.1%)
HVB (1972-76)	244	19 (7.8%)
CARDOSO, J.L.C. (1988)[196]	242	13 (5.4%)

There are two forms of loxoscelism described:

1. Cutaneous

This is the most frequent form of loxoscelism (Table 10). In general the patient seeks help from 12-36 hours after the bite since the evolution of the lesion is slow and progressive.

The moment when the accident took place usually is not mentioned by the patient, since the bite is painless and generally the small spider is crushed within clothes. Bites are more likely to occur inside a house in hot weather[193]. At the bite site there is nonspecific erythema and local edema, which evolves into mottled hemorrhagic areas with regions of ischemia (Figure 35). The pain becomes intensified and general symptoms including fever and generalized erythema may appear. At this stage the diagnosis is usually obvious.

Within 7 days, the lesion evolves into a dry necrosis (Figure 36). Under the necrotic eschar there is an area of ulceration which persists for about 4-8 weeks. The ulcer is slow to heal, with recurrent breakdown, resulting in obvious and often disfiguring scarring. One series from Chile reported an overall rate of scars of 8.3%[193]. There may also be persistent damage to underlying structures such as nerves. Hyalinizing panniculitis and myonecrosis has also been reported[227]. The prognosis may be worse if there is lymphangitis, rash, or the bite is on the thigh or abdomen[228]. Pseudoepitheliomatous hyperplasia and pyoderma gangrenosum may develop as a sequelae of cutaneous loxoscelism[229]. Methaemoglobinaemia is apparently a common secondary phenomenon, reported in 54% of cases in one series, though only of clinical significance in 20% (i.e. >4% methaemoglobin)[200]. In tropical regions the differential diagnosis should include cutaneous leishmaniasis[230].

2. Viscerocutaneous Loxoscelism

Viscerocutaneous loxoscelism is relatively uncommon to rare. In Chile a recent series found 16% of all cases of loxoscelism as viscerocutaneous[193]. When present the systemic signs are observed in the first 24 hours after envenoming. Besides the cutaneous effects, as seen in the purely cutaneous form of loxoscelism, clinical manifestations are due to haematological disturbances such as intravascular hemolysis, thrombocytopenia and disseminated intravascular coagulation[193,227]. There is no established relationship between the intensity of hemolytic and proteolytic (cutaneous) effects; patients with mild cutaneous effects may present with massive hemolysis. Laboratory findings include haemoglobinemia, increased bilirubin, hemoglobinuria and proteinuria.

Acute renal failure is related to systemic effects (principally haemolysis) and is the major cause of death in *Loxosceles* envenoming.

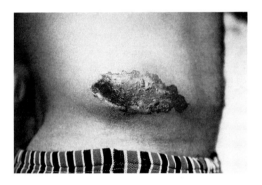

Figure 35. Loxoscelism; generalised exanthema and lesion at the site of the bite, three days later.

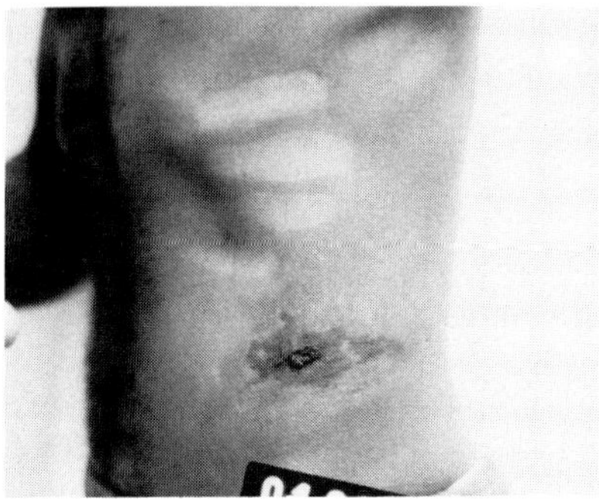

Figure 36. Loxoscelism; local necrosis at the bite site 11 days later.

E. PROPHYLAXIS

Avoidance of bites by *Loxosceles* spiders can be difficult in areas where they are common, though this does not imply that bites themselves are common. Most bites occur at night while the patient is asleep, often unaware of the bite occurring. Reduction of opportunities for the spiders to enter bedding or clothing, such as moving beds away from the walls and careful storage of clothes, may reduce the chance of bites. Maintaining a clean domestic environment, to discourage entry of potential prey for the spiders, may also result in reduction of spider populations in dwellings, thus reducing the chance of bites. However the spiders and their prey may successfully exist in areas difficult to service and clean, such as under the floorboards.

F. FIRST AID

As the bite is often not noticed and the injury only becomes apparent later, when the essential damage has already commenced, first aid for loxoscelism seems problematic. Once a cutaneous lesion is established, the most appropriate first aid advice is to promptly seek medical attention and avoid secondary infection of the lesion by keeping it clean and refraining from further damaging affected skin.

G. TREATMENT

There is controversy about the therapeutic approach to loxoscelism since various methods have been proposed in the literature; surgical excision, systemic corticosteroids, anti-histaminics, dapsone, hyperbaric oxygen therapy and antivenom therapy have all been suggested[27-40,193].

1. Diagnosis

Establishing the diagnosis of loxoscelism is often necessarily based on a clinical picture strongly suggestive of the diagnosis in a region where this condition is known to occur. Only occasionally will a spider be available to confirm the diagnosis. The typical clinical features of loxoscelism have been described elsewhere in this chapter.

2. Laboratory tests

The most specific laboratory test for loxoscelism is detection of either circulating venom or circulating antibodies to the venom. The latter approach has not proved effective so far, possibly due to low levels of antigen circulating, with consequent poor antibody response. Detection of venom has been reported as successful in two cases, using a double "sandwich" enzyme linked immunosorbent assay[16]. The bite area was excised at 29 days and 5 days post bite, respectively, and *Loxosceles gaucho* venom was detected in the excision biopsy supernatant of each patient at a level of 49 ng/ml and 38.5 ng/ml respectively. Slight cross reactivity with the venom of *Phoneutria nigriventer* was shown, though clinically this spider causes a quite different and easily differentiated form of envenoming.

A variety of other tests have been reported to characterise envenoming by *Loxosceles*. These include a lymphocyte transformation test which gave a positive result in 5 out of 6 cases of *L. reclusa* envenoming[17]; a passive haemagglutination inhibition assay (PHAI), again for *L. reclusa* venom[18], which has recently been reported as having 90% sensitivity and 100% specificity at up to 3 days post bite (experimentally in guinea pigs) with positive results in 59 of 62 patients with clinically diagnosed loxoscelism[20]; and radioimmunoassay for *L. reclusa* venom[19]. Of these various tests, the direct detection of venom and the PHAI seem to offer most in positive confirmation of loxoscelism.

Apart from tests confirming loxoscelism, there are a variety of routine laboratory tests which may be applicable. Complete blood examination, serum electrolytes and renal function and analysis of urine for haemoglobin should be performed in all cases of suspected or confirmed loxoscelism if there is any suggestion of systemic involvement, and ideally in all cases, though in many regions logistic and cost considerations may make this impractical.

3. General measures

The wound should be carefully examined and the extent of skin reaction or necrosis accurately documented, to allow ongoing assessment of increasing damage as the lesion evolves. The wound should also be kept clean, and any exudate or discharge cultured for bacterial contamination. Both blood and urine tests should be performed to exclude systemic involvement. Should viscerocutaneous loxoscelism occur, then vigorous supportive measures may be necessary, including blood transfusion and systemic antibiotics. Renal involvement may mandate dialysis.

4. Antivenom

At Hospital Vital Brazil in Sao Paulo, Brazil, the use of specific antivenom has been recommended as routine in patients with acute inflammatory lesions and/or systemic signs of envenoming. However the results of antivenom therapy are disappointing. Most patients are diagnosed more than 24/36 hours after the bite, a treatment delay considered too long to achieve a good therapeutic effect from antivenom[23,231].

At Hospital Vital Brazil, for patients presenting with a characteristic cutaneous lesion, without established necrosis, antiloxoscelic or antiaracnidic antivenom is indicated in a dose of 5 ampoules by the intravenous route. In the viscerocutaneous form the dose varies from 5 to 10 ampoules, assisted by general supporting measures. In most regions where the spiders are found, antivenom is not available.

5. Dapsone

The theoretical basis of dapsone as treatment for loxoscelism rests in the inhibition of polymorphs by this drug, thus reducing the putative local tissue destruction caused by these cells in response to primary venom effects. Rabbits given nitrogen mustard, rendering them neutropenic, showed decreased dermonecrosis in response to venom injection, compared to controls[199]. Dapsone treated guinea pigs also showed smaller skin lesions than controls, in response to venom injection[36]. There have been several reports of the use and apparent effectiveness of dapsone in reducing the extent of skin damage in cases of loxoscelism, though no extensive or control trials[28-36].

Dapsone is a potentially toxic drug, known to induce severe side effects, including haemolysis and agranulocytosis. A case of dapsone hypersensitivity syndrome following its use to treat a case of loxoscelism has been reported[37]. This syndrome consists of fever, headache, nausea, vomiting, lymphadenopathy, hepatitis, haemolysis, leukopenia and mononucleosis, and has previously been described in patients treated with dapsone for leprosy.

6. Hyperbaric oxygen therapy

The use of hyperbaric oxygen therapy for loxoscelism has been suggested as theoretically attractive based on the premise that the necrosis is the result of polymorph cell adhesion to capillary walls, with secondary intravascular coagulation, a mechanism not universally accepted[40]. There is very limited clinical evidence of the use of this therapy in humans. A series of 6 cases of clinically diagnosed loxoscelism, seen at 48 hours to 7 days post bite, were treated with twice daily hyperbaric oxygen at 2 atmospheres absolute for 60 or 90 minutes, with a total of 1 to 6 treatments[39]. All were reported to have prompt healing without skin loss or scarring. It is uncertain what the natural history of these lesions would have been without treatment; thus, the beneficial role of the therapy is unclear. A control study in rabbits using injection of intradermal *L. reclusa* venom extract to simulate cutaneous loxoscelism and treatment with hyperbaric oxygen at 2 atmospheres once or twice daily did not show significant effects on wound healing, as measured by lesion area, between either treatment group or untreated controls[40]. However, the rabbits were sacrificed at day 24 and the lesions examined histologically, which showed evidence of wound healing in rabbits treated twice daily, not seen in either the rabbits treated once daily or the untreated controls. The researchers suggest that if hyperbaric oxygen therapy is to be successful in loxoscelism, then treatment should be commenced at the earliest opportunity. The author's own experience with two cases of loxoscelism in Australia, given hyperbaric oxygen therapy over a week after the bite, is that there was a clear clinical improvement in the lesion, with cessation of expansion and improved healing commencing within 24 hours of starting twice daily hyperbaric oxygen therapy at 2 atmospheres, in case 1, with more dramatic improvement in case 2, treated at 2.8 atmospheres. It is not possible to determine if this improvement was due to the therapy or purely coincidental at this time, though the former seems most likely.

7. Corticosteroids

Corticosteroids have been used on numerous occasions in the past in treatment of loxoscelism, administered by a variety of routes, including systemic, intradermal and even intralesional. Drugs used include methylprednisolone, triamcinalone and dexamethasone. While no controlled studies on effectiveness of corticosteroids in the treatment of loxoscelism are available, there are a number of studies which do not indicate any consistent or reliable benefit[28-31]. In consequence the use of corticosteroids is generally not recommended for loxoscelism.

8. Surgical excision

As in other areas of toxinology, where local tissue damage is a consequence of envenoming, the role of surgery in primary treatment is controversial. Most current advice is that early surgery is at best unhelpful, and at worst may actually extend the area of local damage, by allowing wider venom spread[23-36,38]. Interestingly, a recent paper on loxoscelism in Brazil concluded that because venom was detectable in the wound at up to 29 days post bite, early surgical excision might be advantageous[16]. This does not appear to be supported by advice in recent review articles on management of loxoscelism in North America, where even some plastic surgeons, treating cases, urge caution and withholding surgery until the area of necrosis is fully demarcated. This view is supported by experimental work in animals, showing wound healing following early surgical excision of the bite area, with skin grafting, gave inferior results compared with animals treated conservatively[28].

9. Other treatments

Following recent claims of the effectiveness of directly applied high voltage electric current in treating snakebite, a treatment felt to be quite inappropriate by a number of clinicians with experience treating snakebite, the same method has been suggested for loxoscelism[232]. In two series of 21 and 126 cases of suspected loxoscelism (in 16 cases a spider, *L. reclusa* was identified), electric current was administered using a "stun gun", giving two shocks of about 40-50 KV seconds, with a 5-10 second interval between shocks. A further series of shocks were given over the area surrounding the bite. No patient showed any progression of skin damage beyond the initial blister or area of skin darkening seen prior to treatment. Follow up was for "a minimum of 15 minutes after treatment", though clearly some patients were seen over longer periods and follow up to confirm effectiveness was made by letter or phone in 86% of cases. This form of treatment for spiderbites has not been subjected to controlled laboratory evaluation, but such evaluation for snakebite failed to demonstrate the claimed effectiveness.

XII. THE BANANA SPIDERS: *PHONEUTRIA*

Banana spiders, genus *Phoneutria* (Figure 37), so named because they sometimes are found in shipments of bananas from South America, are members of Family Ctenidae. They are restricted to South America.

A. BIOLOGY AND DISTRIBUTION
1. Biology

Banana spiders are essentially hunting spiders, and so may invade dwellings and other human items, such as boxes of fruit, hence the common name. They have apparently travelled in fruit boxes to areas of the world distant to South America.

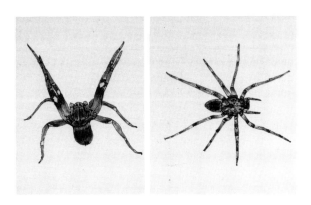

Figure 37. Banana spider, *Phoneutria nigriventer* (photo © Dr. J. White).

2. Taxonomy

These spiders are generally large, adults having body lengths over 30 mm, with a leg span occasionally exceeding 150 mm. There are six named species of *Phoneutria*: *P. boliviensis, P. colombiana, P. fera, P. keyserlingi, P. nigriventer* and *P. reidyi*.

3. Distribution

The banana spiders are largely restricted to the eastern side of South America, particularly the coastal regions of Brazil, where most recorded bites occur (from *P. nigriventer* and *P. keyserlingi*). The genus is represented in the Amazon basin, particularly Brazil, but is also found in Ecuador, Peru, Colombia, Bolivia, the Guyanas and through into Central America as far as Costa Rica.

B. VENOM
1. Venom Composition

Banana spider venom contains histamine, serotonine and other polypeptides[233]. It was found in experimental studies that the venom produces effects by activating Na^+ channels[234]. This leads to depolarization of muscle fibers and sensitive, motor and autonomic end-plates. At least three neurotoxins are reported as present in the venom.

2. Pathophysiology of envenoming

The precise pathophysiology of *Phoneutria* envenoming is not certain, but it appears to involve the release of mediators such as acetylcholine and catecholamines, which are responsible for the systemic effects. Pain is the commonest clinical finding in *Phoneutria* envenoming. It is therefore rather similar to some aspects of latrodectism and envenoming by the Australian funnel web spiders.

C. EPIDEMIOLOGY

Banana spiders are native to South America. They are one of the more common causes of spider bites presenting to hospitals in coastal Brazil, accounting for between 40% and 95% of cases in some series (Table 12). In some hospitals *Phoneutria* bites may be one of the most common causes of presentation; at Hospital Vital Brazil, Sao Paulo (southeastern region of Brazil), in the ten year period 1970 to 1980, of 31,776 medical attendances 7,087 (22.3%) were due to *Phoneutria* bites. Bites may occur at any time of year, but are more common in autumn (April, May).

Table 12
Spider bites presenting to hospital(s) in Brazil (data incomplete as NOT ALL HOSPITALS ARE INCLUDED)

Spider	1954-65		1988-89	
	Number of Cases	% of Total Cases of Spiderbite	Number of Cases	% of Total Cases of Spiderbite
Phoneutria	3,830	94.97	1,857	40.06
Loxosceles	203	5.03	956	20.62
Latrodectus	-	-	10	0.22
Not specified	-	-	1,519	32.77
Other spider	-	-	294	6.34
TOTAL	4,033		4,636	

D. SYMPTOMS AND SIGNS

Pain is the most frequent manifestation in phoneutrism. Almost 100% of cases complain of burning pain at the site of sting that can spread to the whole bitten limb. Other local alterations include: swelling, hiperemia and sudoresis at the site of sting. Due to adrenergic/cholinergic disbalance, systemic clinical picture may range from tachycardia and arterial hypertension to nausea, vomitus, bradycardia, hypotension and cardiac arrhythmia in severe cases. Priapism is observed mainly in children (Figure 38) and is attributed to massive release of acetylcholine. Rarely are observed shock and acute pulmonary edema. Death is extremely rare.

In Brazil, the *Phoneutria* accidents have been classified in three groups in order to establish treatment schedules (Table 13). Mild envenoming is observed in almost 90% of cases, moderate in 9% and severe in less than 1%.

E. PROPHYLAXIS

No specific measures are reported to avoid bites from banana spiders. Care should be exercised in handling goods, such as packed fruit (classically bananas), which have originated in areas where these spiders are native.

F. FIRST AID

There is an apparent lack of information on first aid for banana spider bites and it is unclear if it is best to use a compression immobilisation bandage (as for funnel web spider bite) or use no defined first aid, except, possibly, the use of ice packs for brief periods (as for widow spider bite).

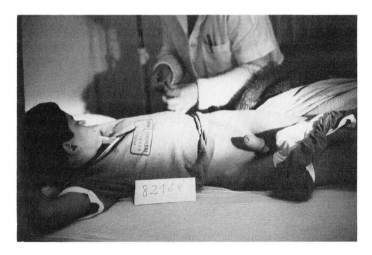

Figure 38. Priapism following *Phoneutria* envenoming in a 14 year old boy.

G. TREATMENT

Symptomatic: anesthesic local block to relieve pain is utilized in Brazil, as a routine, based on local injection of 4 ml of 2% lidocaine by the subcutaneous route (Fleury, 1964). At Hospital Vital Brazil the anaesthetic block has been used extensively (Table 14).

Antivenom therapy has been advocated in moderate/severe cases with systemic envenoming. Less than 5% of patients at Hospital Vital Brazil are treated with antivenom, mainly children under 7 years and elderly people.

Antivenom should be administered by the intravenous route in diluted solution of 2 to 5 vials of "Soro anti-aracnídico polivalente" produced by Butantan Institute (Brazil), which contains anti-*Phoneutria* fraction equine antivenom. Anaphylactic reactions may occur and appropriate treatment (especially adrenaline) should be immediately available.

Table 13
Clinical picture of phoneutrism based on severity

Severity	Local Picture	Systemic Picture
Mild	pain swelling hiperemia	tachycardia agitation
Moderate	pain swelling hiperemia hyperhydrosis	tachycardia arterial hypertension vomiting sialorrhea profuse sudoresis priapism
Severe	pain swelling hiperemia hyperhidrosis	bradycardia arterial hypotension diarrhoea cardiac arrhythmia acute pulmonary edema shock

Table 14
Phoneutrism - schedules for treatment

Treatment	No. of Cases	%
Anaesthetic Block		
1X	326	66.13
2X	42	8.52
3X or more	9	1.64
Antivenom	24	4.87
No treatment	92	18.66
TOTAL	493	100.00

XIII. NECROTIC ARACHNIDISM

Necrotic arachnidism is often vaguely defined and imprecisely used in the literature. Essentially it defines those cases of humans bitten by spiders, where skin damage at the bite site has occurred. This is often assumed to be a primary venom effect, but is more often due to other factors, such as local infection. True necrotic arachnidism is associated with loxoscelism, as noted above. A number of other spiders are variously reported or suspected of causing necrotic arachnidism. They are found in an array of families and it is not possible to equate necrotic arachnidism with a particular taxonomic group at this time, except for loxoscelism. Several species should be noted as associated with tissue damage, particularly *Chiracanthium* sp., *Lycosa* sp. and the Australian spider, *Lampona cylindrata*. For the latter two species, evidence now suggests that, past reputation to the contrary, they do **not** cause significant tissue injury, with the possible exception of individuals "sensitive" to the venom (see comments for each spider, below). There is some experimental evidence to suggest that several other spiders may cause local skin necrosis in at least some cases, either directly due to venom, such as *Argiope* spp., *Phidippus* sp., *Chiracanthium* sp. and *Tegenaria agrestis*, or as a result of wound contamination by digestive juices, such as *Nephila edulis*, *Eriophora transmarina*, *Isopeda immanis* and *Lycosa godeffroyi*.

In Australia there has been a considerable correspondence in the medical literature regarding "necrotic arachnidism"[44,79,86,210-225]. This has failed to resolve the issue, and controversy still surrounds the involvement of several species of spiders. It has been suggested that at least some of the cases of skin damage following spiderbite are due to either the necrotic effect of contaminating salivary secretions[220] or secondary infection, with

315

Mycobacterium ulcerans having been specifically mentioned in regard to the latter causation[223]. The author has seen and treated in excess of 50 cases of "necrotic arachnidism" in the last 15 years, yet in only one of these cases is there a spider species reasonably clearly associated, and in this single case it was *Loxosceles rufescens* (as discussed earlier). At least in Australia, and quite possibly in many inhabited parts of the globe, there is a poorly defined clinical entity consisting of unexplained skin blistering and ulceration, the latter often slow to heal, often associated with a possible spiderbite, though the culprit is virtually never seen. It may be that some of these cases will prove due to spider bite by one or more species. It is quite possible that exotic or native *Loxosceles* spp. are responsible in a proportion of cases, but it seems equally likely that other spiders may also cause skin damage. The possible role of spiders such as *Tegenaria agrestis* has been discussed, though not proven clinically[236,237].

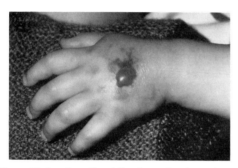

Figure 39. Local swelling, blistering and ecchymosis following a spider bite (photo © Dr. J. White).

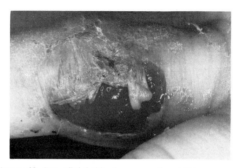

Figure 40. Superficial skin damage under a blister, following a probable spider bite (photo © Dr. J. White).

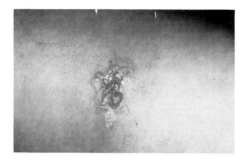

Figure 41. Local blistering and superficial skin damage following a spider bite (photo © Dr. J. White).

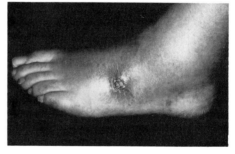

Figure 42. Deep foot ulcer following a spider bite, which took over 4 months to heal (photo © Dr. J. White).

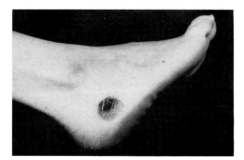

Figure 43. Eschar formation on a foot following a spider bite, with underlying skin damage (photo © Dr. J. White).

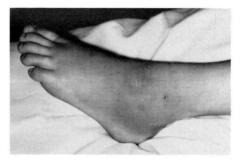

Figure 44. Extensive "cellulitis" of a foot , resistant to iv antibiotic treatment, following a probable spider bite (photo © Dr. J. White).

XIV. OTHER SPIDERS

A wide variety of spiders have variously been reported as causing harm to humans, or causing frequent bites (usually very minor). Some of these are listed in Table 3.

A. OTHER THERIID SPIDERS

A variety of Theriid spiders, other than *Latrodectus* spp., may occasionally bite man. Some, such as the house spider, *Steatoda grossa*, and *Achaearanea tepidariorum* (Figures 45,46,47), are common in urban areas, including in and around dwellings, and bites are possible and have been recorded, though infrequently. None of the non-*Latrodectus* theriids appear capable of causing severe systemic effects, with the exception of species of *Steatoda*. There are several reports of toxic venom from members of this genus. A recent report documents apparent neurotoxicity from a bite of *Steatoda nobilis* in the United Kingdom, where this species is an exotic[244]. There is an Australian report of a likely bite by *Steatoda grossa* which resulted in development of local blisters over 15 hours, with associated lethargy, and healing of the skin lesions by 10 days[238]. Bites by *Achaearanea tepidariorum* appear to be very minor.

B. THE WHITE TAILED SPIDER, *Lampona cylindrata* (AUSTRALIA)

This spider, very common in urban environments in Australia, has unfortunately gained a reputation in that country as the cause of skin necrosis (necrotic arachnidism) following spiderbite[210-225]. It is a distinctive spider (Figure 48), a hunter, found in gaps between objects, such as between furniture and walls. The problem of necrotic arachnidism, though doubtless present for many years, first recieved attention in the Australian medical press in 1983. A case of presumed necrotic arachnidism, culprit unknown, with extensive tissue injury of the bitten limb was published in 1987, and both in this paper[212], and in the accompanying editorial[213], the white tailed spider was mentioned as a possible cause. Since then it has been repeatedly suggested as a likely cause of necrotic arachnidism, both in the lay press, and occasionally in the medical press[214-216]. This has also been questioned[79,86,217,223] and it has been suggested that at least some cases of "necrotic arachnidism" are due to *Mycobacterium ulcerans* infection[223], while others may represent pyoderma gangrenosum. There is now a general belief in a substantial part of the Australian population, and amongst some in the health professions, that this spider is, indeed, the cause of necrotic arachnidism. However, apart from three cases from Tasmania[215,245], there is no clinical evidence published to substantiate this spider with necrotic skin lesions. Indeed, there are case reports published of confirmed bites, where no skin damage has occurred[79]. Furthermore, there is experimental evidence to suggest that *Lampona* venom does not cause skin damage[220]. The author's experience in South Australia has been that bites by this spider are moderately common, that the bite is usually felt, but local discomfort is usually only mild, and that apart from local erythema, of short duration, there are no significant effects from the bite. A few of the many cases seen by or reported to the author have been published. It is also the author's experience that there are a significant number of cases of skin necrosis following presumed bite occurring, and a spider seems the most probable culprit in the majority of cases, though the identity of the spider remains unknown. A recent case in Adelaide (unpublished) showing typical features of blister formation, local pain, mild systemic illness, then development of an area of skin necrosis, resistant to antibiotic therapy, appears likely to have been caused by a bite from *Loxosceles rufescens*. In this case, a spider was seen, then a possible bite in the affected region was felt, followed by discovery of the dead spider close by, subsequently identified as *L. rufescens*. As this species is a member of a group of spiders well known for causing skin necrosis, this case should not be surprising. It is possible that this spider is now widely established in some

317

Australian urban environments[96], as has occurred in other parts of the world, and in time it may prove to be the cause of "necrotizing arachnidism" in Australia. Given the weight of both clinical and experimental evidence, it seems clear that the usual bite of the white tailed spider is harmless. This does not exclude the possibility of rare local "hypersensitivity" reactions resulting in skin damage, though such cases have not been documented.

C. THE BLACK HOUSE SPIDER, *Badumna insignis* (AUSTRALIA)

The black house spider, *Badumna insignis* (Figures 49,50), is another common spider in Australian urban environments, where it builds a ragged web under window sills, around fence posts and similar locations, characterised by a silk tube retreat, from which the spider emerges after dark, to catch prey adjacent to the web. A number of bites have been recorded, none resulting in skin necrosis, but usually associated with local pain of moderate severity and a local erythema and swelling, without significant systemic symptoms, although the latter have occasionally been reported, usually nausea, but also vomiting, abdominal pain, pruritis and swollen, painful joints (knees)[79,239-241].

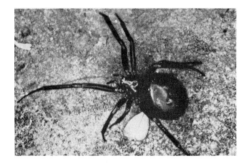

Figure 45. The common therid spider, *Steatoda grossa*, mature female (photo © Dr. J. White).

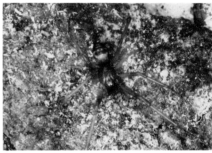

Figure 46. Immature *Steatoda grossa* (photo © Dr. J. White).

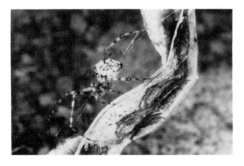

Figure 47. The therid spider, *Archaeranea tepdiarorum* (photo © Dr. J. White).

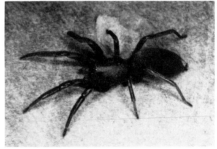

Figure 48. The Australian white tailed spider, *Lampona cylindrata* (photo © Dr. J. White).

D. THE GARDEN ORB WEAVING SPIDERS, *Eriophora* (AUSTRALIA)

The Australian garden orb weaving spider, *Eriophora* sp. (Figures 51,52), is a common large spider found in urban gardens in the warmer months, usually in a web strung between two tall objects, such as across paths. People frequently walk into these webs at night, brushing at the web on their body, causing the spider to bite them. The other common cause of bites is due to the spider's habit of finding a diurnal retreat. Clothes left out overnight on the washing line offer just such a retreat, and the next person to put the clothes on is likely to be bitten. Fortunately the bite of this spider is uniformly minor, causing only mild, short lived pain and mild erythema, even in young children[79].

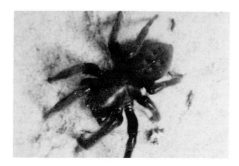

Figure 49. The Australian black house spider, *Badumna insignis* (photo © Dr. J. White).

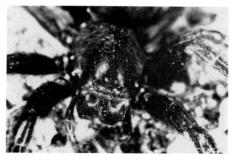

Figure 50. The eye structure of *Badumna* (photo © Dr. J. White).

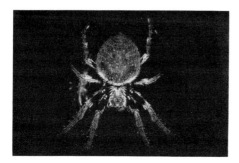

Figure 51. The Australian garden orb weaving spider, *Eriophora* sp., female (photo © Dr. J. White).

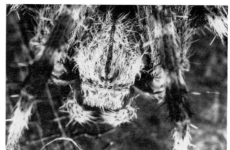

Figure 52. Eye structure of *Eriophora* (photo © Dr. J. White).

E. THE GOLDEN ORB WEAVING SPIDERS, *Nephila* SPP. (FAMILY ARGIOPIDAE)

The large golden orb weaving spiders, *Nephila* sp., have a wide distribution and a distinctive appearance (Figure 53), with a very large untidy orb web, with golden coloured silk, usually with a trail of past prey, silk enclosed, strung in a line above the centre of the web, which is where the female spider is to be found. The male, as in many other orb weavers, is much smaller, and harmless to man. Bites by *Nephila* sp. are poorly documented, but owing to their size, might be expected to cause at least local pain and swelling.

F. THE LYNX SPIDERS (FAMILY OXYOPIDAE)

The green lynx spider, *Peucetia viridans* (Figure 54), has been reported as causing injury to the eye by ejection of venom[93]. Other than this species, lynx spiders appear harmless[242].

G. THE JUMPING SPIDERS (FAMILY SALTICIDAE)

Small hunting spiders with prominent forward facing eyes (Figure 55,56). There are several reports of bites by these common spiders causing injury to man, usually minor, never fatal[6,11,15,79]. In Australia, *Mopsus mormon* is reported to cause local pain and swelling lasting up to one week[239,240]. Other Australian species, *Breda jovialis*, *Opisthoncus* sp. and *Holoplatys* sp. have also caused local pain, and in the case of *Holoplatys*, headache and vomiting as well[79].

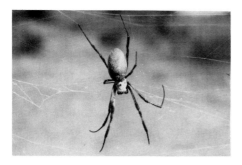

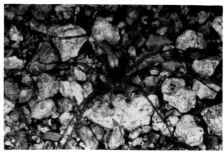

Figure 53. Golden orb weaving spider, *Nephila* sp. (photo © Dr. J. White).

Figure 54. Lynx spider, *Peucetia viridans* (photo © Dr. J. White).

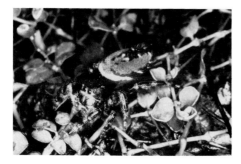

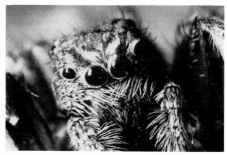

Figure 55. Jumping spider, *Phiippus* sp. (photo © Dr. J. White).

Figure 56. Detail of eye structure of a jumping spider (*Servea* sp.) (photo © Dr. J. White).

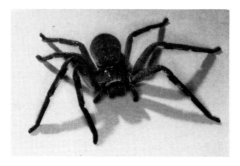

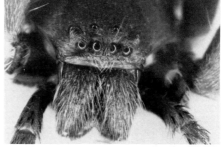

Figure 57. Huntsman spider, *Isopeda pessleri* (photo © Dr. J. White).

Figure 58. Detail of eye structure of huntsman spider (photo © Dr. J. White).

H. THE HUNTSMAN SPIDERS (FAMILY SPARASSIDAE)

The huntsman spiders are large hunting spiders, frequently found in and around dwellings, particularly in Australia (Figures 57,58). They prefer high locations, such as on walls or ceilings, but after dark may venture lower, so may come in contact with resting humans. Despite their size, including moderately large fangs, they are generally reluctant to bite, but when they do bite, slight to moderate local pain, of short duration, is the usual result[79]. A few species, such as *Olios* sp., may also cause a systemic illness, consisting of malaise, headache, nausea, ± vomiting, lasting about 24 hours.

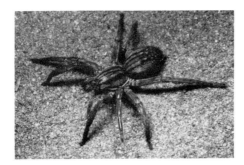

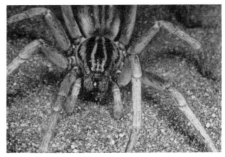

Figure 59. Miturgid spider, *Miturga* sp. (photo ©
Dr. J. White).

Figure 60. Detail of eye structure of *Miturga*
(photo © Dr. J. White).

I. THE MITURGID SPIDERS (FAMILY MITURGIDAE)

Little is known of either the venom or bite effects of these moderate sized spiders, mostly in the genus *Miturga* (Figure 59,60). They were formerly in the same family as *Chiracanthium*. A case of bite by *Miturga* sp. in New Zealand resulted in both local pain and swelling and a systemic illness lasting several days, characterised by malaise, sweating, muscle cramps, and joint pain[243]. A comment from the respected author of a popular book on spiders suggests that these spiders may cause a systemic illness which is "severe" and is associated with a local "necrotic" lesion[240]. No cases are reported to substantiate this.

J. THE WOLF SPIDERS, *Lycosa* SPP. (FAMILY LYCOSIDAE)

Wolf spiders are found worldwide, as hunting spiders, ranging from small to large spiders, with a distinctive eye pattern (Figures 61,62,63). Some species dig burrows, the entrance to which may have a palisade of vegetation or pebbles, or a well concealed silk trapdoor. In some parts of the world, large species of wolf spider are also known as "tarantulas", and it is the bite of these spiders which was thought to be the cause of tarantism, giving rise to the tarantella dance of the afflicted, though it is now generally accepted that bites from *Latrodectus tredecimguttatus* were the actual cause of the "illness". There is some experimental work in animals suggesting a necrotic action in at least some lycosid venoms, as well as hypersalivation and paresis in cats and mice[11]. Reports from Brazil of human cases of wolf spiderbite implicated these spiders as a major cause of local skin necrosis. This reputation has been applied to all wolf spiders, but without supporting evidence. Indeed, more recent reports from Brazil have suggested that those previously reported cases with necrosis were, in fact, due to loxoscelism. A recent series of 515 cases of wolf spider bite seen in Sao Paulo, Brazil, did not find a single case with necrosis, mild pain being the predominant finding[10].

K. THE COMMON HOUSE SPIDERS, *Filistata* SPP. (U.S.) (FAMILY FILISTATIDAE)

There are several dated reports of this spider causing both local tissue injury and systemic illness, including hemoglobinuria and liver damage, but as pointed out by Bucherl[8], this may be a case of mistaken identity, as *Loxosceles* is found in the same regions, and both spiders are frequent invaders of dwellings. This group of spiders continues to be listed as a possible cause of injury to man, though the factual basis for this is uncertain (Figure 64).

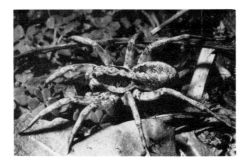

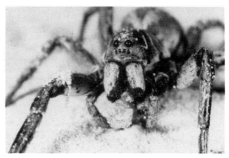

Figure 61. Wolf spider, *Lycosa* sp. (photo © Dr. J. White).

Figure 62. Detail of eye structure of *Lycosa* (feeding on mealworm) (photo © Dr. J. White).

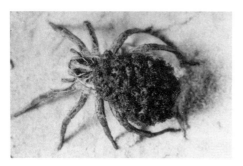

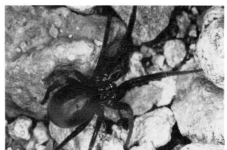

Figure 63. Female wolf spider showing mass of spiderlings on abdomen (photo © Dr. J. White).

Figure 64. American common house spider, *Filistata* sp. (photo © Dr. J. White).

L. THE CLUBIONID SPIDERS, *Clubiona* AND *Chiracanthium* SPP. (FAMILY CLUBIONIDAE)

These spiders have a worldwide distribution and the principal species are cosmopolitan, with frequent association with dwellings, and hence a significant chance of causing bites to humans. Several species of *Chiracanthium* are reported to cause effects in man, usually moderate to severe local pain, with erythema and swelling, lasting up to 24 hours, occasionally longer[8,11,239]. Some reports also mention systemic effects, including fever, malaise, nausea and vomiting. There is one report of five cases of (presumed) *Chiracanthium mildei* bite from Boston, in which local skin necrosis developed over several days, taking up to 8 weeks to heal. A similar pattern of local injury was seen in guinea pigs. The pattern of lesions appears similar to those of loxoscelism, although Boston is not within the accepted range for loxosceles.

M. THE AGELENID SPIDERS (FAMILY AGELINIDAE)

These tent web spiders are mostly small, but at least one large species, *Tegenaria agrestis*, has been implicated in causing local skin necrosis in parts of North America, though not in Europe, where it is probably more common[236,237]. Studies on the venom of this species showed necrotic activity, and a series of cases of loxoscelism-like local tissue damage following presumed spider bite were investigated, revealing *Tegenaria* but no *Loxosceles* in each locality. The states involved were Washington, Oregon and Idaho, not within the expected range of *Loxosceles*. This led to the suggestion that *Tegenaria* was responsible, but this has not been confirmed with definite clinical cases. There are two reports of definite bites by *Tegenaria* without any effects. Two other species of agelenids are reported to cause local pain and muscular spasm after biting, *Coelotes obesus* and *Agelena labyrinthica*.

N. THE SPITTING SPIDERS (FAMILY SCYTODIDAE)

In some texts, this family includes the genus *Loxosceles* (see elsewhere in this chapter). The principle genus, *Scytodes*, encompasses those small spiders known to "spit" a toxic or sticky substance onto potential prey or predators. They do not appear to cause medically significant effects.

O. OTHER SPIDERS

A variety of other Araneomorph spiders have been reported to bite man, yet not have medically significant effects, or significant effects are rarely reported. These were reviewed by Bettini and Brignoli[11] and by Bucherl[8].

1. Dysderid spiders (family Dysderidae)

Of the several hundred species, most of which are palaearctic in distribution, *Dysdera (crocata)*, which has a wider distribution, including Australia and the UK, is the only species consistently reported as biting man. There is considerable doubt about the ability of this spider to cause any effects of medical significance, and it should probably be considered harmless.

2. Segestriid spiders (family Segestriidae)

Worldwide distribution, associated with human habitation, particularly the cosmopolitan species *Segestria florentina*, which at most causes slight local redness and swelling, and not necrosis, as previously suspected.

3. Linyphiid spiders (family Linyphiidae)

Diverse, widely distributed, small spiders, generally considered harmless. There is a report of local redness and swelling following bites by *Leptorhoptrum robustum* in sewage treatment plant workers.

4. Pisaurid spiders (family Pisauridae)

Mostly hunting spiders with a worldwide distribution, some of which are semi-aquatic, such as *Dolomedes*, and have ichythiotoxic venoms, but do not appear to cause significant effects in man.

5. Water spiders (family Argyronetidae)

The common European water spider, *Argyroneta aquatica*, may possibly have a bite which is "not innocuous", but specific and corroborative details are lacking.

6. Crab spiders (family Thomisidae)

Small to medium sized hunting spiders distributed worldwide, with only one species reported as medically significant: "foka", *Phrynarachne rugosa*, from Madagascar, where it causes local, then generalised swelling, and is potentially lethal, although details are lacking to substantiate this.

XV. REFERENCES

1.   **BRISTOE, W.S.** *The World of Spiders.* London:Collins, 1958.
2.   **PETRIE, A.** Poisons information centres. In Eds. Covacevich, J., Davie, P., Pearn, J. *Toxic Plants and Animals: A Guide for Australia* Brisbane:Queensland Museum, pps. 487-491, 1987.
3.   **KIRBY, J.** *1993 Annual Report of the New South Wales Poisons Information Centre.* Sydney:Royal Alexandra Hospital for Children, 1994.
4.   **LITOVITZ, T., VELTRI, C.** 1984 Annual report of the American Association of Poison Control Centres National Data Collection System. *Am. J. Emerg. Med.,* **2**:66-70, 1985.
5.   **PARRISH, H.M.** *Poisonous snakebites in the United States.* New York:Vantage Press, 1980.

6. RUSSELL, F.E. A confusion of spiders. *Emerg. Med., 15*: 6-10, 1988.

8. BUCHERL, W. Spiders. In Eds. Bucherl, W., Buckley, E. *Venomous Animals and their Venoms; Volume III; Venomous Invertebrates.* New York:Academic Press, pps. 197-277, 1971.

9. LUCAS, S. Spiders in Brazil. *Toxicon,* **26**:759-772, 1988.

10. RIBEIRO, L.A., JORGE, M.T., PIESCO, R.V., NISHIOKA, S. DEA. Wolf spider bites in Sao Paulo, Brazil; a clinical and epidemiological study of 515 cases. *Toxicon,* **28**: 715-717, 1990.

11. BETTINI, S., BRIGNOLI, P.M. Review of the spider families, with notes on the lesser known poisonous forms. In Ed.Bettini, S., *Arthropod Venoms.* New York: Springer Verlag, pp. 101-120, 1978.

12. NEWLANDS, G., ATKINSON, P. Review of southern African spiders of medical importance, with notes on the signs and symptoms of envenomation. *Sth. Afr. Med., J.* **73**: 235-239, 1988.

13. NEWLANDS, G., ATKINSON, P. Behavioural and epidemiological considerations pertaining to necrotic araneism in southern Africa. *Sth. Afr. Med. J.,* **77**: 92-95, 1990.

14. NEWLANDS, G., ATKINSON, P. A key for the clinical diagnosis of araneism in Africa south of the equator. *Sth. Afr. Med., J.* **77**: 96-97, 1990.

15. RUSSELL, F.E. Venomous arthropods. *Vet. Hum. Toxicol.,* **33**:505-508,1991.

16. CARDOSO, J.L.C.; FAN HUI WEN: FRANÇA, F.O.S.; WARRELL, D.A., THEAKSTON, R.D.G. Detection by enzyme immunoassay of Loxosceles gaucho venom in necrotic skin lesions caused by spider bites in Brazil. *Trans Royal Soc Trop Med Hyg,* **84**: 608-609, 1990.

17. BERGER, R.S., MILLIKAN, L.E., CONWAY, F. An in vitro test for *Loxosceles reclusa* spider bites. *Toxicon,* **11**:465-470, 1973.

18. FINKE, J.H., CAMPBELL, B.J., BARRETT, J.T. Serodiagnostic test for *Loxosceles reclusa* bites. *Clin. Toxicol.,* **7**:375-382, 1974.

19. REES, R.S., KING, L.E. Therapy for brown recluse spider bites is dependent on venom persistence. *Clin. Res.,* **33**:302, 1985.

20. BARRETT, S.M., ROMINE-JENKINS, M., BLICK, K.E. Passive hemagglutination inhibition test for diagnosis of brown recluse spider bite envenomation. *Clin. Chem.,* **39**:2104-2107, 1993.

21. THEAKSTON, D.K., WARRELL, D.A. Antivenoms:a list of hyperimmune sera currently available for the treatment of envenoming by bites and stings. *Toxicon,* **29**:1419-1470, 1991.

22. BITTERMAN-DEUTSCH, O., BERGMAN, R., FRIEDMAN-BIRNBAUM, R. Brown spider bite. *Harefuah,* **119**:137-139, 1990.

23. FURTRELL, J.M. Loxoscelism. *Am. J. Med. Sci.,* **304**:261-267, 1992.

24. BERGER, R. The unremarkable brown recluse spider bite. *JAMA,* **225**:1109-1111, 1986.

25. WASSERMAN, G.S., ANDERSON, P. Loxoscelism and necrotic arachnidism. *J. Toxicol. Clin. Toxicol.,* **21**:451-472, 1983-84.

26. ANDERSON, P. Necrotizing spider bites. *Am. Fam. Physician,* **26**:198-203, 1982.

27. REES, R., ALTENBERN, P., LYNCH, J., KING, L.E. Brown recluse spider bites; a comparison of early surgical excision versus dapsone and delayed surgical excision. *Ann. Surg.,* **202**:659-663, 1985.

28. JANSEN, J.T., MORGAN, P.N., MCQUEEN, N.N., BENNETT, W.E. The brown recluse spider bite; controlled evaluation of treatment using the white rabbit as an animal model. *South. Med. J.,* **64**:1194-, 1983.

29. CHAN, K.K. A critical look at therapy for brown recluse spider bite. *Arch. Dermatol.,***107**:298-, 1973.

30. FARDON, D.W., WINGO, C.W., ROBINSON, D.W., MASTERS, F.W. The treatment of brown recluse spider bite. *Plast. Reconstr. Surg.,* **40**:482-488, 1967.

31. REES, R., SHACK, B., WITHERS, B., MADDEN, J., FRANKLIN, J., LYNCH, J.B. Management of brown recluse spider bite. *Plast. Recostr. Surg.,* **68**:768-773, 1981.

32. WASSERMAN, G.S. Wound care of spider and snake envenomations. *Ann. Emerg. Med.,* **17**:1331-1335, 1988.

33. YOUNG, V.L., PIN, P. The brown recluse spider bite. *Ann. Plastic. Surg.,* **20**:447-452, 1988.

34. DELOZIER, J.B., REAVES, L., KING, L.E., REES, R.S. Brown recluse spider bites of the upper extremity. *South. Med. J.,* **81**:181-184, 1988.

35. WESLEY, R.E., BALLINGER, W.H., CLOSE, L.W., LAY, A.M. Dapsone in the treatment of presumed brown recluse spider bite of the eyelid. *Ophthal. Surg.,* **16**:116-120, 1985.

36. KING, L.E., REES, R.S. Dapsone treatment of a brown recluse spider bite. *JAMA,* **250**:648, 1983.

37. WILLE, R.C., MORROW, J.D. Case report; dapsone hypersensitivity syndrome associated with treatment of the bite of a brown recluse spider. *Amer. J. Med. Sci.,* **296**:270-271, 1988.

38. REES, R.S., CAMPBELL, D.S., REIGER, E. , KING, L.E. The diagnosis and treatment of brown recluse spider bites. *Ann. Emerg. Med.,* **16**:945-949, 1989.

39. SVENDSEN, F.J. The treatment of problem brown recluse spider bites with hyperbaric oxygen; a clinical observation. *J. Ark. Med. Soc.,* **85**:199-204, 1986.

40. STRAIN, G.M., SNIDER, T.G., TEDFORD, B.L., COHN, G.H. Hyperbaric oxygen effects on brown recluse spider(*Loxosceles reclusa*) envenomation in rabbits. *Toxicon,* **29**:989-996, 1991.

41. GRAY, M. Distribution of the funnel-web spiders. In: Eds COVACEVICH, J., DAVIE, P., PEARN, J. *Toxic Plants and Animals - A Guide for Australia,* Brisbane, Queensland Museum, 1987.

42. **GRAY,   M.R.**   Aspects   of   the   systematics   of   the   Australian   funnel-web   spiders (Araneae:Hexathelidae:Atracinae) based upon morphological and electrophoretic data. In Eds. Austin A.D., Heather N.W. *Australian Arachnology*; Miscl. Publ. No.5, Aust. Entomol. Soc.; 113-125, 1988.

43. **GRAY, M.R., SUTHERLAND, S.K.** Venoms of Dipluridae. In Ed., BETTINI, S., *Arthropod Venoms*, Berlin, Springer Verlag, 1978.

44. **SUTHERLAND, S.K.** *Australian Animal Toxins.* Melbourne: Oxford University Press, 1983.

45. **WIENER, S.** The Sydney funnel-web spider (*Atrax robustus*). 1. Collection of venom and its toxicity in animals. *Med. J. Aust.*, **2**:377-382, 1957.

46. **SUTHERLAND, S.K.** The Sydney funnel-web spider (*Atrax robustus*). 1. A review of published studies on the crude venom. *Med. J. Aust.*, **2**:528-530, 1972.

47. **SUTHERLAND, S.K.** The Sydney funnel-web spider (*Atrax robustus*). Fractionation of the female venom into five distinct components. *Med. J. Aust.*, **2**:593-596, 1972.

48. **SUTHERLAND, S.K.** Isolation, mode of action and properties of the major toxin (Atraxotoxin) in the venom of the sydney funnel web spider (*Atrax robustus*). *Proc. Aust. Soc. Med. Res.*, **3**:172, 1973.

49. **GREGSON, R.P., SPENCE, I.** Isolation and characterization of a protein neurotoxin from the venom glands of the funnel-web spider (*Atrax robustus*). *Comp. Biochem. Physiol.*, **74(1)**:125-132, 1983.

50. **MYELCHARANE, E.J., SPENCE, I., GREGSON, R.P.** *In vivo* actions of atraxin, a protein neurotoxin from the venom glands of the funnel-web spider (*Atrax robustus*). *Comp. Biochem. Physiol.*, **79(2)**: 395-399, 1984.

51. **SHEUMACK, D.D., CARROLL, P.R., HAMPSON, F., HOWDEN, M.E.H., INGLIS, A.S., ROXBURGH, C.M., SKORULIS, A., STRIKE, P.M.** The isolation and n-terminal sequence of the lethal neurotoxin from the venom of the male Sydney funnel-web spider, *Atrax robustus*. *Toxicon*, Suppl. **3**: 397-400, 1983.

52. **SHEUMACK, D.D., BALDO, B.A., CARROLL, P.R., HAMPSON, F., HOWDEN, M.E.H., SKORULIS, A.** A comparative study of properties and toxic constituents of funnel-web spider (*Atrax*) venoms. *Comp. Biochem. Physiol.*, **78(1)**:55-68, 1984.

53. **SHEUMACK, D.D., CLAASSENS, R., WHITELEY, N.M., HOWDEN, M.E.H.** Complete amino acid sequence of a new type of lethal neurotoxin from the venom of the funnel-web spider *Atrax robustus. FEBS Letters*, **181(1)**:154-156, 1985.

54. **SUTHERLAND, S.K., DUNCAN, A.W., TIBBALLS, J.** Local inactivation of funnel-web spider (*Atrax robustus*) venom by first-aid measures. *Med. J. Aust.*, **2**: 435-437, 1980.

55. **SUTHERLAND, S.K., & DUNCAN, A.W.** New first-aid measures for envenomation: with special reference to bites by the Sydney funnel-web spider (*Atrax robustus*). *Med. J. Aust.*, **1**:378-379, 1980.

56. **TIBBALLS, J., SUTHERLAND, S.K., & DUNCAN, A.W.** Effects of male Sydney funnel-web spider venom in a dog and a cat. *Australian Veterinary J.*, **64(2)**:63-64, 1987.

57. **WIENER, S., DRUMMOND, F.H.** Assay of spider venom and antivenene in Drosophila. *Nature (Lond.)*, **178**:267-268, 1956.

58. **MUSGRAVE, A.** Some poisonous Australian spiders. *Rec. Aust. Museum*, **16**:33-46, 1927.

59. **CLELAND, J.B.** Injuries and diseases in Australia attributable to animals (other than insects). *Med. J. Aust.*, **1**:157-166, 1932.

59. **BEAZLEY, R.N.** Death from the bite of a trapdoor spider. *Med. J. Aust.*, **1**:255-256, 1930.

60. **CLELAND, J.B.,** Injuries and diseases in Australia attributable to animals (other than insects). *Med. J. Aust.*, **1**:157-166, 1932.

61. **INGRAM, W.W., MUSGRAVE, A.** Spider bite (arachnidism); a survey of its occurrence in Australia with case histories. *Med. J. Aust.*, **2**:10-15, 1933.

62. **MUSGRAVE, A.** Spiders harmful to man I. *The Aust. Museum Mag.*, **9(11)**:385-388, 1949.

63. **MUSGRAVE, A.** Spiders harmful to man II. *The Aust. Museum Mag.*, **9(12)**:411-419, 1949.

64. **IRWIN, R.S.** Funnel-web spider bite. *Med. J. Aust.*, **2**: 342, 1952.

65. **KAIRE, G.H.** Observations on some funnel-web spiders (*Atrax* species) and their venoms, with particular reference to *Atrax robustus. Med. J. Aust.*, **2**:307-311, 1963.

66. **WIENER, S.** The Sydney funnel-web spider (*Atrax robustus*). II. Venom yield and other characteristics of spider in activity. *Med. J. Aust.*, **2**: 678-682, 1959.

67. **WIENER, S.** Observations on the venom of the Sydney funnel-web spider (*Atrax robustus*). *Med. J. Aust.*, **2**: 693-699, 1961.

68. **WATKINS, A.M.** A bite by *Atrax robustus. Med. J. Aust.*, **1**:710, 1939.

69. **SUTHERLAND, S.K.** The Sydney funnel-web spider (*Atrax robustus*). 3. A review of some clinical records of human envenomation. *Med. J. Aust.*, **2**:642-646, 1972.

70. **FISHER, M.M., CARR, G.A., MCGUINNESS, R., WARDEN, J.C.** *Atrax robustus* envenomation. *Anaesth. Intens. Care*, **8**: 410-420, 1980.

71. **FISHER, M.M., RAFTOS, J., MCGUINNESS, R.G., DICKS, I.T., WONG, J.S., BURGESS, K.R., SUTHERLAND S.K.** Funnel-web spider (*Atrax robustus*) antivenom. 2. Early clinical experience. *Med. J. Aust.*, **2**:525-526, 1981.

72. **TORDA, T.A., LOONG, E., GREAVES, I.** Severe lung oedema and fatal consumption coagulopathy after funnel-web bite. *Med. J. Aust.*, **2**: 442-444, 1980.

73. **HARTMAN, L.J., & SUTHERLAND, S.K.** Funnel-web spider (*Atrax robustus*) antivenom in the treatment of human envenomation. *Med. J. Aust.*, **141**:796-799, 1984.

74. **FISHER, M.M.** Proc. Sydney Allergen Group, 6:30-36, 1989.

75. **FISHER, M.M., BOWEY, C.J.** Urban envenomation. *Med. J. Aust.*, **150**:695-698, 1989.

76. **DIECKMAN, J., PREBBLE, J., MCDONOGH, A., SARA, A., FISHER, M.,** Efficacy of funnel web spider antivenom in human envenomation by *Hadronyche* species. *Med. J. Aust.;* 151:706-707, 1989.

77. **KNIGHT, J., SUTTON, L.** Successful treatment of *Atrax formidabilis* envenomation. *Med. J. Aust.*, **2**: 434-435, 1982.

78. **BROWN, M.R., SHEUMACK, D.D., TYLER, M.I., HOWDEN, M.E.H.** Amino acid sequence of versutoxin, a lethal neurotoxin from the venom of the funnel-web spider *Atrax versutus*. *Biochem. J.*, **250**:401-405, 1988.

79. **WHITE, J., HIRST, D., HENDER, E.** 36 cases of bites by spiders, including the white-tailed spider, *Lampona cylindrata*. *Med. J. Aust.*, **150**: 401-403, 1989.

80. **MORGANS, D., SPIRA, P.J., MYELCHARANE, E.J., GLOVER, W.E.** Effect of funnel-web spider venom in the monkey. *Proc. Aust. Physiol. Phamacol. Soc.*, **5**:234-235, 1974.

81. **MORGANS, D., CARROLL, P.R.** A direct acting adrenergic component of the venom of the Sydney funnel-web spider *Atrax robustus*. *Toxicon*, **14**:185-189, 1976.

82. **DUNCAN, A.W., TIBBALLS, J., SUTHERLAND, S.K.** Effects of Sydney funnel-web spider envenomation in monkeys and their clinical implications. *Med. J. Aust.*, **2**: 429-435, 1980.

84. **SUTHERLAND, S.K.** Treatment of funnel-web spider bites. *Med. J. Aust.*, **1**:1016, 1973.

85. **SUTHERLAND, S.K.** The management of bites by the Sydney funnel-web spider, *Atrax robustus*. *Med. J. Aust.*, **1**:148-150, 1978.

86. **WHITE, J.** Review of clinical and pathological aspects of spider bite in Australia. In: Eds Gopalakrishnakone, P., Tan, C.K. *Progress in Venom and Toxin Research*, Singapore, Univ. Sing, 1987.

87. **NOEL, V., SUTHERLAND, S.K.** Letter to Editor, with reply from S.K. Sutherland. *Med. J. Aust.*, **142**:328, 1985.

88. **WIENER, S., SUTHERLAND, S.K.** Letter to editor, with reply from S.K. Sutherland. *Med. J. Aust.*, **2**:104-106, 1978.

90. **SUTHERLAND, S.K.** Antivenom to the venom of the male Sydney funnel-web spider, *Atrax robustus*. *Med. J. Aust.*, **2**: 437-441, 1980.

91. **SUTHERLAND, S.K., TIBBALLS, J., DUNCAN, A.W.** Funnel-web spider (*Atrax robustus*) antivenom. 1. Preparation and laboratory testing. *Med. J. Aust.*, **2**:522-524, 1981.

93. **MINTON, S.A.** *Venom Diseases*. Springfield: Charles C. Thomas, 1974.

94. **RUSSELL, F.E., WALDRON, W.G.** Spider bites, tick bites. *Calif. Med.*, **106**:248-249, 1967.

95. **RUSSELL, F.E.** Bites of spiders and other arthropods. In Eds. Conn, H.F. *Current Therapy* London:Saunders, pps. 878-879, 1969.

96. **SOUTHCOTT, R.V.** Arachnidism and allied syndromes in the Australian region. *Rec. Adelaide Child. Hosp.* **1**:97-186, 1976.

97. **DAHL, F.** Kann ein Systematiker auch zu sorgfaltig arbeiten? *Zoologischer Anzeige*, **25**:705-708, 1902.

98. **CAMBRIDGE, F.O.P.** On the genus *Latrodectus*. *Annals and Magazine of Natural History*, **(7)10**: 38-40, 1902.

99. **LEVI, H.W.** The spider genus *Latrodectus* (Araneae, Theridiidae). *Trans. Amer. Microscopical Soc.*, **78**: 7-43, 1959.

100. **CAMBRIDGE, F.O.P.** On the spiders of the genus *Latrodectus*, Walckenaer. *Proceed. Zoo. Soc. London*, **1902(1)**:247-261, 1902.

101. **ABALOS, J.W.** The egg-sac in the identification of species of *Latrodectus*. *Psych.*, **69**:268-270, 1962.

102. **LEVI, H.W.** On the value of genetalic structures and colouration in separating species of Widow spiders (*Latrodectus* sp.)(Arachnida: Araneae: Theridiidae). *Verh. naturwiss. Ver. Hamburg*, **26**:195-200, 1983.

103. **PLATNICK, N.** *Advances in spider taxonomy, 1981-1987. A supplement to Brignoli's "A Catalogue of the Araneae Described Between 1940-1981.* Manchester:Manchester Uni. Press, 1990.

104. **JOHNSTON, T.H.** Aboriginal names and utilization of the fauna in the Eyrean region. *Trans. Roy. Soc. South Australia*, **67**:244, 1943.

105. **MARETIC, Z.** Latrodectism in Mediterranean countries, including south Russia, Israel, and north Africa. In Eds. Bucherl, W., Buckley, E. *Venomous Animals and their Venoms; Volume III; Venomous Invertebrates* New York:Academic Press, pps. 197-277, 1971.

106. **MARETIC, Z.** Venoms of Theridiidae, Genus *Latrodectus;* B. Epidemiology of envenomation, symptomatology, pathology and treatment. In Ed. Bettini, S., *Handbook Of Experimental Pharmacology, Vol. 48,Arthropod Venoms* Berlin:Springer Verlag, pps. 185-212, 1978.

107. **NACHI, C.F., KASILO, O.M.** Poisoning due to insect and scorpion stings/bites. *Hum. Exp. Toxicol.* **12**:123-125, 1993.

108. **TORREGIANI, F., LA-CAVERA, C.** Review of latrodectism and malmignatta sting (*Latrodectus tredecimguttatus*) in Italy. *Minerva Med.* **81:**147-154, 1990.

109. **KRASNONOS, L.N., KOVALENKO, A.F., UKOLOV, I.P., ERGASKEV, N.E.** Cases of mass karakurt bites in Uzbekistan. *Med. Parazitol. Mosk.* **July-Aug:**39-42, 1989.

110. **BETTINI, S., MAROLI, M..** Venoms of Theriidae, Genus *Latrodectus*: A. Systematics, distribution and biology of species: chemistry, pharmacology and mode of action of venom. In Ed. Bettini, S., *Handbook Of Experimental Pharmacology, Vol. 48, Arthropod Venoms* Berlin:Springer Verlag, 149-185, 1978.

111. **LONGENECKER, H.E., HURLBUTT, W.P., MAURO, A., CLARK, A.W.** Effects of black widow spider venom on the frog neuromuscular junction. I Effects on end-plate potential, miniature end-plate potential and nerve terminal spike. *Nature,* **225:**701-703, 1970.

112. **CLARK, A.W., MAURO, A., LONGENECKER, H.E., HURLBUT, W.P.,** Effects of black widow spider venom on the frog neuromuscular junction. II. Effects on the fine structure of the frog neuromuscular junction. *Nature,* **225:**703-705, 1970.

113. **IIAMILTON, R.C.** Ultrastructural studies of the action of Australian spider venoms. *30th. Ann. Proc. Electron Microscopy Soc. Amer.,* 1972.

114. **GRANATA, F., PAGGI, P., FRONTALI, N.** Effects of chromatographic fractions of black widow spider venom on in vitro biological systems. *Toxicon,* **10:**551-555, 1972.

115. **HAMILTON, R.C., ROBINSON, P.M.,** Disappearance of small vesicles from adrenergic nerve endings in the rat vas deferens caused by red back spider venom. *J. Neurocytol.,* **2:**465-469, 1973.

116. **TSENG, M.C., SIEKIVITZ, P.** The effect of the purified major protein factor (a-latrotoxin) of black widow spider venom on the release of acetylcholine and norepinephrine from mouse cerebral cortex slices. *Brain Res.* **139:**190-196, 1978.

117. **GRASSO, A., SENNI, N.** A toxin purified from the venom of black widow spider affects the uptake and release of radio-active g-aminobutyrate and N-epinephrine from rat brain synaptosomes. *Eur. J. Biochem.* **102:**337-344, 1979.

118. **DUCHEN, L.W., QUEIROZ, L.S.** Degeneration and regeneration of sensory nerve terminals in muscle spindles; effects of *Latrodectus* spider venoms. *Proc. Physiol. Soc. Cambridge,* June, 1981.

119. **FRONTALI, N., CECCARELLI, B., GORIO, A., MAURO, A., SIEKEVITZ, P., TZENG, M., HURLBUT, W.P.** Purification from black widow spider venom of a protein factor causing depletion of synaptic vesicles at neuromuscular junctions. *J. Cell. Biol.,* **68:**462-479, 1976.

120 **GORIO, A., MAURO, A.** Reversibility and mode of action of black widow spider venom on the vertebrate neuromuscular junction. *J. Gen. Physiol.,* **73:**245-263, 1979.

121. **LEBEZ, D., MARETIC, Z., KRISTAN, J.** Studies on labelled animal poisons. I Distribution of P^{32} labelled *Latrodectus tredecimguttatus* venom in the guinea pig. *Toxicon,* **2:**251-253, 1965.

122. **BOGEN, E.,** Poisonous spider bites. *Ann. Intern. Med.,* **6:**375-388, 1932.

123. **PRESS, J. GEDALIN,** A. Spider bite in a child. *Harefuah,* **116:**466-468, 1989.

124. **SAMPAYO, R.R.L.** *Latrodectus mactans* y latrodectismo. Estudio Experimental y Clinico, Buenas Aires:El Ateno 1942.

124. **LEBEZ, D., MARETIC, Z., GUBENSEK, F., KRISTAN, J.** Studies on labelled animal poisons. II Distribution of the venoms of various spiders labelled with Se^{75} and P^{32} in the guinea pig. *Toxicon,* **5:**261-262, 1968.

125. **MARETIC, Z.** Araneizam u Istri kao prakticini problem. *Lij. vj.* , **73:**203-208, 1951.

126. **LETHBRIDGE, H.O.** Red-back spider bite. *Med. J. Aust.,***1:**113, 1922.

127. **MARETIC, Z.** Latrodectism; Variations in clinical manifestations provoked by *Latrodectus* species of spiders. *Toxicon,* **21(4):**457-466, 1983.

128. **MARETIC, Z.** *Araneizam - sosobitimosvrtom na Istru.* Thesis; Med. Faculty Univ. Zagreb, 1959.

129. **CLARK, R.F., WETHERN-KESTNER, S., VANCE, M.V., GERKIN, R.** Clinical presentation and treatment of black widow spider envenomation: A review of 163 cases. *Ann. Emerg. Med.,* **21(7):**782-787, 1992.

130. **ESTESO, S.C.** Latrodectismo humano en la provincia de Cordoba. *Prensa Med Argent* **72:** 222, 1985.

131. **GRISOLIA, C.S.; PELUSO, F.O.; STANCHI, N.O. FRANCINI, F.** Epidemiologia del latrodectismo en la Provincia de Buenos Aires, Argentina. *Rev Saude Publ SÆo Paulo,* **26 (1):** 1-5, 1992.

132. **HAMBURGER, R.** Mordedura por la "Coya". *Rev Med Cir,* **5 (2):** 11-12, 1938.

133. **MACHADO, O.** *Latrodectus mactans,* sua ocorrência no Brasil. *Bol Inst Vital Brazil,* **5 (4):** 153-160, 1948.

134. **RODRIGUES, D.S. & NUNES, T.B.** Latrodectismo na Bahia. *Rev baiana Saude Publ,* **12 (3):** 38, 1985.

135. **ARTAZA, O.; FUENTES, J.; GOMEZ, P. NORRIS, R.** Lactrodectismo: evaluación clínico-terapéutica de 78 casos. *Parasitol al Día,* **8:** 45, 1984.

136. **JELINEK, G.A., BANHAM, N.D.G., DUNJEY, S.J.** Red back spider bites at Fremantle Hospital, 1982-1987. *Med. J. Aust.,* **150:**693-695, 1989.

137. **SUTHERLAND, S.K., TRINCA, J.C.** Survey of 2144 cases of red-back spider bites; Australia and New Zealand, 1963-1976. *Med. J. Aust.,* **2:**620-623, 1978.

138. **WIENER, S.** The Australian red-back spider (*Latrodectus hasseltii*), preparation of antiserum by the use of venom adsorbed on aluminium phosphate. *Med. J. Aust.*,**1**:739-742, 1956.

139. **MARETIC, Z.** Latrodectism. *Bull. Internat. Yugosl. Acad. Sci. Arts,* **17**:63-87, 1966.

140. **MARETIC, Z.** Medicinsko znacenje ujeda paukova u nasim krajevima. *Med. glas.*, **9**:159-163, 1955.

141. **WEINER, S.** Red back spider bite in Australia; analysis of 167 cases. *Med. J. Aust.*, **2**:44-49, 1961.

142. **WHITE, J., HARBOARD, M.** Latrodectism as mimic. *Med. J. Aust.*, **142**:75, 1985.

143. **WONG, R.C., HUGHES, S.E., VOORHEES, J.J.** Spider bites. *Arch. Dermatol.*, **123**: 98-104, 1987.

144. **STILES, A.D.** Priapism following a black-widow spider bite. *Clin Ped,* **21**: 174, 1982.

145. **MORALES, J.R., CERIONI, L.E., ALVAREZ, A., MASTROGIACOMO, L.D., CERIONI, M.A.** Estudio clinico: aracnoidismo y ofidismo, sobre casuistica en Mendoza. *Rev Nac Cienc Med Univ Nac Cuyo,* **6** (1): 11-20, 1983.

146. **MARETIC, Z. LEBEZ, D.** *Araneism.* Belgrade: Pula-Ljubjana, 253 pp., 1979.

147. **BAERG, W.J.** The effects of the bite of *Latrodectus mactans* Fabr. *J. Parasitol.*, **9**:161-169, 1923.

148. **BANNER, W.,** Bites and stings in the pediatric patient. *Curr. Probl. Pediatr.*, **18**(1):1-69, 1988.

149. **BARTON, C.,** How it feels to be bitten by a black widow. A case history. *Nat. Hist.*, **42**:43-44, 1938.

150. **BETTINI, S., CANTORE, G.,** Quadro clinico del latrodectismo. *Rev. Parassit.*, **20**:49-72, 1959.

151. **BINDER, L.S.,** Acute arthropod envenomation; incidence, clinical features and management. *Med. Toxicol. Adverse Drug Exp.*, **4**:163-173, 1989.

152. **BOGEN, E.,** Arachnidism. A study in spider poisoning. *Arch. Intern. Med.*, **38**:623-634, 1926.

153. **GAJARDO-TOBAR, R.,** El latrodectismo. *Prensa. Med.*, **6**:3-18, 1941.

154. **GAJARDO-TOBAR, R.,** Algo mas sobre lactrodectismo. *Rev. Med. Valparaiso*, **3**:150-159, 1950.

155. **GREER, W.E.R.,** Arachnidism. *New Engl. J. Med.*, **240**:5-8, 1942.

156. **MILLER, D.G.** Bites and stings. *G.P.* ,**4**:35-42, 1951.

157. **BYRNE, G. C., PEMBERTON, P.J.,** Red back spider (*Latrodectus mactans hasselti*) envenomation in a neonate. *Med. J. Aust.*, **2**:665-666, 1983.

158. **JACKSON, E.S.** The red-backed spider bite. *Med. J. Aust.* ,**1**:525, 1927.

159. **BRAUN, G.,** Uber *Latrodectus tredecimguttatus. Wein Med. Presse,* **6**:223-224, 1899.

160. **GUZMAN, C.,** Progr. Med. 1896 (Chile), *An. Admin. Sanit. Asist. Pub.*, **6**:423, 1910.

161. **BELL, J.E., BOONE, J.A.,** Neostigmine methylsulfate an apparent specific for arachnidism (black widow spider bite). *J. Amer. Med. Assoc.*, **129**(15):1016-1017, 1945.

162. **PAMPIGLIONE, S.** Sulla "terapia musicale" dell'evelenamento da punctura di imenotteri (Mutillidae) in Sardegna. *Nuovi Annali Ig. Microbiol.*,**9**:100, 1958.

163. **BARRA, S.,** Su un caso di morte in seguito a morso di *Latrodectus malmigatus. Boll. Soc. Ital. Biol. sper.*, **33**:34, 1957.

164. **SCHENONE, H., NEIDMANN, G., BAHAMONDE, L., BONNEFOY, J.** Algunas alteraciones cardiovasculares observadas en el latrodectismo. *Bol. Chil. Paras.*, **12**:29-30, 1957.

165. **WEITZMANN, S., MARGULIS, G., LEHMANN, E.** Uncommon cardiovascular manifestations and high catecholamine levels due to "black widow" bite. *Amer. Heart J.,* **93**(1):89-90, 1977.

166. **SAMPAYO, R.R.L.T.** Pharmacological action of the venom of *Latrodectus mactans* and other *Latrodectus* spiders. *J. Pharmacol. exp. Ther.* ,**80**:309-322, 1944.

167. **CICARDO, V.H.,** Mechanismo de la hipertension arterial producida por la ponzona de *Latrodectus mactans. Rev. Soc. argent. Biol.*, **30**:19-24, 1954.

168. **LA GRANGE, M.A.C.** Pulmonary oedema from a widow spider bite. *Sth. Afr. Med. J.*, **77**(2):110, 1990.

169. **MARETIC, Z., JELASIC, F.** Uber den Einflus des toxins der spinne *Latrodectus tredecimguttatus* auf das nervensystem. *Acta trop. (Basel),* **10**:209-224, 1953.

170. **THORP, R.W., WOODSEN, W.D.** *Black widow, America's most poisonous spider.* Chapel Hill:Univ. N. Carol. Press, 1945.

171. **KOBERT, R.** *Beitrage zur kenntnis der giftspinnen.* Stuttgart:Ferd. Enke Verl., 1901.

172. **MARETIC, Z., STANIC, M.** The health problem of arachnidism. *Bull. Wld. Hlth. Org.*, **11**:1007-1022, 1954.

173. **BETTINI, S., RAVAIOLI, L., CANTORE, G.,** Nota preliminare sulla preparazione di un siero immune specifico verso il veleno di "*Latrodectus 13-guttatus*" Rosi. *Rend. Ist. Sup. San.*, **17**:192-199, 1954.

174. **TORREGIANI, F., LA CAVERA, C.** (Differential diagnosis of acute abdomen and latrodectism).. *Minerva Chir.*,**45**(5):303-5, 1990.

175. **HAGEN, H.,** Arachnidism. *Kentucky Med. J.*, **36**:120, 1938.

176. **MARZAN, B.** Pathologic reactions associated with the bite of *Latrodectus tredecimguttatus* . Observations on experimental animals. *Arch. Path. (Chicago),* **59**:727-728, 1955.

177. **CONSTANT, Y., GOUERE, P.,** Sur les phenomenes d'araneisme provoques par *Latrodectus menavodi. Bull. Soc. Path. Exot.*, **41**:234-237, 1949.

178. **VANOVSKI, B.** Latrodektizam u Jugoslaviji. *Lij. vj.*, **84**:131-137, 1962.

179. **BOGEN, E.,** The treatment of spider bite poisoning. In Eds. Buckley, E.E., Porges, N., *Venoms, Amer. Ass. Adv. Sci., (Berkeley),* 1956.

180. **RUSSELL, F.E., MARCUS, P., STRENG, J.A.** Black widow spider envenomation during pregnancy. Report of a case. *Toxicon*, **17**:188, 1979.
181. **GALA, S., KATELARIS, C.H.** Rhabdomyolysis due to redback spider envenomation. *Med. J. Aust.*, **157**:66, 1992.
182. **PODGORNY, G.** Consultations in emergency medicine; Spider bites. *Ann. Emerg. Med.*, **10**(3):164, 1981.
183. **KEY, G.F.** A comparison of calcium gluconate and methocarbamol (Robaxin) in the treatment of latrodectism (black widow spider envenomation). *Am. J. Trop. Med. Hyg.*, **30**(1):273-277, 1981.
184. **RAUBER, A.** Black widow spider bites. *J. Toxicol. Clin. Toxicol.*, **21**(4&5):473-485, 1983-84.
185. **KOBERNICK, M.** Black widow spider bite. *Amer. Fam. Physic.*, **29**(5):241-245, 1984.
186. **TIMMS, P.K., GIBBONS, R.B.** Latrodectism - effects of the black widow spider bite. *West. J. Med.*, **144**:315-317, 1986.
187. **REES, R.S., KING, L.E.** Arthropod bites and stings. In Ed. Fitzpatrick, *Dermatology in General Medicine* , New York:McGraw Hill Book Co., pps. 2495-2506, 1986.
188. **MILLER, T.A.** Latrodectis; bite of the black widow spider *Am. Fam. Physician* **45**:181-187, 1992.
189. **GILBERT, E.W., STEWART, C.M.** Effective treatment of arachnidism with clcium salts. Preliminary report. *Amer. J. med. Sci.*, **189**:532-536, 1935.
190. **SCHUMANN, S.H., CALDWELL, S.T.** 1990 South Carolina Physician survey of tick, spider and fire ant morbidity. *J. Sth. Carolina Med. Assoc.*, **87**(8):429-32, 1991.
191. **SCHENONE, H., SUAREZ, G.** Venoms of scytodidae, genus *Loxosceles*. In Ed. Bettini, S., *Arthropod Venoms*, New York, Springer Verlag, pp. 247-275, 1978.
192. **SCHENONE, H.; RUBIO, S.; VILLARROEL, F., ROYAS, A.** Epidemiologia y curso clínico del loxoscelismo. Estudio de 133 casos causados por la mordedura de la araña de los rincones (*Loxosceles laeta*). *Bol Chile Parasitol,* **14**: 17-19, 1975.
193. **SCHENONE, H.; SAVEDRA, T.; ROJAS, A.; VILAROEL, F.** Loxoscelismo en Chile: estudios epidemiologicos, clinicos y experimentales. *Rev Inst Med trop SÆo Paulo,* **36** (1): 403-415, 1989.
194. **GAJARDO-TOBAR, R.** Mi experiencia sobre loxoscelismo. *Mem Inst Butantan,* **33**: 689-698, 1966.
195. **ZAVALETA, A.** Loxoscelismo, un problema de salud en el Perú. *Bol Ofic sanit paname,r* **103**: 378-386, 1987.
196. **CARDOSO, J.L.C.; EICKSTEDT, V.R.D.; BORGES, I.; NOGUEIRA, M.T., FRANÇA, F.O.S.** Loxoscelismo: estudo de 242 casos. *Rev Soc Bras Toxicol,* **1** (1): 58-60, 1988.
197. **BARBARO,K.C.; CARDOSO, J.L.C.; EICKSTEDT, V.R.D., MOTA,I.** IgG antibodies to *Loxosceles sp.* spider venom in human envenoming. *Toxicon,* **30** (9): 1117-1121, 1992.
198. **BARBARO,K.C.; CARDOSO, J.L.C.; EICKSTEDT, V.R.D., MOTA,I.** Dermonecrotic and lethal components of *Loxosceles gaucho* spider venom. *Toxicon,* **30** (3): 331-338, 1992.
199. **SMITH, C.W.; MICKS, D.W.** The role of polymorphonuclear leuckocytres in the lesion caused by the venom of the brown spider, *Loxosceles reclusa*. *Labor Invest,* **22** (1): 90-93, 1979.
200. **BARRETO, O.C.O.; CARDOSO, J.L.C., DE CILLO, D.** Viscerocutaneous form of Loxoscelism and erythrocyte glucose-6-phosphate deficiency. *Rev Inst Med trop SÆo Paulo,* **27** (5): 264-267, 1985.
201. **GATES, C.A., REES, R.S.** Serum amyloid P component: its role in platelet activation stimulated by shingomyelinase D purified from the venom of the brown recluse spider (*Loxosceles reclusa*). *Toxicon,* **28**: 1303-1315, 1990.
202. **BUTZ, W.C.** Envenomation by the brown recluse spider (Aranae, Scytodidae) and related species. A public health problem in the United States. *Clin. Toxicol.*, **4**(4):515-524, 1971.
203. **BALDWIN, G.A., SMITH, D.F., FIKE, S.D.** Loxoscelism in Canada. *Can. Med. Assoc. J,* **138**: 521-522, 1988.
204. **GERTSCH, W.J., ENNIK, F.** The spider genus *Loxosceles* in North America, Central America, and the West Indies. *Bull. Am. Mus. Nat. Hist,*. **175**: 352-360, 1983.
205. **NELSON, J.** Loxoscelism in Canada. *Can. Med. Assoc. J.*, **138**: 888-889, 1988.
206. **ALLEN, P.B.R.** Loxoscelism in Canada. *Can. Med. Assoc. J.,* **138**: 792, 1988.
207. **BOBA, A.** Loxoscelism in Canada. *Can. Med. Assoc. J.* **139**: 98, 1988.
208. **ROSENFELD, G.** Animais peçonhentos e tóxicos do Brasil. In Eds Lacaz, C.S.; Baruzzi, R.G., Siqueira Jr, W. *Geografia Médica do Brasil*. SÆo Paulo: EDUSP, chapter 19: 430-475, 1972.
209. **MARTINO, O.A.; MATHET, H.; MASINI, R.D.; GRASSO, A.I.; THOMPSON, R.M.; GONDELL, C. & BOSH, J.E.** *Emponzoñamiento humano provocado por venenos de origen animal*. Buenos Aires: Ministerio de Bienestar Social de la Nacion, 240 pp, 1979.
210. **SUTHERLAND, S.K.** Spider bites in Australia: there are still some mysteries. *Med. J. Aust.*, **2**: 597, 1983.
211. **SHEPPARD, C.L.** Necrotizing arachnidism. *Med. J. Aust.*, **140**: 504, 1984.
212. **SPRING, W.** A probable case of necrotizing arachnidism. *Med. J. Aust.*, **147**: 605-607, 1987.
213. **SUTHERLAND, S.K.** Watch out, Miss Muffet! *Med. J. Aust.*, **147**: 531, 1987.
214. **MURTAGH, J., SUTHERLAND, S.K.** Venomous spiders of Australia. *Aust. Fam. Physic.*, **16**: 656-657, 1987.
215. **GRAY, M.** A significant illness that was produced by the white tailed spider, *Lampona cylindrata*. *Med. J. Aust.*, **151**: 114-116, 1989.

216. **IBRAHIM, N., MORGAN, M.F., AHMED, M.R.** Arachnidism: a serious new Australian disease. *Aust. NZ J. Surg.*, **59**: 507-510, 1989.

217. **KEMP, D.R.** Inappropriate diagnosis of necrotising arachnidism; watch out Miss Muffet - but don't get paranoid. *Med. J. Aust.*, **152**: 669-671, 1990.

218. **SUTHERLAND, S.K.** Inappropriate diagnosis of necrotising arachnidism. *Med.J. Aust.*, **153**: 499, 1990.

219. **ST. GEORGE, I.** Skin necrosis after white tailed spider bite? *New Zealand Med. J.*, **104**: 207-208, 1991.

220 **ATKINSON, R.K., WRIGHT, L.G.** Studies of the necrotic actions of the venoms of several Australian spiders. *Comp. Biochem. Physiol.* **98**: 441-444, 1991.

221. **BEARDMORE, G.L.** Necrotizing arachnidism in Australia. *Med. J. Aust.*, **155**: 208, 1991.

222. **RAVEN, R.J., HARVEY, M.S.** Necrotizing arachnidism in Australia. *Med. J. Aust.*, **155**:208, 1991.

223. **HARVEY, M.S., RAVEN, R.J.** Necrotizing arachnidism in Australia: a simple case of misidentification. *Med. J. Aust.*, **154**: 856, 1991.

224. **SUTHERLAND, S.K.** Necrotizing arachnidism in Australia. *Med. J. Aust.*, **155**: 136, 1991.

225. **HAYMAN, J.A., SMITH, I.M.** Necrotizing arachnidism in Australia. *Med. J. Aust.*, **155**: 351, 1991.

226. **GROSS, A.S., WILSON, D.C., KING, L.E.** Persistent segmental cutaneous anesthesia after a brown recluse spider bite. *South. Med. J.*, **83(11)**:1321-1323, 1990.

227. **BASCUR, L.; YEVENES, I., BARJA, P.** Effects of *Loxosceles laeta* spider venom on blood coagulation. *Toxicon,* **20 (4)**: 795-796, 1982.

228. **YIANNIAS, J.A., WINKELMANN, R.K.** Persistent painful plaque due to brown recluse spider bite. *Cutis,* **50(4)**:273-5, 1992.

229. **INGBER, A. , TRATTNER, A., CLEPER, R., SANDBANK, M.** Morbidity of brown recluse spider bites; clinical picture, treatment and prognosis. *Acta Derm. Venereol. Stokh.*, **71**: 337-340, 1991.

230. **HOOVER, E.L., WILLIAMS, W., KOGER, L., MURTHY, R., PARSH, S., WEAVER, W.L.** Pseudoepitheliomatous hyperplasia and pyoderma gangrenosum after a brown recluse spider bite. *South. Med. J.*, **83(2)**:243-246, 1990.

231. **VELLARD, J.** *Le venin des araignées.* Paris: Masson Editeurs, 311 p, 1936.

232. **FURLANETTO, R.S.** *Estudos sobre a preparaçÆo do soro antiloxoscélico.* Thesis Faculdade de Farmacia e Odontologia da USP, S.Paulo, 89p. mimeo, 1961.

233. **SCHENBERG, S. & PEREIRA LIMA, F.A.** Venoms of *Ctenidae*. In Eds Born, G.V.R.; Eichler, O.; Farah, A.; Herken, H., Weich, A.D. *Handbook of Experimental Pharmacology.* Berlin: Springer-Velarg, chapter **10**: 217-245, 1978.

234. **FONTANA, M.D., VITAL BRAZIL, O.** Mode of Action of *Phoneutria nigriventer* spider venom at the isolated phrenic nerve-diaphragm of the rat. *Braz J Med Biol Res,* **18**: 557-565, 1985.

235. **OSBORN, C.D.** Treatment of spider bites by high voltage direct current. *J. Okla. State Med. Assoc.*, **84**:257-260, 1991.

236. **VEST, D.K.** Necrotic arachnidism in the northwest United States and its probable relationship to *Tegenaria agrestis* (Walckenaer) spiders. *Toxicon*, **25**: 175-184, 1987.

237. **VEST, D.K.** Envenomation by *Tegenaria agrestis* (Walckenaer) spiders in rabbits. *Toxicon,* **25**: 221-224, 1987.

238. **RUTHERFORD, A.M., SUTHERLAND, S.K.** Large blister formation after a bite by the common cupboard spider, genus *Steatoda*. *Med. J. Aust.*, **151**: 542, 1989.

239. **MAIN, B.Y.** *Spiders.* Sydney; Collins, 1976.

240. **MUSGRAVE, A.** Spiders harmful to man. *Aust. Mus. Magazine.*, **9(12)**:411-419, 1949.

241. **TINGATE, T.R.** Envenomation by the common black window spider. *Med. J. Aust.*, **154**: 291, 1991.

242. **DUFFEY, E., GREEN, M.B.** A linyphiid spider biting workers on a sewage treatment plant. *Bull. Brit. Arachn. Soc.* **3**: 130-131, 1975.

243. **WATT, J.C.** The toxic effects of the bite of a clubionid spider. *New Zealand Entomologist,* **5(1)**:87-90, 1971.

244. **WARRELL, D.A., SHAHEEN, J., HILLYARD, P.D., JONES, D.** Neurotoxic envenoming by an imigrant spider (*Steatoda nobilis*) in southern England. *Toxicon* ,**29(10)**:1263-1265, 1991.

245. **SKINNER, M.W., BUTLER, C.B.** Necrotising arachnidism treated with hyperbaric oxygen. *Med. J. Aust.,* **162**:372-373, 1995.

Chapter 21

BIOLOGY AND DISTRIBUTION OF HYMENOPTERANS OF MEDICAL IMPORTANCE, THEIR VENOM APPARATUS AND VENOM COMPOSITION

Jürg Meier

TABLE OF CONTENTS

I. INTRODUCTION

Representing about two thirds of all animal species known, the insects, with more than one million species, form by far the greatest class of the animal kingdom. The order Hymenoptera with about 250,000 species described to date comprises the most developed forms with regard to anatomy and behaviour[1]. Hymenopterans are a biologically extremely fascinating animal group due to their omnipresence in practically every living space and they comprise the medically most significant venomous animals of the world. In the U.S. and also in Europe, hymenopteran stings are the cause of the majority of deaths due to venomous animals[2]. In this chapter, the phylogenic development (evolution) and mode of action of the hymenopteran sting apparatus is briefly described, since the function of this structure, present only in females, has changed several times during evolution and serves different purposes in the different suborders. Moreover, an overview on the biology and distribution of the hymenopteran groups of medical importance is included and notes on their venom composition are provided.

II. EVOLUTION OF THE STING APPARATUS: FROM OVIPOSITION TO DEFENSE

The order Hymenoptera is divided into two suborders, the Symphyta and the Apocrita; the latter suborder is divided into the sections Terebrantes and the Aculeata[3]. Hymenopteran males develop from unfertilized eggs and are usually simply constituted. All hymenopteran females are characterized by the possession of an ovipositor which serves a variety of different purposes, from being an egg-laying organ, serving as a tool to immobilize prey organisms for the progeniture or as a defense sting in social species, and being present in a more or less rudimentary form in some species.

A. BASIC STRUCTURE OF THE OVIPOSITOR
The body of the insect, which is characterized by the presence of a segmented exoskeleton, can be divided into three main parts, i.e. head, thorax and abdomen. The dorsal (*tergites*) and ventral (*sternites*) plates of the body consist of hard chitin and are bound together by elastic membranes (*pleurae*). In the hymenopteran females, the final abdominal segments are more or less modified and form the ovipositor (Figure 1). The eighth segment is formed by a pair of triangular chitinous plates which are called anterior or first valvifers from each of which a long, movable and backwards bent chitin appendix, the first valve, protrudes. The tergite of the ninth segment extends far towards the abdomen. Close to it, there are two further chitinous plates, the posterior or second valvifers. Each of them bears a second valve, i.e. backwards bent appendices which together with the first valves at the eighth segment form an ovipositor (Figure 1,c). Behind the second valvifers there are finally the third valves which at rest surround the ovipositor formed by the first and second valves. The abdominal segments are thus the main constituents of the hymenopteran ovipositor. Although not only the above mentioned chitinous elements of the skeleton, but also muscles and nerves are integrated components thereof, the term "ovipositor" is restrictively applied to the structural chitinous elements[4]. In this respect, the ovipositor is thus composed of the two pairs of valvifers, three pairs of valves and the ninth tergite, respectively, and the structures deriving therefrom. Within the different suborders and species of the Hymenoptera, the basic construction represented in Figure 1 is subject to modifications.

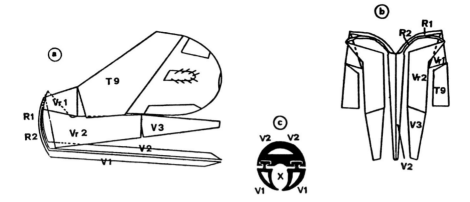

Figure 1. The basic structure of the hymenopteran Ovipositor.

a) Lateral view; b) Dorsal view; c) Cross section of stiger; T..[tergite no...]; S .. [sternite no...]; Vr 1..2 [valvifers 1..2]; V 1..3 [valvula 1..3]; R 1..2 [rami 1..2]; X ..venom duct formed by V1 and V2.

B. MODE OF ACTION OF THE ACULEATE STING APPARATUS

Nearly everybody has experienced at least one painful sting of an aculeate wasp or bee during his or her lifetime. The following explanation, based on different studies, therefore attempts to illustrate in a simple way the principle of the mode of action of the stinger in aculeate wasps and bees[5-9].

Three phases may be recognized as follows:

1. Excavation of the sting apparatus

A wasp or bee preparing to sting moves the whole sting apparatus ventrally by tilting it over a horizontal axis, which lies between tergite 8 and 9, respectively (Figure 2). As a consequence of this movement the stinger formed by the lancets (valvulae 1 [V 1]) and the sting sheath (fused valvulae 2 [V 2 in Figure 1, b+c]) leaves the sheath lobes of the sting (valvula 3 [V 3]).

2. Erection of the sting apparatus

In all members of the *Aculeata* a chitinous structure, the *furcula*, is found at the base of the stinger at which muscles coming from the valvifers 2 [Vr 2 in Figure 2] are attached (Figure 3a). A contraction of these muscles leads to further erection of the stinger into a downward position ready to sting (Figure 3b).

3. Piercing of the stinger

In many cases the movement of the abdomen towards an enemy with simultaneous movement and erection of the sting apparatus leads already to a penetration of the enemy's skin structure[10]. The valvifers 2 and 3 are connected with protractor and retractor muscles, respectively (Figure 4a). Contraction of the protracter muscles leads to a forward movement of the sting lancet [V 1; Figure 4b]. Since barbs at the lancet's top keep the lancet in the tissue while the muscles are retracted, a forward movement of the sting sheath [V 2; Figure 4c] occurs. The following contraction of the retractor muscles leads to a backward movement of the lancet. However, since the barbs prevent this movement, a further forward movement of the sting sheath [V 2; Figure 4d] occurs, which puts the stinger further into the enemy's tissues. The alternate protraction and retraction of the two pairs of muscles leads to a rapid penetration of the enemy's skin. Not only bees (Figure 5), but also wasps (Figure 6) have barbs at the tip of the lancets. Although those of wasps are small compared to the honeybee, they probably contribute towards deeper penetration in much the same way. However, only the sting apparatus of worker bees usually gets lost during the sting act, if a mammalian enemy is stung. This is due to the fact that in worker bees the whole sting apparatus is comparatively small and delicate, the stinger is straight with eight to ten strong barbs at the lancets and a weak and loosely fixed spiracular plate (tergite 8) as a preformed breaking point. Furthermore the barbs are positioned in a direction which strongly enhances the tissue resistance, when the stinger is to be retracted (Figure 7). This is not the case in wasps (Figure 8). Thus, the worker bee loses her life while stinging a big mammalian enemy and the sting apparatus, although removed from the body, is still able to inject venom for quite a while[10]. The preformed breaking point of the sting apparatus in workers of the honey bee may be regarded as a natural reaction, favoured by selection, against their biggest enemies, mammals and birds[9,10].

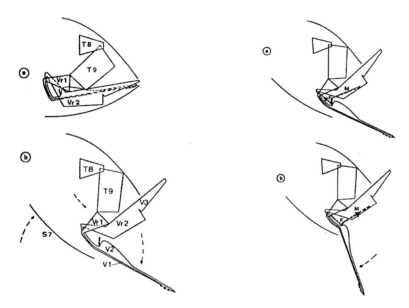

Figure 2. Excavation of the sting apparatus. a) sting apparatus in position of rest; b) sting apparatus excavated.

Figure 3. Erection of the sting apparatus. a) muscle inserting to furcula relaxed; b) muscle contracted. M [muscle], F [furcula].

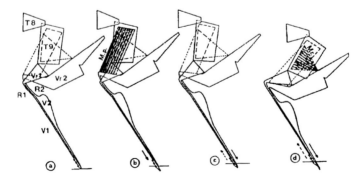

Figure 4. Piercing of the stinger. a) position of rest; b) contraction of the protractor muscle [M.p.]; c) position after relaxation of the protractor muscle; d) contraction of the retractor muscle [M.r.].

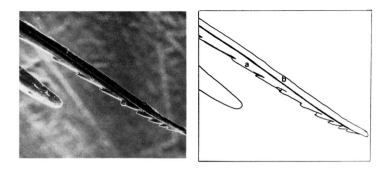

Figure 5. Tip of stinger of a honey bee (*Apis mellifera*). left; scanning electron micrograph, magnification 240x; right; schematic drawing; a ..[valvula 1], b ..[fused valvulae 2].

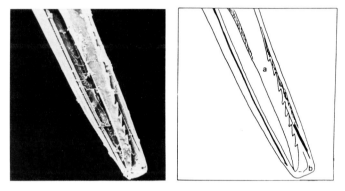

Figure 6. Tip of stinger of a German wasp (*Paravespula germanica*). left: scanning electron micrograph, magnification 260x, right: schematic drawing. a ..[valvula 1], b.. [fused valvulae 2].

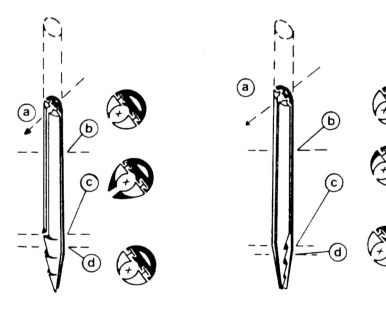

Figure 7. Tip of stinger of a honey bee (*Apis mellifera*). a) total view; b, c, d) cross sections; X ..[venom duct].

Figure 8. Tip of stinger of a German wasp (*Paravespula germanica*). a) total view; b, c, d) cross sections; X ..[venom duct].

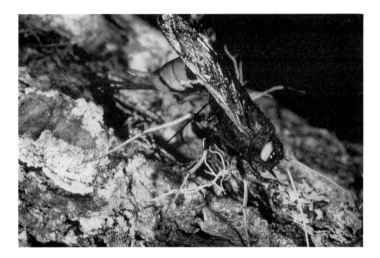

Figure 9. Plant wasp *Sirex gigas*, inserting an egg into a piece of wood (courtesy of Dr. A. Labhardt, Rodersdorf, Switzerland).

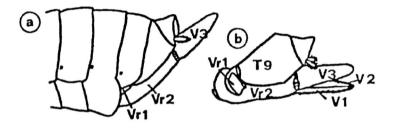

Figure 10. The basic structure of abdominal organisation in *Symphata.*

III. BIOLOGY OF HYMENOPTERA

A. SUBORDER SYMPHYTA

The most significant characteristic of this phylogenetically old group is the absence of the so-called "wasp waist". The abdomen is attached to the full width of the thorax (Figure 9) and the ovipositor (called *serrula*, lat. "saw for oviposition") is relatively well visible at the end of the abdomen (Figure 10). At its base, there are the oviduct as well as accessory glands of the female sex organ, the mucous secretion of which probably allows the easy transport of the eggs through the ovipositor[11,12]. During oviposition, valves 1 as "saw-blades" move against each other and are led into valves 2. Except in some rare cases, the eggs are laid down in leaves, stems or lignified plant parts. Since the solitary female looks for a place for oviposition which provides some protection to the eggs and considerably facilitates the finding of adequate food for the hatched herbivorous larvae, this behaviour is often termed "brood care"[3]. Despite their dangerous aspect, the adult saw-flies are absolutely harmless, since the accessory glands of their female sex organs do not produce any venomous secretions.

B. SUBORDER APOCRITA (APOCRITES)

The second suborder of the Hymenoptera, the "apocrites", are characterized by the presence of a "wasp waist". It is noteworthy that this "waist" is not developed between thorax and abdomen, but that the first abdominal segment is firmly bound with the thorax, whereas the "waist" is formed by a narrowing of the second abdominal segment into a petiole, whereby the abdomen becomes much more movable and allows a considerably wider use of the ovipositor[3].

1. Section *Terebrantes* (Parasitical Hymenoptera)

Due to the common introduction of their offspring in different arthropod hosts (e.g. butterfly caterpillars, saw-fly larvae, spiders, ticks) this species-rich hymenopteran group was often designated as "*parasitica*". The ovipositor is converted into a *terebra* (lat., "sting for oviposition") instead of a *serrula* and, compared to the plant wasps, is more or less retracted in the extremity of the body as long as unused (Figure 11). This functional-anatomical modification is also accompanied by a modification of some accessory glands of the female sex organs, as the "acidic glands" are used for venom production[11,13]. In parasitic hymenoptera four types of oviposition may be distinguished: *1)* the eggs are introduced into the host by stinging, *2)* the eggs are attached to the host's surface, *3)* the eggs are laid in the nearest possible proximity of the host and *4)* a large amount of eggs are laid away from any host organism. The endophagous species parasitise free-living hosts, which are not or only temporarily paralyzed. Exophagous species usually sting their hosts and this results in a complete and permanent or a long-term paralysis. In the superfamily *Ichneumonidae*, the larvae of which feed mainly on larvae of butterflies (Class *Lepidoptera*), there are paralytic venoms which may lead from incomplete to complete, from transient to permanent and even sometimes to delayed paralysis of the host dependent on the species involved. Members of the superfamily *Cynipoidea* have venoms which lead to only transient paralysis of the hosts, which are mainly larvae of flies (Class *Diptera*). The venoms found in the superfamily *Chalcinoidea* lead mainly to transient or incomplete, sometimes also permanent, complete or delayed paralysis of their host, mainly larvae of butterflies (*Lepidoptera*) or beetles (Class *Coleoptera*). The venomous secretions can be highly specific. For example, it has been calculated that 1 mg of venom of the wasp *Microbracon hebetor* should be able to paralyze about 200 kgs of butterfly caterpillars of the species *Galleria mellonella*[14,15]. Very often, the paralyzed host remains alive for a long time and is used by the larva developing inside as a "living tin". Studies on the metabolism of such paralyzed host animals have shown that the paralyzing venom should not be considered as a preservative. In the paralyzed animal, degenerative processes progress quicker than in the uninfluenced host larva[16]. Nevertheless the persistence of elementary living functions in the paralyzed state should have a certain preserving effect. Besides highly specific venoms which can have an action on few host organisms only, venoms of other terebrant species have been found to have a broad spectrum of action. Particularly fascinating from a biologist's point-of-view is the behaviour of wood-boring terebrantes. Thus for example, the wasp *Rhyssa persuasoria* (Figure 11) may inject its eggs in the living larva of the wasp *Sirex gigas* hidden in the wood.

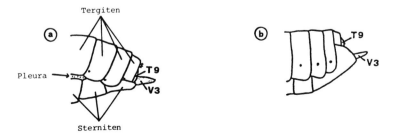

Figure 11. The basic structure of abdominal organisation in *Terebrantes*.

2. Section Aculeata (sting wasps)

Although in many terebrantes the ovipositor has been more or less retracted in the abdomen during evolution, this phenomenon called "internalization" is only typical of aculeates[4] (see Figure. 13). The "law of internalization" says that organs appearing first free on surfaces sink into the body or are covered when further developing[17]. Precisely in relation to the observed invagination of the sting apparatus of Aculeata, the following observation of Remane[17] is of particular importance: "in homologous organs a low degree of internalization is with a high probability to be considered as more primitive than a high degree of internalization". Moreover, in practically all *Aculeata* species the ovipositor is transformed into a defensive venom sting (*aculeus*) and is only rarely connected with the reproductive behaviour. The oviduct opens ventrally into the genital orifice at the ovipositor base (Figure 13).

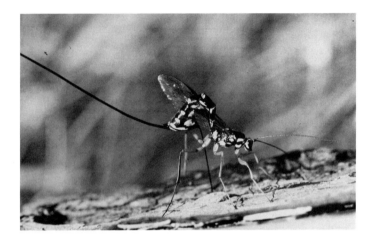

Figure 12. Terebrant wasp *Rhysaa persuasoria*, inserting an egg into the larva of *Sirex gigas* down in a piece of wood (courtesy of Dr. P. Brodmann, Ettingen, Switzerland).

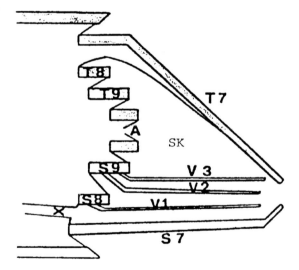

Figure 13. The basic structure of abdominal organisation in *Aculeata*. SK [sting chamber]; A [anus]; X [genital orfice].

The venom of the "acidic glands" is stored in a reservoir. In case of need and according to the animal species, it is extruded either by muscle contraction or, when these muscles are lacking, by a membrane structure located at the inner side of valvulae 1. These structures acting as "pump pistons and valves" have unhappily often been designated as "inhibitory platelets"[4]. Solitary species perform breeding by laying their egg in an arthropod host previously paralysed by sting(s). This host is usually eaten within a week by the hatched larva[3]. Thereafter, either the egg and the animal serving as food remain lying down at the site of attack, or one or more victims are imprisoned together with the egg in a "feeding chamber". A great number of brood parasites are also known, which lay down their eggs in the prepared holes of social sting wasps. According to the species, the hatched larva feeds on additionally introduced, paralyzed feeding insects or on the host larvae. In social aculeates, the sting apparatus serves a defensive role. It is not used for preying, as larvae are generally fed by sexually sterile workers through head gland secretions. When social wasps and bees arrive in the nest, often workers are on guard duty. Each intruder is controlled. If it does not belong to the population of the hive, it is attacked. The odor of released venom has an additional alarm function. Thus, the venom itself may act as a pheromone. In the German wasp *Paravespula germanica*, such an alarm may at any time be triggered off by squeezing an acid gland. Immediately some inhabitants arrive and attack the intruder. It seems that the venom odor also leads to the fact that the victim receives additional stings, mostly in close vicinity to the initial sting. In many ants (family Formicidae) and in the subfamily of "stingless wasps" (Melliponinae), the sting apparatus is more or less atrophied. Instead of the sting, these animals use their extremely well developed mandibles of the mouth as defense. After a bite either venom is instilled in the wound with the still functional venomous gland, or other glands (anal or mandibular glands) are used. In the Formicinae subfamily, however, it has to be spoken of as a transformation rather than a regression. Of course the sting is lacking, but the rest of the sting apparatus allows the ant to spray the venom over long distances. Here too the odor of the released venom is a warning for the environment. Furthermore, the venomous gland secretion might also serve as "trace substance" to rapidly find the nest[1]. To sum up, the hymenopteran ovipositor initially served to introduce eggs in plant tissues. During evolution, it has been used to immobilize arthropod hosts and simultaneously for oviposition and finally, triggered off by reproduction, it has been used for defense. However, and this probably constitutes the most "modern" evolutionary case, it can also be atrophied at the sites where defensive functions are assured by other structures of the organism. Fortunately, all the transitions of this fascinating evolution can be found among the living hymenopteran species.

IV.   DISTRIBUTION OF HYMENOPTERA OF MEDICAL IMPORTANCE

A. SOCIAL WASPS
Most of the social wasps belong to two out of six subfamilies of the family Vespidae, the Vespinae and the Polistinae, respectively. They feed their progeniture with animal prey, mostly arthropods. Their colonies, ranging from 30 to several thousands of individuals in size, live in nests made of vegetable fibers. A colony usually is inititated by one single queen (for review, see[18,19]).

1. Subfamily *Vespinae*
This subfamily includes four genera, the "yellowjackets" *Dolichovespula* (18 species) and *Vespula* (about 25 species), the "hornets", *Vespa* (20 species) and the *Provespa* (3 species). Vespinae are found in Eurasia, North America and North Africa. They may behave

aggressively in defense, especially those species of the Vespinae which form huge colonies, and thus form the predominant stinging problem on a worldwide basis.

2. Subfamily Polistinae

The *Polistinae* are differentiated into three tribes, the Ropalidiini (one genus, *Ropalidia*, with about 130 species, found in Africa south of the Sahara desert, throughout India and the Malaysian peninsula, Indonesia, Papua New Guinea and the northern part of Australia), the Polybiini (26 genera, with about 450 species, distributed from the western part of the United States of America over Central America down to Brazil, in Africa south of the Sahara desert, in the Malaysian peninsula, Japan, Indonesia and Papua New Guinea) and the Polistini, (two genera, *Polistes*, about 200 species, and *Sulcopolistes*, 3 species, distributed in large parts of North, Central and South America, throughout Africa, Europe, most of Asia and Australia), respectively. With the exception of some species of the genus *Polistes* (*P. annularis, P. exclamans, P. fuscatus, P. metricus*) forming huge colonies in the Southern part of the United States, members of this subfamily are not of medical importance.

B. BEES (FAMILY APIDAE)

Out of the superfamily *Apoidea* with its currently distinguished nine families, only the social bumble bees (subfamily *Bombinae*) and honey bees (subfamily *Apinae*) from the family *Apidae* are of medical importance. In contrast to the wasps, bees no longer provision their nests with arthropod prey, but collect pollen and nectar from flowers to feed their progeniture. The bumble bees (*Bombinae*) include the two genera *Bombus* and *Psythurus*, respectively, with about 400 recognized species[21]. In contrast, the honey bees (*Apinae*) only include the following four to six different species, the classification of which is controversial: *Apis mellifera* L. (common honey bee), *A. binghani* Cocherell, *A. cerana* Fab., *A. dorsata* Fab., *A. florea* Fab. and *A. laboriosa* Smith. These species may be further subdivided into subspecies[18]. Bumble bees are found in the temperate regions of Asia, Europe and North America, respectively, extending as far northward as land exists[22,23]. Honey bees are native to Africa, Asia and Europe, respectively. Since the common honey bee, *A. mellifera*, has been domesticated, this species has been introduced in different races and may now be regarded as a cosmopolitan species. A special note has to be devoted to the Brazilian honey bee *A. mellifera scutellata*, a hybridization of the African honey bee, *A. m. adansonii*, which was introduced into Rio Claro, Brazil, in 1956, with the common honey bee, *A. m. mellifera*[27-29]. This particularly aggressive subspecies has spread throughout South America and is referred to as "killer bee" due to its mass sting attacks on humans and livestock. Being sensitive to low temperature, however, there is no risk that this species may extend its distribution into temperate zones.

C. ANTS

With up to 14,000 social species, ants form by far the largest group of social insects. All ants of medical importance belong to the family Formicidae, which is comprised of eleven subfamilies[30,31]. Stings are absent only in the subfamily *Dolichoderinae, Formicinae* and in part in the *Myrmicinae*. However, even in those species lacking a complete sting apparatus, defensive secretions are sprayed from the tip of their abdomen into the wound caused by their bites. Ants are found throughout the world with the exception of high mountain areas, the Arctic and the Antarctic, respectively. Since the sting of most ants is not able to penetrate human skin, only a few species represent a medical problem. The most well-known species in this respect are the fire ants of the genus *Solenopsis*, which occur in the southern part of the United States of America. The site of a sting of a fire ant burns, itches very strongly and white blisters may develop. These signs and symptoms usually disappear within some hours. Thus, ant stings may be regarded as a transient unpleasant experience of rather limited impact. However, anaphylactic phenomena following ant stings may occasionally be observed. Of course, similar sting cases may also occur in other parts of the world. However, the respective reports in the literature are scarce, reflecting the limited medical importance of this animal group with respect to human medicine.

V. VENOM COMPOSITION

A. GENERAL

This review exclusively deals with the venom composition of social wasps and bees of medical importance. The pharmacology and biochemistry of solitary wasps is reviewed elsewhere[12,34,35]. The venoms of social wasps and bees have been extensively investigated throughout the last forty years. However, most pharmacological data are based on experimental systems easily accessible to pharmacologists. This is understandable, since due to their potential for inducing anaphylactic reactions in humans, the investigation of these venoms from an anthropocentric point-of-view has been highly supported. On the other hand, these venoms predominantly serve the purpose of defending the hive against invertebrate intruders and, in the case of the wasps, to immobilize invertebrate prey animals, respectively. Moreover, most honey-loving mammals are nearly extinct and one single sting delivers so small an amount of venom that it usually acts only as a painful deterrent to big animals, whereas it is a deadly challenge for most arthropods. During one single bee or wasp sting a volume of 0.5 to 2 μl venom only is injected. These venoms are colourless proteinaceous liquids with a sharp, bitter taste, an aromatic odor giving an acidic reaction. The dry residue is about 12 percent and dried venoms may have a slightly yellowish colour. In general, three different groups of venom components in a more or less constant quantitative distribution may be distinguished: low molecular weight substances, peptides and enzymes, respectively.

B. WASP VENOMS

A general survey on wasp venom composition and some of their properties is given in Table 1. For detailed reviews, see [8,34].

1. Low molecular weight substances

Histamine , being a powerful pain inducer and leading to dilatation and permeability increase in capillaries at the sting site in vertebrates, is the most common biogenic amine present in wasp venoms. Much more important but less well investigated from a biological point of view is the toxic effect of histamine in invertebrates, where it might release endogenous catecholamines. Other biogenic amines present in wasp venoms are tyramine, dopamine, epinephrine and norepinephrine, respectively. These catecholamines might be responsible for part of the toxicity in invertebrates, since they function as physiological neurotransmitters. Dopamine especially exerts a threefold action: *1)* it functions as an intermediate in the synthesis of quinones, which act as crosslinking agents in the formation and hardening of the arthropode cuticle; *2)* it is the immediate precursor of norepinephrine; and *3)* it is a neurotransmitter in the central nervous system of a number of insects. Thus, catecholamines present in the venom may strongly interact with the central nervous system of an invertebrate victim. Further low molecular weight substances present in at least some wasp venoms are serotonin, acetylcholine and polyamines, like putrescine, spermidine and spermine, respectively.

2. Peptides

A number of wasp kinins, peptides with bradykinin-like activity and, as far as investigated, with a bradykinin domain in their amino acid sequence, have been detected in wasp venoms. These peptides, composed of nine to eighteen amino acids, respectively, lead to mast cell degranulation in vertebrates with release of endogenous smooth muscle reactive mediators (histamine, serotonin) and heparins. These mediators, together with biogenic amines present in the venoms, are responsible for most of the local effects caused by wasp stings in humans. Another group of tetradecapeptide amides, the so-called mastoparans, have a similar effect on mast cell degranulation. A substance known as chemotactic peptide, inducing chemotaxis for macrophages in vertebrates, has been found in *Vespa* venoms. Again, it is not known what role these peptides play in arthropod envenomation.

Table 1
General composition of wasp venoms

Substance	% of Dry Venom	Molecular Mass (D)	Allergenic Activity
Low molecular weight substances	**<10**	**<1,000**	-
Histamine	<6	111	-
Tyramine	<1	137	-
Dopamine	<1	153	-
Epinephrine	<1	183	-
Norepinephrine	<1	169	-
Serotonin	<6	176	-
Acetylcholine	<1	146	-
Putrescine	<1	88	-
Spermidine	<1	145	-
Spermine	<1	202	-
Peptides		**<10,000**	
Wasp kinins		1,000 - 5,000	-
Mastoporans		<1,600	-
Chemotactic peptide		<1,600	-
High molecular weight substances		**>10,000**	**+++**
Phospholipases A & B	<15	~35,000	+++
Hyaluronidases	<5	~45,000	+++
Acidic phosphatases		not known	+
Alkaline phosphatases		not known	+
Proteases		not known	++
Dnase		not known	not known
Cholinesterase		not known	not known
Histidindecarboxylase		not known	not known
"Antigen 5"	<10	25,000	+++
"Vmac 1"		97,000	+
"Vmac 3"		39,000	+

3. High molecular weight substances

Various kinds of enzyme activities have been detected in wasp venoms. Hydrolytic activities may have a digestive effect on tissues, enhance the action of venom peptides and biogenic amines respectively, and increase the overall toxicity by such synergistic actions. Although only poorly characterised, the following enzyme activities may be determined in wasp venoms dependent on the species: phospholipase A_2, phospholipase B, hyaluronidase, acidic phosphatase, alkaline phosphatase, cholinesterase, histidincarboxylase, saccharidase, DNAse and protease, respectively. Phospholipases, hyaluronidases and alkaline phosphatases are potential allergens leading to severe allergic reactions in sensitive people. Some high molecular weight proteins devoid of enzymatic activity have been isolated from wasp venoms. Although the biological activity of such "antigens" remains to be elucidated, some of them have proved to be potent allergens, too.

C. BEE VENOMS

As is shown in Table 2, the composition of bee venoms is quite similar to that of wasp venoms. For detailed reviews, see[8,36,37].

1. Low molecular weight substances

Histamine, dopamine and norepinephrine, respectively, are biogenic amines present in bee venoms. Whereas, as in wasp venoms, these substances in vertebrates may account for the sensation of pain only, in invertebrates they have a deleterious effect on the function of the central nervous system. Amino acids, phospholipids and carbohydrates, respectively, are present in bee venoms in similar quantities as in their hemolymph.

Table 2
General composition of bee venoms

Substance	% of Dry Venom	Molecular Mass (D)	Allergenic Activity
Low molecular weight substances	**<25**	**<1,000**	**-**
Histamine	<1	111	-
Dopamine	<1	153	-
Norepinephrine	<1	169	-
Amino acids	<1	100 -200	-
Oligopeptides	<14	200 -1,000	-
Phospholipids	<5	100 - 400	-
Carbohydrates	<2	<200	-
Peptides	**~60**	**<10,000**	**(+)**
Melittin	<50	2,840	+
		(Tetramer: 12,500)	
Apamin	<2	2,000	-
Mast cell degranulating peptide (401)	<2	2,600	-
Secapin	~0.5	~2,600	-
Tertiapin	<0.1	~2,000	-
Protease inhibitor	<1	~9,000	-
Procamine A & B	<2	~500	-
High molecular weight substances		**>10,000**	**+++**
Phospholipase A	<15	16 - 19,000	+++
Phospholipase B	<1	~22,000	+++
Hyaluronidases	<2	35 - 50,000	+++
Acid phosphomonoesterase	<1	45 - 90,000	+
α-D-Glucosidase	<1	not known	?

2. Peptides

About fifty percent of the dry venom of bees is melittin, a peptide consisting of twenty-six amino acids, free of sulphur. The distribution of the amino acids in the molecule is quite remarkable, since non-polar, hydrophobic and neutral amino acids are found in the N-terminal part, whereas the polar, hydrophilic and basic amino acids are concentrated in its C-terminal part. Thus, the molecule exerts amphiphilic properties and is, like lysolecithin, a natural detergent with a high activity towards membranes. Melittin is responsible for the pain involved in bee stings. In cell membranes, melittin forms tetrameric pores that facilitate ion diffusion. The melittin-tetrameres lead to a breakdown of the resting potential, which initiates the sensation of pain.

Other peptides are found in bee venoms in small concentrations only and probably do not account for much of their toxic action. Oa-Adolapsin is a basic polypeptide consisting of 103 amino acid residues with an inhibitory effect towards microsomal cyclooxygenase and lypoxygenase, and an algesic effect in mice. Apamin, a basic peptide consisting of one chain of eighteen amino acids stabilized by two disulfide bridges, blocks calcium-dependent potassium channels. The Mastcell degranulating peptide (MCD-peptide), a basic peptide of twenty-two amino acids stabilized by two disulfide bridges, leads to massive release of histamine from mastcells and is a potent blocker of voltage-dependent potassium channels.

3. High molecular weight substances

With about twelve percent of the dry weight, phospholipase A_2 is the most prominent enzyme found in bee venoms. Phospholipase A_2 and lysolecithin formed following phospholipase action are very active towards cell membranes and exert this effect in combination with melittin. Moreover, phospholipase is the most important allergen in bee venoms. Hyaluronidase(s) found in bee venoms act as "venom spreading factors" by depolymerizing the mucopolysaccharid hyaluronic acid, which is an important substance in connective tissue.

D. ANT VENOMS

The following substances are found in ant venoms:

1. Low molecular weight substances

A high content of dialkylpiperidines and other alkaloids is found in fire ants of the genus *Solenopsis*, whereas histamine and amino acids are present in the venom of the ant genera *Pogonomyrmex*, *Myrmecia* and *Myrmica*, respectively.

2. Peptides

Kinins and melittin-like peptides have been found in some ant venoms investigated.

3. High molecular weight substances

Phospholipase, hyaluronidase, acidic phosphatase, lipase, esterase and N-acetyl-Beta-glucosaminidase activities have been revealed in some ant venoms.

VI. EPIDEMIOLOGICAL CONSIDERATIONS

A detailed review on epidemiological aspects of hymenoptera stings is provided in[33]. During the warm season, there is the possibility of daily contacts with bees, wasps and ants. These animals are not at all aggressive. However, many people, being afraid of these insects, react with fast movements of their upper extremities to defend themselves. In so doing, they may stimulate aggressive behaviour in the animal, with the aim of defending themselves by stinging. Multiple stings may be the consequence of destroying a bee hive. The smell of venom substances released by a sting acts as a pheromone and initiates stinging attacks of other bees nearby. Bees and wasps in the neighbourhood of soft drinks and cakes sometimes are swallowed by accident. This may lead to larynx oedema, which may occasionally give rise to respiratory problems due to the massive swelling in the upper airway. The highest risk involved with hymenopteran stings, however, is type 1 allergy or anaphylaxis. About two thirds of all fatalities develop after one single sting (Figure 16), within a very short time period (Figure 17), the victim usually being older than 40 years (Figure 18). Most of the fatal stings are inflicted into the head or neck region (Figure 19). For the pathophysiology and treatment of hymenopteran sting anaphylaxis, see the following chapter.

VII. PREVENTION

The prophylactic measures to be taken are a consequence of the biology and behaviour of social wasps and bees: *1)* bees and wasps become aggressive when fast movements are performed; *2)* most bee stings are a consequence of people walking around in rural areas without shoes; *3)* wasp stings often happen when people eat outside or come into close contact with wasp colonies, and in gardens near rotting fruits; *4)* bees and wasps are more active and consequently more aggressive and prepared to sting the higher ambient temperature and humidity are; *5)* The venoms of stinging bees and wasps act as pheromones and attract other specimens nearby to sting, too. The following prophylactic measures to avoid stings from bees and wasps should be taken[38]:

1) **Avoid fast movements if bees or waps are in your vicinity.**
2) **Keep away from flourishing flowers and rotting fruits on the ground.**
3) **Be careful during outside garden work. Wear a hat, shoes, gloves, trousers and shirts or blouses with long sleeves.**
4) **Do not use strong smelling perfumes, hair sprays, sun creams, etc.**
5) **Do not wear wide, fluttering clothes; wear white, green or bright brown instead of dark clothes or dresses with coloured pattern.**
6) **When eating outside, keep sweets, meat and their residues closed from access.**
7) **Perspiration and carbon dioxide attract stinging insects. Thus, be careful during outside sport activities.**
8) **Since bees like clover and many wasps have their nests in the ground, never walk around barefooted.**
9) **Keep wastes in and around your domicile protected from access.**
10) **Keep away from places where animals are fed, since feeding residues attract wasps and bees.**
11) **Do not move around fallen tree-trunks and branches, since wasps may construct their nests inside.**
12) **Keep your windows closed during daytime or install mosquito-nets.**
13) **Notify the fire brigade or a bee-keeper if you observe a swarm of bees in your vicinity.**
14) **If you get annoyed by bees or wasps, protect your head with your upper extremities or articles of clothing and go away from the immediate area using slow motions.**
15) **Wear a helmet and gloves when motor-cycling.**

Persons with a known allergy against bee and wasp venoms, should strictly follow the instructions of their medical doctors.

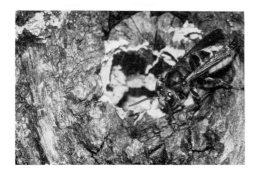

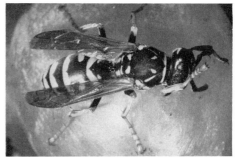

Figure 14. Honey bee, (*Apis mellifera*).   **Figure 15.** German wasp (*Paravespula germanica*).

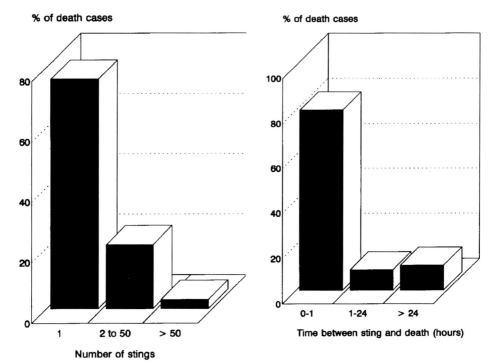

Figure 16. Sting numbers leading to fatalities.

Figure 17. Time interval between sting and death.

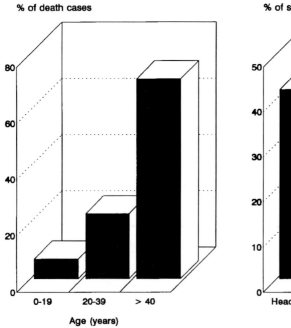

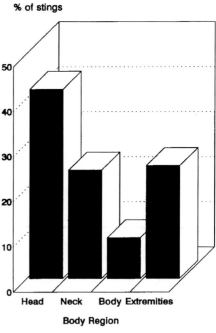

Figure 18. Age of victim in fatal cases.

Figure 19. Region sting inflicted on.

VIII. FIRST AID

If there is no allergy against bee and wasp venoms present, only local signs and symptoms, like burning pain, itching and swelling are seen following a sting. Since in the case of bee stings, the whole sting apparatus usually remains at the sting location, first aid measures consist in a careful removal of the sting apparatus, either by using pincers or the nail of the index finger. The venom sac should by no means be squeezed during this procedure, since this may inject the whole amount of venom present. The sting location may be disinfected, although there is almost no risk of infection following stings from bees and wasps. Special remedies available against hymenopteran stings contain substances like ammonia, menthol or campher. These substances have a cooling and pain relieving effect. Patients who received stings into the region of the mouth or throat should always see a medical doctor, since the risk of life-threatening edema may be present. Patients with multiple stings (in children more than 50 stings, in adults more than 100 stings may be life-threatening) should also be supervised by medical staff for at least 24 hours. Further notes on first aid treatment of non-allergic and allergic patients are given in the following chapter.

IX. REFERENCES

1. **KÄSTNER, E.**, *Lehrbuch der speziellen Zoologie*, Vol. 1, Wirbellose, 3.Teil, Insecta B, Spezieller Teil, G.Fischer, Stuttgart, 1973.
2. **MINTON, S.A.**, *Venom Diseases*, C.C.Thomas, Springfield,1974.
3. **WEBER, H.**, *Grundriss der Insektenkunde*, G.Fischer, Stuttgart, 1974.
4. **OESER, R.**, Vergleichend-morphologische Untersuchungen über den Ovipositor der Hymenopteren, *Mitt. Zool.Mus.Berlin*, 37, 3, 1961.
5. **RIETSCHEL, P.**, Bau und Funktion des Wehrstachels der staatenbildenden Bienen und Wespen, *Z.Morph.Oekol.*,33, 313, 1938.
6. **SNODGRASS, R.E.**, *Anatomy of the Honey Bee*, Constable, London, 1956.
7. **SPRADBERRY, J.P.**, *Wasps*, Sidgwick and Jackson, London, 1973.
8. **EDERY, H., ISHAY, J., GITTER, S. AND JOSHUA, H.**, Venoms of Vespidae, in *Arthropod Venoms*, S. Bettini, Ed., Springer, Berlin,1978, 691.
9. **O'CONNOR, R., PECK, M.L.**, Venoms of Apidae, in *Arthropod Venoms*, S. Bettini, Ed., Berlin, Springer, 1978, 613.
10. **MASCHWITZ, U.W. AND KLOFT, W.**, Morphology and function of the venom apparatus of Insects - Bees, Wasps, Ants and Caterpillars, in *Venomous Animals and Their Venoms*, Vol.3, Bücherl, E.E. Buckley, Eds., Academic Press, New York, 1971.
11. **ROBERTSON, P.L.**, A morphological and functional study of the venom apparatus in representatives of some groups of Hymenoptera, *Aust.J.Zool.*, 16, 134, 1968.
12. **PIEK, T. AND SPANJER, W.**, Chemistry and Pharmacology of solitary wasp venoms, in *Venoms of the Hymenoptera*, T. Piek, Ed., Academic Press, New York, 161, 1986.
13. **VAN MARLE, J. AND PIEK, T.**, Morphology of the venom apparatus, in *Venoms of the Hymenoptera*, T. Piek, Ed., Academic Press, New York, 17, 1986.
14. **BEARD, R.L.**, Insect toxins and venoms, *Ann.Rev.Entomol.*, 8, 1, 1963.
15. **BEARD, R.L.**, Venoms of Braconidae, in *Arthropod Venoms*, S. Bettini, Ed., Springer, Berlin, 773, 1978.
16. **NIELSEN, E.T.**, Über den Stoffwechsel der von Grabwespen paralysierten Tiere, *Videns.Medd.Dansk Naturhist. Foren, Kopenhagen*, 99, 149, 1935.
17. **REMANE, A.**, *Die Grundlagen des natürlichen Systems, der vergleichenden Anatomie und der Phylogenetik*, Geest und Portig, Leipzig, 1952.
18. **AKRE, R.D. AND REED, H.C.**, Biology and distribution of social hymenoptera, in *Handbook of Natural Toxins*, Vol. 2, A.T.Tu, Ed., M.Dekker, New York, 1984, 3.
19. **AKRE, R.D.**, Social wasps, in *Social Insects*, Vol.4, H.R. Herman, Ed., Academic Press, New York, 1982, 1.
20. **VAN DER VECHT, J.**, Bouwproblemen van sociale wespen, *K.Ned.Akad.Wet.Versl.Gewone Vergad. Afd. Natuurkd.*, 76, 59, 1967.
21. **HEINRICH, B.**, *Bumblebee Economics*, Harvard Univ. Press, Cambridge, 1979.
22. **MICHENER, C.D.**, *The Social Behaviour of the Bees: A Comparative Study*, Harvard Univ. Press, Cambridge, 1974.
23. **MICHENER, C.D.**, Biogeography of the bees, *Ann. Missouri Bot. Gard.*, 66, 277, 1979.

24. **SAKAGAMI, S.F., MATSUMARA, T. AND ITO, K.**, *Apis laboriosa* in Himalaya, the little known world largest honeybee (Hymenoptera, Apidae), *Insecta Matsumurana* (N.S.), 19, 47, 1980.
25. **CRANE, E.** (Ed.), *Honey: A Comprehensive Survey*, Crane, Russak, New York, 1975.
26. **FLETCHER, D.J.C.**, The African bee, *Apis mellifera adansonii*, in Africa, *Ann. Rev. Entomol.*, 23, 151, 1978.
27. **TAYLOR, O.R.**, The past and possible future spread of Africanized honey bees in the Americas, *Bee World*, 58, 19, 1977.
28. **TAYLOR, O.R.**, Letters: Africanized bees, *Science*, 210, 248, 1980.
29. **MITCHENER, C.D.**, The Brazilian honeybee - possible problems for the future. *Clin. Toxicol.*, 6, 125, 1973.
30. **WILSON, E.O.**, *The Insect Societies*, Harvard Univ. Press, Cambridge, 1971.
31. **DUMPERT, K.**, *The Social Biology of Ants*, Pitman, London, 1981.
32. **STROM, G.B., BOSWELL, R.N. AND JACOBS, R.L.**, In vivo and in vitro comparison of fire ant venom and fire ant whole body extract, *J.Allergy Clin. Immunol.*, 72, 46, 1983.
33. **MÜLLER, U.R.**, *Insektenstichallergie*, G. Fischer, Stuttgart, 1988.
34. **NAKAJIMA, T.**, Biochemistry of vespid venoms, in *Handbook of Natural Toxins*, Vol. 2, A.T.Tu, Ed., M.Dekker, New York, 1984, 109.
35. **PIEK, T.**, Pharmacology of Hymenoptera venoms, in *Handbook of Natural Toxins*, Vol. 2, A.T.Tu, Ed., M.Dekker, New York, 1984, 135.
36. **SHIPOLINI, R.A.**, Biochemistry of bee venom, in *Handbook of Natural Toxins*, Vol. 2, A.T.Tu, Ed., M.Dekker, New York, 1984, 49.
37. **BANKS, B.E.C. AND SHIPOLINI, R.A.**, Chemistry and Pharmacology of honey-bee venom, in *Venoms of the Hymenoptera*, T. Piek, Ed., Academic Press, New York, 1986.
38. **WORTMANN, F.**, Diagnostik und Therapie der Insektenstichallergie, *Therapiewoche*, 27, 4385, 1977.

Chapter 22

CLINICAL TOXICOLOGY OF HYMENOPTERAN STINGS

Holger Mosbech

TABLE OF CONTENTS

I. INTRODUCTION

As described in the previous chapter the Hymenoptera order contains a large number of species with very different geographic distribution, appearance, way of living and toxic potentials. In this review emphasis will be put on the winged Hymenoptera species, although others - such as the fire ant (*Solenopsis* genus) - may also cause severe reactions[1].

The Hymenoptera species giving rise to most medical problems are those living close to human dwellings either because they are domesticated (honey bees) or because they are attracted by our food such as sweet beverage, pastry, fruit etc. In contrast to other venomous animals, stinging insects occur in nearly all climatic zones. Stings are frequent and most people receive stings by the same species several times during life. Although the amount of venom per sting is rather low, these repeated stings impose a risk of allergic sensitisation to venom components and a subsequent risk of severely enhanced reactions to future stings. The earliest description of such fatal reaction has been found in the tomb of the Egyptian pharaoh Menes who died after an insect sting in 2621 BC.

II. CLINICAL ASPECTS

A. MECHANISMS

The different biologically active components (Chapter 21) in the Hymenoptera venom give rise to toxic reactions in all human beings in a dose dependent manner.

The low molecular weight biogenic amines (histamine, dopamine, noradrenaline etc.) are involved in the local reaction but after a single sting will hardly be able to impose systemic reaction. They act on blood vessels and nerve endings inducing swelling, redness, pain and itching.

Major toxic effects of the venom can be attributed to the larger peptides e.g. melittin, apamin, kinins, haemolysins and mast cell degranulating and chemotactic factors. These peptides can damage the cell membranes leading to liberation of enzymes from lysozymes and of mast cell granula and to cytolysis. They can act as neurotoxins provoking hyperexcitability.

The enzymes (phospholipase A and B, hyaluronidase etc.) have a higher molecular weight and, with the exception of the highly cytotoxic phospholipase A_2, are regarded as less harmful. Hyaluronidase has an indirect effect by increasing the penetration of the active peptides.

The dialkydpiperidines in the venom of the fire ants are highly cytotoxic and account for the major effects of the venoms.

The various enzymes and vasoactive components induce a toxic local inflammation in the sting region. If the sting occurs in a highly vascular area or even intravascularly, the toxic components are spread readily and might give rise to systemic reactions. Several simultaneous stings will cause more severe reactions. In contrast, the allergic patient needs only minute amounts of allergen to initiate a severe reaction.

In a patient with insect allergy the B-lymphocytes have been stimulated to produce IgE antibody directed specifically against components in the venom. Stimulation takes place after a sting, but the factors determining which stings are prone to cause such sensitisation are unknown. The sensitisation takes some time to develop and the allergic reaction is not seen with the sting causing sensitisation but with a subsequent sting by the same insect. Due to memory cells IgE is continuously produced several years after the sensitisation has occurred. The IgE circulates in the blood and is bound to specific receptors on mast cells in the tissue and on basophil granulocytes (white blood cells) in the blood. These cells contain granules with chemotactic, vaso- and neuroactive components (e.g. histamine, serotonin, slow reacting substance), which are released when the allergen cross-binds two adjacent IgE molecules on the cell surface. A cascade reaction is then initiated.

The high molecular weight components of the venoms, i.e. the enzymes, most readily induce IgE production, whereas the smaller molecules are less - if at all - allergenic.

B. SYMPTOMS

The normal reaction to a sting is caused by the toxic substances. It is a painful red swelling of up to 10 cm in diameter lasting up to a few days. Fire ant stings are often more severe with vesicular lesions and subsequent local necrosis.

A broad spectrum of symptoms can occur after an insect sting and in general it is not possible from the clinical history alone to ascertain whether an abnormal reaction is caused by a toxic or an allergic mechanism. Additional diagnostic procedures are necessary.

A systemic reaction caused by multiple stings or by stings to the head and neck or in well vascularized areas might be toxic, especially if the local reaction is small, indicating a rapid spreading of the venom. However, severe reactions to single stings are most often caused by allergic mechanisms.

The abnormal reactions to insect stings are conventionally classified in 4 grades according to H. L. Mueller[2] and slightly modified by Müller[3] (Table 1).

In addition to objective symptoms a variety of subjective and clinically unverifiable symptoms can occur following stings. They can occur alone or accompany objective allergic reactions. As isolated symptoms they might be caused simply by fear or by hyperventilation. Headache, palpitations, paresthesias, heat sensation might be encountered in addition to the symptoms listed in Table 1. The first symptoms often occur within minutes after the sting and last generally for hours to days. In special cases durations of several weeks are seen.

The majority of patients dying from Hymenoptera stings have been stung in the head, throat and neck[4]. The death might - like other less severe reactions - be due to allergy, to toxicity and in addition to local swelling subsequent to stings in throat, on the neck or in the airways causing suffocation. The direct toxic lethal dose in otherwise healthy adults is probably several hundred to thousands of stings. Death often occurs relatively quickly, the majority within the first hour[4,5].

Table 1
Classification of allergic reactions to Hymenoptera stings (From Müller[3])

Large local reactions:	Swelling at site of sting with a diameter > 10 cm, lasting > 24 h
Systemic reactions:	
grade I	Generalized urticaria, itching, malaise, anxiety
grade II	Any of the above, plus two or more of the following:
	angio-oedema (grade II also if alone), constriction in chest, nausea, vomiting, diarrhoea, abdominal pain, dizziness
grade III	Any of the above, plus two or more of the following:
	dyspnoea, wheezing, stridor (any of these alone are grade III), dysphagia, dysarthria, hoarseness, weakness, confusion, feeling of impending disaster
grade IV	Any of the above, plus two or more of the following:
	fall in blood pressure, collapse, loss of consciousness, incontinence (urine, stool), cyanosis
Unusual reactions:	
Serum sickness syndrome, generalized vasculitis	Fever, arthritis, lymphadenopathy, exanthema, vasculitic purpura
Kidney involvement	Glomerulonephritis, nephrotic syndrome
Involvement of the nervous system	Peripheral neuritis, polyradiculitis, epileptic seizures, reversible and irreversible central nervous damage
Blood involvement	Thrombocytopenia, haemolytic anaemia, disseminated intravascular coagulation
Cardiac involvement	Angina pectoris, myocardiac infarction

C. EPIDEMIOLOGY

The less severe symptoms are seen much more frequently than the more serious reactions. Large local reactions have been reported in 2% to 19% in various populations[6,7] and systemic reactions in less than 1% in youngsters[8] and about 1% to 3% in adult studies[6,7,9]. The lower frequency in the young group might reflect a lower accumulated number of stings per individual and thereby a lower risk of developing allergy. Another explanation could be the low frequency of concomitant diseases in this age group, which in elderly persons might lower the tolerance to toxic or allergic reactions.

The frequency of abnormal reactions to Hymenoptera stings increases with the rate of exposure. Bee keepers are at special risk. In this population systemic side effects have been reported in 20 - 35%[10,11].

Mortality from insect stings based on death certificate data is below 0.5 death per year per 1 million inhabitants[4,12,13]. The real figure is probably higher since a certain number of persons found dead may have had an allergic reaction to an insect sting[14].

In large studies the prevalence of atopy seems to be slightly higher in the Hymenoptera allergic patients compared to total population[15,16].

The risk of systemic reactions to future stings is related to previous sting reactions (Table 2). After a systemic reaction 27 - 57% will react systemically to a subsequent sting by the same insect[17-20]. Honey bee allergic patients seem to have a less favourable prognosis than vespid allergic patients[18]. In children following urticarial reactions to stings, only 16% will react similarly on subsequent stings[21] and after large local reactions only 4% will have systemic reaction at reexposure[22,23].

Table 2

Risk (%) of systemic reactions when re-stung in patients with previous systemic reactions to Hymenoptera stings[3]

Treatment	Adults with:		Children with Mild Reaction	Allergy Against:	
	Severe Reaction	Mild Reaction		Bee Venom	Vespid Venom
Immunotherapy	0-29	0-8	0-3	10-29	0-9
Non-treated	43-80	15-44	16	50	24

III. DIAGNOSIS

A. SKIN TEST

In allergological skin tests small amounts of venom are introduced in the superficial layers of the skin - often on the forearm. If the patient is allergic to venom components the mast cells in the skin will release their granules when these components bind to the IgE on the cell surface. A positive reaction would be a weal and flare reaction, similar to a mosquito bite, reaching maximum size within 10 to 20 minutes. The venom extract used for this purpose has to be purified i.e. the low molecular weight components are removed in order to avoid unspecific irritative reactions seen in virtually all persons if a sufficiently high concentration of venom is used. The test can be performed by two different techniques. By skin prick test a needle or a lancet is pricked through a drop of extract placed on the skin surface. By intracutaneous test, a minute volume (0.02 ml) is injected just beneath the skin surface. The latter method is more sensitive, lower concentrations of allergen can be used, but the risk of provoking adverse reactions and the risk of false positive (toxic) reactions are greater when the intracutaneous method is chosen. A titration is performed with doses often applied in a sequential manner until a positive reaction occurs; for skin prick test within the range of 0.001 to 1 mg/ml; for intradermal test concentrations of 0.001 to 1 microgram/ml.

False negative skin test results can occur if the patient has taken antihistamines or certain anti-psychotic drugs. The positive control skin test performed with histamine will disclose such pharmacological effects.

B. SPECIFIC IgE-ANTIBODIES

In the assay the venom antigens are coupled to a carrier. This is incubated with the serum sample to be investigated. If the serum contains IgE molecules with binding sites fitting specifically the epitopes of one or more venom components, these IgE molecules bind to the antigen-carrier complex and can be detected by enzymatic, fluorometric or radiometric assays. The classical method is termed RAST (Radio Allergo Sorbent Test)[24]. Conventionally the results can be given in classes from 0 to 4 or 6. Class 0 and 1 designate no or only very low levels of IgE against venom components.

Like skin tests the IgE measurements might not give valid results within the first few weeks after a sting. The IgE level will decrease over years after the last sting, probably somewhat more rapid than the skin reactivity[25]. It is not known whether this slow decrease is accompanied by a parallel reduction in clinical sensitivity in the individual patients.

False positive detection of specific IgE can occur if the serum contains high concentrations of total IgE as can often be seen in patients with atopic eczema. Depending on the laboratory method specific IgE-antibodies can be detected in 1 to 29% of persons with no previous abnormal sting reaction or even with no reported stings[26-28]. In most such cases the levels are low and of no clinical importance. In some cases however sensitisation might have taken place and more serious reactions will occur to future stings.

C. SPECIFIC IgG-ANTIBODIES

The level of specific IgG-antibodies against venom components is correlated to the number of stings received previously but not to the severity of the sting reactions[11,29]. Measurements are therefore of no value when trying to diagnose allergy. It is of interest since injection of gammaglobulin from beekeepers rich in specific IgG-antibodies seems to protect against reactions in bee sting allergic patients[30,31]. The protection is only of short duration. High levels during immunotherapy might give some protection[32,33] but protection can be accomplished without IgG[18,34] and high levels of specific IgG is no guarantee against systemic reactions[18,35].

D. HISTAMINE RELEASE ASSAY

The basophil granulocytes in the blood will release histamine if allergens bind to IgE molecules on the cell surface. Various assays have been designed to measure this reaction. Blood cells, either the white blood cell fraction or all blood cells, are exposed to the allergen extract in various concentrations and the subsequent histamine release is measured.

The venoms contain several components which can stimulate the release of histamine from the basophil cells even without IgE being involved. This has imposed technical difficulties and the test has not found its place in routine diagnostics. Microtiter methods and highly purified venom extracts might make the method valuable in the future.

E. STING CHALLENGE

Because of the diagnostic difficulties mentioned above some centers have performed in-hospital sting challenges in patients considered for immunotherapy[18,36,37]. In addition the challenge has been used in several studies to check the effect of immunotherapy.

By this method the identity of the insect can be secured. It is often left on the skin for ½ to 1 minute to be sure the venom sac is emptied. Side-effects can be treated readily. However severe reactions have occurred to such sting challenges and they could not be recommended as routine diagnostics.

False negative reactions might occur if the insect has emptied most of the venom sac when captured or during storage. The alternative, the field sting, gives even less valid prognostic results due to less precise identification of the insect and rapid removal of the stinger.

IV. PROPHYLAXIS

Hymenopterans sting humans as a response to threat. The most important prophylactic measures would be to avoid touching or squeezing the insects, to avoid sudden movements close to the insects and to avoid catching the insects in loose-fitting clothes (during bicycling etc.) or in foods or drinks consumed outdoors.

Allergic patients might have to take more extensive precautions. They should not walk barefooted, leave sweet things or meat exposed when eating outdoors or collect sweet fruit themselves. They should have over-ripe fruit removed. Bee hives, dressing and other beekeeping remedies and activities should be removed from the close vicinity of the dwelling.

Repellents used for mosquitos etc. are not effective in the prophylaxis of Hymenoptera stings.

Antihistamine tablets taken prophylactically prior to activities with high risk of stings, e.g. handling honey bees, could be helpful in persons with large local reactions or urticaria after previous stings but can not protect against more severe reactions.

V. TREATMENT

A. FIRST AID TREATMENT

After an insect sting the sting apparatus is often left in the skin together with the venom sac. Muscles on this sac continue to pump out venom through the stinger after the insect has left or has been removed. It is therefore important to scrape off the venom sac rapidly. This can be done with a fingernail avoiding compression of the venom sac. Local anaesthetics are occasionally required for pain and antihistamines may relieve some of the itching and swelling. Immobilisation and elevation of a stung extremity will assist in reducing the swelling.

B. GENERAL PRINCIPLES

A single sting in a non-allergic person in general needs no treatment, but antihistamine tablets are occasionally indicated to reduce itching or swelling.

Persons presenting with large local reactions or generalized urticaria should be treated with antihistamines (H-1) as long as the swelling or itching persists. In cases with severe systemic reactions corticosteroids and adrenaline may be required[38].

Persons stung inside the mouth or on the neck should seek medical assistance immediately, since swelling in these areas could cause suffocation. Similarly multiple stings and generalized reactions usually require additional medical treatment.

In special cases and patients with a past history of major systemic reactions may be supplied with adrenaline for self-medication. Preloaded syringes are available. They facilitate administration and are of value especially for the elderly, children and patients with previous rapid-onset symptoms. Adrenaline should be prescribed for persons with systemic reactions to insect stings not treated with immunotherapy. They should take corticosteroid (e.g. Prednisolone tablets, 50 mg) and a rapid-onset antihistamine tablet when stung, and prepare for adrenaline injection but only take this if systemic reactions develop. When a sufficient maintenance dose has been reached in immunotherapy adrenaline would be superfluous.

Tables 3 and 4 outline proposed European emergency ward treatments of respiratory symptoms and of anaphylactic shock[38].

C. PHARMACOLOGICAL TREATMENT

Adrenaline is the treatment of choice for generalised allergic reactions with cardiovascular involvement or with laryngeal oedema. Adrenaline gives vasoconstriction and bronchodilatation and has positive chronotrop, inotrop and bathmotrop actions on the heart. Treatment should be initiated when slight symptoms occur. An initial dose of 0.3 - 0.5 ml (1 mg per ml) should be given deeply subcutaneously or intramuscularly to secure absorption. A slow intravenous administration might be chosen if peripheral circulation is compromised as in fulminant shock.

Adrenaline in pressurized aerosol is effective for swelling in the throat and larynx and on bronchospasm. Absorption is rapid and the cardiovascular effect is equivalent to subcutaneous administration. In the case of shock injections are preferred.

Table 3
Emergency treatment of respiratory symptoms to stings[38]

Medical treatment	
Bronchial obstruction reaction	Adrenaline[*] 10-20 puffs from aerosol or 0.3-0.5 ml s.c. or beta-2-stimulator 4-10 puffs (e.g. salbutamole, terbutaline)
In severe cases	Beta-2-agonist i.v.
	Corticosteroid (e.g. prednisolone 80-100 mg) i.v.
	Aminophyllin 6 mg/kg over 20 min then 0.9 mg/kg per hr
Laryngeal oedema reaction	Adrenaline[*] 10-20 puffs from aerosol or 0.3-0.5 mg s.c.
	Corticosteroid (e.g. prednisolone 80-100 mg) i.v.
Other measures	Oxygen, medical observation until full recovery
	In severe cases: hospital admission, intubation or cricothyrotomy
Dosage for children	Adrenaline: 0.1 mg/10 kg body weight or 2-4 puffs/10 kg body weight
	Corticosteroid: Prednisolone 20 mg/kg body weight

* With protracted symptoms, adrenaline medication may be repeated every 10-20 min.

Beta-2-agonists (e.g. salbutamol, terbutaline) are effective in the treatment of bronchial obstruction - with less side effects than adrenaline.

Antihistamines could be used as the only treatment for skin symptoms such as local swelling, itching and less severe urticaria. Antihistamines are valuable as a supplement to adrenaline in angio-oedema and anaphylactic shock. The most important antihistamines in this context are the H-1 receptor antagonists. They inhibit the effect of histamine on the smooth muscles of the blood vessels (and in the bronchi) and thereby reduce the swelling and itching. H-2 receptor antagonists are potent antagonists on the acid secretion in the stomach, but both H-1 and H-2 can antagonize the negative effects of histamine on the heart and both should be given in shock as supplements to adrenaline.

Tablets with onset within less than ½ hour and no sedative side effects are now available and would often suffice except in the more severe reactions where injections are necessary.

Corticosteroids are effective in the treatment of the inflammatory reaction with its swelling, pain and redness. They should be used together with antihistamine if a very large local reaction develops or has occurred previously.

The onset of action is slow: several hours after administration even given intravenously. If gastro-intestinal function is not impaired, oral treatment would be sufficient.

Table 4
Emergency treatment of anaphylactic shock to stings[38]

Medication	
Emergency physician	Adrenaline* 0.3-0.5 mg i.m. (s.c.), in severe cases: 0.5 mg in 10 ml over 5 min i.v.
	H-1 and H-2 antihistamine i.v. (e.g. clemastine 2 mg, ranitidine 100 mg)
	Corticosteroids i.v. (e.g. prednisolone 100 mg)
At the hospital	Volume substitution (saline, plasma expanders)
	pH correction (sodium bicarbonate)
	Pressor substances by continuous infusion (e.g. adrenaline 5-20 migrog/min, dopamine 100-1000 microg/min, noradrenaline 8-20 microg/min)
Other measures	Shock position
	Oxygen supply
	I.v. line
	Hospital admission
	Monitoring: ECG, arterial and central venous blood pressure, blood gases
In severe cases	Intubation, assisted ventilation, defibrillation, cardiac massage
Dosage for children	Adrenaline and corticosteroid (see Table 3)
	Antihistamine e.g. Clemastine 1-2 mg i.v.
	Ranitidine 15 mg/10 kg body weight

* With protracted symptoms, adrenaline medication may be repeated every 10-20 min.

D. IMMUNOTHERAPY

In principle immunotherapy is a prophylactic treatment in allergic individuals. It has been used for decades but the mode of action is still unknown. In venom-allergic patients increasing doses of venom extract is administered subcutaneously until a dose equivalent to several stings is reached. The dose is increased at weekly intervals, or with injection regimes, with one to a few hours interval (rush regimen). At maintenance dose the interval is increased to one to two months and therapy is continued generally for 3 to 5 years.

The therapy can be performed in various regimens and choosing the optimum modality is a task for allergy specialists.

The therapy implies administration of substances to which the patient has shown to be allergic. Therefore special precautions have to be taken to avoid and to be able to give early treatment of allergic side effects. Before every injection the patients should be asked about reactions to the previous injection and the present clinical state should be checked. If dose interval has been extended or reaction to a previous injection has occurred, the allergen dose should be reduced. In all cases the patients should be under medical attention for at least ½ hour after the injection.

Immunotherapy has been shown effective in children and adults and in patients allergic to bees as well as to yellow jackets (Table 2). In the first study in which the effect was controlled by sting challenge, one of 19 patients with previous systemic sting reactions had a much weaker reaction; the rest had no systemic reactions to sting[19]. In contrast approx. 60% of the patients treated with placebo or extract made of whole insects (not only the venom) reacted with similar or more severe symptoms to retesting. In studies on children or patients with allergy to yellow jacket 97 - 100% of patients were protected[34,39-41]. In honey bee-allergic patients the effect was nearly as good[42,43]. The standard maintenance dose (100 microgram) is equivalent to 2 stings from a honey bee but to several stings from yellow jackets. In treatment failures the allergen dose might be doubled.

Whereas extract made from whole insects (venom sac and body) is not sufficiently effective in bee and yellow jacket allergy[19] it might be more effective in allergy to fire ants[44].

Reduction in specific IgE has been used as a criterion for stopping treatment[45]. Among such patients only 3 to 8% had systemic reactions when stung from a few months to 5 years after the last immunotherapy injection. Termination of the treatment after 5 years - independently of the immunological parameters - seems to give the same degree of protection[46].

Allergy to insect venom is one of the most important reasons for immunotherapy. Since the treatment is time consuming and not totally without side effects, only patients with a considerable risk of systemic reactions to future stings and a documented IgE related disease should be offered this treatment.

VI. REFERENCES

1. **RHOADES, R. B., STAFFORD, C. T., AND JAMES, F. K. JR.** Survey of fatal anaphylactic reactions to imported fire ant stings, *J. Allergy Clin. Immunol.*, 84, 159, 1989.
2. **MUELLER, H. L.** Diagnosis and treatment of insect sensitivity, *J. Asthma Res.*, 3, 331, 1966.
3. **MUELLER, U. R.** *Insect sting allergy. Clinical picture, diagnosis and treatment*, Gustav Fischer, New York, 1990.
4. **MOSBECH, H**. Death caused by wasp and bee stings, *Allergy*, 38, 195, 1983.
5. **BARNARD, J. H.** Studies of 400 Hymenoptera sting deaths in the United States, *J. Allergy Clin. Immunol.*, 52, 259, 1973.
6. **HERBERT, F. A. AND SALKIE, M. L.** Sensitivity to Hymenoptera in adult males, *Ann. Allergy*, 48, 12, 1982.
7. **GOLDEN, D. B. K., MARSH, D., KAGEY-SOBOTKA, A., FRIEDHOFF, L., SZKLO, M., VALENTINE, M. D., AND LICHTENSTEIN, L. M.** Epidemiology of insect venom sensitivity, *JAMA*, 262, 240, 1989.
8. **SETTIPANE, G. A., NEWSTED, G. J., AND BOYD, G. K.** Frequency of Hymenoptera allergy in an atopic and normal population, *J. Allergy Clin. Immunol.*, 50, 146, 1972.
9. **CHARPIN, D., BIRNBAUM, J., LANTEAUME, A., AND VERVLOET, D.** Prevalence of allergy to hymenoptera stings in different samples of the general population, *J. Allergy Clin. Immunol.*, 90, 331, 1992.
10. **YUNGINGER, J. W., JONES, R. T., LEIFERMAN, K. M., PAULL, B. R., WELSH, P. W., AND GLEICH, G. J.** Immunological and biochemical studies in beekeepers and their family members, *J. Allergy Clin. Immunol.*, 61, 93, 1978.
11. **BOUSQUET, J., COULOMB, Y., BOBINET-LEVY, M., AND MICHEL, F. M.** Clinical and immunological surveys in bee keepers, *Clinical Allergy*, 12, 331, 1982.
12. **PARRISH, H. M.** Analysis of 460 fatalities from venomous animals in the United States, *Amer. J. Med. Sci.*, 245, 129, 1963.
13. **NALL, T. M.** Analysis of 677 death certificates and 168 autopsies of stinging insect deaths, *J. Allergy Clin. Immunol.*, 75, 207, 1985.
14. **SCHWARTZ, H. J., SUTHEIMER, C., GAUERKE, M. B., AND YUNGINGER, J. W.** Hymenoptera venom-specific IgE antibodies in post-mortem sera from victims of sudden, unexpected death, *Clinical Allergy*, 18, 461, 1988.
15. Insect Allergy Subcommittee of the American Academy of Allergy, Insect sting allergy: Questionnaire study 2606 cases, *JAMA*, 193, 109, 1965.
16. **SETTIPANE, G. A., CHAFEE, F. H., KLEIN, D. E., BOYD, G. K., STURAM, J. H., AND FREYE, H. B.** Anaphylactic reactions to Hymenoptera Stings in asthmatic patients, *Clin. Allergy*, 10, 659, 1980.

17. **KAMPELMACHER, J. M. AND VAN DER ZWAN, J. C.** Provocation test with a living insect as a diagnostic tool in systemic reactions to bee and wasp venom: a prospective study with emphasis on the clinical aspects, *Clin. Allergy,* 17, 317, 1987.

18. **BLAAUW, P. J. AND SMITHIUS, L. O. M. J.** The evaluation of the common diagnostic methods of hypersensitivity for bee and yellow jacket venom by means of an in-hospital insect sting, *J. Allergy Clin. Immunol.,* 75, 556, 1985.

19. **HUNT, K., VALENTINE, M. D., SOBOTKA, A. K., BENTON, A. W., AMODIO, F. J., AND LICHTENSTEIN, L. M.** A controlled trial of immunotherapy in insect hypersensitivity, *N Engl J Med,* 299, 257, 1978.

20. **REISMAN, R. E.** Natural history of insect sting allergy: Relationship of severity of symptoms of initial sting anaphylaxis to re-sting reactions, *J. Allergy Clin. Immunol.,* 90, 335, 1992.

21. **SCHUBERTH, K. C., LICHTENSTEIN, L. M., KAGEY-SOBOTKA, A., SZKLO, M., KWITEROVICH, K. A., AND VALENTINE, M. D.** Epidemiologic study of insect allergy in children. II Effect of accidental stings in allergic children, *J. Pediatr.,* 102, 361, 1983.

22. **MAURIELLO, P. M., BARDE, S. H., GEORGITIS, J. W., AND REISMAN, R. E.** Natural history of large local reactions from stinging insects, *J. Allergy Clin. Immunol.,* 74, 494, 1984.

23. **GRAFT, D. F., SCHUBERTH, K. C., KAGEY-SOBOTKA, A., KWITEROVICH, K. A., YAFFA, B. S. N., LICHTENSTEIN, L. M., AND VALENTINE, M. D.** A prospective study of the natural history of large local reactions after Hymenoptera stings in children, *J. Pediatr.,* 104, 664, 1984.

24. **CESKA, M., ERIKSSON, R., AND VARGA, J. M.** Radioimmunosorbent assay of allergens, *J. Allergy Clin. Immunol.,* 49, 1, 1972.

25. **MOSBECH, H., CHRISTENSEN, J., DIRKSEN, A., AND SØBORG, M.** Insect allergy. Predictive value of diagnostic tests: a three-year follow up study, *Clin. Allergy,* 16, 433, 1986.

26. **BISCHOF, M., MÜLLER, U., AND VOLKART, H. D.** How important are Dolichovespula (DV) in insect sting allergy ? *J. Allergy Clin. Immunol.,* 77, 142, 1986.

27. **KEMENY, D. M., LESSOF, M. H., AND TRULL, A. K.** IgE and IgG antibodies to bee venom as measured by a modification of the RAST method, *Clin. Allergy,* 10, 413, 1980.

28. **SETTIPANE, G. A. AND CARLISLE, C. C.** A critical evaluation of RAST to venoms of Hymenoptera, *Clin. Allergy,* 10, 667, 1980.

29. **MÜLLER, U., SPIESS, J., AND ROTH, A.** Serological investigations in Hymenoptera sting allergy: IgE and haemagglutinating antibodies against bee venom in patients with bee sting allergy, beekeepers and non-allergic blooddonors, *Clin. Allergy,* 7, 57, 1977.

30. **LESSOF, M. H., SOBOTKA, A. K., AND LICHTENSTEIN, L. M.** Effects of passive antibody in bee venom anaphylaxis, *The Johns Hopkins Medical Journal,* 142, 1, 1978.

31. **MÜLLER, U. R., MORRIS, T., BISCHOF, M., FRIEDLI, H., AND SKARVIL, F.** Combined active and passive immunotherapy in honeybee-sting allergy, *J. Allergy Clin. Immunol.,* 78, 115, 1986.

32. **GOLDEN, D. B. K., MEYERS, D. A., KAGEY-SOBOTKA, A., VALENTINE, M. D., AND LICHTENSTEIN, L. M.** Clinical relevance of the venom-specific immunoglobulin G antibody level during immunotherapy, *J. Allergy Clin. Immunol.,* 69, 489, 1982.

33. **GOLDEN, D. B. K., LAWRENCE, I. D., HAMILTON, R. H., KAGEY-SOBOTKA, A., VALENTINE, M. D., AND LICHTENSTEIN, L. M.** Clinical correlation of the venom-specific IgG antibody level during maintenance venom immunotherapy, *J. Allergy Clin. Immunol.,* 90, 386, 1992.

34. **MOSBECH, H., MALLING, H. J., BIERING, I., BOEWADT, H., SOBORG, M., WEEKE, B., AND LOWENSTEIN, H.** Immunotherapy with yellow jacket venom. A comparative study including three different extracts, one adsorbed to aluminium hydroxide and two unmodified, *Allergy,* 41, 95, 1986.

35. **MÜLLER, U., THURNHEER, U., PATRIZZI, R., SPIESS, J., AND HOIGNE, R.** Immunotherapy in bee sting sensitivity, *Allergy,* 34, 369, 1979.

36. **PARKER, J. L., SANTRACH, P. J., DAHLBERG, M. J. E., AND YUNGINGER, J. W.** Evaluation of Hymenoptera-sting sensitivity with deliberate sting challenges: inadequacy of present diagnostic methods, *J. Allergy Clin. Immunol.,* 69, 200, 1982.

37. **VAN DER LINDEN, P. -W. G., HACK, P. E., POORTMAN, J., VIVIÉ-KIPP, Y. C., STUYVENBERG, A., AND VAN DER ZWAN, J. K.** Insect-sting challenge in 138 patients: Relation between clinical severity of anaphylaxis and mast cell activation, *J. Allergy Clin. Immunol.,* 90, 110, 1992.

38. **MÜLLER, U., MOSBECH, H., BLAAUW, P., DREBORG, S., MALLING, H. J., PRZYBILLA, B., URBANEK, R., PASTORELLO, E., BLANCA, M., AND BOUSQUET, J.,** Emergency treatment of allergic reactions to Hymenoptera stings, *Clin. Exp. Allergy,* 21, 281, 1991.

39. **MALLING, H. -J., DJURUP, R., SONDERGAARD, I., AND WEEKE, B.** Clustered immunotherapy with Yellow Jacket venom. Evaluation of the influence of time interval on in vivo and in vitro parameters, *Allergy,* 40, 373, 1985.

40. **NATAF, P., GUINNEPAIN, M. T., AND HERMAN, D.** Rush venom immunotherapy: a 3-day programme for hymenoptera sting allergy, *Clin. Allergy,* 14, 269, 1984.

41. **CHIPPS, B. E., VALENTINE, M. D., KAGEY-SOBOTKA, A., SCHUBERTH, K. C., AND LICHTENSTEIN, L. M.** Diagnosis and treatment of anaphylactic reactions to Hymenoptera stings in children, *J. Pediatr.*, 97, 177, 1980.

42. **YUNGINGER, J. W., PAULL, B. R., JONES, R. T., AND SANTRACH, P. J.** Rush venom immunotherapy program for honeybee sting sensitivity, *J. Allergy Clin. Immunol.*, 63, 340, 1979.

43. **GILLMAN, S. A., CUMMINS, L. H., KOZAK, P., AND HOFFMAN, D. R.** Venom immunotherapy: comparison of "rush" vs "conventional" schedules, *Ann. Allergy*, 45, 351, 1980.

44. **FREEMAN, T. M., HYLANDER, R., ORTIZ, A., AND MARTIN, M. E.** Imported fire ant immunotherapy: Effectiveness of whole body extracts, *J. Allergy Clin. Immunol.*, 90, 210, 1992.

45. **URBANEK, R., FORSTER, J., KUHN, W., AND ZIUPA, J.** Discontinuation of bee venom immunotherapy in children and adolescents, *J. Pediatr.*, 107, 367, 1985.

46. **GOLDEN, D. B., ADDISON, B. I., GADDE, J., KAGEY-SOBOTKA, A., VALENTINE, M. D., AND LICHTENSTEIN, L. M.** Prospective observations on stopping prolonged venom immunotherapy, *J. Allergy Clin. Immunol.*, 84, 162, 1989.

Chapter 23

CLINICAL TOXICOLOGY OF HELODERMATIDAE LIZARD BITES

Dietrich Mebs

TABLE OF CONTENTS

I. INTRODUCTION

Besides the snakes there exist only two venomous lizard species in the reptile order Squamata: *Heloderma suspectum* and *Heloderma horridum* which belong to the unique family Helodermatidae. Commonly named Gila monster, beaded lizard or escorpión (Spanish) they are restricted to the New World where they inhabit some areas of the southern part of North-America[1]. The lizards produce a powerful venom which has lethal potency. In humans their bite may cause severe symptoms of envenoming; however, fatal cases have not been reported during the last 50 years[2].

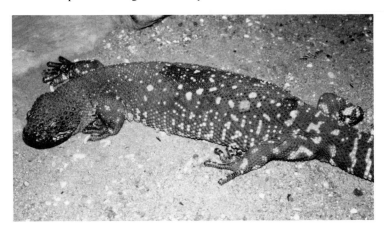

Figure 1. *Heloderma suspectum* (photo © Dr. J. White).

II. EPIDEMIOLOGY AND CIRCUMSTANCES OF ENVENOMING

Bites by *Heloderma* are rare. In almost all cases of human envenoming the lizard had been provoked or handled carelessly. Therefore, most bites occur on fingers or the hand[1,2]. The rather shy animal usually tries to escape when disturbed and bites only when attempts are made to catch it. Its defensive behaviour includes hissing and open mouth threats, but the lizard attacks quickly and bites when the offender gets too close; it holds on which facilitates the introduction of venom into the wound.

Few cases of human envenoming are reported in the literature[1]. They occurred in areas where the lizards live, but also in other parts of the world, where the animals are kept as pets. From an epidemiological point of view *Heloderma* bites are negligible and have no public health implications.

III. BIOLOGY AND VENOM OF HELODERMATIDAE LIZARDS

A. BIOLOGY AND DISTRIBUTION

Both *Heloderma* species, *Heloderma suspectum* and *Heloderma horridum*, are large (maximum length: *H. suspectum* about 50 cm, *H. horridum* about one meter), stout lizards with a fat tail. The body is covered with thick scales like beads (beaded lizard). Whereas *Heloderma suspectum* shows an irregular black band pattern over the body and tail on a yellow, orange to pink background, *Heloderma horridum* tends to have a more brown or black pattern, but some subspecies (*alvarezi*) are virtually devoid of pattern and are almost uniformly black. The coloration pattern varies during growth. Juveniles are generally more distinctly marked[1-4].

The geographical distribution of *Heloderma suspectum* (the Gila monster) ranges from the southern border of Utah and Nevada (U.S.) into Mexico. *H. horridum* is distributed along the Pacific coast of Mexico. Both species comprise five subspecies such as *H. suspectum suspectum* and *H. s.cinctum; H. horridum horridum, H. h.exasperatum* and *H. h.alvarezi.*

The habitats of *Heloderma* are generally arid areas, deserts with rocks, shrubs and cacti, but the lizards may also be found in dry forests. They are mostly diurnal during spring and autumn, but are active at night in summer. The lizards retreat most of the time to burrows or rocky shelters to avoid the heat of the day. They are oviparous and lay clutches of up to 12 eggs. Their diet consists of eggs of groundnesting birds and of small mammals.

B. VENOM APPARATUS

In contrast to venomous snakes the two venom glands of *Heloderma* are located on each anterior side of the lower jaw[1,5,6] (Figure 2). Ducts of the gland, which is composed of several lobes, open at the base of lance-sharp teeth (2 to 6 mm long) which are grooved on both the anterior and posterior side. The venom is discharged at the base of the teeth where it is eventually mixed with saliva entering the wound by capillary action along the grooves of the teeth[1,7]. Holding on during the bite facilitates the introduction of the venom into the puncture wound; the longer the bite the more severe is the envenoming.

The venom seems to be used more for defense than for subduing the prey, which is easily crushed by the biting force.

C. VENOM: CHEMISTRY AND PHARMACOLOGY

The venom of *Heloderma* is similar in composition and lethality for both species and represents a mixture of proteins and peptides. Besides a factor named gilatoxin, which is lethal to mice, it consists mainly of enzymes such as hyaluronidase, kallikrein, phospholipase A_2 and arginine esterase[8-10]. Moreover, peptides like helodermin and helospectin, which are similar in structure and activity to vasoactive intestinal peptides (VIP), have been identified[11-14]. However, the venom lacks typical neurotoxins or enzymes which interfere with blood coagulation. Heloderma venom exhibits very high hyaluronidase activity. This enzyme, also considered to be a "spreading factor", has been suggested to promote the introduction of venom components into the tissue[15].

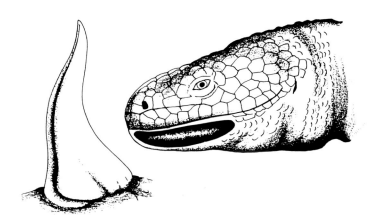

Figure 2   Location of the venom gland along the lower jaw of *Heloderma* (right); grooved tooth of the lower jaw (left).

Very active kallikreins have been isolated from both *Heloderma* suspectum[16] and *Heloderma horridum* venom[17]; the enzyme from the latter venom was named helodermatine. The enzymes possess arginine ester hydrolase activity and release vasoactive kinins (most probably bradykinin) from a plasma precursor, kininogen. Another arginine ester hydrolase was shown to produce massive haemorrhage of the eyeball, the intestines, the kidneys and occasionally bleeding in the lungs[18,19].

A phospholipase A_2 was isolated from *Heloderma horridum* venom. Surprisingly the N-terminal sequence of the acidic protein shows 56% homology with bee venom phospholipase A_2 [20].

A lethal factor called gilatoxin was isolated from both *Heloderma* venoms and found to be an acidic glycoprotein of 35 kD and 37 kD molecular mass, respectively[21]. It appears to be a minor component in the venom (the yield is between 3 to 5%). Its lethality is almost the same as that of crude venom; therefore, a synergistic action with other venom components has been proposed.

Helothermine is a toxin with a molecular mass of 25,500 which was isolated from *Heloderma horridum* venom. It has no effects on excitable membranes, but causes lowering of body temperature beside lethargy and partial paralysis of hind limbs in mice. Its N-terminal amino acid sequence has no similarity to any other protein[22].

In mice the medium lethal dose (LD_{50}) of *Heloderma* venom is in the range of 0.4 to 2.7 mg/kg (i.v. injection)[8,9,21,23]. Envenomed animals generally exhibit restlessness, cyanosis due to dyspnea or apnea, and convulsions preceding death.

In dogs and rats the intravenous injection of *H. suspectum* venom causes reduced carotid blood flow followed by a rapidly developing hypotension, tachycardia, and ventilatory irregularities such as gasping, rapid and shallow breathing or apnea[24]; but the electrocardiogram is essentially normal. The release of kinins in the blood may contribute to the shock-like symptoms seen in experimental animals as well as in humans. The venom fails to alter the blood coagulation *in vivo* and *in vitro*. It produces considerable local edema, but is not haemorrhagic locally. Mice when injected with sublethal doses exhibit massive haemorrhage of the eyeball and intestinal bleeding, an effect which is caused by an arginine ester hydrolase of the venom[18,19].

IV. CLINICAL SIGNS AND SYMPTOMS OF ENVENOMING

Bites of *Heloderma* produce small puncture wounds, which vary in extent due to the number of teeth involved. By attempts to remove the animal from the bite site, where it holds on firmly, teeth may break off and remain in the wound.

The first sign of envenoming is intense pain. It occurs usually within minutes and spreads to involve the entire arm or leg. Depending on the amount of venom injected pain ranges from burning to more severe excruciating or stabbing sensations reaching its greatest intensity within 30 to 60 minutes, but may persist for several (till 12) hours.

Swelling and edema at the bite site appear within 15 minutes and progress slowly over the next hours. The extent of edema may be considerable and appears to contribute to the local pain; however, there is no indication or danger of a compartment syndrome. Tenderness about the wound site is common, in some cases with cyanosis and blueish discoloration, but no haemorrhage or necrosis follow. Lymphadenitis and lymphadenopathy may also be associated with extensive edema.

General weakness, dizziness, faintness and increased perspiration are common symptoms and seem to be due to primary hypotension which may persist for hours. But in severe cases rapid fall of blood pressure and severe shock symptoms may occur within minutes after the bite; however, this is rather rare.

Except for mild leukocytosis, blood parameters are generally within the normal range[1,2].

Fatalities have been reported in the older literature[1], which have been rather uncritically evaluated[25,26]. Death after *Heloderma* bite is rather unlikely, but may occur under certain unfavourable conditions (general health situation of the patient, shock etc.).

V. PROPHYLAXIS

As the lizards bite only when attacked, bites can easily be avoided by leaving them alone. Attempts to catch the animal or grasping into burrows or under rock crevices (which are also inhabited by rattlesnakes) should be avoided. Animals kept in captivity should be carefully handled; they are usually "tame", but become suddenly aggressive when placed in a new environment. Thick gloves at least prevent venom introduction.

VI. FIRST AID TREATMENT

The most important measure, which is often difficult to achieve, is to remove the lizard from the bite site where it firmly holds on. A strong stick or bar may be put into the mouth behind the bitten part to open the jaws. Pulling the animal away usually results in breaking of the teeth and laceration of the wound.

No measures other than those applied in snakebite are recommended. The patient who suffers severe pain should be reassured to avoid panic. Rings, bangles etc. should be immediately removed from the bitten limb, because of the rapidly spreading edema. No incisions at the bite site, no ice or heat, no tourniquet or bandage should be used. However the bitten limb should be immobilized (applying a splint etc.) and the patient should be transported to medical care as quickly as possible.

VII. CLINICAL MANAGEMENT

There is no antivenom available, and snake antivenoms do not crossreact with *Heloderma* venom[27]. Treatment of envenoming has to be essentially symptomatic and supportive. There is no need for surgical intervention (edema etc.)[2].

Hypotensive crisis is the most likely symptom of severe envenoming and should be treated appropriately by infusions of electrolyte solutions and application of antishock drugs (adrenaline etc.). Vital signs (blood pressure, heart rate etc., but also hematocrit when severe edema or shock symptoms develop) should be constantly checked. Pain is not easy to control; common analgesics (aspirine, metamizole or even morphine derivatives) may be tried. The bitten limb should not be packed in ice, but left at heart level. The puncture wound should be probed for broken teeth and cleaned. Antibiotics may be considered in case of tissue laceration. Tetanus prophylaxis has to be performed. Antihistaminics or corticosteroids are of no therapeutic value except if the patient develops allergic symptoms. There is no danger of venom induced coagulopathy.

VIII. REFERENCES

1. **BOGERT, C.M. & DEL CAMPO, R.M.** The Gila monster and its allies. The relationships, habits, and behavior of the lizards of the family Helodermatidae. *Bull.Am.Mus.Nat.Hist.* **109**, 1-238, 1956.
2. **RUSSELL, F.E. & BOGERT, C.M.** Gila monster: its biology, venom and bite - a review. *Toxicon* **19**, 341-359, 1981.
3. **LOWE, C.H., SCHWALBE, C.R. & JOHNSON, T.B.** The Venomous Reptiles of Arizona. *Arizona Game and Fish Dept.*, Phoenix, AZ, 1986.
4. **ERNST, C.H.** *Venomous Reptiles of North America.* Smithsonian Inst. Press, Washington,DC, 1992.
5. **STAHNKE, H.L., HEFFRON, W.A. & LEWIS, D.L.** Bite of the Gila monster. *Rocky Mountain Med.J.* **67**, 25-30, 1970.
6. **KOCHVA, E.** Oral glands of the reptilia. In: *Biology of the Reptilia* (C.GANS & K.A.GANS eds.) vol.8, pp 49-161, Academic Press, London, 1978.
7. **TINKHAM, E.R.** The biology of the Gila monster. In: *Venomous Animals and Their Venoms,* vol.2 Eds. Bucherl, W. & Buckley, E.E. pp 387-413. Academic Press, New York, 1971.
8. **MEBS, D. & RAUDONAT, H.W.** Biochemical investigations of *Heloderma* venom. *Mem.Inst.Butantan*, Sao Paulo, **33**, 907-912, 1966.
9. **MEBS, D. & RAUDONAT, H.W.** Biochemie des Giftes der Krustenechse, *Heloderma suspectum* und *Heloderma horridum. Naturwissenschaften* **54**, 494, 1967.
10. **TU, A.T. & MURDOCK, D.S.** Protein nature and some enzymatic properties of the lizard *Heloderma suspectum suspectum* (Gila monster) venom. *Comp. Biochem. Physiol.***22**, 389-396, 1967.
11. **PARKER, D.S., RAUFMANN, J.P., O'DONOHUE, T.L., BLEDSOE, M., YOSHIDA, H. & PISANO, J.J.** Amino acid sequence of helospectins, new members of the glucagon superfamily found in Gila monster venom. *J. Biol. Chem.* **259**, 11751-11755, 1984.
12. **HOSHINO, M., YANAHARA, C., HONG, Y.M., KISHIDA, S., KATSUMARU, Y., VANDERMEERS, A., VANDERMEERS-PIRET,M.C., ROBBERECHT, P., CHRISTOPHE, J. & YANAIHARA, N.** Primary structure of helodermin, a VIP-secretin-like peptide isolated from Gila monster venom. *FEBS Lett.* **178**, 233-239, 1984.
13. **VANDERMEERS, A., VANDERMEERS-PIRET, M.C., ROBBERECHT, P., WAELBROECK, M., DEHAYE, J.P. & CHRISTOPHE, J.** Purification of a novel pancreatic secretory factor (PSF) and a novel peptide with VIP- and secretin-like properties (helodermin) from Gila monster venom. *FEBS Lett.* **166**, 273-276, 1984.
14. **VANDERMEERS, A., GOURLET, P., VANDERMEERS-PIRET, M.C., CAUVIN, A., DENEEF, P., SVOBODA, M., ROBBERECHT, P. & CHRISTOPHE, J.** Chemical and biological properties of peptide-like vaso-active-intestinal peptide and peptide-histidine isoleucimidine extracted from the venom of *Heloderma horridum horridum* and *Heloderma suspectum. Eur. J. Biochem.* **164**, 321-327, 1987.
15. **TU, A.T. & HENDON, R.A.** Characterization of lizard venom hyaluronidase and evidence for its action as a spreading factor. *Comp. Biochem. Physiol.***76B**, 377-383, 1983.
16. **MEBS, D.** Isolierung und Eigenschaften eines Kallikreins aus dem Gift der Krustenechse *Heloderma suspectum. Hoppe-Seyler´s Z. Physiol. Chem.***350**, 821-826, 1969.

17. **ALAGON, A.C., POSSANI, L.D., SMART, J. & SCHLEUNIG, W.D.** Helodermatine, a kallikrein-like hypotensive enzyme from the venom of the *Heloderma horridum horridum* (Mexican beaded lizard). *J. Exp. Med.* **164**, 1835-1845, 1986.

18. **MEBS, D.** Biochemistry of *Heloderma* venom. In: *Toxins of Animal and Plant Origin* In Eds. De Vries, A. & Kochva, E., vol.2, pp. 499-513, Gordon & Breach, New York, 1972.

19. **NIKAI, T., IMAI, K., SUGIHARA, H. & TU, A.T.** Isolation and characterization of horridum toxin with arginine ester hydrolase activity from *Heloderma horridum* (beaded lizard) venom. *Archs Biochim. Biophys.* **264**, 270-280, 1988.

20. **SOSA, B.P., ALAGON, A.C., MARTIN, B.M. & POSSANI, L.D.** Biochemical characterization of the phospholipase A_2 purified from the venom of the Mexican beaded lizard (*Heloderma horridum horridum* Wiegmann). *Biochemistry* **25**, 2927-2933, 1986.

21. **HENDON, R.R. & TU, A.T.** Biochemical characterization of the lizard gilatoxin. *Biochemistry* **20**, 3517-3522, 1981.

22. **MOCHCA-MORALES, J., MARTIN, B.M. & POSSANI, L.D.** Isolation and characterization of helothermine, a novel toxin from *Heloderma horridum horridum* (Mexican beaded lizard) venom. *Toxicon* **28**, 299-309, 1990.

23. **STYBLOVA, Z. & KORNALIK, F.** Enzymatic properties of *Heloderma suspectum* venom. *Toxicon* **5**, 139-140, 1967.

24. **PATTERSON, R.A.** Some physiological effects caused by venom from the Gila monster, *Heloderma suspectum*. *Toxicon* **5**, 5-10, 1967.

25. **WOODSON, W.D.** Toxicity of *Heloderma* venom. *Herpetologica* **4**, 31-33, 1947.

26. **GRANT, M.L. & HENDERSON, L.J.** A case of Gila monster poisoning with a summary of some previous accounts. *Proc.Iowa Acad.Sci.* **64**, 686-697, 1957.

27. **MEBS, D.** Untersuchungen über die Wirksamkeit einiger Schlangengiftseren gegenüber *Heloderma-Gift*. *Salamandra* **6**, 135-136, 1970.

Chapter 24

BIOLOGY AND DISTRIBUTION OF VENOMOUS SNAKES OF MEDICAL IMPORTANCE AND THE COMPOSITION OF SNAKE VENOMS

Jürg Meier and Kurt F. Stocker

TABLE OF CONTENTS

* This chapter is based in part on review articles published by CRC Press under the following titles:

MEIER, J. (1990): Venomous Snakes. In: Medical Use of Snake Venom Proteins (K.F. Stocker, Ed.), pp. 1-32. Boca Raton: CRC Press.

MEIER, J. and STOCKER, K. (1991) Effects of Snake Venoms on Haemostasis. CRC Critical Reviews in Toxicology 21, pp. 171-182.

The authors thank CRC Press for its permission to include parts of these publications in this chapter.

I. INTRODUCTION

This chapter deals with venomous snakes, the composition and mode of action of snake venoms, their distribution and some more general aspects of snake biology. Medical aspects and the clinical toxicology of snakebite are covered in the different chapters written by physicians experienced with snakebite. As a consequence of the cryptic life habits and the defensive behaviour of snakes, snakebite is mainly a rural and occupational hazard. Furthermore, reliable observations confirm that at least half of all victims bitten by snakes escape with little or even no envenomation, since often only small amounts of venom are injected when the snake strikes in defense. However, snakebite is unpredictable in its early stage and therefore needs medical observation to assess the severity of envenomation and to ensure adequate treatment.

II. SNAKES AND THE BIOLOGICAL SIGNIFICANCE OF THEIR VENOMS

A. SHORT HISTORY OF SNAKES

During the Cretaceous period the first obviously snake-like forms came into existence. Although the fossil record is meagre, there is evidence that snakes passed a burrowing stage in their early history. This theory[1-3] is particularly supported by the structure of the eyes which differs from that of typical lizards. Thus, a redevelopment of the eye from the degenerate condition characteristic of a burrowing ancestor has been suggested. The theory may be further supported by the quite extraordinary evolution of the Jacobsons's organ, which is the dominant organ of smell in snakes. The paired saccular structures are situated in the anterior part of the mouth roof. The very long tongue obviously picks up airborne substances, which are brought into these ducts by the tips when the tongue is drawn back into the mouth. The olfactory epithelium is connected to the brain by a branch of the olfactory nerves. In burrowing species the chemical sense seems to be of important value. Also in higher developed snakes this sense is of special significance, since the first sign of activity is always the protrusion of the tongue. The systematic classification of snakes is controversial and presents difficulties even at higher taxonomic levels[4-6]. However, these systematic problems are of no interest in the context of this chapter. The blind snakes (Typhlopidae) and the thread snakes (Leptotyphlopidae) belong to the infraorder Scolecophidia. Both snake families consist of burrowing species with primitive characteristics. Whereas in Typhlopidae teeth are typically absent in the lower jaw, they are absent in the upper jaw in Leptotyphlopidae. Members of both families feed on earthworms and insects. A transition from the more primitive forms found in the Aniliidae to more or less advanced forms, as represented e.g. by the Acrochordidae, is seen in the infraorder Henophidia. The cylinder snakes (Aniliidae) are burrowing animals found in South America, Sri Lanka, Indonesia and Malaysia. They feed on small preys including vertebrates. The shieldtail snakes (Uropeltidae) are also burrowing species restricted to Sri Lanka and southern India, feeding on earthworms and insects. The sunbeam snake *Xenopeltis unicolor*, the only species of the family Xenopeltidae, is another burrowing species occurring in southeastern Asia from southern India to Indonesia and feeding on small vertebrates. Two species are present in the wart snake family (Acrochordidae). These are large water snakes occurring in rivers, estuaries and coastal waters from southeastern India to New Guinea and Australia. They feed on fish. The well-known pythons and boas are representatives of the family Boidae which includes the largest snakes, which may reach a length of 10 metres or more. This family, however, also includes small burrowing forms which are modified accordingly. Boas and pythons mainly feed on birds and mammals, the burrowing species on earthworms and insects. Members of the family Boidae are found worldwide, especially in wooded areas although desert species and semiaquatic forms are also known. The higher snakes are included in the infraorder Caenophidia. Venomous species are present in this infraorder only. The snake family Colubridae including about two thirds of all living snake species belongs to this infraorder. Their distribution is worldwide; terrestrial, arboreal, burrowing and aquatic snakes are found in this family. As will be shown later, there are different degrees of venomosity existing in this family. The venomous snakes *sensu stricto* are grouped in three families: the family Elapidae includes well-known snakes, like cobras, mambas and coral snakes which form the subfamily Elapinae, as well as the sea snakes (subfamilies Hydrophiinae and Laticaudinae; these two subfamilies are placed in a separate family, Hydrophiidae, by some authors) which are all marine, except a Philippine fresh water lake species. Sea snakes are found in all warmer seas, except the Atlantic Ocean. They feed mainly on fish (See Chapter 13). The terrestrial or arboreal

Elapinae snakes are also found throughout the warmer parts of the world, except Madagascar; their main prey are vertebrates. They are all venomous. The well-known vipers and pit vipers including the rattlesnakes form the family Viperidae which is subdivided into the Viperinae (true vipers) and the subfamily Crotalinae (pit vipers). All members of the latter group possess facial pit organs located on either side of the head between the eye and the nostril. These are temperature-sensitive receptors which face forward and allow the pit viper to localize nearby objects that have a higher temperature than surrounding objects. These thermal receptors have been shown to respond to temperature changes of less than 0.003°C[7]. All viperid snakes mainly feed on vertebrates; they are all venomous. Snakes of the Viperinae are found throughout the Old World north to the polar circle; they are absent in America and Australia, whereas Crotalinae snakes occur in North and South America and southern Asia, but not in Australia and Africa. The family Atractaspididae includes only one genus with about 15 species distributed over central Africa and reaching South Africa in the south and Israel in the north.

B. FEEDING STRATEGIES OF SNAKES

With the exception of some egg-eating colubrine snakes (the African genus *Dasypeltis* with five species and the Indian *Elachistodon westermanni*), all snakes are strictly carnivorous. Due to their elongated body form, however, their mouth is small and narrow compared to their body volume. Furthermore, since snakes lack cutting or grinding teeth to reduce their prey to small pieces before swallowing, one would expect them to continuously eat large amounts of small and feeble animals. Most snakes, on the contrary, feed on relatively big animals with long time intervals in between. This feeding behaviour is advantageous, since the less frequent the food intake takes place in free nature, the rarer are the risks involved, and it also saves energy. Special adaptations in skull anatomy allow snakes to swallow large prey animals. Possibly as a consequence of fossoriality, their brain is enclosed in a firm brain case. In contrast to lizards all the bones of the jaws are no longer rigidly connected to the brain pan, but kinetically attached to the latter, thus forming a highly mobile jaw organization[8]. Left and right parts of the jaws may be independently moved and alternatively protracted and retracted, thus leading to the typical swallowing sequence called "unilateral feeding"[9] observed in most snakes (Figure 1). These adaptations allow snakes to considerably widen their mouth opening and advance their skull in unilateral sequences over the prey organism to be swallowed. In this context, it is worth noting that a ten per cent increase of the mouth orifice allows snakes to swallow a prey animal of a twenty per cent bigger body volume[10]. In contrast to this obvious advantage, the highly kinetic skull also shows disadvantages: vulnerability. Consequently, feeding strategies to immobilize prey animals prior to ingestion had to be developed.

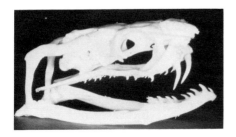
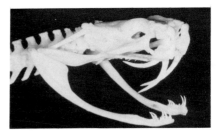

Figure 1. Skulls of venomous snakes
1a. Cobra (*Naja naja kaouthia*).   **1b.** Pit viper (*Bothrops moojeni*).

1. Biting, grasping

Quite a number of snakes feed on small and feeble animals which they swallow without any preliminary subjugation. This (probably very old) type of feeding strategy is seen in ancient snakes such as blind, thread and cylinder snakes (Typhlopidae, Leptotyphlopidae, Aniliidae) as well as in many modern colubrid species (Colubridae).

2. Constriction

A well-known feeding strategy found in ancient and modern snakes (Acrochordidae, Xenopeltidae, Aniliidae, Boidae, Colubridae) is constriction[11]. In this behaviour pattern, a prey organism is immobilized by pressure exerted from two or more loops of the snake's body encircling it. The coil surrounding the prey normally leads to strangulation, since the victim is unable to breathe as a consequence of the pressure on its respiratory tract. Constriction is certainly an effective strategy for subduing prey and therefore a feeding behaviour widespread in snakes.

3. Venom

Another highly effective strategy for subduing prey animals is the parenteral injection of venom produced in specialized, complex dental glands located in the upper jaw of snakes[12-15,40]. It is evident that this subduing technique has the advantage of reducing the hazards of holding onto a relatively large prey capable of self-defence[14]. Thus, the primary function of snake venoms has to be seen in this context. However, as will be shown later, the full development of an efficient venom apparatus not only requires the production of toxic substances able to immobilize prey organisms but also more or less specialized tooth structures able to deliver them. Snake venom also serves functions other than prey immobilization. For a long time, beginning with Fontana's statements in the 18th century, snake venoms have also been suspected of promoting digestion[16-18]. However, only few experimental data are available on this topic to date[19,101]. A recent study using X-rays to compare the digestive progress with and without the influence of venom in five different snake species failed to show any difference[20]. There is no doubt that snake venoms play a role also in defensive behaviour. To be seen in the context of snake coloration and behaviour, the skin coloration and ornamental pattern is of special value as a camouflage in the natural environment. When a snake is threatened, the first active reaction in the presence of a potential enemy is to try to escape notice. The next step is escape to some inaccessible retreat. If this is not possible or circumvented, various kinds of warning devices, either visual or audible, may be used. In the last resort the snake counterattacks, normally by biting, or, in the case of the so-called spitting cobras, by squirting out venom through pressure of the muscles surrounding the venom glands[21,22]. This is a special defence behaviour facilitated by modified fangs. In contrast to other elapid venoms, human encounters with spitting cobras can result in eye damage or serious local reactions following a spitting act[23-25].

C. "VENOMOUS" VS. "NON VENOMOUS" SNAKES

Snakes are usually called venomous, when envenomations or human fatalities after their bites are known. Since the members of the Elapidae, Viperidae and Atractaspididae snake families all possess a venom apparatus able to produce and efficiently inject venom, they are also referred to as genuinely venomous snakes[15]. Since colubrid snakes are usually of no medical importance, they are generally termed to be "nonvenomous". However, as quite a number of colubrid snakes are able to produce highly toxic secretions and to inject them more or less efficiently, this popular terminology has to be critically revised. Human fatalities are known after bites of the two African opisthoglyphous species, the boomslang

(*Dispholidus typus*) and the vine snake (*Thelothornis kirtlandii*)[75,76,78] as well as of the Japanese aglyphous Yamakagashi (*Rhabdophis tigrinus*)[79,84]. Quite a number of other colubrids are known to produce at least local symptoms after a bite[77,93,94]. In consequence, as has been stated before, about two thirds of all living snake species are venomous although much fewer are of medical importance.

D. DISTRIBUTION OF SNAKES OF MEDICAL IMPORTANCE

Snakes of medical importance are found in temperate, but predominantly in tropical areas throughout the world. Viperidae snakes are even present in the arctic region, where the Common Viper (*Vipera berus*) is found up to 69° N latitude, and in the alpine region, where they may be found up to 3,000 meters altitude. Table 1 provides information on those regions, where venomous snakes of medical importance are not found.

Table 1
Geographic Regions without Venomous Snakes of Medical Importance

Geographic Region	Countries
Africa	Canary Islands
	Cape Verde Islands
	Madagascar
America	
- North	northern from 55° N latitude
	Greenland
- Central	West Indies (excl. Trinidad, Tobago, Sta. Lucia, Martinique)
- South	Chile
	Galapagos Islands
Asia	northern from 60° N latitude
Atlantic Ocean	free from sea snakes
Australia	New Zealand
Europe	northern from the polar circle
	Balearic Islands
	Corsica
	Crete
	Ireland
	Iceland
	Sardinia
Pacific Ocean	Hawaii
	New Hebrides
	Loyality Islands
	Micronesia
	Polynesia

III. THE VENOM APPARATUS

A. THE FOUR TYPES OF VENOM APPARATUS

An efficient venom apparatus consists of two parts: a pair of glands for the production of toxic substances (venom capable of immobilizing prey organisms), and modified teeth, the so-called fangs as a means to deliver it. The more harmonious the evolution of these two elements, the more efficient the resulting venom apparatus. Four main principles of the venom apparatus are distinguished in snakes. According to the morphological status of the maxillary teeth, the venom apparatus may be termed "aglyphous", "opisthoglyphous", "proteroglyphous" and "solenoglyphous", respectively. Unfortunately, these terms have been used as a scheme for taxonomic classification of snakes, which should be strictly avoided since it is now generally accepted that the venom apparatus of the different groups of venomous snakes has developed independently along several lines[14,15]. However, as a nomenclature of the morphological pattern, these terms are quite convenient and will be used here.

1. Venom apparatus with aglyphous dentition (Figure 2)

Quite a number of colubrine snakes have Duvernoy's glands located at the sides of the head and extending sometimes to the angle of the mouth[12]. These glands consist of serous or seromucous cells and are sometimes able to produce effective toxic proteinaceous substances[26] (Figure 2a). The glands' single ducts lined with mucous cells open into the oral mucosal sheath of the posterior maxillary teeth. Since there are no specialized muscles of the glands, their secretion is probably infiltrated into the prey rather slowly during feeding. Muscle fibers connected to the sheet of Duvernoy's glands have so far only been found in the boomslang (*Dispholidus typus*) and in the genus *Mehelya* (file snakes)[27]. It has been found that of 300 investigated species in the family Colubridae, about 250 have Duvernoy's glands of appreciable size[28]. Thus an estimated two third of all colubrids might produce toxic secretions. In those cases where the ducts of these glands open nearby simple, ungrooved teeth (Figure 2b), a venom apparatus with aglyphous dentition is present ("aglyphous" = fangless). It seems obvious that this venom apparatus is not very efficient as a prey-immobilizing device, although it has been shown that the duct of the glands terminates at the posterior end of the upper jaw in a dental pocket which, together with the back maxillary teeth, may form an application system[29] (Figure 2c). This may especially be the case when there are two or more enlarged teeth in the region of the gland's duct. Since these snakes firmly hold onto a prey organism, making chewing movements, toxic secretions may enter the body, thus promoting digestion.

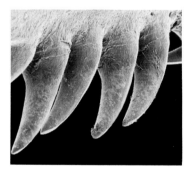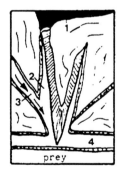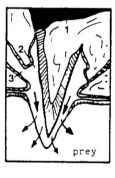

B   C

Figure 2. Venom apparatus with aglyphous dentition. 1= maxillary bone; 2= dental pocket; 3= venom duct; 4= oral cavity.

2a. Example of a simple, ungrooved "aglyphous" tooth occurring in "aglyphous" colubrid snakes.

2b. Scheme of the dental pocket formed in *Natrix tessellata* and, **2c.**, its mode of venom injection[29].

2. Venom apparatus with opisthoglyphous dentition (Figure 3)

There are colubrid snakes in which the Duvernoy's glands terminate in a duct at the posterior end of the maxillary bone nearby one or more (generally two) enlarged grooved teeth (Figure 3b). Some species even possess three fangs on each maxillary bone, e.g. *Dispholidus typus*, *Thelotornis kirtlandii* and snakes of the genera *Boiga* and *Chrysopelea*[43,46]. Such fangs lead to much more efficient injection of the venom than aglyphous teeth do. However, since these fangs are located behind the eye at the back of the maxillary bone, they are only effective when the snake firmly holds on to its prey.

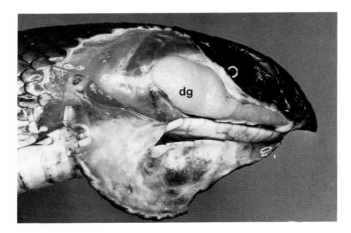

Figure 3. Venom apparatus with opisthoglyphous dentition. dg= Duverny's gland; lg= labial gland; d= duct; s= adductor superficialis muscle.
3a. Lateral view of the head of *Rhamphiophis oxyrrhyncus* (courtesy of Prof. E. Kochva, Tel Aviv).

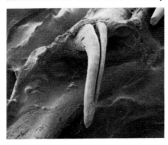

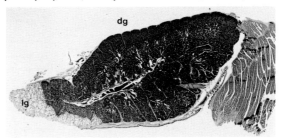

3b. Opisthoglyphous fang of *R. oxyrrhynchus* (x30).

3c. Sagittal section through Duvernoy's gland of *R. oxyrrhynchus* (courtesy of Prof. E. Kochva, Tel Aviv).

3. Venom apparatus with proteroglyphous dentition (Figure 4)

The venom fangs of all elapid snakes (Fam. Elapidae) are located at the anterior end of the maxillary bone ("proteroglyphous" = front-fanged). In contrast to the fangs of the opisthoglyphous colubrid snakes, their overall diameter is greater and their venom groove may be almost entirely enclosed (Figure 4b). The secretory cells of the elapid-type venom gland (Figure 4c) are somehow similar to those of the Duvernoy's glands of the colubrid snakes[15]. The secretion is mainly stored intracellularly and there is but a small central lumen. Besides the serous venom gland, which is of elongated structure continuing in a narrow duct, there is an accessory mucous gland the function of which still remains to be clarified, and that completely surrounds the duct[13,30]. This equally applies to Elapinae and Hydrophiinae as the structure of the venom glands of sea snakes (Hydrophiinae) follows the general pattern of the elapid-type venom gland[31].

4. Venom apparatus with solenoglyphous dentition (Figure 5)

Both vipers (Viperinae) and pit vipers (Crotalinae) are able to swallow prey organisms as large as about 35% of their own body mass due to their wide heads, long jaws, comparatively stout bodies[32,33] and an extreme mobility of their skull bones. Their fangs have a completely enclosed venom channel forming an injection needle and, due to the very great shortening of the maxillary bones which can rotate on a horizontal axis transversally to the head, they can be folded back when the mouth is closed (Figure 5c,d). Thus, a substantial increase in fang length is attained. The fang erection movements are under voluntary muscular control, and the fangs point nearly straight forward when the snake is about to strike; in so doing, the prey organism is stabbed with the fangs and venom injected before the mouth is closed. The venom glands are also very similar in both subfamilies of the Viperidae[13]. The viperid-type venom glands are roughly of triangular shape, being shorter and having a longer duct than the elapid-type glands. The accessory gland, which is globular and may be divided into an anterior and a posterior part, surrounds the anterior end of the venom duct. A secondary duct connects the lumen of the accessory gland to the pocket formed by the fang sheath[34]. Furthermore, the venom gland has a large lumen in which most of the venom is stored. In conclusion, the solenoglyphous, viperid-type venom apparatus with its syringe-like, hollow fangs may be considered as the most efficient with regard to speed as well as to the amount of venom injected[13,35-37].

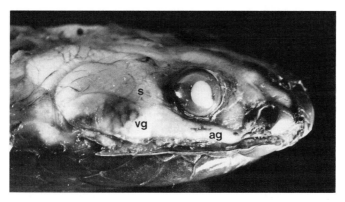

Figure 4. Venom apparatus with proteroglyphous dentition. sl= supralabial gland; ag= accessory gland; vg= venom gland; d= duct; s= adductor superficialis muscle.
4a. Lateral view of the head of *Walterinnesia aegyptia* (courtesy Prof. E. Kochva, Tel Aviv).

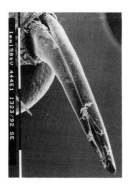
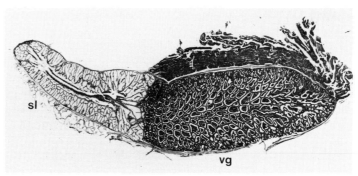

4b. Proteroglyphous fang of *Naja melanoleuca* (x45).   **4c.** Sagittal section through the venom gland of *W. aegyptia* (courtesy of Prof. E. Kochva, Tel Aviv).

5. Some special cases (Figure 6)

The burrowing asps (Atractaspididae) are now considered to form a separate snake family[38,39]. Their venom apparatus may be distinguished from the viperid-like venom apparatus by the lack of a differentiated accessory gland, by the radial arrangement of the secretory tubules surrounding the lumen-like duct of the venom gland, and by the variety of cell types found[13]. Due to their fossorial life habits, the burrowing asps also exhibit quite a peculiar striking pattern. They strike with an almost closed mouth, one single fang at a time moving sideways, downwards and backwards[39]. This striking pattern is made possible by the connection between the maxillary and the prefrontal bones which are linked in a ball-and-socket articulation[41,42]. Thus, although their fang canal is completely closed as it is in all solenoglyphous snakes, the term *Atractaspis*-like venom apparatus is quite appropriate due to the differences found[14,15]. Together with a number of other snakes, *Atractaspis engaddensis* possesses a blade-like ridge at the back of the fang's distal orifice[41,43-45]. Such edge structures which may be found either on the mesial or distal side of the teeth might function to free the teeth from the prey during jaw opening[44] and/or to diminish tissue resistance[43] (Figure 6). Some species of the genus *Atractaspis*, as well as two of the night adder genus *Causus* (Viperidae) and the Malayan banded coral snake (*Maticora intestinalis*; Elapidae) possess elongated venom glands extending far beyond the head into the body[47,48].

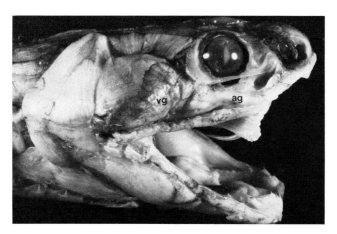

Figure 5. Venom apparatus with solenoglyphous dentition. vg= venom gland; ag= accessory gland; pp= posterior part; ap= anterior part; lu= lumen.
5a. Lateral view of the head of *Vipera palestinae* (courtesy of Prof. E. Kochva, Tel Aviv).

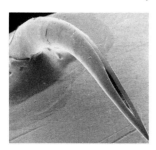
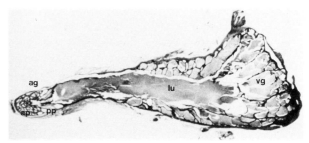

5b. Solenoglyphous fang of jeuvenile *Bothrops atrox* (x26).

5c. Sagittal section through the *Vipera* type venom gland.

IV. SNAKE VENOM COMPOSITION

A. GENERAL CONSIDERATIONS ON VENOM COMPOSITION AND VENOM ACTIONS

Snake venoms are unique mixtures with reference to their biochemical and pharmacological properties. They are either colourless or yellowish, depending on the amount of L-amino acid oxidase present, an enzyme with riboflavin as part of its prosthetic group[19]. Since freshly collected venoms are not stable, drying is essential for maintaining their biological activity[50-53]. However, it has been shown that different drying procedures also influence venom activity and some activities present in fresh venom might even be destroyed during drying[83].

Since all snake venoms contain multiple components with different mechanisms of action, the pathogenesis of reactions developing after a bite is of a very complex nature. It is not only dependent on the qualitative composition, that is what kinds of components are involved, but also on their quantitative distribution, since it is well known that snake venom composition shows great variability due to individual, regional, and age-dependent differences[64-68,83]. Some general principles of the most important pharmacologically active constituents of snake venoms, the proteins, are to be briefly discussed. There are two groups to be distinguished: enzymes and non-enzymic polypeptides. It has already been pointed out that proteolytic enzymes may contribute in one way or another (e.g. by leading to tissue damage) to the digestion of prey organisms. However, the way immobilization of the prey is achieved is of special interest. Although immobilization does not necessarily lead to death, the best way is to kill the prey organism rapidly by inducing either respiratory paralysis or circulatory failure[54]. Snake venom components therefore are discussed in the following sections according to their local effects and their ability to affect the nervous system and the cardiovascular system, respectively.

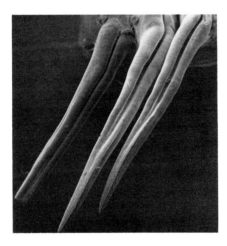

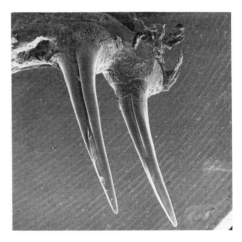

Figure 6. Fangs with special structure.
6a. Fangs of the boomslang (*Dispholidus typus*), an opisthoglyphous colubrid snake of medical importance. Note the blade-like ridges.

6b. Fangs of the vine snake (*Thelatornis kirtlandii*), another opisthoglyphous colubrid snake of medical importance.

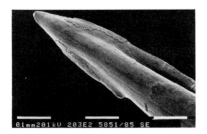

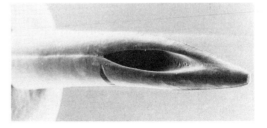

6c. Fang tip of the burrowing asp (*Atractaspis enggadensis*), with blade-like structure opposite the venom orifice.

6d. Venom exit point near tip of fang.

B. VENOM COMPONENTS WITH LOCAL ACTION

For a detailed review, see Ownby, 1990[58], Tu, 1991[59].

1. Enzymes

A general remark on the nomenclature of proteolytic enzymes should be added in this context: all those enzymes that participate in protein degradation are included under the general term "protease" (E.C. 3.4). Those enzymes which act as endopeptidases, that means acting on the interior of peptide chains, are termed "proteinases". The latter group includes the serine proteinases (E.C.3.4.21), the cysteine proteinases (E.C.3.4.22), the aspartic proteinases (3.4.23) and the metalloproteinases (E.C.3.4.24), respectively. In contrast to the proteinases or endopeptidases, the "exopeptidases" attack peptide chains at their terminal ends[248]. A great number of enzymes with either proteolytic action or acting on other substrates have been isolated from snake venoms of different origin[49]. In Table 2, the different enzyme groups found are listed. Every group may comprise several individual enzymes with distinct species-related properties. Proteolytic enzymes may act at the local level, thus serving digestive purposes by leading e.g. to tissue breakdown. Hyaluronidases (E.C. 3.2.1.35), widely found in animal venoms[123,128], catalyze the cleavage of internal glycosidic bonds of several acid mucopolysaccharides, e.g. sodium hyaluronic acid and sodium chondroitinsulfate A and C, respectively. Since the hydrolysis of hyaluronic acid facilitates venom diffusion into the tissues of a prey animal, hyaluronidase is also termed "spreading factor"[139]. Hyaluronidase is present in all snake venoms in varying amounts[140].

2. Myotoxins

Small, basic proteins devoid of detectable enzymatic activity with a molecular weight of about 5 kD and large, basic proteins possessing phospholipase A_2 activity with a molecular weight of about 12 to 16 kD, respectively, which act on muscle cells, are termed myotoxins[58,59]. It should be noted that some phospholipase A_2 presynaptic acting "neurotoxins" also have powerful myotoxic actions in man. Myonecrotic events provoked by these myotoxins may cause a permanent tissue damage resulting even in the loss of parts of the extremity in the case of a severe envenomation[60], whereas in less severe cases, the muscles may be regenerated[61]. Although a common feature in many cases of snakebite envenomation, myonecrosis is most pronounced with viper and pit viper venoms and a few elapid venoms, particularly some Australian elapids.

a. Low-molecular weight myotoxins

All basic low-molecular weight myotoxins known to date were isolated from venoms of the rattlesnake genus *Crotalus* (Table 3). The precise mode of action of the small myotoxins is not yet elucidated. However, it has been shown that crotamine[62] and myotoxin a[63] lead to a permeability increase of the sodium channel or its modulator for sodium ions.

b. Myotoxins with phospholipase A_2 activity

Phospholipases A_2 (PLA_2) seem to occur generally in snake venoms. Meanwhile, the amino acid sequence of over 50 different PLA_2 enzymes and toxins has been determined[69]. Thus, PLA_2 form a group of venom components with a wide range of pharmacological actions, from membrane damage, inhibition of blood coagulation, hemolysis and myonecrosis to cardiotoxicity and neurotoxicity, dependent on the PLA_2 under investigation. For some of these actions, the enzymatic activity of the PLA_2 may even be irrelevant[57]. Chemically, PLA_2 may consist of one, two or more different polypeptide chains, which are non-covalently bound. Myotoxins with PLA_2 activity were found in pit viper venoms, in the venoms of Australian elapids and in one sea snake species (Table 4).

The pathogenesis of myonecrosis induced by PLA$_2$ myotoxins may be summarized as follows (cf.[58]):

1) The plasma membrane of the muscle is ruptured accompanied by hypercontraction of the myofibrills,

2) within the cytoplasm the formation of dense clumps of myofibrills is observed,

3) some areas in the cytoplasm are left empty from myofibrills, the basal lamina, however, being unaffected,

4) within about 24 hours, mitochondrial damage, dispersion of myofibrills and disintegration of myofilaments takes place,

5) phagocytes within the basal lamina are observed phagocytosing the cellular debris.

3. Haemorrhagic Toxins

The haemorrhagic toxins (Table 5) also are usually divided according to their molecular weights into a low-molecular weight group (22 to 26 kD) and into a high-molecular weight group (60 to 90 kD). Although some earlier investigations dealt with haemorrhagic toxins said not to be of enzymic nature, it has meanwhile been shown that all haemorrhagic toxins are proteolytic enzymes[58]. Many of these haemorrhagic toxins have also been shown to be fibrinogenases, since they are able to digest fibrinogen to unclottable material[99]. Haemorrhagic toxins rapidly induce haemorrhage at the site of venom injection. Dependent on their origin, haemorrhagic toxins may induce haemorrhage either "by diapedesis", which means that the erythrocytes leave the intact endothelium through intercellular junctions, or "per rhexis", which means that the endothelial cell is lysed.

C. VENOM COMPONENTS AFFECTING THE NERVOUS SYSTEM

Venoms, especially of elapid snakes, lead predominantly to neurotoxic manifestation in both prey animals and human bite victims. Five types of neurotoxins are known, which cause muscle paralysis in different ways, schematically shown in Figure 7. Excellent reviews on snake venom neurotoxicity are available[73,80].

1. Neurotoxins affecting the postsynaptic membrane

The postsynaptically acting neurotoxins (also called "curare-mimetic toxins") or "a-toxins" are small, basic molecules with a single polypeptide chain. More than 100 of these toxins have been isolated from elapid venoms and their amino acid sequences elucidated. Consequently, these toxins are the best documented molecules present in snake venoms to date. According to their polypeptide chain length, two groups of a-toxins are distinguished: "short" neurotoxins possessing 60 to 62 amino acid residues, cross-linked by four disulphide bonds, and "long" neurotoxins with 70 to 74 amino acid residues, cross-linked with five disulphide bonds. Despite their different chain length, short and long neurotoxins are highly homologous, sharing a number of invariant residues. All postsynaptic neurotoxins prevent the interaction between acetylcholine released at the presynaptic membrane and the α-subunit of the nicotinic cholinergic receptor at neuromuscular junctions, since they bind to the α-subunit with high affinity[81]. As a consequence of this action, muscle contraction is no longer possible. If the muscles of the respiratory system are affected, respiratory paralysis may lead to death.

Table 2
Types of enzymes found in snake venoms

IUB Classification	Enzyme Type	Action	Origin	Characteristics	Ref.
1.	*Oxydoreductases*				
1.11.1.6.	Catalase	$H_2O + H_2O_2 \rightarrow O_2 + 2H_2O$			172
1.1.1.27	Lactat dehydrogenase	$L\text{-Lactat} + NAD^+ \rightarrow$ pyruvate + NADH	Elapidae		172
1.4.3.2.	L-amino acid oxidase	$L\text{-amino acid} + H_2O + O_2 \rightarrow 2\text{-oxoacid} + NH_3 + H_2O_2$	all species	heat labile, flavoprotein	172
	F.XIII inactivating enzyme	catalyzes oxidation of SH groups in F.XIII	*Echis coloratus*		150
2.	*Transferases*				
2.6.1.2.	Alanine amino transferase	L-Ala + 2-oxoglutarate -> pyruvate + L-Glu			172
3.	*Hydrolases*				
3.1.	- acting on ester bonds				
3.1.1.4.	Phospholipases A_2	Lecithin + H_2O -> unsat. fatty acid + lysolecithin	all species	heat stable	69, 172
3.1.1.5.	Lysophospholipase	Lysolecithin + H2O -> fatty acid + glycero-phosphocholine	Elapidae, Viperidae	heat stable	167, 172, 256
3.1.1.7.	Acetylcholinesterase	Acetylcholine + H_2O -> choline + acetate	Elapidae	inhibited by DFP	172
3.1.3.1.	Alkaline phosphatase phosphoric acid	Phosphoric ester + H_2O -> alcohol + phosphate	*Bothrops atrox*	Zn^{++} and EDTA	167, 172

381

Table 2
Types of enzymes found in snake venoms (continued)

IUB Classi- fication	Enzyme Type	Action	Origin	Characteristics	Ref.
3.1.3.2.	Acid phosphatase		*Agkistrodon acutus*	Zn^{++} sensitive	172
3.1.3.5.	5'-Nucleotidase	5-Ribonucleotide + H2O -> ribonucleoside + phosphate	all species	heat labile, $Zn++$ and EDTA sensitive	167, 172
3.1.4.1.	Phosphodiesterase	removes 5'-nucleotides from oligonucleotides	all species		167, 172
3.1.21.1.	Desoxyribonuclease	endonucleolytic cleavage of DNA	all species		167,
3.1.27.5.	Ribonuclease 1 (venom RN-ase)	endonucleolytic cleavage of RNA	all species		167, 172
3.2.	*- acting on glycosyl bonds*				
3.2.1.1.	Amylase	Endohydrolysis of 1,4-α-D-glycoside linkages			172
3.2.1.35.	Hyaluronidase	cleavage of hyaluronate into subunits	all species	heat labile	172, 250
	Heparinase	elimination of 4,5-D-glucuronate from polysaccharides	Crotalinae	heat stable	172
3.2.2.6.	NAD-nucleosidase	NAD+ + H_2O -> nicotinamide+ADP-ribose	all species	heat labile, inhibited by nicotinamide	172

Table 2
Types of enzymes found in snake venoms (continued)

IUB Classification	Enzyme Type	Action	Origin	Characteristics	Ref.
3.4.	*- acting on peptide bonds* unspecific Proteinases	hydrolysis of casein, hemoglobin, gelatin	Viperidae	heat labile Zn metalloenzymes	172
3.4.21.8.	Kininogenases	plasma kininogen -> bradykinin/kallidin	Viperidae	serine proteinases	172, 232, 251
3.4.21.11.	Elastase	hydrolysis of elastin	Viperidae	metalloproteinases	257
3.4.21.23.	Factor X activator	F. X -> F. Xa	*Vipera russelli*	metalloproteinases	137, 253
	Protein C activator	Prot. C -> Prot. Ca	*Agkistrodon* species	serine proteinases	152, 254
	Hemorrhagic proteinases	lysis of collagen	Crotalinae	metalloproteinases	176
	Collagenase	proteolytic degradation	Viperidae	metalloproteinases	255

fibrinogen-coagulating enzymes (see also Table 8)

Table 2
Types of enzymes found in snake venoms (continued)

IUB Classi-fication	Enzyme Type	Action	Origin	Characteristics	Ref.
3.4.21.28.	Ancrod	cleavage of fibrinopeptide A from fibrinogen	*Calloselasma rhodost.*	serine proteinase	218
3.4.21.29.	Batroxobin	cleavage of fibrinopeptide A from fibrinogen	*Bothrops* species	serine proteinase	232, 241
3.4.21.30.	Crotalase	cleavage of fibrinopeptide A from fibrinogen	*Crotalus adamanteus*	serine proteinase	220
		fibrinogen-degrading enzymes (see Table 9)			
		enzymes inhibiting platelet functions (see Table 7)			
		enzymes activating platelet functions (see Table 6)			
	Proteinases affecting plasma proteinase inhibitors				
	CR-Serpinase	cleavage of AT III	*Causus* species	serine proteinase	154
	Proteinase II and similar enzymes	cleavage of AT III, proteolytic degradation	*Crotalus adamanteus* Viperidae	metalloproteinase metalloproteinases	155 155
4.3.	***Carbon-nitrogen lyases***				
4.3.1.9.	Glucosaminate ammonia lyase (ß-glucosaminidase)	2-aminodeoxygluconate-> 2-keto-deoxygluco-nate + NH$_3$			167, 172

Table 3
Low-molecular weight myotoxins

Trivial Name	Snake Species	Sequence, Mol.wt. AA = Amino Acid	LD50 (Route) (mg/kg)	Reference
CAM	*Crotalus adamanteus*	45 AA, 5202	0.9 (*s.c.*)	281
Crotamine	*Crotalus durissus terrificus*	42 AA, 4890	1.5 (*i.v.*)	282
Myotoxin I	*Crotalus viridis concolor*	43 AA, 5061		283
Myotoxin II	*Crotalus viridis concolor*	43 AA, 5034		283
Peptide C	*Crotalus viridis helleri*	43 AA, 4989	1.96 (*i.v.*)	284
Myotoxin a	*Crotalus viridis viridis*	42 AA, 4828	3.0 (*i.m.*)	285
Myotoxins 2 and 3	*Crotalus viridis viridis*	42 AA, 5246		286

Table 4
Myotoxins with phospholipase A$_2$ activity

Toxins	Origin	Structure (AA=Amino Acids)	Mol.Weight	Reference
Myotoxin	*Agkistrodon bilineatus*	129 AA	15'070	287
Myotoxin	*Agkistrodon c. mokeson*	125 AA	14'570	288
Myotoxin	*Agkistrodon p. piscivorus*	121 AA	13'961	289
Bothrops asper Myotoxin	*Bothrops asper*	122 AA	13'886	290
Crotoxin	*Crotalus durissus terrificus*	Crotoxin A:		291,
		three polypeptide chains, linked by disulfide bonds:		292
		A) 40 AA	4'274	
		B) 34 AA	3'658	
		C) 14 AA	1'558	
		Crotoxin B: 122 AA	14'500	
Mojavetoxin	*Crotalus scutulatus scutulatus*	Acidic Chain: 88 AA	9'400	293
		Basic Chain: 122 AA	14'199	294
Myotoxin VI:5	*Enhydrina schistosa*	119 AA	13'446	295
Notexin	*Notechis scutatus scutatus*	119 AA	13'578	296
Notechis II-5	*Notechis scutatus scutatus*	119 AA		297
Taipoxin	*Oxyuranus scutellatus scutellatus*	Alpha-Chain: 119 AA	13'829	298
		Beta-Chain: 118 AA	13'236	299
		Gamma-Chain: 133 AA	14'603	300
Mulgotoxin A	*Pseudechis australis*	122 AA	13'000	301
Pseudechis australis VIII-A	*Pseudechis australis*	122 AA		301
Pseudechis colletii II	*Pseudechis colletii*	127 AA	14'170	301
Pseudechis colletii IV	*Pseudechis colletii*	130 AA	14'200	301
Pseudexin; I-B	*Pseudechis porphyriacus*	143 AA	16'659	301
Myotoxin	*Trimeresurus flavoviridis*	123 AA	13'914	302

Table 5
Haemorrhagic Metalloproteinases

Name	Origin	Properties Mol.weight	Metal	Ref.
Ac1-proteinase	*Agkistrodon acutus*	24,500	Ca, Zn	260
Ac2-proteinase	*Agkistrodon acutus*	25,000	Ca, Zn	260
Ac3-proteinase	*Agkistrodon acutus*	57,000	Ca, Zn	260
Ac4-proteinase	*Agkistrodon acutus*	33,000		260
Ac5-proteinase	*Agkistrodon acutus*	24,000		260
AaH I	*Agkistrodon acutus*	22,000		261
AaH II	*Agkistrodon acutus*	22,000		261
AaH III	*Agkistrodon acutus*	22,000		261
HR I	*Agkistrodon h. blomhoffi*	85,000		262
HR II	*Agkistrodon h. blomhoffi*	95,000		262
Hemor. factor	*Atractaspis engaddensis*	50,000		263
HF 2	*Bothrops jararaca*	49,100		264
HF 3	*Bothrops jararaca*	62,000		264
Bothropasin	*Bothrops jararaca*	48,000		265
Moojeni Protease A	*Bothrops moojeni*	22,500		265
NHFa	*Bothrops neuwiedi*	46,000		266
NHFb	*Bothrops neuwiedi*	58,000		266
Proteinase H	*Crotalus adamanteus*	85,700		267
HTa	*Crotalus atrox*	68,000	Zn	268
HTb	*Crotalus atrox*	24,000	Zn	268
HTc	*Crotalus atrox*	24,000	Zn	268
HTd	*Crotalus atrox*	24,000	Zn	268
HTe	*Crotalus atrox*	25,700	Zn	268
HTf	*Crotalus atrox*	64,000	Zn	268
HTg	*Crotalus atrox*	60,000		268
HP IV	*Crotalus horridus horridus*	56,000	Zn	269
HT-1	*Crotalus ruber ruber*	60,000	Zn	270
HT-2	*Crotalus ruber ruber*	25,000	Zn	270
HT-3	*Crotalus ruber ruber*	25,500	Zn	270
VT	*Crotalus viridis viridis*	115,000		271
VT_m	*Crotalus viridis viridis*	69,000		272
VT_{wo}	*Crotalus viridis viridis*	69,000		272
LHF-1	*Lachesis muta muta*	100,000		273
LHTa	*Lachesis muta muta*	22,000	Zn	274
LHTb	*Lachesis muta muta*	23,000	Zn	274
HR-1A	*Trimeresurus flavoviridis*	60,000		275
HR-1B	*Trimeresurus flavoviridis*	60,000		275
HR-1a	*Trimeresurus flavoviridis*	23,500		276
HR-2b	*Trimeresurus flavoviridis*	23,700		276
HR-1	*Trimeresurus gramineus*	23,500	Zn	277
HR-2	*Trimeresurus gramineus*	23,700	Zn	277
HF-a	*Trimeresurus mucrosquamatus*	15,000		278
HF-b	*Trimeresurus mucrosquamatus*	27,000		278
Mucrotoxin A	*Trimeresurus mucrosquamatus*	94,000	Zn,Ca	279

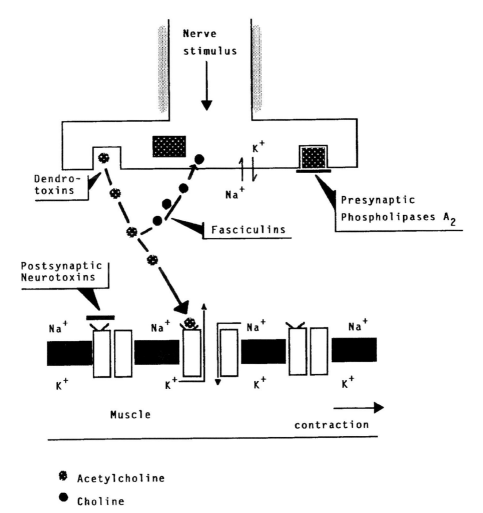

Figure 7. Scheme of the neuromuscular endplate and locations of attack of different snake venom neurotoxins.

2. Neurotoxins affecting the presynaptic membrane

Three groups of snake neurotoxins acting at the presynaptic level have to be distinguished: the PLA_2-toxins, the dendrotoxins and the fasciculins (see Figure 7). All PLA_2-toxins found in elapid and some viperid snake venoms have a basic phospholipase A_2 in common that may be complexed with acidic, basic or neutral protein units. PLA_2-Toxins may consist of a single chain (e.g. Caudoxin from *Bitis caudalis* venom, Notexin from *Notechis scutatus* venom, Ammodytoxin from *Vipera ammodytes* venom), of two chains (ß-Bungarotoxin from *Bungarus multicinctus* venom), they may form a two protein complex (e.g. Crotoxin from *Crotalus durissus terrificus* venom, Mojave toxin from *Crotalus scutulatus* venom) or they may consist of a multiple protein complex (e.g. Taipoxin from *Oxyuranus scutellatus* venom, Textilotoxin from *Pseudonaja textilis* venom). They all act in a complex, usually triphasic manner[55,56,70]. Probably due to their binding at the presynaptic nerve membrane, a short inhibition of neurotransmitter release is observed. In a second phase there is an increasing neurotransmitter release due to the action of the phospholipase, finally followed by a block, when all neurotransmitter is released[74]. For crotoxin, a two component neurotoxin, it has been shown that the non-enzymatic component

A increases the pharmacological efficacy of the PLA$_2$-component B, since component A directs component B onto its acceptor at the neuromuscular junctions. In so doing component A prevents the PLA$_2$-component B from being bound onto inefficient binding sites[249]. For detailed reviews on PLA$_2$-toxins, see[82,85]. Dendrotoxins are very basic single chain polypeptides consisting of 57 to 60 amino acid residues, cross-linked by three disulphide bridges. They are devoid of enzymatic activity and block certain potassium channels in nerve membranes, thus facilitating the release of neurotransmitters (for a review, see[86]). Dendrotoxins have only been found in venoms of the African mambas (*Dendroaspis* species). Dendrotoxins share structural homology with the bovine pancreatic trypsin inhibitor (aprotinin, BPTI), although they neither inhibit trypsin nor other trypsin-like serine proteinases. Fasciculins are again neurotoxins, which are only found in Mamba venoms (*Dendroaspis* species). They belong to a toxin group, which was named "angusticeps-type" toxins (from *Dendroaspis angusticeps*, the Common Mamba). These toxins share structural homology with postsynaptic neurotoxins and snake cardiotoxins, although they are immunologically distinct from all other snake toxins. Fasciculins are potent inhibitors of cholineesterases from different sources. Therefore, they potentiate the action of acetylcholine and cause a generalized muscle fasciculation *in vivo* (for a review, see[87]).

D. CARDIOTOXIC VENOM COMPONENTS
1. Cardiotoxins
Elapid venoms contain, besides postsynaptic neurotoxins, molecules with 60 to 62 amino acid residues and high structural similarity to the "short" neurotoxins, which, however, do not bind to the nicotinic acetylcholine receptor at the postsynaptic membrane. Their toxicity is primarily associated with direct effects on the heart. Therefore they are often referred to as cardiotoxins. However, they also have lytic effects on a wide range of cells. Therefore other names include e.g. "direct lytic factors", "cytotoxins", "cobramine", "membrane toxins". However, the heart still appears to be the main target tissue of cardiotoxins. The mechanism of action of cardiotoxins to date remains unclear. Generally the first observed effect of cardiotoxin action is a cellular depolarization. In *in vitro* test systems, cardiotoxins induce a prolonged depolarization leading to muscular contraction with loss of ability to contract to normal stimuli. (For a review, see[85].)

2. Sarafotoxins
The venom of the burrowing asp *Atractaspis engaddensis* exerts an apparent direct action on the heart[89]. It has been shown that this venom contains three single-chain isopeptides with 21 amino acid residues cross-linked by two disulfide bridges, and called sarafotoxins. The sarafotoxins are highly homologous to the endothelin from porcine aortic endothelium. Sarafotoxins lead to 1) a rapid and marked vasoconstriction of the coronary vessel, 2) a severe atrioventricular block, and 3) a slower, but very strong positive inotropic effect, which may neither be blocked by a- nor by ß-adrenergic receptor blocker[90]. As revealed in rats, sarafotoxins bind specifically and with high affinity to the membranes of the atrium and the brain, where they induce a hydrolysis of phosphatidylinosito[124,138].

E. VENOM COMPONENTS AFFECTING THE CARDIOVASCULAR SYSTEM
Circulatory shock is the main cause of death following viper and pit viper bites. The induction of shock is usually a multifactorial event. Indeed, a general scheme of the interactions of humoral and cellular factors leading to circulatory shock might be used as a basis to explain the action of many snake venom components present in viperid and crotalid snake venoms to a species-dependent extent (Figure 8). Of special importance are all the

different possibilities for interaction between different snake venom components and the haemostatic system. In all vertebrates, the haemostatic system is based on a vulnerable interaction between blood platelets, endothelial cells, subendothelial structures and plasma proteins. By using this vulnerability, the evolution of venomous snakes and their venoms has produced many venom proteins that exert an activating or inactivating effect on nearly all the phases of human haemostasis. Such venom proteins often act in the same way as the corresponding physiological clotting factors, with the difference that there are no inhibitors present against these exogenous clotting factors in the prey organism or bitten victim, respectively. Consequently, the respective action may reach fatal proportions. The human haemostatic system is better investigated than any other. However, those cell, plasma and tissue proteins that lead to haemostasis in man may be assumed to also be present in a species-specific form in all other mammals. The haemostatic systems of lower vertebrates, in contrast, are often characterized by the absence of platelets, a contact phase activation pathway, intrinsic prothrombin activation or fibrinolysis, respectively. These particularities explain the different sensitivity of the various animal species to blood-coagulating snake venom proteins. Indeed, animals such as birds and reptiles, which do not possess a fibrinolytic system, react more sensitively to fibrinogen-coagulating snake venom enzymes than mammals, since they are not able to prevent massive fibrin deposition in their vessels. Thus, the fibrinogen-coagulating snake venom enzymes might be potently lethal for lower vertebrates, whereas in mammalian prey the additional action of haemorrhagic venom components is necessary for lethality. The more we learn about the haemostatic systems of natural prey animals of snakes, the better will be our understanding of snake venom toxicology. However, since there is a major medical interest in thrombosis and haemostasis, snake venoms which affect the haemostatic system in man have been relatively well investigated and a considerable number of venom components acting on haemostasis have been isolated and characterized. Many of these substances are used as experimental tools in basic research, whereas others have found a current practical application in diagnosis and even in therapy. Recently, a subcommittee of the International Committee of Thrombosis and Haemostasis has been charged to establish a nomenclature system for exogenous clotting factors. The inventories of these substances have been published[95-99].

1. Venom components affecting blood pressure

Most Viperidae venoms exert kallikrein-like (kininogenase or kinin-releasing) activity[91,92]. The molecular weight of these single-chain glycoproteins is in the range of 22 to 63 kD. Some of these venom kallikreins so far investigated are homologous with porcine kallikrein (cf.[100]). Most of the venom kallikreins are serine proteinases, which liberate the vaso-active and smooth muscle stimulating nonapeptide bradykinin. Released bradykinin causes vasodilatation of peripheral arterioles. It has been shown that the very fast decrease in blood pressure observed in experimental animals after e.g. *Bothrops atrox* envenomation is due to venom kallikrein[71]. In this way, venom kallikreins may contribute to the immobilization of prey animals. The bradykinin effects, however, are only of a comparatively short duration (15 to 30 min.), since plasma kininases have an inactivating effect on bradykinin[63,71].

2. Venom components affecting the vessel wall

Cutaneous or subcutaneous bleeding at the bite site as well as generalized bleeding may be provoked by haemorrhagic proteins found in Viperidae snake venoms. Most of these proteins are metalloproteinases containing zinc as an essential cofactor[176]. They attack components of the basal membrane of the vessel wall with different substrate specificity. Although some haemorrhagins were said to have no proteolytic activity[177], more recent data have shown that all of them exert proteolytic activity on casein and dimethylcasein, respectively[58].

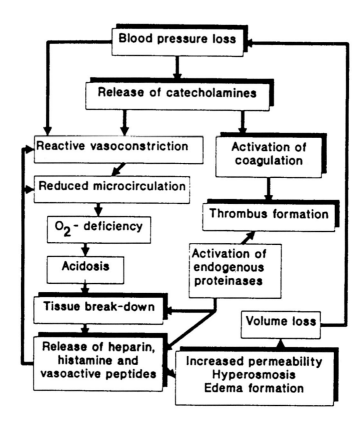

Figure 8. Interactions between humoral and cellular factors in the pathogenesis of circulatory shock. The effects in the shadowed frames may be directly induced by components present in Viperidae snake venoms.

3. Venom components affecting endothelial cells

Thrombocytin, the platelet aggregating serine proteinase from *Bothrops atrox* venom, stimulates, similarly to thrombin, the liberation of prostaglandin I2 of endothelial cells from human umbilical cord[119]. Moreover, thrombocytin induces an endothelium-dependent relaxation of porcine coronary artery segments precontracted with prostaglandin F2α[120]. The thrombin-like serine proteinase Batroxobin from *Bothrops atrox moojeni* venom has been shown to liberate tissue-type plasminogen activator in an *in vitro* test system using a perfused isolated pig ear[121]. The venoms of some rattlesnakes (*Crotalus* sp.) have been shown to release plasminogen activators from human erythrocytes, platelets, polymorphonuclear leukocytes, venous endothelial and smooth muscle cells in culture[122].

4. Venom components affecting blood platelets

Platelet aggregation, release reactions and clot retraction are induced by a number of proteins, predominantly present in Viperidae snake venoms[126] (Table 6). Enzymatic and non-enzymatic inhibitors of platelet aggregation are also found in venoms of this snake family (Table 7). Moreover, a non-enzymatic cardiotoxin from the cobra *Naja naja atra* venom has been described as potentiating ADP, collagen or thrombin-induced platelet aggregation[127]. Platelet agglutination is a physical phenomenon in which protein or glycoprotein ligands with two or more binding domains interact with platelets, independent of their metabolic state. In pit viper venoms, particularly of the South American lanceheads (genus *Bothrops*), potent non-enzymatic inducers of agglutination, the so-called venom coagglutinins, are present. Botrocetin[R], the co-agglutinin of *Bothrops* venoms, is used to differentiate between human variants of von Willebrand factor[128,129]. In the venoms of some pit vipers and of the elapid mambas, lectins are present, which also cause platelet agglutination as well as aggregation[130].

5. Venom components affecting the contact phase of coagulation

To date, little is known about snake venom components activating the contact phase of blood coagulation. However, numerous Viperidae venoms contain kallikrein-like proteinases which may interact with the contact phase by activating coagulation factor XII.

6. Venom components affecting the exogenous and endogenous activation of prothrombin

A highly specific activator of clotting factor V (RVV-V) has been isolated and characterized from Russell's Viper (*Vipera russelli*) venom[131]. The complete amino acid sequence of this serine proteinase has recently been elucidated[132]. The platelet activator thrombocytin from *Bothrops atrox* venom also activates factor V by limited proteolysis. However, in contrast to RVV-V, thrombocytin also activates factors VIII and XIII[131]. An activator of factor X (RVV-X) detected in the venom of *Vipera russelli* has also been shown to activate clotting factor IX[133,136]. Activation of factor IX is achieved by cleavage of an Arg-Val bond[133]. A proteinase which hydrolyses the vitamin K dependent clotting factors IX, X, prothrombin and protein C to inactive products has recently been isolated from Malayan pit viper (*Calloselasma rhodostoma*) venom[134]. Activators of factor VII have not been isolated from snake venoms until now. Nevertheless, the venom of the spitting cobra *Naja nigricollis crawshawii* contains a phospholipase A_2, which leads to a prolonged thrombin time by hydrolysis of the phospholipid component of tissue thromboplastin[135]. Clotting factor X may be activated by a number of Viperidae venoms. The activators of factor X from *Vipera russelli* (RVV-X)[136], *Bothrops atrox*[137], *Cerastes cerastes*[138] and *Echis carinatus*[139] have been isolated and characterized. RVV-X is used to determine the factor X content of plasma either in a clotting assay or in a chromogenic substrate method. Numerous snake venoms contain activators of prothrombin. According to their properties, three types of snake venom activators may be distinguished[140].

Type 1: Activators, the activity of which is not influenced by the non-enzymatic cofactors (factor Va and phospholipid) of the prothrombinase complex and which convert prothrombin into enzymatically active meizothrombin. The most well-known activator of this type is "ecarin" from *Echis carinatus* venom[141]. Similar activators are common in the venoms of South American lanceheads (*Bothrops* spp.)[142], in the venom of *Trimeresurus okinavensis*[143] and in those of the medically important colubrid snakes *Dispholidus typus*[144], *Thelotornis kirtlandi capensis*[145] and *Rhabdophis tigrinus*[146].

Type 2: The activity of these activators from venoms of the Tiger snakes (*Notechis* sp.) and other Australian elapid snakes is greatly enhanced by the presence of phospholipids plus Ca ions and by factor V. Their properties strongly resemble those of clotting factor Xa.

Type 3: The activity of the prothrombin activators found in the venoms of the Australian Taipans (*Oxyuranus* sp.) and brown snakes (*Pseudonaja* sp.) is increased by the presence of phospholipids plus Ca ions. Finally, some thrombin-like snake venom enzymes are able to cleave peptide bonds in prothrombin, leading to inactive prothrombin fragments[147].

7. Venom components affecting fibrinogen

Many Viperidae venoms contain serine proteinases which convert fibrinogen into fibrin by splitting off fibrinopeptides. As this phenomenon corresponds to the best known action of thrombin, these snake venom components are generally termed "thrombin-like snake venom enzymes". Such serine proteinases have been isolated and characterized from one Colubridae and several Viperidae snake venoms (Table 8). Parts of the primary structure of some of them, the complete cDNA sequence coding for batroxobin from *Bothrops atrox moojeni* venom and the complete amino acid sequence of flavoxobin from *Trimeresurus flavoviridis* venom have been determined[107,149]. Due to their primary structure and to the organization of their genes, these enzymes may be allocated to serine proteinases of the trypsin-kallikrein family. Some of these enzymes, like crotalase, also split kininogens and synthetic kallikrein substrates and they are also inhibited by selective kallikrein inhibitors[109]. The numerous characteristics of fibrinogen-coagulating snake venom enzymes reflect a broad and flexible development of these proteins. There are enzymes, like gabonase from the venom of the Gaboon viper (*Bitis gabonica*), which like thrombin catalyze the release of fibrinopeptides A and B from fibrinogen. A selective splitting off of fibrinopeptide A is catalyzed e.g. by batroxobin from *Bothrops atrox moojeni* venom, whereas a preferential fibrinopeptide B release is catalyzed e.g. by an enzyme from *Agkistrodon contortrix* venom. All the thoroughly investigated proteinases of this group act with a pronounced species specificity on fibrinogen of different mammals, and the serum proteinase inhibitors (serpines and α2-macroglobulin) of various species react with a species-dependent preference with these enzymes, the majority of which is not inhibited by natural thrombin inhibitors. Numerous Viperidae and some Elapidae venoms contain proteinases with fibrin(ogen)olytic activity[151]. According to the fibrinogen chain, which is preferentially or exclusively attacked, a-fibrinogenases and b-fibrinogenases, respectively, are distinguished (Table 9). It has been shown that several haemorrhagic proteinases also exert fibrin(ogen)olytic activity[58]. This is just mentioned to point out how difficult it is to categorize venom components according to their pharmacological action since often they are multifunctional proteins.

8. Venom components affecting protein C

Recently, protein C activators with similar physicochemical properties have been isolated and characterized from the venom of the copperhead (*Agkistrodon contortrix*) and closely related pit viper species[152]. These activators, independent from any cofactors, directly activate the zymogen protein C into protein Ca, which is a potent physiological anticoagulant. A slow protein C activating effect of RVV-X has also been reported[153] and, as recently observed in our laboratory, the fibrinogen coagulant proteinase batroxobin from *Bothrops atrox moojeni* venom causes a thrombomodulin-dependent activation of protein C (unpublished results).

9. Venom components affecting antithrombin III

Recently, a serine proteinase from Night Adder (*Causus rhombeatus*) venom, which is able to cleave human antithrombin III at the Arg 393 - Ser 394 bond, thus leading to inactivation of this physiological serine proteinase inhibitor (serpin) has been isolated and purified[154]. Some other snake venoms have been shown to exert serpin destroying activity[155].

Table 6
Platelet activators from snake venoms

Name	Source	Aggregation Reaction	Release	Retraction	Ref.
ENZYMES					
Phospholipase A2	*Trimeresurus mucrosquamatus*	+			88
Phospholipase A2	*Agkistrodon c. contortrix*	+			181
Thrombocytin	*Bothrops atrox*	+	+	+	182
Crotalocytin	*Crotalus horridus horridus*	+	+		183
Ecarin	*Echis carinatus*	+			202
NON-ENZYMATIC VENOM PROTEINS					
Platelet aggregating factor	*Trimeresurus okinavensis*	+	+		184
Convulxin	*Crotalus durissus terrificus*	+			185
Convulxin	*Crotalus durissus cascavella*	+			186
Aggregoserpentin	*Trimeresurus mucrosquamatus*	+			187
Aggregoserpentin	*T. mucrosq.* (Hunan province)	+			188
Aggregoserpentin	*Trimeresurus gramineus*	+			189
Aggregoserpentin	*Calloselasma rhodostoma*	+			190
Triwaglerin	*Trimeresurus wagleri*	+	+		191

Table 7
Platelet inhibitors from snake venoms

Name	Source	Ref.
ENZYMES		
Phospholipase A_2	*Agkistrodon halys*	192
Phospholipase A_2	*Vipera russelli*	193
Phospholipase A_2	*Vipera r. siamensis*	194
Phospholipase A_2	*Naja nigricollis crawshawii*	135
Fibrinogenase	*Vipera palaestinae*	195
Fibrinogenase	*Vipera aspis*	196
α-Fibrinogenase	*Trimeresurus mucrosquamatus*	197
α-Fibrinogenase	*Calloselasma rhodostoma*	198
F1-proteinase	*Naja nigricollis crawshawii*	199
(Â-Fibrinogenase) ADPase/5'-nucleotidase	*Vipera aspis*	196
5'-nucleotidase	*Trimeresurus gramineus*	200
5'-nucleotidase	*Agkistrodon acutus*	200
ADPase	*Agkistrodon acutus*	200
l-Amino acid oxidase	*Crotalus adamanteus*	201
NON-ENZYMATIC VENOM PROTEINS		
Carinatin	*Echis carinatus*	202
Platelet inhibitor	*Calloselasma rhodostoma*	203
Trigramin	*Trimeresurus gramineus*	204
Echistatin	*Echis carinatus*	205
Applaggin	*Agkistrodon p. piscivorus*	206
Bitistatin	*Bitis arietans*	207
Cardiotoxins CTX-1 to CTX-4	*Naja nigricollis crawshawii*	208

Table 8
Fibrinogen - coagulating snake venom components

Source (Snake Species)	Trivial Name	Fibrinopeptide Released	Ref.
Agkistrodon acutus	Acutin		230
Agkistrodon caliginosus			209
Agkistrodon c. contortrix	Venzyme	B,(A)	210
Agkistrodon halys blomhoffi		A,B	211
Agkistrodon halys pallas		B>A	212
Bitis gabonica	Gabonase	A,B	213
Bothrops asper	Asperase		214
Bothrops atrox	Batroxobin	A,(B)	215
Bothrops atrox moojeni	Batroxobin	A,(B)	216
Bothrops insularis			217
Bothrops jararaca		A,(B)	215
Calloselasma rhodostoma	Ancrod	A,(B)	218
Cerastes vipera	Cerastobin		219
Crotalus adamanteus	Crotalase	A,(B)	220
Crotalus atrox	Catroxobin	A,(B)	221
Crotalus durissus terrificus	Gyroxin		222
Crotalus h. horridus	Defibrizyme	A,(B)	223
Crotalus viridis helleri			224
Crotalus v. oreganus			225
Dispholidus typus			226
Lachesis muta muta		A,(B)	227
Lachesis m. noctivaga	Clotase		228
Trimeresurus flavoviridis	Flavoxobin	A	149
Trimeresurus gramineus			229

Table 9
Fibrinogen - degrading snake venom components

Source (Snake species)	Trivial Name	Haemorrhagic Activity	Fibrinogenolytic Activity	Fibrinolytic Activity	Reference
α - Fibrinogenases					
Agkistrodon acutus		+	AÂ	+	231
Agkistrodon c. contortrix	Fibrolase	+	AÂ	+	232
Agkistrodon c. mokasen		-	AÂ	+	233
Agkistrodon piscivorus conanti		n.d.	AÂ>Bβ	+	234
Bothrops asper		-	AÂ>Bβ	n.d.	235
Calloselasma rhodostoma		n.d.	AÂ	+	198
Cerastes cerastes	Cerastase F-4	-	AÂ>Bβ	+	236
Crotalus atrox	Protease-I	n.d.	AÂ>Bβ	n.d.	237
	Protease-IV	n.d.	AÂ>Bβ	n.d.	237
		-	AÂ>Bβ	-	238
	Atroxase		AÂ>Bβ	+	239
Naja nigricollis	Proteinase F-1	n.d.	AÂ	+	240
Trimeresurus gramineus	Haemorrhagic Proteinase 1	+	AÂ	+	241
Trimeresurus mucrosquamatus		+	AÂ	+	242
	P-2	-	AÂ>Bβ	n.d.	243
	P-3	-	AÂ>Bβ	n.d.	243
	Haemorrhagic Factor b	+	aÂ	n.d.	244
ß - Fibrinogenases					
Agkistrodon p. piscivorus		n.d.	Bβ	n.d.	245
Crotalus atrox	Protease II	n.d.	Bβ	n.d.	237
	Protease III	n.d.	Bβ	n.d.	234
		n.d.	Bβ>AÂ	-	246
Trimeresurus gramineus		-	Bβ>AÂ	weak	231
Trimeresurus mucrosquamatus		-	Bβ>AÂ	weak	242
	P-1	-	Bβ>AÂ	n.d.	243
	ME-1,2	-	Bβ>AÂ	+	247
	ME-3,42	-	Bβ=AÂ	+	247
	HF a	+	Bβ	n.d.	244

n.d. = not determined

F. VENOM COMPONENTS WITH MISCELLANEOUS ACTIONS

In the following section, snake venom components are listed, the contribution of which to the overall toxicity of the venoms is not yet fully understood.

1. Lectins

Lectins are proteins able to bind specifically to carbohydrate residues of e.g. other glycoproteins. Such interactions are of special importance in membrane to membrane interactions. However, lectins are also found in some Viperidae venoms and in the venom of the Mamba *Dendroaspis jamesoni*[130,156,157]. Whether these components have a protecting action for the venom gland remains to be investigated.

2. Nerve growth factors

A number of Viperidae and Elapidae snake venoms contain nerve growth factors (NGFs), which are able to induce growth of nerve tissues (trophic effect) and support their well-being (trophic effect)[158]. Since, for example, the venom of the cobra (*Naja naja*) contains quite high amounts of NGFs, the question arises why snake venoms could contain such factors. Since NGFs are multifunctional proteins with further actions (e.g. on the immune system), and NGFs, according to recent experimental findings, are very strong mast cell degranulating agents, this may lead to the conclusion that such effects from snake venom derived NGFs may contribute to the toxicological action of snake venoms.

3. Phospholipase inhibitors

A low molecular weight polypeptide (MW 1,500-5,000) with PLA_2 inhibiting activity has been isolated from *Bothrops neuwiedi* venom[159] and a further PLA_2-inhibitor has been found in *Naja naja* venom[160]. Similar inhibitors are probably present in *B. jararaca*, *B. jararacussu* and *B. atrox* venoms[159]. The presynaptic neurotoxin Vipoxin from *Vipera a. ammodytes* venom is composed of a toxic basic protein with weak PLA_2 activity and a nontoxic acidic inhibitor protein. The latter stabilizes the basic PLA_2[160].

4. Proteinase inhibitors

Some Elapidae and some Viperidae venoms have been shown to contain polypeptides with 52 to 62 amino acid residues, cross-linked by two or three disulphide bridges, which either act as proteinase inhibitors or show structural homology with known proteinase inhibitors[161]. The dendrotoxins (see IV. C.2.) are also homologous with the bovine pancreatic trypsin inhibitor, although they do not inhibit proteolytic enzymes.

5. Venom components affecting the complement system

Some proteolytic enzymes from Viperidae venoms have been shown to inactivate the complement activity of serum and to degrade purified complement factors. These degradations, however, seem to be nonspecific[162,163]. Cobra (*Naja* spp.) venoms contain cobra venom factor (CVF), a glycoprotein consisting of three peptide chains linked by disulfide bridges. CVF participates in the generation of different complement fragments (C3a, C3b, C5a and C5b). To date, it is speculated that the biological function of CVF is to locally activate the complement system at the bite site. This local complement activation leads to a release of the anaphylatoxins C3a and C5a. Thus, mast cell degranulation with subsequent increase of vascular permeability might help the toxic venom components to enter the bloodstream. For reviews, see[164,165].

G. NONPROTEIN SNAKE VENOM COMPONENTS

Since they do not represent the pharmacologically active constituents, nonprotein venom components are not investigated in great depth. They may, however, contribute in one way or another indirectly to venom toxicity e.g. by stabilizing different pharmacologically active venom components.

1. Amino acids

Free amino acids are present in snake venoms in various amounts[166]. Obviously, these amino acids do not contribute to the toxicity of the venoms and it remains to be investigated whether these amino acids are formed by autolysis of peptidic venom components or by so far unknown proteolytic activation processes of venom components.

2. Biogenic amines

Acetylcholine and other cholamines are constituents of Elapidae and Viperidae venoms[167]. Where present, they might contribute to the development of pain at the bite site.

3. Carbohydrates

The monosaccharides glucose, galactose and mannose have been detected in some snake venoms. Polysaccharides have not been detected in snake venoms, although it is well-known that basic mucopolysaccharides have been detected in snake venom glands[166]. It has been speculated that lectins present in the venom might serve to attach mucopolysaccharides as a tissue protecting layer covering the lumen in viperid-type venom glands[130].

4. Lipids

In crotalid (*Agkistrodon c. contortrix, A. c. mokasen, A. p. piscivorus, Crotalus atrox, C. v. viridis, C. adamanteus, C. h. horridus, Sistrurus miliarius barbourix*) and an Elapidae (*Naja naja*) venom, the analysis of lipid fractions revealed the presence of caprylic, capric, lauric, linoleic, myristic, oleic, palmitic, palmitoleic, stearic and arachidonic acids[168,175]. Removal of the lipid fraction in *Naja naja* venom is said to give a decrease in venom lethality of about 50%[169]. The activity of *Vipera palaestina* neurotoxin, a two-component PLA_2-toxin, is substantially decreased, when venom lipids are removed[170].

5. Nucleosides and nucleotides

Substantial amounts of adenosine, guanosine and inosine have been detected in several Elapidae and Viperidae snake venoms[166,167].

6. Riboflavin

The yellow colour of many snake venoms is due to riboflavin, which is present in the form of flavine mononucleotide (FMN) and forms the prosthetic group of venom L-amino acid oxidase[171,172]. Recently, it has been shown that the L-amino acid oxidase present in many snake venoms has antibacterial activity [173,174].

7. Organic acids

The organic acids in snake venoms are usually present as triglycerides and phospholipids[169]. However, it has recently been shown that citrate is the major organic acid found in venoms of *Agkistrodon c. contortrix, A. c. mokasen, A. p. piscivorus, Bothrops asper, Crotalus adamanteus, C. atrox, C. h. horridus, C. v. viridis* and *Sistrurus miliarius barbouri*, respectively. It was estimated that the citrate content of *C. atrox* and *B. asper* venom is higher than 5 percent of their dry residue[175].

8. Anions

As inorganic anions, phosphate, sulphate and chloride have been described from various snake venoms[167]. Whereas the pyrophosphate found in venom ash results from inorganic and organic hydrolyzable phosphates, the major part of sulphate found in venom ash originates from cysteine and cystine sulphur.

9. Cations

The content of cations detected in different venoms by different authors varies within a wide range, probably depending on the method of analysis and on venom sample condition. As already recognized during early snake venom research, relatively high amounts of zinc are present in probably all snake venoms[178]. A hypothesis of Fleckenstein and colleagues suggests that zinc is present in snake venom as a reversible enzyme inhibitor which might protect the venom gland from destruction by its own venom, whereas reactivation could take place upon venom injection into a prey organism, where the zinc concentration is diluted into an inactive level[179,180]. Likewise, zinc might switch on and switch off the activity of some snake venom enzymes.

V. EVOLUTIONARY CONSIDERATIONS

A. EVOLUTION OF THE VENOM APPARATUS

Since the fossil record of snakes is meagre, the origin of venomous snakes is highly speculative. Although it should not be used as an element of taxonomic value, dentition provides a more or less natural and convenient way to differentiate venomous snakes[102]. Based on morphological and biochemical findings, it is now also accepted that the families of venomous snakes evolved in different lines. However, in a very simplified way, the following trends may be observed: within the colubrid snakes, the evolution of the maxillary bone proceeds from an aglyphous to an opisthoglyphous condition. Furthermore, the elapid snakes with their proteroglyphous venom apparatus have been shown to be closer to the Colubridae than the snakes of the family Viperidae[15]. The viperid snakes with their extremely mobile maxillary bone and their extremely prolonged fangs have the most specialized venom apparatus. The same trends can also be seen in the evolution of the venom glands, the Duvernoy's glands of the Colubridae being the evolutionary predecessor of the venom glands[13]. The elapid-type venom gland again is more closely related to the Duvernoy's gland than the viperid-type venom gland is, with its wide lumen containing large amounts of stored venom.

B. EVOLUTION OF THE VENOM

As has been stated before, venoms of the Viperidae and Colubridae usually contain high amounts of different enzymes, whereas in the venoms of the Elapidae non-enzymatic toxins are present besides enzymes. With the elucidation of the primary structure of an increasing number of venom toxins, a comparison with known protein structures became possible. The more details available, the stronger the evidence that the non-enzymatic toxins found in elapid snake venoms evolved from digestive enzymes[15,103,104]. As a consequence, it is hypothetized that the evolving venom glands first produced enzymes that were already secreted by the pancreas of the respective snake ancestor and against which inhibitors were present in the blood[104]. There is a surprisingly high sequence homology between mammalian pancreatic phospholipase A_2 and certain elapid venom components. It is thus postulated that the phospholipase A_2 containing toxins with a presynaptic action found at least in some snake species of all families of venomous snakes as well as the postsynaptic neurotoxins found in the Elapidae have evolved from an ancestral protein dimer with both phospholipase and ribonuclease activity (Figure 9)[103]. Snake venom proteinases affecting the circulatory system and haemostasis to date are less well investigated in this respect. However, at least partial amino acid sequences have been reported for the enzymes crotalase from the eastern diamondback rattlesnake (*Crotalus adamanteus*)[105], gabonase from the Gaboon viper (*Bitis gabonica*)[106] and the complete sequence of batroxobin from the fer-de-lance (*Bothrops atrox moojeni*)[107]. It has been shown that these sequences are homologous to the B-chain of thrombin (29%, 31% and 26%, respectively)[100], a highly advanced serine proteinase. These enzymes share homologies with many other serine proteinases. Of special interest in this context is the fact that crotalase showed the most pronounced homology with porcine pancreatic kallikrein[105] and was shown to have kallikrein-like activity[109]. Again, a homology to a pancreatic enzyme is seen, further supporting the hypothesis that enzymes of pancreatic origin were subsequently produced by oral glands of reptiles[104]. This hypothesis furthermore provides an elegant explanation for the well-known resistance of snakes to their own venoms: the ancestors of snakes had a pancreas secreting a phospholipase and other enzymes and they had also corresponding enzyme inhibitors in their blood to prevent noxious effects[110]. Recently, it has been shown that the acetylcholine receptor of snakes differs in several crucial amino acid residues from other muscle acetylcholine receptors, which bind a-toxins. This again may explain the resistance of snakes to their own venom components[177]. In consequence, a molecular co-evolution of enzymes and their inhibitors seems plausible. That regulating serine proteinases affecting blood coagulation and fibrinolysis are related to digestive enzymes is now generally accepted although different hypotheses are in discussion[111]. Another snake venom component of special interest in inflammation research is the so-called cobra venom factor (CVF), a complement-activating protein with a molecular weight of 140,000 D. There is a structural homology between CVF and the third component of human complement (C3), suggesting that both molecules, CVF and C3, may have derived from a common ancestor molecule[112]. Indeed, a component homologous to C3 of the mammalian complement system is already present in lampreys (*Lampetra japonica*) which belong to the most primitive existent vertebrates[113]. The antigenic relationship between human and cobra complement factors C3 and CVF is also known[114]. The final proof that CVF is a slightly modified derivative of cobra complement factor C3 secreted by the snake venom glands may be expected soon, since the elucidation of the primary structure of both proteins is in progress[117]. Thus, the fascinating story of molecular evolution might, in the near future, bring up quite a number of interesting relationships between snake venom components and other body proteins present in the respective snake species.

C. EVOLUTIONARY ASPECTS OF THE PREDATOR-PREY RELATIONSHIP

When working with snake venoms, we are often faced with the fact that a certain purified venom component may have no visible contribution to the overall toxicity of the venom in the animal experiments usually performed. Batroxobin, the purified thrombin-like serine proteinase from *Bothrops atrox moojeni* venom, is an example in this respect. Its acute toxicity in mice and rats is extremely low, suggesting that batroxobin is of almost no toxicological significance as a venom component. This suggestion is further supported by the fact that the addition of a high amount of antibatroxobin IgG to a lethal dose of *Bothrops atrox moojeni* venom did not at all affect the lethal effect of the latter, although its clotting activity was completely inhibited. However, batroxobin was shown to exert a comparatively high lethality in pigeons, because these birds do not possess a fibrinolytic system as efficient as that of mammals. In organisms devoid of a potent fibrinolytic system, batroxobin could thus cause harmful intravascular coagulation which could only be poorly controlled by phagocytosis[115]. It will be a challenge to also take such phenomena into consideration, when trying to better understand the evolutionary aspects of venomous snakes and snake venoms. Of special interest will be species-specific differences in the coagulation and fibrinolytic systems, the kallikrein-kinin system and the complement system, since these systems are connected to each other by a number of feedback mechanisms, and activating or inhibiting events may lead to dramatic disturbances in the cardiovascular system. Furthermore, multi-domain molecules are present in these systems and slight differences in their molecular structure may be of great consequence in respect of both their specificity and sensitivity[111,116,118]. In conclusion, the evolutionary aspects of the predator-prey relationship have to be taken into consideration in the future. This was hardly the case until now, since our understanding of the molecular structure of snake venom components is still incomplete and since most of the studies performed were restricted to the experimental animals easily available. There is no doubt that a lot of so far unanswered questions concerning the biological significance of snake venom components will easily find an answer as soon as we know more about the physiology of the natural prey organisms of snakes.

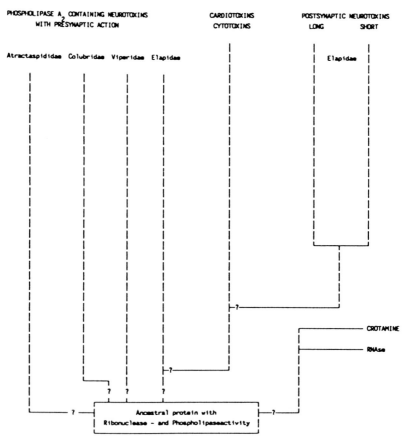

Figure 9. The possible evolution of snake venom neurotoxins from a common ancestor protein with phospholipase/RNase function.

VI. CONCLUSIONS FOR MEDICAL DOCTORS

The accumulated knowledge on snake venom chemistry and pharmacology briefly described in section IV. of this chapter is of course quite impressive. The physician facing snakebite victims and interested in snakebite, however, should always keep in mind that research results obtained by *in vivo* and *in vitro* experiments should be interpreted with great caution. Extrapolation from such experiments to the situation in humans often leads to wrong conclusions. Moreover, for the treatment of snakebite patients, this knowledge is of rather limited importance, since it should be kept in mind that 1) snake venoms do not consist of single, purified substances, but are complex mixtures of many different components, which differ on a qualitative as well as quantitative basis from specimen to specimen within the same snake species, 2) the development of signs and symptoms may strongly be influenced by parameters inherent to the patient and 3) the mode of first aid and clinical management. Some of these parameters are shown in Figure 10. However, the physician involved in snakebite treatment hopefully has found in this chapter some theoretical background to the signs and symptoms seen in his or her practice and described by the different authors in the chapters on clinical toxicology of snakebite, respectively.

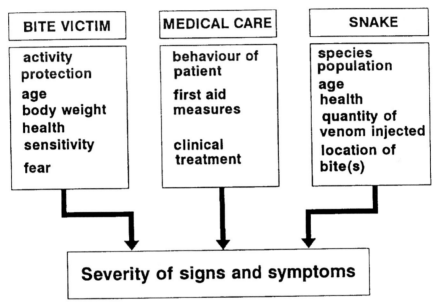

Figure 10. Factors influencing the pathogenesis of snakebite.

VII. REFERENCES

1. **WALLS, G.L.,** The vertebrate eye and its adaptive radiation cranbrook, *Inst. Sci. Bull.*, 19, 1, 1942.
2. **UNDERWOOD, G.,** On lizards of the family Pygopodidae: a contribution to the morphology and phylogeny of the Squamata, *J. Morphol.*, 100, 207, 1957.
3. **NORTHCUTT, R.G., AND BUTLER, A.B.,** Retinal projections in the northern water snake Natrix sipedon sipedon (L.), *J. Morphol.*,142, 117, 1974.
4. **UNDERWOOD, G.,** *A contribution to the classification of snakes*, The British Museum (Nat. Hist.), London, 1967, 179.
5. **UNDERWOOD, G.,** Classification and distribution of venomous snakes in the world, in *Snake Venoms*, Lee, C.Y., Ed., Springer, Berlin, 1979, 15.
6. **GREENE, H.A.,** *Phylogeny, Convergence, and Snake Behaviour*, Doctoral thesis, University of Tennessee, 1977, 112.
7. **BARRETT, R., MADESSON P.F.A., AND MESZLER, R.M.,** The pit organs of snakes, in *Biology of the Reptilia*, Vol. 8, Gans,C., Ed., Academic Press, New York, 1978, 277.
8. **SAVITZKY, A.H.,** The role of venom delivery strategies in snake evolution, *Evolution*, 34, 1194, 1980.
9. **GANS, C.,** The feeding mechanism of snakes and its possible evolution, *Amer. Zool.*, 1, 217, 1961.
10. **GANS, C.,** Reptilian venoms: some evolutionary considerations, in *Biology of the Reptilia*, Vol. 8, Gans, C., Ed., Academic Press, New York, 1978, 1.
11. **GREENE, H.W., AND BURGHARDT, G.M.,** Behaviour and phylogeny: constriction in ancient and modern snakes, *Science*, 200, 74, 1978.

12.   **TAUB, A.M.**, Ophidian cephalic glands, *J. Morphol.*, 118, 529, 1966.

13.   **KOCHVA, E.**, Oral glands of the reptilia, in *Biology of the Reptilia*, Vol. 8, Gans, C., Ed., Academic Press, New York, 1978, 43.

14.   **KOCHVA, E.**, Phylogeny of the oral glands in reptiles as related to the origin and evolution of snakes, in *Toxins: Animal, Plant and Microbial*, Rosenberg, P., Ed., Pergamon Press, Oxford, 1978, 29.

15.   **KOCHVA, E.**, The origin of snakes and evolution of the venom apparatus, *Toxicon*, 25, 65, 1987.

16.   **FONTANA, F.**, Ricerche fisiche sopra il veleno della vipera Lucca, *J. Giusti*, 1767.

17.   **REICHERT, E.**, *Bothrops jararacussu*, Bl. *Aquarien- und Terrarienkunde*, 47, 228, 1936.

18.   **RIEPPEL, O.**, A review of the origin of snakes, in *Evolutionary Biology*, Vol. 22, Hecht, M.K., Wallace, B., and Prance, G.T., Eds., Plenum Press, New York, 1988, 37.

19.   **THOMAS, R.G., AND POUGH, F.H.**, The effect of rattle snake venom on digestion of prey, *Toxicon*, 17, 221, 1979.

20.   **BODIO, M.**, Röntgenographische Untersuchung über den Einfluss von Schlangengiften auf die Zeitdauer der Verdauung bei den Arten *Naja mossambica, Bitis arietans, Vipera aspis, Crotalus viridis* und *Python reticulatus*, Basle University, unpublished, 1987.

21.   **BOGERT, C.M.**, Dentitional phenomena in cobras and other elapids with notes on adaptive modifications of fangs, *Bull. Amer. Mus. Nat. Hist.*, 81, 285, 1943.

22.   **FREYVOGEL, T.A., AND HONEGGER, C.G.**, Der Speiakt von *Naja nigricollis*, *Acta Tropica*, 22, 289, 1965.

23.   **WARRELL, D.A., AND ORMEROD, L.D.**, Snake venom ophthalmia and blindness caused by the spitting cobra (*Naja nigricollis*) in Nigeria, *Am. J. Trop. Med. Hyg.*, 25, 525, 1976.

24.   **GRÜNTZIG, J., JAMBROWSKI, R., BERHEMEIER, B., AND MEBS, D.**, Experimental studies on spitting cobra ophthalmia (*Naja nigricollis*) (Abstract), in *Proc. 6th Europ. Symp. Animal, Plant and Microbial Toxins*, Meier, J., Stocker, K., and Freyvogel, T.A., Eds., Basle, 1984, 93.

25.   **WARRELL, D.A., GREENWOOD, B.M., DAVIDSON, W.MC.D., ORMEROD, L.M., AND PRENTICE, C.R.M.**, Necrosis, haemorrhage and complement depletion following bites by the spitting cobra (*Naja nigricollis*), *Q. J. Med.*, 45, 1, 1976.

26.   **ROSENBERG, H.I., BDOLAH, A., AND KOCHVA, E.**, Lethal factors and enzymes in the secretion from Duvernoy's gland of three colubrid snakes, *J. Exp. Zool.*, 233, 5, 1985.

27.   **KOCHVA, E., AND WOLLBERG, M.**, The salivary glands of Aparallactinae (Colubridae) and the venom glands of *Elaps* (Elapidae) in relation to the taxonomic status of this genus, *Zool. J. Linn. Soc.*, 49, 217, 1970.

28.   **TAUB, A.M.**, Comparative histological studies on Duvernoy's gland of colubrid snakes, *Bull. Amer. Mus. Nat. Hist.*, 138, 1, 1967.

29.   **GYGAX, P.**, Entwicklung, Bau und Funktion der Giftdrüse (Duvernoy's gland) von *Natrix tessellata*, *Acta Tropica*, 28, 226, 1971.

30.   **ROSENBERG, H.J.**, Histology, histochemistry and emptying mechanism of the venom glands of some elapid snakes, *J. Morph.*, 123, 133, 1967.

31.   **GOPALAKRISHNAKONE, P.**, Structure of the venom glands of sea snakes (Hydrophiinae) (Abstract), *Toxicon*, 23, 571, 1985.

32.   **GREENE, H.W.**, Dietary correlates of the origin and radiation of snakes, *Amer. Zool.*, 23, 431, 1983.

33.   **POUGH, F.H., AND GROVES, J.D.**, Specializations of the body form and food habits of snakes, *Amer. Zool.*, 23, 443, 1983.

34.   **KOCHVA, E., AND GANS, C.**, The venom gland of *Vipera palaestinae* with comments on the glands of some other viperines, *Acta Anat.*, 62, 365, 1966.

35.   **KOCHVA, E.**, A quantitative study of venom secretion by *Vipera palaestinae*, *Am. J. Trop. Med. Hyg.*, 9, 381, 1960.

36.   **MORRISON, J.J., PEARN, J.H., AND COULTER, A.R.**, The mass of venom injected by two Elapidae: the Taipan (*Oxyuranus scutellatus*) and the Australian tiger snake (*Notechis scutatus*), *Toxicon*, 20, 739, 1982.

37.   **MORRISON, J.J., PEARN, J.H., CHARLES, N.T., AND COULTER, A.R.**, Further studies on the mass of venom injected by elapid snakes, *Toxicon*, 21, 279, 1983.

38.   **KOCHVA, E., VILIJOEN, C.C., AND BOTES, D.P.**, A new type of toxin in the venom of snakes of the genus *Atractaspis* (Atractaspidinae), *Toxicon*, 20, 581, 1982.

39.   **KOCHVA, E., GOLANI, J., AND WOLLBERG, Z.**, The burrowing asp of the genus *Atractaspis*, a separate group of venomous snakes, in *Proc. 6th Europ. Symp. Animal, Plant and Microbial Toxins*, Meier, J., Stocker, K., and Freyvogel, T.A., Eds., IST, Basel, Switzerland, 1984, 102.

40.   **KOCHVA, E., AND GANS, C.**, Salivary glands of snakes, *Clinical Toxicol.*, 3, 363, 1970.

41.   **KOCHVA, E., AND MEIER, J.**, The fangs of *Atractaspis engaddensis* Haas (Serpentes: Atractaspididae), *Revue Suisse Zool.*, 93, 749, 1986.

42.   **GOLANI, I., AND KOCHVA, E.**, Striking and some other offensive and defensive behaviour in *Atractaspis engaddensis* (Atractaspididae, Ophidia), *Copeia*, 792, 1988.

43. **MEIER, J.**, The fangs of *Dispholidus typus* Smith and *Thelothornis kirtlandii* Smith (Serpentes: Colubridae), *Revue Suisse Zool.*, 88, 897, 1981.

44. **FRAZETTA, T.H.**, Studies on the morphology and function of the skull in the Boidae, *J. Morph.*, 118, 217, 1966.

45. **WRIGHT, D.L., KARDONG, K.V., AND BENTLEY, D.L.**, The functional anatomy of the teeth of the western terrestrial garter snake, *Thamnophis elegans, Herpetologica*, 35, 223, 1979.

46. **PHISALIX, M.**, *Animaux Venimeux et Venins*, Vol. 2, Masson et Cie, Paris, 1922.

47. **KOCHVA, E.**, An extended venom gland in the Israel mole viper *Atractaspis engaddensis* Haas 1950, *Bull. Res. Counc. Israel*, B8, 31, 1959.

48. **SHAYER-WOLLBERG, M., AND KOCHVA, E.**, Embryonic development of the venom apparatus in *Causus rhombeatus* (Viperidae, Ophidia), *Herpetologica*, 4, 249, 1967.

49. **ZELLER, E.A.**, Enzymes of snake venoms and their biological significance, *Advances in Enzymology*, 8, 1948, 459.

50. **KLAUBER, L.M.**, *Rattlesnakes - Their Life Habits, Life Histories and Influence on Mankind*, 2 Vols., Univ. of California Press, Berkeley, 1972.

51. **TAN, N.H., AND TAN, C.S.**, Thermal stability of snake venom enzymatic activities, in *Progress in Venom and Toxin Research*, Gopalakrishnakone, P., and Tan, C.K., Eds., Nat. Univ. of Singapore, Singapore, 1987, 188.

52. **RAMSEY, H.W., AND GENNARO, J.F.**, An analysis of the toxicity and haemolytic properties of stored dessicated venoms of two Crotalidae, *Am. J. Trop. Med. Hyg.*, 8, 552, 1959.

53. **RUSSELL,F.E., EMERY, J.A., AND LONG, T.E.**, Some properties of rattlesnake venom following 26 years storage, *Proc. Soc. Exp. Biol. Med.*, 103, 737, 1960.

54. **LEE, Z.Y., LIN, V.V., CHEN, Y.M., AND LEE, S.Y.**, On the causes of acute death produced by animal venoms and toxins, in *Progress in Venom and Toxin Research*, Gopalakrishnakone, P., and Tan, C.K., Eds., Nat. Univ. of Singapore, Singapore, 1987, 3.

55. **CHANG, C.C., AND LEE, C.Y.**, Isolation of neurotoxins from the venom of *Bungarus multicinctus* and their mode of neuromuscular blocking action, *Arch. Int. Pharmacodyn. Ther.*, 144, 241, 1963.

56. **FOHLMAN, J., EAKER, D., KARLSSON, E., AND THESLEFF, S.**, Taipoxin, an extremely potent presynaptic neurotoxin from the venom of the Australian snake taipan (*Oxyuranus scutellatus scutellatus*) - Isolation, characterization, quaternary structure and pharmacological properties, *Europ. J. Biochem.*, 68, 457, 1976.

57. **ROSENBERG, P.**, The relationship between enzymatic activity and pharmacological properties of phospholipases in natural poisons, in *Natural Toxins - Animal, Plant and Microbial*, Harris, J.B., Ed., Clarendon Press, Oxford, 1986, 129.

58. **OWNBY, C.**, Locally acting agents: myotoxins, hemorrhaghic toxins and dermonecrotic factors, in *Handbook of Toxinology*, Shier, W.T., and Mebs, D., Eds., Marcel Dekker, New York, 1990, 601.

59. **TU, A.T.**, Tissue damaging effects by snake venoms: hemorrhage and myonecrosis, in *Handbook of Natural Toxins,* Vol. 5, Tu, A.T., Ed., Marcel Dekker, New York, 1991, 297.

60. **KITCHENS, C.S., HUNTER, S., AND VAN MIEROP, L.H.S.**, Severe myonecrosis in a fatal case of envenomation by the canebrake rattlesnake (*Crotalus horridus atricaudatus*), *Toxicon*, 25, 1987, 455.

61. **GUTIERREZ, J.M., CHAVES, F., MATA, E., AND CERDAS, L.**, Skeletal muscle regeneration after myonecrosis induced by *Bothrops asper* (Terciopelo) venom, *Toxicon*, 24, 1986, 223.

62. **CHANG, CC., AND TSENG, K.H.**, Effect of crotamine, a toxin of South American rattlesnake venom, on the sodium channel of murine skeletal muscle, *Br. J. Pharmac.*, 63, 551, 1978.

63. **MEIER, J., AND STOCKER, K.**, Beeinflussung der Toxizität von *Bothrops atrox*-Gift durch Eingriffe in das Gerinnungs- und Kallikreinsystem von Beutetieren, *Folia Haematol.*, 111, 877, 1984.

64. **TABORSKA, E.**, Intraspecies variability of the venom of *Echis carinatus*, *Physiol. bohemoslov.*, 20, 307, 1971.

65. **TABORSKA, E., AND KORNALIK, F.**, Individual variability of *Bothrops asper* venom, *Toxicon*, 23, 612, 1985.

66. **MEIER, J.**, Individual and age-dependent variations in the venom of the fer-de-lance (*Bothrops atrox*), *Toxicon*, 24, 395, 1986.

67. **MINTON, S.A., AND WINSTEIN, S.A.**, Geographic and ontogenic variation in venom of the western diamondback rattlesnake (*Crotalus atrox*), *Toxicon*, 24, 71, 1986.

68. **CHIPPAUX, J.P., WILLIAMS, V., AND WHITE, J.**, Snake venom variability: methods of study, results and interpretation, *Toxicon*, 29, 1279, 1991.

69. **ROSENBERG, P.**, Phospholipases, in *Handbook of Toxinology*, Shier, W.T., and Mebs, D., Eds., Marcel Dekker, New York, 1990, 67.

70. **ADEM, A., ASBLOM, A., AND KARLSSON, E.**, Muscarinic toxins from green mamba venom (Abstract), in *Proc. 7th Europ. Symp. Animal, Plant and Microbial Toxins*, Kornalik, F., and Mebs, D. Eds., IST, Prag, 1986, 91.

71. **MEIER, J.**, Study on the toxicity of *Bothrops atrox* venom and its modification after interventions in the coagulation, fibrinolytic and kallikrein-kinin system of prey animals (Abstract), in *Proc. 6th Europ. Symp.*

on *Animal, Plant and Microbial Toxins*, Meier, J., Stocker, K., and Freyvogel, T.A., Eds., IST, Basle, 1984, 112.

72. **JAYANTHI, G.P., AND VEERAKASAPPA GOWDA, T**., Geographical variation in India in the composition and lethal potency of Russell's viper (*Vipera russelli*) venom, *Toxicon*, 26, 257, 1988.

73. **MEBS, D., AND HUCHO,F**., Toxins acting on ion channels and synapses, in *Handbook of Toxinology*, Shier, W.T., and Mebs, D., Eds., Marcel Dekker, New York, 1990, 493.

74. **CARATSCH, C**., Die Bedeutung peripher wirkender Neurotoxine zur Erforschung neurophysiologischer Prozesse, *Viertel- jahrsschrift Natf. Ges. Zürich*, 132, 191, 1985.

75. **BROADLEY, D.G**., Fatalities from bites of *Dispholidus* and *Thelothornis* and a personal case history, *J. Herp. Ass. Rhodesia*, 1, 5, 1957.

76. **FITZSIMONS, D.C., AND SMITH, H.M**., Another rear-fanged South African snake lethal to humans, *Herpetologica*, 14, 198, 1958.

77. **MEBS, D**., Bissverletzungen durch "ungiftige" Schlangen, *Dt. Med. Wschr.*, 102, 1429, 1977.

78. **MEBS, D., SCHARRER, J., STILLE, W., AND HANK, H**., A fatal case of snakebite due to *Thelotornis kirtlandii*, *Toxicon*, 16, 477, 1978.

79. **MITTLEMAN, M.B., AND GORIS, R.C**., Death caused by the bite of the Japanese colubrid snake *Rhabdophis tigrinus* (Boie), *J. Herpetol.*, 12, 109, 1978.

80. **MEBS, D**., Snake venom toxins: structural aspects, in *Neurotoxins in Neurochemistry*, Dolly, J.O., Ed., Ellis Horwood, Chichester, 1988, 3.

81. **LOW, B.W., AND CORFIELD, P.W.R**., Acetylcholine receptor a-toxin binding site - theoretical and model studies, *Asia Pacific J. Pharmacol.*, 2, 115, 1987.

82. **ROSENBERG, P**., Phospholipase A2 toxins, in *Neurotoxins in Neurochemistry*, Dolly, J.O., Ed., Ellis Horwood, Chichester, 1988, 27.

83. **MEIER, J., ADLER, CH., HÖSSLE, P., AND LOCASCIO R**., The influence of three different drying procedures on some enzymatic activities of three Viperidae snake venoms, *Mem.Inst.Butantan*, 53, 119, 1991.

84. **OGAWA, H., AND SAWAI, Y**., Fatal bite of the Yamakagashi (*Rhabdophis tigrinus*), *Snake*, 18, 53, 1986.

85. **HARRIS, J**., Phospholipases in snake venoms and their effects on nerve and muscle, in *Snake Toxins*, Harvey, A.L., Ed., Pergamon Press, Oxford, 1991.

86. **HARVEY, A.L., AND ANDERSON, A.J**., Dendrotoxins: snake toxins that block potassium channels and facilitate neurotransmitter release, in *Snake Toxins*, Harvey, A.L., Ed., Pergamon Press, Oxford, 1991, ..

87. **CERVENANSKY, C., DAJAS, F., HARVEY, A.L., AND KARLSSON, E**., Fasciculins, anticholinesterase toxins from mamba venoms: biochemistry and pharmacology, in *Snake Toxins*, Harvey, A.L., Ed., Pergamon Press, Oxford, 1991.

88. **HARVEY, A.L**., Cardiotoxins from cobra venom, in *Handbook of Natural Toxins*, Vol. 5, Tu, A.T., Ed., Marcel Dekker, New York, 1991, 85.

89. **WEISER, E., WOLLBERG, Z., KOCHVA, E., AND LEE, S.Y**., Cardiotoxic effects of the venom of the burrowing asp *Atractaspis engaddensis* (Atractaspididae, Ophidia), *Toxicon*, 22, 767, 1984.

90. **WOLLBERG, Z., SHABO-SHINA, R., INTRATOR, N., BDOLAH, A., SHAVIT, G., ORON, Y., VIDNE, B.A., AND GITTER, S.A**., A novel cardiotoxic polypeptide from the venom of *Atractaspis engaddensis* (burrowing asp): cardiac effects in mice and isolated rat and human heart preparations, *Toxicon*, 26, 525, 1988.

91. **MEBS, D**., A comparative study of enzyme activities in snake venoms, *Int. J. Biochem.*, 1, 335, 1970.

92. **OSHIMA, G., SATO-OHMORI, T., AND SUZUKI, T**., Proteinase, argininester hydrolase and a kinin releasing enzyme in snake venoms, *Toxicon*, 7, 229, 1969.

93. **MINTON, S.A., AND MEBS, D**., Vier Bissfälle durch Colubriden, *Salamandra*, 14, 41, 1978.

94. **GONZALES, D**., Bissverletzungen durch *Malpolon monspessulanus*, *Salamandra*, 15, 266, 1979.

95. **SMITH, S.V., AND BRINKHOUS, K.M**., Inventory of exogenous platelet-aggregating agents derived from venoms, *Thromb. Haemostas.*, 66, 259, 1991.

96. **TENG, C.M., AND HUANG, T.F**., Inventory of exogenous inhibitors of platelet aggregation, *Thromb.Haemostas.*, 65, 624, 1991.

97. **PIRKLE, H., AND STOCKER, K**., Thrombin-like enzymes from snake venoms: an inventory, *Thromb.Haemostas.*, 65, 444, 1991.

98. **ROSING, J., AND TANS, G**., Inventory of exogenous prothrombin activators, *Thromb.Haemostas.*, 65, 627, 1991.

99. **MARKLAND, F.S**., Inventory of a- and b-fibrinogenases from snake venoms, *Thromb.Haemostas.*, 65, 438, 1991.

100. **PIRKLE, H., AND THEODOR, I**., Thrombin-like enzymes in the study of fibrin formation, in *Hemostasis and Animal Venoms*, Pirkle, H., and Markland, F.S., Eds., Marcel Dekker, New York, 1988, 121.

101. **MEIER, J., ADLER, C., AND SURBER-CUENI, G**., A simple method to evaluate the digestive effect of snake venom. (Abstract). *Toxicon*, 29, 290, 1991.

102. **MINTON, S.A.**, Origins of poisonous snakes: evidence from plasma and venom proteins, in *Natural Toxins - Animal, Plant and Microbial*, Harris, J.B., Ed., Clarendon Press, Oxford, 1986, 3.

103. **STRYDOM, D.J.**, The evolution of toxins found in snake venoms, in *Snake Venoms*, Lee, C.Y., Ed., Springer-Verlag, Berlin, 1979, 258.

104. **KOCHVA, E., NAKAR, O., AND OVADIA, M.**, Venom toxins: plausible evolution from digestive enzymes, *Amer. Zool.*, 23, 427, 1983.

105. **PIRKLE, H., MARKLAND, F.S., THEODOR, J., BAUMGARTNER, R., BAJWA, S.S., READDY, N.N., AND KIRAKOSSIAN, H.**, The primary structure of crotalase, a thrombin-like venom enzyme, exhibits closer homology to kallikrein than the other serine proteases, *Biochem. Biophys. Res. Commun.*, 99, 715, 1981.

106. **PIRKLE, H., THEODOR, J., MIYADA, D., AND SIMMONS, G.**, Thrombin-like enzyme from the venom of *Bitis gabonica*, *J. Biol. Chem.*, 261, 8830, 1986.

107. **ITOH, N., TANAKA, N., MIHASHI, S., AND YAMASHINA, J.**, Molecular cloning and sequence analysis of cDNA for batroxobin, a thrombin-like snake venom enzyme, *J. Biol. Chem.*, 262, 3132, 1987.

108. **KAISER, E., AND MICHL, H.**, *Die Biochemie der tierischen Gifte*, Franz Deuticke, Wien, 1958, 192.

109. **MARKLAND, F.S., KETTNER, C., SCHIFFMANN, S., SHAW, E., BAJWA, S.S., READDY, N.N., KIRAKOSSIAN, H., PATKOS, G.B., THEODOR, J., AND PIRKLE, H.**, Kallikrein-like activity of crotalase, a snake venom enzyme that clots fibrinogen, *Proc. Natl. Acad. Sci.*, 79, 1688, 1982.

110. **KOCHVA, E., ORON, U., OVADIA, M., SIMON, T., AND BDOLAH, A.**, Venom glands, venom synthesis, venom secretion and evolution, in *Natural Toxins,* Eaker, D., and Wadström, T., Eds., Pergamon Press, Oxford, 1980, 3.

111. **PATTHY, L.**, Evolution of the proteases of blood coagulation and fibrinolysis by assembly from modules, *Cell*, 41, 657, 1985.

112. **VOGEL, C.W., SMITH, G.A., AND MÜLLER-EBERHARD, H.J.**, Cobra venom factor: structural homology with the third components of human complement, *J. Immunol.*, 133, 3235, 1984.

113. **NONAKA, M., FUJII, T., KAIDOH, T., NATSUUME-SAKAI, S., YAMAGUCHI, N., AND TAKAHASHI, M.**, Purification of a lamprey complement protein homologous to the third component of the mammalian complement system, *J. Immunol.*, 133, 3242, 1984.

114. **EGGERTSEN, G., LUNDWALL, A., HELLMANN, U., AND SJOQUIST, J.**, Antigenetic relationships between human and cobra complement factors C3 and cobra venom factor (CVF) from the Indian cobra (*Naja naja*), *J. Immunol.*, 131, 1920, 1983.

115. **STOCKER, K.**, Use of snake venom proteins in the diagnosis and therapy of haemostatic disorders, in *Proc. 7th Europ. Symp. Animal, Plant and Microbial Toxins*, Kornalik, F., and Mebs, D., Eds., Int. Soc. Toxinology, Prag, 1986, 9.

116. **MÜLLER-ESTERL, W., KELLERMANN, J., LOTTSPEICH, F., AND HENSCHEN, A.**, Structural diversity and evolutionary origin of the mammalian kininogenases, in *Kininogenases 7*, Haberland, D.L., Rohen, J.W., and Fritz, H., Eds., F.K. Schattauer, Stuttgart, 1986, 1.

117. **LAMBRIS, J.**, Institute of Immunology, Basle, personal communication, 1988.

118. **MORAN, J.B., PANG, S.Y.Y., MARTIN, D.W., AND GEREN, C.R.**, Fractionation of northern copperhead venom by ion-exchange chromatography: primary characterization of the primary lethal fraction, *Toxicon*, 17, 499, 1979.

119. **CZERVIONKE, R. L., SMITH, J. B., HOAK, J. C., FRY, G. L., AND HAYCRAFT, D. L.**, Use of a radioimmunoassay to study thrombin induced release of PGI2 from cultured endothelium, *Thromb. Res.*, 14, 781, 1979.

120. **GLUSA, E., BRAUNS, H., AND STOCKER, K.**, Endothelium-dependent relaxant effect of thrombocytin, a serine proteinase from *Bothrops atrox* snake venom, on isolated pig coronary arteries, *Toxicon*, 29 , 725, 1991.

121. **KLÖCKING, H. P., HOFFMANN, A., AND MARKWARDT, F.**, Release of plasminogen activator by batroxobin, *Haemostasis*, 17, 235, 1987.

122. **KIRSCHBAUM, N. E., RECZKOWSKY, R.S., AND BUDZINSKY, A.Z.**, Secretion of cellular plasminogen activators upon stimulation by Crotalinae snake venoms, in *Hemostasis and Animal Venoms*, Pirkle, H., and Markland, F.S., Eds., New York; Marcel Dekker 1988, 191.

123. **MEYER, K., HOFFMANN, P., AND LINKER, A.**, Hyaluronidases, in *The Enzymes*, Boyer, P.D., Lardy, H., Myrbäck, K., Eds., New York; Academic Press, 1960, 447.

124. **KLOOG, Y., AMBAR, J., SOKOLOVSKY, M., KOCHVA, E., WOLLBERG, Z., AND BDOLAH, A.**, Sarafotoxin, a novel vasoconstrictor peptide: phosphoinositide hydrolysis in rat heart and brain, *Science*, 242, 268, 1988.

125. **GAUR, D., BDOLAH, A., WOLLBERG, Z., AND KOCHVA, E.**, Homology between snake venom sarafotoxins and mammalian endothelins, *Israel J. Zool.*, 35, 171, 1988/89.

126. **BRINKHOUS, K.M., AND SMITH, S.V.**, Platelet-aggregating noncoagulant snake venom fractions, in *Hemostasis and Animal Venoms*, Pirkle, H., and Markland, F.S., Eds., New York; Marcel Dekker, 1988, 363.

127. **TENG, C.M., CHEN, Y.H., AND OUYANG, C.**, Cardiotoxin from *Naja naja atra* venom: a potentiator of platelet aggregation. *Toxicon*, 22, 463, 1984.

128. **READ, M.S., SHERMER, R.W., AND BRINKHOUS, K.M.**, Venom coagglutinin: an activator of platelet aggregation dependent on von Willebrand factor, *Proc. Nat. Acad. Sci. U.S.A.*, 75, 4514, 1978.

129. **BRINKHOUS, K.M., READ, M.S., FRICKE, W.A., AND WAGNER, R.H.**, Botrocetin (venom coagglutinin): reaction with a broad spectrum of multimeric forms of factor VIII macromolecular complex, *Proc. Nat. Acad. Sci. U.S.A.*, 80, 1463, 1983.

130. **OGILVIE, M.L., AND GARTNER, T.K.**, Identification of lectins in snake venoms, *J. Herpetol.*, 18, 285, 1984.

131. **KISIEL, W., AND CANFIELD, W.M.**, Snake venom proteases that activate blood coagulation factor V., in *Methods in Enzymology*, Vol. 80, Lorand, L., Ed., New York; Academic Press, 1981, 275.

132. **TOKUNAGA, F., NAGASAWA, K., TAMURA, S., MIYATA, T., IWANAGA, S., AND KISIEL, W.**, The factor V-activating enzyme (RVV-V) from Russell's viper venom. Identification of isoproteins RVV-V_, Vß and V_ and their complete amino acid sequences, *J. Biol. Chem.*, 263, 17471, 1988.

133. **ENFIELD, D.L., AND THOMPSON, A.R.**, Cleavage and activation of human factor IX by serine proteases. *Blood*, 64, 821, 1984.

134. **LOLLAR, P., PARKER, C.G., KAJENSKI, P.J., LITWILLER, R.D., AND FASS, D.N.**, Degradation of coagulation proteins by an enzyme from Malayan pit viper (*Agkistrodon rhodostoma*) venom. *Biochemistry*, 26, 7627, 1987.

135. **KINI, R.M., AND EVANS, H.J.**, Mechanism of platelet effects of cardiotoxins from *Naja nigricollis crawshawii* (spitting cobra) snake venom. *Thromb. Res.*, 52, 185, 1988.

136. **FURIE, B.C., AND FURIE, B.**, Coagulant protein of Russell's viper venom. In: *Methods in Enzymology*, Vol. 45, Lorand, L., Ed., New York: Academic Press, 1976, 191.

137. **HOFMANN, H., AND BON, C.**, Blood coagulation induced by the venom of *Bothrops atrox*. 2. Identification, purification, and properties of two factor X activators. *Biochemistry*, 26, 780, 1987.

138. **FRANSSEN, J.H., JANSSEN-CLAESSEN, T., AND VAN DIEIJEN, G.**, Purification and properties of an activating enzyme of blood clotting factor X from the venom of *Cerastes cerastes*, *Biochim. Biophys. Acta* 747, 186, 1983.

139. **DURAN-REYNALS, F.**, A spreading factor in certain snake venoms and its relation to their mode of action. *J. Exp. Med.*, 69, 1939, 69.

140. **FAVILLI, G.**, Occurrence of spreading factors and some properties of hyaluronidases in animal parasites and venoms, in *Venoms*, Buckley, E.E., and Porges, N., Eds., Washington, D.C.: Amer.Assoc.Adv.Sci., 1956, 281.

141. **SCHIECK A., KORNALIK, F., AND HABERMANN, E.**, The prothrombin- activating principle from *Echis carinatus* venom. I.Preparation and biochemical properties. *Naunyn Schmiedeberg's Arch. Pharmacol.*, 272, 402, 1972.

142. **NAHAS, L., KAMIGUTI, A.S., AND BARROS, M.A.R.**, Thrombin-like and factor X-activator components of *Bothrops* snake venoms. *Thromb. Haemost.*, 41, 314, 1979.

143. **SAKURAGAWA, N., AND TAKAHASHI, K.**, Coagulation studies on Habu (*Trimeresurus okinavensis*) venom, in *Hemostasis and Animal Venoms*, Pirkle, H., and Markland, F.S., Eds.,. New York: Marcel Dekker, 1988, 515.

144. **GUILLIN, M.C., BEZEAUD, A., AND MENACHE, D.**, The mechanism of activation of human prothrombin by an activator isolated from *Dispholidus typus* venom. *Biochim. Biophys. Acta*, 537, 160, 1978.

145. **KORNALIK, F., TABORSKA, E., AND MEBS, D.**, Pharmacological and biochemical properties of a venom gland extract from the snake *Thelotornis kirtlandi*. *Toxicon*, 16, 535, 1978.

146. **MORITA, T., MATSUOMOTO, H., IWANAGA, S., AND SAKAI, A.**, A prothrombin activator found in *Rhabdophis tigrinus tigrinus* (yamakagashi snake) venom. In: *Hemostasis and Animal Venoms*, Pirkle, H., and Markland, F.S., Eds., New York: Marcel Dekker, 1988, 55.

147. **PIRKLE, H., MARKLAND, F.S., AND THEODOR, I.**, Thrombin-like enzymes of snake venoms: action on prothrombin. *Thromb. Res.*, 8, 619, 1976.

148. **GEIGER, R., AND KORTMANN, H.**, Esterolytic and proteolytic activities of snake venoms and their inhibition by proteinase inhibitors, *Toxicon*, 15, 257, 1977.

149. **SHIEH, T.C., TANAKA, S., KIHARA, H., OHNO, M., AND MAKISUMI, S.**, Purification and characterization of a coagulant enzyme from *Trimeresurus flavoviridis* venom. *J. Biochem.*, 98, 713, 1985.

150. **DJALDETTI, M., COHEN, I., JOSHUA, H., BESSLER, H., LORBEERBAUM, O., AND DE VRIES A.**, In vivo and in vitro inactivation of fibrin stabilizing factor by *Echis colorata* venom, *Hemostase*, 5, 121, 1965.

151. **MARKLAND, F.S.**, Fibrin(ogen)olytic enzymes from snake venoms, in *Hemostasis and Animal Venoms*, Pirkle, H., and Markland, F.S., Eds., New York: Marcel Dekker, 1988, 149.

152. **MEIER, J., AND STOCKER, K.**, Snake venom protein C activators, in *Handbook of Natural Toxins*, Vol. 5, Tu, A.T., Ed., New York: Marcel Dekker, 1991, 265.

153. KISIEL, W., Human plasma protein C: isolation, characterization and mechanism of activation by _-thrombin. *J. Clin. Invest.*, 64, 761, 1979.

154. JANSSEN, M., MEIER, J., AND FREYVOGEL, T.A., Purification and characterization of an antithrombin III inactivating enzyme from the venom of the African night adder (*Causus rhombeatus*), *Toxicon,* 30, 985, 1992.

155. KRESS, L.F., The action of snake venom metalloproteinases on plasma proteinase inhibitors, in *Hemostasis and Animal Venoms*, Pirkle, H., and Markland, F.S., Eds., New York: Marcel Dekker, 1988, 335.

156. MASTRO, A.M., HURLEY, D.J., WINNING, R.K., FILIPOWSKI, R., OGILVIE, M.L., AND GARTNER, T.K., Mitogenic activity of snake venom lectins, *Cell Tissue Kinet.*, 19, 557, 1986.

157. GARTNER, T.K., STOCKER, K., AND WILLIAMS, D.C., Thrombolectin: a lectin isolated from *Bothrops atrox* venom. *FEBS Lett.*, 117, 13, 1980.

158. HOGUE-ANGELETTI, R.A., AND BRADSHAW, R.A., Nerve growth factors in snake venoms, in *Snake Venoms*, Lee, C.Y., Ed., Berlin, Springer, 1979, 276.

159. VIDAL, J.C., AND STOPPANI, A.O.M., Isolation and properties of an inhibitor of phospholipase A from *Bothrops neuwiedii* venom, *Arch. Biochem. Biophys.*, 147, 66, 1971.

160. BRAGANÇA, B.M., SAMBRAY, Y.M., AND SAMBRAY, R.Y., Isolation of polypeptide inhibitor of phospholipase A from cobra venom, *Eur. J. Biochem.*, 13, 410, 1970.

161. HOKAMA, Y., IWANAGA, S., TATSUKI, T., AND SUZUKI, T., Snake venom proteinase inhibitors. III. Isolation of five polypeptide inhibitors from venoms of *Haemachatus haemachatus* (Ringhal's cobra) and *Naja nivea* (Cape cobra) and the complete amino acid sequence of two of them. *J. Biochem. (Tokyo)*, 79, 559, 1976.

162. MAN, D.P., AND MINTA, J.O., Purification, characterization and analysis of the mechanism of action of four anti-complementary factors in *Crotalus atrox* venom. *Immunochemistry*, 14, 521, 1977.

163. EGGERTSEN, G., FOHLMAN, J., AND SJÖQUIST, J., In vitro studies on complement inactivation by snake venoms. *Toxicon*, 18, 87, 1980.

164. VOGT, W., Snake venom constituents affecting the complement system, in *Medical Use of Snake Venom Proteins*, Stocker, K., Ed., Boca Raton, CRC Press, 1990, 79.

165. VOGEL, C.W., Cobra venom factor: the complement-activating protein of cobra venom, in *Handbook of Natural Toxins*, Vol. 5, Tu, A.T., Ed., New York, Marcel Dekker, 1991, 147.

166. BIEBER, A.L., Metal and nonprotein constituents in snake venoms, in *Snake Venoms*, Lee, C.Y., Ed., Berlin, Springer, 1979, 295.

167. ELLIOTT, W. B., Chemistry and immunology of reptilian venoms, in *Biology of the Reptilia*, Vol. 8, Gans. C., Ed., New York: Academic Press, 1978, 163.

168. COOKE, M.E., ODELL, G.V., HUDIBURG, S.A., AND GUTIERREZ, J.M., Analysis of fatty acids in the lipid components of snake venom (Abstr.), in *Proc. 2nd American Symp. on Animal, Plant and Microbial Toxins*, Tempe, 1986.

169. KABARA, J.J., AND FISCHER, G.H., Chemical composition of *Naja naja*: extractable lipids, *Toxicon*, 7, 223, 1969.

170. MOROZ, C., DE VRIES, A., AND SELA, M., Isolation and characterization of a neurotoxin from *Vipera palaestinae* venom. *Biochim.biophys.Acta*, 124, 136, 1966.

171. INAMASU, Y., NAKANO, K., KOBAYASHI, M., SAMESHIMA, Y., AND OBO, F., Nature of the prosthetic group of the L-amino acid oxidase from habu snake (*Trimeresurus flavoviridis*) venom, *Acta Med. Univ. Kagoshima*, 16, 23, 1973.

172. IWANAGA, S., AND SUZUKI, T., Enzymes in snake venoms, in *Snake Venoms*, Lee, C.Y., Ed., Berlin, Springer, 1979, 61.

173. STILES, B.G., SEXTON, F.W., AND WEINSTEIN, S.A., Antibacterial effects of different snake venoms: purification and characterization of antibacterial proteins from *Pseudechis australis* (Australian king brown or mulga snake) venom, *Toxicon*, 29, 1129, 1991.

174. SVOBODA, P., ADLER, CH., AND MEIER, J., Antimicrobial activity of several Elapidae and Viperidae snake venoms, in *Proc. Xth World Congress on Animal, Plant and Microbial Toxins*, Gopalakrishnakone, P., and Tan, C.K., Eds., 1992.

175. FREITAS, M.A., GENO, P.W., SUMNER, L.W., COOKE, M.E., HUDIBURG, S.A., OWNBY, C.L., KAISER, I.I., AND ODELL, G.V., Citrate is a major component of snake venoms, *Toxicon*, 30, 461, 1992.

176. TU, A. T., Local tissue damaging (hemorrhage and myonecrosis) toxins from rattlesnake and other pit viper venoms, *J. Toxicol. - Toxin Rev.*, 2, 205, 1983.

177. NEUMANN, D., BARCHAN, D., HOROWITZ, M., KOCHVA, E., AND FUCHS, S., Snake acetylcholine receptor: cloning of the domain containing the four extracellular cysteines of the α subunit, *Proc.Natl.Acad.Sci.*US, 86, 7255, 1989.

178. DELEZENNE, C., Le zinc, constituant cellulaire de l'organisme animal. Sa présence et son rôle dans le venin de serpents, *Ann. Inst. Pasteur Paris*, 33, 68, 1919.

179. **FLECKENSTEIN, A., AND GERKHARDT, H.,** Über die biologische Bedeutung des hohen Zink-Gehalts in Schlangengiften. Zink als Schlangengift-Inhibitor, *Arch. Exp. Pathol. Pharmakol.*, 214, 135, 1952.

180. **FLECKENSTEIN, A., AND JÄGER, W.,** Weitere Ergebnisse über die Blockierung der Bienengift- und Schlangengift-Wirkung durch Zinksalze, *Arch. Exp. Pathol. Pharmakol.*, 215, 163, 1952.

181. **TAKAGI, J., SEKIYA, F., KASAHARA, K., INADA, Y., AND SAITO, Y.,** Venom from southern copperhead snake (*Agkistrodon contortrix contortrix*). II. A unique phospholipase A2 that induces platelet aggregation, *Toxicon*, 26, 199, 1988.

182. **KIRBY, E.P., NIEWIAROWSKI, S., STOCKER, K., KETTNER, C., SHAW, E., AND BRUDZYNSKI, T.M.,** Thrombocytin, a serine proteinase from *Bothrops atrox* venom. 1. Purification and characterization of the enzyme. *Biochemistry*, 18, 3564, 1979.

183. **SCHMAIER, A.H., CLAYPOOL, W., AND COLMAN, R.W.,** Crotalocytin: recognition and purification of a timber rattlesnake platelet activating protein, *Blood*, 56, 1013, 1980.

184. **DAVEY, M.G., AND ESNOUF, M.P.,** The isolation of a component of the venom of *Trimeresurus okinavensis* that causes the aggregation of blood platelets. *Biochem. J.*, 111, 733, 1969.

185. **PRADO-FRANCESCHI, J., TAVARES, D.Q., HERTEL, R., AND DE ARAUJO, A.L.,** Effects of convulxin, a toxin from rattlesnake venom, on platelets and leucocytes of anesthetized rabbits. *Toxicon*, 19, 661, 1981.

186. **MARLAS, G.,** III - Isolation and characterization of the a and b subunits of the platelet-activating glycoprotein from the venom of *Crotalus durissus cascavella*. *Biochimie*, 67, 1231, 1985.

187. **OUYANG, C., WANG, J.P., AND TENG, C.M.,** A potent platelet aggregation inducer purified from *Trimeresurus mucrosquamatus* snake venom. *Biochim. Biophys. Acta*, 630, 246, 1980.

188. **CHEN, J.H., WAN, H., AND RUAN, C.,** Activation of human platelets induced by the aggregoserpentin of *Trimeresurus mucrosquamatus* venom (TMVA), in *Hemostasis and Animal Venoms*, Pirkle, H., and Markland, F.S., Eds., New York, Marcel Dekker, 1988, 411.

189. **OUYANG, C., AND HUANG, T.F.,** Potent platelet aggregation inhibitor from *Trimeresurus gramineus* snake venom. *Biochim. biophys. Acta*, 757, 332, 1983.

190. **OUYANG, C., YEH, H.I., AND HUANG, T.F.,** Purification and characterization of a platelet aggregation inducer from *Calloselasma rhodostoma* (Malayan pit viper) snake venom, *Toxicon*, 24, 633, 1986.

191. **TENG, C.M., HUANG, M.L., HUANG, T.F., AND OUYANG, C.,** Triwaglerin: a potent platelet aggregation inducer purified from *Trimeresurus wagleri* snake venom, *Biochim. Biophys. Acta*, 992, 258, 1989.

192. **OUYANG, C., YEH, H.I., AND HUANG, T.F.,** A potent platelet aggregation inhibitor purified from *Agkistrodon halys* (mamushi) snake venom, *Toxicon*, 21, 797, 1983.

193. **IATRIDIS, S.G., IATRIDIS, P.G., MARKIDOU, S.G., AND RAGATZ, B.H.,** Inhibition of human platelets by phospholipase-A.*Thromb. Res.*, 9, 335, 1976.

194. **LI, Y.S., LIU, K.F., WANG, Q.C., RAN, Y.L., AND TU, G.C.,** A platelet function inhibitor purified from *Vipera russelli siamensis* (Smith) snake venom. *Toxicon*, 23, 895, 1985.

195. **GROTTO, L., JERUSHALMY, Z., AND DE VRIES, A.,** Effect of purified *Vipera palestinae* hemorrhagin on blood coagulation and platelet function. *Thromb. Diathes. Haemorrh.*, 22, 482, 1969.

196. **BOFFA, M.C., AND BOFFA, G.A.,** Correlation between the enzymatic activities and the factors active on blood coagulation and platelet aggregation from the venom of *Vipera aspis*. *Biochim. Biophys. Acta*, 354, 275, 1974.

197. **OUYANG, C., AND TENG, C.M.,** Fibrinogenolytic enzymes of *Trimeresurus mucrosquamatus* venom. *Biochem. biophys. Acta*, 420, 298, 1976.

198. **OUYANG, C., HWANG, L.J., AND HUANG, T.F.,** α-Fibrinogenase from *Agkistrodon rhodostoma* (Malayan pit viper) snake venom. *Toxicon*, 21, 25, 1983.

199. **EVANS, J.H.,** Purification and properties of a fibrinogenase from the venom of *Naja nigricollis. Biochim. Biophys. Acta*, 802, 49, 1984.

200. **OUYANG, C., AND HUANG, T.F.,** Platelet aggregation inhibitors from *Agkistrodon acutus* snake venom, *Toxicon*, 24, 1099, 1986.

201. **NATHAN, I., DVILANSKY, A., YIRMIYAHU, T., AHARON, M., AND LIVINE, A.,** Impairment of platelet aggregation by *Echis colorata* venom mediated by L-amino acid oxidase or H2O2. *Thromb. Haemos.*, 48, 277, 1982.

202. **OUYANG, C., MA, Y.H., JIH, H.C., AND TENG, C.M.,** Characterization of the platelet aggregation inducer and inhibitor from *Echis carinatus* snake venom. *Biochim. biophys. Acta*, 841, 1, 1985.

203. **HUANG, T.F., WU, Y.J., AND OUYANG, C.,** Characterization of a potent platelet aggregation inhibitor from *Agkistrodon rhodostoma* snake venom. *Biochim. Biophys. Acta*, 925, 248, 1987.

204. **HUANG, T.F., HOLT, J.C., LUKASIEWICZ, H., AND NIEWIAROWSKI, S.,** Trigramin. A low molecular weight peptide inhibiting fibrinogen interaction with platelet receptor expressed on glycoprotein IIb-IIIa complex. *J. Biol. Chem.*, 262, 16157, 1987.

205. **GAN, Z.R., GOULD, R.J., JACOBS, J.W., FRIEDMAN, P.A., AND POLOKOFF, M.A.,** Echistatin. A potent platelet aggregation inhibitor from the venom of the viper, *Echis carinatus, .J. Biol. Chem.,* 263, 19827, 1988.

206. **CHAO, B.H., JAKUBOWSKI, J.A., SAVAGE, B., CHOW, E.P., MARZEC, U.M., HARKER, L.A., AND MARAGANORE, J.M.,** *Agkistrodon piscivorus piscivorus* platelet aggregation inhibitor: a potent inhibitor of platelet activation, *Proc. Nat. Acad. Sci., U.S.* 86, 8050, 1989.

207. **SHEBUSKI, R.J., RAMJIT, D.R., BENCEN, G.H. AND POLOKOFF, M.A.,** Characterization and platelet inhibitory activity of bitistatin, a potent arginine-glycine-aspartic acid-containing peptide from the venom of the viper *Bitis arietans, J. Biol. Chem.,* 264, 21550, 1989.

208. **KINI, R.M., STEFANSSON, S., AND EVANS, H.J.,** Non-phospholipase anticoagulants in *Naja nigricollis* venom, in *Progress in Venom and Toxin Research,* Gopalakrishnakone, P., and Tan, C.K., Eds., Singapore, National University of Singapore, 1987, 175.

209. **SUZUKI, T., AND TAKAHASHI, H.,** Purification of two thrombin-like enzymes from the venom of *Agkistrodon caliginosus* (kankoku-mamushi), *Toxicon,* 22, 29, 1984.

210. **HERZIG, R.H., RATNOFF, O.D., AND SHAINOFF, J.R.,** Studies on a procoagulant fraction of Southern copperhead snake venom: the preferential release of fibrinopeptide B. *J. Lab. Clin. Med.* 76, 451, 1970.

211. **SATO, T., IWANAGA, S., MIZUSHIMA, Y., AND SUZUKI, T.,** Studies on venoms. XV. Separation of arginine ester hydrolase of venom of *Agkistrodon halys blomhoffii* into three enzymatic entities: "bradykinin releasing", "clotting" and "permeability increasing". *J. Biochem.,* 57, 380, 1965.

212. **GUAN, L.F., CHI, C.W., AND YUAN, M.,** Study on the thrombin- like enzyme preferentially releasing fibrinopeptide B from the snake venom of *Agkistrodon halys* Pallas. *Thromb. Res.,* 35, 301, 1984.

213. **GAFFNEY, P.J., MARSH, N.A., AND WHALER, B.C.,** A coagulant enzyme from Gaboon-viper venom: some aspects of its mode of action. *Biochem. Soc. Transactions,* 1, 1208, 1973.

214. **ARAGON-ORTIZ, F., AND GUBENSEK, F.,** Isolation and some properties of blood clotting enzyme from the venom of *Bothrops asper, Bull. Inst. Pasteur,* 74, 145, 1976.

215. **BLOMBÄCK, B., BLOMBÄCK, M., AND NILSSON, I.M.,** Coagulation studies on "Reptilase", an extract of the venom from *Bothrops jararaca. Thromb. Diath. Haemorrh.,* 1, 76, 1957.

216. **ITOH, N., TANAKA, N., FUNAKOSHI, I., KAWASAKI, T., MIHASHI, S., AND YAMASHINA, I.,** Organization of the gene for batroxobin, a thrombin-like snake venom enzyme, *J. Biol. Chem.,* 263, 7628, 1988.

217. **SELISTRE, H.S., AND GIGLIO, J.R.,** Isolation and characterization of a thrombin-like enzyme from the venom of the snake *Bothrops insularis* (jararaca ilhoa), *Toxicon,* 25, 1135, 1987.

218. **HATTON, M.W.C.,** Studies on the coagulant enzyme from *Agkistrodon rhodostoma* venom. Isolation and some properties of the enzyme. *Biochem. J.,* 131, 799, 1973.

219. **FARID, T.M., TU, A.T., AND FARID EL-ASMAR, M.,** Characterization of cerastobin, a thrombin-like enzyme from the venom of *Cerastes vipera* (Sahara sand viper). *Biochemistry,* 28, 371, 1989.

220. **MARKLAND, F.S., AND DAMUS, P.S.,** Purification and properties of a thrombin-like enzyme from the venom of *Crotalus adamanteus* (Eastern diamondback rattlesnake). *J. Biol. Chem.,* 246, 6460, 1971.

221. **PIRKLE, H., THEODOR, I., AND LOPEZ, R.,** Catroxobin, a weakly thrombin-like enzyme from the venom of *Crotalus atrox.* NH2-terminal and active site amino acid sequences. *Thromb. Res.,* 56, 159, 1989.

222. **ALEXANDER, G., GROTHUSEN, J., ZEPEDA, H., AND SCHWARTZMAN, R.J.,** Gyroxin, a toxin from the venom of *Crotalus durissus terrificus,* is a thrombin-like enzyme. *Toxicon,* 26, 953,1988.

223. **SHU, Y.Y., MORAN, J.B., AND GEREN, C.R.,** A thrombin-like enzyme from timber rattlesnake venom, *Biochim. Biophys. Acta,*748, 236, 1983.

224. **BAJWA, S.S., MARKLAND, F.S., AND RUSSELL, F.E.,** Fibrinolytic and fibrinogen clotting enzymes present in the venoms of Western diamondback rattlesnake, *Crotalus atrox,* Eastern diamondback rattlesnake, *Crotalus adamanteus,* and Southern Pacific rattlesnake, *Crotalus viridis helleri. Toxicon,* 19, 53, 1981.

225. **MACKESSY, S.P.,** Isolation of a thrombin-like protease from the venom of the Northern Pacific rattlesnake, *Crotalus viridis oreganus. Toxicon,* 27, 61, 1989.

226. **HIESTAND, P.C., AND HIESTAND, R.R.,** *Dispholidus typus* (boomslang) snake venom: purification and properties of the coagulant principle. *Toxicon,* 17, 489, 1979.

227. **CAMPOS, S., ESCOBAR, E., LAZO, F., YARLEQUE, A., MARSH, N.A., PEYSER, P.M., WHALER, B.C., CREIGHTON, L.J., AND GAFFNEY,P.J.** Partial separation and characterization of a thrombin-like enzyme from the venom of the Peruvian bushmaster snake, *Lachesis muta muta,* in *Hemostasis and Animal Venoms,* Pirkle, H., and Markland, F.S., Eds., New York, Marcel Dekker, 1988, 107.

228. **MAGALHAES, A., DE OLIVEIRA, G.J., AND DINIZ, C.R.,** Purification and partial characterization of a thrombin-like enzyme from the venom of the bushmaster snake, *Lachesis muta noctivaga. Toxicon,* 19, 279, 1981.

229. **OUYANG, C., AND YANG, F.Y.**, Purification and properties of the thrombin-like enzyme from *Trimeresurus gramineus* venom. *Biochim. Biophys. Acta*, 351, 354, 1974.

230. **OUYANG, C., HONG, J.S., AND TENG C.M.**, Purification and properties of the thrombin-like principle of *Agkistrodon acutus* venom and its comparison with bovine thrombin, *Thromb. Diath. Haemorrh.*, 26, 224, 1971.

231. **OUYANG, C., AND HUANG, T.F.**, Purification and characterization of the fibrinolytic principle of *Agkistrodon acutus* venom, *Biochim. Biophys. Acta*, 439, 146, 1976.

232. **MARKLAND, F.S.**, Rattlesnake venom enzymes that interact with components of the hemostatic system. *J. Toxicol.- Toxin Rev.*, 2, 119, 1983.

233. **MORGAN, J.B., AND GEREN, C.R.**, Characterization of a fibrinogenase from Northern copperhead (*Agkistrodon contortrix mokasen*) venom. *Biochim. Biophys. Acta*, 659, 161,1981.

234. **RETZIOS, A.D., AND MARKLAND, F.S.**, Two-step HPLC purification of a fibrinolytic enzyme from Florida cottonmouth venom, *The Protein Society 2nd Symposium*, 77, 1988.

235. **ARAGON-ORTIZ, F., KOPILAR, M., BABNIK, J., AND GUBENSEK, F.**, Some properties of two fibrinolytic enzymes of *Bothrops asper. Period. biol.*, 80 (Suppl. 1), 90, 1978.

236. **DAOUD, E., TU, A.T., AND FARID EL-ASMAR, M.**, Isolation and characterization of anticoagulant proteinase, cerastase F-4, from *Cerastes cerastes* (Egyptian sand viper) venom. *Thromb. Res.*, 42, 55, 1986.

237. **PANDYA, B.V., AND BUDZYNSKI, A.Z.**, Anticoagulant proteases from Western diamondback rattlesnake (*Crotalus atrox*) venom, *Biochemistry*, 23, 460, 1984.

238. **NIKAI, T., KITO, R., MORI, N., SUGIHARA, H., AND TU, A.T.**, Isolation and characterization of fibrinogenase from Western diamondback rattlesnake venom and its comparison to the thrombin-like enzyme, crotalase. *Comp. Biochem. Physiol.*, 76B, 679, 1983.

239. **WILLIS, T.W., AND TU, A. T.**, Purification and characterization of atroxase, a nonhemorrhagic fibrinolytic protease from western diamondback rattlesnake venom. *Biochemistry*, 27, 4769, 1988.

240. **EVANS, J.H., AND BARRETT, A.J.**, The action of proteinase F1 from *Naja nigricollis* venom on the Aa-chain of human fibrinogen, in *Hemostasis and Animal Venoms*, Pirkle, H., and Markland, F.S., Eds, New York, Marcel Dekker, 1988, 213.

241. **OUYANG, C., AND HUANG, T.F.**, a- and b-fibrinogenases from *Trimeresurus gramineus* snake venom. *Biochem. Biophys. Acta*, 571, 270, 1979.

242. **OUYANG, C., TENG, C.M., AND CHEN, Y.C.**, Physicochemical properties of a- and b-fibrinogenases of *Trimeresurus mucrosquamatus* venom. *Biochem. biophys. Acta*, 481, 622, 1977.

243. **SUGIHARA, H., MORI, N., NIKAI, T., KISHIDA, M., AND AKAGI, M.**, Comparative study of three proteinases from the venom of the Chinese habu snake (*Trimeresurus mucrosquamatus*). *Comp. Biochem. Physiol.*, 82B, 29, 1985.

244. **NIKAI, T., MORI, N., KISHIDA, M., KATO, Y., TAKENAKA, C., MURAKAMI, T., SHIGEZANE, S., AND SUGIHARA, H.**, Isolation and characterization of hemorrhagic factors a and b from the venom of the Chinese habu snake (*Trimeresurus mucrosquamatus*). *Biochim. Biophys. Acta*, 838, 122, 1985.

245. **NIKAI, T., KATANO, E., KOMORI, Y., AND SUGIHARA, H.**, ß- fibrinogenase from the venom of *Agkistrodon p. piscivorus*, *Comp. Biochem. Physiol.*, 89B, 509, 1988

246. **SAPRU, Z.Z., TU, A.T., AND BAILEY, G.S.**, Purification and characterization of fibrinogenase from the venom of Western diamondback rattlesnake (*Crotalus atrox*), *Biochim. Biophys. Acta*, 747, 225, 1983.

247. **SUGIHARA, H., KISHIDA, M., NIKAI, T., AZUMA, H., YAMAMOTO, F., AND MORI, N.**, Comparative study of four arginine ester hydrolases, ME-1, 2, 3 and 4 from the venom of *Trimeresurus mucrosquamatus* (the Chinese habu snake), *Comp. Biochem. Physiol.*, 83B, 743, 1986.

248. **BARRETT, A.J.**, The classes of proteolytic enzymes, in *Plant Proteolytic Enzymes*, Dalling, M.J., Ed., Boca Raton, CRC Press, 1986, 1.

249. **BON, C., CHOUMET, V., FAURE, G., JIANG, M.S., LEMBEZAT, M.P., RADVANYI, F., AND SALIOU, B.**, Biochemical analysis of the mechanism of action of crotoxin, a phospholipase A2 neurotoxin from snake venom, in *Neurotoxins in Neurochemistry*, Dolly, J.O., Ed., Chichester, Ellis Horwood, 1988, 52.

250. **XU, X., WANG, X., XI, X., LIU, J., HUANG, J., AND LU, Z.**, Purification and partial characterization of hyaluronidase from five pace snake (*Agkistrodon acutus*) venom, *Toxicon*, 20, 973, 1982.

251. **OHTANI, Y., YABUKI, Y., MIMURA, M., AND TAKAHASHI, H.**, Some properties of a kininogenase from the venom of *Agkistrodon caliginosus* (kankoku mamushi), *Toxicon*, 26, 903, 1988.

252. **COPLEY, A.L., BASU, D., AND DEVI, A.**, Biochemical and light scattering studies of the action of partially purified *Bothrops atrox* venom fibrinolysin on fibrin gels, *Coagulation*, 4, 47, 1971.

253. **DI SCIPIO, R.G., HERMONDSON, M.A., AND DAVIE, E.W.**, Activation of human factor X (Stuart factor) by a protease from Russell's viper venom, *Biochemistry*, 16, 5253, 1977.

254. **STOCKER, K., FISCHER, H., MEIER, J., BROGLI, M., AND SVENDSEN, L.**, Characterization of the protein C activator ProtacR from the venom of the southern copperhead (*Agkistrodon contortrix*) snake, *Toxicon*, 25, 239, 1987.

255. **SIMPSON, J.W.,** Distribution of collagenolytic enzyme activity among snake venoms. *Comp. Biochem. Biophys. B*, 51, 425, 1975.

256. **BERNHEIMER, A.W., WEINSTEIN, S.A., AND LINDER, R.,** Isoelectric analysis of some Australian elapid snake venoms with special reference to phospholipase B and hemolysis, *Toxicon*, 24, 841, 1986.

257. **BERNICK, J.J., AND SIMPSON, J.W.,** Distribution of elastase- like enzyme activity among snake venoms, *Comp. Biochem. Physiol. B*, 54, 51, 1976.

258. **MORRIS, B.J., AND LAWRENCE, C.H.,** Activation of inactive renin during the selective destruction of proteinase inhibitors in human plasma by a metalloproteinase in *Bitis arietans* venom, *Biochim. Biophys. Acta*, 612, 137, 1980.

259. **KURECKI, T., LASKOWSKI, M., AND KRESS, L.F.,** Purification and some properties of two proteinases from *Crotalus adamanteus* venom that inactivate human a1-proteinase inhibitor, *J. Biol. Chem.*, 253, 8340, 1978.

260. **MORI, N., NIKAI, T., AND SUGIHARA, H.,** Biochemical characterization of a proteinase (AC5-proteinase) and characterization of hemorrhagic toxins from the venom of the hundred-pace snake (*Agkistrodon acutus*), *Toxicon*, 22, 451, 1984.

261. **XU, X., WANG, C., LIU, J., AND LU, Z.,** Purification and characterization of hemorrhagic components from *Agkistrodon acutus* (hundred pace snake) venom, *Toxicon*, 19, 633, 1981.

262. **OSHIMA, G., IWANAGA, S., AND SUZUKI, T.,** Some properties of proteinase b in the venom of *Agkistrodon halys blomhoffi*, *Biochim. biophys. Acta*, 250, 416, 1971.

263. **OVADIA, M.,** Isolation and characterization of a hemorrhagic factor from the venom of the snake *Atractaspis engaddensis* (Atractaspididae), *Toxicon*, 25, 621, 1987.

264. **MANDELBAUM, F.R., REICHEL, A.P., AND ASSAKURA, M.T.,** Isolation and characterization of a proteolytic enzyme from the venom of the snake *Bothrops jararaca* (Jararaca), *Toxicon*, 20, 955, 1982.

265. **MANDELBAUM, F.R., AND ASSAKURA, M.T.,** Antigenic relationship of hemorrhagic factors and proteinases isolated from the venoms of three species of *Bothrops* snakes, *Toxicon*, 26, 379, 1988.

266. **MANDELBAUM, F.R., ASSAKURA, M.T., AND REICHL, A.P.,** Characterization of two hemorrhagic factors isolated from the venom of *Bothrops neuwiedi* (Jararaca pintada), *Toxicon*, 22, 193, 1984.

267. **KURECKI, T., AND KRESS, L.F.,** Purification and partial characterization of the hemorrhagic factor from the venom of *Crotalus adamanteus* (eastern diamondback rattlesnake), *Toxicon*, 23, 657, 1985.

268. **BJARNASON, J.B., AND TU, A.T.,** Hemorrhagic toxins from western diamondback rattlesnake (*Crotalus atrox*) venom: isolation and characterization of five toxins and the role of zinc in hemorrhagic toxin e, *Biochemistry*, 17, 3395, 1978.

269. **CIVELLO, D.J., DUONG, H.L., AND GEREN, C.R.,** Isolation and characterization of a hemorrhagic proteinase from timber rattlesnake venom, *Biochemistry*, 22, 749, 1983.

270. **MORI, N., NIKAI, T., SUGIHARA, H., AND TU, A.T.,** Biochemical characterization of hemorrhagic toxins with fibrinogenase activity isolated from *Crotalus ruber ruber* venom, *Arch. Biochem. Biophys.*, 253, 108, 1987.

271. **FABIANO, R.J., AND TU, A.T.,** Purification and biochemical study of Viriditoxin, tissue damaging toxin, from Prairie rattlesnake venom, *Biochemistry*, 20, 21, 1981.

272. **GLEASON, M.L., ODELL, G.V., AND OWNBY, C.L.,** Isolation and biological activity of Viriditoxin and a Viriditoxin variant from *Crotalus viridis viridis* venoms, *J. Toxicol. - Toxin Reviews*, 2, 235, 1983.

273. **SANCHEZ, E.F., MAGALHAES, A., AND DINIZ, C.R.,** Purification of a hemorrhagic factor (LHF-1) from the venom of the bush- master snake, *Lachesis muta muta*, *Toxicon*, 25, 611, 1987.

274. **RAN, Y.L., ZHENG, S., AND TU, A.T.,** Biochemical characte- rization of two hemorrhagic proteases from the venom of *Lachesis muta* (bushmaster), *Chem. Res. Toxicol.*,1, 337, 1988.

275. **OHSAKA, A.,** Hemorrhagic, necrotizing and edema-forming effects of snake venoms, in *Snake Venoms*, Lee, C.Y., Ed., Springer, Berlin, 1979, 480.

276. **NIKAI, T., NIIKAWA, M., KOMORI, Y., SEKOGUCHI, S., AND SUGIHARA, H.,** Proof of proteolytic activity of hemorrhagic toxins, HR-2a and HR2b, from *Trimeresurus flavoviridis* venom, *Int. J. Biochem.*, 19, 221, 1979.

277. **HUANG, T.F., CHANG, J.H., AND OUYANG, C.,** Characterization of hemorrhagic principles from *Trimeresurus gramineus* venom, *Toxicon*, 22, 45, 1984.

278. **NIKAI, T., MORI, N., KISHIDA, M., KATO, Y., TAKENAKA, C., MURAKAMI, T., SHIGEZANE, S., AND SUGIHARA, H.,** Isolation and characterization of hemorrhagic factors a and b from the venom of the Chinese habu snake (*Trimeresurus mucrosquamatus*), *Biochim. Biophys. Acta*, 838, 122, 1985.

279. **KISHIDA, M., NIKAI, T., MORI, N., KOHMURA, S., AND SUGIHARA, H.,** Characterization of Mucrotoxin A from the venom of *Trimeresurus mucrosquamatus* (the Chinese habu snake), *Toxicon*, 23, 637, 1985.

280. **MÉNEZ, A.,** Les venins de serpents, *La Recherche*, no. 190, 886, 1987.

281. **SAMEJIMA, Y., AOKI, Y., AND MEBS, D.,** Amino acid sequence of a myotoxin from venom of the Eastern Diamondback Rattlesnake (*Crotalus adamanteus*), *Toxicon*, 29, 461, 1991.

282. **LAURE, C.J.,** Die Primärstruktur des Crotamins, *Hoppe Seyler's Z. Physiol. Chem.*, 356, 213, 1975.

283. **BIEBER, A.L., MCPARLAND, R.H., AND BECKER, R.R.,** Amino acid sequences of myotoxins from *Crotalus viridis concolor* venom, *Toxicon*, 25, 677, 1987.

284. **MAEDA, N., TAMIYA, N., PATTABHIRAMAN,T.R., AND RUSSELL, F.E.,** Some chemical properties of the venom of the rattlesnake *Crotalus viridis helleri*, *Toxicon*, 16, 431, 1978.

285. **FOX, J.W., ELZINGA, M., AND TU, A.T.,** Amino acid sequence and disulfide bond assignment of myotoxin a isolated from the venom of prairie rattlesnake (*Crotalus viridis viridis*), *Biochemistry*, 18, 678, 1979.

286. **GRIFFIN, P.R., AND AIRD, S.D.,** A new small myotoxin from the venom of the prairie rattlesnake (*Crotalus viridis viridis*), *FEBS Lett.*, 274, 43, 1990.

287. **MEBS, D., SAMEJIMA, Y.** Isolation and characterization of myotoxic Phospholipases A2 from crotalid venoms. *Toxicon*, 24, 161, 1986.

288. **MORAN, J.B., HILL, D., GEREN, C.R.,** Comparison of three phopholipases isolated from copperhead venoms. *Comp. Biochem. Physiol.*, 68B, 561, 1981.

289. **AUGUSTYN, J.M., ELLIOT, W.B.,** Isolation of a phospholipase A from *Agkistrodon piscivorus* venom. *Biochim. Biophys. Acta*, 206, 98, 1970.

290. **KAISER, I.I., GUTIERREZ, J.M., PLUMMER, D., AIRD, S.D., AND ODELL, G.V.,** The amino acid sequence of a myotoxic phospholipase from the venom of *Bothrops asper*, *Arch. Biochem. Biophys.*, 278, 319, 1990.

291. **BREITHAUPT, H., RUBSAMEN, K., AND HABERMANN, E.,** Biochemistry and pharmacology of the crotoxin complex. Biochemical analysis of crotapotin and the basic *Crotalus* phospholipase A, *Eur. J. Biochem.*, 49, 333, 1974.

292. **BOUCHIER, C., BOULAIN, J.C., BON, C., AND MÉNEZ, A.,** Analysis of cDNAs encoding the two subunits of crotoxin, a phospholipase from rattlesnake venom: the acidic non enzymatic subunit derives from a phospholipase A2-like precursor, *Biochim. Biophys. Acta*, 1088, 401, 1991.

293. **BIEBER, A.L., BECKER, R.R., MCPARLAND, R., HUNT, D.F., SHABANOWITZ, J., YATES, J.R.III, MARTINO, P.A., AND JOHNSON, G.R.,** Studies of the sequence of mojave toxin: the acidic subunit, *Biochim. Biophys. Acta*, 1037, 413, 1990.

294. **AIRD, S.D., KRUGGEL, W.G., AND KAISER, I.I.,** Amino acid sequence of the basic subunit of mojave toxin from the venom of the Mojave Rattlesnake (*Crotalus s. scutulatus*), *Toxicon*, 28, 669, 1990.

295. **LIND, P., AND EAKER, D.,** Amino acid sequence of a lethal myotoxic phospholipase A2 from the venom of the common sea snake (*Enhydrina schistosa*), *Toxicon*, 19, 11, 1981.

296. **HALPERT, J., AND EAKER, D.,** Amino acid sequence of a presynaptic neurotoxin from the venom of *Notechis scutatus scutatus* (Australian Tiger Snake), *J. Biol. Chem.*, 250, 6990, 1975.

297. **HALPERT, J., AND EAKER, D.,** Isolation and the amino acid sequence of a neurotoxic phospholipase A from the venom of the Australian Tiger Snake *Notechis scutatus scutatus*, *J. Biol. Chem.*, 251, 7343, 1976.

298. **LIND, P., AND EAKER, D.,** Amino-acid sequence of the alpha- subunit of taipoxin, an extremely potent presynaptic neurotoxin from the Australian snake Taipan (*Oxyuranus scutellatus scutellatus*), *Eur. J. Biochem.*, 124, 441, 1982.

299. **LIND, P.,** Amino-acid sequence of the beta1 isosubunit of taipoxin, an extremely potent presynaptic neurotoxin from the venom of the Australian snake Taipan (*Oxyuranus scutellatus scutellatus*), *Eur. J. Biochem.*, 128, 71, 1982.

300. **FOHLMAN, J., LIND, P., AND EAKER, D.,** Snake venom neurotoxin. Elucidation of the acidic carbohydrate containing taipoxin subunit, a phospholipase homolog, *FEBS Lett.*, 84, 367, 1977.

301. **MEBS, D, AND SAMEJIMA, Y.,** Purification from Australian elapid venoms and properties of phospholipase A2 which cause myoglobinuria in mice, *Toxicon*, 18, 443, 1980.

302. **MEBS, D., AND SAMEJIMA, Y.,** Isolation and characterization of myotoxic phospholipase A2 from crotalid venoms, *Toxicon*, 24, 161, 1986.

Chapter 25

CLINICAL TOXICOLOGY OF SNAKEBITE IN EUROPE

Hans Persson

TABLE OF CONTENTS

I. EPIDEMIOLOGY

A. SNAKE SPECIES DISTRIBUTION

In Europe most naturally occurring venomous snakes belong to the family Viperidae, genus *Vipera*, and this chapter will only deal with the European vipers. A few venomous colubrid species also occur in Europe, and especially *Malpolon monspessulanus* might be of medical importance. This snake species is discussed separately at the end of this chapter. The approximate geographical distribution of the most common species is presented in Figures 1 and 2[1]. *Vipera berus*, *Vipera aspis* and *Vipera ammodytes* are the most widely distributed venomous snakes in Europe.

Vipera aspis (Figure 1) occurs in vast regions of France and Italy, in the Pyrenees and the Alps, but it has also been reported from other parts of South Europe and southern Germany. *Vipera ammodytes* is widespread in south-eastern Europe and is also found in northern Italy, Austria and Turkey. *Vipera ursinii* occurs in restricted areas in central and eastern Europe.

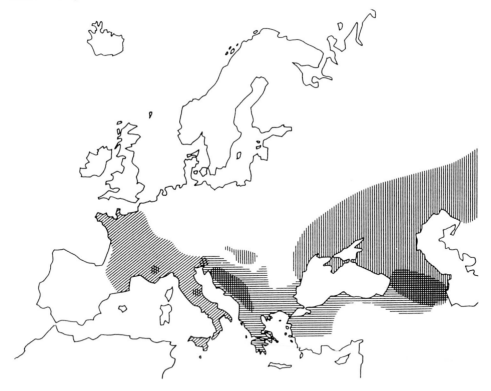

Figure 1. The distribution of *Vipera ammodytes* (horizontally hatched), *Vipera aspis* (obliquely hatched) and *Vipera ursinii* (vertically hatched). (*From Venomous Animals and their Venoms, Volume 1*, Bücherl W., Buckley, E.E., and Deulofeu, V., Eds, Academic Press, New York, 1968, chap. 12.)

Vipera berus (Figure 2) is considered to occupy more land area than any other poisonous snake[2]. It occurs almost in the whole of Europe below the arctic circle except for Ireland, the more southerly parts of the continent and the larger Mediterranean islands. It extends eastwards through Asia to the Pacific Ocean. *Vipera latasti* is common on the

Iberian peninsula. *Vipera lebetina* and *Vipera xanthina* are not indicated on the map but are found in Cyprus, Turkey, West Asia and North Africa. *Vipera palestinae* occurs in the Middle East.

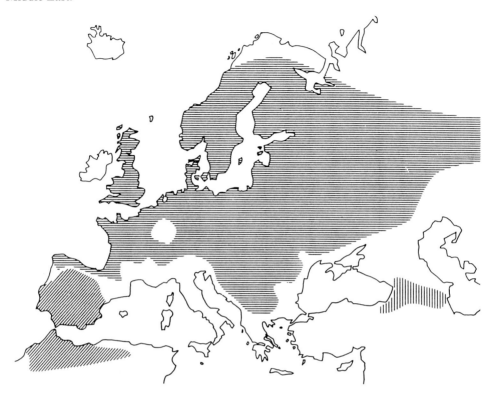

Figure 2. The distribution of *Vipera berus* (horizontally hatched), *Vipera kaznakoni* (vertically hatched) and *Vipera latasti* (obliquely hatched). (*From Venomous Animals and their Venoms, Volume 1*, Bücherl W., Buckley, E.E., and Deulofeu, V., Eds, Academic Press, New York, 1968, chap. 12.)

B. INCIDENCE OF BITES

The incidence of viper bites in Europe is difficult to assess. Existing reports are often local and they are widely spread, both geographically and timewise. Statistics from poison centres do not seem to be complete, as many cases apparently are not reported to the centres. However, a few larger reports have been published from various parts of Europe, giving at least some idea about occurrence, morbidity and mortality of venomous snakebites.

An investigation from Italy undertaken by Pozio[3] shows that 2,329 patients were admitted to 292 hospitals because of snakebite during the period 1980-1984, and 286 of these could be studied in detail. In this Italian material bites by *Vipera aspis* dominated heavily. Moderate or severe poisoning occurred in 22% of the cases and there were three fatalities (0.1%).

In a Swiss report recorded over 16 years Stahel et al[4] studied 113 cases of *Vipera berus* and *Vipera aspis* bite. Altogether 33% of these patients developed moderate or severe envenomation. There were no fatalities. In France the number of viper bites has been estimated at around 2,000 per year with a few fatalities[5]. Claud et al[6] found that 80 patients had been treated for viper bite in one French hospital between 1980-1987 and this further confirms that bites are not infrequent. In another French publication seven serious envenomation reactions in children are presented (period 1976 - 1986), three of whom died[7]. In the U.K. the number of bites was estimated in the seventies to be lower, around 100 per year, with only a few deaths during the last decades[8].

In a study from Sweden[9] it was found that around 150-200 people are hospitalized annually because of *Vipera berus* bites. Also in this material the clinical course was studied in detail and 27% of the patients developed signs of moderate or severe envenomation. Children dominated in this hospital material. The total incidence of bites in Sweden was estimated in the 1950s to be around 1,300 per year[10], and as a little more than 10% of the cases are estimated to be hospitalized, the magnitude of this figure might still be relevant. In Sweden 45 deaths due to *Vipera berus* bites have been officially registered during the period 1911 - 1991, but only seven of these deaths have occurred since 1950.

According to González[11] the number of venomous snakebites in Spain was 1,500-2,000 per year in the mid-1980s and there were 6-8 fatalities annually during the same period. According to the same author (quoting Maretic, 1989) the number of cases in former Yugoslavia was 700 - 800 per year and there were 10 - 15 deaths annually.

In conclusion it can be stated that the statistics are incomplete but that bites seem to be rather common in some areas on the European continent and in Scandinavia, especially in mountain districts and along the coasts. Fatalities occur but seem nowadays to be rare. Estimations made by Gonzalez[11] of a total incidence of 15,000-20,000 venomous snakebites and 50 deaths annually in Europe as a whole may be accurate, but are difficult to assess.

II. SYMPTOMS AND SIGNS

A. TOXINS AND MECHANISMS OF ACTION

The venoms from Viperid snakes have been less studied than many venoms from snakes belonging to the families Elapidae and Hydrophidae. In this respect there are also differences among the European vipers, and *Vipera ammodytes* and *Vipera aspis* seem to have been more extensively investigated as regards the toxins than *Vipera berus*. In contrast, the clinical aspects of *Vipera berus* envenomation seem to be better reflected in the literature.

Although differing considerably in size, the European vipers are closely related to each other and there are only minor differences in venom composition and symptoms of envenoming. However, there are a few specific characteristics for some of the species and the intensity of the symptoms may also vary between smaller and larger snake species.

The composition of snake venoms is dealt with in more detail elsewhere in this book. Venom contains a mixture of mainly proteins with enzymatic and toxic activity such as proteolytic enzymes, peptide hydrolases, hyaluronidase, phospholipases A_2, phosphodiesterases and L-amino acid oxidase. In addition, there are amino acids, carbohydrates, toxic polypeptides and metallo proteins.

Local spread of the venom is facilitated by the action of hyaluronidase. Proteolytic enzymes cause damage to subcutaneous tissue structures including capillary endothelium with leakage of plasma and erythrocytes. This will, depending on the amount of venom injected, lead to a more or less extensive oedema that gradually will take on a hemorrhagic discoloration. Local and systemic hemolysis and coagulopathies may also be induced through enzymatic action.

A spectrum of systemic effects may follow the release of highly active endogenous substances like histamine, bradykinin, prostaglandins and serotonin. Also this release is mediated through an enzymatic, possibly kallikrein-like activity.

The existence of specific cardio-, neuro- and nephrotoxic components in the venom of European vipers has been discussed. ECG-changes involving T-wave flattening and inversion as well as arrhythmias have been described after bites by European vipers, and this could perhaps partly be due to a direct cardiotoxic action.

For *Vipera ammodytes* a neurotoxin has been isolated, but it is questionable whether this has any clinical significance[12]. For *Vipera aspis* there is evidence of a neurotoxic component as certain neurological symptoms have been observed after bites[3,13]. The more dramatic central nervous system symptoms occasionally seen in envenoming by European vipers, like somnolence, unconsciousness, urine and faeces incontinence and convulsions, have mostly been attributed to sudden and profound hypotension.

Although the venom from certain Asian vipers, e.g. *Vipera (Daboia) russelli*, have a most obvious nephrotoxic action, renal impairment and renal damage after European viper bites is generally considered to be a secondary phenomenon, related to hypotension and shock.

B. CIRCUMSTANCES. ROUTE OF EXPOSURE

Bites by European vipers most commonly occur outdoors and when people come across the snakes in their natural habitat. Of course, European vipers may also be kept by private collectors as pets in their homes, and bites may ensue from too brave behaviour and careless handling of the snakes.

Most bites occur in the extremities (the hand or foot region). In some reports the lower extremity is more commonly involved[6,9], especially in children. In adults the dominance is not so clear, because many bites occur in the upper extremities in connection with picking wild berries and mushrooms or during gardening. In other studies the upper extremity clearly dominates among men of all ages, whereas bites in women occur more often in the legs[3]. There is in almost all reports a heavy dominance for men. Bites are also regularly, although much more seldom, observed on the trunk, neck and head. This may happen during swimming, when laying down on the grass on a sunny day or when looking the snake too closely in the eyes[9,14]. In addition some snakes, like *Vipera latasti*, may sometimes be found in trees, with a consequent increase in bites to the head or trunk, e.g. in farmers harvesting fruits[15].

The snake releases the victim directly after the bite. Bites can occur at any time of the day and the year, however, not outdoors during the winter season in northern countries. Bites occur most commonly in warm and dry weather and the snakes are mostly found in sunny, rocky parts of forests, in meadow-land, in mountain districts (even at high altitude) and along the coasts. Vipers can both swim and climb.

The route of exposure is, for obvious reasons, mostly intra- or subcutaneous. More rarely it is intramuscular. Intravenous injection has been reported[9]. The venom can not penetrate intact skin.

C. SEVERITY OF ENVENOMING. VARIATIONS

The toxic effects caused by various European vipers are, as already mentioned, rather similar for the different species. The symptomatology may vary in intensity and some of the more robust snakes in southern and south-eastern Europe are claimed to cause more severe reactions. This is, however, not apparent from the literature and it is not easy to define these differences with any certainty. In a previous section of this chapter some fairly large hospital reports were compared. An Italian report with mainly *Vipera aspis* bites[3], a Swedish report with only *Vipera berus* bites[9] and a Swiss report with a mixture of both[4] did not reveal any remarkable differences as concerns severity. The smaller species, like *Vipera ursinii*, seem, however, to give milder reactions.

More generally any of the four following reactions is possible, namely (a) none except for fang marks and fright, (b) local reaction, (c) local reaction and systemic effects, and (d) only systemic effects with no local findings except for fang marks.

Both the local reaction and the systemic symptoms may vary considerably in intensity. One extreme situation is when no venom has been injected, as indicated above under item (a). Of course, in these cases no toxic reaction at all is to be expected. Such dry bites are not infrequent, and it is claimed that no venom is injected in 30-50% of all snakebites. This is important to understand, as the absence of symptoms after snakebites often has led to the misconception that the venom is of low toxicity and that bites are harmless.

The great variations in severity of envenoming and hence clinical symptomatology are due to some basic conditions as indicated in Table 1. The two most important factors are probably the amount of venom injected, which may vary from zero to full dose, and the age and weight of the patient. Small children and old people are more sensitive. Physical activity is an important factor that, if too energetic, may be most deleterious. There are, in fact, two cases reported where cardiac arrest followed intensive physical activity directly after snakebite (*Vipera aspis* and *berus* respectively)[3,9]. Bites on the trunk, head and neck and in highly vascularized areas are generally considered more dangerous than bites on the extremities. There is, however, no clear evidence of this either in the literature or when considering local experience. Besides, bites on areas other than the extremities are relatively so few that any reliable comparisons are difficult to make.

Table 1
Factors of importance for the development of symptoms after bite by European vipers

Amount of venom injected
Age and weight of the patient
Location of the bite
Previous state of health
Physical activity after the bite
Psychological reactions

It is a common conception that heavy physical activity in general, and of the bitten limb in particular, has an unfavourable influence on the clinical course. Part of the explanation could be a quicker spread of the venom to the systemic circulation due to an enhanced lymphatic flow in moving limbs. This is the rationale of first aid immobilization. It is also well known that strong psychological reactions may occur, particularly at an early stage, and fright and anxiety may certainly influence the symptomatology, at least for some time.

D. SYMPTOMATOLOGY
1. General aspects

Most patients bitten by European vipers will present with a relatively mild clinical course, but severe cases are constantly found in every clinical report of magnitude. For the European vipers the main features of envenoming are local tissue damage, gastrointestinal symptoms and systemic circulatory disturbances. In addition there is a wide variety of symptoms, many of which are related to the main features just mentioned. The symptomatology is briefly summarized in Table 2 and described in more detail below.

Mostly symptoms of systemic envenomation develop rapidly, often within minutes. They may also be delayed many hours after the bite. The local reaction starts slowly and may continue to develop for two to three days. Many of the serious complications, like severe anaemia, hemolysis, renal impairment, pulmonary oedema and bleeding are late complications.

Table 2
Envenoming by European vipers. Overview of symptoms

Psychological reactions
Local symptoms
Gastrointestinal symptoms
Circulatory disturbances
Central and peripheral nervous system disturbances
Renal dysfunction
Respiratory symptoms
Angioneurotic oedema, etc.
Haematological changes
Coagulopathy
Others
Late symptoms

The symptomatology of European viper envenomation has been described in numerous case reports, but it has also been analysed more thoroughly in a number of larger clinical reports[3-9,16-20]. A systematic description of symptoms observed after bites by European vipers is given below together with comments on the pathogenesis.

2. Psychological reactions

The impact of psychological reactions after snakebites can be confirmed by every clinician treating these patients. Fright and anxiety with concomitant vegetative symptoms are common and early symptoms of short duration.

3. Local symptoms

Fang marks, pain and gradual centripetal development of the oedema is typical. The pain may vary considerably, from very mild to almost intolerable. The initial pain is in most cases minimal, although there are exceptions. On the other hand the secondary pain, related to the development of oedema, is often intense and provoked by movements and contact, rather than being spontaneous[20]. The swelling may be extensive and involve not only the bitten limb, but also adjacent parts of the trunk[7,9,19,20]. In some cases the whole trunk will become involved and the swelling could even extend to other extremities[9,21,22]. A typical example of extensive swelling after *Vipera berus* bite is shown in Figure 3. After about 24 hours the oedema becomes hemorrhagic with a bluish discolouration[16]. The swelling may not reach its maximum until after 48-72 hours. The oedema will normally vanish within one to two weeks, but it may remain longer, especially in adults, with subsequent difficulties in use of the affected limb. There may also be blisters, ecchymosis and involvement of lymphatic vessels and regional lymph nodes. In a series of 42 children Bouqwier *et al*[20] noticed a thrombosis of the saphenous vein (palpated as a tender cord) in half of the patients. The local symptoms are mainly caused by enzymatic effects on subcutaneous tissues and capillary endothelium.

Although rare, bites to the face or neck occur and may cause considerable swelling, threatening the airways. Bites even on the lips and tongue have been observed under abnormal circumstances[14], resulting in lifethreatening conditions. See also below, under angioneurotic oedema, etc.

It has been claimed that necrosis and gangrene is rare after *Vipera berus* bites[8]. This is certainly true, but a few cases have been described where necrosis of skin and underlying tissues developed[16,23], in one patient even requiring extensive skin transplants[16]. Furthermore, Gonzalez[11] states that these complications are not infrequent in severe envenoming, necessitating amputation in some cases of *Vipera aspis*, *V. latasti* and *V. ammodytes* bites. Compartment syndrome with risk of gangrene has occasionally been described[23-25]. It has also been reported that local symptoms may reappear after months, especially in connection with weather changes[26]. It may finally be remarked that if the venom happens to be injected intravenously, systemic envenoming may ensue in the absence of any local reaction at all, except for fang marks[9].

If there is no swelling at all after six hours and there have been no signs of systemic envenomation, it can be assumed that no venom has been injected[8].

4. Gastrointestinal symptoms

Gastrointestinal symptoms, including abdominal pain, vomiting and diarrhoea, are the most commonly observed systemic effects after European viper bites[3,4,8,9,17,19,27]. These symptoms normally start rather early, within a few minutes to a couple of hours, but they may occasionally be delayed until after four to six hours. The abdominal pain may be very intense, mimicing acute surgical abdomen. However, gastric perforation and bleeding because of acute stress ulcer is extremely rare, although it has been reported after bites by European vipers[11]. Both haematemesis and melaena have occurred. There is also one case of acute pancreatitis diagnosed through laparotomy[28]. The symptoms from the gastrointestinal tract may, at least partly, be caused by histamine release with subsequent contractions of the intestinal smooth musculature[12,27]. Involuntary defaecation has been observed in a number of cases with severe envenoming (see also below under Neurological Disturbances). Both ascites and paralytic ileus have been observed in severe cases[9,14].

5. Circulatory disturbances

The circulatory disturbances are normally the most threatening features[9,20]. Predominant in the early phase of envenoming is tachycardia, hypotension and shock of multiple origin: 1) vasodilatation caused by release of endogenous vasoactive agents like bradykinin and histamine, 2) hypovolemia because of leakage of plasma and erythrocytes through the damaged capillary endothelium, 3) fluid loss through vomiting, diarrhoea and sweating, and 4) finally perhaps also a specific effect on the central blood pressure regulation[29]. Rarely arterial hypertension has been described in *Vipera latasti* bites[11].

A cardiotoxin has been discussed as an explanation for the typical ECG-changes and arrhythmias described. T-wave flattening or inversion is the most commonly observed ECG-change[8,9,16,19,30,31], but is not invariably associated with severe envenomation[16]. Myocardial infarction has been described in some exceptional cases of *Vipera berus*, *V. latasti* and *V. seoanei* bite[11,32,33]. Arvanis et al[34] described myocardial infarction and cerebrovascular accident in a young girl after a viper bite in Greece. More recently a second degree heartblock associated with *Vipera berus* envenoming was reported[35]. Karlson-Stiber et al[19] have observed ST-elevation, atrial fibrillation and episodes of both brady- and tachyarrythmias after *Vipera berus* bites. The risk of cardiac arrest after physical exhaustion in connection with snakebite also deserves special attention[3,9].

The circulatory failure often rapidly resolves, either spontaneously or with treatment. In severe cases it may be protracted or recurring. The patients often develop circulatory symptoms rapidly after the bite, presenting with palor, weakness, CNS-depression, tachycardia, peripheral coolness and hardly measurable blood pressure. Secondarily there may also be oliguria and acidosis. Rarely the circulatory failure may not occur until after four to six hours.

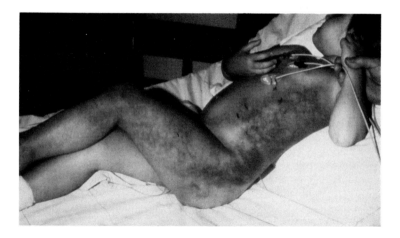

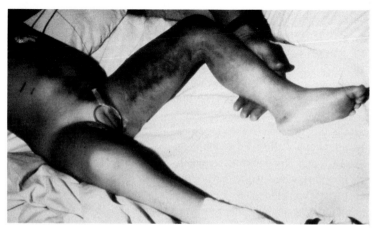

Figure 3 (top) and **Figure 4** (bottom). A 4 year old girl bitten by *Vipera berus* on the left big toe and not treated with antivenom. After 4 days the edema involved the whole leg, the left side of the trunk and the axillary region. There was pleural exudate, ascites and paralytic ileus. (Courtesy of Karlskrona hospital, Sweden.)

6. Neurological disturbances

Symptoms from the central nervous system include dizziness, vertigo, anxiety, fatigue, somnolence and coma[3,4,8,9,19]. Convulsions and involuntary defaecation and urination have occurred[9,36] and might be attributed to central nervous system excitation. Whether these symptoms are related to a primary toxic action or secondary to profound hypotension with subsequent hypoxia is an open question. Drowsiness and irritability has been observed in children during the initial days and even a pathological EEG has been registered[36].

More striking evidence of a direct neurotoxic action is provided by cranial nerve symptoms and peripheral nervous system symptoms. Thus, ophthalmoplegia, partial or total ptosis, swallowing and speaking difficulties, paralysis and paraesthesias of the bitten limb have been observed after bites by some southern European vipers, particularly *Vipera aspis* but also *V. latasti* and *V. ursinii*[3,11,13,20].

7. Renal dysfunction

Kidney disturbances in envenoming by European vipers are normally mild and manifested as proteinuria and haematuria. More rarely, elevated serum creatinine and development of oliguria or anuria are seen[6,8,9,20]. The renal complications are considered to be secondary to circulatory failure and shock, rhabdomyolysis and haemolysis, and they are normally transient and spontaneously resolving. It has not, however, been possible to entirely exclude the existence of a primary nephrotoxic component in the venom of the European vipers, as is the case with certain Asian relatives like *Vipera (Daboia) russelli*[37]. There is also one report in the literature about the development of glomerulonephritis two days after a *Vipera berus* bite[38].

8. Respiratory symptoms and complications

Early respiratory symptoms may be bronchospasm induced by histamine release, or mucous membrane swelling in the pharynx or upper respiratory tract. This swelling may be pronounced and threaten the airways[13,27]. An often reported striking feature is oedema of the face, lips, gums and tongue[4,8,13,27].

A most dreaded pulmonary complication is certainly the development of a late pulmonary oedema[6,7,14,21,22,36]. This may happen in small children with extensive local swelling when, after three to five days, all the extravascular fluid starts to get reabsorbed. There may temporarily be a critical, transient phase of overhydration and the lung vessels, vulnerable from systemic envenoming, may not be able to resist this. Other late pulmonary complications described are interstitial pulmonary bleeding[39], hemothorax and pleural exudate[14].

Respiratory distress seems, on the whole, to be more common in *Vipera aspis* and *Vipera ammodytes* envenomation[3] than after *Vipera berus* bites[9,19].

9. Angioneurotic oedema, etc.

Symptoms mimicking "allergic" reactions are glottis oedema, exanthema, urticaria, bronchospasm, rash and angioneurotic oedema. In some reports swelling of eyelids, lips, face and tongue are reported to be fairly frequent[4,8,13,19,27], and such symptoms may be serious as they constitute a threat to the airway (see also above). These manifestations of envenoming seem to appear more often in *Vipera aspis* and *V. ammodytes* bites than in *V. berus* bites. The swelling may cause both breathing and swallowing difficulties, and the patient may be unable to speak.

10. Hematological changes

Early hemoconcentration because of plasma loss is typical. Later on anemia develops because of extravasation of erythrocytes and hemolysis. The systemic hemolysis is usually mild but may occasionally be severe. An early and pronounced leucocytosis ($>20 \times 10^9$/L) is often present in severe envenoming and may be of great prognostic value[8,9]. Thrombocytopenia is also a surprisingly common finding in severe envenomation[3,9,19] and the thrombocyte count may reach very low levels[19,40]. Figure 5 displays the local reaction in a patient whose thrombocyte count dropped to 11×10^9/L and where the local bleeding was unusually prominent[40].

11. Coagulopathy

Bites by European vipers rarely result in systemic bleeding. There are, however, a few exceptional cases reported. More recently a 9-year-old girl developed massive hematuria and pulmonary bleeding after a *Vipera berus* bite[39], and there is a report of a lethal case due to massive hemothorax after a similar bite[14]. Severe coagulation disturbances with bleeding have been observed in *Vipera latasti* and Vipera *ammodytes* bites[15,41], and disseminated intravascular coagulation has also been reported in severe cases[11].

Mostly the coagulation disturbances are detected only incidentally through laboratory findings, and generalized bleeding is unusual. Local bleeding in the oedematous area around the bite is, however, common. Pronounced thrombocytopenia may develop and prothrombin time or equivalent tests may be slightly to moderately abnormal.

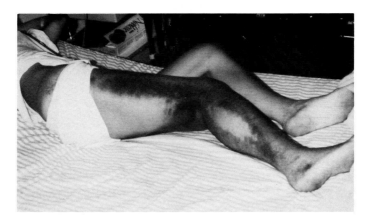

Figure 5. *Vipera berus* bite at the right malleolus medialis in a 46 year-old woman. There was a very pronounced thrombocytopenia in this case and because of excessive local bleeding the oedema has an unusually dark discolouration (From *Läkartidningen* 90, 62, 1993).

12. Others

Metabolic acidosis, fever, profuse perspiration, hyponatraemia and hypoalbuminemia are other signs observed in severe envenoming.

Deep venous thrombosis has been reported in a few cases[11,42] but this complication is probably not as common as has been suspected. On the other hand, as already mentioned, thrombosis of the saphenous vein has been observed in children bitten in the leg and developing significant swelling[20]. An exceptional complication was noted in a woman who died after a *Vipera aspis* bite and where autopsy revealed cerebral thrombosis[3].

13. Late symptoms

Late sequelae have been reported, especially in adults. Among symptoms observed are remaining swelling, stiffness, lymphoedema, pain and restricted mobility in both minor and major joints[14,17]. Also sensory disturbances have been reported[14]. Also reappearance of local symptoms after many months has been reported, usually during weather changes[26]. These symptoms may occasionally have a long duration, from months to years. Another late complication is serum sickness as a side effect of antivenom treatment.

14. Intrauterine death of foetus

It is quite likely many pregnant women have been bitten by snakes but there are few reports of any exceptional risk connected with pregnancy. However, there are three cases known, where *Vipera berus* bites in pregnant women resulted in severe systemic envenoming and where the foetus died[19,14]. In all these three cases the women were bitten in late pregnancy. Similar observations were made by James[43] who described four pregnant women bitten by poisonous (non-European) snakes, and in all cases there was an evident slowing of foetal movements and weakening of foetal heart sounds. One of these women was delivered of a stillborn baby. Apparently the venom crosses the placenta, and pregnancy imposes a special risk situation.

Table 3
Laboratory analyses of value for evaluation of severity and choice of treatment in bites by European vipers

- Hemoglobin concentration, hematocrit (EVF), leucocyte and thrombocyte count, urine analyses.

   Initially in all patients and repeatedly in those developing systemic symptoms and/or progressive oedema.

- Acid-base and electrolyte balance, tests for hemolysis (free hemoglobin, LD), coagulation tests, CPK, serum creatinine.

   Initially and repeatedly in patients with systemic symptoms and/or progressive oedema.

- ECG in systemic envenomation.

- EEG in persisting CNS disturbances.

E. LABORATORY INVESTIGATIONS

Relevant laboratory analyses for diagnosis and monitoring of bites by European vipers are summarized in Table 3. The analyses are intended for severity grading and treatment guidance. For interpretation of laboratory analyses, see under Prognostic Indications below.

F. PROGNOSTIC INDICATIONS

Some symptoms and signs that are of prognostic value have already been mentioned; a short summary of such indications is given below.

A patient who has not, within six hours, developed either local or systemic signs of envenoming is not likely to do so. In such cases there has probably been a 'dry bite'.

Signs of severe envenoming are rapid onset of circulatory disturbances, unconsciousness, severe gastrointestinal symptoms and rapid progress of the local oedema. The occurrence of an early, pronounced leucocytosis ($>20 \times 10^9$/L), early hemoconcentration, metabolic acidosis and signs of systemic hemolysis will support the diagnosis of severe envenoming. High CPK and pathological ECG are among parameters to be taken into account when estimating the risk, but these findings seem to be less reliable in this context.

Especially in small children the swelling may be very extensive and involve not only the bitten extremity but also parts of or the whole trunk. The oedema may even extend to other extremities via the trunk. This imposes a serious risk of fluid and electrolyte disturbances with subsequent renal involvement and later on pulmonary oedema.

III. PROPHYLAXIS

A. AVOIDANCE OF BITES

The primary goal must be to avoid bites as far as possible. The general public, especially children, should be advised to use boots when walking through long grass and told not to walk barefoot where snakes are known or supposed to be found. But it is also relevant to warn against careless handling of snakes. The habit of picking up snakes with the hands, common and popular among males of all ages, should be condemned. Many bites occur through thoughtless and foolishly brave interaction with venomous snakes.

B. PUBLIC EDUCATION

The aspects given above should be considered in public education activities. It is, however, also important to give some information about relevant first aid measures in case of snakebite, as there are many myths and misconceptions in this particular field.

Poison centres have an important role here. The centres have experience of producing printed material for the general public about prevention and first aid of poisoning, and they also collaborate with the media in various information campaigns. They should use these channels also for spreading information on first aid and prevention of snakebite.

IV. FIRST AID TREATMENT

A. GENERAL ASPECTS

The first aid treatment is in a way part of prevention. It aims at (a) minimizing the local damage, (b) slowing down the spread of the venom from the bite area, (c) protecting the patient from exhaustion and (d) ensuring life support whenever necessary.

Immobilization of the bitten limb, preferably in an elevated position, is advisable to reduce the extent of the local damage. In addition, as the spread of venom to the systemic circulation is enhanced by muscular activity of the bitten limb, immobilization will be helpful in reducing the risk of systemic symptoms.

Systemic envenoming may be less pronounced if the patient is resting and avoids physical exhaustion[3,9].

Psychological reactions may be severe, requiring reassurance.

B. FIRST AID PRINCIPLES IN BITES BY EUROPEAN VIPERS

- The patient should lay down and rest
- Reassurance
- The bitten limb should be immobilized in a simple way e.g. using a splint, and preferably in an elevated position
- Take off any rings, watches, bangles etc. from the bitten limb
- The site of the bite should not be manipulated in any way (no sucking, cutting, cooling, heating or electricity!)
- Torniquet should not be used
- Any need for support of vital functions should be met as soon as possible
- Avoid peroral intake, absolutely no alcohol. No sedatives outside hospital
- If the offending snake has been killed it should be brought with the patient for identification (only relevant in areas where there are more than one naturally occurring venomous snake species)
- The patient should always be transported (not run or go by bicycle himself) to the nearest hospital or physician in the following circumstances:
  - Children below the age of 15 years, elderly people or persons with preexisting serious disease
  - Bites on the trunk, head or neck
  - Signs of systemic envenoming
  - Evident progress of the local reaction
  - Lack of tetanus protection

Adult, healthy people could stay at home if the reaction after six to eight hours is restricted to a mild, non-progressive local oedema without any previous or ongoing systemic symptoms. They should, however, keep in contact with a hospital or physician and tetanus protection should be ascertained.

If there is any doubt the patient should seek medical care!

V. CLINICAL MANAGEMENT

A. DIAGNOSIS

Mostly the diagnosis of snakebite is quite obvious from circumstances and history, but occasionally it may be overlooked. It may happen that people are found confused, unconscious, with generalized weakness and shock, being unable to tell what has happened. In one reported case a swollen limb in combination with convulsions and somnolence was interpreted as traumatic sprain and commotio, being in reality a *Vipera berus* bite[36].

Once the diagnosis of snakebite is clear, the question might be which snake is involved. In many places in Europe this is not a problem as only one *Vipera* species is found in the area. In those areas where more than one viper occurs, treatment principles are very similar for the different European species. Antivenom prepared for one of the European vipers seems to work for most of the others. However, it is advisable to have the biting snake killed and brought with the patient for identification. In the future it is probable that more specific antivenoms might be available and then a more precise diagnosis could be advantageous.

Venom detection through analytical procedures has recently become a reality in some countries. The clinical benefit of determining exactly the actual venom might be considerable in areas where many different, highly venomous snakes are at hand[44]. The treatment may, under those circumstances, vary considerably, and the choice of antivenom may be critical. This is less relevant when considering the European vipers at present.

Diagnosis also aims at assessing the degree of poisoning. An enzyme-linked immunosorbent assay (ELISA) principle to detect venom from European vipers has been developed and also tested in patients. Audebert et al[45] have shown that in 102 patients bitten by *Vipera aspis* there was a good correlation between clinical signs and the level of venom antigens in blood and urine. Therefore there is evidence that the ELISA test may be helpful in severity grading of snakebites and in deciding treatment, especially antivenom. In the management of snakebite there is one critical step about which there is always a lot of discussion: to give, or not to give antivenom.

Furthermore, diagnosis, including estimation of severity grade, is based on wound inspection, development of local and general symptomatology, laboratory data and complications.

B. TREATMENT
1. Initial management
Initial management in hospital overlaps with the First Aid Principles as indicated above. A brief summary is given here:
   - Support of vital functions
   - Reassurance, the patient should rest
   - Immobilization of the bitten limb, preferably in an elevated position
   - The site of the bite should not be manipulated in any way
   - Tetanus prophylaxis should be given
   - All patients admitted to hospital should be observed for 24 hours or more. The patient should be hospitalized if there is a prominent or progressive local reaction and/or if there are any signs of systemic envenoming. All children should be observed in hospital.

2. Antivenom treatment
a. General aspects
Antivenoms were introduced in clinical practice for European viper bites in the 1920s and were used extensively. However, these fairly crude horse sera were often associated with serious adverse effects, and antivenom treatment gradually fell into disrepute. Therefore, when corticosteroids were introduced in the 1950s this 'miraculous medicine' more or less replaced antivenom. So a fairly effective but dangerous treatment was replaced by a therapy that till now has no proven benefit in snakebite.

During the last two decades there has, however, been a gradual change in the attitude to the use of antivenom in European viper bites. This has mainly been due to the fact that antivenoms have been produced with new techniques, allowing more purified products of F(ab)$_2$-type with lower contents of antigenic horse protein components. These newer antivenoms are more effective and less antigenic[4,8,19,21,46]. In a recent study[19] antivenom significantly reduced the occurrence of extensive oedema and pronounced anaemia in 30 patients with severe envenomation from *Vipera berus*. Acute symptoms resolved quickly and the total hospital stay has shortened almost 50%. In this report, Zagreb antivenom was used in the majority and Behring antivenom in some of the cases. There were three early or delayed hypersensitivity reactions (10%). Very similar observations have been made in other reports[4], and even less frequent side effects have been observed[20,47]. It seems, however, that there are differences in quality between various antivenoms currently used in Europe[7], and both efficacy and safety may therefore differ. This is also reflected by a more reluctant attitude to the use of antivenom supported by some authorities[6]. The purpose of using antivenom is certainly not only to reduce mortality, which is already low, but to reduce morbidity which is not negligible.

b. Indications

The indications for antivenom treatment in European viper bites could be summarized as follows:
- Circulatory shock that is responding poorly to treatment, or recurring
- Protracted or recurring or gastrointestinal symptoms
- Evident progress of the local reaction with likelihood of involving the trunk
- Less severe circulatory disturbances together with one or more of the following signs
  - leucocytosis ($>20 \times 10^9$/L)
  - metabolic acidosis
  - increased CPK
  - hemolysis
  - ECG-changes
  - coagulopathy
- Neurological symptoms, like CNS-depression, pareses

Note that small children and pregnant women seem to be risk groups that should be given antivenom liberally (see below Special Cases).

Allergy to animals, especially horses, is a relative contraindication, but antivenom should be given in a critical situation, provided that the patient is carefully observed and that there is an immediate readiness to treat anaphylactic reactions[48]. In such instances pretreatment with corticosteroids should be considered.

c. Dose, administration

The patient's history is checked for possible allergic disposition, and if considered appropriate a skin test may be performed. The latter should not be a routine measure but used selectively. Some authorities do not, however, advocate serum sensitivity tests at all, claiming that they are unreliable and may be misleading[8,49]. Pretreatment with corticosteroids and epinephrine, especially in allergic patients, has been discussed but it seems preferable to keep these medications easily available during the antivenom infusion. Antivenom should only be given under intensive care conditions.

Antivenom should be given intravenously, preferably diluted and as an infusion. The dosage may vary between different preparations and the recommended initial dose is normally indicated on the package. The infusion rate should initially be slow but then increased so that the whole dose is given within 30-60 minutes. The dose is the same irrespective of the patient's age and body weight. Antivenom might have to be given repeatedly, if the clinical response is unsatisfactory or if symptoms recur.

The earlier the antivenom is given the better is the effect. Although most beneficial within the first four hours, antivenom is effective also if given within 18 hours. After this time the effect of antivenom gradually seems to vanish. The progression of the oedema, that at this stage often is considerable, might, however, slow down but this is difficult to assess with certainty. Furthermore, in one *Vipera berus* bite, severe coagulopathy normalized promptly when antivenom was given after 30 hours[19], and it appears that late antivenom treatment is especially rewarding in coagulation disorders. Thus, there are some startling examples where clinical bleeding stopped promptly on antivenom administration seven and eight days respectively after bites by *Vipera ammodytes*[41] and an Asian viper[50].

Finally it must be remembered that there is always, after administration of foreign proteins, a risk of acute or delayed hypersensitivity reactions. Therefore patients given antivenom must be checked for this during the following weeks. Serum sickness is in general successfully treated with cortisone.

d. Future perspectives

Although the majority of bites by European vipers result in mild or moderate poisoning, a number of patients develop severe acute illness with risk of complications and sequelae. To reduce suffering from this most unpleasant type of poisoning it is necessary to improve treatment. To achieve this, the use of antivenoms is unavoidable. The unpredictable risk of allergic reactions in every single case will, however, continue to influence the decision whether to use antivenom or not and a certain hesitation will always be there. Therefore the future development of this area is a challenge to toxinology. It is not acceptable that the only effective treatment of severe snake envenomation still is associated with such a high risk of adverse effects.

Access to safer antivenoms is highly desirable, and toxinology must take into account the progress in immunotherapy during recent years. It is natural to try to apply existing techniques to develop pure Fab fragments in other animals than horses (sheep, goats). The application of these principles in digitalis poisoning has been eminently successful[51]. For *Vipera berus* venom specific sheep Fab fragments have also recently been produced and tested experimentally[52]. The initial clinical experiences of this new principle for immunotherapy of snake envenomation are promising[53] (Beritab; Therapeutic Antibodies Inc.).

3. Symptomatic treatment
a. Circulation

Hypotension and shock due to vasodilation and fluid loss should be treated with intravenous rehydration as required. Preferably a combination of crystalloid and colloid solutions should be given. Inotropic support may sometimes be necessary, at least for some period. An initial dose of epinephrine may be of benefit in profound hypotension, and dopamine may be a suitable choice for continuous infusion as both peripheral α-adrenergic effect and inotropic support might be of value. Any electrolyte and acid-base balance disturbances should be corrected. In patients not given antivenom the swelling may be very extensive and necessitate extra fluids for two to four days. Continuous ECG-monitoring is advisable in severe envenoming, and a central venous catheter as well as an arterial line may be useful in monitoring pronounced circulatory failure. However, the risk of bleeding must be assessed before invasive methods are applied.

b. Respiration

Initial respiratory distress, e.g. due to bronchospasm, usually resolves quickly on epinephrine administration as do other symptoms of 'allergic' character, like urticaria, rash and angioneurotic oedema. Antihistamines and corticosteroids may be of value for prevention and treatment of these kinds of symptoms. Occasionally pronounced swelling may occur in the oropharynx and laryngeal regions, necessitating prompt measures to secure an adequate airway (intubation, tracheotomy).

One late and dreaded respiratory complication is the development of pulmonary oedema. This has been observed in small children three to five days after the bite, when the extensive oedema is being absorbed with subsequent overhydration of the vulnerable circulatory system. In these situations vigorous treatment including controlled mechanical ventilation is urgent and often lifesaving.

c. Kidney function

Severe renal dysfunction is rare in envenomation by European snakes. Slight rises in serum creatinine, proteinuria and hematuria are observed, but are usually transient. Occasionally oliguria and anuria are seen. It is thought that the etiology is mainly prerenal and related to dehydration and hypotension. The rational treatment is therefore adequate hydration, control of the diuresis and use of diuretics when required. In severe hemolysis or rhabdomyolysis it is advisable to provide an alkaline diuresis to protect the kidneys. Occasionally dialysis must be instituted.

d. Blood disorders

The most prominent derangement in the blood is the development of anaemia due to extravasation of erythrocytes and sometimes also hemolysis. This anaemia may be pronounced and require blood transfusions. Coagulation disturbances are normally restricted to laboratory abnormalities and very rarely need any therapeutic interventions apart from antivenom treatment. Occasionally fresh frozen plasma and specific coagulation factors are needed.

e. Infections

Tetanus prophylaxis should always be provided in snakebite. Otherwise local infections are generally not to be expected in bites by European vipers and prophylactic antibiotics should normally not be given routinely. However, these conditions seem to vary a lot geographically and for some of the South European vipers infections seem to be more frequent and antibiotics are used more often, even routinely. In case of evident local or systemic infection antibiotics should, of course, be given as required and after appropriate cultures.

f. Local symptoms

Apart from immobilization no local treatment is normally required, and as stated above most manipulations at the site of the bite discussed in the past are useless or dangerous. The only way to "treat" the swelling effectively is to prevent its further development - through administration of antivenom. Very rarely a compartment syndrome has been reported requiring fasciotomy. Such treatment should be avoided unless absolutely necessary as complications and sequelae may ensue if surgery is applied to the extensively damaged tissues[22].

Pain and itching may occur and should, when appropriate, be alleviated by analgesics and antihistamines, preferably without sedating properties.

4. Other aspects and controversies

a. Heparin

Deep venous thrombosis is not common after viper bites but has been reported[42]. Children generally have a low tendency of developing deep venous thrombosis, whereas thrombophlebitis of the saphenous vein has been described[20]. One could, however, consider giving adults with extensive swelling prophylactic heparin in a low dose. The former practice of giving higher doses of heparin as a kind of antidote to slow down the local reaction seems abandoned nowadays. There is strong evidence that energetic heparin treatment might worsen the situation and increase the risk of bleeding[40].

b. Cortisone

The role of cortisone in the treatment of European viper bites, and of snakebites more generally, is unclear and opinions are diverging. In some places cortisone has, since it was introduced, been given routinely in all cases of snakebite, although convincing scientific evidence about its effectiveness in snakebite is lacking. The morbidity of snakebite is considerable in spite of the fact that cortisone is used extensively and in many places routinely. There is no case reported where cortisone has cured the symptoms of severe envenoming.

As cortisone might be of some benefit for protecting against and alleviating certain snake venom reactions of 'allergic' type, it might, however, be reasonable to use it in moderate doses as part of the symptomatic treatment. Under these circumstances it might be beneficial and, at least, it will not do any harm. But on the other hand, cortisone should not, by any means, be expected to be of vital importance in curing severe envenomation and its role as a kind of general 'antidote' in snakebites belongs to the past. Another issue is whether high dose cortisone is of any benefit more generally in severe shock as seen also in snake envenomation but this discussion falls outside the scope of this presentation.

5. Special cases

It has already been mentioned that small children are specially sensitive to viper bites and therefore might benefit from a more liberal attitude to antivenom therapy.

Pregnancy is another difficult issue, as was also discussed in a previous section. In accordance with this antivenom should always be considered early in pregnant women who suffer from systemic reactions or if there is a slowing of the foetal movements, irrespective of the mother's general condition.

6. Follow up

While discussing the clinical aspects of snakebite, follow up of the patients seems to be a sadly neglected area. Whenever a follow up has been undertaken more systematically, it has proven to be a most rewarding activity.

In many mild or moderate cases there is certainly no need for a follow up, but those patients who have been severely envenomated really need to see a doctor more than once after discharge from hospital. There may be remaining symptoms, and some patients have problems for a long time. Also the risk of serum sickness must be taken into account so that adequate treatment can be given. Moreover, the follow up is of academic interest. As relatively few patients seem to be brought back for medical evaluation after a snakebite, the knowledge of longlasting and late symptoms is very incomplete. To be able to judge about the whole problem of snake envenoming and its complications, and to assess the efficacy of treatment given, a better and more systematic follow up seems indispensable. It is clear that patients, having suffered a snake envenomation, deserve more attention and devotion also after the acute phase, and a careful follow up actually seems to be a corner-stone as concerns the development of better treatment principles for snake envenoming.

VI. COLUBRID SNAKES AND THEIR BITES IN EUROPE

Although the vipers dominate heavily in Europe from a medical point of view, also some venomous species of colubrid snakes occur in the more southerly parts of the continent.

Malpolon monspessulanus (Montpellier snake) is a large and active snake occurring in Morocco, Portugal, Spain, coastal France and northwestern Italy[54]. Gonzalez[15] has reported 60 bites by this snake, and in 10 cases there were signs of envenoming.

Typical symptoms were local swelling, parasthesia around the site of the bite, lymphangitis and lymphadenitis. In severe cases neurological symptoms were also observed, such as CNS depression, ptosis, and paresis of the affected limb. Dyspnoea and dysphagia has been reported. The treatment is symptomatic and supportive, following the general principles as indicated above for viper bites, and there is no specific antivenom available.

Also bites by *Elaphe* spp., e.g. *Elaphe longissima* (aesculapian snake) are occasionally observed but are not associated with significant envenoming.

VII. REFERENCES

1. **KLEMMER, K.**, Classification and Distribution of European, North African, and North and West Asiatic Venomous Snakes, in *Venomous Animals and their Venoms*, Volume 1, Bücherl, W., Buckley, E. E., and Deulofeu, V., Eds, Academic Press, New York, 1968, chap. 12.
2. **STEWARD, J. W.**, *The Snakes of Europe*, David and Charles Ltd, Plymouth, 1971, 159.
3. **POZIO, E.**, Venomous snake bite in Italy: epidemiological and clinical aspects, *Trop. Med. Parasit.*, 39, 62, 1988.
4. **STAHEL, E., WELLANER, T., AND FREYVOGEL, T. H.**, Vergiftungen durch einheimische Vipern (Vipera berus und Vipera aspis), *Schweiz. med.Wschr.*, 115, 890, 1985.
5. **CHIPPAUX, J.P. AND GOYFON, M.**, Les morsures accidentalles des serpents en France metropolitaine, *Presse Med.* 18: 794, 1989.
6. **CLAUD, B., CHAGUE, A., AND TOURRET, J.**, Morsures de vipères, *Cahiers d'Anésthésiologie*, 37, 259, 1989.
7. **ROWSSELOT, J.C., BERTHIER, J.C., ROZE, J.C., FLORET, D., AND VIDAILHET, M.**, Envenomation viperine grave, *Arch. Fr. Pediatr.*, **48**: 589, 1991.
8. **REID, H. A.**, Adder Bites in Britain, *Br. Med. J.*, 2, 153, 1976.
9. **PERSSON, H., AND IRESTEDT, B.**, A study of 136 cases of adder bite treated in Swedish hospitals during one year, *Acta. Med. Scand.*, 210, 433, 1981.
10. **MARQUARD, H.**, Recherches statistiques sur les accidents par morsure de serpents au Danemark et en Suède de 1900 à 1947, *Presse Med.*, 59, 1110, 1951.
11. **GONZÁLEZ, D.**, Snakebite problems in Europe, in *Reptile Venoms and Toxins, Handbook of Natural Toxins, Volume 5*, Tu, A. T., Ed., Marcel Dekker, Inc., New York, 1991, chap 22.
12. **HARRIS, J. B.**, Toxic constituents of animal venoms and poisons, *Adv. Drug React. Ac. Pois. Rev. 1.*, 65, 1982.
13. **SCHOLER, H., AND WÜTHRICH, W.**, Klinische und toxikologische Probleme der Bisse durch Giftschlangen, *Sweiz. Med. Wschr.*, 100, 1761, 1970.
14. **KARLSON-STIBER, C.**, Swedish Poison Centre, unpublished data (1992).
15. **GONZALEZ, D.**, Epidemiological and clinical aspects of certain venomous animals in Spain, *Toxicon*, **20**: 925, 1982.
16. **HAWLEY, A.**, Adder bite in the British army 1979-1988: a decade of experience, *J. R. Army Med. Corps.*, 136, 114, 1990.
17. **WALKER, C. W.**, Notes on adder-bite (England and Wales), *Br. Med. J.*, 2, 13, 1945.
18. **WILD, R. N.**, Adder bites in children, *Arch. Dis. Child.*, 54, 392, 1979.
19. **KARLSON-STIBER, C., AND PERSSON, H.**, Antivenom treatment in *Vipera berus* envenomating - report of 30 cases, *J. Internatl. Med.*, **235**:57, 1994.
20. **BOWQUIER, J. J., GUIBERT, J., DUPONT, C. L., AND UMDENSTOCK, R.**, Les piqûres de Vipère chez l'enfant. Etude de 43 cas, *Arch. Fr. Pediatr.*, 31, 285, 1974.
21. **CEDERHOLM, I., AND LENNMARKEN, C.**, Vipera berus bites in children - experience of early antivenom treatment, *Acta. Paediatr. Scand.*, 76, 682, 1987.

22. **BØRRESEN, H. C., AND WAGNER, K.**, Huggormbitt, lungeskade og antiserum, *Tidsskr. Nor. Laegeforen.*, 102, 840, 1982,

23. **WAGNER, H. E., BARBIER, P., FREY, H. P., JANGGEN, F. M., AND ROTHEN, H. U.**, Akutes Compartment - Syndrom nach Schlangenbiss, *Chirurg*, 57, 248, 1986.

24. **HAWLEY, A.**, Adder bites in Aldershot, *J. R. Army Med. Corps.*, 134, 135, 1988.

25. **STYF, J., AND KÖRNER, L.**, Akut Compartmentsyndrom orsakat av ormbett, *Läkartidningen*, 82, 1059, 1985.

26. **GONZALEZ, D.**, Clinical aspects of bites by vipers in Spain, *Toxicon*, **20**: 349, 1982.

27. **JACKSON, O. F.**, Effects of a bite by a sand viper (Vipera ammodytes), *Lancet*, 2, 686, 1980.

28. **KJELLSTRÖM, B. T.**, Acute pancreatitis after snake bite, *Acta Chir. Scand.*, 155, 291, 1989.

29. **BICHER, H. I., ROTH, M., AND GITTER, S.**, Neurotoxic activity of Vipera palaestinae venom. Depression of central autonomic vasoregulatory mechanisms, *Med. Pharm. Exp.*, 14, 349, 1966.

30. **MARETIC Z.**, Electrocardiographic changes following bites and stings of venomous animals, *Arch. Hyg. Rada Toksikol*, 33, 325, 1982.

31. **CHADHA, J. S., ASHBY, D. W., AND BROWN, J. O.**, Abnormal electrocardiogram after adder bite, *Br. Heart J.*, 30, 138, 1968.

32. **BROWN, R., AND DEWAR, H. A.**, Heart damage following adder bite in England, *Br. Heart J.*, 27, 144, 1965.

33. **RASMUSSEN, J. T., AND PETERSEN, P.**, Hugormebid, *Ugeskr. Laeger.*, 147, 2078, 1985.

34. **ARVANIS, C., IOANNIDIS, P. J., AND KTENAS, J.**, Acute myocardial infarction and cerebrovascular accident in a young girl after a viper bite, *Br. Heart J.*, 47, 500, 1982.

35. **MOORE, R. S.**, Second-degree heart block associated with envenomation by *Vipera berus*, *Arch. Emerg. Med.*, 5, 116, 1988.

36. **REVENÄS, B., STJERNSTRÖM, H., AND WASSÉN, C.**, Huggormsbett hos   sexårig pojke, *Läkartidningen*, 75, 2484, 1978.

37. **SITPRIJA, V., BENYAJATI, C., AND BOON-PUCKNAVIG, V.**, Further observations of renal failure in snake bite, *Nephron*, 13, 396, 1974.

38. **SCHABEL, F., MITTERSTIELER, G., AND NIRK, S.** Glomerulonephritis nach Schlangenbiss, *Paediatrie und Padologie*, **15**: 61, 1980.

39. **GERRARD, M., AND PUGH, R.**, An adder bite with unusual consequences, *Practitioner*, 226, 527, 1982.

40. **SVENSSON, H.**, Huggormsbett gav grav trombocytopeni, *Läkartidningen*, 90, 62, 1993.

41. **TIWARI, I., AND JOHNSTON, W. J.**, Blood coagulability and viper envenomation, *Lancet*, 2, 613, 1986.

42. **KARELD, L., AND PETTERSSON, P.**, Vådan av ormbett: Trombos och dödsfall efter en månad, *Läkartidningen*, 78, 2228, 1981.

43. **JAMES, R. F.**, Snake bite in pregnancy, *Lancet*, 2, 731, 1985.

44. **PUGH, R. N. H., AND THEAKSTON, R. D. G.**, A clinical study of viper bite poisoning, *Annals of Tropical Medicine and Parasitology*, 81, 135, 1987.

45. **AUDEBERT, F., SORKINE, M., AND BON, C.**, Envenoming by viper bites in France: clinical gradation and biological quantification by ELISA, *Toxicon*, 30, 599, 1992.

46. **THEAKSTON, R. D. G., AND REID, H. A.**, Effectiveness of Zagreb antivenom against envenoming by the adder, Vipera berus, *Lancet*, 2, 121, 1976.

47. **CURRO, V., STABILE, A., AND MICHETTI, V.**, Antivenom treatment in snake bites, *Acta Pediatr. Scand.*, 77, 597, 1988.

48. **PERSSON, H., AND ZETTERSTRÖM, O.**, Serumterapi vid huggormsbett, *Läkartidningen*, 81, 2752, 1984.

49. **MALASIT, P., WARRELL, D. A., CHANTHAVANICH, P., VIRAVAN, C., MONGKOLSAPAYA, J., SINGHTHONG, B., AND SUPICH, C.**, Prediction, prevention, and mechanism of early (anaphylactic) antivenom reactions in victims of snake bite, *Br. Med. J.*, 292, 17, 1986.

50. **DWIVEDI, S., SHUBHA SHESHADNI, D'SOUZA, C.**, Time limit for anti-snake venom administration, *Lancet*, 2, 622, 1989.

51. **HICHEY, A. R., WENGER, T. L., CARPENTER, V. P., TILSON, H. H., HLATKY, M. A., FURBERG, C. D., ET AL**, Digoxin immune Fab therapy in the management of digitalis intoxication: Safety and efficacy results of an observational surveillance study, *J. Am. Coll. Cardiol.*, 17, 590, 1991.

52. **SMITH, D. C., REDDI, K. R., LAING, G., THEAKSTON, R. G. D., AND LANDON, J.**, An affinity purified ovine antivenom for the treatment of Vipera berus envenoming, *Toxicon*, 30, 865, 1992.

53. **KARLSON-STIBER, C., PERSSON, H., HEATH, A., SMITH, D., AND AL ABDULLAH, I.**, Clinical experiences with specific sheep Fab fragments in the treatment of *Vipera berus* bites: A preliminary report, *Vet. Hum. Toxicol.* , **35**:333, 1993.

54. **MEHRTENS, J.M.**, *Living Snakes of the World*, Sterling Publishing Co. Inc:New York, 1987.

Chapter 26

CLINICAL TOXICOLOGY OF SNAKEBITE IN AFRICA AND THE MIDDLE EAST / ARABIAN PENINSULA

David A. Warrell

TABLE OF CONTENTS

I. INTRODUCTION

This chapter covers the whole continent of Africa including Madagascar and "the Arabian Peninsula" bounded to the north by Syria and to the northeast by Iraq. Turkey is included in Chapter 25 (Europe) and Iran and the other Asian countries to the north and east of it in Chapter 27 (Asia). Deserts cover the northernmost third of Africa, much of the Arabian peninsula, the coastal regions of the Horn of Africa and the southwestern corner of the continent. Sub-Saharan steppe merges towards the south with the savanna of western Central Africa which surrounds the equatorial block of tropical rain forest. There are mountainous areas in the northwest (Morocco and Algeria) and in East and east Central Africa. The distribution of the various species of venomous snake is governed by the extent of the different climatic and vegetational zones. Typical desert species are the desert black cobra (*Walterinnesia aegyptia*) and the Cerastes vipers. Saw-scaled or carpet vipers (*Echis*), puff adders (*Bitis arietans*), spitting cobras (*Naja nigricollis, N. katiensis, N. pallida* etc) and Egyptian cobras (*N. haje*) are found in steppe and savanna. Rain forest species include the gaboon viper (*Bitis gabonica*), rhinoceros horned viper (*B. nasicornis*) and the western green mambas (*Dendroaspis viridis* and *D. jamesoni*).

In Africa, snakes have for millenia been the subject of fear and loathing but also of awe and reverence. The earliest treatise on snake bite and its treatment is in the Brooklyn Museum Papyri, written before 2200 BC[1]. The cobra was a prominent theme in pharaonic religion and art[2]. Early European travellers to West Africa, such as Bosman in Nigeria in 1705, Adanson in Senegal in 1759, Winterbotham in Sierra Leone in 1803 and Hutchinson in Fernando Po Island in 1858, found that snakes were venerated. An enormous body of observations, beliefs and superstitions surrounds the subject of snakes and snakebites in many parts of Africa and in most regions there is a range of traditional remedies which are usually preferred to western medicine. Paterson (1789)[3], in his four voyages to the "southern extremity of Africa" ("Hottenttot country and Caffraria"), learned of the local venomous snakes from the indigenous natives and Dutch settlers. These included a horned snake (either *Bitis caudalis* or *B. cornuta*), puff adder (*B. arietans*), night adder (*Causus rhombeatus*), Cape cobra (*Naja nivea*) and rinkhals (*Hemachatus haemachatus*).

Despite urbanization and destruction of the environment, venomous snakes are plentiful in most parts of Africa and there are no countries free from the risk of snake bite. In some rural areas, such as the Benue Valley of northern Nigeria, snake bite is a leading cause of morbidity and mortality among farmers, pastoralists and hunters. Snakes, such as puff adders (*B arietans*), also kill and injure many domestic grazing animals. However, the essential role of snakes in the balance of nature must not be forgotten. They protect crops and food stores by destroying large numbers of rodents. The larger species such as pythons are frequently eaten, both as delicacies and valuable protein supplements, but also as part of various ju ju rituals in West Africa. The prevalence of this practice is indicated by the discovery of calcified nymphs of *Armillifer armillatus*, a parasite of the respiratory tract of snakes, in abdominal radiographs of 2-4% of Nigerians in Ibadan.

II. THE VENOMOUS SNAKES OF AFRICA AND THE MIDDLE EAST/ARABIAN PENINSULA AND THEIR DISTRIBUTIONS

All five families of venomous snakes, Colubridae, Atractaspididae, Hydrophiidae, Elapidae and Viperidae, are represented in this region (Table 1).

Table 1
Venomous snakes of Africa and the Middle East/Arabian Peninsula

Family/Species	Common Name
Colubridae	**back fanged and other snakes**
Capable of fatal envenoming	
Dispholidus typus	boomslang
Thelotornis capensis	bird, twig, vine snake
T kirtlandi	
Capable of severe envenoming	
M monspessulanus	Montpellier snake
Capable of mild envenoming	
Amplorhinus multimaculatus	many-spotted snake
Boiga blandingii	Blanding's tree snake
Coluber rhodorachis	racer
Crotaphopeltis hotamboeia	herald, red- or white-lipped snake
Malpolon moilensis	hooded malpolon
Madagascarophis meridionalis	
Psammophis biseriatus	
P phillipsii	olive grass snake
P sibilans	
Psammophylax rhombeatus	spotted or rhombic skaapsteker
P tritaeniatus	striped skaapsteker
Telescopus semiannulatus	eastern tiger snake
Atractaspididae	**burrowing asps (burrowing or mole vipers or adders, side stabbing or stiletto snakes), Natal black snake etc**
Atractaspis aterrima	
A battersbyi	
A bibronii	southern or Bibron's burrowing asp
A boulengeri	
A coalescens	
A congica	eastern Congolese burrowing asp
A corpulenta	Hallowell's burrowing asp
A dahomeyensis	brown or Dahomeyan burrowing asp
A duerdeni	Duerden's burrowing asp

Family/Species	Common Name
A engaddensis	Ein Geddi or Israeli burrowing asp
A engdahli	
A fallax	
A irregularis	variable or Reinhardt's burrowing asp
A leucomelas	
A microlepidota	small-scaled burrowing asp
A micropholis	
A reticulata	
A scorteccii	
Macrelaps microlepidotus	Natal black snake
Elapidae	**cobras, mambas, coral snakes and garter snakes**
Aspidelaps lubricus	South African coral snake
A scutatus	shield or shield-nose snake
Boulengerina annulata	ringed water cobra
B christyi	Christy's water cobra
Dendroaspis angusticeps	common or eastern green or white-mouthed mamba
D jamesoni	Traill's, Jameson's or western green mamba
D polylepis	black or black-mouthed mamba
D viridis	Hallowell's or western green mamba
Elapsoidea chelazzi	
E guntheri	
E laticincta	
E loveridgei	Loveridge's garter snake
E nigra	
E semiannulata	
E sundervallii	Sundervall's garter snake
Hemachatus haemachatus	rinkhals
Homoroselaps lacteus	spotted harlequin or dwarf garter snake
Naja haje	Egyptian cobra
N katiensis	western brown spitting cobra
N melanoleuca	black and white lipped or forest cobra
N mossambica	Moçambique spitting cobra, m'Fezi
N nigricollis	black-necked spitting cobra
N nivea	Cape cobra
N pallida	red spitting cobra
Paranaja multifasciata	burrowing cobra
Pseudohaje goldii	Gold's, false or tree cobra
Walterinnesia aegyptia	Walter Innes's snake or black desert cobra
Hydrophiidae	**sea snakes**
Astrotia stokesii	Stoke's sea snake
Enhydrina schistosa	beaked sea snake
Hydrophis sp	
Lapemis curtus	
Microcephalophis gracilis	
Pelamis platurus	pelagic or yellow-bellied sea snake
Thalassophina viperina	
Viperidae	**adders and vipers**
Adenorhinos barbouri	Barber's bush viper
Atheris ceratophorus	horned or Usambara forest viper
A chlorechis (A chloroechis)	West African or Schlegel's green tree viper
A desaixi	Mount Kenya bush viper
A hindii (Vipera hindii)	montane viper
A hispidus	rough-scaled, prickly or hairy bush viper
A katangensis	
A laeviceps	
A nitschei	Great lakes bush viper
A squamiger	Hallowell's green tree or bush viper
A superciliaris	lowland, swamp or domino-bellied viper

Family/Species	Common Name
Bitis arietans	puff adder
B atropos	berg adder or cape mountain adder
B caudalis	horned or sidewinding adder
B cornuta	hornsman or many-horned adder
B gabonica	Gaboon viper or adder
B heraldica	
B inornata	plain mountain adder
B nasicornis	rhinoceros-horned or nose-horned viper or river jack
B parviocula	
B peringueyi	Péringuey's desert or side-winding adder
B schneideri	Namaqua dwarf adder
B worthingtoni	Kenyan horned viper or Worthington's viper
B xeropaga	desert mountain adder
Causus bilineatus	
C defilippi	snouted night adder
C lichtensteini	forest, small, Lichtenstein's or olive night adder
C maculatus	western rhombic night adder
C resimus	velvety green night adder
C rhombeatus	eastern rhombic night adder
Cerastes cerastes	horned or desert viper
C gasperettii	Gasperetti's horned or desert viper
C vipera	Sahara desert viper
Echis coloratus	Burton's carpet viper
E leucogaster	white-bellied carpet viper
E ocellatus	West African or ocellated carpet viper
E pyramidum	Egyptian carpet viper
E sochureki	Sochurek's saw-scaled viper
Pseudocerastes persicus	Field's or false-horned viper
Vipera bornmuelleri	Bornmueller's viper
V latasti	Lataste's or snub-nosed viper
V (Macrovipera) lebetina	Levantine or blunt-nosed viper
V palaestinae	Palestine viper

A. BACK-FANGED SNAKES (FAMILY COLUBRIDAE)

The grooved back fangs or enlarged solid maxillary teeth of these snakes convey the venomous secretions of Duvernoy's glands which empty into a fold of buccal mucosa. All the back fanged colubrids should be regarded as potentially dangerous to man and must be handled with caution. Three species of African colubrid, the boomslang (*Dispholidus typus*) and the vine, twig, tree or bird snakes (*Thelotornis kirtlandii* and *T capensis*) are capable of killing humans; the Montpellier snake (*Malpolon monspessulanus*) may produce severe systemic symptoms, while bites by a dozen or more other species have been reported to cause local and in some cases transient mild systemic symptoms.

1. Colubrids capable of fatal envenoming

*a. Boomslang (*Dispholidus typus*) (Figure 1)*

This slender snake, which grows up to a length of 2 metres, has very large eyes. Its coloration is variable (grey, brown, green with black markings). It is swift, agile, arboreal but also terrestrial and inflates its throat and body in defence. It inhabits open bush and savanna through sub-Saharan Africa. This species is often confused with mambas (*Dendroaspis*).

*b. Vine, twig or bird snakes (*Thelortornis kirtlandii *and* T capensis)*

These exceptionally slender snakes can reach 1.5 metres in length. They have large eyes. They are fast-moving and arboreal. They inflate their throats in defence. The habitat is rain forests of western Central Africa (*T kirtlandii*) and savanna and coastal forests of Eastern and Southern Africa (*T capensis*).

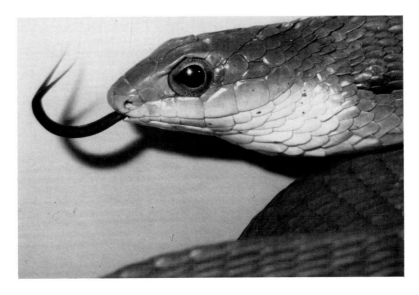

Figure 1. Boomslang (*Dyspholidus typus*). A specimen from Zimbabwe inflating its throat in defence (photo © Dr. D.A. Warrell).

2. Colubrids capable of severe systemic envenoming

*a. Montpellier snake (*Malpolon monspessulanus*)*

This snake has large eyes with an "eyebrow" ridge. The colouring is blackish, greyish, brown or olive. Maximum length up to 2.5 metres. It is terrestrial, inhabiting dry, open or stony country with low bushy vegetation or semi-desert along the Mediterranean coast and up to altitudes of more than 2000 metres in the Atlas Mountains.

3. Colubrids capable of mild envenoming

Species include -

1. Many-spotted snake (*Amplorhinus multimaculatus*): Zimbabwe and South Africa.
2. Blanding's tree snake (*Boiga blandingii*): rain forest areas of West, East and Central Africa.
3. Racer (*Coluber rhodorachis*): North Africa and the Middle East.
4. Herald, red- or white-lipped snake (*Crotaphopeltis hotamboeia*): sub-Saharan Africa except rain forest and western South Africa.
5. *Madagascarophis meridionalis* (and other species of this genus): Madagascar[4].
6. Hooded malpolon (*Malpolon moilensis*): North Africa and the Middle East.
7. *Psammophis biseriatus*: North and East Africa.
8. Olive grass snake (*Psammophis phillipsii*): sub-Saharan Africa.
9. *Psammophis sibilans*: throughout Africa outside rain forest areas.
10. Spotted or rhombic skaapsteker (*Psammophylax rhombeatus*): Central and Southern Africa.
11. Striped skaapsteker (*Psammophylax tritaeniatus*): Central and Southern Africa.
12. Eastern tiger snake (*Telescopus semiannulatus*): Eastern, Central and Southern Africa.

B. BURROWING ASPS, STILETTO SNAKES, BURROWING/ MOLE ADDERS/ VIPERS, SIDE-STABBING SNAKES AND NATAL BLACK SNAKE (FAMILY ATRACTASPIDIDAE)[4a]

Some 18 species of burrowing asps of the genus Atractaspis and *Macrelaps microlepidotus* have been described in sub-Saharan Africa and the Middle East but only the eight species proven to have been responsible for biting humans will be discussed here.

They are glossy, cylindrical snakes with the head indistinct from the neck and short, pointed tails, giving a "two-headed" appearance (reflected in some local names and myths). Most are uniformly blackish or brown with some pale flecks on the subcaudals, but the southern or Bibron's burrowing asp has a white or grey belly. The eyes are extremely small. Atractaspis possess very long, erectile front fangs which are protruded from the corner of the partially closed mouth to impale their prey which they meet in burrows (Figure 2a). Macrelaps (and other genera in this family such as Aparallactus) have large grooved fixed posterior fangs. Length usually 30-50 cm but may exceed 1 metre (*A. microlepidota*). These snakes are fossoreal, and are seen on the surface only at night after heavy rains.

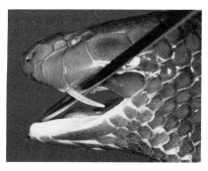

Figure 2.Burrowing asp

2a. *Atractaspis aterrima* from Nigeria showing long erectile front fang (photo © Dr. D.A. Warrell).

2b. Small scaled burrowing asp (*A. microlepidota*) specimen from Kenya (photo © Dr. D.A. Warrell).

1. *Atractaspis*: medically-important species

1.   *A. aterrima* (Figure 2a): maximum length 700 mm. It inhabits the rain forest and savanna of West Africa to northwest Uganda. It is easily confused with the harmless *Calamelaps unicolor*.

2.   Southern or Bibron's burrowing asp (*A. bibronii*): maximum length 650 mm. It occurs in Kenya and Southern Africa. It is easily confused with the harmless purple-glossed snakes (*Amblyodipsas*) and wolf snakes (*Lycophidion*).

3.   Hallowell's burrowing asp (*A. corpulenta*): maximum length 700 mm. It inhabits rain forest and savanna in West Africa.

4.   Brown or Dahomeyan burrowing asp (*A. dahomeyensis*): maximum length 550 mm. It is found in the savanna region of West Africa.

5.   Israeli or Ein Geddi burrowing asp (*A. engaddensis*): maximum length 800 mm. It inhabits desert areas of Egypt, Israel, Palestine and Arabia.

6.   Variable or Reinhardt's burrowing asp (*A. irregularis*): maximum length 787 mm. It occurs in forest regions of West and East Africa.

7.   Small-scaled burrowing asp (*A. microlepidota*) (Figure 2b): maximum length exceeding 1000 mm. It is found in the savanna region, from Mauritania to the Horn of Africa and south to Kenya.

2. *Macrelaps microlepidotus*

There are two very large fixed grooved fangs at the posterior end of the maxilla (beneath the eye). This is a uniformly black, relatively thick snake with no discernible neck, maximum length 1.15 m. It occurs in damp localities along the east coast of South Africa.

C. COBRAS, MAMBAS, RINKHALS, GARTER SNAKES, CORAL SNAKES AND SHIELD-NOSE SNAKES (FAMILY ELAPIDAE)

Among the 27 species of elapid snake in this region is Africa's longest and most feared venomous snake, the black mamba (*Dendroaspis polylepis*) and a number of other large species of major medical importance such as the black-necked spitting cobra (*Naja nigricollis*), Moçambique spitting cobra or m'Fezi (*N. mossambica*), Egyptian cobra (*N. haje*) and Cape cobra (*N. nivea*). Compared to vipers, elapids possess relatively short (up to about 10 mm long), fixed, front (proteroglyphous) fangs. However, in the case of mambas, the fang is mounted at the very front of the maxilla which can rotate at its articulation with the pre-frontal bone (Figure 3). There are reliable reports of fatal bites by 11 species of African/Middle Eastern elapids and another five species are highly likely to be capable of fatal envenoming.

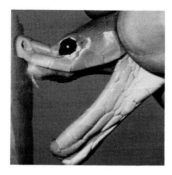 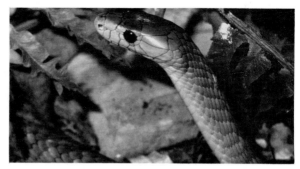

Figure 3. Green mambas.

3a. Eastern green mamba (*Dendroaspis angusticeps*) showing fang and rotation of maxilla on the pre-frontal bone (photo © Dr. D.A. Warrell).

3b. Western green mamba (*D. jamesoni kaimosae*). Specimen from Kakamega forest, Kenya (photo © Dr. D.A. Warrell).

1. Shield-nose/shield and coral snakes (genus *Aspidelaps*)

1. South African coral snake (*A. lubricus*): it has a relatively thick body and grows up to 80 cm in length. It is coloured black and orange (*A. l. lubricus* - Cape coral snake) or greyish with blackish bands (*A. l. infuscatus* - western coral snake). It rears up, spreads a narrow hood and hisses in defence. Coral snakes occur in dry sandy or rocky regions in southwestern Angola and northwestern Namibia (*A. l. cowlesi* - Angolan coral snake) and the western part of Southern Africa. *A. l. lubricus* is often confused with the eastern tiger snake (*Telescopus semiannulatus*).

2. Shield-nose/shield snake (*A. scutatus*): a relatively thick set snake with broad head and very large rostral shield, coloured greyish or reddish-brown with dark dorsal saddle markings, a pale throat and dark neck. Maximum length 60-70 cm. It rears up, flattens its neck and hisses in defence and will feign death. Found in western Zimbabwe and Southern Africa, where it burrows in sandy soil.

2. Water cobras (genus *Boulengerina*)

Two species of aquatic elapids occur in lakes and rivers in the rain forest area of Central Africa.

1. Ringed water cobra (*B. annulata*): this species is heavily built and coloured a uniform greyish-brown with a pale belly and several narrow black bands, some forming complete rings anteriorly (*B. a. stormsi* from Lake Tanganyika); or brown or reddish with 20 or more black rings, many in pairs (*B. a. annulata* found in Cameroon, Zaire and Gabon). Maximum length 2.5 metres. It rears up and spreads a narrow hood in defence. *B. annulata* could be mistaken for Gray's water snake (*Grayia smithii*).

2. Christy's water cobra (*B. christyi*): this species is black with yellow cross bands in the anterior quarter of its body. The throat and chin are yellow. Maximum recorded length 2 metres. It occurs in western Zaire and southern Congo.

3. Mambas (genus *Dendroaspis*)

Mambas are very long, thin, alert, nervous and agile, arboreal or (*D. polylepis*) terrestrial, highly dangerous venomous snakes.

1. Common or eastern green, or white-mouthed mamba (*D. angusticeps*) (Figure 3a): it is uniformly bright green. It rarely exceeds 2.5 metres in length. It is strictly arboreal and is found in thick forest or bush down the eastern coast of Africa from Kenya to South Africa. It can be confused with harmless bush snakes (genus Philothamnus) and green boomslangs (*Dispholidus typus*).
2. Traill's, Jameson's, green forest or western green mamba (*D. jamesoni*) (Figure 3b): the colouring is bright green to yellowish green, with the scales edged with black. Maximum length 3.66 metres. It is mainly arboreal. In defence it spreads a hood or inflates its throat. It inhabits rain forests from Ghana east to western Kenya.

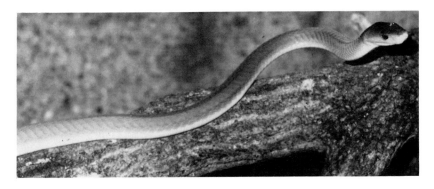

Figure 4. Black mamba, (*Dendroaspis polylepis*) (photo © Dr. D.A. Warrell).

3. Black or black-mouthed mamba (*D. polylepis*) (Figure 4): it is coloured greyish brown or olive brown with a black buccal lining. It is more heavily built than other mambas; maximum length 4.3 metres (fang length up to 6.5 mm). In defence, it rears up distending a small hood, opening its mouth and hissing. It occurs in dry woodland and scrub but not in rain forest or desert, throughout sub-Saharan Africa. There are few records of it in West Africa.
4. Hallowell's or western green mamba (*D. viridis*): its colouring is like *D. jamesoni*. Maximum length 2.4 metres. It inflates its throat and spreads a small hood in defence. This mamba is both arboreal and terrestrial and occurs in coastal rain forests of West Africa from Senegal to Nigeria and on São Tomé Island.

4. African garter snakes (genus *Elapsoidea*)

A genus of seven small fossoreal snakes with very short tails, cylindrical bodies, with no distinct neck and a bluntly rounded rostral scale as in other burrowing species. Bites and envenoming by only the following three species have been reported. There have been no fatalities.

1. Loveridge's garter snake (*E loveridgei*): young snakes have a series of white bordered brown, grey or reddish bands which in adults are marked by pairs of narrow white transverse lines. Maximum length 65 cm. This burrowing snake emerges from the ground only at night or after heavy rain. It inhabits evergreen forests and montane grassland regions around the Great Lakes up to altitudes of more than 2000 metres in Ethiopia, Kenya,

Uganda, Rwanda, Zaire and Tanzania.

2. *E. semiannulata*: as in *E. loveridgei*, the pale bands of juvenile snakes develop dark centres, leaving pairs of white transverse lines. The maximum length is 705 mm. This is a burrowing snake of dry savanna throughout sub-Saharan Africa. Three subspecies have been described: *E. s. moebiusi* in West and Central Africa; the Angolan garter snake (*E. s. semiannulata*) in Central Africa and Namibia and Boulenger's garter snake (*E. s. boulengeri*) in Tanzania and Southern Africa.

3. Sundevall's garter snake (*E. sundevallii*): the juveniles are banded pinkish and dark brown, darkening in adults as in the above species. Maximum length almost 1 metre. A burrowing snake of drier areas of Southern Africa.

5. Rinkhals (*Hemachatus haemachatus*)

In the fangs of the rinkhals, the venom canal bends sharply upwards before its exit orifice so the venom can be squeezed out in a fine stream under pressure forward from the front of the fang. The body is relatively thick set and flattened compared with cobras, and is speckled black/brown and white with dark and light bands. It has a uniformly dark belly with anterior narrow and posterior broad pale bands on the front of the neck. Maximum length 1.5 metres. It rears and "spits" its venom about 2 metres towards the eyes of an aggressor or similarly reflecting objects and also feigns death. It inhabits grasslands from the coast up to 2500 metres in South Africa and eastern Zimbabwe.

6. Spotted harlequin or dwarf garter snake (*Homoroselaps lacteus*)[4a]

A small, brightly coloured, slender snake growing up to 60 cm long. The colour is variable, yellowish with black spots or cross bands, a reddish-orange dorsal band and pale or black belly with black-edged ventrals. Occurs in dry areas of southern South Africa.

7. Cobras (genus *Naja*)

Seven species of this familiar genus are found in the region. They are generally large, relatively heavy-bodied snakes whose most notable characteristic is their habit of rearing up and, by elevating their long cervical ribs, spreading a hood in defence. The effect of this manoeuvre is to make the snake appear large and threatening. The display is accompanied by hissing, inflation of the body and, in the case of four species, "spitting" venom towards the eyes of the adversary. All seven species are capable of life-threatening envenoming.

1. Egyptian or, in the case of some forms, banded cobra (*N. haje*) (Figure 5): the colour is extremely variable; black, brown, grey, reddish or yellow on the dorsal surface with paler grey, brownish or yellowish ventral surface with bands or blotches of darker colour and commonly a dark band below the neck. Albino, lutino, speckled and banded variants also occur. Anchieta's cobra (*N. h. anchietae*) from Central and Southern Africa is dark brownish or blackish above and pale below with a broad, dark anterior neck band. The banded cobra (*N. h. annulifera*) is found in the eastern part of Southern Africa. It has broad pale-coloured annular bands often divided by a narrower dark band. The Arabian cobra (*N. h. arabica*), found in southwestern Arabia and Dhofar, is black, copper coloured, brown or yellow with a black head and tail. Egyptian cobras are ground dwelling, nocturnal, aggressive snakes popular with snake charmers in many parts of Africa. They inhabit dry savanna and semi-desert up to an altitude of 2000 metres in many parts of Africa. Maximum length 2.5 metres, with fangs up to 10 mm long.

2. West African brown spitting cobra (*N. katiensis*): chestnut brown, paler on the ventral surface with one or two reddish, brownish or black bands below the neck. Maximum length 1 metre. It inhabits Sudan and the savanna of northern Ghana, Mali, Burkina Fasso and northern Nigeria.

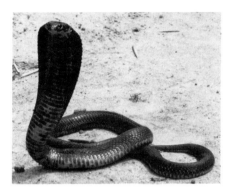 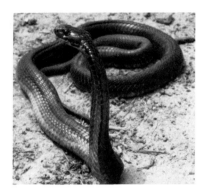

Figure 5. Egyptian cobra, (*Naja haje*). Specimens from northern Nigeria (photo © Dr. D.A. Warrell).

3.   Black and white-lipped or forest cobra (*N. melanoleuca*): it is glossy black, dark grey or dark brown above with a paler belly. The supra- and infra-labial scales are cream edged with black (hence "black and white-lipped cobra"). There is a black and yellow banded variety in West Africa. This is the largest African cobra which may exceed 3 metres in length. A 2.6 metre specimen had a girth of 159 mm and weighed 3.2 kg. It inhabits forested and formerly forested areas of West and Central Africa, São Tomé island, southern East Africa and an eastern coastal strip of South Africa. This is an active, alert, fast-moving, inquisitive but non-aggressive snake which is equally at home in trees, on the ground or swimming in lakes and rivers.

4.   Moçambique spitting cobra or m'Fezi (*N. mossambica*) (Figure 6): the colour is grey, olive or brown above with black edged scales and black skin, and a pale belly with black bars on the neck.   Maximum length 1.5 metres. It inhabits savanna from southeastern Tanzania and southern Angola southwards.

5.   Black-necked spitting cobra (*N. nigricollis*) (Figure 7): the scales are not glossy. The colour is variable throughout the range. In West Africa it is dark grey, black or brown above with a broad dark band below the neck and pink or reddish patches above and below, this colour being replaced by yellowish or pale brown in East Africa. Maximum length 2.2 metres (West Africa), 2.7 metres (Kenya). The western barred spitting cobra (*N. n. nigricincta*) grows to a maximum length of only 1.5 metres and is greyish or pinkish with black bands. The black spitting cobra (*N. n. woodi*) is uniform black. *N. nigricollis* inhabits grassland, savanna and cleared forest throughout sub-Saharan Africa. It is mainly terrestrial and nocturnal.

6.   Cape cobra (*N. nivea*): the colour is yellow, brown, or black with speckling. Maximum length 1.7 metres. It inhabits dry areas of western South Africa.

7.   Red spitting cobra (*N. pallida*): it is pinkish or reddish above and yellowish below with a black throat band. Maximum length 1.5 metres. It inhabits semi-desert areas of upper Egypt, Ethiopia, Sudan, Somalia and Kenya.

8. Burrowing cobras (genus *Paranaja*) and Gold's, hoodless, false or tree cobras (genus *Pseudohaje*)

These are rare, elusive, rain forest-dwelling elapids which are unlikely to be of any medical importance.

9. Black desert cobra or Walter Innes's snake (*Walterinnesia aegyptia*) (Figure 8)

This species is uniformly glossy jet black with bluish black-underparts. Maximum length 1.3 metres. It lives underground in rodent burrows in desert areas of lower Egypt, the Arabian peninsula and Iran. It is said to be aggressive, rearing its head without spreading a hood and hissing in defence.   It is easily mistaken for a large burrowing asp (*Atractaspis*).

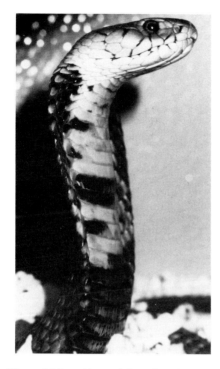

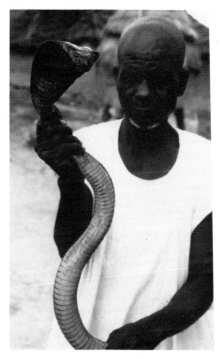

Figure 6. Moçambique spitting cobra (*Naja mossambica*). Specimen from Zimbabwe (photo © Dr. D.A. Warrell).

Figure 7a. Black necked spitting cobra (*Naja nigricollis*). Specimen from Nigeria (photo © Dr. D.A. Warrell).

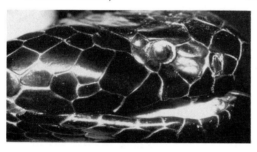

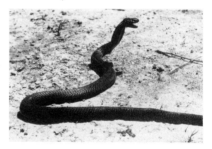

7b. Black necked spitting cobra, (*Naja nigricollis*). Head of specimen from Ghana showing fang (photo © Dr. D.A. Warrell).

7c. Specimen from Nigeria in the act of "spitting" venom (photo © Dr. D.A. Warrell).

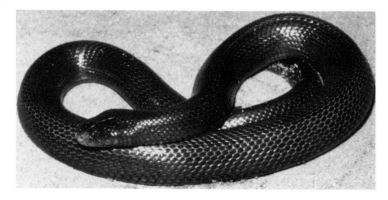

Figure 8. Black desert cobra, (*Walterinnesia aegyptia*). (photo © Dr. D.A. Warrell).

10. Sea snakes (family Hydrophiidae)
The following species of sea snakes have been reported along the east coast of Africa and in Arabian waters.
1. Stoke's sea snake (*Astrotia stokesii*): Gulf of Oman.
2. Beaked sea snake (*Enhydrina schistosa*): Gulf of Oman.
3. *Hydrophis cyanocinctus, H. lapemoides, H. ornatus* and *H. spiralis*: Gulf of Oman and Arabian/Persian Gulf.
4. *Lapemis curtus*: Gulf of Oman, Arabian/Persian Gulf.
5. *Microcephalophis gracilis*: Gulf of Oman and Arabian/Persian Gulf.
6. Yellow bellied, parti-coloured or pelagic sea snake (*Pelamis platurus*): Gulf of Oman, Arabian/Persian Gulf, Arabian Sea, Gulf of Aden, east and southern coast of Africa as far as Cape Town, Seychelles and Madagascar.
7. *Thalassophina* (formerly *Praescutata viperina*): Gulf of Oman, Arabian/Persian Gulf.

Sea snakes are most likely to be encountered stranded in rock pools or on beaches. They are fully discussed elsewhere (Chapter 13).

D. VIPERS AND ADDERS (FAMILY VIPERIDAE)
Vipers and adders are relatively thick bodied, sluggish, mainly terrestrial snakes which have long, curved, cannulated and fully erectile fangs which fold down against the upper jaw in a sheath of mucous membrane when the snake is not striking. Some 45 species inhabit the region, including some of immense medical importance such as the saw-scaled or carpet vipers (genus *Echis*) and the puff adder (*Bitis arietans*).

1. Bush, tree or sedge vipers (genera *Adenorhinos* and *Atheris*)
About 10 species of these small, mainly arboreal snakes inhabit forests of tropical Africa at altitudes between 600 and 2800 metres. Most species have small, rough, overlapping scales and prehensile tails.
Bites by only the following four species have been reported and only *A. squamiger* has proved capable of fatal envenoming.
1. Horned or Usambara forest viper (*A. ceratophorus*): this arboreal snake has three horn-like scales above each eye. The scales are strongly keeled. The colour is dark olive green above with black spots forming crossed bands. The belly is pale olive, speckled with black. It is found in the Usambara Mountains of Tanzania.
2. West African or Schlegel's green tree viper (*A. chlorechis* or *A. chloroechis*): the colour is pale green, darker on the sides and towards the tail and paler below with paired yellow spots along the dorsal surface. Maximum length 720 mm. These vipers are arboreal in the rain forests of West Africa from Guinea west to Cameroon.
3. Hallowell's green tree or bush viper (*A. squamiger*) (Figure 9): the colour is very variable; green brown or reddish. Maximum length 780 mm. They are arboreal in rain forest from Ghana east to Cameroon, Uganda and western Kenya.
4. Lowland, swamp or domino-bellied viper (*A. superciliaris*, formerly *Vipera superciliaris*): the colouring is greyish brown with three rows of dorsal blackish spots separated by yellow bars. Maximum length over 60 cm. They are terrestrial in marshy land in Mozambique, Malawi and southern Tanzania.

2. African adders and vipers (genus *Bitis*)
There are currently 13 species in this genus of adders or vipers which are endemic to Africa and the Arabian peninsula. All have relatively thick bodies with flattened heads and upward-pointing nostrils, keeled scales and very short tails. They range in size from the Namaqua dwarf adder (*B. schneideri*), maximum length 28 cm, to the gaboon viper (*B.*

gabonica) which may exceed 2 metres in length. Bites have been reported by the following nine species.

1. Puff adder (*B. arietans*) (Figure 10): this is a very large, heavy bodied snake. Its colour is almost black, brown, reddish or even orange above with pale, black-edged, "U" or "V" marks along the dorsum becoming annular rings around the tail. The belly is pale with blackish marks. Maximum length exceeds 1.9 metres. One specimen, 1.626 metres long, had a girth of 318 mm, a head 64 mm broad and fangs nearly 5 mm in length. A 1.549 metre long specimen weighed almost 4.2 kg. It inflates its body and hisses loudly when threatened. It inhabits savanna, scrub and semi-desert up to 2500 metres altitude, throughout sub-Saharan Africa, southern Morocco, western Algeria, West Sahara, Mauritania, coastal southwest Arabia (above 1500 metres) and Dhofar. It is sluggish, mainly terrestrial and nocturnal.

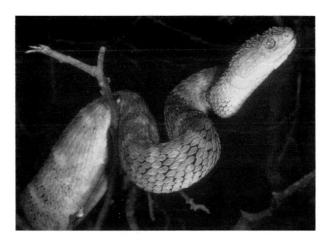

Figure 9. Green bush viper (*Atheris squamiger*). Specimen from Kenya (photo © Dr. D.A. Warrell).

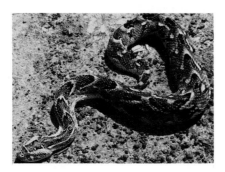

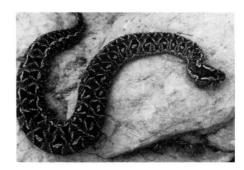

Figure 10. Puff adder (*Bitis arietans*). Specimen from Nigeria (photo © Dr. D.A. Warrell).

Figure 11. Berg adder (*Bitis atropos*). Specimen from eastern Zimbabwe (courtesy of J. Akester, Harare, Zimbabwe).

2. Berg adder or Cape mountain adder (*B. atropos*) (Figure 11): this stoutly built snake is greyish olive to dark brown with two rows of triangular black dorsal markings and lateral rows of square markings. Some snakes are uniformly coloured. Maximum length 60 cm. It inhabits mainly mountainous regions but also down to sea level (e.g. at Port Elizabeth, South Africa), on the eastern border of Zimbabwe and Mozambique and in eastern and southern South Africa.

3. Horned adder (*B. caudalis*): it has a single horn above each eye and is coloured grey to brown with a dorsal row of dark square/oval markings. Maximum length more than 50 cm. A "sidewinder", which buries itself in the sand. It inhabits dry, sandy regions of southern Africa.

4. Hornsman or many-horned adder (*B. cornuta*): this snake has 2-7 horn-like scales up to 4.5 mm long above each eye. The colour is grey-brown or reddish with two dorsal rows of large and two lateral rows of smaller, dark spots with white edges. Maximum length 60 cm. The habitat is rocky mountainsides and sandy areas. The western subspecies (*B. c. cornuta*) occurs in southern Namibia and the western Cape; the eastern subspecies (*B. c. albanica*), which has smaller horns, occurs in the southern Cape; a third subspecies, the plain mountain adder (*B. c. inornata*), lacks horns and inhabits two small areas in the Cape. The maximum length is 34 cm.

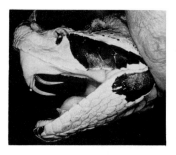 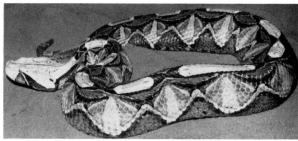

Figure 12. Gaboon viper (*Bitis gabonica*) (photos © Dr. D.A. Warrell).
12a. West African subspecies (*B.g. rhinoceros*) showing fangs.   **12b.** Eastern race (*B.g. gabonica*). There are two dark subocular triangles.

5. Gaboon viper or adder or forest puff adder (*B. gabonica*) (Figure 12): this is one of the heaviest venomous snakes in the world. It has "nose horn" scales. The colouring is brilliant, like an oriental carpet. There is a dorsal series of pale brownish or yellowish elongated rectangles with rounded or pointed ends, with dark triangles at their anterior and posterior ends. The flanks bear a complicated series of lozenge-shaped yellow or pale brownish areas edged with dark scales and separated by brown, purple and yellow areas. The belly is yellowish blotched with brown or black. The dorsum of the head is pale apart from a narrow, dark, median line. The western race (*B. g. rhinoceros*) has one dark sub-ocular triangle (Figure 12a), whereas the eastern race (*B. g. gabonica*) has two (Figure 12b). This species inhabits rain forest and forest fringes up to an altitude of more than 2000 metres. It is sluggish, nocturnal and inoffensive. Maximum length exceeds 2 metres, with a girth of 470 mm and fangs 55 mm long. A specimen 1.8 metres long weighed 11.4 kg. It inhabits East, West and Central Africa and the eastern part of southern Africa (eastern Zimbabwe, Mozambique and coastal northeastern South Africa).

6. Rhinoceros-horned, nose-horned viper or riverjack (*B. nasicornis*): a heavily built snake with long "nose-horn" scales. Its overall pattern is similar to that of *B gabonica*, but with darker colours and more red and blue. The dorsum of the head bears a large dark arrow-shaped marking. Maximum length 1.2 metres. It inhabits rain forest of West and Central Africa, extending into western Kenya. It is often found in trees.

7. Péringuey's desert or side-winding adder (*B. peringueyi*): this is a small, orangey brown snake with a series of dark dorsal spots, some with pale centres. Maximum length 29 cm. It is found in the deserts of coastal Namibia and south Angola.

8. Namaqua dwarf adder (*B. schneideri*): this is the smallest venomous snake with a maximum length of 28 cm. It is pale greyish or brown with three rows of dark dorsal markings with pale centres. Its eyes are on the top of the head, close together. It inhabits

dunes of southern Namibia and northern Namaqualand.

9. Kenyan horned viper (*B. worthingtoni*): this is a small, stoutly-built snake with prominent supraorbital "horns". Its colour is usually darkish-brown or olive with two lighter undulating lines along each flank. There is a dorsal series of dark triangular blobs and a dark arrow-shaped marking on the back of the head. Length about 300 mm. It is predominantly terrestrial and occurs in east central Kenya and the Rift Valley above an altitude of 1500 metres.

3. African night adders (genus *Causus*)

The five species of endemic African snakes in this genus are small and nocturnal. They differ from other African viperine snakes in having large smooth symmetrical scales on top of the head, a circular pupil, relatively short fangs, unusually long venom glands extending into the neck and little demarcation between the head and neck. Bites have been reported by all the species except *C. bilineatus* from Central Africa.

1. Snouted night adder (*C. defilippi*): it has a relatively thick body and pointed upturned snout. The colour is brownish, greenish or greyish with a prominent dark V-shaped mark on the top of the head and a dorsal series of dark rhomboidal or "V"-shaped markings extending to dark stripes on the flanks. Maximum length 44 cm. It is found in Eastern Africa from Kenya, south to Natal.

2. Forest, small, Lichtenstein's or olive green night adder (*C. lichtensteini*): the colour is green, olive, yellowish or grey without a marking on the head. There is a "V" on neck and dorsal black chevrons. Maximum length 58 cm. It inhabits rain forests of western Central Africa, southeastern Sudan, Uganda and western Kenya.

3. Western rhombic night adder (*C. maculatus*) (Figure 13): the colour is greyish, brownish or olive green with large dark edged V-marking on its head and neck. The dorsal pattern is of darkish rhomboidal marks with narrow jagged extensions down the flanks. Maximum length 65 cm. It inflates its body and hisses in defence. It inhabits savanna and forest clearings of West and western Central Africa.

4. Green or velvety-green night adder (*C. resimus*): a vivid grass green snake with yellowish or whitish belly and upturned snout. Maximum length 75 cm. It inhabits moist, warm, low-lying localities up to an altitude of 2000 metres, from Nigeria, east to Somalia and south to Zaire and Mozambique.

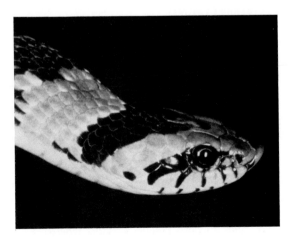

Figure 13. Snouted night adder (*Causus defilippi*). Specimen from Zimbabwe (photo © Dr. D.A. Warrell).

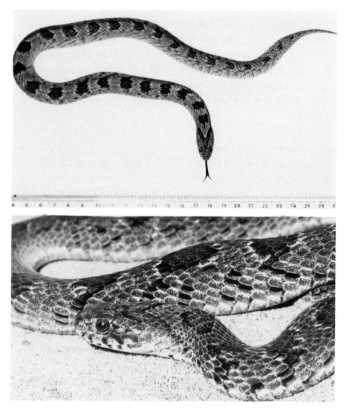

Figure 14. Night adders (photos © Dr. D.A. Warrell).
Upper: Western rhombic night adder (*Causus maculatus*). Specimen from
Nigeria. **Lower:** Eastern rhombic night adder (*C. rhombeatus*).

5. Eastern rhombic night adder (*C. rhombeatus*) (Figure 14): there is a solid dark "V" marking on the head and dark, white-edged dorsal rhomboid markings. Maximum length more than 90 cm. It inhabits savanna throughout sub-Saharan Africa, eastern Nigeria, south of Eritrea through Central Africa and in the eastern half of Southern Africa.

4. Sand or desert vipers (genus *Cerastes*)

The genus contains three species of relatively small, thick-bodied side-winding desert snakes with markedly keeled and serrated scales, found in North Africa and the Middle East.

1. Horned or desert viper (*C. cerastes* - formerly known as *C. cornutus* and *Aspis cerastes*): a whitish, greyish, yellow or brown snake with a dorsal series of paired or confluent darkish blobs and three dark spots on the cheeks. The distinctive supraorbital "horns", up to 5-6 mm long, are sometimes absent in males and females. Maximum length 92 cm. It inhabits the Sahara Desert from Morocco east to Israel, Egypt, Sudan and southwestern Arabia.

2. Gasperetti's horned or desert viper (*C. gasperettii*) (Figure 15): it is very similar to *C. cerastes*, but the head is broader and flatter and the cheek markings are less prominent. Maximum length 86 cm. It is found in the deserts of the Arabian Peninsula, west into Israel and east to western Iran.

3. Sahara desert viper (*C. vipera*) (also known as *Aspis vipera*): a yellowish or pinkish snake with dorsal pairs or alternating brownish spots. There is no supraocular "horn". Maximum length 49 cm. It is found throughout the Sahara Desert from Morocco and Mauritania, east to Egypt and Israel.

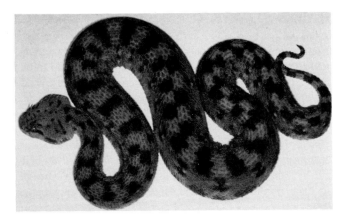

Figure 15. Gasperetti's horned or desert viper (*Cerastes gasperettii*). Specimen from Saudi Arabia (photo © Dr. D.A. Warrell).

5. Saw-scaled or carpet vipers (genus *Echis*)

This genus of snakes of great medical importance is extensively distributed, except in arid desert and mountains, throughout the North of Africa, from Senegal in the west, the Mediterranean coast in the north, the Tana River in Kenya in the south, throughout the Middle East and western Asia north as far as the Aral Sea and throughout the Indian subcontinent including Sri Lanka. In the 1970s, only two species (*E. carinatus* and *E. coloratus*) were recognised and it was appropriate to describe *E. carinatus* as the most important species of snake in the world from the medical point of view. However, since then, a number of new species have been created and, in the recent taxonomic revision by Cherlin and Borkin,[5,6] 12 species are recognised in three subgenera. However, there is still uncertainty about the status of some of these "species" and for the purposes of this account, two West African species will be discussed: *E. ocellatus* and *E. leucogaster* (which includes Cherlin's *A. .a arenicola* and the southern population of his *E. a. leucogaster*); one North and East African and a southwest Arabian species: *E. pyramidum* (including the northern population of Cherlin's *E. a. leucogaster* and his *E. varia* and *E. khosatzkii*); one Middle Eastern species: *E coloratus* (Cherlin's *E. froenatus*) and one southeast Arabian species, *E. sochureki*. Other species described from small areas within this region, *E. jogeri*, *E. megalocephalus* and *E. hughesi*, have not been reported to be responsible for envenoming in humans.

Echis are relatively small, slender-bodied snakes with overlapping keeled scales. The scales on the flanks have serrated keels so that when the snake rubs its coils together when irritated, a rasping sound is produced.

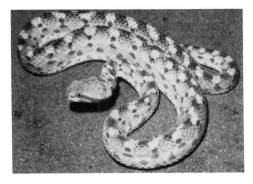

Figure 16. Burton's carpet viper (*Echis coloratus*) (photo © Dr. D.A. Warrell).

1. Burton's carpet viper (*E. coloratus*) (Figures 16, 17): the colouring is variable; ground colour grey, brown, blue or pink with a series of large, pale, oval patches along the dorsum with dark edges connected to a row of dark spots on each flank. Maximum length more than 80 cm. It is found in rocky, boulder-strewn sites on hard ground up to an altitude of 1500 metres in Egypt (east of the Nile), Israel, Jordan, mountainous areas of western Arabia, south to Hadramawt and east to Riyadh, and in Oman from Musandam south to Dhofar.

2. White bellied carpet viper (*E. leucogaster*): the colour and dorsal pattern resemble *E. pyramidum*. The undulating pale line on the flanks is usually incomplete producing a series of inverted "U"-shaped or crescentic marks either side of the dorsal series of pale patches which sometimes form a zig-zag pattern as in *E. sochureki*. The belly is pure white. Maximum length 87 cm. It is found in semi-desert and Sudan savanna, in Mauritania, Senegal, Burkina Faso, northeastern Nigeria, Niger and the Hoggar Mountains of Algeria.

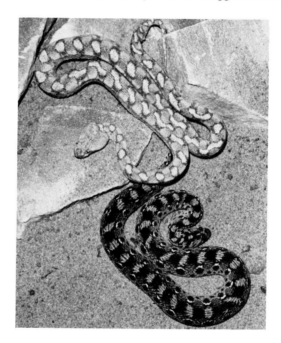

Figure 17. **Upper:** Burton's carpet viper (E. coloratus). Specimen from Israel. **Lower:** West African ocellated carpet viper (E. ocellatus). Specimen from Nigeria.(photos © Dr. D.A. Warrell).

3. West African or ocellated carpet viper (*E. ocellatus*) (Figures 17, 18): a reddish brown snake with pale oval or rhomboidal dorsal markings connected by a dark median band and flanked by white spots ("eyes") bordered with black scales. The belly is white, heavily spotted with black. Maximum length more than 70 cm. This species can be confused with the egg-eating snake (*Dasypeltis scabra*) which mimics its colour, pattern and coiling and rasping defensive display, and the western cat or tiger snake (*Telescopus variegatus*) which occurs in the Sudan and Guinea savanna of West Africa from Senegal to Chad, the Central African Republic, Cameroon and possibly western Sudan.

4. Egyptian carpet viper (*E. pyramidum*): the colour is greyish, brownish or reddish brown (*E. p. aliaborri*) with white dorsal oval markings connected by a dark band and flanked by a more or less complete pale undulating line. The belly is pale. Maximum length 85 cm. It occurs in northeast Algeria, Tunisia (Figure 20), the coast of western Libya, Egypt, the Sudan, Ethiopia, Somalia and the northern half of Kenya (Figure 19) and in southwest Arabia, east to the Hadramawt and in Dhofar.

5. Sochurek's saw-scaled viper (*E. sochureki*) (Figure 21): a reddish brown snake with a dorsal series of pale, dark-edged spots, sometimes connected to form a zig-zag. There is an incomplete, undulating pale line along the flanks. The pattern may be indistinct and the overall colour almost uniform. Maximum length about 62 cm. It occurs in the northeastern tip of the Arabian Peninsula from north of Dhofar to the Musandam Peninsula, the eastern United Arab Emirates and Masirah Island, from sea level to 500 metres' elevation. It is rarely found far from water and some vegetation.

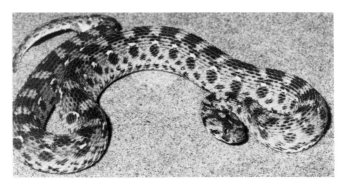

Figure 18. West African ocellated carpet viper (*E. ocellatus*). Specimen from Nigeria (photo © Dr. D.A. Warrell).

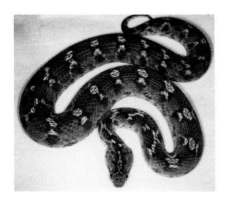

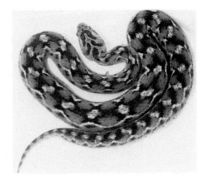

Figure 19. Kenyan carpet viper (*E. pyramidum leakeyi*). Specimen from Kenya (photo © Dr. D.A. Warrell).

Figure 20. *Echis "pyramidum"*. Specimen from Tunisia (courtesy of Dr. Adrian Gillissen, Bochum).

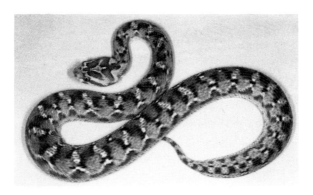

Figure 21. Sochurek's saw-scaled viper (*E. sochureki*) (photo © Dr. D.A. Warrell).

6. Field's or false-horned viper (*Pseudocerastes persicus*)

Colouring generally greyish or brownish with four series of dark spots, the dorsal pair often joined to form cross bands. There is a horn composed of several overlapping scales above each eye. The head is very broad. Maximum length 89 cm. It is found in Egypt, Israel, Jordan, northern Saudi Arabia, the mountains of Oman (and in Iran, Afghanistan and Pakistan).

7. Typical old world vipers (genus *Vipera*)

1. Bornmueller's viper (*V. bornmuelleri*): the ground colour is greyish or brownish with a darker dorsal pattern of short cross bars sometimes edged with white, either meeting at the vertebral line or alternating, and a line of smaller spots on the flanks. The belly is greyish with fine speckling. There is a dark postocular stripe. Maximum length 80 cm. It is found between altitudes of 1400 and 2000 metres in restricted areas of Lebanon, Syria and Israel.

2. Lataste's or snub-nosed viper (*V. latasti*): the colour is greyish or reddish brown with a dorsal pattern of connected grey or brown, black-edged rhomboids connected and sometimes coalescing to produce a zig-zag. On the flanks are darkish blobs in line with the recesses of the dorsal pattern. The snout is upturned. In North Africa, there are two species:

V. l. monticola (regarded by some as a separate species *L. monticola*) is found only in the high Atlas Mountains of Morocco (Troubkal) at altitudes of between 2200 and 4000 metres. Average length 60 cm.

V. l. gaditana occurs in Morocco at altitudes below 1500 metres and along the Algerian and Tunisian coast. Maximum length 40 cm.

Both species are nocturnal and climb well. They inhabit dry, rocky, wooded or open country.

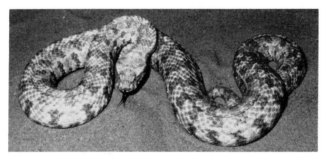

Figure 22. Levantine viper (*Vipera (Macrovipera) lebetina*) (photo © Dr. D.A. Warrell).

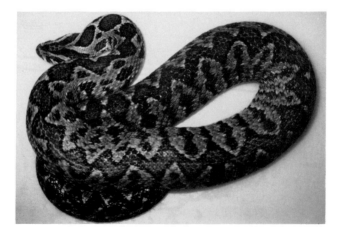

Figure 23. Palestine viper (*Vipera palaestinae*). Specimen from Israel (photo © Dr. D.A. Warrell)

3. Levantine, Levant, Lebetine or blunt-nosed viper (*V. (Macrovipera) lebetina*) (Figure 22): this snake is greyish or reddish with two rows of black or brown dorsal spots which may alternate or coalesce to produce a zig-zag stripe. A series of smaller, darkish spots is distributed along the flanks. There is a "V" marking on the head. In desert areas the markings may be absent or indistinct and the general colour is palish brown. Maximum length 1.5 metres. It inhabits dry rocky areas of North Africa, the Middle East and beyond. There are two subspecies in the region:

V. l. deserti (regarded by some as a separate species *V. (Macrovipera) mauritanica*) occurring in Algeria, south of the Atlas Mountains, Tunisia and Libya.

V. l. obtusa occurring in the Middle East: Israel, Lebanon, Syria, Iraq and elsewhere.

4. Palestine viper (*V. palaestinae*) (Figure 23): the ground colour is grey, yellowish or reddish with a dorsal zig-zag pattern of dark reddish brown edged with black and outside that white. There are several rows of dark spots on the flanks which may coalesce into vertical stripes. The dorsal pattern may break up into separate rhomboid blotches. There is a dark "V" shaped mark on the top of the head. Maximum length more than 1.3 metres and weight more than 1.5 kg. It inhabits agricultural areas in Syria, Jordan, Israel and Lebanon.

III. VENOMS OF AFRICAN AND MIDDLE EASTERN SNAKES

Snake venoms contain a rich variety of enzymes (proteases, phospholipases etc.), non-enzymatic polypeptide toxins (post-synaptic neurotoxins, cardiotoxins, sarafotoxins etc.), amino acids, biogenic amines, carbohydrates, lipids, nucleosides and nucleotides and metals (see Chapter 24). Most of these components have no obvious role in the pathogenesis of envenoming in human patients. This discussion will concentrate on those constituents of the venoms of African and Middle Eastern snakes which seem to contribute to the clinical manifestations of envenoming in humans.

A. COLUBRIDAE

The venoms of the dangerous African colubrids, *D. typus* and *Thelotornis* sp., have low intravenous mouse median lethal doses (LD$_{50}$) of 0.07 and 1.23 mg/kg respectively. Both venoms contain enzymes which activate prothrombin and possibly Factor X which explains the disseminated intravascular coagulation with deposition of microthrombi observed in human victims of envenoming. A human victim of *D. typus* showed activation of the alternative complement pathway. The venoms of a number of other African colubrid snakes such as the Natal green snake (*Philothamnus natalensis*) demonstrate powerful procoagulant activity which, in unusual circumstances, might prove clinically significant. Nothing is known about the venoms of Malpolon species.

B. ATRACTASPIDIDAE

Lethal toxicity (mouse iv LD$_{50}$) of the venom of burrowing asps varies from 0.075 (*A. engaddensis*) to more than 3 mg/kg (*A. micropholis*)[7]. The venoms of at least two species contain sarafotoxins, 21 amino acid peptides which are homologous to the endothelins found in vertebrate endothelium. So far, five sarafotoxins (SRTX A-C) have been isolated and characterised from *E. engaddensis* venom and one (bibrotoxin) from the venom of *A bibroni*. Sarafotoxins are potent coronary artery vasoconstrictors leading to myocardial ischaemia, they decrease atrioventricular conduction but have a powerfully inotropic effect on the heart. These effects explain ECG changes resembling Printzmetal's angina and AV block with cardiovascular collapse in human victims of envenoming by these species. The venom of *A. microlepidota*, a species which resembles *A. engaddensis* morphologically and overlaps its range in the Middle East, lacks sarafotoxins. Envenomed patients show no haemostatic disturbances; the venom contains no procoagulant activity but a haemorrhagin was demonstrable in mice. Necrotic activity has been demonstrated experimentally and is one of the principal clinical effects of the venom. Despite earlier suggestions of neurotoxicity, *A. engaddensis* venom showed no activity on conventional nerve muscle preparations.

C. ELAPIDAE

Clinically, the most common and important effect of elapid envenoming in Africa is, perhaps surprisingly, local tissue necrosis rather than neurotoxicity. The mechanism of local necrosis resulting from elapid and viper bites may be different. Elapid venoms are generally less rich in enzymes, particularly proteases, thought to be responsible for tissue damage following viper bites. Necrotic effects of bites by the African spitting cobras could, however, be explained by the 60-70 amino acid polypeptides known as cytotoxins or in some cases cardiotoxins and to phospholipases A_2 (myotoxins). Polypeptide cytotoxins/cardiotoxins are confined to the venoms of *Naja* and *Hemachatus*. Venoms of African "spitting cobras" also have a locally cytotoxic effect when applied to the cornea. There is not yet a clear correlation between the composition of elapid venoms and the incidence of local necrosis after their bites. The dose of venom injected may be an important variable. Cobra venom factor (which is probably the cobra's own C_{3b}), which activates the complement system by the alternative pathway, is present in the venoms of *Naja* species and *Hemachatus*. Complement activation could contribute to pathological effects including tissue damage[8]. African elapid venoms generally lack significant antihaemolytic activity but the venom of *N. nigricollis* contains a PLA_2-like anticoagulant and there is defective clot retraction *in vitro*.

Elapid venoms are best known for their neurotoxic activity. Among African and Middle Eastern elapids, the following classes of neurotoxins have been identified.
1. Post-synaptic "alpha-toxins". "Long" (70-74 amino acids) and/or "short" (60-62 residues) neurotoxins have been found in the venoms of mambas (*D. jamesoni, D. polylepis, D. viridis*), cobras (*N. haje, N. melanoleuca, N. mossambica, N. nigricollis* and *N. nivea*) and the desert black cobra (*W. aegyptia*). Surprisingly, the venoms of African spitting cobras (*N. nigricollis* etc.) do not appear to be neurotoxic in humans.
2. Pre-synaptic neurotoxins: (a) Phospholipase A_2 toxins prevent release of acetylcholine from the presynaptic nerve membrane. They are found in venoms of *N. mossambica* and *N. nigricollis*, but appear to have little or no neurotoxic activity in humans; (b) Dendrotoxins, containing 59 amino acids, which block potassium channels in nerve membranes and hence facilitate the release of neurotransmitters. They are unique to mamba venoms (*D. angusticeps, D. polylepis* and *D. viridis*); (c) Fasciculins ("angusticeps-type" toxins) are also unique to mamba venoms. Fasciculins from the venoms of *D. angusticeps* and *D. polylepis* inhibit cholinesterases and so potentiate the effects of the neurotransmitter acetylcholine causing generalised muscle fasciculation.

D. VIPERIDAE

The principal clinical features of envenoming by Africa and Middle Eastern vipers are haemostatic disturbances, hypotension and local tissue necrosis.

1. Haemostatic effects[9,10]

Fibrinogen clotting activity has been found in the venoms of the gaboon viper (*B. gabonica*) ("Gabonase"), which splits off fibrinopeptides A and B from fibrinogen and also activates Factor XIII, and *Cerastes vipera* ("Cerastobin"). Ecarin, a metalloproteinase from the venom of "*Echis carinatus*", activates prothrombin. Venoms of "*E. carinatus*", *E. coloratus* and *Cerastes cerastes* activate Factor X. Procoagulant activity has also been demonstrated in the venoms of *C. rhombeatus, Pseudocerastes persicus* and *Vipera lebetina*.

E. sochureki venom activates protein C. *C. rhombeatus* venom contains a serine protease which inactivates antithrombin III. Venoms of *B. gabonica, C. cerastes* and "*E. carinatus*" have direct fibrino(gen)olytic activity. Echistatin and Echicetin from "*E. carinatus*" venom inhibit platelet activation and the venom of *B arietans* contains botrocetin-like activity which causes platelet aggregation. Echistatin also inhibits bone resorption and may be useful in the treatment of osteoporosis. Echis venoms also contain a fibrinogenolysin. Haemorrhagins such as the zinc metalloproteinase from "*E. carinatus*" venom damage vascular endothelium. Haemorrhagin activity is also exhibited by venoms of *E. coloratus, B. gabonica, B. arietans* and *Causus rhombeatus*.

2. Cardiovascular effects

Viper venoms can cause shock (fall in blood pressure) by increasing vascular permeability leading to hypovolaemia, by direct effects on the heart (*B. gabonica, B. arietans*), by splanchnic vasodilatation (*B. arietans*) and by autopharmacological release of vasodilators such as bradykinin (*V. palaestinae*).

The tissue necrosis caused by viper venoms is usually attributed to their abundant proteolytic enzymes and phospholipases A_2. Neurotoxicity has been observed clinically in patients envenomed by the berg adder (*B. atropos*) and Tunisian "*E. pyramidum*". PLA_2 neurotoxins have been found in the venoms of the horned adder (*B. caudalis*) and *B. atropos*. A neurotoxic polypeptide "viperotoxin" from the venom of the Palestine viper (*V. palaestinae*) is said to cause circulatory failure by acting directly on medullary centres.

IV. EPIDEMIOLOGY OF SNAKEBITE IN AFRICA AND THE MIDDLE EAST/ARABIAN PENINSULA

In their famous review of "Snakebite mortality in the world", Swaroop and Grab concluded that it was difficult to make even an approximate estimate for Africa but that an annual total of snakebite deaths of 400-1000 seemed likely[11].

Because this figure was based on reporting by hospitals to national centres, it was certainly an underestimate. For example, they record 166 snakebites and nine deaths from the northern region of Nigeria during the period 1947 to 1952, yet between 1964 and 1969, 953 bites and 50 deaths were reported by one mission hospital (Bambur) and its network of dispensaries in Muri Division, a community of about a quarter of a million people in this northern region[12]. This disparity is explained by the fact that snakebite is largely a problem of rural areas, where hospitals and dispensaries tend to be understaffed and overworked and find it difficult regularly to provide accurate returns. Even reliable hospital returns will underestimate the problem of snakebite in the community because, in most parts of the world, many snakebite victims will prefer traditional herbal methods of treatment. Pugh et al[13] using a questionnaire method found that in Malumfashi, also in northern Nigeria, only 8.5% of 106 victims of presumed spitting cobra bite had been treated in hospital. In this area, the apparent incidence of snakebite based on hospital attendances was 1 per 100,000 per year, whereas the true incidence revealed by the survey was 15-20 per 100,000 per year. Pugh and Theakston[14] used enzyme immunoassay to survey the prevalence of venom antibodies in a population, but this technique is now known to produce many false positives in sera from rural communities in the tropics[15]. By unwarranted extrapolating from snakebite data obtained from a few areas of notoriously high incidence they produced the preposterously unlikely figure of 23,000 snakebite deaths per year in the West African savanna region.

In Kilifi district, on the coast of Kenya, few patients are admitted to hospital with snakebite but a population survey revealed that there are 15 adults deaths from snakebite per 100,000 population per year (Snow R, personal communication). Before the advent of reliable venom antigen detection by EIA[15,16], precise identification of the biting snake was possible only if the snake had been killed and brought to hospital. Inferring the species diagnosis from the clinical manifestations has proved misleading. In Chapman's classical study of 1067 cases of snakebite in Natal, South Africa (1957-63), patients with local envenoming were classified as viperid bites (mainly *B. arietans*) because, at that time, it had not been widely recognised that spitting cobras (*N. mossambica*) could produce similar effects[17].

A. INCIDENCE OF SNAKEBITE IN AFRICAN COUNTRIES

Precise figures for the incidence of snakebite and resulting morbidity and mortality are not available for any country in this region but some idea of the relative importance of snakebite can be gained from the literature. The highest incidence of snakebite is in the West African savanna region where saw-scaled or carpet vipers (*Echis*), spitting cobras (*N. nigricollis* and possibly *N. katiensis*) and puff adders (*B. arietans*) are most often involved. In the Ivory Coast, the estimated annual mortality from snakebite is 191[18]. In northern Ghana, the incidence of bites (predominantly by *E ocellatus*) is 86 per 100,000 per year with 24 deaths per 100,000 per year[19]. Among rubber plantation workers in Liberia, the incidence of symptomatic snakebites was 420 per 100,000 in field workers and 170 per 100,000 per year in factory workers. Most bites were caused by night adders (*C maculatus*)[20]. In Muri Division, northeastern Nigeria, it was estimated that 120 bites and eight deaths occurred per 100,000 population per year, mainly caused by *E ocellatus*[12]. Echis bites are particularly common in the valleys of the Niger and Benue Rivers and northern areas of Nigeria and Cameroon. In Burkina Fasso, 3,576 snakebites were reported in 1968 (Roman 1980) and, in one sector of the country, the incidence was 40 per 100,000 per year[21]. Echis is responsible for most snakebites in northern Sudan, Somalia (Hargeisa), Eritrea, Ethiopia, Djibouti and in northern Kenya (Turkana and Wajir)[12,22]. In East Africa, the only reliable figures for snakebite mortality are those referred to above from Snow's study in Kilifi, Kenya. In this area, most serious bites are attributed to *B arietans*, *N nigricollis* and, in the few cases of neurotoxic envenoming, to mambas (*D. polylepis* and *D. angusticeps*). In Central Africa, the incidence of bites was estimated at 20 per 100,000 per year in urban Brazzaville and 125 and 430 per 100,000 per year in two rural areas of the Congo[23].

In Zimbabwe, there were hospital records of 995 snakebite cases during the 10 year period 1980-1989 with at least 18 deaths[24]. In Botswana, 108 cases of snakebite were reported in 1980 and 595 in 1982[25]. In South Africa, the incidence of snakebite was estimated as 24 and deaths as 0.35 per 100,000 in Natal[17] and 34 and 0.53 per 100,000 in Kangwane in the Transvaal[26] with a mortality of about 2%[27]. Throughout Eastern and Southern Africa, *B. arietans* is thought to be responsible for most cases of severe envenoming followed by spitting cobras (*N. nigricollis*, *N. mossambica*). Mambas, especially *D polylepis*, are responsible for relatively few bites but with a high case fatality. Bites by *Causus* and *Atractaspis* species are common in some areas but rarely prove serious.

In the Middle East, few snakebite cases are reported. In Israel, bites by *E. coloratus* and *V. palaestinae* are most often mentioned with a few reports of severe envenoming by *A. engaddensis* and rare accounts of proven envenoming by *W. aegyptia*. In the Arabian peninsula, *Cerastes* species are the venomous snakes most often seen, but *Echis* species (*E. coloratus, E. pyramidum* and *E. c. sochureki*) are thought to be responsible for most serious bites with sporadic reports of severe envenoming by *A. engaddensis/microlepidota*[28]. Snakebite appears to be most common in southwestern Arabia and Oman. In Israel, 300-500 bites are reported each year with a mortality of 4-8%[29].

B. SEASONAL VARIATION IN INCIDENCE

In most countries, snakebite incidence increases with the start of the rainy season or in association with the increased agricultural activity anticipating that event. In northern Ghana and northern Nigeria, snakebites increase in about March and April just before the start of the rains. In Southern Africa the peak incidence is from October to March. Snakebites decrease when the temperature falls. The incidence of snakebite is determined by the diurnal and seasonal activity patterns of humans and snakes. Most snakebites occur during daylight hours or shortly after dusk as people walk to or from the fields. More than 50% of bites by spitting cobras (*N. nigricollis* and *N. mossambica*) occur at night while the victims are asleep in their huts[30,31]. In Africa, more than 80% of bites are inflicted on the feet and legs. Young adult male farmers, herdsmen and hunters and children are the most likely to be bitten. Virtually all the reported cases of severe envenoming by back fanged colubrid snakes (*D. typus* and *Thelotornis* species) have occurred in people who were handling the snakes, such as herpetologists.

V. CLINICAL FEATURES OF SNAKEBITE IN AFRICA AND THE MIDDLE EAST/ARABIAN PENINSULA

Not all patients bitten by venomous snakes, with puncture marks on the skin indicating penetration by the fangs, will develop envenoming. Apart from the effects of injected venom, fear and first aid treatment will determine the symptoms and signs. Anxiety may cause tachycardia, palpitations, trembling, flushing, sweating, a feeling of constriction of the chest and hyperventilation leading to dizziness, faintness, carpopedal spasms and acroparaesthesiae. Tourniquets and constriction bands may produce congested, swollen and even ischaemic limbs; incisions, bleeding and sensory loss; and herbal medicines, vomiting. The earliest symptoms are pain at the site of the bite, which may be intense; pain, swelling, tenderness and inflammation spreading up the bitten limb and tender enlargement of regional lymph nodes. Nausea, vomiting and headache are common symptoms of severe envenoming. Patients envenomed by *Vipera* and *Atractaspis* species and those suffering anaphylactic reactions to venom as a result of previous sensitization may collapse within minutes of the bite and remain unconscious for up to 30 minutes. Associated symptoms include vomiting, colic, diarrhoea, angio-oedema and wheezing.

A. ENVENOMING BY COLUBRIDAE
1. Boomslang (*D typus*) and vine snake (*Thelotornis* species)
The clinical and laboratory effects of bites by these species are indistinguishable. South of the distribution of Echis species in Africa, the finding of incoagulable blood in a snakebite victim strongly suggests envenoming by *D. typus* which appears to bite much more readily than Thelotornis species whose venoms also cause defibrinogenation. Although most reported bites have been on the hands of people attempting to pick up the snakes, bites by *D. typus* have occurred when the snake was touched inadvertently while the victim was climbing a palm tree or when snakes were trodden on in long grass. Characteristically these back fanged snakes attempt to hang on and chew after the bite and may have to be removed forcibly.

Symptoms may develop very soon after the bite or be delayed for 12-48 hours. Persistent bleeding from the fang marks is the earliest symptom. Within a few hours, nausea, vomiting, colicky abdominal pain and headache may develop with bleeding from old and recent wounds such as venepunctures, spontaneous bleeding from the gums, nose and external auditory meatus, haematemesis, rectal bleeding or melaena, subarachnoid and intracranial haemorrhages, haematuria and extensive superficial ecchymoses. Petechial haemorrhages are widespread in serosal cavities, heart, walls of the great vessels and elsewhere. Intravascular haemolysis and microangiopathic haemolysis have been described. Some of the fatal cases died of renal failure from acute tubular necrosis many days after the bite. Local effects of envenoming are usually trivial, but several patients showed some local swelling and one, bitten by *D. typus*, had massive swelling with blood-filled bullae. Local tender lymphadenopathy may develop. Investigations reveal incoagulable blood, defibrinogenation, elevated serum fibrin(ogen) degradation products, severe thrombocytopenia and anaemia.

2. Montpellier snake (*M. monspessulanus*)

Extensive local oedema, local paraesthesia at the site of the bite, lymphangitis, local lymphadenitis and some ill-defined symptoms ("nervous troubles" and "paresis of the affected limb") have been described from Spain and Algiers. One patient developed symptoms of systemic neurotoxic envenoming, ptosis and weakness of the muscles of deglutition and respiration, which resolved within 48 hours.

3. Minor syndromes of colubrid envenoming

At least a dozen other species of colubrid, other than those discussed above, have proved capable of causing mild envenoming. All these species can produce mild local swelling and in some cases inflammation, discoloration, transient local bleeding, pain, smarting, numbness or stiffness at the site of the bite. Lymphangitis with or without tender enlargement of local lymph nodes has been reported after bites by *Coluber rhodorachis, Madagascarophis meridionalis*[4], *Psammophis biseriatus* and *Psammophylax rhombeatus*. Systemic symptoms such as nausea, headache and rigors were described after bites by *Amplorhinus multimaculatus, Psammophis phillipsii* and *Psammophylax tritaeniatus*, and blood clots in the urine after a bite by *Psammophis phillipsii* (S. Durrant, personal communication). The most serious local effects were produced by *Madagascarophis meridionalis*; swelling, bruising, blistering and necrosis of the bitten digit[4].

B. ENVENOMING BY ATRACTASPIDIDAE[34]

1. Burrowing asps (genus *Atractaspis*)

Bites by seven species of Atractaspis have been reported to cause local symptoms such as pain, swelling, blistering, local necrosis, especially when bites are on the fingers of herpetologists who inadvisedly pick up the snakes, and painful lymphadenopathy. Systemic symptoms include fever, nausea, headache, faintness and generalised weakness. Severe life-threatening and fatal symptoms have been described in patients bitten by *A. engaddensis, A. irregularis* and *A. microlepidota*. Some victims of *A. engaddensis* developed nausea, vomiting, diarrhoea, dyspnoea, acute respiratory failure and collapse. ECG abnormalities show evidence of atrioventricular conduction abnormalities (prolonged PR interval) and myocardial ischaemia (ST segment depression or elevation and flattening of the T waves). Deaths have occurred less than 45 minutes after the bite. Prolongation of the prothrombin time (*A. corpulenta* and *A. engaddensis*) and elevated serum alkaline phosphatase and aspartate aminotransferase with abnormal liver histology (*A. engaddensis*) have been described. Patients envenomed by *A. dahomyensis* and *A. microlepidota* in Nigeria showed no haematological, biochemical or haemostatic abnormalities apart from mild peripheral leucocytosis.

2. Natal black snake (*Macrelaps microlepidotus*)

According to Visser and Chapman[32] "complete loss of consciousness and collapse for up to 30 minutes has resulted in the two incidences recorded when the species has inflicted a bite". FitzSimons and Smith reported that a bite by this species produced a severe reaction and that the bite "might have been fatal had the patient not received antivenin and hospital treatment"[33].

C. ENVENOMING BY ELAPIDAE

Bites by the African spitting cobras (*N. katiensis, N. mossambica, N. nigricollis, N. pallida*) cause almost immediate severe local pain and tenderness. Swelling usually develops early and spreads rapidly; blistering may appear at the site of the bite within a few hours and superficial necrosis with "skip" lesions may extend to affect the whole limb. Bites by the other elapids of Africa and the Middle East produce little more than pain and mild local swelling but several species, notably the mambas (*Dendroaspis*), Egyptian cobra (*N. haje*) and Cape cobra (*N. nivea*), can cause severe neurotoxic effects. Early symptoms, before there are objective neurological signs, include vomiting, "heaviness" of the eyelids, blurred vision, paraesthesiae around the mouth, headache and dizziness. Paralysis, first detectable as ptosis and external ophthalmoplegia, may be evident as early as 15 minutes after the bite but can be delayed for 10 hours or more. Progression of neurotoxicity involves the palate, jaws, tongue, vocal cords, neck muscles and muscles of deglutition. Respiratory failure may be precipitated by airway obstruction at this stage, or later after paralysis of intercostal muscles and diaphragm. Patients may develop generalised flaccid paralysis but may retain their ability to flex fingers or toes and so signal their response to questions. Neurotoxic effects are completely reversible, either acutely in response to antivenom or after spontaneous resolution in 1-7 days. It is doubtful whether elapid venoms have central effects in humans and, if their respiratory and circulatory failure is corrected, patients with generalised neurotoxicity will be fully conscious.

1. Snake venom ophthalmia caused by spitting cobras[35]

Venom can be "spat" into the eyes, and onto nasal and buccal membranes from a distance of several metres. There is intense pain in the eye, blepharospasm, palpebral oedema and leucorrhoea. Corneal erosions can be seen by slit lamp or fluorescein examination in more than half of those spat at by *N. nigricollis*. Rarely, venom is absorbed into the anterior chamber, causing hypopyon and anterior uveitis. Secondary infection of corneal abrasions may lead to permanent blinding opacities or panophthalmitis. Venom absorbed through the conjunctivae may spread by the lymphatics and cause transient facial nerve paralysis.

2. Shield nose and coral snakes (genus *Aspidelaps*)

Neurotoxic and fatal envenoming has been reported, very rarely, after bites by shield nosed snakes (*A. scutatus*)[36-38] and western coral snakes (*A. lubricus infuscatus*)[39]. These species are clearly potentially dangerous especially if a large specimen bites a child. Bites by *Aspidelaps scutatus* cause pain, swelling, inflammation and tender enlargement of local lymph glands, all of which are slow to resolve.

3. Water cobras (genus *Boulengerina*)

There are no documented cases of envenoming by water cobras but, in Lake Tanganyika[40] and the Ivindo River of Gabon[41], *B. annulata* has the reputation of inflicting fatal bites on fishermen.

4. Mambas (*Dendroaspis*)
a. Black mamba (D. polylepis)
   Case history
   A 41 year old snake keeper was bitten on the base of the right middle finger by his 3.06 metre long black mamba when he put his hand into the cage. The snake let go immediately,

leaving seven bleeding puncture marks, but after the initial prick there was only mild burning pain. This man, who was a mild asthmatic, had been bitten on a number of occasions by viperid snakes and once by *Thelotornis capensis* but never by elapids. About one minute after the bite he noticed transient tingling of the tip of his tongue and the outside of his lips. While being driven by his wife to hospital he felt lightheaded, noticed tingling all over his body and dull pain in the pit of his stomach, but there was no ptosis and he was able to talk normally. When he arrived at the hospital about 20 minutes after the bite he was sweating profusely. He was unable to get out of the car unaided because his lower limbs were weak. Coordination of his upper arms was impaired and the light seemed brighter than usual. He was moved to the emergency unit by wheelchair and, despite irritating delays, remained calm and was able to talk. About 30 minutes after the bite, he felt nauseated and then vomited. He wanted to urinate but could not do so. He was sweating profusely all over his body. His eyelids felt heavy but he could open his eyes by puckering his brow. The vision was normal. His throat became blocked by thick saliva which was increasingly difficult to cough up and he began to experience difficulty in breathing; the sensation was of tightness of the chest like asthma. He was seen by a consultant surgeon with a special interest in snakebite 40 minutes after the bite and was able to discuss the problem. At this stage there was pain and swelling of the whole bitten finger. His skin was cold to touch and had the appearance of gooseflesh; his conjunctivae and eyelids were congested and he was unable to open his mouth fully and protrude his tongue. Intravenous infusion of 20 ml of antivenom was started 1¾ hours after the bite and the patient was moved to the intensive care unit. He was still conscious, retched occasionally and felt alternately hot and cold. About 42 minutes after the start of antivenom treatment he developed urticaria over his back. Chest tightness increased, he experienced rigors and retched repeatedly, and his level of consciousness deteriorated. About four hours after the bite, he was sedated, intubated and, 20 minutes later, mechanical ventilation was begun. Five and a half hours after the bite 70 ml of antivenom was infused and, 20 hours after the bite, 50 ml of antivenom was given. Twelve hours after the bite he developed some pulmonary oedema; 18 hours after the bite he felt considerably better but developed diffuse fasciculations. He was extubated after 40 hours' mechanical ventilation. At this stage he felt well apart from slight residual tenderness in the bone near the site of the bite. About three days after the antivenom treatment he developed itching over the back which persisted for three days; he then made a complete recovery (S. Durrant, personal communication; see also[42]).

This case report illustrates the rapid development of life-threatening neurotoxicity following bites by what is justifiably the most dreaded African venomous snake. There is a high risk of severe envenoming after *D. polylepis* bite, even if only one fang penetrates the skin, but cases of proven *D. polylepis* bites with negligible local swelling and no neurotoxic symptoms have been described. Some patients describe severe local pain but local swelling is usually mild or absent and local necrosis was seen in only one patient and was attributable to injection of antivenom into the finger pulp. Early symptoms include paraesthesiae, a strange taste in the mouth, nausea, retching, vomiting, abdominal pain, diarrhoea, sweating, salivation, "gooseflesh" and conjunctival congestion. Neurotoxic symptoms may develop as early as 15 minutes after the bite or they may be delayed for seven hours or more. They include ptosis, diplopia, dysphagia, slurred speech and dyspnoea attributable to respiratory muscle paralysis. Skeletal muscles may contract involuntarily or fasciculate. Paralytic episodes may recur for two days or more after the bite despite antivenom treatment. Because these large snakes can rear high off the ground before striking, bites may be inflicted on the upper part of the body, but in most of the published cases, bites were either on the hands of people attempting to handle the snakes or on the lower limbs. The seven cases attributed to this species by Campbell all died[17], but in a series of 20 cases at Shongwe Hospital, Kangwane, South Africa, including eight in which the dead snake was brought and identified, only one patient died (in the ambulance on the way to hospital)[26].

b. Eastern green mamba (D. angusticeps)

This appears to be the least venomous of the four species of mamba. A number of cases of bites without envenoming have been reported, but there has been at least one fatal case, an 11 year old boy in Natal, South Africa, who was bitten on the face[43]. Local symptoms include mild swelling and pain which may spread up the arm. Local necrosis at the site of the bite has been described. Systemic symptoms include alteration in speech, hyperacusis, sweating, increased salivation, colicky abdominal pain, chest pain and dizziness, together with the usual symptoms of neurotoxic envenoming.

c. Western green mambas (D. jamesonii and D. viridis)

The severity of bites by these species is intermediate between those of *D. polylepis* and *D. angusticeps*. Local swelling may involve the entire limb. Symptoms include vomiting, numbness of the tongue, lower jaws and body, blurred vision, slurring of speech, nausea, epigastric pain, salivation, cold, sweaty skin with "gooseflesh" and fatal respiratory paralysis.

5. African garter snakes (genus *Elapsoidea*)

Bites by these species are extremely rare and there have been no fatalities. Local pain with or without swelling or tender enlargement of regional lymph nodes has been described after bites by *E. loveridgei*, *E. sundevallii* and *E. semiannulata*.

6. Rinkhals (*H. haemachatus*)

In a series of eight patients bitten by this species, two developed mild local swelling and bruising and five systemic symptoms: drowsiness, nausea, vomiting, vertigo, mild pyrexia and atrial fibrillation in one elderly patient. Neurotoxic symptoms were seen in only one of these: diplopia with some degree of dyspnoea[44]. FitzSimons described immediate local tingling and burning, followed within half a minute by tightness of the throat, paralysis of the tongue and vocal cords, nausea, blurring of vision, weakness of the arms and legs and, two minutes later, unconsciousness which lasted for four hours[45]. When he recovered consciousness, he noticed chest tightness, dyspnoea, blurred vision and vomiting. A two year old child was reported to have died of respiratory paralysis two hours after being bitten by a rinkhals[46]. Spitting of venom into the eyes by the rinkhals causes the symptoms described above for spitting cobras. The incidence of corneal abrasions, secondary infections and blindness after these accidents has not been investigated.

7. Spotted harlequin snake (*Homoroselaps lacteus*)

Bites are very rare, but in two cases there was mild to severe local swelling, mild (presumably local) bleeding, lymphangitis and tender lymphadenopathy resolving in 3-4 days and headache lasting 24 hours[39].

8. Cobras (genus *Naja*)

Bites by the four species of spitting cobras (*N. katiensis, N. mossambica, N. nigricollis* and *N. pallida*) cause severe local envenoming: swelling, blistering and necrosis with general symptoms of systemic envenoming but rarely if ever neurotoxic signs. *N. haje, N. melanoleuca* and *N. nivea* cause neurotoxic envenoming with variable amounts of local swelling without necrosis at the site of the bite.

"Neurotoxic cobras"
a. Egyptian cobra (N. haje)[47]

This species is widely distributed in Africa and the Middle East but bites are uncommon. There is local pain and swelling which may involve more than half the bitten limb and be associated with blistering at the site of the bite but it resolves without necrosis. Vomiting is an early systemic symptom. Neurotoxic symptoms develop within a few hours, but transient ptosis was first noticed 20 hours after the bite in one mildly envenomed patient. Deaths have occurred 6-16 hours after bites by large snakes despite the use of antivenom and mechanical ventilation. Many snake charmers and even members of their audiences have been killed by this species.

b. Forest cobra (N. melanoleuca)

This species is reclusive and reluctant to bite and scarcely more than a dozen cases of bites have been reported. In at least four there was no envenoming, but five died between one hour and three days after the bite. Symptoms included local swelling, tender regional nodes, giddiness, ptosis, slurring of speech, muscular spasms, dyspnoea, tremor of the extremities and fever.

c. Cape cobra (N. nivea)

Some ten cases of envenoming, one fatal, have been reported. Local symptoms were pain, numbness, swelling and enlargement of regional lymph nodes. Systemic symptoms included nausea, vomiting, dry mouth or excessive salivation, sweating, headache, fever and dizziness. Early neurotoxic symptoms were visual disturbance (as early as 30 minutes after the bite), a feeling of heaviness of the eyelids, ptosis, external ophthalmoplegia and slurring of speech. Respiratory weakness can develop as early as two hours or up to 12 hours after the bite and, in two cases, mechanical ventilation was necessary for 4½ and 7 days despite antivenom treatment[44,48,49].

"Cytotoxic cobras"
a. N. katiensis

There are no reports of bites by this small West African spitting cobra.

b. Black necked spitting cobra (N. nigricollis)[8,50]

Among 17 cases of proven bites in northern Nigeria, 14 occurred at night. Eleven patients were bitten inside their homes, 10 while they were asleep. All patients complained of feeling pain at the site of the bite immediately. Five began to vomit within six hours of the bite. Signs of local envenoming developed in all cases with swelling of the entire bitten limb or beyond in more than half, local blistering in 60% and local tissue necrosis in 70% (Figure 24). Tissue necrosis usually involves the skin and subcutaneous connective tissues only (Figure 25). The commonest signs of systemic envenoming were leucocytosis, fever and absence of clot retraction in vitro. Classical signs of elapid neurotoxicity were not seen. Evidence of complement activation, principally by the alternative pathway, was found in the majority of patients, and a minority showed biochemical abnormalities suggestive of a transient hepatocellular abnormality. Spontaneous bleeding and failure of clot retraction sugggested a haemostatic defect in some patients. Subspecies of *N. nigricollis* in other parts of Africa (for example, by the "zebra snake" (*N. n. nigricincta*) of northern Namibia and southwestern Angola) can cause just as severe local effects as *N. nigricollis* in West and East Africa. Chronic ulcers at the site of these injuries may eventually show malignant change (Figure 26).

c. Moçambique spitting cobra (N. mossambica)

Despite earlier impressions[30] the clinical effects of *N. mossambica* venom are very similar to those of *N. nigricollis*. Seventeen cases of bites by *N. mossambica*, six of them confirmed by identifying the dead snake, were seen in two hospitals in Zululand[31]. Sixteen of the bites occurred in the patients' homes, 13 while the victims were asleep. Local discoloration or blistering at the site of the bite developing as soon as three hours after the bite, presaging the development of tissue necrosis. Four patients were drowsy and in three of these there was evidence of hypovolaemic shock. No convincing evidence of neurotoxicity was observed. Some more recent case reports have suggested that, in children at least, *N. mossambica* may be capable of causing neurotoxic envenoming[51,52]. However, the evidence is not conclusive. In one patient undoubted neurotoxic symptoms were associated with a tensely-swollen hand, but the snake was not identified and the local effects do not rule out envenoming by *N. haje*[51]. In the other patient who developed extensive necrosis typical of *N. mossambica* envenoming, the neurological symptoms could have been the result of severe hypovolaemic shock[52].

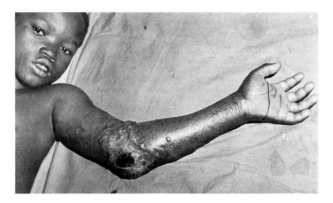

Figure 24. Swelling, blistering and early necrosis in a Nigerian boy bitten on the elbow while sleeping, by a black-necked spitting cobra (*N. nigricollis*) 16 hours previously (photo © Dr. D.A. Warrell)..

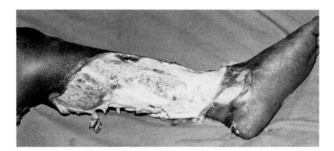

Figure 25. Sloughing of necrotic skin and subcutaneous tissue in a woman bitten eight days earlier by a black-necked spitting cobra (*N. nigricollis*) in Nigeria (photo © Dr. D.A. Warrell)..

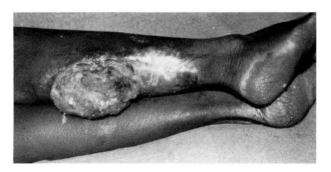

Figure 26. Squamous cell carcinoma arising in a chronic ulcer following a bite by a black-necked spitting cobra (*N. nigricollis*) several years previously (photo © Dr. D.A. Warrell)..

d. Red spitting cobra (N. pallida)
Bites by this species in Kenya have caused fluctuant swelling and local necrosis.

Ophthalmia resulting from "spitting" of venom
a. Black-necked spitting cobra (N. nigricollis)
Thirteen cases were reported from northern Nigeria[35,50,53]. One received venom in both eyes, one in one eye and up one nostril and the others into one eye. In all cases there were symptoms of acute chemical conjunctivitis: intense pain, watering of the eye, spasm and swelling of lids, congestion and oedema of the conjunctivae and cornea and a whitish discharge (Figure 27). Five patients developed nothing more than a simple conjunctivitis but in six there was evidence, by fluorescein staining, slit lamp biomicroscopy or by development of complications, of corneal ulceration. One patient developed hypopyon, suggesting that venom had entered the anterior chamber[53]. One showed signs of anterior uveitis (Figure 28). One presented with a perforating corneal ulcer with gross endophthalmitis requiring enucleation (Figure 29). One patient was found to have a dense opacity causing blindness, the result of having venom spat into that eye five years before. Pugh et al examined 19 patients spat at between six months and 53 years before[13]. Eight had superficial punctate corneal nebulae, two epithelial punctate staining of the lower periphery of the cornea and three others had other keratopathies.

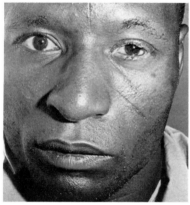

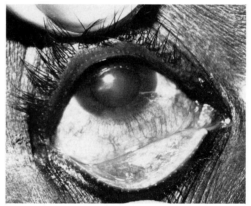

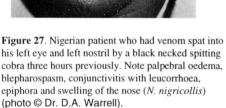

Figure 27. Nigerian patient who had venom spat into his left eye and left nostril by a black necked spitting cobra three hours previously. Note palpebral oedema, blepharospasm, conjunctivitis with leucorrhoea, epiphora and swelling of the nose (*N. nigricollis*) (photo © Dr. D.A. Warrell).

Figure 28. Anterior uveitis (note circumcorneal injection) in a patient who had venom spat into his eye by a black necked spitting cobra (*N. nigricollis*) two days previously. The pupil has been dilated with atropine (photo © Dr. D.A. Warrell).

b. Moçambique spitting cobra (N. mossambica)
Lath and Patel (1984) examined 34 patients in Livingstone, Zambia[54]. Two-thirds had been spat into both eyes, a third had evidence of superficial keratitis and three patients had iritis. In Zimbabwe, 37 cases developed no corneal ulceration or any other form of morbidity, but in another case there were numerous corneal ulcers[55].

c. Red spitting cobra (N. pallida)
In one case, symptoms were similar to those described for *N. nigricollis*.

9. Burrowing cobras (genus *Paranaja*) and tree cobras (genus *Pseudohaje*)
No bites have been reported.

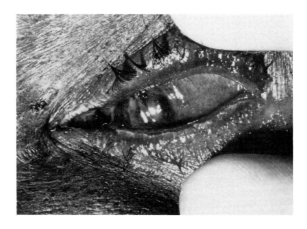

Figure 29. Panophthalmitis in a spitting cobra injury incurred two weeks previously and not treated (photo © Dr. D.A. Warrell).

10. Black desert cobra (*Walterinnesia aegyptia*)

This snake has a bad reputation in some parts of its range. In Iraq, two fatal cases were ascribed to this species; one because the snake was said to be black and in the other because the victim developed paralysis of the legs[56]. However, a recent report of four proven cases from Israel describes local pain and swelling with fever, general weakness, headache, nausea and vomiting. All patients recovered within several days without specific treatment[57].

D. ENVENOMING BY VIPERS AND ADDERS (*VIPERIDAE*)

The venoms of most Viperidae produce marked local effects. Swelling may become detectable within 15 minutes but is sometimes delayed for several hours. It spreads rapidly and may involve the entire bitten limb and adjacent areas of the trunk. Superficial lymphatics may become visible as red or ecchymotic lymphangitic lines and there is pain and tenderness of regional lymph nodes and bruising of the skin overlying them. Bruising, blistering and necrosis at the site of the bite may appear within 24 hours of the bite. Necrosis is common after bites by *Bitis* and *Echis* species, *Vipera lebetina* and *V. palaestinae*. Compartmental syndromes, especially of the anterior tibial compartment, may arise when tissues contained within a tight fascial compartment are envenomed. Haemostatic abnormalities are characteristic of envenoming by many of the Viperidae. Persistent bleeding from fang puncture wounds, venepuncture sites and other new and partially-healed wounds is a clinical indication that blood has become incoagulable through defibrinogenation. Spontaneous systemic haemorrhage is most often detected in the gingival sulci and may also be seen as epistaxis, haematemesis, cutaneous ecchymoses, haemoptysis, subconjunctival, retroperitoneal, intracranial and uterine bleeding. Hypotension and shock, mainly as a result of hypovolaemia, is seen in patients with massive swelling resulting from bites by *Bitis* species. Direct myocardial involvement is suggested by an abnormal ECG or cardiac arrhythmia (for example with *Bitis* and *Echis* species). Patients envenomed by some species of *Vipera*, notably *V. palaestinae*, experience transient recurrent syncopal attacks associated with features of an auto-pharmacological or anaphylactic reaction such as vomiting, sweating, colic, diarrhoea, shock and angio-oedema. Renal failure may develop in severely envenomed patients. Mild neurotoxic symptoms (ptosis, ophthalmoplegia) have been described in patients envenomed by *B atropos* and Tunisian *E. "pyramidum"*. The venom of *B. caudalis* contains a neurotoxin.

1. Bush vipers (genus *Atheris*)

Bites by these species appear to be rare. The green bush viper (*A. squamiger*) has proved capable of fatal envenoming. In the Central African Republic a 37 year old man developed massive swelling of the bitten limb and incoagulable blood 10 hours after a bite by a 71 cm long *A. squamiger*. There is no specific antivenom and his blood remained incoagulable. On the fifth day he had a haematemesis and developed haemorrhagic shock from which he died on the sixth day[58]. In other cases of bites by this species, there was swelling, local bruising, immediate severe pain with dizziness, shivering, nausea and local lymphadenopathy. In Kumasi, Ghana, several patients developed incoagulable blood after bites by unidentified green tree vipers (probably *A. chlorechis*). A bite by a 55.4 cm long horned tree viper (*A. ceratophorus*) caused transient local pain and bruising.

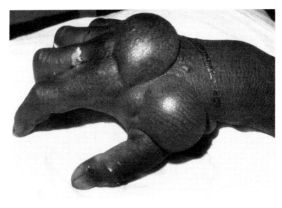
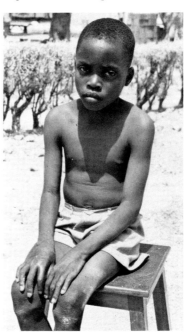

Figure 30. Seven year old boy bitten by a 1.18m long puff adder (*Bitis arietans*) in Nigeria.(photos © Dr. D.A. Warrell).

30a. Gross swelling and blistering of the bitten hand (the bite was in the first interdigital cleft) 22 hours after the bite.

30b. The same patient four weeks later showing complete recovery without necrosis. He was treated with antivenom 5½ hours after the bite.

2. African adders and vipers (genus *Bitis*)

a. Puff adder (B. arietans)

Among 11 proven cases studied in Nigeria, local swelling involved the entire limb in seven, and extended on to the trunk in two[59]. Local blistering developed in six (Figure 30) and local necrosis in four of these patients. In one patient, the bitten leg became cold, anaesthetic and pulseless below the knee, suggesting a popliteal artery thrombosis. Compartmental syndromes, especially involving the anterior tibial compartment, may develop. Shock (hypotension with evidence of impaired peripheral circulation) is an important feature of *B. arietans* envenoming. Hypovolaemia, resulting from the leakage of circulating volume into the bitten limb, is an important cause[17], but direct myocardial effects of the venom, for example causing sinus bradycardia, may contribute. Dramatic clinical responses to intravenous antivenom treatment in patients with hypotension and sinus bradycardia also suggest a direct myocardial effect. Spontaneous bleeding from the gums and nose, extensive bruising of the bitten limb and the discovery of haemorrhages in the walls of the small intestine and into the adventitia of the aorta was observed in victims of *B. arietans* in West Africa[59]. However, these patients' blood was coagulable but a number of them had thrombocytopenia (27-10 x 10^9/l). However, in Uganda, two patients, one of them a professional snake catcher, bitten by snakes which they identified as puff adders, developed incoagulable blood with depleted levels of clotting factors II, VII, X and V, hypofibrinogenaemia and thrombocytopenia[60]. It seems possible that these two very interesting patients may have been bitten by *B. gabonica* since, in a number of the local languages, the name for the two species is the same[61] and their haemostatic disturbances were more consistent with envenoming by *B. gabonica*. Mild abnormalities in blood coagulation have been reported in two proven cases of puff adder bite. Many patients develop a neutrophil leucocytosis.

Although the systemic effects, such as hypotension, hypovolaemia, bradycardia, shock and extensive haemorrhage may be life-threatening in some patients, local effects of envenoming predominate in the majority. Extensive and massive swelling, bruising, regional lymphadenopathy, blistering and necrosis are common and in some patients local thrombosis and intracompartmental syndromes may be additional causes of tissue damage. Secondary infection of necrotic tissue is always a risk and spontaneous separation of necrotic tissue may give rise to severe bleeding. Despite these formidable effects of envenoming, fewer than 20 fatal cases have been reported. Deaths have occurred up to 16 days after the bite with a median interval between bite and death of 24 hours.

b. Gaboon viper (B. gabonica)

In some parts of the West African rain forest, this is the commonest venomous species and the cause of most snakebites. However, it is surprising in view of its wide distribution and prodigious size that only about 20 cases of envenoming have been reported[62]. There is immediate severe pain at the site of the bite and rapid painful swelling of the bitten area, appearing as early as five minutes after the bite. Local effects of envenoming are perhaps less severe than those produced by *B. arietans*, but extensive swelling, bruising (Figure 31), blistering (Figure 32) and necrosis are common. Dizziness, chest tightness, dyspnoea, hyperventilation, nausea, vomiting, blurred vision, impaired visual accommodation and other symptoms may develop within minutes or up to one hour after the bite. One patient developed blurring of vision with clear paralysis of accommodation and progressive deafness[63]. However, although neurotoxicity is mentioned or inferred in published reports, typical neurotoxicity (ptosis etc) has not been convincingly demonstrated. Cardiovascular abnormalities include hypotension and shock, arrhythmias such as bradycardia and atrial tachycardia with ectopics, and ECG changes indicating myocardial damage[63]. Spontaneous systemic bleeding is a common feature of severe envenoming; haematemesis, bleeding from the gastrointestinal and urinary tracts and blood in saliva have been reported. Haemostatic abnormalities were investigated in three patients. Thrombocytopenia, prolongation of prothrombin and partial thromboplastin times and increased fibrin(ogen) degradation products were observed. In one patient studied in detail, there was progressive prolongation of the thrombin time associated with a fall in fibrinogen and Factor XIII levels, increasing FDP (D-dimer) levels and mild thrombocytopenia three days after the bite[62]. There was no parallel fall in Factor V, Factor VIII, anti-thrombin III or protein C levels. Hypofibrinogenaemia was attributed to the direct thrombin-like (gabonase) and plasmin-like activities of the venom. Two patients described by Sezi et al with severe haemostatic abnormalities may have been envenomed by this species[60]. Neutrophil leucocytosis may be marked. Compared with *Bitis arietans* envenoming, *B. gabonica* can be expected to produce more severe systemic bleeding, haemostatic abnormalities, cardiovascular effects and early and potentially life-threatening autopharmacological symptoms but perhaps less severe local effects.

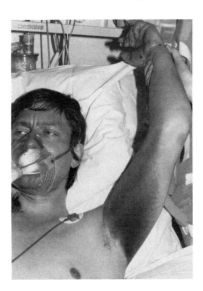
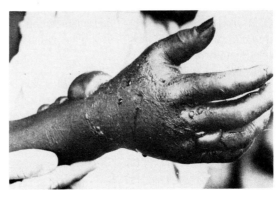

Figure 31. Thirty five year old man bitten on the left wrist by a 1m long Gaboon viper (*Bitis gabonica*) 51 hours previously, showing swelling and bruising (photo © Dr. D.A. Warrell).

Figure 32. Fifteen year old patient bitten by a Gaboon viper (*B. gabonica*) in Ivory Coast 24 hours previously (courtesy of Dr. Jean Doucet, Basel).

c. Rhinoceros-horned viper (B. nasicornis)

A few cases of bites have been mentioned in the literature but there are no details of symptoms except that local necrosis has developed requiring amputation.

d. Berg adder (B. atropos)

Cases have been reported from Zimbabwe and South Africa. Local pain and swelling at the site of the bite develop early, followed after an interval of 30-60 minutes by paraesthesia of the tongue and lips, blurring of vision, loss of taste and smell, hyperacusis, nausea and vomiting. Heaviness of the eyelids develops followed by complete ophthalmoplegia, facial weakness and slurring of speech. The pupils are found to be dilated and fixed to light. Nausea, vomiting and abdominal colic may occur. One patient developed generalised painful and tender muscles.

The local swelling may extend to involve the forearm after bites on the fingers and in one patient there was swelling of the entire limb and adjacent area of the trunk without development of local necrosis. Another patient developed necrosis of the bitten finger. In the absence of specific antivenom, neurotoxic symptoms may resolve within a few hours or persist for up to a week. There may be a mild neutrophil leucocytosis. No haemostatic disturbances have been reported. One fatal case has been reported without any other clinical details[64].

e. Bites by other Bitis species

Horned adder (*B. caudalis*) bites have ranged in severity from swelling of the bitten hand with painful axillary lymphadenopathy without development of local necrosis, to more extensive swelling with shock, nausea, vomiting and development of blistering and necrosis at the site of the bite. The few bites known to have been caused by the hornsman adder (*B. cornuta*) are said to have produced symptoms similar to those for *B. caudalis*. Péringuey's adder (*B. peringueyi*) bites have resulted in pain and local swelling and the one reported bite by a Namaqua dwarf adder (*B. schneideri*) produced a painful, swollen finger with a blood blister at the site of the bite and tender axillary nodes. Envenoming by a Kenyan horned viper (*B. worthingtoni*) caused moderate pain and swelling with systemic effects including weakness, coldness accompanied by sweating, a dry mouth, abdominal pain, diarrhoea and vomiting.

3. Night adders (genus *Causus*)[34]

In many parts of the region, the small snakes of this genus are responsible for the majority of snakebites. Local envenoming, with pain, swelling and lymphadenopathy, is usually the only effect. Bites by the snouted night adder (*C. defilippi*) produce local swelling, lymphadenopathy and mild fever without development of local necrosis. Forest night adders (*C. lichtensteini*) are said to be responsible for most bites in Makokou, Gabon, but the results are never serious. One of two patients bitten by green night adders (*C. resimus*) in the Sudan developed fever.

The western rhombic night adder (*C. maculatus*) is responsible for many bites in the West African savanna region. Most patients suffer no more than pain, limited local swelling and painful regional lymphadenopathy. Of 13 cases reported from northern Nigeria, three had fever and one, a five year old boy bitten by a 60 cm long specimen, became hypotensive and drowsy but recovered rapidly[34]. Mild neutrophil leucocytosis but no evidence of haemostatic disturbances was found. There are no reliable reports of fatal cases.

The eastern rhombic night adder (*C. rhombeatus*) causes pain, local swelling and fever. Local necrosis and fatalities have not, reliably, been attributed to this species.

4. Sand vipers (genus *Cerastes*)

The horned viper (*C. cerastes*) is said to have caused severe envenoming in some parts of North Africa. This seems unlikely but there are a few reports of fatal cases in the French colonial literature at the end of the nineteenth century. Envenoming usually results in local pain and swelling, complicated by necrosis in some cases. In Israel, nausea, vomiting, haemorrhages into the skin, haematuria, reduced fibrinogen concentration, increased prothrombin time and other evidence of mild disseminated intravascular coagulation have been described[65]. In Saudi Arabia, Aramco Medical Department treated 26 cases of presumed *C. gasperettii* bites in 10 years. Less than half needed hospital admission and there were no fatalities. Sahara Desert viper (*C. vipera*) bites have been reported from Algeria and Israel. There was local pain and swelling with or without a haematoma at the site of the bite and regional lymphadenopathy. A minority of patients show evidence of mild coagulopathy (prolonged prothrombin time, low fibrinogen concentration and evidence of increased fibrinolytic activity). Spontaneous bleeding has not been described.

5. Saw-scaled or carpet vipers (genus *Echis*)

Snakes of this genus produce moderately severe local swelling, blistering and necrosis with severe systemic haemostatic disorders (spontaneous systemic bleeding and incoagulable blood) and more rarely shock and renal failure.

a. Burton's carpet viper (*E. coloratus*)

There are reports of some 80 cases from Israel in the literature[66] and a few from elsewhere[12]. Pain at the site of the bite and rapidly developing local swelling are common symptoms. In severe cases, local swelling may involve the whole limb, bruising and haemorrhagic blisters may appear at the site of the bite and necrosis may develop (requiring surgery in 9% of cases in Israel). Systemic symptoms develop from 15 minutes to 1-2 hours after the bite: nausea, vomiting, headache and spontaneous bleeding from the gums, nose and gastrointestinal and urinary tracts, and bleeding from partly healed and recent wounds. Most patients have incoagulable blood when they are admitted to hospital. There is hypofibrinogenaemia, elevated fibrin(ogen) degradation products and in about one-fifth of patients there is thrombocytopenia (less than 100 x 10^9/l). Biochemical evidence of renal impairment is seen in less than a fifth of patients. A few, including one of the fatal cases, developed acute renal failure[67,68]. Anaemia is attributed either to microangiopathic haemolysis or haemorrhage. Haemostatic dysfunction may persist for up to nine days in the absence of treatment. Other abnormalities include hypotension and shock with loss of consciousness and electrocardiographic abnormalities, neutrophil leucocytosis, proteinuria, microscopic haematuria and casts in the urine. Histopathological changes in two cases suggested "acute haematogenous interstitial nephritis", focal mesangial proliferation and tubular necrosis. Only four deaths have been reported in the literature; three by PH Manson-Bahr in the Jordan Valley in 1918[69] and one in Israel in 1961[67]. There is an impression that, compared with bites by other Echis species, *E coloratus* envenoming is more likely to cause thrombocytopenia and renal dysfunction but less likely to cause fatalities.

b. White bellied carpet viper (E. leucogaster)

Bites by this species have not yet been reported. Its venom is now used in the commercial production of Pasteur-Mérieux "IPSER Afrique" antivenom.

c. West African or ocellated carpet viper (E. ocellatus)

This species is the most important cause of snakebite morbidity and mortality in West Africa. Clinical studies have been reported from Ghana, Nigeria and Togo[12,22]. In northern Nigeria 137 proven cases of *E ocellatus* bite were investigated[50,70]. Only 4% of this series of patients admitted to hospital had no signs of envenoming. The remaining 96% showed evidence of both local and systemic envenoming. Local swelling involved more than half the bitten limb in 37% and spread to the trunk in 4% (Figure 33). Twelve per cent showed local blistering and 9% developed necrosis. Bites on the digits were more likely to result in necrosis than those elsewhere (6 out of 13 cases). All patients with local swelling showed laboratory evidence of haemostatic disturbance such as elevated fibrin(ogen) degradation products or circulating soluble fibrin. Eighty-eight per cent had incoagulable blood and 55% showed spontaneous systemic bleeding, usually from the gums (65%) (Figure 34). Other bleeding sites were subconjunctival, sublingual (Figure 35), intramuscular, subcutaneous, retroperitoneal, gastrointestinal tract, urinary tract (Figure 36), subarachnoid space and respiratory tract. The degree of local swelling was not a reliable indicator of the severity of systemic envenoming. Incoagulable blood (20 minute whole blood clotting test) was a sensitive sign of systemic envenoming. Despite almost total defibrinogenation with high levels of FDP, thrombocytopenia (less than 103 x 10^9/l) was observed in only 7% of cases. Severe hypotension (systolic blood pressure <60 mmHg) developed in five patients, three of whom died. Haemorrhage was responsible in all cases. Electrocardiographic abnormalities (transient atrial arrhythmias) were found in only one of 27 patients studied. Only one patient developed acute renal failure, following a period of prolonged haemorrhagic shock and a transfusion reaction. However, granular casts were found in the urine of 37% of patients and proteinuria in 41% on admission to hospital. All five deaths were attributed to haemorrhage; three into the gastrointestinal tract and other tissues and in two intracerebrally. Among 121 patients treated with specific antivenom, the mortality was 2.5% compared with an estimated untreated mortality of about 20%.

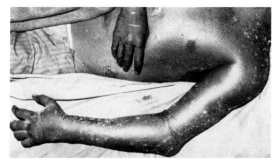

Figure 33. Nigerian man bitten by *Echis ocellatus* four days previously, showing swelling of the whole bitten limb and adjacent areas of the trunk. The limb is plastered with a traditional remedy, "gadali" (*Crinum yuccaeflorum* Amaryllidaceae)
(photo © Dr. D.A. Warrell).

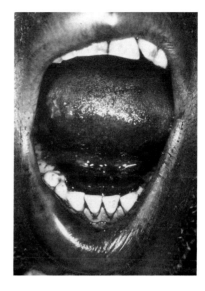

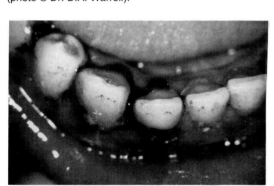

Figure 35 (above). Bleeding from the gums and into the floor of the mouth in a Nigerian patient bitten by *E. ocellatus* several hours previously (photo © Dr. D.A. Warrell).

Figure 34 (left). Bleeding from the gingival sulci in a Nigerian patient bitten by *E. ocellatus* two hours previously (photo © Dr. D.A. Warrell*)*.

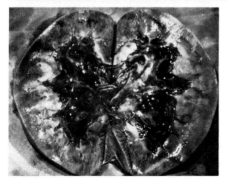

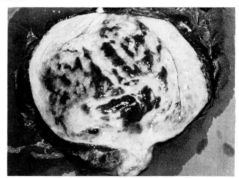

Figure 36. Autopsy appearances in a 50 year old man who died seven hours after admission to hospital, six days after a bite by *E. ocellatus* in Nigeria (photos © Dr. D.A. Warrell)..
36a. Bleeding into the pelvicalyceal system of the   **36b.** Bleeding into the wall of the bladder.
kidney.

d. Egyptian carpet viper (E. pyramidum)

This species is regarded as the commonest cause of snakebites and resulting deaths in northern Sudan. In one series, five out of 26 patients died[71]. Symptoms included bleeding gums, haematuria and fever. In Somalia, the species is said to be the principal venomous snake[22]. At Hargeisa in the north, envenomed patients develop local pain, swelling and blistering, abdominal pain, vomiting, haematuria, bleeding from the gums and fever. In northern Kenya, bites have been reported in Turkana in the northwest (presumed *E. p. leakeyi*)[72] and around Wajir in the northeast (presumed *E. p. aliabori*)[22,73,74]. Clinical features included swelling, haematomas at the sites of intramuscular injection and recent injury, epistaxis, severe haematuria, haematemesis, melaena, menorrhagia, generalised bruising, peri-orbital bleeding, fever, vomiting, shock, anaemia and leucocytosis. In a 50 year old European woman, renal failure resulted in bilateral contracted calcified kidneys[72]. A patient bitten by a Tunisian "*E. pyramidum*" showed transient bilateral ptosis. Intravascular haemolysis, most probably the result of microangiopathic haemolysis, was well documented in this patient and in several cases of bites by other Echis sp/subsp.

e. Echis sochureki
    No proven cases of bites have been reported from this region (but see Chapter 27 (Asia) for accounts from northern India and elsewhere).

6. False-horned viper (*Pseudocerastes persicus*)
    The few clinical cases showed only local symptoms[75].

7. Typical old world vipers (genus *Vipera*)
    Of the four species which occur in this region, two (*V. lebetina* and *V. palaestinae*) are capable of causing severe local and systemic envenoming.

a. Bornmueller's viper (V. bornmuelleri)
    "The only bite known was uneventful and caused only very slight local swelling."[75]

b. Lataste's viper (V. latasti):
    No bites have been reported in this region but, in Europe, the following symptoms have been reported: early anaphylactic symptoms (angio-oedema, nausea, vomiting, abdominal pain, shock and tachycardia), local pain and swelling with persistent morbidity, regional lymphadenopathy and rarely renal failure. Reports of local necrosis and rare fatalities have not been substantiated.

c. Blunt-nosed viper (V. (Macrovipera) lebetina)
    A few cases have been reported from the region, but it is generally regarded as a dangerous species. There is local pain and swelling which may extend to involve the whole bitten limb and trunk with bruising, lymphangitic markings and regional lymphadenopathy. Local blistering and necrosis may develop. Systemic symptoms include nausea, vomiting, trembling, hypotension, shock, tachycardia, syncope, cold sweats and spontaneous bleeding (haemoptysis, melaena, subconjunctival haemorrhage). Anaemia, with evidence of haemolysis, thrombocytopenia and leucocytosis, was observed. In Iraq, Corkhill considered it the most important cause of snakebite casualties and cited a 50% mortality[76]. Fatal cases have been reported in Cyprus and the U.S.S.R. Horses, mules, cattle and camels have also been killed by *V. lebetina* bites in Central Asia.

d. Palestine viper (V palaestinae)
    Large series of bites have been reported from Israel[65,77], where this species is responsible for 100-300 bites each year. The clinical picture is dominated by a dramatic severe early anaphylactic syndrome. Within 15-20 minutes of noticing the initial pain at the site of the bite, the patient suddenly feels weak and restless and begins to vomit and sweat. There is abdominal pain with diarrhoea which may be watery and bloodstained. Angio-oedema affects the upper lip and face, the tongue may be swollen to "several times its normal size" and patches of urticaria appear on the trunk. Blood pressure falls, there is tachycardia and evidence of peripheral circulatory failure. The patient may collapse unconscious. Massive tender swelling ascends up the bitten limb with local blistering,

bruising, lymphangitic lines and regional lymphadenopathy. In untreated patients, hypovolaemic shock may develop within a few days of the bite. There is progressive anaemia, thrombocytopenia and leucocytosis but the blood remains coagulable although the clot formed is said to lyse after an hour or so. Patients are initially haemoconcentrated. There may be bleeding from the gastrointestinal tract and transient proteinuria. Deaths occurred 2-48 hours after the bite. At autopsy extensive haemorrhages were found in the heart, serous membranes, gastrointestinal mucosa, and urinary tract.

VI. PREVENTION OF SNAKEBITE

The people most exposed to snakebite are those who live and work in snake-infested areas of the tropics. A better understanding of diurnal and seasonal patterns of snake activity and their preferred habitats, avoidance of unnecessarily high risk activities and the use of protective clothing, such as shoes or boots, would reduce the risk of bites. Educating the community in correct methods of first aid, dissuading them from wasting valuable time indulging in useless and potentially dangerous traditional treatments and improving the understanding and treatment of snakebite at primary health care posts, rural dispensaries and district hospitals in the tropics could reduce the incidence of severe envenoming. In western countries, amateur herpetologists and others should be dissuaded from picking up dangerous or potentially dangerous species as most bites result from this behaviour. Snakes should never be disturbed, attacked, cornered or handled even if they are thought to be harmless species or appear to be dead. Venomous species should never be kept as pets or as performing animals. In high risk areas, boots, socks and long trousers should be worn for walks in undergrowth or deep sand and a light should always be carried at night. Collecting firewood, dislodging logs or boulders with bare hands, pushing sticks or fingers into burrows, holes and crevices, climbing rocks and trees covered with dense foliage and swimming in overgrown lakes and rivers are particularly hazardous activities. Unlit paths and gutters are particularly dangerous at night after heavy rains. It is difficult to exclude snakes from fields and gardens. It is futile and ecologically undesirable to attempt the extermination of venomous snakes and at present there is no "snake repellant" that is effective without poisoning the snake. These compounds include naphthalene, sulphur, nicotine sulphate, strichnine, insecticides (such as DDT and dieldrin), organophosphates and fumigants such as calcium cyanide, formaldehyde, tetrachloroethane and methyl bromide.

Prophylactic immunization against snake venom has been experimented with in several Asian countries and even taken as far as field trials in Japan, but there are theoretical and practical problems which make it unlikely that this will provide the answer to rural snakebite in Africa.

VII. FIRST AID TREATMENT OF SNAKEBITE IN AFRICA AND THE MIDDLE EAST

Patients bitten by snakes need urgent medical assessment but, especially in the rural tropics, where most bites occur, rural health stations or district hospitals serve large areas and many agricultural areas infested with snakes may be relatively inaccessible by road, especially during the rainy season. It may take a patient hours or even days to reach the nearest medical facility. Education of rural communities in good first aid practice may prevent time-wasting and dangerous practices and could prolong a patient's life until they reach medical care.

The principles of first aid are:

1. The delivery of snakebite victims as quickly as possible to a place where they can be

seen by medical staff.
2. The use of methods to delay the evolution of life-threatening envenoming at least until the patient reaches a place where they can receive medical care.
3. The alleviation of severe and possibly life-threatening early symptoms of envenoming.

Advice about first aid must take into account the fact that it can only be carried out by the snakebite victim or by those who are nearby or arrive quickly on the scene. In most cases, first aid procedures can not be carried out by people who have been medically trained. Only in zoos, snake farms, research stations and organised expeditions is it possible to provide equipment, even as simple as splints and crepe bandages, to be used soon after the accident has occurred. First aid treatment of snakebites is an appropriate subject for health education in the community, especially among high risk groups such as agricultural workers and their families.

1. General recommendations for first aid
1. The bitten person should be reassured. Many will be terrified, fearing sudden death and, in this mood, they may behave irrationally or even hysterically. The basis for reassurance is the fact that many venomous bites do not result in envenoming, the relatively slow progression to severe envenoming (hours following elapid bites, days following viper bites) and the effectiveness of modern medical treatment.
2. The bite wound should not be tampered with in any way. Wiping it once with a damp cloth to remove surface venom is unlikely to do much harm (or good) but the wound must not be massaged.
3. The bitten limb should be immobilised as effectively as possible using an extemporised splint or sling; if available, crepe bandaging of the splinted limb is an effective form of immobilisation.
4. The snakebite victim should be transported as quickly and as passively as possible to the nearest place where they can be seen by a medically-trained person (health station, dispensary, clinic or hospital). The bitten limb must not be exercised as muscular contraction will promote systemic absorption of venom. If no motor vehicle or boat is available, the patient can be carried on a stretcher or hurdle, on the pillion or crossbar of a bicycle or on someone's back. Most traditional, and many of the more recently fashionable, first aid measures are useless and potentially dangerous. These include local cauterization, incision, excision, amputation, suction by mouth, vacuum pump or syringe, combined incision and suction ("venom-ex" apparatus), injection or instillation of compounds such as potassium permanganate, phenol (carbolic soap) and trypsin, application of electric shocks or ice (cryotherapy), use of traditional herbal, folk and other remedies including the ingestion of emetic plant products and parts of the snake, multiple incisions, tattooing and so on.
5. If the snake responsible for the bite has been killed, it should be taken along with the patient for identification, but it should not be touched with bare hands even if it appears dead and no attempt should be made to pursue the snake into the undergrowth as this will risk further bites.

2. Dangers of tourniquets, ligatures and compression bands
Systemic envenoming by some elapid snakes (for example *D. polylepis, N. haje, N. nivea*) may develop so rapidly that fatal respiratory paralysis may ensue, exceptionally, within 30 minutes of the bite. In these cases there is a strong argument for attempting to impede the systemic uptake of venom to allow more time to transport the patient to hospital. Tourniquets of some sort are still the most popular first aid method in developing countries and most medical staff working in areas where snakebite is common will have been

impressed by the damaging effects of this technique; ischaemia and gangrene, damage to superficial peripheral nerves, increased fibrinolytic activity and congestion and swelling in the occluded limb leading to increased bleeding, shock or acute development of systemic envenoming after release of the tourniquet and intensification of local effects of venom in the occluded limb. A majority of tourniquets applied in rural South East Asia were shown to be ineffective in preventing the systemic spread of venom. *For all these reasons, the use of tourniquets, ligatures and pressure bands is not recommended.*

3. Sutherland's compression immobilisation method

In animals, arterial-occlusive ligatures or tourniquets have been shown to prevent the absorption of venom and to prolong survival after the injection of elapid and viper venoms[78-80]. Immobilisation of the injected limb without occlusion was shown to delay the absorption of higher molecular weight toxins (eg in *Notechis scutatus* and *Daboia russelii* venoms) spread through the lymphatics, but not smaller molecular weight toxins (eg in cobra venom) absorbed directly into the bloodstream[81]. Venom procoagulants in some venoms seem to be permanently localised (perhaps through local thrombosis) or inactivated in occluded limbs[78]. Sutherland et al found that in restrained monkeys compression and immobilisation of the injected limb in a pneumatic chamber at 55 mmHg and crepe bandaging and splinting judged to exert the same compressive effect delayed the movement of labelled venom from the injected limb without causing the ischaemia inevitable with conventional tourniquets[82]. In monkeys, this method was effective with 13 Australasian elapid venoms, and the venoms of the Indian cobra (*N. naja*) and the eastern diamond back rattlesnake (*Crotalus adamanteus*). The method was formally endorsed by the Australian National Health and Medical Research Council in 1979 and has been enthusiastically promoted in Australasia, Southern Africa and elsewhere. However, even in Australia it is still used in only 18-45% of snakebite cases[83]. Unfortunately, there have been few clinical reports of the use of this method and no attempt at comparative or controlled studies. The rapid development of systemic envenoming with increasing systemic venous venom antigen concentration has been observed in several cases after the release of crepe or Esmarch bandages. In Australia, the method has proved safe, but prolonged application of pressure immobilisation has produced evidence of intensification of local effects of neurotoxic and cytotoxic venom components in a few patients. Compared with the venoms of African vipers and spitting cobras, Australasian elapid venoms produce little or no tissue damage at the site of the bite. Pressure immobilisation is likely to cause the intensification of locally necrotic effects of African snake venoms with secondary ischaemic effects resulting from increased pressure in tight fascial compartments, especially the anterior tibial compartment. *For this reason pressure immobilisation is not recommended in patients bitten by African and Middle Eastern vipers and spitting cobras.*

For victims of snakebite in rural areas of Africa and the Middle East, the pressure immobilisation method raises difficult practical problems. Long stretchy bandages are unlikely to be available except to wealthy outsiders such as campers, hikers and expedition members. It is difficult to judge the pressure applied by a crepe bandage. If it is too loose it will be ineffective and if too tight it could produce the same risk of ischaemia and gangrene as an arterial tourniquet. Finally, the application of the bandage may prove difficult or impossible if the victims are on their own, especially if the bite is on the dominant arm.

However, Sutherland's pressure immobilisation method, when correctly applied, is undoubtedly far more tolerable and less dangerous than tight tourniquets or ligatures. *The method is recommended after bites by dangerous neurotoxic species such as mambas (Dendroaspis) and cobras (N. haje, N. melanoleuca, N. nivea).*

4. Treatment of early symptoms of envenoming before the patient reaches hospital

a. Anaphylaxis

As early as a few minutes and up to several hours after bites by *V palaestinae* and more rarely other Vipera species and *Atractaspis engaddensis*, patients may develop symptoms of anaphylaxis and stimulation of the autonomic nervous system: hypotension, tachycardia, shock, impaired consciousness, angio-oedema of the tongue, mouth, gums, lips and face, urticaria, abdominal colic, nausea, retching, vomiting and diarrhoea (sometimes repeated and profuse), sweating and "gooseflesh" and in some cases breathlessness and bronchospasm. These features are attributable to autopharmacological effects of venom, releasing endogenous mediators or activating precursors such as bradykinin. On rare occasions, people (usually herpetologists or snake handlers) who have been bitten or exposed in other ways to a specific snake venom may become sensitized and develop true immediate-type I hypersensitivity after a bite or contact of mucosae such as the lips and mouth with venom when applying suction to a wound. ***The treatment of all these anaphylactic syndromes is subcutaneous or intramuscular injection of 0.1% adrenaline, followed by an intravenous injection of an antihistamine H_1 antagonist*** (see below). Hypotensive patients should be tipped head downwards and those with severe bronchospasm, dyspnoea or cyanosis should be given oxygen by any available means.

b. Pain in the bitten limb

This may be severe. Oral paracetamol is preferable to aspirin which commonly causes gastric erosions even in healthy people and could lead to persistent gastric bleeding in patients with incoagulable blood.

c. Vomiting

This is a common early symptom of severe systemic envenoming by any species of snake. Patients should lie on their side to prevent aspiration of vomit. Persistent vomiting can be treated with an injection[*] of chlorpromazine (25-50 mg for adults, 1 mg/kg for children).

d. Respiratory distress and cyanosis

This may indicate paralysis of the respiratory muscles or blockage of the airway in a patient with respiratory or circulatory failure. The patient should be laid on their side, the airway cleared by elevating the jaw, removing foreign bodies and inserting oral airway if available. If respiratory distress and cyanosis persist, oxygen should be given and, if there are still signs of respiratory failure, ventilation will have to be assisted. In the absence of any special equipment, mouth-to-mouth or mouth-to-nose ventilation can be life-saving. If the patient is unconscious and no femoral or carotid pulse can be felt, external cardiac massage and mouth-to-mouth ventilation should be started without delay.

Community first aid workers can be trained to place snakebite victims in the correct position, maintain the airway and even to do cardiopulmonary resuscitation. In some countries dispensers, nurses and ambulancemen can be trained to give adrenaline, antihistamines, chlorpromazine and other drugs, to insert oral airways, administer oxygen and carry out CPR.

---

[*]Patients with incoagulable blood may develop massive haematomas after intramuscular and subcutaneous injections. Except in the case of adrenaline, the intravenous route should be used whenever possible.

VIII. MEDICAL TREATMENT IN HEALTH STATIONS, DISPENSARIES AND HOSPITALS

Snakebite is a medical emergency. Ideally, all patients bitten by snakes should be assessed by medically trained staff. In most patients, uncertainties such as the species responsible, the amount of venom injected and the variable time course for development of signs require that patients should be kept under observation for at least 24 hours. Exceptions are those cases in which the bite was by an unequivocally non-venomous species such as legless lizards (Amphisbaenids or worm lizards - Amphisbaenia; legless skinks - Acontiinae; slow worms - Anguidae in northwest Africa), legless amphibians (Caecilians) and non-venomous snakes (blind snakes - Typhlopidae and Leptotyphlopidae; boas and pythons - Boidae) and those colubrid snakes known to be non-venomous. Medical staff must decide quickly whether the patient has been bitten by a snake, whether there are signs of envenoming and whether antivenom or ancillary treatment is needed.

A. HISTORY
Three important initial questions are:
1. On which part of your body were you bitten?
2. How long ago were you bitten?
3. Have you brought the snake and, if not, can anyone describe it?

Patients should be asked to describe their symptoms and then questioned directly about local pain, swelling, tenderness, regional lymph nodes, bleeding, motor and sensory symptoms, vomiting, fainting and abdominal pain. The time after the bite when these symptoms appeared and their progression should be noted. Details of pre-hospital treatment (tourniquets, herbal remedies etc) should also be recorded as these may, themselves, cause symptoms.

B. EXAMINATION
The absence of discernible fang marks does not exclude snakebite, but the discovery of two or more discrete puncture marks suggests a bite by a venomous snake. The pattern of fang punctures is rarely helpful as there may be marks by accessory fangs, other teeth and multiple bites. The distance between the fang marks is proportional to the size of the snake. Local swelling and enlargement and tenderness of regional lymph nodes are often the earliest signs of envenoming, but factitious swelling may be caused by a tourniquet. Most cases of significant envenoming by African vipers and spitting cobras are associated with the development of local swelling within two hours of the bite but there have been exceptions to this rule and symptoms and signs of severe systemic envenoming from colubrids (*D. typus*, *Thelotornis* species) have been delayed for 15 hours or more after the bite. Systemic envenoming by most African species is associated with local swelling, although in the case of some bites by colubrids, mambas and neurotoxic cobras, this may be negligible. Persistent bleeding from the fang marks, other recent wounds and venepuncture sites suggest that the blood is incoagulable. The gums should be examined thoroughly as these are usually the first site of spontaneous systemic bleeding. The signs of shock are fall in blood pressure; collapse; cold, cyanosed and sweaty skin and impaired consciousness. The foot of the bed should be raised and an intravenous infusion of isotonic saline or a plasma expander such as haemaccel, gelofuse, dextran or fresh frozen plasma should be started immediately. The earliest symptoms of neurotoxicity after elapid bites is often blurred vision, a feeling of heaviness of the eyelids and drowsiness. The frontalis muscle is contracted, raising the eyebrows and puckering the forehead, even before ptosis can be demonstrated. Respiratory muscle paralysis with imminent respiratory failure is suggested

by dyspnoea, restlessness, sweating, exaggerated abdominal respiration, central cyanosis and coma. If there is any suggestion of respiratory muscle weakness, objective monitoring should be attempted by measuring peak expiratory flow, vital capacity or expiratory pressure using the mercury manometer of a sphygmomanometer. Coma is usually the result of respiratory or circulatory failure. Patients with widespread flaccid paralysis may seem deeply comatose because they are unresponsive and arreflexic but, provided they are adequately ventilated, they are likely to be fully conscious. Enough distal motor function may be retained to allow them to signal by flexing a finger or toe in response to questions.

C. MONITORING OF SNAKE-BITTEN PATIENTS

Patients bitten by snakes should, ideally, be observed in hospital for at least 24 hours after the bite. The following should be checked at least once an hour:
1. level of consciousness
2. presence or absence of ptosis
3. pulse rate and rhythm
4. blood pressure
5. respiratory rate
6. extent of local swelling
7. new symptoms or signs.

D. DIAGNOSIS

In most patients, the history of snakebite will be clear-cut and the clinician will have to decide which species was likely to be responsible and whether there are signs of envenoming. However, some patients may only suspect that they have been bitten by a snake because they experienced a sharp pricking pain while walking in the dark or in undergrowth, collecting firewood or even while asleep on the floor in their hut. Thorns, rodent bites and bites and stings by arthropods could produce immediate local pain and one or more puncture marks. Bites and stings by venomous African arthropods (for example, scorpions, spiders, centipedes) can cause mild local swelling and severe systemic symptoms. Local swelling and inflammation, sometimes resulting in a hot, red, swollen limb with enlarged regional nodes, can result from secondary infection (cellulitis) following penetrating wounds from thorns or rodent bites. The interval between the accident and the development of inflammatory swelling is usually more than 24 hours, but in the case of *Pasteurella multocida* infection following mammal bites, this interval may be as short as 6-12 hours.

1. Species diagnosis

Descriptions of snakes by snakebite victims and onlookers, and the use of local names for snakes, are often misleading and so, unless the snake has been brought for identification, the clinician will have to rely on the clinical picture and the results of laboratory tests to make a species diagnosis. Unfortunately, clinical features are rarely diagnostic. The circumstances of the bite can be helpful. Spitting cobras are most likely to be responsible for bites inflicted at night on people asleep on the floor of their huts[8,31]. In and near rivers, lakes and marshy areas, cobras are most likely to be responsible.

In most parts of Africa and the Middle East there are four main clinical syndromes of envenoming:
1. Severe local swelling, blistering and necrosis with coagulable blood - spitting cobras or puff adders are usually responsible.
2. Moderately severe local envenoming (as above) with incoagulable blood and spontaneous systemic bleeding (in the northern third of Africa) - *Echis* species are usually responsible.

3. Mild or negligible local envenoming with incoagulable blood and spontaneous systemic bleeding - boomslangs (rarely vine snakes) are usually responsible.
4. Mild local swelling with neurotoxic symptoms - mambas, Egyptian cobras (in South Africa, Cape cobras) are usually responsible.

2. The 20 minute whole blood clotting test

This is a simple and rapid "bedside" test which must be carried out, on admission and repeated subsequently, in all patients with suspected snakebite. A few ml of venous blood are placed in a new, clean, dry, glass test tube and left upright and undisturbed at room temperature for 20 minutes. The tube is then tipped. If the blood is still liquid and runs out of the tube, the patient is defibrinogenated, suggesting systemic envenoming by *Echis* species (in the northern third of Africa) and, more rarely and in other parts of Africa, by boomslangs, vine snakes, Gaboon vipers and *Atheris* species.

3. Immunodiagnosis[15,16]

Specific snake venom antigens can be detected in wound aspirate, swabs or biopsies, serum urine, cerebrospinal fluid and other body fluids. Enzyme immunoassay has been the most widely used. For the Africa/Middle East region, there is no commercial test available, but immunoassay has proved a valuable tool in the clinical investigation of snakebite. Nonspecific ("heterophile") reactions are common with sera from rural populations. In the case of venom antigen detection, this problem can be partly overcome by technique and by using a large number of unenvenomed controls from the same population to establish the background absorbence. Detection of venom antibodies in patients bitten by snakes in the past remains too unreliable to be useful for individual diagnosis or epidemiological studies.

D. ANTIVENOM TREATMENT

The most important and urgent decision to be made in any patient bitten by a snake is whether or not to give antivenom, the only specific antidote to venom. Antivenom is the hyperimmune serum or plasma of animals, usually horses or sheep, which have been immunized with snake venoms. Most commercial antivenoms consist largely of F(ab)$_2$ fragments of immunoglobulin obtained by pepsin digestion and ammonium sulphate precipitation. For the following reasons, antivenom should never be used routinely and indiscriminately, but only when indicated.
1. All commercial antivenoms carry a risk of potentially dangerous serum reactions.
2. Antivenom is not always necessary: some patients are bitten by non-venomous snakes and 10-50% of those bitten by venomous snakes are not envenomed.
3. Antivenoms have a range of specific and paraspecific neutralizing activity but are useless for venoms outside that range. Specific antivenoms are not available for treatment of envenoming by some species (eg *Thelotornis* species and other colubrids except *D. typus*; *Atractaspis* species; elapid species which rarely bite - *Aspidelaps, Boulengerina, Elapsoidea* etc; *Atheris* species and *Bitis atropos*).
4. Antivenom is very expensive, usually in short supply and has a limited shelf life. Scarce and valuable supplies must not be wasted.

1. Indications for antivenom

Antivenom is indicated in all cases of systemic and severe local envenoming (Table 2).

2. Contraindications to antivenom

There is no absolute contraindication to antivenom when a patient has life-threatening systemic envenoming. However, patients with an atopic history (asthma, hay fever etc) and those with a history of reactions to equine antisera have an increased risk of severe reactions. In those cases, pretreatment with subcutaneous adrenaline and intravenous antihistamine and hydrocortisone may prevent or diminish the reaction. There is not time for desensitization.

Table 2
Indications for antivenom treatment after bites by African and Middle Eastern snakes

Systemic envenoming
1. Neurotoxicity
2. Spontaneous systemic bleeding
3. Incoagulable blood (20 minute whole blood clotting test)
4. Cardiovascular abnormality: hypotension, shock, arrhythmia, abnormal electrocardiogram
5. Impaired consciousness

Local envenoming by species known to cause local necrosis*
1. Swelling involving more than half the bitten limb
2. Rapidly progressive swelling
3. Bites on fingers and toes

*Bitis, Echis and Vipera species and spitting cobras

3. Hypersensitivity testing

Intradermal, subcutaneous or intraconjunctival tests with diluted antivenom have no predictive value for early anaphylactic or late serum sickness type antivenom reactions and should no longer be used[84].

4. Timing of antivenom treatment

Antivenom should be given as soon as possible once signs of systemic or severe local envenoming are evident (Table 2). It is almost never too late to try antivenom treatment; it has proved effective in reversing coagulopathy 10 days or more after Echis bites. When patients arrive in hospital with a tourniquet or other constricting band in place, antivenom treatment, if it is thought necessary, should be started before these are loosened or there is a risk of severe envenoming when the venom in the occluded limb is released into the general circulation.

5. Antivenom specificity

If the species responsible for the bite is known, monospecific antivenom is the optimal treatment. However, in areas where the venoms of a number of different species produce similar clinical effects, polyspecific antivenoms must be used in the majority of patients who do not bring the dead snake for identification. Polyspecific antivenoms are specific for the range of venoms which they cover, but a larger dose is required to provide the same specific neutralizing power as a monospecific antivenom.

6. Antivenom administration

Ideally, antivenom should be used before its expiry date, but these stated dates are usually very conservative, partly for commercial reasons. It has been found that most liquid antivenoms retain 90% of their activity for years even when stored at high ambient temperatures (25 or 30°C) and that lyophilized antisera are even more stable[19]. However, antivenom solutions which have become opaque should not be used as protein precipitation is associated with loss of activity and an increased risk of reactions. Antivenom is most effective when given intravenously. Freeze-dried (lyophilized) antivenom is dissolved in sterile water. Antivenom can be given by intravenous injection at a rate of about 5 ml per minute, or diluted in isotonic fluid and infused over 30-60 minutes. The incidence and severity of antivenom reactions was the same with these two methods[84]. The advantage of intravenous infusion is ease of control, but intravenous "push" injection requires less expensive equipment, is quicker to set up and ensures that someone remains at the patient's side during the crucial first 10-15 minutes after the start of treatment, when early reactions are most likely to occur.

When intravenous administration is impossible, antivenom can be given by deep intramuscular injection at multiple sites in the anterior and lateral aspects of the thighs, followed by massage to promote absorption. Absorption from intragluteal injection is unreliable. There is a limit to the volume of antivenom that can be given by this route and there is a risk of haematoma formation in patients with incoagulable blood.

7. Dosage of antivenom

Guidelines for initial dosage based on clinical studies are available for some important antivenoms used in the African and Middle Eastern region (Table 3). In most cases, manufacturer's recommendations given in the "package insert" are based on mouse assays which may not correlate with clinical findings. The initial dose of antivenom, however large, may not completely neutralize the depot of venom at the site of injection. Patients should therefore be observed for several days even if they show a good clinical response to the initial dose of antivenom. Continuing absorption of venom may cause recurrent neurotoxicity or haemostatic problems after the serum antivenom concentration has declined[15].

Children must be given the same dose of antivenom as adults.

Table 3
Guide to initial dosage of some important antivenoms for bites by African and Middle Eastern snakes

Species Scientific Name	English Name	Manufacturer, Antivenom	Approximate Initial Dose
Bitis arietans	Puff adder	SAIMR,[1]Behringwerke P-M[2] polyspecific	80 ml
B gabonica	Gaboon viper		
Dendroaspis sp	Mambas	SAIMR, P-M Dendroaspis	50-100 ml
Dispholidus typus	Boomslang	SAIMR, Boomslang	20 ml
Echis coloratus	Burton's carpet viper	SAIMR, Echis monosp	20 ml
E ocellatus	West African/ ocellated carpet viper	SAIMR, Echis monosp	20 ml
		P-M "IPSER Afrique" polysp	40 ml
		Behringwerke "North Africa" polysp	100 ml
Naja haje	Egyptian cobra	SAIMR, Behringwerke, P-M polysp	50-100 ml
N mossambica	Moçambique spitting cobra/m'Fezi	SAIMR polysp	100 ml
N nigricollis	Black-necked spitting cobra	SAIMR, Behringwerke, P-M polysp	80 ml
N nivea	Cape cobra	SAIMR polysp	80-100 ml
Vipera palaestinae	Palestine viper	Israel Min Hlth "anti-*V palaest*"	50-80 ml

[1] South African Institute for Medical Research
[2] Pasteur-Mérieux serums et vaccins

8. Response to antivenom treatment

Neurotoxic signs often respond slowly, after several hours, or unconvincingly. Cardiovascular effects such as hypotension and sinus bradycardia (for example after bites by Bitis and Vipera species) may respond within 10-20 minutes. Spontaneous systemic bleeding usually stops within 15-30 minutes and blood coagulability is restored within about six hours if an adequate dose of antivenom has been given. The 20 minute whole blood clotting test (see above) should be used to monitor the dose of antivenom in patients with coagulopathy. If the blood remains incoagulable six hours after the first dose, the dose should be repeated and so on, every six hours, until blood coagulability is restored.

Antivenom treatment has undoubtedly reduced snakebite mortality: in northern Nigeria, mortality was reduced from approximately 20% to less than 3% following bites by *Echis ocellatus*[50,70]. Some antivenoms are capable of rapidly eliminating venom antigenaemia and haemostatic and cardiovascular abnormalities. Efficacy against neurotoxicity, even against the predominantly post-synaptic neurotoxins of African elapids, is less convincing. The efficacy of antivenoms against local necrosis is controversial. Laboratory studies have shown that the antivenom must be given very early after envenoming to prevent these changes, but clinical observations suggest that antivenom may prevent local necrosis after bites by *Bitis arietans*[59] and *Naja mossambica*[31] if given in adequate doses within three to six hours of envenoming.

9. Antivenom reactions
Early (anaphylactic), pyrogenic and late (serum sickness type) reactions may occur.

a. Early reactions

These begin 10-60 minutes after starting intravenous administration of antivenom. Cough, tachycardia, itching (especially of the scalp), urticaria, fever, nausea, vomiting and headache are common symptoms. More than 5% of patients with early reactions develop systemic anaphylaxis - hypotension, bronchospasm and angio-oedema; but there are few reports of deaths reliably attributed to these reactions. The incidence of these reactions varies from 3-54% depending on manufacturer, refinement, dose and route of administration. *The vast majority of early anaphylactic antivenom reactions are not immediate type I hypersensitivity reactions but result from complement activation by IgG aggregates present in the antivenom.* Adrenaline (epinephrine) 0.1% (1 in 1,000) should be given subcutaneously or intramuscularly in a dose of 0.5-1.0 ml for adults, 0.01 mg/kg for children. This should be followed by an intravenous injection of an H_1 antagonist (antihistamine) such as chlorpheniramine maleate (10 mg for adults, 0.2 mg/kg for children).

b. Pyrogenic reactions

These result from pyrogen contamination of the antivenom during manufacture. They begin 1-2 hours after treatment. There is an initial chill with cutaneous vasoconstriction, gooseflesh and shivering. Temperature rises sharply during the rigors and there is intense vasodilatation, widening of the pulse pressure and eventual fall in mean arterial pressure. In children, febrile convulsions may occur at the peak of the fever. Patients should be laid flat to prevent postural hypotension. Their temperature should be reduced by fanning, tepid sponging and antipyretic drugs such as paracetamol (15 mg/kg) given by mouth, suppository or via nasogastric tube.

c. Late (serum sickness type) reactions

They occur 5-24 (average 7) days after treatment. There is itching, urticaria, fever, arthralgia, proteinuria and sometimes neurological symptoms. Antihistamines are used for milder attacks, but in severe cases, including those with neurological symptoms, a short course of prednisolone should be given.

E. ANCILLARY TREATMENT
1. Treatment of local envenoming
Although most local effects of snakebite are attributable directly to cytolytic and other activities of the venom itself, the bite may introduce bacteria and the risk of local infections greatly increases if the wound has been incised with an unsterile instrument or tampered with in some other way. The pattern of bacterial flora may vary in different countries[85]. It is

appropriate to give prophylactic antimicrobials and a booster dose of tetanus toxoid. The wound should be cleaned with antiseptic. Blisters and bullae should be aspirated to dryness with a fine sterile needle rather than allowing them to rupture. Snake-bitten limbs should be nursed in the most comfortable position. The wound should be examined frequently for evidence of necrosis: blistering, blackening or depigmentation of the skin, loss of sensation and a characteristic smell of putrefaction. Necrotic tissue should not be left to slough spontaneously but should be debrided by a surgeon under general or local anaesthesia as soon as possible to reduce the risk of secondary infection and to promote eventual healing. Skin appearances may be deceptive, for necrosis can undermine apparently normal skin. Large areas may be denuded of skin; recovery can be accelerated by applying split skin grafts immediately after debridement provided that the wound is not infected. Debrided tissue, serosanguinous discharge and pus should be cultured and the patient treated with appropriate antimicrobials. Fluctuant areas, suggestive of an underlying abscess, should be aspirated and opened for drainage.

Severe pain, especially in the lower leg, may indicate an intracompartmental syndrome or thrombosis of a major artery. Fasciotomies are performed far too readily by many surgeons impressed by tensely swollen limbs, pale, tight, cool skin and difficulty in palpating peripheral arteries. These clinical signs may be misleading; the limb may be cool only because of the insulating layer of extravasated fluid; normal arterial flow may be detectable with a doppler ultrasound probe and measurement of intracompartmental pressure may reveal reassuringly normal pressures, well below the figure of 45 mmHg (60 cmH$_2$0) associated with a high risk of ischaemic necrosis. Fasciotomy may be disastrous if it is performed while the patient's blood is still incoagulable and there is severe thrombocytopenia. Animal studies showed that fasciotomy was not effective in saving envenomed muscles[86]. Provided that adequate antivenom treatment is given as soon as possible after the bite, fasciotomy is rarely if ever needed. However, bites involving the finger pulps are frequently complicated by necrosis. Expert surgical advice should be sought, especially if the thumb or index finger is involved.

Arterial thrombosis is a rare complication, reported after bites by *B. arietans*[59] and *V. palaestinae*[65]. It should be suspected in a patient who rapidly develops severe pain in a limb with a sharply demarcated cold distal area and arterial pulses that are undetectable by doppler. Once any haemostatic abnormality had been corrected, this could be investigated by arteriography and the possibility of angioplasty, thrombectomy or reconstructive arterial surgery considered.

2. Haemostatic abnormalities

Once adequate doses of antivenom have been given to neutralize venom antihaemostatic factors, recovery of normal haemostatic function may be accelerated by giving fresh whole blood, fresh frozen plasma, cryoprecipitates or platelet concentrates. ***Heparin and antifibrinolytic agents should not be used.***

3. Neurotoxic envenoming

The airway must be protected in patients developing bulbar and respiratory paralysis. Once secretions begin to pool in the pharynx, a cuffed endotracheal tube should be introduced. Mechanical ventilation is usually required for only a few days but patients have recovered after 10 weeks of mechanical ventilation and 30 days of manual ventilation by ambu bag or anaesthetic bag. Antivenoms cannot be relied upon to reverse neurotoxicity or prevent its progression to respiratory paralysis.

a. Anticholinesterases

Neuromuscular blockade by post-synaptic neurotoxins may be partly overcome by the use of anticholinesterase drugs. For example, in this region, prostigmine was used successfully to treat patients with severe neurotoxic envenoming following bites by *N. melanoleuca*[20] and *Dendroaspis viridis* and in a patient envenomed by *N. nivea* there was an improvement in motor response to command and electromyographic responses after administration of prostigmine[48].

All patients with neurotoxic symptoms should be given a "Tensilon" (edrophonium) test as in the case of patients with suspected myasthenia gravis. Atropine sulphate (0.6 mg for adults, 50 µg/kg for children) is given by intravenous injection to block the muscarinic effects of acetylcholine. This is followed by edrophonium chloride (10 mg in adults, 0.25 mg/kg in children) by slow intravenous injection. The response should be assessed objectively. Those who respond convincingly can be maintained on neostigmine, methyl sulphate and atropine sulphate.

4. Hypotension and shock

Specific antivenom can reverse the direct myocardial and vasodilating effects of some venoms, but in patients who have leaked large amounts of blood and plasma into the bitten limb and elsewhere, a plasma expander is needed to correct hypovolaemia. The foot of the bed should be raised in an attempt to improve cardiac filling while an intravenous infusion is set up. Central venous pressure should be monitored to prevent fluid overload. Other causes of hypotension, such as a massive concealed haemorrhage or an autopharmacological effect of the venom, should be considered.

5. Renal failure

Acute renal failure may be caused by haemorrhage, ischaemia resulting from hypotension, disseminated intravascular coagulation and renal vasoconstriction, pigment nephropathy caused by haemoglobinuria, direct nephrotoxicity and immune complex glomerulonephritis caused by serum sickness reactions. Renal failure is not a common complication of envenoming by any African and Middle Eastern snake but cases of renal failure have been reported after bites by *E. coloratus, E. ocellatus, E. pyramidum, B. arietans, Thelotornis* species and *D. typus*, and this complication can occur in any case of severe envenoming. If the urine output falls below 400 ml in 24 hours, central venous pressure should be monitored and a urethral catheter inserted. Cautious rehydration with isotonic fluid (to increase the central venous pressure to +10 cmH$_2$0) can be followed by high dose frusemide (up to 100 mg intravenously) and finally dopamine (2.5 µg/kg/minute) by continuous infusion into a central vein. If these measures fail to increase urine output, patients should be managed conservatively until dialysis is indicated.

F. SNAKE VENOM OPHTHALMIA

The five "spitting" elapids in this region (*H. haemachatus, N. nigricollis, N. pallida, N. katiensis* and *N. mossambica*) can cause intense conjunctivitis, corneal erosions, complicated by secondary infection, anterior uveitis and permanent blindness[13,35,54,55]. First aid treatment consists of irrigating the eye or other affected mucous membrane as soon as possible using large volumes of water or any other available bland fluid. Unless a corneal abrasion can be excluded by slit lamp examination or fluorescein staining, the patient should be treated as for a corneal injury with a topical antimicrobial agent (tetracycline and chloramphenicol). Topical or systemic antivenom treatment is not indicated. 1 in 1000 adrenaline eye drops are said to relieve the burning sensation instantaneously.

G. TREATMENT OF BITES BY PARTICULAR SPECIES IN THE AFRICAN AND MIDDLE EAST REGION

1. Colubridae

Antivenom is available for the treatment of bites by only one African colubrid - the boomslang (*D. typus*). A small stock is held by the South African Institute of Medical

Research, Johannesburg, and is available on special request. Envenoming by other species, for which there is no antivenom, such as *Thelotornis* species, is conservative, aimed at the control of bleeding and prevention of renal failure. Heparin should not be used. Platelets and clotting factors can be replenished, but since the procoagulant venom factors from the venom may persist for days or even weeks, patients may continue to bleed.

2. Atractaspididae

No antivenoms are available. Early anaphylactic reactions should be treated with adrenaline and effects on the heart should be treated symptomatically.

3. Elapidae

Aspidelaps: No specific antivenom is available.

Boulengerina: No specific antivenom is available.

Dendroaspis: Five commercial antivenoms are available, for which activity is claimed against the venoms of all four species ([87] nos 6, 9, 119, 122 and 128). These include SAIMR "polyvalent antivenom" and "*Dendroaspis* antivenom", Pasteur-Mérieux "IPSER Afrique", Behringwerke "Central Africa" and Pasteur-Mérieux "*Dendroaspis*". The main therapeutic problem is the prevention or treatment of rapidly developing respiratory paralysis. Pressure immobilisation is recommended as first aid. The initial dose of antivenom should be not less than 50 ml, which should be repeated in 30-60 minutes if there has been a deterioration in neurotoxic signs. There is at least one anecdotal report of a response to anticholinesterase in a victim of *D. viridis* envenoming in Sierra Leone. Assisted ventilation may be needed in severe cases.

Elapsoidia species: No antivenom is available but severe envenoming seems unlikely.

Hemachatus haemachatus: Four polyspecific antivenoms are available, including SAIMR "polyvalent antivenom".

Naja - cytotoxic species: *(N. katiensis, N. nigricollis, N. mossambica, N. pallida)*: In this group only the venoms of *N. nigricollis* and *N. mossambica* are used for antivenom production. Cross neutralization of *N. pallida* and *N. katiensis* venoms by commercial antivenoms has not been studied. Polyspecific antivenoms are available for the treatment of envenoming by *N. mossambica* ([87] no 6) and *N nigricollis* ([87] nos 6, 118, 119, 127, 128) envenoming. Patients who develop local swelling should be given generous amounts of antivenom as early as possible. It is doubtful whether antivenoms are effective against the local necrosis caused by these venoms unless it is given very soon after the bite. In Nigeria, eight patients bitten by *N. nigricollis* developed local necrosis despite receiving 20-80 ml of polyspecific antivenom 6-24 hours after the bite[8]. However, in South Africa, four patients bitten by *N. mossambica* who received 80-100 ml of SAIMR antivenom 25 minutes to three hours after the bite escaped with negligible or no local necrosis[31]. Extensive superficial necrosis may develop in the subcutaneous tissues, occasionally affecting deeper tissues such as muscle. Antimicrobial treatment, early debridement and split skin grafting may be required.

In humans, neurotoxic envenoming by species in this group has not been convincingly demonstrated but it might occur if an unusually large dose of venom were injected, for example into a child. Hypovolaemic shock may develop within 24 hours in patients with extensive local swelling, especially children[31].

Naja - neurotoxic species: Polyspecific antivenoms are available for the treatment of envenoming by *N. haje* ([87] nos 5, 6, 118-120, 127, 129), *N. melanoleuca* ([87]nos 6, 118, 119, 127, 128) and *N. nivea* ([87]nos 6, 10, 118, 128). The main clinical problem is respiratory paralysis. Pressure immobilisation is recommended. An initial dose of not less than five ampoules of antivenom should be given at the earliest sign of neurotoxic envenoming. In the case of *N. nivea* envenoming, an initial dose of eight to ten ampoules has been recommended[48]. Anticholinesterase proved effective in a patient envenomed by *N. melanoleuca*[20] and produced some electrical and clinical improvement in a patient envenomed by *N. nivea*[48]. Assisted ventilation may be required in severely envenomed patients.

***Paranaja* and *Pseudohaje*:** Envenoming seems unlikely. Paraspecific cover of *Pseudohaje goldii* venom is claimed for SAIMR "polyvalent antivenom".

***Walterinnesia*:** A monospecific antivenom is available, but only by special request, from the Department of Zoology, Tel Aviv University, and paraspecific cover is claimed for SAIMR "polyvalent antivenom".

3. Viperidae

***Atheris* species:** No specific antivenom is available, but there was good paraspecific neutralization of *A. squamiger* venom by SAIMR "*Echis* antivenom".

***Bitis*:** Of the 13 species in this region, only four, *B. arietans*, *B. atropos*, *B. gabonica* and *B. nasicornis*, are likely to produce significant medical problems. No antivenom is available for *B. atropos* envenoming. Six polyspecific antivenoms are active against *B. arietans* and *B. gabonica* venoms ([87] nos 6, 10, 118, 119, 127, 128) and three against the venom of *B. nasicornis* ([87] nos 6, 118 and 128). In the case of *B arietans* bites, experience in northern Nigeria suggested that a starting dose of not less than eight ampoules of polyspecific antivenom should be given if there were any signs of systemic envenoming (such as spontaneous bleeding, thrombocytopenia, hypotension, bradycardia or leucocytosis) or if local swelling involved more than half the bitten limb. Antivenom appeared to prevent the development of local necrosis in severely envenomed patients when given between two and six hours after the bite. Patients with hypotension and bradycardia may respond rapidly to antivenom treatment. Hypovolaemia must be corrected in patients who have extravasated into massively swollen limbs[17]. Local necrosis may result in extensive skin loss with exposure of tendons and secondary infection. A rare complication, especially following bites on the lower leg, is anterior tibial compartment syndrome with ischaemic necrosis of the peroneal muscles. *B. gabonica* is capable of producing very severe envenoming: profound shock, cardiac arrhythmias and other ECG changes, coagulopathy, diffuse spontaneous bleeding and severe local swelling, blistering and necrosis. The approach to treatment should be the same as with *B. arietans* envenoming. A temporary cardiac pacemaker was inserted in a patient with marked atrial arrhythmia and prolonged QTc interval who also developed ARDS[63].

***Causus* species:** These snakes are a common cause of mild envenoming (local swelling with regional lymphadenopathy). SAIMR "polyvalent antivenom" produces slight paraspecific neutralization.

***Cerastes* species:** A number of mono- and polyspecific antivenoms are produced by institutes in North Africa and elsewhere[87]. Bites by these species rarely produce severe envenoming. Systemic bleeding, incoagulable blood and secondary infection of local necrosis at the site of the bite are all uncommon.

***Echis* species:** Several monospecific and a large number of polyspecific antivenoms manufactured in Europe, Africa, Iran, Russia, India and Pakistan are claimed to be effective against venoms of "*E. carinatus*" and *E. coloratus*[87]. However, antivenom raised against venom from geographically distant snakes has proved ineffective: for example Iranian antivenom in northern Nigeria[12] and SAIMR, Behringwerke and Pasteur-Mérieux specific antivenoms against the venom of a Tunisian *E. "pyramidum"*[88]. Comparative clinical trials have been carried out in Nigeria. SAIMR "*Echis* antivenom" proved more effective than Behringwerke "North Africa". An average of 15.2 ml of SAIMR antivenom permanently restored normal haemostasis[89]. Pasteur Paris "*Echis* monospecific antivenom" (not commercially available) proved more effective than Behringwerke "North Africa antivenom"; 20-40 ml of the Pasteur antivenom restored blood coagulability in all cases[9]. Pasteur-Mérieux "IPSER Afrique" antivenom proved effective in a dose of 20 ml in patients with mild systemic envenoming by *E. ocellatus*, but 30-60 ml were required for severely envenomed patients[91]. Based on this experience, the recommended dose of antivenom for victims of *E. ocellatus* in West Africa with incoagulable blood would be 20 ml of SAIMR or 40 ml of Pasteur-Mérieux "Ipser Afrique" and 100 ml of Behringwerke "North Africa antivenom". A new ovine Fab fragment antivenom raised against Nigerian *E. ocellatus* venom will be available soon from Therapeutic Antibodies Inc.

Patients bitten by *Echis* species should be admitted to hospital and examined repeatedly for evidence of systemic envenoming for at least 48 hours. Patients may start to bleed as late as 13 hours after the bite and their blood may not become incoagulable until 27 hours after the bite. Recurrent coagulopathy, after its initial correction by antivenom, was detected after an interval of up to 65 hours. Patients should, therefore, be followed for at least four days in hospital irrespective of their initial response to antivenom. Patients with evidence of systemic envenoming should be given antivenom even if they arrive at hospital many days after the bite. Patients rarely die before 23 hours after the bite but fatal cerebral haemorrhage has been described up to 12 days later. Cardiac arrhythmias, shock and renal failure occur very rarely after *Echis* bites. The effects of local envenoming should be treated as described above. Intramuscular injections must be avoided, and persistent oozing from venepuncture sites prevented by the application of pressure dressings.

For *E coloratus* envenoming, a monospecific antivenom is manufactured in Israel ([87] nos 55 and 57) and SAIMR "*Echis* antivenom" shows good neutralization. In the Israeli literature, there has been much discussion about the value of antivenom and the indications for its use. Heparin and antifibrinolytic agents have been preferred to antivenom by some, while others have recommended that the use of antivenom should be restricted to patients with persistent severe bleeding. Those who use antivenom appear to give a single initial dose without monitoring the effect on haemostasis and giving further doses where necessary. As a result, antivenom treatment appears to have had only a modest effect on the duration of coagulopathy[66,92].

Pseudocerastes persicus: Mono- and poly-specific antivenoms are manufactured in Iran ([87] nos 60, 62-64) but bites have rarely been reported.

Vipera species: Mono- and poly-specific antivenoms are available, but significant envenoming must be very rare. For *V. (Macrovipera) lebetina* envenoming, a number of mono- and poly-specific antivenoms are available[87]. Since geographical variation in the venom's antigenicity and composition can be expected, it would be wise to choose an antivenom raised against venoms from the appropriate country. The few case reports of bites by this species contain little information about the efficacy of antivenom. For *V. palaestinae*, a monospecific antivenom is manufactured in Israel and polyspecific antivenoms are available including Pasteur-Mérieux and Behringwerke "Near and Middle East". In Israel, use of the locally produced antivenom is indicated only in cases in whom symptoms of systemic envenoming such as hypotension, vomiting and diarrhoea appear soon after the bite. The initial dose is 50-80 ml. After antivenom treatment, bleeding ceased, blood pressure was restored in shocked patients and the period in hospital was reduced[65]. Mortality rate of *V. palaestinae* bites has been reduced from 6-10% before antivenom was available to virtually zero.

IX. REFERENCES

1. **SAUNERON S.** Un traité egyptien d'ophiologie. Cairo: Institut Francais d'Archeologie Orientale, 1989.
2. **KEIMER L.** Histoires de serpents dans l'Egypte ancienne et moderne. Cairo: L'Institut Francais d'Archeologie Orientale, 1947.

3. **PATERSON W.** A narrative of four voyages into the country of the Hottenttot and Caffraria. London: J.Johnson, 1789.
4. **DOMERGUE CA.** Un serpent venimeus de Madagascar. Observation de deux cas de morsure par *Madagascarophis* (Colubride opisthoglyphe). *Arch Inst Past Madagascar;* **56 (1):**299-311, 1989.
4a. **UNDERWOOD G, KOCHVA E.** On the affinities of the burrowing asps *Atractaspis* (Serpentes: Atractaspididae). *Zool J Linn Soc;* **107:** 3-64, 1993.
5. **CHERLIN VA, BORKIN LJ.** Taxonomic revision of the snake genus *Echis* (Viperidae). I An analysis of the history of study and synonymy. *USSR Academy of Sciences Proc Zool Inst Leningrad;* **207:**175-192, 1990.
6. **CHERLIN VA.** Taxonomic revision of the snake genus *Echis* (Viperidae). II An analysis of taxonomy and description of new forms. *USSR Academy of Science Proc Zool Inst, Leningrad;* **207:**193-223, 1990.
7. **KOCHVA E, BDOLAH A, WOLLBERG Z.** Sarafotoxins and endothelins: evolution, structure and function. *Toxicon;* **31 (5):**541-568, 1993.
8. **WARRELL DA, GREENWOOD BM, DAVIDSON NMcD, ORMEROD LD, PRENTICE CRM.** Necrosis, haemorrhage and complement depletion following bites by the spitting cobra (*Naja nigricollis*). **QJM; 45:**1-22, 1976.
9. **KORNALIK F.** The influence of snake venom problems on blood coagulation. In: Harvey AL, ed. *Snake Toxins.* New York: Pergamon Press,323-383, 1991
10. **HUTTON RA, WARRELL DA.** Action of snake venom components on the haemostatic system. *Blood Rev;* **7:**176-189, 1993.
11. **SWAROOP S, GRAB B.** Snakebite mortality in the world. *Bull Wld Hlth Org;* **10:**35-76, 1954.
12. **WARRELL DA, ARNETT C.** The importance of bites by the saw-scaled or carpet viper (*Echis carinatus*). Epidemiological studies in Nigeria and a review of the world literature. *Acta Tropica (Basel);* **33 (4):**307-341, 1976.
13. **PUGH RNH, THEAKSTON RDG, REID HA, BHAR IS.** Malumfashi endemic diseases research project *XIII. Ann Trop Med Parasitol;* **74 (5):**523-530, 1980.
14. **PUGH RNH, THEAKSTON RDG.** Incidence and mortality of snake bite in savanna Nigeria. *lan;* **Nov 29:**1181-1183, 1980.
15. **HO M, WARRELL MJ, WARRELL DA, BIDWELL D, VOLLER A.** Review. A critical reappraisal of the use of enzyme-linked immunosorbent assays in the study of snake bite. *Toxicon;* **24 (3):**211-221, 1986.
16. **THEAKSTON RDG, LLOYD-JONES MJ, REID HA.** Micro-Elisa for detecting and assaying snake venom and venom-antibody. *lan;* **ii:**639-641, 1977.
17. **CHAPMAN DS.** The symptomatology, pathology and treatment of the bites of venomous snakes of Central and Southern Africa. In: Bucherl W, Buckley EE, Deulofeu V, eds. *Venomous Animals and their Venoms Vol 1.* New York: Academic Press,463-527, 1968.
18. **CHIPPAUX J-P, BRESSY C.** L'endemie ophidienne des platations de Cote-d'Ivoire. *Bull Soc Path Exot et Fil;* **74 (4):**458-467, 1981.
19. **WORLD HEALTH ORGANIZATION.** Progress in the characterization of venoms and standardization of antivenoms. *WHO Offset Publication No 58.* Geneva: World Health Organization, 1981.
20. **STAHEL E.** Epidemiological aspects of snake bites on a Liberian rubber plantation. *Acta Tropica;* **37:**367-374, 1980.
21. **LANKOANDE SALIFOU T.** Envenimations par morsure de serpents. *Med Afr Noire;* **28:**143-146, 1981.
22. **PITMAN CRS.** The saw-scaled viper or carpet viper (*Echis carinatus*) in Africa and its bite. *J Herpetol Ass Afr;* **9:**6-34, 1973.
23. **CARME B, TRAPE JF, KUMBA LL.** Les morsures de serpent au Congo. Estimation de la morbidite a Brazzaville et en zone rurale de la region du Pool et du Mayombe. *Annals Soc Belge Med Trop;* **66:**183-189, 1986.
24. **KASILO OMJ, NHACHI CFB.** A retrospective study of poisoning due to snake venom in Zimbabwe. *Hum & Exper Toxicol;* **12:**15-18, 1993.
25. **AUERBACH RD.** *The amphibians and reptiles of Botswana.* Gaborone: Mokwepa Consultants, 1987.
26. **McNALLY SL, REITZ CJ.** Victims of snakebite. A 5-year study at Shongwe Hospital, Kangwane, 1978-1982. *S Afr Med J;* **72:**855-860, 1987.
27. **CHRISTENSEN PA.** Snakebite and the use of antivenom in southern Africa. *S Afr Med J;* **59:**934-938, 1981.
28. **WARRELL DA.** Venomous bites and stings in Saudi Arabia. *Saudi Med J;* **14 (3):**196-202, 1993.
29. **EFRATI P.** Symptomatology, pathology and treatment of the bites of viperid snakes. In: Lee CY, ed. *Snake Venoms.*: Berlin, Springer Verlag, 956-977, 1979.
30. **CHRISTENSEN PA.** African snake venoms. In: Gear JHS, ed. *Medicine in a Tropical Environment.* Cape Town: South African Medical Research Council, 310-322, 1977.
31. **TILBURY CR.** Observations on the bite of the Mozambique spitting cobra (*Naja mossambica mossambica*). *S Afr Med J;* **61:**308-313, 1982.
32. **VISSER J, CHAPMAN DS.** Snakes and snakebite. *Venomous snakes and management of snakebite in Southern Africa.* Cape Town, Johannesburg, London: Purnell, 1978.

33. **FITZSIMONS DC, SMITH HM.** Another rear-fanged South African snake lethal to humans. *Herpetologica*; **14:**198-202, 1958.
34. **WARRELL DA, ORMEROD LD, DAVIDSON NMcD.** Bites by the night adder (*Causus maculatus*) and burrowing vipers (genus Atractaspis) in Nigeria. *Am J Trop Med Hyg*; **25 (3):**517-524, 1976.
35. **WARRELL DA, ORMEROD LD.** Snake venom ophthalmia and blindness caused by the spitting cobra (*Naja nigricollis*) in Nigeria. *Am J Trop Med Hyg*; **25 (3):**525-529, 1976.
36. **BROADLEY DG, COCK EV.** *Snakes of Rhodesia.* Rhodesia: Longman, 1975.
37. **VAN EGMOND KC.** A fatal bite by the shield-nose snake (*Aspidelaps scutatus*). *S Afr Med J*; **66:**714, 1984.
38. **ZALTMAN M, RUMBAK M, RABIE M, ZWI S.** Neurotoxicity due to the bite of the shield-nose snake (*Aspidelaps scutatus*). *S Afr Med J*; **66:**111-112, 1984.
39. **BRANCH WR.** *Field Guide to the Snakes and Other Reptiles of Southern Africa.* London: New Holland Publ, 1988:
40. **LOVERIDGE A.** On two amphibious snakes of the Central African Lake Region. *Bull Antiven Inst Am*; **5 (1):**7-12, 1931.
41. **KNOEPFFLER LP.** Faune du Gabon (Amphibien et Reptiles). I Ophidiens de l'Ogooue-Ivindo et du Woleu N'tem. *Biologia gabonica*; **2 (fasc 1):**1-23, 1966.
42. **DURRANT S.** Snake bite - case history. *Herp Assoc Zimbabwe; Newsletter No*; **11:** 33-4, 1992.
43. **HERPETOLOGICAL ASSOCIATION OF AFRICA.** Schoolboy dies from mamba bite. *Herpetological Association of Africa Newsletter*; **12:**9, 1990.
44. **RIPPEY JJ, RIPPEY E, BRANCH WR.** A survey of snakebite in the Johannesburg area. *S Afr Med J*; **50 (46):**1872-1876, 1976.
45. **FITZSIMONS VFM.** *Snakes of Southern Africa.* London: MacDonald, 1962.
46. **GEAR JHS.** Non-polio causes of polio-like paralytic syndrome. *Rev Inf Dis*; **6 Suppl 2:**S379-S384, 1984.
47. **WARRELL DA, BARNES HJ, PIBURN MF.** Neurotoxic effects of bites by the Egyptian cobra (*Naja haje*) in Nigeria. *Trans R Soc Trop Med Hyg*; **70 (1):**78-79, 1976.
48. **BLAYLOCK RS, LICHTMAN AR, POTGIETER PD.** Clinical manifestations of Cape cobra (*Naja nivea*) bites. Two cases. *S Afr Med J*; **68 (5):**342-344, 1985.
49. **CHRISTENSEN PA.** *South African Snake Venoms and Antivenoms.* Johannesburg: South African Institute for Medical Research, 1955.
50. **WARRELL DA.** Clinical snake bite problems in the Nigerian savanna region. *Technische Hochschule Darmstadt Schriftenreihe Wissenschaft und Technik*; **14:**31-60, 1979.
51. **HOFFMANN LAC, DE WETPOTGIETER S.** *Naja mossambica* Mozambique spitting cobra or M'fezi envenomation. *J Herpetol Ass Afr*; **35:**41-42, 1988.
52. **DELPORT SD, SCHMID EV, FARRANT PJ.** Delayed neurotoxic and cytotoxic complications after snake envenomation. *S Afr Med J*; **79:**169, 1991.
53. **PAYNE T, WARRELL DA.** Effects of venom in eye from spitting cobra. *Archs Ophth*; **94 (10):**1803, 1976.
54. **LATH NK, PATEL MM.** Treatment of snake venom ophthalmia. *Centr Afr J Med*; **30 (9):**175-176, 1984.
55. **BLAYLOCK RSM.** Snake bites at Triangle Hospital January 1975 to June 1981. *Centr Afr J Med*; **28:**1-11, 1982.
56. **CORKILL NL.** *Snakes and snake bite in Iraq.* London: Baillier Tindall Cox, 1932.
57. **YAYON E, SIKULAR E, KEYNAN A.** Desert black snake (*Walterinnesia aegyptia*) bites - a presentation of four cases. *Harefuah*; **115:**269-270, 1988.
58. **LANOIE LO, BRANCH WR.** Venoms and snakebite. *J Herpetol Ass Afr*; **39:**29, 1991.
59. **WARRELL DA, ORMEROD LD, DAVIDSON NMcD.** Bites by puff adder (*Bitis arietans*) in Nigeria and value of antivenom. *BMJ*; **4:**697-700, 1975.
60. **SEZI CL, ALPIDOVSKY VK, REEVE MI.** Defibrination syndrome after snake bite. *E Afr Med J*; **49:**589-596, 1972.
61. **PITMAN CRS.** *A Guide to the Snakes of Uganda.* Codicote: Wheldon & Wesley, 1974.
62. **McNALLY T, CONWAY GS, JACKSON L, ET AL.** Accidental envenoming by a Gaboon viper (*Bitis gabonica*): the haemostatic disturbances observed and investigation of *in vitro* haemostatic properties of whole venom. *Trans R Soc Trop Med Hyg*; **87:**66-70, 1993.
63. **EDWARDS IR, FLEMING JB, JAMES MF.** Management of a Gaboon viper bites: a case report. *Centr Afr J Med*; **25 (10):**217-221, 1979.
64. **ROSE W.** *Snakes - mainly South African.* Cape Town: Maskew Miller Ltd, 1955.
65. **EFRATI P.** Clinical manifestations of snake bite by *Vipera xanthina palestinae* (Werner) and their pathophysiological basis. *Mem Inst Butantan*; **32:**189-191, 1966.
66. **BENBASSAT J, SHALEV O.** Envenomation by *Echis coloratus* (Mid-East saw-scaled viper): a review of the literature and indications for treatment. *Israel J Med Sci*; **29:**239-250, 1993.
67. **MANN G.** *Echis colorata* bites in Israel: an evaluation of specific antiserum use on the base of 21 cases of snake bite. *Toxicol Eur Res*; **1 (6):**365-369, 1978.

68. **TILBURY CR, MADKOUR MM, SALTISSI D, SULEIMAN M.** Acute renal failure following the bite of Burton's carpet viper *Echis coloratus* Gunther in Saudi Arabia: case report and review. *Saudi Med J*; **8** (1):87-95, 1987.

69. **FLOWER SS.** Notes on the recent reptiles and amphibians of Egypt. *Proc Zool Soc Lond*; 735-851, 1933.

70. **WARRELL DA, DAVIDSON NMcD, GREENWOOD BM, ET AL.** Poisoning by bites of the saw-scaled or carpet viper (*Echis carinatus*) in Nigeria. *QJM*; **46**:33-62, 1977.

71. **CORKILL NL.** Sudan Thanatophidia. *Sudan Notes and Records*; **30**:101-106, 1949.

72. **ORAM S, ROSS G, PELL L, WINTELER J.** Renal cortical calcification after snake bite. *BMJ*; **1**:1647-1648, 1963.

73. **HALL L.** Investigations in a case of snake bite. *E Afr Med J*; **39** (2):66-68, 1962.

74. **DREWES RC, SACHERER JM.** A new population of carpet vipers *Echis carinatus* from northern Kenya. *J E Afr Nat Hist Soc*; **145**:1-7, 1974.

75. **KOCHVA E.** Venomous snakes of Israel. In: Gopalakrishnakone P, Chou LM, eds. *Snakes of Medicinal Importance (Asia-Pacific region)*. National University of Singapore; 311-321, 1990.

76. **CORKILL NL.** An inquiry into snake bite in Iraq. *Ind J Med Res*; **20**:599-696, 1932.

77. **EFRATI P, REIF L.** Clinical and pathological observations on sixty-five cases of viper bite in Israel. *Amer J Trop Med Hyg*; **2**:1085-1108, 1953.

78. **HAMILTON-FAIRLEY N, KELLAWAY CH.** Symposium on snake bite. *Med J Austr*; **Mar 9**: 296-377, 1929.

79. **GRASSET E.** Concentrated African antivenom serum: its preparation, standardization and use in the treatment of snake bite. *S Afr Med J*; **7**:35-39, 1933.

80. **CHRISTENSEN PA.** The treatment of snake bite. *S Afr Med J*; **43** (41):1253-1258, 1969.

81. **BARNES JM, TRUETA J.** Absorption of bacteria, toxins and snake venoms from the tissues. Importance of the lymphatic circulation. *lan*; **1**:623-626, 1941.

82. **SUTHERLAND SK, COULTER AR, HARRIS RD.** Rationalisation of first-aid measures for elapid snake bite. *lan*; **i**:183-186, 1979.

83. **CURRIE B.** Pressure-immobilization first aid for snakebite - fact and fancy. *Toxicon*; **31** (8):931-932, 1993.

84. **MALASIT P, WARRELL DA, CHANTHAVANICH P, ET AL.** Prediction, prevention and mechanism of early (anaphylactic) antivenom reactions in victims of snake bites. *BMJ*; **292**:17-20, 1986.

85. **THEAKSTON RDG, PHILLIPS RE, LOOAREESUWAN S, ECHEVERRIA P, MAKIN T, WARRELL DA.** Bacteriological studies of the venom and mouth cavities of wild Malayan pit vipers (*Calloselasma rhodostoma*) in southern Thailand. *Trans R Soc Trop Med Hyg*; **84**:875-879, 1990.

86. **GARFIN SR, CASTILONIA RR, MUBARAK SJ, HARGENS AR, RUSSELL FE, AKESON WH.** Rattlesnake bites and surgical decompression: results using a laboratory model. *Toxicon*; **22**:177-182, 1984.

87. **THEAKSTON RDG, WARRELL DA.** Antivenoms: a list of hyperimmune sera currently available for the treatment of envenoming by bites and stings. *Toxicon*; **29** (12):1419-1470, 1991.

88. **GILLISSEN A, THEAKSTON RDG, BARTH J, MAY B, KRIEG M, WARRELL DA.** Neurotoxicity and haemostatic disturbances after a bite by a Tunisian saw-scaled or carpet viper (*Echis "pyramidum"* complex). *Toxicon*;**32**(8):937-944, 1994.

89. **WARRELL DA, DAVIDSON NMcD, ORMEROD LD, ET AL.** Bites by the saw-scaled or carpet viper (*Echis carinatus*): trial of two specific antivenoms. *BMJ*; **4**:437-440, 1974.

90. **WARRELL DA, WARRELL MJ, EDGAR W, PRENTICE CRM, MATHISON JH, MATHISON J.** Comparison of Pasteur and Behringwerke antivenoms in envenoming by the carpet viper (*Echis carinatus*). *BMJ*; **280** (6214):607-609, 1980.

91. **DAUDU I, THEAKSTON RDG.** Preliminary trial of a new polyspecific antivenom in Nigeria. *Anns Trop Med Parasitol*; **82** (3):311-313, 1988.

92. **SCHULCHYNSKA-CASTEL H, DVILANSKY A, KEYNAU A.** *Echis colorata* bites: clinical evaluation of 42 patients. A retrospective study. *Israel J Med Sci*; **22**:880-884, 1986.

Chapter 27

CLINICAL TOXICOLOGY OF SNAKEBITE IN ASIA

David A. Warrell

TABLE OF CONTENTS

I. INTRODUCTION

This chapter covers the whole of Asia: limited in the west by the Ural'skiy Khrebet (Russian Federation), Kazakhstan, the Caspian Sea and Iran; and in the east and southeast by the Japanese, Philippine and Indonesian islands but excluding Irian Jaya and the islands of eastern Indonesia inhabited by Australasian elapids (e.g. Obi, Seram, Kep. Tanimbar, Kep. Kai and Kep. Aru) (see Chapter 28). Climate and vegetation vary enormously throughout this vast region. In Asia, no venomous snakes are found within the Arctic Circle, but species such as *Vipera berus* and *Vipera ursinii* are found in the boreal forests of Siberia. Further south is desert and steppe in Kazakhstan, Mongolia and northern China and rocky desert and mountainous country in southwestern Asia (Uzbekhistan, Turkmenistan, Iran and Afghanistan and the high Tibetan plateau with the Himalayan range to the south). The tropical rain forest, rapidly dwindling, occurs throughout South East Asia, southern China, Indonesia and along the west coast of India and in parts of Sri Lanka. Monsoon forest exists in eastern India, Bangladesh, parts of Sri Lanka and areas of Southeast Asia. Much of northeastern and southern India is dry tropical scrub forest and thorn forest.

The distribution of the various species of venomous snake is largely determined by their preferences for climate and habitat, together with changes in sea levels and climate during the pleistocene era. Two medically-important species, Russell's viper (*Daboia russelii*) and the Malayan pit viper (*Calloselasma rhodostoma*), show a puzzling discontinuity in their distribution. In the case of Russell's viper, Wüster et al[1] have attempted to explain this first by this species' preference for partially open habitats with dry areas and avoidance of rain forests, and secondly by rising sea levels and an increasingly humid climate which might have eradicated the species between central Thailand and eastern Java. In the case of *C rhodostoma*, Gloyd and Conant[2] explain its distribution by a need for a dry season, which does not occur between northwestern Malaysia and Java. Since ancient times, snakes have been worshipped, feared, loathed, eaten and used for the production of medicines and leather in many parts of Asia. For example, the architect of the Great Stupa (Ruwanweli Seya) at Anuradhapura in Sri Lanka was said to have been killed by a cobra in the 2nd Century BC. Snakes, especially the sacred cobra or "nag", feature in many of the traditional stories about Hindu deities and the Buddah. In India, the cult of serpent worship has survived for at least 3000 years, its living tradition being Naga-panchami, a festival celebrated throughout India. Serpents are associated with fertility and rain-making. In southern India, serpents are worshipped under the name of the god Subramani, whose shrine is situated in Mysore[3]. In China, venomous snakes were mentioned by Confucius in his "Shih Ching" of the 6th Century BC[4]. The medicinal use of *Agkistrodon blomhofii brevicaudus* ("fu she") was described in Chinese pharmacopoeias of the 8th Century AD and in "The Great Pharmacopoeia" of Shi-zhen Li of the 16th Century. Today, the Chinese still use snakes as food and almost every organ and tissue of the snake finds some place in traditional Chinese medicine[5]. European visitors to Asia, such as Baldaeus (17th Century) and the Portuguese physician Garcia da Orta (16th Century), were impressed by the danger of snakebite and advocated traditional remedies such as "snakewood" and the "snake stone"[6]. Today, the market for snake meat, leather and other constituents is threatening the survival of some species in countries such as Thailand, India, Vietnam and the Philippines.

II. THE VENOMOUS SNAKES OF ASIA AND THEIR DISTRIBUTIONS

Four families of venomous snakes, Colubridae, Hydrophiidae, Elapidae and Viperidae, are represented in this region (Table 1). The Hydrophiidae are dealt with in Chapter 13 and will not be discussed here.

Table 1
Snakes of medical importance in Asia

Family/Species	Common Name
Colubridae (back-fanged snakes)	
Capable of causing fatal envenoming	
Rhabdophis subminiatus	red-necked keelback
R tigrinus	yamakagashi
Capable of causing severe envenoming	
Malpolon monspessulanus	Montpellier snake
Capable of causing mild envenoming	
Ahaetulla nasuta	common green or long-nosed whip snake
Balanophis ceylonicus	Sri Lankan keelback or blossom krait
Boiga ceylonensis	Sri Lankan cat snake
B dendrophila	mangrove snake
B forsteni	Forsten's cat snake
Cerberus rhynchops	dog-faced water snake
Coluber ravergieri	mountain racer
C rhodorachis	Jan's desert racer
Enhydris enhydris	rainbow water snake
Malpolon moilensis	hooded malpolon
Elapidae (kraits, cobras, coral snakes)	
Bungarus bungaroides	northeastern hill krait
B caeruleus	common (Indian) krait
B candidus	Malayan krait
B ceylonicus	Sri Lankan krait, karawala
B fasciatus	banded krait
B flaviceps	red- or yellow-headed krait
B javanicus	Javan krait
B lividus	lesser black krait
B magnimaculatus	Burmese krait
B multicinctus	Chinese or many banded krait
B niger	greater black krait
B sindanus (= B walli)	Sind (Wall's) krait
Calliophis beddomei	Beddome's coral snake
C bibroni	Bibron's coral snake
C calligaster	red-bellied coral snake
C gracilis	slender coral snake
C japonicus	hyan, hai
C kelloggi	Kellog's coral snake
C macclellandi	Macclelland's coral snake
C maculiceps	small-spotted coral snake
C melanurus	black-tailed coral snake
C nigrescens	common (Indian) coral snake
C sauteri	Sauter's coral snake
Maticora bivirgata	blue long-glanded coral snake
M intestinalis	banded long-glanded coral snake
Naja atra	Chinese cobra
N kaouthia	monocellate cobra
N naja	Indian spectacled cobra
N oxiana	Oxus cobra
N philippinensis	Philippine cobra
N samarensis	Samar cobra
N siamensis	Thai spitting cobra
N sputatrix	Javan spitting cobra
N sumatrana	Sumatran spitting cobra
Ophiophagus hannah	king cobra or hamadryad
Walterinnesia aegyptia	black desert cobra
Viperidae (vipers and pit vipers)	
Viperinae (old world vipers)	
Azemiops feae	Fea's viper
Cerastes gasperettii	Gasperetti's horned sand viper

Family/Species	Common Name
Daboia russelii	Russell's viper or daboia
Echis carinatus	Indian saw-scaled viper or phoorsa
E multisquamatus	Central Asian saw-scaled viper
E sochureki	Sochurek's saw-scaled viper
Eristocophis mcmahoni	McMahon's viper
Pseudocerastes persicus	Persian horned viper
Vipera xanthina complex	(Middle Eastern mountain vipers)
V albicornuta	white-horned viper
V latifii	Latifi's viper
V raddei	Raddi's viper
V wagneri	Wagner's viper
V xanthina	Ottoman viper
V berus	European viper or adder
V (Macrovipera) lebetina	Levantine or blunt-nosed viper
V ursinii	Orsini's or steppe viper
Crotalinae (Asian pit vipers)	
Agkistrodon (Gloydius) blomhoffii blomhoffii	Japanese mamushi
A b brevicaudus	Chinese mamushi
A halys	Siberian pit viper
A himalayanus	Himalayan pit viper
A intermedius	Central Asian pit viper
A saxatilis	rock mamushi
A shedaoensis	snake island (Shedao) mamushi
A ussuriensis	Ussuri mamushi
A monticola	Likiang pit viper
A strauchi	Tibetan pit viper
Calloselasma rhodostoma	Malayan pit viper
Deinagkistrodon acutus	sharp-nosed pit viper or hundred-pacer
Hypnale hypnale	Merrem's hump-nosed viper
H nepa	Sri Lankan hump-nosed viper
H walli	Wall's hump-nosed viper
Ovophis chaseni	Chasen's pit viper
O convictus	Penang pit viper
O monticola	mountain pit viper
O okinavensis	Hime-habu or kufah
Trimeresurus albolabris	white-lipped green pit viper
T borneensis	Bornean pit viper
T brongersmai	Brongersma's pit viper
T cantori	Cantor's pit viper
T cornutus	horned pit viper
T elegans	Sakishima-habu
T erythrurus	red-tailed green pit viper
T fasciatus	banded pit viper
T flavomaculatus	yellow-spotted pit viper
T flavoviridis	habu
T gracilis	slender pit viper
T gramineus	Indian bamboo pit viper
T hageni	Hagen's pit viper
T huttoni	Hutton's pit viper
T jerdoni	Jerdon's pit viper
T kanburiensis	Kanchanaburi pit viper
T kaulbacki	Kaulback's pit viper
T labialis	lipped pit viper
T macrolepis	large-scaled pit viper
T macrops	dark green pit viper
T malabaricus	Malabar rock pit viper
T mangshanensis	Mount Mang pit viper
T medoensis	Medog pit viper
T mucrosquamatus	Chinese habu, Taiwanese pit viper
T popeiorum	Pope's pit viper
T puniceus	flat-nosed pit viper
T purpureomaculatus	mangrove pit viper
T schultzei	Schultze's pit viper

Family/Species	Common Name
T stejnegeri	Chinese bamboo pit viper
T strigatus	horse-shoe pit viper
T sumatranus	Sumatran pit viper
T tibetanus	Tibetan pit viper
T tokarensis	Tokara-habu
T tonkinensis	Tonking pit viper
T trigonocephalus	Sri Lankan green pit viper
T xiangchengensis	Xiangcheng pit viper
Tropidolaemus wagleri	Wagler's or temple pit viper

A. BACK FANGED SNAKES (FAMILY COLUBRIDAE)

The grooved back fangs or enlarged solid maxillary teeth (Figure 1a) of these snakes convey the venomous secretions of Duvernoy's glands which empty into a fold of buccal mucosa. All the back-fanged colubrids should be regarded as potentially dangerous to man and must be handled with caution. Two species of Asian colubrid, the Yamakagashi (*Rhabdophis tigrinus*) and the red-necked keelback (*R subminiatus*) (Figure 1), are capable of killing humans; the Montpellier snake (*Malpolon monspessulanus*) of western Iran can produce severe systemic symptoms, while bites by at least seven other species are reported to have caused mild local swelling and in some cases transient mild systemic symptoms.

1. Colubrids capable of fatal envenoming

1. Red-necked keelback (*Rhabdophis subminiatus*) (Figure 1b): the last two maxillary teeth are greatly enlarged (Figure 1a). The colour is brownish green above with thin broken lines of black and white/yellow on the interstitial skin and edges of the scales. The belly is pale with a yellowish gular region. There is an oblique black bar beneath the eye. The interstitial skin on the neck is red. The maximum length is 80 cm. This snake is mainly terrestrial and diurnal. It occurs widely from Sikkim, Bhutan and Assam in the west, throughout Southeast Asia and east to southern China and the Indonesian islands as far east as Sulawesi.

2. Yamakagashi or Japanese garter snake (*R tigrinus*): the two last maxillary teeth are greatly enlarged and curved with a sharp posterior cutting ridge but no venom groove. The coloration is variable from almost uniform greenish-brown with a pale belly, to a striped pattern with black, pale-flecked, bands on a ground colour which is generally red in the anterior third of the body and greenish-brown in the posterior two-thirds. There are black flecks on the supralabial scales. The maximum length can exceed 1 metre. It is a very common snake in Japan, inhabiting fields and mountain forests. It is found in Honshu, Shikoku, Kyushu, Osumi and some of the smaller islands and, outside Japan, in Korea, southern Primorskiy (Russian Federation), China and Taiwan. The nuchal glands of this species release their defensive secretions when pressure is applied to the skin. They contain Bufo-like steroid toxins which can damage the eye on contact[7].

2. Colubrids capable of severe systemic envenoming

Montpellier snake (*Malpolon monspessulanus*): this species occurs in western Iran. It is discussed in the chapter on African and Middle Eastern snakes.

3. Colubrids capable of mild envenoming

Species include -

1. Common green or long-nosed whipsnake (*Ahaetulla nasuta*): India (except the northwest), Sri Lanka, Burma, Thailand, Cambodia and Vietnam.

2. Sri Lanka keelback or blossom krait (*Balanophis ceylonensis*): endemic to Sri Lanka.

3. Sri Lanka cat snake (*Boiga ceylonensis*): Sri Lanka and southwest India (Western Ghats).

4. Mangrove snake (*B. dendrophila*): southern Thailand, Malaysia, Singapore, Indonesia as far east as Sulawesi.

5. Forsten's cat snake (*B. forsteni*): Sri Lanka and India north to Sikkim.

6. Dog-faced water snake (*Cerberus rhynchops*): coast of the Indian subcontinent, Andaman and Nicobar Islands, Southeast Asia, Indonesian islands and Philippines.

7. Mountain racer (*Coluber ravergieri*): Iran, Afghanistan, Pakistan, northwestern India, eastern Turkmenistan, Uzbekistan, eastern Kazakhstan, western Mongolia, Xinjiang China.

8. Jan's desert racer (*C. rhodorachis*): southern Iran east to Pakistan (North Africa and the Middle East).

9. Rainbow water snake (*Enhydris enhydris*): India, Bangladesh, Southeast Asia and southern China.

10. Hooded malpolon (*Malpolon moilensis*): southern Iran (North Africa and the Middle East).

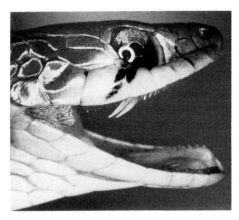 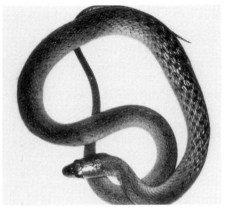

Figure 1. Red necked keelback (*Rhabdophis subminiatus*). Specimen from Thailand (photos © Dr. D.A. Warrell).

1a. Showing large posterior maxillary teeth.   **1b.** Whole snake, 38cm long.

B. COBRAS, KRAITS AND CORAL SNAKES (FAMILY ELAPIDAE)

Six genera and thirty species of elapid snakes inhabit this region including the world's largest venomous snake, the king cobra (*Ophiophagus hannah*) and the familiar cobras and kraits. All are potentially dangerous. Compared to vipers, elapids possess relatively short (but up to about 10 mm long) fixed, front (proteroglyph) fangs which are mounted at the anterior end of the maxilla.

1. Kraits (genus *Bungarus*)

The species of this genus are found in the Indian subcontinent, Southeast Asia, southern China and Indonesia. They are relatively long, slender snakes with highly polished scales and with the vertebral row of scales usually enlarged. They feed largely on snakes and lizards and frequently enter human dwellings at night in pursuit of their prey. All 12-14 species should be regarded as potentially dangerous, but there are reports of bites by only six species.

1. Common (Indian) krait (*B. caeruleus*) (Figure 2): black, brownish-black or bluish-black above crossed by pairs of narrow white stripes. The belly is white. The length may exceed 1.5 metres. It is found from sea level up to an altitude of 1600 metres in Pakistan, India, Bangladesh, Nepal and Sri Lanka.

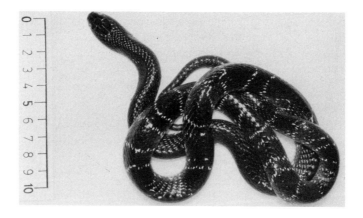

Figure 2. Common (Indian) krait (*Bungarus caeruleus*). Specimen 70cm long
from Anuradhapura, Sri Lanka (photo © Dr. D.A. Warrell).

2. Malayan krait (*B. candidus*) (Figure 3): the belly is pure white (Figure 3b). There is a
series of black or brownish-black saddle-shaped markings along the back separated by
broad white or yellowish cross bars, speckled with black (up to 25 on the body and up to 10
on the tail). The body is circular in cross section and the tail ends in a sharp tip. It is easily
confused with harmless "mimics" such as *Lycodon laoensis* and *Dryocalamus davisonii*[8]
(Figure 4). The maximum length is 1.6 metres. This cryptic species inhabits lowland forests
throughout Thailand and is widely distributed in Thailand, other Southeast Asian countries
(Laos, Cambodia, Malaysia) and in Indonesia (Sumatra, Java, Sulawesi and some smaller
islands) and possibly in southeastern Burma.

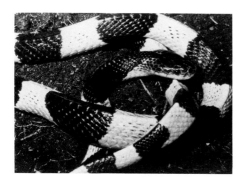
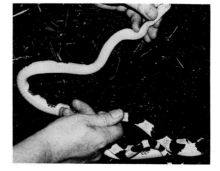

Figure 3. Malayan krait (*Bungarus candidus*). Specimen from Thailand (photo © Dr. D.A. Warrell).
3a. Showing black saddle-shaped patches.   **3b.** Showing pure white belly.

3. Sri Lankan krait (*B ceylonicus*) (Figure 5): black above, greyish below with a series of
complete white rings which are narrow on the vertebral line and broaden laterally.
Maximum length is 1,346 mm. It is endemic to Sri Lanka where its range overlaps with that
of *B caeruleus*.
4. Banded krait (*B. fasciatus*) (Figure 6): this large snake, which may reach a length of
more than 2 metres, is easily recognised by its alternating circumferential bands of yellow
and black (Figure 6b), its triangular body cross section and blunt tail. It occurs in lowland
forests in northeastern India, throughout Southeast Asia, southern China (south of latitude
25°N, including Hong Kong and Hainan) and in Indonesia (Sumatra, Java and Borneo).
5. Red- or yellow-headed krait (*B. flaviceps*) (Figure 7): blue-black above and below with
a bright red head, neck and tail. A whitish stripe on the flanks is present in juveniles but

usually fades with age. Maximum length 1.6 metres. It inhabits forests in southern Thailand, (possibly southern Burma), Malaysia, Cambodia and Indonesia (Sumatra, Java, Borneo and some smaller islands).

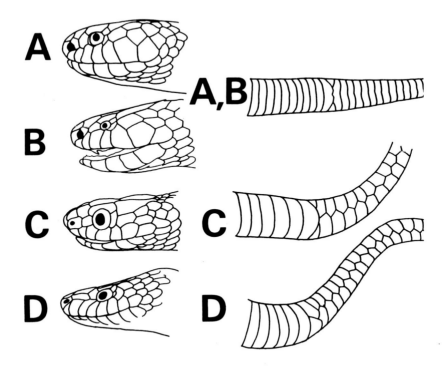

Figure 4. Head scales and ventral surface of the tails of:
A. Banded krait (*Bungarus fasciatus*);
B. Malayan krait (*Bungarus candidus*);
and two of their non-venomous mimics;
C. *Dryocalamus davisonii*;
D. *Lycodon laoensis*.
Note the relatively large nasal scales in the kraits, large eye of *Dryocalamus* and flattened head of *Lycodon*, which, unlike the other species, has two scales (loreal and pre-ocular) between the nasal scale and the eye. The kraits, which have front fangs and unpaired subcaudal scales, grow much larger than their mimics[8].

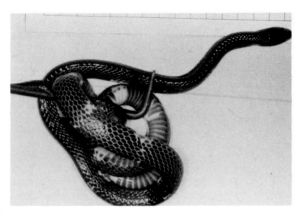

Figure 5. Sri Lankan krait (*B. ceylonicus*), showing dark and white bands encircling the body. Scale in cm. (photo © Dr. D.A. Warrell).

503

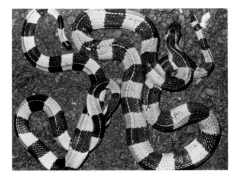 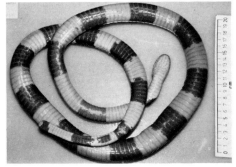

Figure 6. Banded krait (*Bungarus fasciatus*) (photos © Dr. D.A. Warrell).
6a. Two specimens from eastern Thailand   **6b.** Ventral view showing that the black bands encircle the body.

6. Javan krait (*B. javanicus*): the top of the head, neck and tail are blue-black; supralabial scales whitish with darker spots; white specks on the enlarged vertebral scales becoming larger towards the tail. Lateral scales white edged. Belly whitish-yellow. Length 860 mm. Known only from Java, in the neighbourhood of Cheribon, Indramaju and Linggardjati.

7. Chinese or many-banded krait (*B. multicinctus*) (Figure 8): this species resembles *B. candidus*. The belly is pure white. Along the back is a series of black, bluish-black or dark brown saddle-shaped markings separated by 30-50 narrow white bands sprinkled with dark spots. The maximum length is 1.84 metres. It inhabits low plains and hilly regions up to an altitude of 1300 metres, ranging throughout southern China south of the Yangtze River, Taiwan, Hong Kong and Hainan and west to northern Laos and Burma.

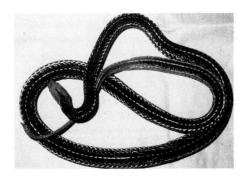 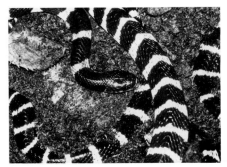

Figure 7. Red headed krait (*B. flaviceps*). 1.1m long specimen from southern Thailand (photo © Dr. D.A. Warrell).

Figure 8. Chinese krait (*B. multicinctus*). Specimen from Hong Kong (photo © Dr. D.A. Warrell).

2. Asian coral snakes (*Calliophis*) (Figure 9)

Ten or 11 species of long, slender, strikingly-marked snakes of this genus have been described from India, Sri Lanka, Nepal, Southeast Asia, China, Taiwan, Japan and Sumatra. They are cryptic and nocturnal, and have rarely been responsible for bites. One case of fatal envenoming by *C. maclellandii univirgatus* has been described[9].

3. Long-glanded coral snakes (genus *Maticora*)

This genus comprises two species of very long, thin, brilliantly-coloured snakes whose venom glands extend for almost a third of the length of the body but which bite very rarely. They have proved capable of severe and fatal envenoming.

1. Blue Malaysian or long-glanded coral snake (*M. bivirgata*) (Figure 10): dark blue-black above with pale blue lateral lines. The head, entire belly and tail are bright red. In defence, it raises and coils its tail revealing the red, ventral surface. The length may exceed 1.5 metres. They are found on the ground near forest streams in southern Thailand, Cambodia, peninsula Malaysia, Singapore and Indonesia (Java, Borneo and smaller islands).
2. Banded or brown long-glanded coral snake (*M. instestinalis*): brown with longitudinal black, yellow and whitish lines; belly alternately black and white, red and black sub-caudals. Maximum length 50 cm. In defence it raises its tail to display the brightly-coloured ventral surface. It is found under rocks and vegetation in forested areas up to elevations of 1100 metres. It ranges from southern Thailand through peninsula Malaysia and Singapore to Indonesia (Borneo, Sumatra, Sulawesi and some smaller islands) and the Philippines.

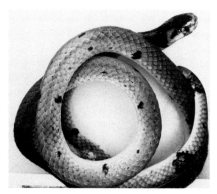 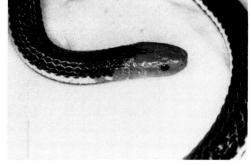

Figure 9. Coral snake (*Calliophis maculiceps*). Specimen from Thailand (photo © Dr. D.A. Warrell).

Figure 10. Blue coral snake (*Maticora bivirgata*). 90cm long specimen from southern Thailand (photo © Dr. D.A. Warrell).

4. Cobras (genus *Naja*)

This is the most important genus of venomous snakes in Asia from the medical point of view[10]. Recent studies by Wüster and Thorpe have provided support for nine or 10 species, previously regarded as subspecies or varieties of *N. naja*[11-15]. Cobras are large heavy-bodied snakes whose most notable characteristic is their habit of rearing up and, by elevating long cervical ribs, spreading a hood in defence. This display, accompanied by hissing and inflation of the body, serves to make the snake appear large and threatening. At least six species of Asian cobra are capable of "spitting" venom towards the eyes of adversaries, and at least three (*N. kaouthia*, *N. naja* and *N. oxiana*) seem unable or unwilling to "spit" their venom in defence. Two of the "non-spitters" (*N. naja* and *N. oxiana*) have long venom orifices in their fangs, while some of the "spitters" have short fangs with short orifices[14].

1. Chinese/Taiwan cobra (*N. atra*) (Figure 11): the colour is variable grey-brown or black with a paler coloured belly. The back of the hood may be unmarked but often bears a pale, black-edged band with a central dark spot or spectacle marking. Anteriorly there is often a dark band across the throat. Along the body are narrow white transverse lines especially prominent in juveniles. The maximum length is about two metres. It is capable of "spitting" its venom in defence. It inhabits all kinds of countryside including rice fields, marshy areas, forest and human settlements. It occurs in China south of the Yangtze River including Taiwan, Hong Kong and Hainan, west to northern Vietnam and northern Laos.
2. Monocellate cobra (*N. kaouthia*)[10] (Figure 12): the colour varies from pale olive brown to black. The commonest nuchal pattern is a white annular marking with a black centre and rim; the single "eye" or monacle (Figure 12b). Some specimens have a transverse band with a central eye like *N. atra*; others lack the marking altogether. The ventral surface of the neck

is paler or yellowish with a broad, dark band. The maximum length may exceed 1.5 metres. It is distributed from northeastern India through Bangladesh, Burma including islands of the Mergui archipelago, southwestern China (northwestern Guangxi, western Yunnan, southwestern Sichuan) and Southeast Asia, south to northwestern peninsular Malaysia and east to Vietnam. This is the commonest species of cobra in most parts of Southeast Asia.

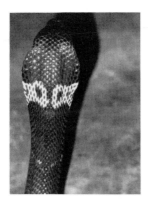 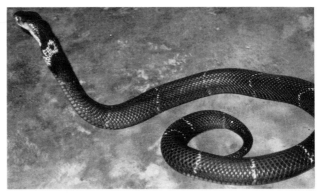

Figure 11. Chinese cobra (*Naja atra*). Specimen from Hong Kong.(photos © Dr. D.A. Warrell).
11a. Showing typical nuchal marking.   **11b.** Showing narrow white cross stripes on the body.

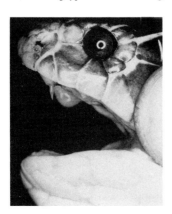 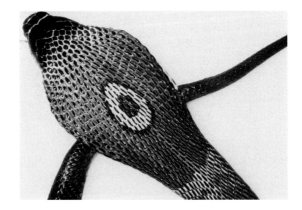

Figure 12. Monocellate cobra (*Naja kaouthia*). Specimens from Thailand (photos © Dr. D.A. Warrell).
12a. Showing fang.   **12b.** Showing typical "eye" nuchal marking.

3. Indian spectacled cobra (*N. naja*) (Figure 13): the colour is greyish, brownish or blackish above with a paler belly. There is a speckling of pale markings on the scales and interstitial skin sometimes forming transverse bands. The most typical nuchal pattern is the white spectacles edged with black (Figure 13b); on the front of the hood are two dark patches, either side of the throat and two or more transverse dark bands with white areas in between. Rarely, the length may exceed two metres. This species occurs in Pakistan, India, Nepal and Sri Lanka.

4. Trans-Caspian, Central Asian or Oxus cobra (*N. oxiana*): the hood is narrower than in other Asian Naja species. The colour is uniform yellowish, brownish, greyish or black with darkish circumferential bands, marked in juveniles. There is no nuchal pattern. On the anterior part of the neck are two dark bands. The belly is usually yellowish. The length may exceed 1.8 metres. It inhabits stony, rocky, shrub-covered foothills up to an altitude of 2,300 feet in northeastern Iran, southern Turkmenistan and southern Uzbekistan (north to

Samarkand and Aristan-Bel-tau Mountains) and southwestern Tajikistan, Afghanistan, northeastern Pakistan and the extreme northwest of India (Kashmir and the Punjab).

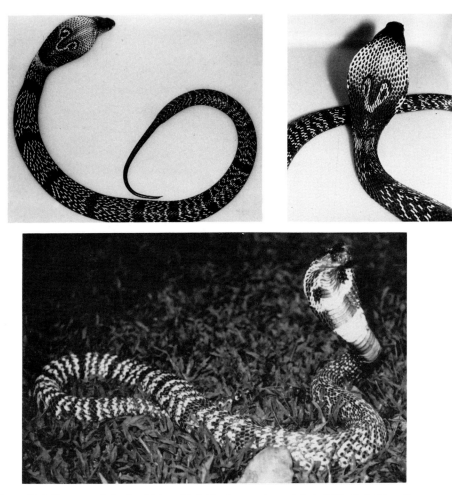

Figure 13. Indian spectacled cobra (*Naja naja*). Sri Lankan specimens (photo © Dr. D.A. Warrell).
13a. (top left) Specimen 1.1m long showing speckled cross-bands. **13b.** (top right) Showing typical "pair of spectacles" nuchal marking. **13c.** (bottom) Showing markings on the throat.

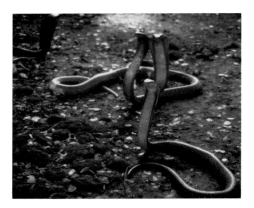

Figure 14. Philippine cobras (*N. philippinensis*)
(photo courtesy of Dr. George Watt).

5. Philippine cobra (*N. philippinensis*) (Figure 14): the colour is yellowish to olive brown above becoming paler on the outer scale rows. The belly is yellowish white. There are no markings in adult specimens. Maximum length 1.3 metres. Occurs in Luzon, Mindoro and Marinduque Islands, the Philippines.

6. Samar cobra (*N. samarensis*): the colour is iridescent brownish black above with yellowish reticular pattern on the scales and interstitial skin. The chin and upper neck are yellowish with a broad black band starting at about the ninth ventral. The maximum length exceeds 1 metre. It inhabits the islands of Samar, Leyte, Bohol and Mindanao, the Philippines.

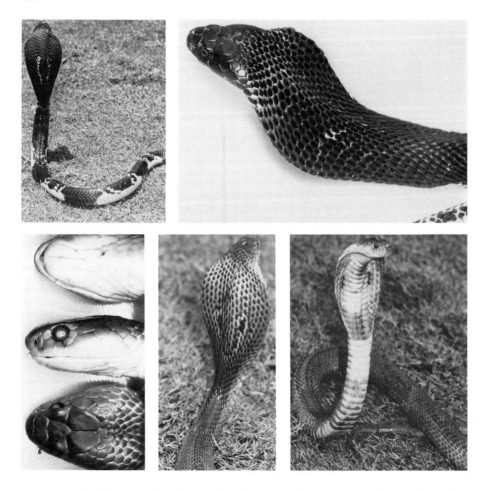

Figure 15. Thai spitting cobra (*Naja siamensis*). Specimens from Thailand (photos © Dr. D.A. Warrell).
15a. (top left) Black and white pattern with vague "spectacle" nuchal marking.
15b. (top right) Black and white pattern with no nuchal markings.
15c. (bottom right) Brown pattern showing throat markings.
15d. (bottom middle) Brown pattern showing "spectacle" nuchal marking.
15e. (bottom left) Brown pattern showing details of head scales. Scale in cm.

7. Thai, black and white, black, brown or Isan spitting cobra (*N. siamensis*)[15] (Figure 15): the colour is variable; entirely black or brown, or largely white with black dorsal surface of the hood and vertebral markings (Figure 15a) or pale brown with a whitish yellow anterior neck with a dark band below (Figure 15c-e). The nuchal pattern may consist of whole or partial "spectacles" (Figure 15a,d) or may be completely absent (Figure 15b). This species

is smaller than *N kaouthia*, growing to a maximum length of less than 1 metre. It readily "spits" its venom in defence. It is found in Thailand (except in the peninsula), Cambodia, southern Vietnam, Laos and probably in parts of eastern Burma[15].

8. Javan and Sunda Island spitting cobra (*N. sputatrix*): grey, brown or black above, belly greyish-black, supralabials and throat whitish. This species inhabits Java and the lesser Sunda Islands in Indonesia (Bali, Lombok, Sumbawa, Flores east to Alor). It readily "spits" in defence.

9. Black, golden, Sumatran, Malayan or equatorial spitting cobra (*N. sumatrana*) (Figure 16): in southern Thailand the colour is usually uniform yellow or yellowish-green and this phase (? lutino) is also found in peninsular Malaysia. However, south of Thailand this species is usually uniform jet black with a bluish-black belly and some pale markings on the supralabials, chin and neck. The maximum length is about 1.5 metres. It occurs in jungles in southern Thailand, peninsular Malaysia, Singapore, Sumatra, Borneo and the island of Palawan in the Philippines. It "spits" readily in defence.

5. King cobra or hamadryad (*Ophiophagus hannah*) (Figure 17)

This is the world's largest venomous snake, growing to a length of more than 5.7 metres. Adults vary in ground colour from grey to olive greenish-brown with a yellowish chin and throat, dark and paler striped belly and dark interstitial skin. Juvenile snakes are strikingly striped with black and white or black and yellow. In Thailand, adults lose all but vague traces of these markings, but in Burma even adults can be strikingly banded, these bands tending to angle forward like chevrons along the dorsum. This species rears up and spreads a long narrow hood in defence and "growls". It inhabits jungle areas but also open agricultural lands. It is found throughout India, Southeast Asia including King Island in the Mergui archipelago, southern China (generally south of latitude 25°N, including Hong Kong and Hainan), southeastern Tibet, Indonesia (Sumatra, Java, Borneo, Sulawesi and some smaller islands) and on many of the Philippine islands.

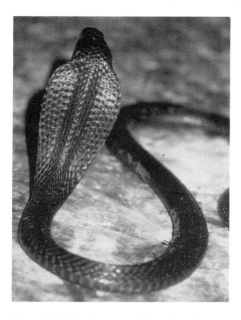 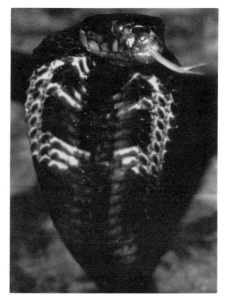

Figure 16. Malay-Sumatran spitting cobra (*N. sumatrana*). Black specimen from Singapore (photos © Dr. D.A. Warrell).

16a. Showing absence of nuchal markings.   **16b.** Showing pattern on throat.

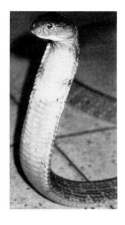 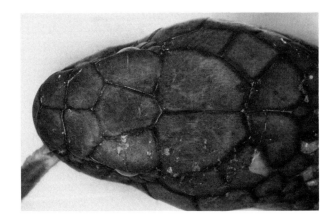

Figure 17. King cobra (*Ophiophagus hannah*) (photos © Dr. D.A. Warrell).
17a. Specimen from southern   17b. Dorsal head scales showing enlarged parietal scales (compare
Thailand   with Figure 15e).

6. Black desert cobra or Walter Innes' snake (*Walterinnesia aegyptia*)

This Middle Eastern species occurs in southwest Iran. It is discussed in the chapter on African and Middle Eastern snakes.

C. VIPERS (FAMILY VIPERIDAE)

With some exceptions, the Asian vipers are relatively short, thick-bodied, sluggish and terrestrial snakes. They have long, curved, cannulated and fully erectile fangs which fold down against the upper jaw in a sheath of mucous membrane when the snake is not striking. The two subfamilies, typical vipers (Viperinae) and pit vipers (Crotalinae), are represented by a total of almost 70 species in 14 genera in this region. The pit vipers have a heat sensitive organ housed in an obvious depression in the loreal scale between the eye and the nostril. Many species of vipers, such as Russell's viper in the Indian subcontinent and Southeast Asia, the mamushis (genus *Agkistrodon (Gloydius)*) of the Far East, the habus (genus *Trimeresurus*) of Japan and pit vipers (genera *Calloselasma* and *Trimeresurus*) of Southeast Asia, are responsible for many bites and much morbidity and mortality.

1. Typical vipers (subfamily Viperinae)

a. Fea's viper (Azemiops feae)
The colour is glossy blue-black with a series of narrow orange-yellow circumferential bands. The head is orange with a pair of dark, longitudinal bands on the dorsum. Maximum length about one metre. It is found in hilly regions of northern Burma (Kakhyen hills, east of Bhamò), southern and central China and north Vietnam.

b. Horned sand viper (Cerastes gasperettii)
This species occurs in Khuzistan Province of western Iran and in the Middle East. It is discussed in the chapter on snakes of Africa and the Middle East.

c. Russell's viper, Daboia, chain viper, cobra monil or necklace snake (Daboia russelii)[17,18]
This species or species complex occurs throughout the Indian subcontinent from the Indus Valley of Pakistan and Kashmir, India in the northeast, the foothills of the Himalayas in northern India, Nepal and Bhutan in the north, Assam and Bangladesh in the east and Sri Lanka in the south. A second population is found in the central rice-growing area of Burma and may be continuous with the population in northeastern and central Thailand and the far west of Cambodia. It also occurs in China south of latitude $25°N$ (Guangdong, Guangxi,

south Fujian and Taiwan but not Hainan). Relict populations are found in Indonesia: in Java on the limestone hills west of Surabaya and in the east of the island, in Komodo, Endeh Island (where it may now be extinct), Flores and Lomblen Islands and some of the adjacent smaller islands. Five subspecies have been recognised

1. *D. r. formosensis* (Taiwan)
2. *D. r. limitis* (Indonesia)
3. *D. r. pulchella* (Sri Lanka) (Figure 18)
4. *D. r. russelii* (Indian subcontinent)
5. *D. r. siamensis* (Southeast Asia and southern China) (Figure 19)

A recent morphological analysis indicates clear differences between western (*D. r. russelii* and *D. r. pulchella*) and eastern forms[1]. Differences between *D. r. pulchella* and *D. r. russelii*, and between *D. r. formosensis, D. r. siamensis* and Javan *D. r. limitis*, were not thought to be significant. Russell's vipers are nocturnal and predominantly terrestrial in paddy fields and other agricultural land, open, rocky, bushy or grassy terrain up to altitudes of 3,000 metres. In defence it coils up in a striking position, inflates its lungs and emits loud sustained hisses through the unusually large trumpet-shaped nostrils. The maximum length is up to 2 metres in India.

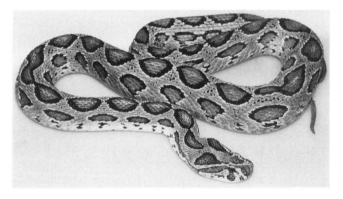 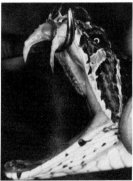

Figure 18. Sri Lankan Russell's viper or Tic Polonga (*Daboia russelii pulchella*) (photos © Dr. D.A. Warrell)
18a. Specimen 1.3m long from Anuradhapura.   **18b.** Fangs (right fang sheathed).

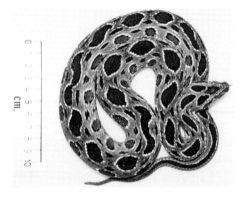 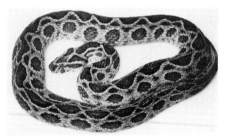

Figure 19. Eastern Russell's viper (*Daboia russelii siamensis*) (photos © Dr. D.A. Warrell).
19a. Specimen from Thailand.   **19b.** Specimen from Burma.

The ground colour above varies from pale greyish-brown to reddish-brown. There are dorsal and lateral series of round or oval spots of darker brown which may have pale centres (of the same hue as the ground colour) and white edging (especially prominent in Thai specimens). The dorsal series may coalesce. In the eastern forms there is an extra row of roughly triangular spots between the large vertebral and lateral series of blotches. The belly is white with large black spots. Despite its distinctive pattern, several harmless species are regularly confused with Russell's viper, notably the spotted cat snake (*Boiga multomaculata*) throughout the range of *D. russelii* which is probably a mimic[8].

d. Saw-scaled or carpet vipers (genus Echis)

Echis species, which are of great medical importance, are relatively small, slender-bodied snakes with overlapping keeled scales. The scales on the flanks have serrated keels so that when the snake rubs its coils together, when irritated, a rasping sound is produced. Two or three species and up to four subspecies have been described in this region.

1. Indian saw-scaled viper or phoorsa (*E. carinatus*) (Figure 20): the colour above is a shade of brown (greyish, greenish or yellowish); the white belly is speckled with brown or black. There is a series of white markings along the dorsum edged with black, bridging to the undulating continuous white line along each flank. There is a cruciform white marking on the dorsum of the head. Maximum length 80 cm but averages only 20 cm in Sri Lanka and rarely exceeds 30 cm in southern India. It inhabits open, dry or semi-desert country in India, south of latitude 24° north (but excluding Bengal) and Sri Lanka (arid coastal areas around the island).

2. Central Asian saw-scaled viper (*E. multisquamatus*) (Figure 21): the colouring is similar to other Echis species but the pattern is bolder with a wide well-defined pale continuous undulating line along the flanks and a cruciform mark on the dorsum of the head. There are scattered dark spots on the belly. Maximum length 86 cm. It inhabits open scrubby, dry, sandy and rocky areas in Uzbekistan (as far north as the Aral Sea), Turkmenistan, northern and eastern Iran, northwestern Tajikistan (west of the Vakhsh Valley) and south to southern Afghanistan and western Pakistan (Baluchistan)[19].

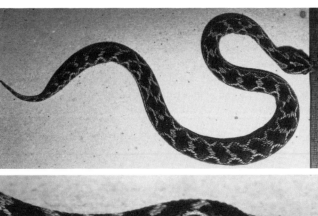

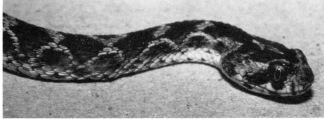

Figure 20. Indian saw-scaled viper (*Echis carinatus*). Specimen from Sri Lanka (photos © Dr. D.A. Warrell).
20a. (top) Whole snake (scale in inches).
20b. (bottom) Detail of head.

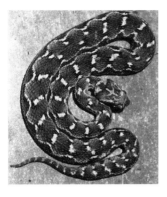 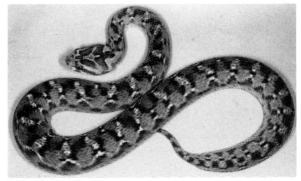

Figure 21. Central Asian saw-scaled viper (*Echis multisquamatus*) (photo © Dr. D.A. Warrell).

Figure 22. Sochurek's saw-scaled viper (*Echis sochureki*) (photo © Dr. D.A. Warrell).

3. Sochurek's saw-scaled viper (*E. sochureki*) (Figure 22): the background colour is grey-beige with a series of white transverse dorsal spots mostly divided into two, partly connected by a diagonal black band and bordered with black, in contact with inverted "U" of the lateral white stripes. These arcs enclose a series of dark lateral spots. The belly is white with grey flecks. There is a light grey cruciform pattern on the dorsum of the head. Maximum length about 76 cm. Open, dryish, rocky or scrubby areas where it is mainly terrestrial but sometimes climbs into low bushes and trees. Found in the Ad Diwaniyah area of Iraq (Arabian Peninsula), southern Iran, southern Afghanistan, eastern Pakistan[19], northern India (Jammu and Kashmir south of the Ganges as far south as approximately latitude 23°N but excluding Bengal). Astola island on the Makran coast of Pakistan is inhabited by a dark coloured subspecies (*E. s. astolae*). It has a dorsal series of large dark brown blotches separated by paler interspaces. There are smaller dark brown spots on the flanks. Most individuals lack the undulating white line of the mainland subspecies.

e. McMahon's viper (Eristocophis mcmahoni) (Figure 23)

This species has a relatively large broad head and has large "butterfly"-shaped scales on the snout. The colour is brownish-khaki with lateral rows of dark spots with pale edges. Maximum length 70-80 cm. It occurs in Iran (Kerman Province), Pakistan (Chagai Desert, northwestern Baluchistan) and the southern desert of Afghanistan. It inhabits deserts up to an altitude of 1200 metres.

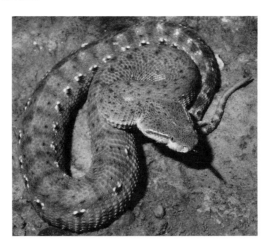

Figure 23. McMahon's viper (*Eristocophis mcmahoni*) (photo © Dr. D.A. Warrell).

f. Persian horned viper (Pseudocerastes persicus)

This species, which has been described in the chapter on African and Middle Eastern snakes, is widely distributed in sandy, rocky and hilly country up to an altitude of 2,000 metres in southwestern and eastern Iran, western Pakistan and southern Afghanistan.

Typical Asian vipers (genus *Vipera*)

1. Middle Eastern mountain vipers of the *Vipera xanthina* complex (*V. albicornuta, V. latifii, V. raddei, V. wagneri* and *V. xanthina*)[20]: these five species are found in restricted areas of rocky, grassy or sparsely wooded mountainous country, up to almost 3,000 metres altitude in the north and northwest of Iran. All have some sort of zig-zag dorsal pattern, in the case of *V. xanthina* black or brown against a pale white grey or brownish background, in the case of *V. raddei* reddish-orange against a dark brownish or blackish background. *V. albicornuta, V. latifii* and *V. raddei* have a raised and angled supraocular plate separated from the eye by a ring of circumocular scales. Maximum length exceeds one metre[20] (see also chapter on snakes in Europe).

2. European adder or viper (*V. berus*) (Figure 24): this species is found in forest, forest steppe and mountainous country across the Russian Federation east to its Pacific coast and Sakhalin Island, north to latitude 61°N and south into northern Kazakhstan, northern Mongolia, northern China (extreme northern Xinjiang and Jilin) and the northern part of North Korea. It is discussed in the chapter on European snakes.

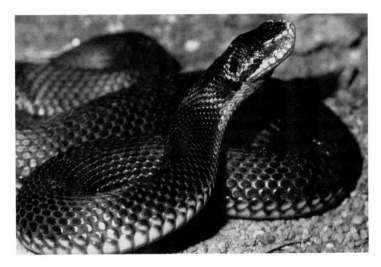

Figure 24. European adder or viper (*Vipera berus*). Melanistic specimen from Russia (photo © Dr. D.A. Warrell).

3. Levantine, Levant, lebetine or blunt-nosed viper (*V. (Macrovipera) lebetina*): the ground colour is pale to dark grey with an olive or brownish tinge with a paler belly speckled with darker markings. There is a dorsal series of two rows of darker markings which may fuse or alternate. The eastern subspecies (*V. l. turanica*) has brownish-red or brownish-yellow dorsal markings, often with dark edges which may fuse to form a zig-zag; its abdomen has dense dark speckles. Maximum length 1.7 metres. The West Asian subspecies (*V. l. obtusa*) is found in western Iran, eastern Afghanistan and Pakistan (southern Waziristan and Quetta district). The eastern subspecies (*V. l. turanica*) occurs in Turkmenistan, Uzbekistan, northeast Iran, northern Afghanistan, northern Pakistan and India (Kashmir).

4. Orsini's or steppe viper (*V. ursinii*): the colour is brownish-grey above with a dark dorsal zig-zag line which may be broken into spots. Maximum length about 60 cm. The eastern

subspecies (*V. u. renardi*) occurs in northern China (western Xinjiang), western Mongolia (Mount Altai), Kazakhstan, Uzbekistan, Kyrgyzstan and northwestern Iran. It is described in the chapter on European snakes.

II. ASIAN PIT VIPERS (SUBFAMILY CROTALINAE)
This subfamily is characterized by the loreal pit organ which is occupied in a hollow of the maxillary and pre-frontal bones. About 50 species occur in this region but only those reported to have inflicted bites or likely to be of medical importance will be discussed.

1. Asian pit vipers and mamushis (genus *Agkistrodon (Gloydius)*)
These pit vipers have nine enlarged symmetrical scales on the dorsum of the head. The nomenclature of *Agkistrodon* species is particularly confusing. Names such as Pallas' pit viper or *A. halys* (Pallas) found in the older literature and especially in the snakebite literature, are difficult to reconcile with the species described in more recent herpetological literature. Here, the schemes of Gloyd and Conant[2] and Zhao and Adler[4] are followed, and the differences between these two accounts are indicated (Table 2).

Table 2
Equivalence of nomenclature of some Asian *Agkistrodon* (*Gloydius*) species

Zhao & Adler (1993)[4]	Gloyd & Conant (1990)[2]
A blomhoffii brevicaudus*	*A b siniticus*
	A b dubitatus
	A b brevicaudus
A intermedius	*A intermedius*
	A halys cognatus
A saxatilis	*A intermedius saxatilis*
A ussuriensis	*A blomhoffii ussuriensis*
	A caliginosus

*Commonly referred to in older literature as Pallas' pit viper or *A halys* Pallas

1. Mamushi (*A. blomhoffii*): there are at least two subspecies[4]; the Japanese mamushi (*A b blomhoffii*) (Figure 25) which occurs in all the main islands of Japan and in many of the smaller offshore islands including those of northern Ryukyu and in the far eastern part of the Russian Federation in Sakhalin Island and Kunashir Island of the Kuril Archipelago; and the Chinese mamushi (*A. b. brevicaudus*), which comprises the two other subspecies described by Gloyd and Conant (1990), *A. b. siniticus* and *A. b. dubitatus*. *A. b. brevicaudus* occurs in China (southern Liaoning around Beijing and in Central China west to Guizhou and Sichuan) and Korea including Cheju-do Island[4]. The colouring is variable, but most specimens have a dark brownish or blackish post-ocular stripe with a white line above it and white supralabial scales below. The ground colour above is greyish, brownish or reddish. There is a row of large circular markings on each flank: like inverted "U"s, in *A. b. brevicaudus*, and in the form of an almost complete annular ring with a central dark "bullseye" spot in *A. b. blomhoffii*. The belly is lighter with darker markings of variable density. The tail tip is pale or yellowish, especially in juveniles, in *A. b. brevicaudus*. The maximum length is about 70 cm. This species is found on the edge of forests and agricultural areas. In Japan, *B. b. blomhoffii* is often mistaken for *Elaphe climacophora*, the aodaisho.
2. Siberian and Central Asian pit viper (*A. halys*): like *A. blomhoffii*, this species has a dark post-ocular stripe with a white line above it and pale supralabials below. The ground colour is pale grey, olive or darker brown with pale cross bands sometimes with dark edges. The maximum length is about 80 cm. The range of this species extends across Central Asia from the Caspian Sea in the west through Kazakhstan, Uzbekistan, Kyrgyzstan, the Russian Federation (southern Siberia), Mongolia, Afghanistan and China (Yellow River Basin).

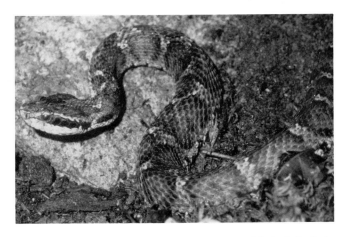

Figure 25. Japanese mamushi (*Agkistrodon blomhoffii*) (photo © Dr. D.A. Warrell).

3. Himalayan pit viper (*A. himalayanus*): the colour is darkish brown with a dark post-orbital streak continuous with longitudinal lines on the neck. On the dorsal surface of the body is a series of interrupted dark longitudinal lines interrupted by paler cross bands. The maximum length is about 90 cm. This species inhabits forest and rocky areas in high mountains at some of the highest altitudes recorded for any species of snake (1500-5,300 metres)[9]. It occurs in northeastern Pakistan, in the western Himalayas from Kashmir through Nepal to Darjeeling in the east.

4. Central Asian pit viper (*A. intermedius*): the post-ocular stripe is less well-defined than in the above species and lacks the white line superiorly. The colour is whitish, greyish, brownish, reddish or olive with pale dorsal cross bands with dark edges, which may be in two halves not meeting exactly at the vertebral line. The maximum length is up to 80 cm, but the Caucasian subspecies (*A. i. caucasicus*) rarely exceeds 60 cm. Found in grasslands and shrublands in mountainous country in northern Iran, southern Turkmenistan, northwestern Afghanistan and in Europe (Azerbaydzhan) (*A. i. caucasicus*); and Kyrgyzstan, eastern Kazakhstan, northwestern China (from Xinjiang east to Shanxi), Mongolia and the Russian Federation (southern Siberia) (*A. i. intermedius*). Zhao and Adler[4] include with *A. intermedius, A. h .cognatus*[2].

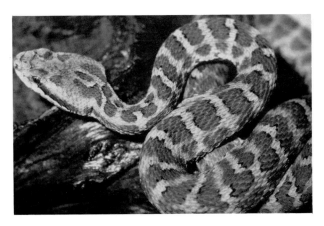

Figure 26. Rock mamushi (*Agkistrodon saxatilis*). Specimen from the Far Eastern Russia Federation (photo © Dr. D.A. Warrell).

5. Rock mamushi (*A. saxatilis*) (Figure 26): the ground colour is whitish or pale greyish, brownish or yellowish with dark cross bands of various shades of brown sometimes edged with black and a ventrolateral series of small brown spots. The belly is light brownish or pinkish. The top of the head has some asymmetrical darkish spots. There is a darkish post-ocular stripe, ill-defined above but scalloped and bordered below with white. Maximum length 85 cm. It is found on rocky slopes and woodland in the far east of the Russian Federation (eastern Siberia east of Selemdzha River), in northeastern China south to Shandong and in Korea excluding Cheju-do Island.

6. Snake island (Shedao) mamushi (*A. shedaoensis*): this arboreal species is confined to Shedao (Snake Island) northwest of Lushun (Port Arthur), Liaoning Province, China.

7. Ussuri mamushi (*A. ussuriensis*): the ground colour varies from pale to darkish brown or reddish with a row of large dark "bullseye" markings (darkish brown ring with a central dark spot) along both flanks. Between these paired markings there may be a palish transverse stripe. There is a dark post-ocular stripe extending down on to the supralabials and limited above by a white line. The belly is greyish. Maximum length 65 cm. It is found in open fields, forest edges and marshes in northeastern China (northern Liaoning to Heilongjiang), Far Eastern Russian Federation and Korea, including Cheju-do Island. This species comprises *A. b. ussuriensis* and *A. caliginosus* of Gloyd and Conant[2].

8. High mountain pit vipers (*A. monticola* and *A. strauchi*): *A. monticola* is found at altitudes of 3,600 to 4,000 metres near Likiang in northern Yunnan, China. *A. strauchi* occurs at altitudes between 2,800 and 4,300 metres on the Tibetan Plateau.

2. Malayan pit viper (*Calloselasma rhodostoma*) (Figure 27)

This snake causes many bites with much morbidity and some mortality especially among rubber and coffee plantation workers in Southeast Asia. It is a relatively short, thick-set snake with a flattened body and a large triangular-shaped head with a pointed and slightly upturned snout. There is a well-defined dark post-ocular patch, sometimes with a white edge above and below. Its lower limit, on the supralabials, is scalloped. The top of the head is covered by nine large smooth symmetrical scales and is normally dark. The ground colour of the body varies from very dark brownish-black to various shades of reddish, yellowish and greyish. The dorsal pattern is of alternating dark, triangular markings with their apices towards the vertebral line and below these, a series of dark spots on the flanks. The belly is pale with darker mottlings. The tail is very short and thin. Its favoured habitat is low secondary growth on the floor of rubber, coffee and other plantations and in forested, hilly country. It is found throughout the whole of Thailand, possibly in southern Burma, and in Laos, Cambodia, southern Vietnam and northwest Malaysia (Kedah, Perak and possibly as far south as Kuala Lumpur) including Penang and other offshore islands, in western Java, especially near Bogor, and on some smaller islands north and northeast of Java.

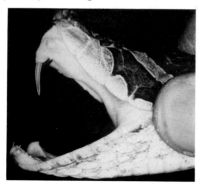 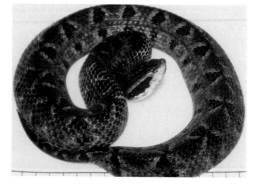

Figure 27. Malayan pit viper (*Calloselasma rhodostoma*) (photo © Dr. D.A. Warrell).
27a. Showing fang.   **27b.** Whole snake (scale in cm).

517

3. Sharp-nosed pit viper or hundred-pacer (*Deinagkistrodon acutus*) (Figure 28)

This is a relatively thick-bodied snake which has a very large triangular head with nine enlarged symmetrical shields on the dorsum (as in *Agkistrodon* and *Calloselasma*) and a long upturned snout. There is a dark, straight post-ocular streak and the top of the head is usually darkish, but the lower part of the head and chin are pale. The dorsal ground colour is greyish, brownish or yellowish, sometimes with an indistinct dark vertebral stripe. There is a row of striking dark triangular marks on each side with their apices meeting at the vertebral line. These triangles may have pale centres containing two dark spots. The belly is whitish or yellowish with large black ventrolateral blotches below and between the bases of the triangular markings. The maximum length is 1.6 metres. It is found in rocky or wooded hilly country in China (between latitudes 25° and 31^ON and east of longitude 104^OE), Taiwan (but not Hainan Island) and the extreme north of north Vietnam and possibly Laos.

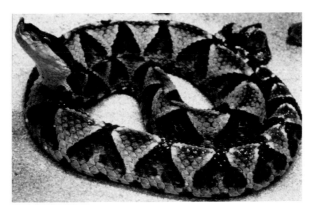

Figure 28. Sharp-nosed pit viper (*Deinagkistrodon acutus*) (photo © Dr. D.A. Warrell).

4. Hump-nosed vipers (genus *Hypnale*)

These small pit vipers resemble *Calloselasma* in their general appearance, upturned snouts, flattened bodies and very short, narrow tails. Like the preceding three genera, they have large parietal, supraorbital and temporal scales, but anterior to these they have a number of smaller scales.

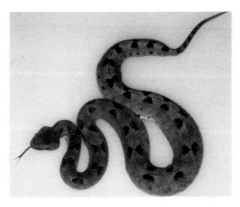 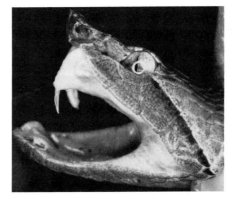

Figure 29. Merrem's hump-nosed viper (*Hypnale hypnale*) (photo © Dr. D.A. Warrell).
29a. 35 cm long specimen from Sri Lanka.   **29b.** Showing fangs.

1. Merrem's hump-nosed viper (*H. hypnale*) (Figure 29): the head colour is usually paler above and darker below a pale post-ocular line. The top of the head may be uniform or with a dark pattern. The dorsal ground colour of the body ranges from greyish, brownish, yellowish to reddish-brown. The dorsal pattern consists of dark tips of triangles, their apices meeting or alternating at the vertebral line. The belly is darkish. Maximum length 55 cm. It is found in leaf litter, beneath undergrowth, especially in plantations throughout Sri Lanka and in the western Ghats of India north to latitude 16°N (Belgaum) up to an altitude of 1,525 metres in Sri Lanka and 600 metres in India.

2. Sri Lanka or Millard's hump-nosed viper (*H. nepa*): this species is smaller than *H hypnale* (maximum length 39.2 cm) and has a wart-like hump composed of numerous small scales at the tip of its snout. The colour is similar to *H. hypnale*. It is found in forests up to an altitude of 1800 metres in the wet zone of southwest Sri Lanka. A third species, *H. walli*, even smaller and with the same warty protuberance on the tip of the snout, has been described from southwest Sri Lanka.

5. Indo-Chinese mountain vipers (genus *Ovophis*)

The members of this genus, formerly included in the genus *Trimeresurus*, are distinguished by a number of morphological features of which the most obvious is their undivided anterior sub-caudal scales. The top of the head is covered by numerous small, smooth, slightly overlapping scales. There are four species.

1. Mount Kinabalu or Chasen's mountain viper (*O. chaseni*) (Figure 30): brownish above with irregular blackish, light-edged blotches which become transverse bands posteriorly. Yellowish below heavily powdered with grey; an oblique black stripe behind the eye bordered below with white. Maximum length about 70 cm. It was found in the village of Kiau at an altitude of 900 metres at the base of Mount Kinabalu, Sabah, Borneo. It probably also occurs in eastern Brunei.

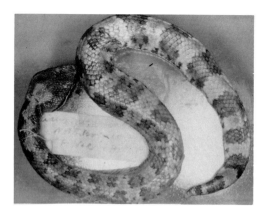 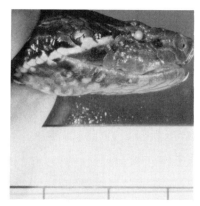

Figure 30. Chasen's pit viper (*Ovophis chaseni*). Paratype in National University of Singapore collection (photo © Dr. D.A. Warrell).
30a. Dorsal view.   **30b.** Lateral view of the head (scale in cm).

2. Mountain pit viper (*O. monticola*): a relatively thick-set snake with a distinct triangular head which is dark brown or blackish above. The body is light olive, reddish or orangey-brown above with squarish or irregularly-shaped black marks meeting or alternating at the vertebral line. There is usually a pale post-ocular line. The belly is palish spotted with brown. The maximum length is 1.1 metres. It is found in mountain forests and cultivated areas at altitudes between 1,000 and 2,000 metres in southern China, Hong Kong, Taiwan, Hainan Island (?), Southeast Asia, Sumatra, the eastern Himalayas (Assam and Sikkim) as

far west as Nepal, Bhutan and southeastern Tibet. A separate species, *O. convictus*, was described from Penang.

3. Hime-habu or kufah (*O. okinavensis*): a relatively short, thick-set snake with a prominent canthus rostralis. The colour is brownish, greyish or olive brown with rectangular or irregular dark markings either side of the vertebral line which may alternate or coalesce. A lateral row of similar-shaped darkish markings along the flanks. There is a post-ocular darkish stripe bordered above and below with white. The ventral scales are dark in the centre and whitish at their lateral edges. The maximum length may exceed 70 cm. It inhabits mountain forests in the Amami and Okinawa Islands.

6. Asian arboreal pit vipers (genus *Trimeresurus*)

The morphological features separating the different species are sometimes subtle and misidentifications are very common in the literature. Compared with other vipers, they are relatively long and thin with a triangular-shaped head, the dorsum of which is covered with many small scales. Many are arboreal and some have prehensile tails. Some 30 species have been described, excluding those now placed in the genera *Ovophis* and *Tropidolaemus*. Only 20 species, with proven or likely medical importance, will be discussed.

1. White-lipped green pit viper (*T. albolabris*) (Figure 31): the head is relatively narrow and more elongated than in *P popeiorum* and there is no marked canthus rostralis. Above, the colour is uniformly green, varying from olive yellowish green to bright grass green. Some specimens have darker cross bands on the scales and interstitial skin. A narrow lateral white line bordering the ventrals is present in some specimens. The reddish-brown colour on the tail is concentrated on its dorsal surface. The belly is pale yellowish white to dark green as are the supralabials and chin. The nasal scale is undivided and wholly or partially fused with the first supralabial. The iris is amber-yellow. This is a common snake which is found on the ground as well as in trees, even in the centre of Bangkok. Three subspecies are described, in the Himalayas from Kashmir to Nepal (*T. a. septentrionalis*); northwestern Assam eastwards through Burma to southern China including Hainan Island and Hong Kong, the whole of Thailand, the Malayan peninsula as far south as Penang, Laos, Cambodia, Borneo, Sulawesi, Sumatra, Java and Madura and the Nicobar Islands (*T. a. albolabris*); and the lesser Sunda Islands east of Bali (*T. a. insularis*). Maximum length about 90 cm.

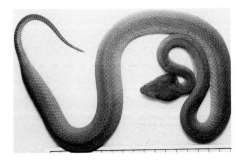

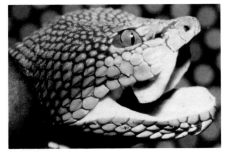

Figure 31. White-lipped green pit viper (*Trimeresurus albolabris*). Specimen from Thailand (scale in cm) (photo © Dr. D.A. Warrell).

Figure 32. Red-tailed green pit viper (*T. erythrurus*). Specimen from Burma. Note the heavily keeled temporal scales (photo © Dr. D.A. Warrell).

2. Cantor's pit viper (*T. cantori*): the colouring of this species is variable. It may be generally dark brown in colour with some whitish or yellowish scales or olive-brownish above with or without brownish spots, a white streak extending from the snout below the eye to the angle of the jaw and a palish line along the first lateral scale rows from the neck

to the base of the tail. The belly is greenish, whitish or yellowish with or without brown spots. Length up to 123 cm. Some regard this species as a subspecies of *T. purpureomaculatus*. It is only found in the Nicobar Islands.

3. Sakishima-habu (*T. elegans*): a long, slender snake with a thin neck and broadly triangular head, closely resembling the Taiwan habu (*T. mucrosquamatus*). There is a dark post-ocular stripe. The supralabials, chin and ventral surface are pale, peppered with grey spots. The dorsal colour of the body is greyish, brownish or yellowish with a series of irregular octagonal or semi-circular dark markings touching, coalescing or alternating at the vertebral line. A smaller series of dark spots lines the flanks. There is an orangeish hue to the top of the head and a vertebral stripe between the dark markings. The maximum length is 1.2 metres. It is found in rocky or wooded country in the Yaeyama Islands, the southwesternmost group in Japan (Ishigaki, Kuroshima, Iriomote and Taketomi).

4. Red-, burnt- or dry-tailed green pit viper (*T. erythrurus*) (Figure 32): this species closely resembles *T. albolabris* except that it has heavily keeled temporal scales (smooth in *T. albolabris*), raised tubercle-like dorsal head scales (flat in *T. albolabris*) and more lateral scale rows. The colour is uniformly green, various shades from olive to bright grass green above, becoming yellow on the flanks, with or without a thin white line bordering the ventrals and darker cross stripes on scales and interstitial skin. The belly is whitish or yellowish and the tail is spotted with reddish-brown. The maximum length exceeds one metre. It is found in lowlands, low hills, orchards and plantations. It occurs in Sikkim, possibly Bhutan, Assam (especially in the Naga Hills), Mizoram, Bangladesh (the Ganges Delta), Burma as far south as Moulmein and the Mergui archipelago and possibly in northwestern Thailand.

5. Yellow-spotted pit viper (*T. flavomaculatus*) (Figure 33): this species has a broad triangular head. The colour is bright or olive green with or without a row of irregular brown blotches or cross bands on the back. A broken or continuous line of yellow dots extends along the flanks close to the ventral scales. The subspecies from Polillo Island, *T. f. halieus*, has yellow dorsal blotches, and the subspecies from Batan (*T. f. mcgregori*) is uniformly bright yellow with a darker yellow streak along its sides and a few small reddish brown spots near the end of the tail. Maximum length exceeds 90 cm. This species is arboreal in low vegetation and is also terrestrial by streams. It occurs in a number of the Philippine islands (Camiguin, Jolo, Luzon, Mindanao, Batan, Polillo and Patnanongan).

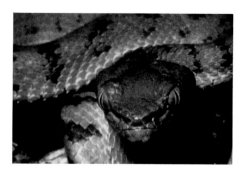
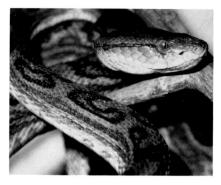

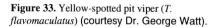

Figure 33. Yellow-spotted pit viper (*T. flavomaculatus*) (courtesy Dr. George Watt).

Figure 34. Japanese habu (*T. flavoviridis*) (photo © Dr. D.A. Warrell).

6. Habu, Okinawa habu or yellow-green pit viper (*T. flavoviridis*) (Figure 34): this is the longest of the Asian pit vipers growing, exceptionally, to a length of 2-3 metres. It is a slender snake with a relatively thin neck and broad triangular head. The colouring is variable; light brown, yellowish brown or reddish. The dorsal pattern varies from bold

distorted dark, sometimes black annular markings, with pale centres set against a dorsal background which is paler than the flanks, to specimens with paler markings in the Tokara and Kume-jima Islands. This species inhabits the vicinity of palm trees, farms and traditional rural dwellings in 25 of the Amami and Okinawa (northern Ryukyu) Islands including Amami-oshima, Tokunoshima, Okinawa-jima and Kume-jima. These are all mountainous islands of ancient origin. This species does not inhabit flat coral-reef islands or new volcanic islands[21].

7. Bamboo pit viper or common Indian pit viper (*T. gramineus*): the colour is uniformly dull green or brownish green above with a pale whitish, yellowish or greenish belly. A narrow, longitudinal whitish, yellowish or bluish line runs close to the ventrals. The iris is yellow. The tail is mottled reddish-brown. Vague, darkish cross bars may be visible along the dorsal surface of the body. The maximum length is 1,117 mm. It is found in bamboo and low vegetation in low hills. It is confined to the northeastern ghats and hills of central and eastern India south of latitude 22°N. However, the name *T. gramineus* has been used indiscriminately to describe arboreal green pit vipers throughout Southeast Asia, including those (*T. stejnegeri*) occurring in Taiwan.

8. Jerdon's pit viper (*T. jerdonii*): greenish yellow or greenish brown above with a dorsal series of transverse irregularly-shaped blackish or reddish-brown spots with darker edges and series of vertical dark spots along the flanks. There is a black post-ocular stripe. The top of the head is marked with symmetrical black markings against a yellowish background. Maximum length 1.4 metres. It is found only at high altitudes, between 1,400 and 2,800 metres, in Assam, Nepal, Burma north of Mandalay, southeastern Tibet, southwest China (Yunnan, Szechwan and Hubei) and north Vietnam.

9. Kanchanaburi pit viper (*T. kanburiensis*) (Figure 56): this small snake is olive green above with brownish spots forming vague cross bands along the body. The top of the head is spotted brown, the belly is pale with dark flecks on the lateral ends of the ventral scales and flecking of the adjacent lateral scale rows with black and white. Maximum length about 70 cm. It is found in hilly country, especially where bamboos grow in eastern Thailand, at about latitude 14°N. Very similar snakes have been found in the south of Thailand and possibly in Malaysia and described as a separate species "*T. venustus*". *T. kanburiensis*, which is not rare, has been widely misidentified and mislabelled as a juvenile *T. purpureomaculatus*[22].

10. Large-scaled pit viper (*T. macrolepis*): the scales on the top of the head are, for this genus, unusually large, smooth and symmetrical. The colour is bright green above, paler beneath with a whitish or yellowish line along the most lateral scale rows. Some specimens have a black post-ocular stripe. Maximum length about 60 cm. This arboreal species is found in hill country in the southwestern Ghats of India between 600 and 2,200 metres altitude.

11. Dark green pit viper (*T. macrops*) (Figure 35): compared with *T. albolabris*, whose range it overlaps, this species is smaller with a shorter, broader head with larger supraocular scales (Figure 35B), paler yellow iris, and darker colouring. The dorsal surface of the head and body is uniform dark bluish green, the labials bluish green, chin and throat bluish white and the belly blue, the scales becoming greenish at their lateral margins and on the most lateral row or dorsal scales. In some specimens there is a suggestion of darker cross bands on the scales and interstitial skin. The maximum length exceeds 70 cm. It is arboreal in central, northern and northeastern Thailand (including urban Bangkok), Cambodia, southern Vietnam and possibly Laos. This species has been frequently misidentified as *T. popeiorum* in the literature[23].

12. Malabar rock pit viper or Anamally pit viper (*T. malabaricus* = *T. anamallensis*): the colour is variable; greenish, olive-yellow or brownish above with darker brown or blackish blotches or cross bands, separate or confluent with yellowish spots along the flanks. The

belly is yellow, pale green or whitish. This species rarely grows longer than 80 cm but 105 cm has been recorded. It is found in the branches of small trees and shrubs and on rocks in the Western Ghats and other hills of southwestern India, south of the Krishna River, at altitudes between 600 and 2,200 metres.

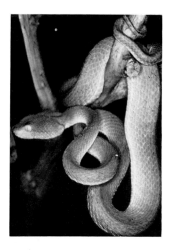 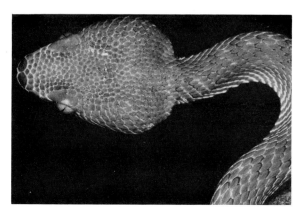

Figure 35. Dark green pit viper (*T. macrops*) (photos © Dr. D.A. Warrell).
35a. Specimen from Thailand.   **35b.** Dorsal head scales showing large supraoculars.

13. Taiwan or Chinese habu (*T. mucrosquamatus*): a long, relatively slender, snake with a thin neck and large triangular head. The body is light brown, greyish brown or brown above with a vertebral row of large purplish brown or chocolate coloured spots sometimes edged with a pale line. Some divided at the vertebral line, fusing or alternating (giving the impression of a wavy dorsal dark line). A lateral row of dark circular blotches. Whitish below with brownish dots. The top of the head is brown with dark markings. There is a dark post-ocular line to the angle of the jaw with a pale mark above it. Labials and chin whitish. Maximum length 1.3 metres. It is found in open agricultural country and forests up to an altitude of 1,400 metres. It occurs in the far northeast of India (Assam), northern Bangladesh, Burma, southern China, Taiwan, Hainan Island and north Vietnam.

14. Pope's pit viper (*T. popeiorum*) (Figure 36): unlike *T. albolabris*, this species has a more triangular head, a more pointed snout with an overhanging ridge above the nostril and pit organ, a brownish orange iris and a nasal scale which is completely separate from the first supralabial. The dorsal surface of the head and body is uniform apple green and the belly pale green. There may be a white post-ocular stripe and a thin white stripe which may be bordered below with red. The tail is brownish with darker transverse stripes. The maximum length approaches one metre. It is found in hilly forested country in northeastern India (Sikkim, Assam), Burma, Thailand, Laos, Vietnam, Cambodia, northern peninsula Malaysia, Borneo, Java, Sumatra and Pagay Island. Particularly in the Thai literature, the name of this species has been wrongly applied to *T. macrops*[23].

15. Flat-nosed pit viper (*T. puniceus*) (Figure 37): this small arboreal snake has a flattened, slightly upturned snout. The colour is greyish, greenish or brownish red with darker irregular transverse markings which may be fragmented into three separate spots There is a pale post-ocular streak. The belly is darker with brown mottlings. Maximum length about one metre. It is found in lowland forests in southern Thailand, peninsular Malaysia, Sumatra, Java and the Natuna Islands, Simeuluë and Mentawai Islands. The "species" described as *T wiroti* in the Thai literature may prove to be *T. puniceus* or *T. borneensis*.

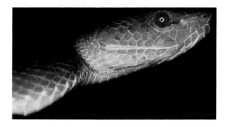

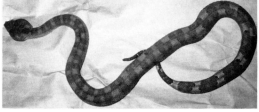

Figure 36. Pope's pit viper (*T. popeiorum*) showing separate nasal and first supralabial scales (photo © Dr. D.A. Warrell).

Figure 37. Flat-nosed pit viper (*T. puniceus*). Specimen from Malaysia (photo © Dr. D.A. Warrell).

16. Shore, mangrove, Gray's or purple-spotted pit viper (*T purpureomaculatus*) (Figure 38): the colour varies from almost uniform dark purplish brown (especially in peninsular Malaysia) to paler patterned forms with a background colour of greyish, whitish or yellowish and a series of large brownish saddle-shaped markings with smaller spots on the flanks. The belly is whitish. The maximum length may exceed one metre. It is found along coasts, in mangrove swamps and marshy areas, more commonly on offshore islands than on the mainland. It has also been reported from inland bamboo jungles up to an altitude of 2,000 feet. It is found in southern Burma (south of latitude 17°N), western Thailand (Kanchanaburi) and the west coast, peninsular Malaysia, Sumatra and its offshore islands and the Andaman and Nicobar Islands. This species has often been misidentified as "*T. kanburiensis*" in the literature[22].

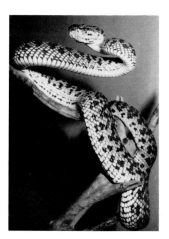

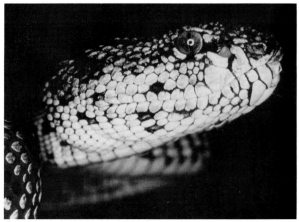

Figure 38. Mangrove pit viper (*T. purpureomaculatus*) (photo © Dr. D.A. Warrell).
38a. Specimen from Kanchanaburi, Thailand.   **38b.** Detail of head scales.

17. Bamboo pit viper or Chinese green tree viper (*T. stejnegeri*): this species is superficially identical to *T. popeiorum*. The species are distinguishable only by the form of the hemipenes (spinose in *T. stejnegeri*). Maximum length exceeds 80 cm. It is found in shrubs and bamboos in hilly country in northeastern India (Sikkim, Assam, Darjeeling), northern Burma, southern China including Hainan Island, Taiwan, Vietnam, Cambodia and Thailand.
18. Horseshoe pit viper (*T. strigatus*): the colouring is brown above with large dark brown spots, often confluent, producing a zig-zag stripe. The belly is whitish, heavily spotted with brown and with spots on the lateral margins of the ventral scales. There is a dark temporal stripe and a horseshoe-shaped mark on the nape of the neck. Maximum length 45 cm. It is

found in the Western Ghats and other hills of southern India between altitudes of 900 and 2,500 metres.

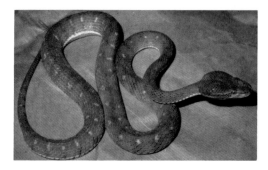 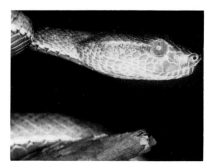

Figure 39. Hagen's pit viper (*T. hageni*) (photo © Dr. D.A. Warrell).
39a. Specimen from Malaysia.   **39b.** Details of head scales.

19. Sumatran pit viper (*T. sumatranus*): this long, relatively slender, snake is bright green above with darker cross bands, a row of pale brownish or pinkish spots both sides of the vertebral line, a lateral white stripe along the first two rows of dorsal scales and a greenish belly. There is a pale post-ocular streak. The scales on the top of the head are relatively large and flat. A separate species, Hagen's pit viper (*T. hageni*) (Figure 39) has been described, differing in minor respects. In southern Thailand, all specimens conform to the description of *T. hageni*. It is the longest Trimeresurus species found on the Asian mainland; maximum length is 1.6 metres. It is found in lowland forests in Thailand, peninsular Malaysia, Singapore, Sumatra, Borneo and their smaller offshore islands.

20.   Tokara-habu (*T. tokarensis*) (Figure 40): this snake's proportions are similar to *T. flavoviridis*. A paler form is greyish-brown with two dorsal rows of blackish-brown spots with pale centres and lateral dark linear extensions. The darker form is uniform dark brown with the ring-shaped dorsal markings scarcely discernible. The maximum length is 1.5 metres. It is found in the Tokara Islands south of Kyushu.

21. Sri Lankan green pit viper (*T. trigonocephalus*) (Figure 41): pale yellowish-green above, the scales edged with black. A dorsal series of paired triangular yellowish-green markings enclosed in blackish areas. There is a dark pre- and post-ocular stripe. Labials yellowish, ventrals light greenish-yellow, tail tipped with black. Maximum length 1.3 metres. It is found in forested areas throughout Sri Lanka.

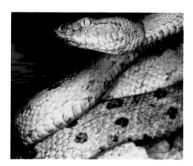 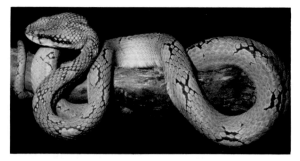

Figure 40. Tokara-habu (*T. tokarensis*) (photo © Dr. D.A. Warrell).

Figure 41. Sri Lankan green pit viper (*T. trigonocephalus*) (photo © Dr. D.A. Warrell).

A number of other species of *Trimeresurus* have been described, some of uncertain taxonomic status, all of uncertain medical importance. These include species with very localised geographical distributions such as *T. labialis* from the Andaman and Nicobar Islands, *T. brongersmai* from the Simeuleü Islands off Sumatra, *T. fasciatus* from Tanajampea Island off Sulawesi, *T. kaulbacki* only from its terra typica in northern Burma, *T. huttoni* from southern India, *T. schultzei* from Balabac and Palawan Islands in the Philippines, *T. cornutus* and *T. tonkinensis* from Vietnam, *T. borneensis* from Borneo, *T. gracilis* from Taiwan and several unfamiliar species described from China or Tibet (*T. mangshanensis, T. medoensis, T. tibetanus* and *T. xiangchengensis*).

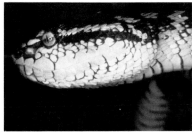 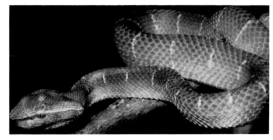

Figure 42. Wagler's pit viper (*Tropidolaemus wagleri*) (photo © Dr. D.A. Warrell).
42a. Specimen from southern Thailand.   **42b.** Juvenile from the Philippines (courtesy Dr. George Watt).

7. Wagler's or temple pit viper (*Tropidolaemus wagleri*) (Figure 42)
This species is relatively short and thick-set. Adults are greenish or bluish-green. Each scale has a black edging, broadest in the scales closest to the vertebral line. There is a series of narrow transverse bright yellow or greenish-yellow stripes. The top of the head is blackish with some yellowish-green markings. There is a yellowish-green post-ocular streak edged above with black; below this the labials and chin are yellowish. Juvenile snakes look quite different. They are bright green with a row of half-white, half-red spots or short vertical lines along each flank (Figure 38b). An arboreal species found in lowland forests up to an altitude of 600 metres in the extreme south of Thailand, peninsular Malaysia, Sumatra, Sulawesi, Borneo and surrounding smaller islands of Indonesia and in the Philippines.

III. VENOMS OF ASIAN SNAKES

Snake venoms contain a large variety of enzymes (proteases, phospholipases etc), non-enzymatic polypeptide toxins (post-synaptic neurotoxins, cardiotoxins etc), amino acids, biogenic amines, carbohydrates, lipids, nucleosides, nucleotides and metals (see Chapter 24). Most of these components have no obvious role in the pathogenesis of envenoming in human patients. This discussion will concentrate on those constituents of the venoms of Asian snakes which seem to contribute to the clinical manifestations of envenoming in humans.

A. COLUBRIDAE
Venoms of the two Asian species capable of fatal envenoming (*Rhabdophis subminiatus* and *R. tigrinus*) have relatively high median lethal doses in mice (130 μg and 5.3 μg per 20g mouse respectively). Both venoms contain a prothrombin activator similar in action to Ecarin, rather than the Factor X activating activity which was originally described.
Nothing is known of the venom of *Malpolon* species.

B. ELAPIDAE
The most important effects of elapid envenoming in Asia are neurotoxicity (kraits, cobras, king cobra and coral snakes) and local tissue necrosis (cobras). The mechanism of local necrosis resulting from elapid and viper venoms may be different. Elapid venoms are

generally less rich in enzymes, particularly proteases, thought to be responsible for tissue damage following viper bites. Necrotic effects of bites by Asian cobras could, however, be explained by the 60-70 aminoacid polypeptides known as cytotoxins or in some cases cardiotoxins and phospholipases A_2 (myotoxins). Polypeptide cytotoxins/cardiotoxins are found in Asian *Naja* venoms, but also in the venom of the Chinese krait (*B. multicinctus*) whose venom does not cause local tissue necrosis. There is not yet a clear correlation between the composition of elapid venoms and the incidence of local necrosis after their bites. The dose of venom injected may be an important variable. Philippine cobra (*N. philippinensis*) venom seems the least likely to cause local tissue damage. Cobra venom factor (which is probably the cobra's own C_{3b}) which activates the complement system by the alternative pathway was first found in Indian cobra (*N. naja*) venom and has also been found in the venom of the king cobra (*Ophiophagus hannah*) but not in krait (*Bungarus*) venoms. Asian elapid venoms show negligible haemostatic effects in humans but, in vitro, phospholipases in the venom of *N. kaouthia* ("*N. n. siamensis*") were anticoagulant and the venom of *O. hannah* contains a species-specific haemorrhagin "hannahtoxin".

Elapid venoms are best known for their neurotoxic activity. Among Asian elapids, the following classes of neurotoxins have been identified.

1. Post-synaptic "alpha-toxins". "Long" (70-74 amino acids) and/or "short" (60-62 residues) neurotoxins have been found in the venoms of *N. atra, N. oxiana, N. philippinensis, N. kaouthia* ("*N. n. siamensis*") and *N. sumatrana* ("*N. n. sputatrix*"). "Long" neurotoxins have been found in the venoms of *Bungarus multicinctus* and *O. hannah*.

2. Toxic phospholipases A_2 which have presynaptic neurotoxic activity have been found in the venoms of kraits (*Bungarus fasciatus* and *B. multicinctus*) and cobras (*N. atra, N. kaouthia, N. sumatrana*).

C. VIPERIDAE

The principal clinical features of envenoming by Asian vipers and pit vipers are haemostatic disturbances, hypotension and local tissue injury.

1. Haemostatic effects

Procoagulants: fibrinogen clotting (thrombin-like) enzymes have been isolated from the venoms of many Asian pit vipers. Ancrod ("Arvin") is a serine protease from the venom of *Calloselasma rhodostoma* which splits fibrinopeptide A from the alpha (A) chain of fibrinogen. It has been used therapeutically as an antithrombotic agent and to reduce blood viscosity in patients with peripheral vascular disease. Other examples are from the venoms of *Trimeresurus flavoviridis, Agkistrodon blomhoffii brevicaudis* (described as "*A. halys* Pallas"), *Deinagkistrodon acutus* ("Acutin"), *Ovophis okinavensis* (= *T. okinavensis*), Taiwanese *T. stejnegeri* (= "*T. gramineus*") and *A. ussuriensis* (= "*A. caliginosus*"). Prothrombin-activating activity (Ecarin) has been found in the venom of *Echis "carinatus"*.

Factor X activity has been found in the venom of Russell's viper (*Daboia russelii*), *E. "carinatus"* and *Cerastes cerastes*. Russell's viper venom also activates Factor V. Anticoagulants, specific inhibitors of coagulation factors, have been found in the venoms of *D. acutus*, Taiwanese *T. stejnegeri* (*T. "gramineus"*), *Vipera berus, A b brevicaudus* (*A. "halys"*) and *T. mucrosquamatus*. Direct fibrinolysins have been found in the venom of *T. mucrosquamatus, D. russelii* and *C. cerastes*. Platelet aggregation is stimulated by the venoms of *T. mucrosquamatus, C. rhodostoma* (Aggregoserpentin) and platelet activation is inhibited by venoms of *E. "carinatus"* ("Echistatin" and "Echicetin"), *C. rhodostoma* (rhodostomin), *D. russelii* and *D. acutus*. Vessel wall damaging and haemorrhage-inducing principles (haemorrhagins) have been found in venoms of *T. flavoviridis, D. acutus* and *Echis* species.

2. Cardiovascular effects

Viper venoms can cause shock (fall in blood pressure) by increasing vascular permeability leading to hypovolaemia, by direct effects on the heart, by splanchnic vasodilatation and by autopharmacological release of vasodilators such as bradykinins. In experimental animals, venoms of *T. flavoviridis* and *T. mucrosquamatus* cause a fall in systemic blood pressure and sometimes a rise in pulmonary artery pressure and bradycardia, which have been attributed to peripheral vasodilatation and to effects on the myocardium. In the case of *D. russelii* venom, hypotension is the result of peripheral vasodilatation, especially in the splanchnic area. A similar effect was shown by the venom of Indian *Echis carinatus*. A bradykinin releasing enzyme and bradykinin-potentiating peptide were found in the venom of *A. b. brevicaudus*.

3. Other venom components

The tissue necrosis caused by viper venoms is usually attributed to their abundant proteolytic enzymes and phospholipases A_2. Neurotoxicity has been observed clinically in patients envenomed by Sri Lankan and south Indian Russell's vipers and Chinese and Japanese mamushis (*A. b. brevicaudus* and *A. b. blomhoffii*) and has been found experimentally in the venom of *A intermedius* from Sinjiang Province. Phospholipases A_2 with presynaptic neurotoxic activity have been found in these venoms. Phospholipases A_2 are also thought to be responsible for the generalised rhabdomyolysis observed in victims of Sri Lankan Russell's vipers (*V. r. pulchella*).

IV. EPIDEMIOLOGY OF SNAKEBITE IN ASIA

A. DETERMINANTS OF SNAKEBITE INCIDENCE AND SEVERITY

The incidence of snakebite in a particular area will depend on the density and activity of snake and human populations in that area and hence the frequency of contact between humans and snakes. Seasonal and diurnal fluctuations in snake and human activity will also determine the likelihood of physical contact between the two. Among indigenous human populations of rural areas of Asia, contact with snakes is likely to be inadvertent except in the case of the relatively few snake catchers and snake charmers and, in China, those who handle snakes for trade and cooking. Usually the human victim steps on a snake while walking or working in the fields or picks up the snake in a handful of rice paddy or other vegetation. When this happens, the risk of a bite depends on the snake's "irritability" or readiness to strike. This varies from species to species. Species such as Russell's vipers and saw-scaled vipers (Echis) seem very likely to strike. The severity of envenoming following a bite will depend on the species of snake and on the various factors which will affect the quantity and quality of venom injected, such as the mechanical efficiency of the bite, the age and size of the snake and, in some cases, the season and the geographical area (in those species whose venoms show wide variation within their geographical range). However, whether the snake has eaten recently or not has no effect on the severity of envenoming[24]. The immune status of the human victim could be important. Snakebite can induce persisting low levels of neutralizing antibody but it seems unlikely that people other than professional snake handlers would be bitten frequently enough to develop any useful immunity. Severity of envenoming also depends on the speed and quality of first aid and medical treatment.

B. EPIDEMIOLOGICAL TECHNIQUES

Most data on the incidence of snakebites, including those in the famous review by Swaroop and Grab[25], are derived from hospital records or official returns to government ministries. These are well known to be unreliable. The following methods, though more demanding in planning, are likely to provide more accurate data for snakebite morbidity and mortality.

1. Population surveys

Questions on past snakebites, personal and in the family and neighbourhood and their outcome, can be added to larger surveys such as those carried out by the World Bank and FAO and in studies of rural morbidity and mortality in Kilifi, Kenya (R. Snow, personal communication 1994).

2. Combining data from western and traditional therapists

In some countries, such as Sri Lanka, China and Taiwan, traditional medicine is licensed and may be preferred to western medicine by a majority of patients. Ayurvedic hospitals in Sri Lanka keep records which can be used in snakebite surveys[26].

3. Eliciting data from anthropologists and rural community workers

Some of the populations which suffer the highest morbidity and mortality from snakebite are geographically isolated (such as the Orang Asli and other indigenous tribes in the Thai-Malay Peninsula and certain of the "tribals" in India) that are well known to anthropologists. For example, among the Phi Tang Luang, a nomadic tribe in northeastern Thailand/Laos, fatal attacks by wild animals including cobras were not uncommon[27].

4. Checking government mortality data at the village or hamlet level

In the dry zone of Sri Lanka, near Anuradhapura, Sawai et al discovered that records of some cases of death from snakebite, which had been reported to village officials, had not been passed on to the provincial authorities and thence to the Registrar General[28].

5. Measurement of the prevalence of snake venom antibodies

At one time, it seemed that this method might be a valuable means of deriving snakebite incidence[29]. Unfortunately, sera of rural populations are notoriously liable to produce false positive reactions in enzyme immunoassay and other serological tests as a result of cross reactions by heterophile antibodies. This so-called "sticky serum" phenomenon has defeated attempts to employ this epidemiological method[30].

C. DIFFICULTIES WITH SNAKEBITE EPIDEMIOLOGY

The inadequacies of available data on snakebite epidemiology are increasingly recognised. The numbers of cases reported to central government departments underestimate the true problem. For example, Table 3 illustrates the discrepancies between figures published by the Division of Epidemiology, the Ministry of Public Health and clinical research studies in Thailand. These problems arise for the following reasons:

1. Snakebite usually has its highest incidence in areas of the rural tropics where personnel and resources for record keeping and reporting may be rudimentary.

2. The incidence of snakebite varies greatly, both geographically and seasonally. To be representative data must therefore be obtained from all parts of the country throughout the year.

3. Traditional treatments are preferred in many areas of high snakebite incidence. Patients attending traditional practitioners, herbalists, bomas (Malaysia), mor glang baan (Thailand), ozhas, hakims, dukuns and vaids (India), vedarala (Sri Lanka), chu-i (China) or monks or priests in temples will rarely be included in official statistical returns.

4. Snakebite cases may be concealed for superstitious reasons. This was certainly the case when H.A. Reid undertook his survey of sea snakebites in northwest Malaysia in the 1950s[31].

Table 3
Thailand: reported snakebites[a]

Year	Bites	Deaths	Notes
1979	1527	14	Hospitals + health stations 9217[b]
1980	1411	16	
1981	1809	13	
1982	2407	18	
1983	2776	4	
1984	2673*	6[+]	*includes only 2 from Trang, but 161 found in 3 months[c]
			[+]5 deaths found
1985	3377	8[x]	[x]11 deaths found
1986	4498	16	
1987	4877	24	
1988	5368	13	

a   Thailand. Division of Epidemiology, Annual Summaries (1981-1990).
b   Thailand. Ministry of Public Health Statistics (1981).
c   Looareesuwan et al[76]

D. EPIDEMICS OF SNAKEBITE

1. Seasonal epidemics

These result from increases in the numbers and level of activity of humans and snakes in a particular area. Snakebite is usually most frequent just before or during seasonal rains because of increases in human agricultural activity. High ambient temperatures and seasonal changes in the snake's reproductive activity may contribute.

2. Heavy flooding

This can result in epidemics of snakebite when populations of snakes and humans are concentrated on diminishing areas of high ground. This has happened in Pakistan, India, Bangladesh and most recently following flooding of the Irrawaddy River in Burma.

3. Invasion of the snake's habitat

This happens during road building, logging and seasonal farming activities.

4. Irrigation schemes

The former dry zone of Sri Lanka became watered and fertile as a result of the Mahaweli Irrigation Scheme. This attracted many farmers to this heavily snake infested area. As a result, there was a sharp increase in the number of snakebite cases.

E. INCIDENCE OF SNAKEBITE IN ASIAN COUNTRIES

Swaroop and Grab[25] estimated, from government data, that between 25,000 and 35,000 people died each year from snakebite in Asia.

1. The Indian subcontinent

With its huge human population and profusion of venomous snakes, the Indian subcontinent has long been recognised to have a large snakebite problem. Writing in 1892,

Sir Joseph Fayrer reported that in 1889 and 1890, 22,480 and 21,412 humans and 3,793 and 3,948 cattle respectively had been killed by snakes in "India" which would then have included Pakistan and Burma[32]. In the 1940s, between 7,396 and 15,876 snakebite deaths were reported each year in India with an overall mortality of about 5.4 per 100,000 population per year. Since the case fatality rate was thought to be about 8%, an estimated 200,000 people were bitten by snakes each year in India[25]. West Bengal was worst affected; in Dinajpur in the period 1949-52, the mortality rate was 12.6 per 100,000 population per year. In more recent times it has proved impossible to estimate the incidence of snakebite morbidity and mortality in India. In Maharashtra State from 1954-8, snakebite deaths ranged from 1237-1788 (average 1496) per year, 3.1 per 100,000 population per year, whereas, from another source, there were said to be only 922 bites with 14 deaths in that year.

2. Pakistan
There are an estimated 40,000 snakebites each year with possibly as many as 20,000 deaths per year (15-18 per 100,000 population per year)[33].

3. Sri Lanka
3,000 snakebite deaths were reported between 1939 and 1949, an incidence of 4.2 per 100,000 population per year[25]. In 1978, 820 deaths were reported to the Registrar General (5.6 per 100,000 population). In a study in Anuradhapura in 1982, a total of 110 deaths from snakebite were discovered, but 63 had not been reported. Forty-four per cent were attributed to *B. caeruleus*, 31% to Russell's vipers and 24% to cobras[28].

4. Burma
Annual snakebite mortality exceeded 2,000 (15.4 per 100,000 population) in the 1930s, and is still thought to exceed 1,000 per year (3.3 per 100,000), attributed mainly to Russell's vipers[34]. Snakebite has been the country's fifth most important cause of death.

5. Thailand
The average number of bites reported each year was 224 in the 1940s, 2,316 (bites) and 179 (deaths) in the 1950s, 3,058 and 80 in the 1960s and 3,244 and 13 in the 1980s respectively. The reported number of cases of snakebite per 100,000 population per year increased from less than 4 (1979 to 1981) to 10 in 1988 (Figure 43). It seems likely that this increase was the result of better reporting rather than more snakebites in the country.

6. China
Zhao wrote that "no statistical data on incidence of snakebite in China is available due to the country's size"[35]. The area south of latitude 25°N and between latitudes 25° and 31°N, east of longitude 105°E, including Hainan and Taiwan Islands, has the worst snakebite problem. In Guangxi Zhuang autonomous region, the average snakebite incidence was 11.67 per 100,000 population per year during the period 1973 to 1984, attributed mainly to *N. atra* and *B. multicinctus*. In 1990, 974 cases of snakebite were recorded in this region with 23 deaths, 14 of which were caused by *O. hannah* and *B. multicinctus*[36]. In this survey, the commonest causes of bites were *N. atra* (27.4%), *T. stejnegeri* (20.9%) and *T. mucrosquamatus* (13.4%). In 1982 in Wujin County, Jiangsu Province, 9.7 cases of snakebite per 100,000 population were attributed to *A blomhoffii brevicaudus*[35].

Reported cases of snake bite per 100,000 population by year   Thailand 1979-1988

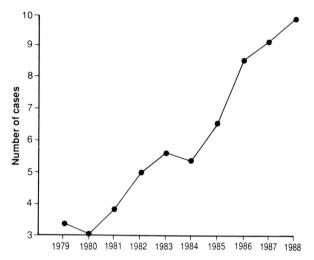

Figure 43. Reported cases of snakebite in Thailand per 100,000 population per year, 1979-1988.

7. Taiwan

12,645 snakebites with 839 deaths (case fatality 6.6%) were reported from 1904 to 1938. In 1931, the mortality was 11.3 per 100,000 population. More recently, there have been approximately 20 deaths per year. In a study of 901 cases of snakebite from 1964 to 1968, 45.5% were caused by *T. mucrosquamatus*, 19.6% by *T stejnegeri* and 17% by *B multicinctus*[37].

8. Laos and Cambodia

Snakebites have rarely been reported from Laos and Cambodia.

9. Peninsular Malaysia

There were 2,114 bites with 34 deaths in 1958 and 1959. Seventy-five per cent of the bites occurred in the northwestern states of Perlis, Kedah and Penang and more than 60% were caused by *C. rhodostoma*[38]. From 1960 to 1968 there were 15,919 reported cases with 122 deaths and, in 1969, of 1,519 cases reported, 27.5% were caused by *C. rhodostoma*, 2.4% by cobras and 3.4% by sea snakes[39]. There was an average of about 6,600 bites each year from 1980 to 1983 with a 0.1% fatality rate[40]. *C. calloselasma*, cobras and *T. purpureomaculatus* were responsible for most of the venomous bites.

10. Philippines

An average of 183 deaths each year, mainly caused by cobras, were reported before 1940 but, in 1968, 294 deaths were recorded, 237 in Luzon and 36 in Mindanao[39].

11. Japan

In the islands of the Ryukyu Archipelago of Japan, there were 5,488 cases with 50 deaths from habu bites (*T. flavoviridis*) between 1962 and 1970, a fatality rate of 0.9%[7]. From 1971-1984 there was an average of 467 bites each year with a fatality rate of 0.54% (incidence of morbidity and mortality 240 and 26 per 100,000 population per year). In the larger islands where it is found, the mamushi (*A. b. blomhoffii*) bites more than 500 people each year with a mortality rate of 0.9%.

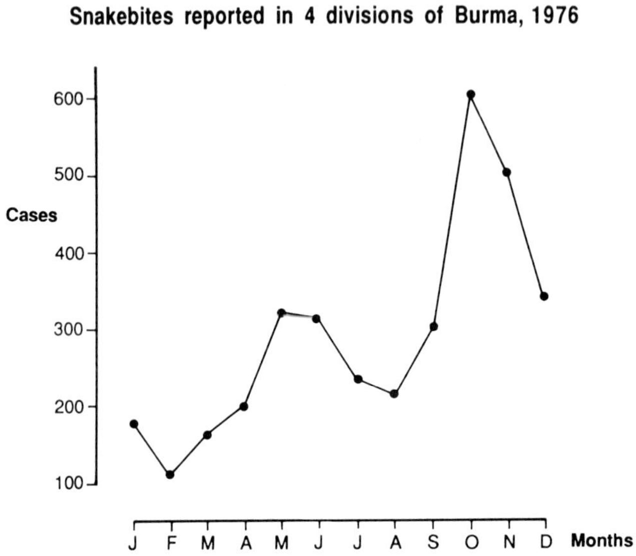

Snakebites reported in 4 divisions of Burma, 1976

Figure 44. Incidence of snakebites in four divisions of Burma, 1976, showing two peaks of incidence.

12. South Korea

Bites by *A. ussuriensis*, *A. blomhoffii brevicaudus* and *A. saxatilis* have been reported. One hundred and twenty-six cases were seen in five hospitals during two years (1976 and 1977)[41].

13. Vietnam

No data are available, but bites by *C. rhodostoma* are common, especially in the rubber and coffee plantations of southwestern Vietnam (for example in Song-be Province). Cobra bites cause a number of deaths.

14. Indonesia

No recent data on snakebite bite are available. In Java, *C. rhodostoma* bites plantation workers. Fatal bites by other species were reported in the 1930s[42]. In Komodo and Flores, Russell's vipers (*D. r. limitis*) are said to be the commonest cause of snakebite deaths. Snakebite is apparently rare in Sumatra, Sulawesi and Borneo. Approximately 16 patients with snakebites were admitted each year to Kuching Hospital, Sarawak, East Malaysia[39].

15. Iran

Judging by its production of antivenoms, more than 35,000 vials each year, Iran must have many snakebite cases but no data are available[43]. Little is known of snakebite in Afghanistan, except that, in Waziristan, *V. lebetina* was greatly feared by humans and caused much mortality among camels[44].

16. Nepal

More than 20,000 people are bitten by snakes; 1,000 of them die[45]. Among a group of 3,189 cases studied from 1980 to 1985, the case fatality rate was 4.5%.

F. SEASONAL VARIATION IN INCIDENCE

In most countries in this region, snakebite incidence increases with the start of the rainy season or in association with the increased agricultural activity anticipating that event. A striking seasonal variation in snakebite incidence occurs in Burma (Figure 44). The first smaller peak in May to July coincides with the beginning of the rainy season when the farmers start planting paddy, while the second larger peak is from October to December when the paddy is being harvested. During these two periods of intense agricultural activity in the rice growing areas of Burma and Thailand, tens of thousands of farmers go into the fields barefooted and barehanded. Most bites are inflicted by Russell's vipers on the feet and ankles of these farmers. In the States of Delhi, Maharashtra and West Bengal, India, the seasonal peak of snakebite incidence in June-October is related to rainfall rather than temperature[48]. In the Amami and Okinawa islands of Japan, 97% of habu (*T. flavoviridis*) bites occur during the warm weather from March until October. The habu lives close to human dwellings and 22% of bites are inflicted in people's homes especially at night. Detailed analysis of 3,782 habu bites with 25 deaths on Amamioshima and Tokunoshima during the 16 years 1967-82 revealed that 7% of victims were bitten 2-7 times during this period. In Tokunoshima, 15% of all males aged 15-64 years were bitten. The seasonal peak of bites in June was related to maximal snake and human activity. Meteorological optima were a temperature of 25°C and humidity of 80%. The risk of bites was significantly related to the time spent in sugar cane fields[21,46]. In southern China, snakebite is most common during the warm months from April to August. In some parts of Sri Lanka there is a peak of incidence from March to May coinciding with the paddy harvest. In the case of bites by *B. caeruleus*, it has been suggested that the peak incidence observed from September to November is the result of increased activity of these snakes during their annual mating season[47]. Most victims of krait bites (*B. caeruleus, B. candidus, B. ceylonicus*) are bitten while asleep on the floor of their huts at night in India, Sri Lanka, Pakistan and Thailand. It seems likely that these snakes enter human dwellings at night in pursuit of their natural prey of other snakes and skinks. They bite when inadvertently rolled on or touched by sleeping humans. Snakebite is an occupational hazard of rice farmers in Southeast Asia who are at risk from Russell's vipers and cobras, plantation workers in Thailand, Malaysia, Vietnam and elsewhere who are frequently bitten by Malayan pit vipers, tea pickers in Sri Lanka (bitten by *H. hypnale*) and in southern India (bitten by *T. macrolepis*), by fish farmers in Thailand and the Philippines (cobras) and by those who handle snakes for food and production of traditional medicines in China (cobra, king cobra and *D. acutus*).

V. CLINICAL FEATURES OF SNAKEBITE IN ASIA

Not all patients bitten by venomous snakes, with puncture marks on the skin indicating penetration by the fangs, will develop evidence of envenoming. In the states of Perlis and Kedah in northwestern peninsula Malaysia, among 824 patients bitten by vipers, cobras or sea snakes, 53% developed slight or no envenoming[38]. In patients bitten by *C. rhodostoma* and cobras the incidence of slight or no envenoming was 50% and 61% respectively. In a detailed study of 250 patients with proven bites by *C. rhodostoma*, 19% developed no symptoms or signs, not even pain; 10% developed pain only and 22% developed slight local swelling only[49]. In Burma, 28% of a group of 123 proved cases of Russell's viper bite did not develop envenoming[34]. In Sri Lanka, 27% of patients bitten by Russell's vipers developed no signs of envenoming[50].

Even if no venom is injected by the bite, fear and first aid treatment may give rise to symptoms and signs. Anxiety can cause tachycardia, palpitations, trembling, flushing, sweating, a feeling of tightness of the chest and hyperventilation leading to dizziness, faintness, carpopedal spasm and acroparaesthesiae. Tourniquets and constriction bands may produce congested, swollen and even ischaemic limbs; incisions, bleeding and sensory loss; and herbal medicines, vomiting. In Sri Lanka, the repertoire of traditional ayurvedic treatments for snakebite comprises incisions (including deep incisions into the vertex of the scalp), instillation of irritant liquids into the eyes (which may cause severe chemical conjunctivitis or even blindness), forceful insufflation of oil through a tube introduced into the nasopharynx (which may lead to ruptured ear drums and aspiration lipid pneumonia) and heating over a fire (which may cause severe burns)[50-52].

The earliest symptoms of snakebite are the mechanical pain of the fangs penetrating the skin (which may be insufficient to wake those who are bitten while asleep by kraits) followed by the pain of envenoming, which may be intense. Pain, swelling, tenderness and inflammation spread up the bitten limb, in the case of bites by vipers and some elapids. Lymph nodes draining the bitten limb may become enlarged and tender. Nausea, vomiting and headache are common symptoms of severe systemic envenoming. Patient envenomed by Daboia and Vipera species and those suffering anaphylactic reactions to venom as a result of hypersensitization may collapse within minutes of the bite and remain unconscious for up to 30 minutes. Associated symptoms include vomiting, colic, diarrhoea, angio-oedema and wheezing.

A. ENVENOMING BY COLUBRIDAE
1. Asian keelbacks (genus *Rhabdophis*)
a. Red necked keelback (R subminiatus)

No cases of envenoming have been reported from any of the countries where this species occurs naturally. In a national hospital-based survey of snakes responsible for bites in Thailand, five patients who had trodden on or touched the snakes accidentally were bitten but suffered negligible effects[8]. However, four cases of severe envenoming have been reported from England, Germany, the United States and the Netherlands[53-57]. These cases were remarkably similar. All four victims were young men (aged 20-25 years) who were handling the pet snake when they were bitten on the fingers or thumb. In two cases, two bites were inflicted and in the others the bites were sustained for 30 seconds or more. The bites were painless and local swelling was slight or minimal in two of the cases. Symptoms began 30 minutes to many hours after the bite with headache, nausea and vomiting. Symptoms of a bleeding diathesis developed between a few hours and a few days after the bite: bleeding from the fang marks, venepunctures, pimples and other signs of trauma and spontaneous bleeding from the gums, nose, gastrointestinal and urinary tracts and ecchymoses. All four patients had incoagulable blood when admitted to hospital five hours to five days after the bite. There was defibrinogenation and depletion of other clotting factors, evidence of increased fibrinolytic activity, elevated FDPs, thrombocytopenia and microangiopathic haemolysis. Two patients showed neutrophil leucocytosis. In the absence of a specific antivenom the coagulopathy persisted for up to four weeks, but fibrinogen usually became detectable after seven days. One patient showed a transient increase in serum creatinine. All made a complete recovery. Apparently, large numbers of these snakes have been imported into Europe and the United States as "harmless" pets. Their resemblance to familiar and innocuous natricine snakes such as the European ringed snake or grass snake (*Natrix natrix*) gave a false sense of security!

b. Yamakagashi (R tigrinus)

Cases of envenoming have been described only in Japan although the species also occurs in Korea, the far east of the Russian Federation, China and Taiwan. Bites by this species are common in Japan. Clinical features are similar to those of *R. subminiatus* envenoming, but are generally more severe. Envenoming was first described by Sakamoto in 1932[58].* All the victims have been male, several of them boys, who were bitten on the thumb, fingers or hand while handling the snake. One was a professional snake catcher who had been bitten by yamakagashis 10 times before receiving the double bites which caused severe envenoming. Early symptoms, which could start within 20 minutes of the bite, included local swelling, collapse with transient loss of consciousness, headache, nausea, retching, vomiting and evidence of a bleeding diathesis which could be delayed for several hours after the bite. There was bleeding from the fang marks and other recent sites of trauma including venepunctures and intramuscular injection sites, bleeding gums, epistaxis, bleeding from the gastrointestinal and urinary tracts, skin petechiae and extensive subcutaneous and intramuscular ecchymoses and haematomas.

Local swelling was more extensive than with *R. subminiatus* bites, extending to the forearm in several cases. Laboratory abnormalities included peripheral neutrophil leucocytosis, thrombocytopenia, incoagulable blood with depletion of clotting factors, and evidence of increased fibrinolytic activity with elevated FDP. Two patients developed resistant renal failure. One of the two fatal cases, the 61 year old professional snake catcher, died of pulmonary oedema while being dialysed for renal failure 62 days after the bite. Earlier renal biopsies had showed severe tubular necrosis and at autopsy the kidneys were atrophic[60]. The other fatal case was a 14 year old boy who became unconscious 16 hours after the bite, was found on CT scan to have bleeds in the left temporal and occipital lobes and died 10 days later[61].

2. Other colubrids capable of severe envenoming

Clinical features of envenoming by the Montpellier snake (*Malpolon monspessulanus*) are described in the chapter on African and Middle Eastern snakes.

3. Minor syndromes of colubrid envenoming

At least eight other species of colubrid, other than those discussed above, have proved capable of causing mild envenoming, and it is likely that bites by many more species would produce similar symptoms. Most colubrids will have the opportunity to bite humans only when being handled and, under these circumstances, may be provoked to bite repeatedly or to sustain the bite long enough (and to "chew") so that venom can be injected by the back fangs or enter wounds made by enlarged posterior maxillary teeth. Herpetologists, snake catchers, those who handle snakes for culinary and medicinal purposes and people, often children, who keep snakes as pets, are therefore most likely to be bitten. Local pain ("stinging") and swelling with or without numbness, redness, lymphangitis and tender enlargement of local lymph nodes have been reported after bites by *Balanophis ceylonensis*[62], *Boiga ceylonensis*[63], *B. dendrophila*[64], *Ahaetulla (Dryophis) nasuta*[62], *Coluber ravergieri*[65], *C. rhodorachis*[67], *Cerberus rhynchops*[62], *Enhydris enhydris*[66], and *Malpolon moilensis*[67]. Mild systemic symptoms such as headache and giddiness were reported after bites by *Balanophis ceylonensis* and *Boiga forsteni*[62].

B. ENVENOMING BY ELAPIDAE

Envenoming by Asian cobras (Naja) and the king cobra (*Ophiophagus hannah*) causes almost immediate severe local pain and tenderness. The incidence and extent of swelling and necrosis varies among the different species, being lowest in the case of bites by Philippine cobras (*N. philippinensis*)[68]. Envenoming by other Asian elapids, notably the

---

*Two of the cases reported by Mittleman and Goris[58] (JWL and WSA) were republished by Mandell et al[59] "Cases 2 and 1" respectively, but with the misleading attribution of the bite in Case 1 to the "Aodaisho" (*Elaphe climacophora*), but with a description of the snake's dentition which rejects this diagnosis and makes it more likely that the patient was bitten by *R. tigrinus*.

kraits (*Bungarus*), is virtually painless (the bite may fail to rouse the victim from sleep), swelling is trivial or absent and no local necrosis develops. Most species of Asian elapid are capable of producing neurotoxic symptoms in human victims. Early symptoms, before there are objective neurological signs, include vomiting, "heaviness" of the eyelids, blurred vision, drowsiness and sometimes paraesthesiae of the mouth, tongue or lips, headache and dizziness. Paralysis, first detectable as ptosis and external ophthalmoplegia, may be evident minutes after the bite[68] but is more often delayed for many hours. Neurotoxicity progresses to involve the palate, jaws, tongue, vocal cords, neck muscles and muscles of deglutition. Respiratory failure may be precipitated by airway obstruction at this stage, or later after paralysis of intercostal muscles and diaphragm. It may progress to generalised flaccid paralysis but patients may retain their ability to flex fingers or toes in response to questions confirming that they are fully conscious. Neurotoxic effects are completely reversible, either acutely in response to antivenom, or in some cases anticholinesterases, or after spontaneous resolution over several days or weeks. Generalised rhabdomyolysis has not been shown to be clinically important after bites by Asian elapids. It is doubtful whether elapid venoms have central effects in humans. Clinically significant bleeding and clotting problems have not been reliably reported after bites by Asian elapids. Abdominal pain is a common and unexplained symptom of bites by some species of kraits such as *B caeruleus*[51].

1. Snake venom ophthalmia caused by spitting cobras

All the species of Asian cobra except *N. kaouthia, N. naja* and *N. oxiana*, are capable, in defence, of "spitting" their venom into the eyes and onto nasal and buccal membranes of a supposed aggressor for a distance of several metres. There is intense pain in the eye, blepharospasm, palpebral oedema and leucorrhoea and a risk of corneal erosions and others complications observed in patients with venom ophthalmia caused by African spitting cobras.

2. Envenoming by kraits (genus *Bungarus*)

a. Common (Indian) krait (B caeruleus)

B caeruleus has long been regarded, with *N. naja*, as the most dangerous species of venomous snake in the Indian subcontinent[69]. In Anuradhapura, Sri Lanka, surveys indicate that this species accounts for 22-44% of snakebite deaths[28,70]. In west Bengal, *B. caeruleus* was blamed for 33% of all venomous snakebites[71]. Most patients are bitten while asleep on the floor of their huts, shelters or jhuggis, in India and Sri Lanka[51,69-72]. Patients may be bitten when they roll over or move in their sleep, especially when they are particularly restless during the time of rapid eye movement sleep, touching or trapping a snake which is prowling around their home in search of its natural prey. Because they are bitten while lying down, the target may be any part of the body including the head, neck and shoulders. These bites usually produce invisible or scarcely perceptible puncture marks, no local symptoms apart from mild pain, itchiness, numbness or some other paraesthesia and negligible or no local swelling. As a result, snakebite may not be suspected and patients commonly present to hospital after waking in the morning with paralysis of the muscles innervated by cranial nerves III, IV, VI, V, VII, IX and X and excessive salivation (Figure 45)[51,72]. In patients presenting with progressive paralysis, initially of muscles innervated by the cranial nerves, envenoming may be misdiagnosed as acute idiopathic inflammatory polyneuropathy (Guillain-Barré syndrome, especially its variants Miller-Fisher syndrome[**] and polyneuritis cranialis, or myasthenia gravis). Rarely, local lymph nodes may be painfully enlarged. Abdominal pain has been described in up to a third of cases. Paralysis can develop within two hours but may be delayed for 7-12 hours. Severe generalised muscle pains were

---

[**]Ophthalmoplegia, ataxia, areflexia and facial and bulbar weakness.

complained of by a few patients and moderately elevated plasma myoglobin concentration raises the possibility of generalised rhabdomyolysis. Cardiovascular effects of *B caeruleus* venom have been described in dogs, but in patients these are observed only as a consequence of respiratory failure or antivenom reactions. Marked neutrophil leucocytosis has been described[69]. The mortality rate of *B. caeruleus* bites in patients not treated with antivneom is high; 77% of 35 cases in India[69] and 100% of 27 cases in Sri Lanka[70]. Fayrer describes a bizarre incident in which two prisoners forced a large *B. caeruleus* to bite four labourers. Three of them died within hours and the fourth was severely envenomed but recovered[73].

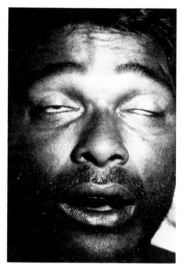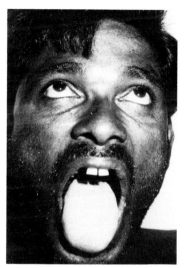

Figure 45. Forty year old Sri Lankan rice farmer who slept in the paddy fields and awoke with inability to open his eyes, swallow, speak and protrude his tongue (photo © Dr. D.A. Warrell).
45a. On admission on the morning his symptoms had developed.
45b. 24 hours later after antivenom treatment showing full recovery from neurotoxic symptoms. Envenoming by *Bungarus caeruleus* was proved by enzyme immunoassay[51].

b. Malayan krait (B candidus)

The older literature is confusing because the common (Indian) krait (*B. caeruleus*) is sometimes incorrectly referred to as *B. candidus*[44]. Proven cases of bites by *B. candidus* were identified in Malaya in the 1950s and in Thailand in the 1980s[74,75]. Surprisingly for a species that had been regarded as rare, it was found to be one of the three commonest causes of fatal snakebite in Thailand[76]. Like *B. caeruleus*, it usually bites at night while the victims are asleep on the floor of their homes. However, two out of five patients reported from Malaya and Thailand[75], although bitten by large snakes, 1.4 and 1.1 metres long, developed no signs of envenoming. Most of the envenomed patients developed no signs or symptoms at the site of the bite (Figure 46a) or in the draining lymph nodes. One patient noticed slight local pain and bleeding at the time of the bite with numbness 30 minutes later and another developed slight swelling, redness, tenderness and numbness at the site, 30 minutes after the bite. Other early symptoms included abdominal discomfort, headache and giddiness. One patient became breathless 30 minutes after the bite but in most cases neurotoxic symptoms, beginning with ptosis, developed within a few hours of the bite. Patients developed ptosis, external ophthalmoplegia, facial paralysis, inability to open the mouth, swallow or protrude the tongue and eventually respiratory and flaccid paralysis (Figure 46b). In one patient fasciculations were evident in the legs, another had dilated pupils and evidence of autonomic paralysis. Among 13 fatal cases, the interval between bite and death was 3-288 (median 96) hours[76]. Survivors showed complete recovery in 6-14 days. A peripheral neutrophil leucocytosis was found in most of the envenomed patients.

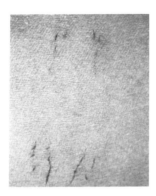 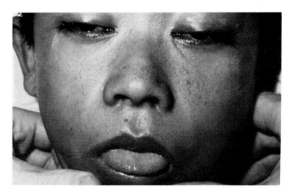

Figure 46. Thirteen year old Thai boy bitten while asleep on the floor of his hut in eastern Thailand by a 1.1m long *Bungarus candidus* (British Museum Natural History, London, Accession number 1982.457) (photo © Dr. D.A. Warrell).
46a. Site of the bite on his thigh, showing marks of the fangs and tooth marks from the upper and lower jaw. Note the absence of local reaction.
46b. Third day after the bite, showing persistent ptosis, facial paralysis, inability to open the mouth and protrude the tongue. He had been treated with mechanical ventilation since no specific antivenom was available[75].

c. Sri Lankan krait (B ceylonicus)

Although common in several areas of Sri Lanka, this species has been reliably implicated in only a few cases of snakebite. A woman who was bitten by a 1.05 metre long specimen while sleeping on a mat on the floor of her house felt slight transient local pain at the site of the bite, she developed blurred vision and difficulty in swallowing within about 30 minutes and, when admitted to hospital about six hours after the bite, she was drowsy with bilateral ptosis, blurred vision, hypersalivation, difficulty in swallowing, protruding the tongue, opening the mouth, speaking and breathing. This patient died as a result of complications of traditional treatment and antivenom, three days after the bite[52]. In a case of probable *B. ceylonicus* envenoming, the patient developed respiratory paralysis about six hours after the bite. When weaned off the mechanical ventilator 78 hours later, she showed evidence of a distal motor neuropathy which could have been explained by the damaging effect of some presynaptic bungarotoxins on motor nerve terminals[77].

d. Banded krait (B fasciatus)

This species is very widely distributed but is responsible for very few bites. It seems extremely reluctant to bite, even when aggravated, but, in one published report of systemic envenoming, the snake was provoked to bite a man who was attempting to bite off its tail[78]. 2.7% of a series of 974 cases of snakebites in Guangxi, China were attributed to this species. Twenty-three per cent developed paralytic symptoms and the fatality rate was 7.7%[36]. A fatal case was identified by enzyme immunoassay in a survey of suspected cobra bites[29]; the patient died of respiratory failure a few hours after being bitten at night by a snake which she did not see. In another five published cases of bites, there was no envenoming, but in a sixth, sequelae of envenoming were said to be severe, leading to shock but the patient recovered[29]. It has been frequently stated in the Thai literature that envenoming by *B fasciatus* is associated with petechial haemorrhages, bleeding gums, haemoptysis and gastrointestinal bleeding causing abdominal pain. No basis for such disturbances has been discovered in proven cases of envenoming by *B. fasciatus* or in studies of its venom.

e. Red headed krait (B. flaviceps)

Only one case of a bite by this species has been reported[79]. No clinical details are given. The patient was said to have been given specific antivenom and he recovered.

f. Javan krait (B. javanicus)[32]

At Matanghadji, Soember, about 20 km south of Cheribon (Ceribon) on the north coast of Java, three farmers were sleeping in a small open shelter in the fields during the rice harvest. One awoke to find a snake crawling over his hand, made a sudden movement and was bitten on the finger. He shouted out "a snake has bitten me" and, unfortunately, threw the snake on to his father who was bitten on the calf. Soon after the bites, both men pointed to their throats and developed laboured breathing. Neither could speak or move. The father died about 30 minutes after the bite while being carried home and his son died about 16 hours after the bite. Small bite wounds were visible on the bodies but there was no swelling or other changes. The snake, 86 cm long, was the type specimen of the new species[32].

g. Chinese krait (B. multicinctus)

This species is an important cause of snakebite mortality in southern China. In Guangxi Zhuang autonomous region, 8.4% of snakebites were caused by *B. multicinctus*; 36.3% developed paralytic symptoms and the case fatality was 10%[36]. In Taiwan, 8% of bites were caused by this species between 1904 and 1971 with 23% case fatality[80]. Bites occur mainly at night, but only 16% were inflicted in the home[36]. Local symptoms are negligible. The bite is felt as a prick followed by slight itching, numbness or redness but with minimal swelling. Nausea and vomiting may develop about 30 minutes later and neurotoxic symptoms within 1-4 hours of the bite. These include ptosis, inability to speak and swallow, "trismus" (inabilty to open the mouth), chest tightness, breathlessness, generalised aching and weakness of the limbs. Other symptoms include headache, dizziness, thirst, confusion, throat pain, laryngeal spasm and drowsiness. In patients not treated with antivenom, the interval between bite and death ranges from 6-23 hours.

3. Envenoming by Asian coral snakes (*Calliophis*)

In Nepal, H. Schnurrenberger was bitten by a juvenile specimen of *C. macclellandii univirgatus* approximately 30 cm long and as thick as a pencil. He was symptom-free for two hours and ignored the bite, but six hours after the bite he developed pain on movement and he died of respiratory paralysis eight hours after the bite[9].

4. Envenoming by long-glanded coral snakes (genus *Maticora*)

In Borneo "there are many stories among the Iban of deaths from bites from these snakes, and they should be accounted dangerous"[81].

a. Blue coral snake (M. bivirgata)

Reid reported two cases with no envenoming[74]. A two year old Malay girl bitten at the base of the thumb by an 85 cm long specimen near Malacca died two hours later on her way to hospital[82]. This species was also suspected of being responsible for the death of a man in Singapore in 1985 who died five minutes after being bitten twice on his toes while taking a shower[83].

b. Banded coral snake (M. intestinalis)

While collecting snakes in Java in 1937, Dr Jacobson was bitten by a 49 cm long specimen. One fang penetrated the web of the fingers. There was slight local pain and swelling and, after 2¼ hours, attacks of giddiness and breathlessness with vomiting and diarrhoea which lasted about four hours[84].

5. Envenoming by cobras (genus *Naja*)

The various species of Asian *Naja* are probably responsible for more human mortality and morbidity than any other genus of venomous snakes. Cobras have been regarded as "the commonest and most deadly of all Indian poisonous snakes"[85]. "There can be little doubt that it contributes very largely to the mortality from snake-bite, especially in northern and western India"[85].

a. Chinese cobra (N atra)

In Guangxi, China, this species is the most important cause of identified snakebites but with a low case fatality of 0.7%[36]. 40.9% of patients develop local necrosis and in 10.7% there was persistent dysfunction of the affected limb. In Taiwan, between 1904 and 1971, 5% of bites were caused by *N. atra* with a case fatality of 14.4%[80]. Among 471 cases of snakebite from Guangxi, Yunnan and Guangdong Provinces, 27% were caused by *N. atra*[86]. In Guangxi, 70.8% of bites were inflicted on the upper limbs, because 50% of the patients were bitten while catching or handling the snakes, for commercial, culinary or medicinal purposes[36]. Envenomed patients noticed pain and swelling at the site of the bite almost immediately. Swelling may extend to involve the whole limb and, within 24 hours, blistering and dark discoloration appear at the site of the bite. Later there is necrosis and sloughing of skin and superficial fascia down to the level of the tendons with "skip" lesions further up the limb. Even if amputation of a gangrenous digit is avoided, scarring and ankylosis may result in permanent disability. Peripheral neutrophil leucocytosis is common and serum aspartate and alanine aminotransferases are elevated in patients with necrosis. In the minority of patients who develop neurotoxic symptoms, vomiting and abdominal pain start within a few hours of the bite followed by the usual progression of drowsiness, ptosis, ophthalmoplegia, inability to open the mouth, speak, protrude the tongue and eventually respiratory paralysis in some.

2. Monocellate cobra (N. kaouthia)

In 45 of Alistair Reid's series of 47 patients bitten by cobras in northwestern Malaya, *N. kaouthia* was responsible[88]***. Forty-five per cent of patients in this classical study developed no envenoming and in 8% there was only slight local swelling lasting a few days. In envenomed patients, pain started immediately after the bite and persisted for an average of 10 days in those who developed extensive necrosis (more than 100 cm^2). Swelling usually started 2-3 hours after the bite and was maximal in 24-48 hours; it rarely involved the whole limb. "A constant feature of local swelling from cobra-bites is a dusky discoloration around the bite marks, extending in area and deepening in colour each day. About the third or fourth day the grey-black area becomes encircled by a red raised rim, sometimes studded with small blisters. In about half the cases sanguineous blisters developed over the middle of the dusky area: they were usually small, rarely exceeding 3-5 cm diameter, but in two cases they involved the whole dorsum of the foot. After 4-5 days fluctuation was often evident: incision revealed red-yellow material and necrosis of subcutaneous tissue. The extent of sloughs was invariably much wider than the surface changes suggested"[88]. Some patients develop extensive necrosis without any neurotoxic signs. Some patients with extensive necrosis showed a persistent fever. Neurotoxic envenoming presented with drowsiness, starting 1-5 hours after the bite. Ptosis and difficulty with speaking, opening the mouth, moving the lips and swallowing followed 3-4 hours later and in some patients there was progression to general weakness. Paresis of muscles innervated by the facial nerve and the neck flexors (giving rise to "broken neck

---

***Unfortunately this paper is misleading. In Figure 1A *N. kaouthia* is mislabelled
N. n. leucodira and in B yellow *N. sumatrana* is mislabelled *N. n. kaouthia.*

syndrome") was seen in some cases. Other systemic symptoms included headache, vomiting and abdominal pain. Four patients became hypotensive, perhaps as a result of hypovolaemia. ECGs were normal. Investigations were normal apart from leucocytosis, evidence of mild haemolysis and a transient rise in blood urea in one patient. Some of the necrotic wounds were infected. Severely necrotic wounds (more than 100 cm^2) took an average of 15 weeks to heal. Two patients died, probably of respiratory failure, 3¾ and 8 hours after being bitten. In 14 fatal cases of cobra bite in northwest Malaya from 1955 to 1961, the time from bite to death ranged from 1¼ to 60 (mean 12.6) hours[88].

In a national survey of snakes responsible for bites in Thailand, 7.2% were found to be *N. kaouthia*[8]. This species was also responsible for 12 of 46 cases of fatal snakebite in Thailand[76]. At Insein Hospital, Burma, 5% of snakebite cases had been bitten by cobras; 32% developed no signs of envenoming. Mortality rate was 4%[87]. At Bang Phli Hospital, southeast of Bangkok, 58 patients with proven bites by *N. kaouthia* were studied prospectively. Most were rice farmers (82%) or fishermen (15%) who had been bitten on their feet or ankles (74%). Local pain and swelling developed within 15 minutes and was eventually detected in 83% of the patients. Blistering and necrosis developed in 10% (Figure 47). Systemic symptoms developed from 30 minutes to several hours after the bite. Three per cent of patients felt nauseated and vomited and some became drowsy. Ptosis was the commonest sign followed by dysphagia, dysphonia and respiratory distress. The case fatality in this series was 7%. A group of children with proven or suspected *N kaouthia* bites were studied at Chulalongkorn Hospital in Bangkok[89]. Most had been bitten on their feet in the back yard of their homes. Seventy-seven per cent developed swelling and 49% pain usually noticeable within 30 minutes of the bite. Neurotoxic symptoms began as early as 30 minutes and as late as 17-19 hours after the bite. Ptosis and drowsiness were seen in 64%. Laboured breathing, respiratory arrest, frothy saliva, slurred speech and flaccid skeletal muscles were also noted. Associated symptoms included nausea, vomiting, thirst, abdominal pain and diarrhoea. Necrosis was first evident as dark red discoloration and blistering on about the second day after the bite. By the end of the first week, necrosis was evident in 40% of cases. Bacterial infection was detected in 58% (*Proteus rettgeri, P. morgani, E. coli, Pseudomonas aeruginosa* and *Enterobacteriaceae*). Healing took 1-2 months. A neutrophil leucocytosis was the only consistent laboratory abnormality. The mortality in this series was 4.3%[89]. Among a group of 20 Thai farmers admitted to a rural health centre east of Bangkok, local pain and swelling began 1-3 hours after the bite, reaching a peak within 48 hours. Most developed local necrosis, usually four days later. The earliest symptom of systemic envenoming was drowsiness (60%) starting 30 minutes to three hours after the bite. Features include ptosis, inability to speak, open the mouth, move the lips and swallow. Ptosis was seen in all cases of systemic envenoming, beginning 1.6 to six hours after the bite. In three patients there was progression to respiratory paralysis. The mortality was 5%[90].

c. Indian spectacled cobra (N. naja)

Cobra bites are very common in many parts of India and hundreds of individual case reports have been published in books and journals over the past 130 years. It is amazing, however, that no large prospective study of patients with proven bites by *N. naja* has been undertaken and reported. In a survey of snakebites in India, 91.4% of cases were bitten by an unidentified snake. Of the 6.1% of identified venomous snakes responsible for bites, 40% were *N. naja*[91]. As with bites by *N. kaouthia*, patients may show manifestations of systemic neurotoxic envenoming or local envenoming or both. Local necrosis was described after cobra bites in India in the 1860s and up to the 1920s[88,92] but this was apparently forgotten until Reid's work in Malaysia. Severe local pain and swelling may begin almost immediately after the bite. The pain persists while swelling and tenderness extend up the bitten limb (Figure 48a), sometimes spreading to the adjacent trunk. Darkening of the necrotic area of skin and blistering are apparent by about the third day (Figure 48b) with a characteristic putrid smell typical of necrotic cobra bites in Africa and Asia. Early systemic symptoms include headache, nausea, vomiting, dizziness and a feeling of lassitude, drowsiness and intoxication. "Many subjects describe their drowsiness as if they had imbibed large quantities of some potent intoxicant."[69] Neurotoxic symptoms begin with ptosis (the patient puckers their brow, contracting the frontalis muscle, attempting to raise the eyelids or tilts the head back so as to see beneath the drooping upper lids), profuse viscid saliva, inability to clear secretions, sagging of the jaw or inability to open the mouth and progression to respiratory paralysis[51]. It is not clear from the available literature whether the proportion of patients developing neurotoxicity and necrosis is different from that in patients bitten by *N. kaouthia*. The clinical syndromes following bites by the two species seem identical. Fatal envenoming can occur as soon as 15 minutes after a bite by *N. naja*.

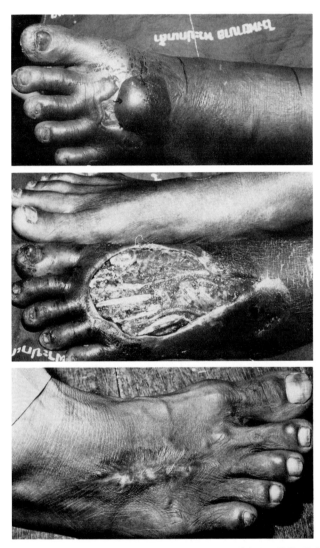

Figure 47. Thai woman bitten on the dorsum of the foot by *Naja kaouthia* (photos © Dr. D.A. Warrell).
47a. (top) Swelling of the foot, blistering and early signs of necrosis 4 days after the bite.
47b. (middle) Sloughing of superficial tissues 14 days after the bite.
47c. (bottom) Scarring after bite by *N. kaouthia* many years earlier.

d. Oxus cobra (N. oxiana)

No precise information is available from the large area of West Asia where this species occurs. In Iran, the only neurotoxic species is *N oxiana*. According to Latifi[43] weakness, drowsiness and paralysis of the throat are important symptoms which appear in less than one hour after the bite and progress rapidly to respiratory distress and death. This author also mentions "haemorrhages and lack of blood coagulation" which is hard to explain. There is no reference to local necrosis.

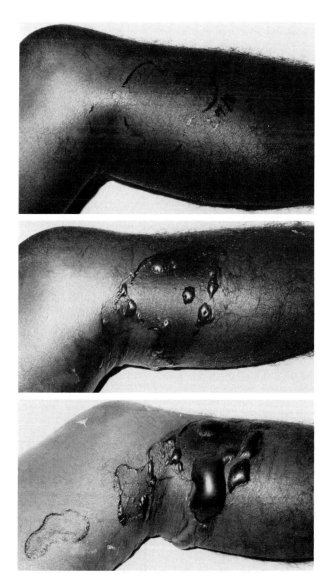

Figure 48. Thirty five year old Sri Lankan man bitten on the shin by *Naja naja* (photos © Dr. D.A. Warrell).
48a. (top) Swelling 36 hours after the bite.
48b. (middle) Blistering and darkening of the skin (suggestive of early necrosis) 3 days after the bite.
48c. (bottom) Extensive blistering and early necrosis 4 days after the bite.

e. Philippine cobra (N. philippinensis)

Cobras are responsible for about half of the snakebites in the Philippines[39]. Watt and his colleagues studied snakebites in the central rice-growing area of Luzon Island north of Manila where only one species of cobra occurs (*N. philippinensis*) and is responsible for almost all cases of envenoming. Of 39 patients bitten by cobras, 38 developed neurotoxicity. The first symptom, occurring as early as three minutes or as late as 24 hours after the bite (median 1 hour), was usually ptosis (87%) or slurred speech, dysphonia or breathlessness in the remainder[68]. Respiratory paralysis occurred within 10 minutes of the bite in one case and three patients became apnoeic within 30 minutes. Thirty-six per cent of patients developed no local swelling, including six with respiratory muscle paralysis. Only 8% of patients developed local necrosis. These clinical findings are consistent with animal studies in which .*N. philippinensis* venom was found to be more lethal and less necrotic than other *Naja* venoms.

f. Samar cobra (N. samarensis)

There have been no formal reports of bites by this species, but case 11 described by Sawai et al[39] occurred in Mindanao Island where this is the only species of cobra. The patient developed severe pain, swelling and dyspnoea but recovered fully in four days after antivenom treatment.

g. Thai spitting cobra (N. siamensis)

In a national hospital based survey of snakes responsible for bites in Thailand, 10% of all dead snakes brought by snake-bitten patients were of this species (described as "*Naja atra* northern spitting cobra")[8]. Neurotoxic signs (ptosis and difficulty in breathing) were observed in 12 of the 114 cases (10.5%). Local swelling and necrosis were common, but many of the patients were followed up for too short a time to allow precise assessment of the incidence of these effects. We have seen swelling and necrosis, comparable in all respects with that following bites by *N. kaouthia*, in patients envenomed by *N. siamensis* in Ubon and Kanchanaburi in Thailand (Looareesuwan S, Phillips RE and Warrell DA, personal communication) (Figure 49). This species also spits its venom and can cause venom ophthalmia (Figure 50).

h. Javan and Sunda Island spitting cobra (N. sputatrix)

In Java, neither Kopstein nor his colleagues had seen any cases of envenoming by bites of this species, but, in the course of 55 years, they had heard of a few cases of fatal envenoming in children[93]. Venom ophthalmia after "spitting" seemed to be mild[93].

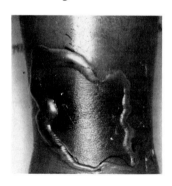 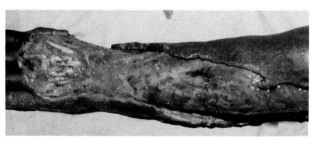

Figure 49. Envenoming by the Thai spitting cobra (*Naja siamensis*).
49a. (left) Darkening of an area of necrotic skin at the site of the bite, with surrounding blisters and a putrid smell 3 days after the bite. (courtesy of Dr. R.E. Phillips, Oxford).
49b. (right) Extensive necrosis of skin and subcutaneous tissues 10 days after the bite. (courtesy of Prof. Sornchai Looareesuwan, Bangkok).

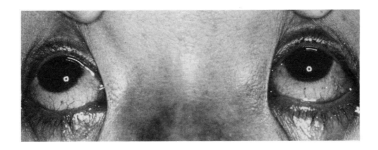

Figure 50. Thai woman who had venom "spat" into both eyes by a Thai spitting cobra (*Naja siamensis*), showing intense conjunctivitis and some oedema of the lids (photo © Dr. D.A. Warrell).

i. Sumatran-Malay spitting cobra (N. sumatrana)

One of 198 cobras responsible for bites in Thailand was of this species (near Pattani in the extreme south of the country)[8]. Two of Reid's 47 cases were caused by this species (wrongly identified as yellow *N. n. kaouthia* in the paper)[88]. Reid's case 43 was bitten on the ankle by a 92 cm yellow *N sumatrana* and developed moderately severe local pain. Five-and-a-quarter hours after the bite he became drowsy and found it difficult to open his mouth. Nine hours after the bite he appeared apathetic, had severe ptosis and could not open his eyes although eye and facial movements were unimpaired. He could not open his mouth, swallow or protrude his tongue. Flaccid paresis affected the neck, trunk and proximal limb muscles. Breathing was shallow and diaphragmatic. He responded within an hour to antivenom treatment and recovered from the neurotoxic symptoms in three days. However, the entire bitten limb became swollen and, two weeks after the bite, there was necrosis of the skin from ankle to mid thigh (600 cm^2). After skin grafting the wound healed completely 146 days after the bite[88].

In north Sumatra, cobra bites were common but transient mild oedema was the usual result. Necrosis, never extensive, was sometimes seen in the area of the bite[94].

6. Envenoming by the king cobra (*Ophiophagus hannah*)

Fortunately, bites by this formidable species are rare. Its reputation for aggressiveness is unwarranted. Two out of 13 bites which occurred in Guangxi in 1990 were inflicted while the captive snake was being handled[36]. Three cases of bites in people involved in the famous snake dance in Rangoon Zoological Gardens, Burma, were described and 32 other cases reviewed[95]. Many of these patients were bitten by snakes which they had greatly provoked. When the king cobra bites its natural prey, a snake or monitor lizard, it retains its grip sometimes for 10-30 minutes until the prey is immobile or dead. In one case, the snake held on to the human it had bitten for at least eight minutes. Sixty-three per cent of these 35 patients died but two of them showed no signs of envenoming. The snakes ranged in length from 2-4.9 metres and up to 2.5 kg in weight. Local envenoming has rarely been mentioned in reports of bites by *O. hannah*, but in two of the patients observed in Rangoon, swelling was extensive, involving the entire bitten limb and adjacent areas of the trunk and neck in one of them[94]. Local swelling was described in six of the 32 cases from the literature and blistering and small areas of local necrosis in five out of 35 cases[94] and in three of 13 patients in Guangxi[36]. Despite its high enzyme (especially hyaluronidase) content, the venom of *O. hannah* is clearly less necrotic than those of the Asian *Naja*, perhaps because of its low content of proteases. Neurotoxicity is the most prominent feature of envenoming, reputedly leading to death "soon" or in a "few minutes". A 30 year old reptile house keeper in Rangoon who was bitten by a 2 metre long specimen began to feel dizzy 15 minutes after the bite. Thirty minutes after the bite his speech was slurred and his breathing difficult; 10

minutes later he had developed bilateral ptosis and his respirations were shallow. There was a gradual deterioration in his breathing which became slow and diaphragmatic. He could open his mouth only slightly and, 90 minutes after the bite, he had respiratory arrest and required 38½ hours of mechanical ventilation. Two-and-a-half hours after the bite he had congested conjunctivae, ptosis, complete external ophthalmoplegia, areflexia and generalised flaccid paralysis but was fully conscious (shown by his ability to answer "yes" or "no" to questions by flexing his fingers) (Figure 51). The pupils were normal and reactive to light. There was slight improvement in neurological signs before specific antivenom could finally be given 38 hours after the bite. Recurrent hypotension (also mentioned in two other cases) could have been the result of hypovolaemia as he had extensive local swelling (Figure 52b). No bleeding or clotting disorders have been reliably reported in victims of *O. hannah*. Neutrophil leucocytosis and elevated aspartate aminotransferase and creatine phosphokinase were found in the patient described above[94].

A wandering juggler was bitten by a 3m long *O. hannah* at Tasikmalaja, Java in 1928. There was mild local swelling (from the bitten hand to the elbow), he became dyspnoeic and nauseated, retched, developed cramps and asphyxiated ¾ hour after the bite[93].

Proteus vulgaris was cultured from infected wound sites in four of 35 cases[94]. The interval between bite and death has ranged from a few minutes to 12 hours. In Guangxi, two-thirds of the patients developed paralytic symptoms and seven out of 13 (54%) died[36].

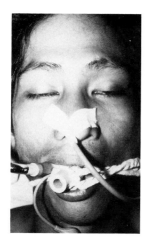 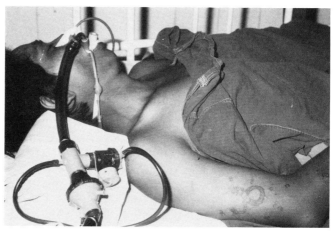

Figure 51. Thirty year old Burmese zoo keeper bitten on the right forearm by a 2m long king kobra (*Ophiophagus hannah*) (photos © Dr. D.A. Warrell).
51a. (left) 2½ hours after the bite showing generalised flaccid paralysis, including bilateral ptosis, ophthalmoplegia and respiratory paralysis.
51b. (right) 15 hours after the bite showing multiple fang and tooth marks near the elbow and tense swelling of the bitten limb. Necrosis did not develop[95].

7. Envenoming by the black desert cobra (*Walterinnesia aegyptia*)
This is discussed in the chapter on African and Middle Eastern snakes.

8. Ophthalmia resulting from "spitting" of venom
Of the nine species of Asian cobra currently recognised, three do not spit their venom (*N. naja, N. oxiana, N. kaouthia*), two rarely do so (*N. samarensis, N. atra*) and four do so frequently (*N. sumatrana, N. sputatrix, N. philippinensis, N. siamensis*)[14,94]. No detailed studies have been published and few patients have been examined by ophthalmologists. Pain, conjunctivitis and palpebral oedema have resulted from spitting by *N. sputatrix* in Java,[95] *N. sumatrana* in west Malaysia and *N. siamensis* in Thailand (Figure 50). In

Sumatra, *N. sputatrix* spit causes gross conjunctivitis and chemosis in dogs, invariably resulting in blindness[94]. In Guangxi, five cases of spitting of venom into human eyes by *N. atra* were reported in 1990[36].

Severe venom ophthalmia (corneal ulceration, anterior uveitis, secondary panophthalmitis and permanent blindness) of the type described in Africa has not been observed in Asia. Accidental introduction of *N. naja* venom into one eye caused painful conjunctivitis, palpebral oedema and a transient VII nerve palsy on that side, probably due to the tracking of venom absorbed through the conjunctiva and lymphatics to the superficial course of the VIIth cranial nerve in the cheek (D.A. Warrell, unpublished).

C. ENVENOMING BY VIPERS (FAMILY VIPERIDAE)

Venoms of most Viperidae produce marked local effects. Swelling, sometimes detectable within 15 minutes or delayed for several hours, may spread rapidly to involve the entire bitten limb and adjacent areas of the trunk. Superficial lymphatics may become visible as red or ecchymotic lymphangitic lines. There is pain, tenderness and enlargement of regional lymph nodes with bruising of the overlying skin. Bruising, blistering and necrosis at the site of the bite may be evident within 24 hours. Necrosis develops after bites by most species of Viperinae and Crotalinae and is the main cause of persistent morbidity in survivors of snakebite. Compartmental syndromes, especially of the anterior tibial compartment, may arise when tissue contained within a tight fascial compartment are envenomed (for example after bites by Deinagkistrodon, Calloselasma and *Trimeresurus flavoviridis*). Haemostatic abnormalities are characteristic of envenoming by many of the vipers. Persistent bleeding from fang puncture wounds, venepuncture sites and other new and partially healed wounds suggests that blood has become incoagulable through defibrinogenation. Spontaneous systemic haemorrhage is most often detected in the gingival sulci or as epistaxis, haematemesis, cutaneous ecchymoses, haemoptysis, subconjunctival, retroperitoneal, intracranial or uterine bleeding. Hypotension and shock, mainly as a result of hypovolaemia, is seen in patients with massive swelling. Direct myocardial involvement is suggested by an abnormal ECG or cardiac arrhythmia. Patients envenomed by some species of Vipera and *Daboia russelii* experience transient recurrent syncopal attacks associated with features of an autopharmacological or anaphylactic reaction such as vomiting, sweating, colic, diarrhoea, shock and angio-oedema. Renal failure may develop in severely envenomed patients but is particularly common after bites by *Daboia russelii*. Mild neurotoxic symptoms (ptosis, ophthalmoplegia) have been described in patients envenomed by *Daboia russelii pulchella* (Sri Lanka and south India), Japanese mamushi (*Agkistrodon b blomhoffii*) and Chinese mamushi (*A. b. brevicaudus*). Acute and chronic endocrine abnormalities (pituitary, adrenal failure) may occur as a result of infarction of the anterior pituitary (Sheehan's-like syndrome) in victims of Russell's vipers in Burma and India.

1. Envenoming by typical vipers (subfamily Viperinae)

a. Envenoming by Fea's viper (Azemiops feae)

The venom of this rare species has been little studied. In mice it produced flaccid paralysis, respiratory depression and clonic convulsions with negligible local reaction and no obvious haemostatic disturbances[95]. The mouse intravenous LD_{50} was 0.52 mg/kg. However, in the only three reported cases of human bites there was only local pain and swelling[36].

b. Envenoming by the horned sand viper (Cerastes gasperettii)
This is discussed in the chapter on snakes of Africa and the Middle East.

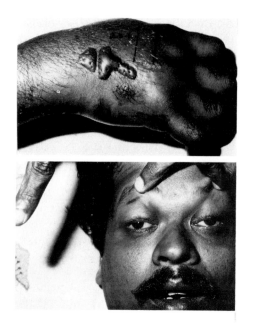
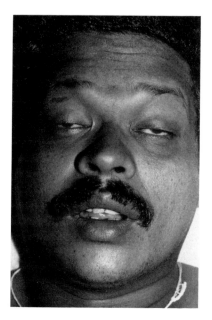

Figure 52. Envenoming by the Sri Lankan Russell's viper (*Daboia russelii pulchella*).
52a. (top left) Local swelling and blistering 24 hours after the bite (photos © Dr. D.A. Warrell).
52b. (right) Ptosis, external ophthalmoplegia and inability to open the mouth 18 hours after the bite.
52c. (bottom left) External ophthalmoplegia: the patient is attempting to look to his right (same patient as in Figure 52b)[50].

c. Envenoming by Russell's vipers (Daboia russelii)

Throughout its discontinuous distribution, Russell's viper is an important cause of snakebites and resulting mortality, especially among rice farmers. There is an intriguing geographical variation in the clinical manifestations of envenoming, doubtless reflecting differences in venom composition (Table 4)[10,17].

Table 4
Geographical variation in the clinical manifestations of Russell's viper bite

	Sri Lanka	India	Burma	Thailand	China	Taiwan
Blood coagulability	+	++	++	++	++	+
Renal failure	++	+	++	+	+	+
"Sheehan's" syndrome	-	+	++	-	?	?
Intravascular haemolysis	++	+	-	+	+	?
Neuro-myotoxicity	++	+	-	-	-	?
Generalized capillary permeability	-	-	++	-	?	?
Shock / hypotension	-	+	++	-	+	?

Note. No data available from Pakistan, Nepal, Bangladesh or Indonesia

1. Taiwan Russell's viper (D. r. formosensis)

In Taiwan, few cases of Russell's viper bite are reported. Most occur among the aboriginal populations in mountainous areas. Between 1904 and 1971, 65 cases were reported with four deaths (0.5% of all snakebite cases)[80]. In Ping Tung prefecture, in the south of the island, 20 cases with three fatalities were recorded during the seven years 1965-71, 6% of all snakebites[39]. Two patients bitten by small (20 cm long) snakes developed acute renal failure despite being given antivenom within three hours of the bite. Renal biopsies confirmed acute tubular necrosis and in one of the cases, there was deposition of fibrin thrombi in glomerular capillaries. Symptoms included nausea, vomiting, oliguria and jaundice (bilirubin direct/indirect 0.3/5.4 mg/dl). Both patients were thrombocytopenic, one showed mild coagulopathy and both had heavy proteinuria. One developed gangrene requiring amputation of the bitten toe. Both recovered after prolonged courses of haemodialysis[96].

Another patient, bitten on the thumb, noticed pain, slight swelling, sleepiness and dizziness starting 10 minutes later. There was tender swelling of an axillary lymph node and mild leucocytosis. He recovered without evidence of bleeding or clotting problems. Suggestions that *D. r. formosensis* produced "neurotoxic" effects in humans are unsupported by clinical evidence, unless the "sleepiness" of the case described above was actually ptosis[80] (their Figure 13). The venom of *D. r. formosensis* is rich in phospholipases (RV-4 and RV-7 complex, mouse LD_{50} 0.15 mg/kg) which constitute about 40% of the protein. RV-4 potentiated by RV-7 is a powerful presynaptic neurotoxin.[97]

2. Indonesian Russell's viper (D. r. limitis)

No clinical descriptions of bites by this subspecies have been published. "Komodo villagers greatly fear this snake (which they call *misa*), for it has caused more snakebite deaths on this island than any other species."[98]

3. Sri Lankan Russell's viper or Tic polonga (D. r .pulchella)

This species is responsible for 17.5% of bites and about a half of all snakebite fatalities in Sri Lanka. In Anuradhapura, 36 cases of proven *D. r. pulchella* bites were investigated, 73% of all snakebite cases[50]. Twenty-eight per cent showed no clinical evidence of envenoming. Most were young male farmers bitten on the lower limbs while working in the fields. In the 23 envenomed patients, pain was almost immediate and severe and two fainted within a few minutes of the bite. Early symptoms included blurred vision, ptosis (30 minutes to 7.25 hours - mean 2.3 - after the bite), double vision, difficulty swallowing (1.5-19 - mean 5.4 - hours after the bite) and aching in the proximal limb girdle muscles and trunk. Seventy-three per cent of envenomed patients developed local swelling, two blistering followed by necrosis (Figure 52a). The most striking signs were of neuromyotoxicity: ptosis (77%), external ophthalmoplegia (82%), inability to open the mouth (23%), to swallow and protrude the tongue, generalised muscle tenderness (32%) and black urine (27%) (Figure 52B,C). Most patients showed evidence of intravascular haemolysis (falling haematocrit, low serum haptoglobin and elevated plasma haemoglobin without red cell glucose-6-phosphate-dehydrogenase deficiency). A third of patients bled spontaneously from the upper gastrointestinal tract, gums, nose, urinary tract, skin or into the brain. Fifty-nine per cent had incoagulable blood on admission and most had evidence of moderate coagulopathy with thrombocytopenia (61%). There was a peripheral leucocytosis. Plasma and urine myoglobin concentrations and serum aspartate aminotransferase concentrations were greatly elevated. Two of the patients developed oliguric renal failure requiring peritoneal dialysis. Three patients died 2.5 to 20.8 hours after the bite. Neurotoxic features have been recognised in Sri Lankan victims of Russell's viper since the early years of the century. Generalised flaccid paralysis and respiratory paralysis leading to cyanosis and respiratory failure, are rare. Paralytic features are usually confined to muscles innervated by cranial nerves III, IV, VI, X, XI and XII.

4. Indian Russell's viper or Daboia (D. r. russelii)

Among 1,231 cases of snakebite from all parts of India, 5% were attributed to Russell's vipers with a case fatality of 11%[69]. In five states of India, Russell's vipers were responsible for 27% of identifiable bites[91], but in Jammu in the northeast of India, only four out of 310 identified viperine bites were caused by this species[99]. Some authors have considered that there is essentially no difference in the clinical picture of patients bitten by Russell's viper and of those bitten by *Echis* species. A patient bitten by a 1.1 metre long Russell's viper developed pain and swelling, vomited and had abdominal discomfort and diarrhoea. The blood was found to be incoagulable on admission to hospital four hours after the bite. He developed haematemesis, bleeding from the nose and mouth and into the urine. Swelling and discoloration involved the whole bitten limb. He developed hiccups, lost consciousness and died 36 hours after the bite[69]. At Angamally, Kerala, south India, eight patients were seen with neurotoxic signs such as ptosis and ophthalmoplegia and with evidence of a bleeding disorder and were thought to have been bitten by Russell's vipers[100]. In the same hospital, two men and one woman developed bleeding from the site of bites thought to have been inflicted by Russell's vipers and from the gums, gastrointestinal and urinary tracts. Other acute problems included subarachnoid haemorrhage, anaemia requiring blood transfusion, hypotension and renal failure. Local necrosis was not uncommon, but was rarely extensive. One month to one year later they came back to hospital complaining of loss of libido, impotence, loss of secondary sexual hair, hypotension and amenorrhoea. Panhypopituitarism was confirmed in all three cases. Among 1,000 cases of snakebite in that hospital, seven developed hypopituitarism and one diabetes insipidus[101]. Other cases of hypopituitarism following presumed or proven Russell's viper bites have been reported from Pune and Trichur in India, and in Burma (see below).

In parts of India, especially in the south, Russell's viper bite is the most common cause of acute renal failure in adults and children. At a hospital at Kottayam, Kerala, 2.2% of all admissions were for snakebite which was the cause of 40% of all cases of acute renal failure[102]. This complication is relatively more frequent and severe in children than in adults. In the children local pain and swelling develops almost immediately. Local changes were maximal at 72 hours and subsided over 10 days. Bleeding began within two or three hours (gums, upper gastrointestinal tract, skin and urinary tract). All the cases with renal failure developed anuria within 48 hours of the bite, 19% of them within three hours. Renal failure lasted 10-25 days. Jaundice appeared 5-6 days after the bite in 19%. Almost all had evidence of coagulopathy with thrombocytopenia, and all had a peripheral leucocytosis[102]. Almost 80% required dialysis. The mortality was 14%, attributed to shock, pulmonary oedema, hyperkalaemia, septicaemia and haemorrhage from a peritoneal cannula. Adult patients with renal failure after proven or presumed Russell's viper bites have been studied in Calcutta[105], Chandigarh[104] and southern India[105,106]. Among 45 patients transferred to a hospital in Calcutta with acute renal failure, all had local swelling; five developed necrosis of superficial tissues. Spontaneous systemic haemorrhage was common (ecchymoses, subconjunctival haemorrhages, haematemesis, melaena, epistaxis and retinal haemorrhages causing visual defect in five cases). Oliguria developed almost immediately in some cases but up to four days after the bite in others (mean 2 days) and lasted 1-9 (mean 2) days. Clinical findings in the patients referred to Vellore[105] and Chandigarh[104] were essentially similar but, in the latter study, six of the eight patients had evidence of intravascular haemolysis and two of microangiopathic haemolytic anaemia[104]. The triad of acute renal failure, thrombocytopenia and haemolytic anaemia with fragmented erythrocytes after snakebite has misleadingly been described as "haemolytic-uraemic syndrome"[107]. Renal histopathological studies are described below (renal changes in patients envenomed by Russell's vipers).

5. Southeast Asian and Chinese (mainland) Russell's vipers (D. r. siamensis)

Although the populations of Russell's vipers from Burma, Thailand and southern mainland China are morphologically similar, there are important clinical differences in the effects of envenoming, at least between Burmese Russell's vipers and the other eastern forms[10,17].

6. Russell's viper bites in Burma

Two populations of Russell's vipers were found to be responsible for bites during the rice harvest from November to January in Tharrawaddy, 130 km north of Rangoon; one population measured 125-375 mm and had probably been born that year. The other measured 500-1,125 mm[24]. The presence of prey, usually a rodent, in the snake's stomach, indicating that it had eaten recently, did not influence the severity of envenoming. The length of the biting snake correlated with the extent and degree of local swelling[34]. Bites by longer snakes were more likely to result in systemic envenoming[24].

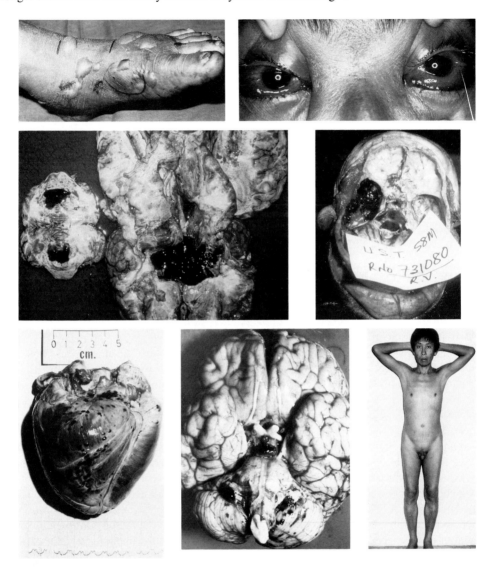

Figure 53. Envenoming by Russell's viper (*Daboia russelii siamensis*) in Burma (photo © Dr. D.A. Warrell).

53a. (top left) Swelling and blistering 24 hours after a bite (the 2 fang marks are circled).

53b. (top right) Bilateral intense conjunctival oedema 48 hours after the bite.

53c. (middle left) Extensive intraventricular haemorrhage (courtesy of Dr. U Hla Mon).

53d. (middle right) Intracerebral haemorrhage (courtesy of Dr. U Hla Mon).

53e. (bottom left) Extensive subepicardial haemorrhages in a patient who had a paroxysmal supraventricular tachycardia during life[112].

53f. (bottom centre) Haemorrhagic infarction of the anterior pituitary in a patient who died with intractable shock 18 hours after the bite (courtesy of Dr. U Hla Mon).

53g. (bottom right) 34 year old Burmese man bitten by a Russell's viper 3 years previously, showing loss of secondary sexual hair and gonadal atrophy[113].

The classical studies of Burmese Russell's viper bite were carried out at Insein by Maung-Maung-Aye[78,87]. His 226 cases described sharp pricking pain with slight burning when bitten. Discoloration, blister formation and swelling appeared (Figure 53a) and in some cases there was necrosis. However, patients with little or no local evidence of envenoming could suffer severe systemic effects. Spontaneous bleeding (gums, epistaxis, haemoptysis, haematemesis, haematuria) developed in a few hours. A unique sign, orbital oedema with subconjunctival haemorrhages (Figure 53b), appeared in severe cases. Some patients developed shock (hypotension, tachycardia and impaired peripheral circulation). Other symptoms included a burning sensation in the epigastrium or chest. Blood was incoagulable, platelet count fell from the day after the bite and red blood cells and granular casts were found in the urine. Within three or four days acute renal failure evolved with anuria, drowsiness, vomiting, hiccuping, acidotic breathing and occasionally convulsions. There was bilateral loin tenderness and hypertension. In some cases, spontaneous diuresis started in 7-10 days and there was complete recovery without residual renal defect. A proportion of patients developed a late haemorrhagic syndrome with recurrent shock. At post mortem haemorrhages of the pituitary and sometimes of the adrenal glands, intracranial haemorrhage (Figure 53c,d) and swollen haemorrhagic kidneys were found[87]. At Tharrawaddy Township Hospital, 123 cases of proven Russell's viper bite were studied (1983-1985)[34]. Eighty-two per cent were male, 93% rice farmers and 82% bitten while farming, usually on the lower leg or foot (79%). Local pain, the commonest symptom, started within minutes of the bite and spread and intensified during the next few hours, becoming localised in regional lymph nodes. Vague abdominal or epigastric pain, loin pain and vomiting sometimes developed within six hours of the bite. Two patients fainted within 90 minutes of the bite but recovered consciousness within minutes. Twenty-eight per cent of patients showed no clinical evidence of envenoming at any stage. Swelling rarely involved more than half the bitten limb and blistering and local necrosis were rare. Patients with systemic envenoming had incoagulable blood, present on admission to hospital or developing up to 15 hours later. Thirty-nine per cent of these patients with systemic envenoming bled from the gums, gastrointestinal tract, conjunctivae or nose. Microscopic haematuria was found in 72%. No retinal haemorrhages were seen. Only a quarter of the patients were thrombocytopenic on admission. Platelet counts reached their lowest point on the third day after the bite. Peripheral leucocytosis was common. Hypotension developed in 35%. There was clinical evidence of increased capillary permeability in 26% of the systemically envenomed patients. This was manifested as conjunctival, periorbital or facial oedema, pleural effusion, ascites, pulmonary oedema and transient proteinuria and hypoalbuminaemia[34,108,109]. Conjunctival oedema (chemosis) evolved from early clear oedema fluid, appearing within 24 hours of the bite, to intense congestion with extravasation of erythrocytes about 12 hours later, resolving to leave residual subconjunctival haemorrhages several days later. Oliguria was evident as early as one day after the bite and eventually developed in 44% of systemically envenomed patients. Hypertension was observed in a few patients. Renal angle tenderness predicted the development of oliguria (sensitivity 0.7, specificity 0.9)[34]. In a study of 52 patients whose serum creatinine exceeded 1.3 mg/dl, 65% became oliguric, but the remainder maintained a urine output of more than 400 ml/24 hours. Gastrointestinal haemorrhage, renal angle tenderness and conjunctival oedema occurred more commonly and peak serum creatinine, blood urea nitrogen and fractional excretion of sodium were significantly higher in oliguric than non-oliguric patients[109]. Among 24 patients whose blood was coagulable when first admitted to hospital, 15 went on to develop incoagulable blood, 10 developed mild renal dysfunction and five acute renal failure. Albuminuria, detected on admission, predicted the development of systemic envenoming[108]. Plasma renin activity was elevated in patients who were hypertensive, had loin pain and developed acute renal failure[109].

Russell's viper venom contains a number of components which influence haemostasis, including procoagulants (one which activates Factors X, IX and protein C and another which activates Factor V), a fibrinolytic agent, platelet aggregation stimulating and inhibiting factors, an anticoagulant and a haemorrhagin. In patients, the most striking laboratory features of the coagulopathy are depletion of fibrinogen, Factors V, X and XIIIa, plasminogen, anti-plasmin, protein C and platelets. Fibrinolytic activity is intense resulting in high levels of FDP, mostly cross-linked[110]. Among 20 patients admitted to hospital within four hours of the bite, at which time their blood was coagulable, six developed mild and nine severe haemostatic abnormalities. Serum FDP concentration predicted the development of defibrination[111].

Post mortem studies have shown widespread congestion and bleeding of the lungs, gastrointestinal and renal tracts, adrenals, heart (Figure 53e), brain and anterior pituitary (Figure 53f). Histopathological evidence of focal haemorrhage and fibrin deposition was found at the site of the bite and in the pituitary, lungs and kidneys and there was acute tubular necrosis[112]. In a group of patients who developed symptoms of panhypopituitarism years after severe envenoming, this diagnosis was confirmed by insulin stress tests[113].

7. Envenoming by Russell's vipers in China

There are few reports of bites in this region. In Guangxi, 50 bites occurred in 1990 with one death. Most occurred in the fields or mountains and were inflicted on the feet with a peak of incidence in July and August[36]. In Hong Kong, a snake shop employee was bitten while handling a Russell's viper imported from China. He deteriorated while receiving herbal treatment and was admitted to hospital 40 hours after the bite, unconscious and with CT scan evidence of a massive left frontal lobe cerebral haemorrhage and subarachnoid haemorrhage. He was severely defibrinated and already in renal failure. He died six weeks later despite evacuation of the cerebral blood clot, antivenom treatment, haemofiltration and peritoneal dialysis[114]. In China, a man was admitted to hospital one hour after being bitten by a Russell's viper. He was bleeding from the fang marks, was in pain and headache, rigors, cold sweats, malaise, swelling of lymph nodes, bleeding from the nose and gums and swelling and bruising of the bitten limb. He was hypotensive[86]. Other symptoms include local blistering and necrosis followed by severe ulceration, early haematuria, haemolytic anaemia, jaundice and acute renal failure[35].

8. Envenoming by Russell's vipers in Thailand

Among 68 cases of Russell's viper bite, 28% had incoagulable blood on admission to hospital[8]. Seven rice farmers died 2.5-264 (median 72) hours after bites by Russell's vipers; these deaths were attributed to shock, cerebral haemorrhage and renal failure[76].

In Prachinburi, in the central rice-growing area of Thailand, 55 cases of definite Russell's viper bites were studied in 1982[115]. All patients had local pain and swelling but this did not spread to involve more than half the bitten limb and none developed necrosis. Swelling resolved in 5-7 days. Bruising and blood-filled blisters were common at the site of the bite. One patient bled profusely from six fang marks. There was tender enlargement of regional lymph nodes. About one-fifth of the patients developed hypotension and a few had mild fever before antivenom treatment. Ten per cent of the patients became comatose 2-3 hours after the bite, regaining consciousness 6-7 hours later. Forty per cent developed systemic bleeding from gums, gastrointestinal and urinary tracts, 5% developed acute renal failure; all had suffered from systemic bleeding - haematuria, haematemesis, haemoptysis, melaena and bleeding from the gums. There were two deaths, 13 and 14 hours after the bite. Reports from a rural area near Chainat[116] and from a referral hospital in Bangkok[117] suggest that local envenoming after Russell's viper bites is less severe than after bites by green pit vipers. Other symptoms include nausea, vomiting, abdominal pain, chest discomfort, bleeding from venepuncture sites and subconjunctival haemorrhage. Laboratory tests showed neutrophil leucocytosis, coagulopathy with depletion of fibrinogen Factor X and Factor V and evidence of fibrinolysis, intravascular haemolysis (massive in one case) and appearance of fragmented erythrocytes. Haematuria, haemoglobinuria and albuminuria were common.

9. Renal changes in Russell's viper envenoming [102-109,112,118]

A variety of glomerular, tubular, vascular and interstitial lesions have been observed, of which acute tubular necrosis is the most common. Glomerular lesions include mesangial proliferation, proliferative glomerulonephritis and deposition of fibrin thrombi in glomerular capillaries. The most severe changes of bilateral cortical necrosis have also been seen in a minority of cases.

4. Envenoming by saw-scaled or carpet vipers (genus *Echis*)

1. Indian/Sri Lankan saw-scaled viper (E. carinatus)

In parts of its range such as Ratnagiri District, Maharashtra and Tamil Nadu, this is the commonest snake. In the 1880s, 115,921 Echis were killed in eight days in Ratnagiri District and there were records of 62 fatal cases of envenoming treated at the local hospital in one year[119]. Recently, a practitioner near Deogad, Ratnagiri District, has treated 300 cases of Echis bites in 15 years[121] and so this species is still a common cause of bites, but the effects of envenoming are thought to be far less severe than those of the larger *E sochureki* in northern India and Pakistan. This is partly attributable to the small size of most *E carinatus*; in India specimens rarely exceed 25 cm in length and in Sri Lanka the average length is 20 cm. Pain and swelling develop in 80% of cases, but the swelling rarely spreads to involve more than half of the bitten limb. Enlarged tender lymph glands are often palpable in the popliteal, inguinal or axillary regions, depending on the site of the bite. After 10-12 hours patients may begin to bleed from their gums and later develop gastrointestinal, urinary tract or vaginal bleeding and some collapse[119-121].

2. Central Asian saw scaled viper (E. multisquamatus)

No clinical details are available about envenoming by this species in any part of its range. In the former U.S.S.R. it was regarded as less venomous than *Vipera (Macrovipera) lebetina*, but fatalities had been reported.

3. Sochurek's saw scaled viper (E. sochureki)

This species has long been regarded as the most deadly snake in Sind (Pakistan). In the 1850s there was a report of 306 cases with a mortality of 21% during a six month period. Bites are also a serious problem in parts of Rajasthan and Jammu[119]. In Jammu, northern India, *E. sochureki* is the commonest cause of envenoming; 117 of 121 recognisable dead snakes brought by patients were *E. sochureki*[99]. Peak incidence was in July and August. All the patients with proven *E. sochureki* bites developed systemic envenoming. Pain and swelling started soon after the bite and the swelling was maximal within the first 24 hours. Systemic bleeding started between six and 72 hours after the bite and coagulopathy was detectable within six hours of the bite in two-thirds of the patients. Other symptoms included vomiting (38%), abdominal pain (37%), regional lymph node enlargement (27%) and shock (2%). Sites of bleeding were ecchymoses, haematuria, haemoptysis, gums, haematemesis, epistaxis, rectal and subarachnoid. Although 42% of the patients developed local blistering, necrosis did not occur in any of them. Abortion with severe bleeding occurred in all three of the pregnant women in this series. Seventy-eight per cent of the patients had incoagulable blood on admission to hospital and 22% had defective coagulation. Haemoglobin concentration fell in many of the patients but there was no evidence of haemolysis. Neutrophil leucocytosis occurred only in patients with secondary local infections who were feverish. Microscopic or frank haematuria was present in the majority. There was a transient rise in blood urea in a few of the patients but none developed acute renal failure. ECG T wave inversion was seen in 23 seriously ill patients with reversion to normal in the 17 survivors. The mortality rate in the whole series was 2%. The six patients died 3-6 days after the bite with shock, subarachnoid haemorrhage or massive gastrointestinal bleeding.

Severe haemostatic disturbances were described in an American envenomed by a large *E. sochureki* from Pakistan (see below)[122].

Although the clinical picture of envenoming by Daboia and Echis species is similar, the former generally have more severe symptoms and are far more likely to become shocked and to develop acute renal failure.

e. Envenoming by McMahon's viper (Eristocophis mcmahoni)

Five cases of bites were described from Baluchistan[123]. Two died several hours after the bite after developing local swelling and inflammation, abdominal pain and distention and, in one of them, inability to swallow and open the eyes suggesting possible neurotoxicity. In a third case there was swelling of the bitten arm which lasted for three days and subsequent ulceration. One of the two fatal cases, a boy of 15, was bitten in the pubic region while asleep. There was serosanguinous discharge from the urethra and from local incisions made at the site of the bite.

f. Envenoming by Persian horned viper (Pseudocerastes persicus)

This is described in the chapter on African and Middle Eastern snakes.

g. Envenoming by typical Asian vipers (genus Vipera)
1. Middle Eastern mountain vipers (Vipera xanthina complex)

Little is known of the clinical effects of envenoming by most of these species. *V, raddei* is capable of killing domestic animals. Envenoming by *V, xanthina* is described in the chapter on European snakebites.

2. European adder or viper (V. berus)

Envenoming by this species is described in the chapter on European snakebites.

3. Levantine viper (V. lebetina)

Envenoming by this dangerous species is described in the chapters on African and Middle Eastern snakebites and European snakebites.

4. Orsini's viper (V. ursinii)

Envenoming by this species is described in the chapter on European snakebites.

2. Envenoming by Asian pit vipers (subfamily Crotalinae)
a. Envenoming by Asian pit vipers and mamushis (genus Agkistrodon)
1. Mamushi (A. blomhoffii)

The Japanese mamushi (A. b. blomhoffii) is thought to bite about 3,000 people with two deaths each year in the Japanese islands. Unlike bites by most other species, more than 70% are inflicted on the fingers and hands. In urban areas this is explained by handling of mamushis in the production of "mamushi whisky". Painful swelling develops in the bitten part and in two or three hours may extend from the bitten finger to the forearm with painful tenderness of the axillary node 1-2 hours after the bite. In severe cases, which are unusual, there may be swelling of the entire bitten limb with local blistering, nausea, vomiting, fever, headache, abdominal and lumbar pain, shock, acute renal failure, bleeding gums and ecchymoses. Rare manifestations include retinal haemorrhages, diplopia usually resulting from paralysis of the medial rectus muscles but occasionally affecting accommodation and causing ptosis. These neurotoxic signs can develop 1-48 hours after the bite[124].

The Chinese mamushi (A. blomhoffii brevicaudus) is the commonest cause of snakebite in the oriental region of China, north of latitude 25°N. Five hundred and thirty patients were studied in Kiangsu (= Jiangsu) and Chekiang (= Zhejiang) Provinces[125]. Seventy-three per cent of bites were inflicted on the feet and legs. Local symptoms were pain and slight bleeding at the site of the bite, swelling, rapid tender enlargement of local lymph nodes and local bruising in children. Local swelling rarely extended to involve more than half of the bitten limb; in 40% of upper limb bites swelling extended to the shoulder and in 5% of lower limb bites swelling extended to the hip. Early systemic symptoms included blurring of vision, ptosis and development of dyplopia within 24 hours of the bite. Breathlessness, dysphagia and difficulty opening the mouth also suggested neurotoxic activity of the venom, while generalised myalgia, chest tightness, neck rigidity and "haemoglobinuria" suggested the possibility of generalised rhabdomyolysis. Other symptoms were headache, dizziness, chills, fever, cold sweats, palpitations, nausea, vomiting, thirst, abdominal pain and distention and, in a few severe cases, convulsions, lethargy and coma. Six patients, admitted more than 26 hours after the bite, died of respiratory (4) or renal (2) failure. Lethal systemic symptoms could arise without signs of local envenoming[125].

At a United States military dispensary near Daechon, Choong Nam Province, on the west coast of south Korea, 48 patients presented with painful local swelling attributed to the "Doksa" or mamushi[126]. These bites could have been caused by any of the three species of Agkistrodon (*A. blomhoffii brevicaudus, A. saxatilis* and *A. ussuriensis*). Twenty-three of the patients (46%) developed systemic envenoming, notably dyplopia (12), nuchal rigidity with or without signs of severe meningism (17), ileus (5), dysphagia and dysarthria (3), distended bladder (2), acute renal failure with hyperkalaemia (2) and coma (1). The urine was described as maroon-coloured, initially without erythrocytes and reacting positively to stix tests for blood. The author makes the interesting suggestion that this might have been myoglobinuria which could have been responsible for the two cases of renal failure[126]. As in the study from China[125] nuchal rigidity, painful distended abdomen with ileus and vomiting and a distended bladder were observed in the six severe cases[126].

At Wonju Union Christian Hospital in South Korea 12 bites by *A. blomhoffii brevicaudus* were identified among 82 historical records of mamushi bites (1959 to 1973)[127]. Unfortunately, the clinical features of these cases were not distinguished from those resulting from bites by the other two species of mamushi (*A. saxatilis* and *A. ussuriensis*) except in two of the figures. Local effects of envenoming were much more severe than those reported above. There was pain, bleeding from wounds, swelling, blistering, subcutaneous haemorrhage, lymphadenopathy and necrosis of skin, subcutaneous tissue, muscle and bone in 43% of cases. Two-thirds of the patients who developed necrosis had applied tourniquets. Systemic symptoms occurred in 22% of patients. They included blurred vision, ptosis, dyspnoea, dizziness, drowsiness, vomiting, abdominal pain, diarrhoea and fever. The four deaths occurred 4-9 days after the bite and were associated with shock, respiratory muscle paralysis and pulmonary oedema.

Respiratory paralysis, requiring assisted ventilation, has been described in nine cases of bites by this species in China[128].

2. Central Asian pit viper (A. halys)

This name has been used widely in the medical and herpetological literature, often referring to *A. blomhoffii brevicaudus*. Restricted to its definition by Gloyd and Conant[2], it refers to a species found in Central Asia from the Caspian Sea to Lake Baikal and central Mongolia. No precise clinical data are available. People bitten by this species usually recover but it has been responsible for the deaths of domestic animals, particularly horses, in eastern Kazakhstan. In Kiel, Germany, a snake-keeper was bitten and, within two hours, had developed incoagulable blood with afibrinogenaemia, elevated fibrin(ogen) degradation products (10% crosslinked), thrombocytopenia and mildly reduced plasminogen concentration. At the site of the bite he developed blood-filled blisters and necrosis requiring surgery[129].

3. Himalayan pit viper (A. himalayanus)

In Kashmir, bites by this species were said to be common but recovery took only a couple of days[92]. Frank Wall's brother was bitten on the ankle. There was almost immediate lancinating burning pain, a blood blister developed, the limbs swelled up to the groin and pain continued. There was no systemic bleeding or persistent bleeding from the wound and he recovered after two days. Tissues in the vicinity of the wound were much discoloured for some time. Another patient, bitten on the finger, developed painful swelling up to the elbow and in the armpit which persisted for four days. Four other patients developed only pain or swelling which passed off in two or three days.

4. Central Asian pit viper (A. intermedius)

No clinical data are available. The venom is neurotoxic and has a lower mouse LD_{50} than other Chinese crotalid venoms[130]. Clinical effects similar to those produced by bites of *A. blomhoffii brevicaudus* may be expected.

5. Rock mamushi (A. saxatilis)

Some cases of bites by this species were included in the reports from Korea discussed above[126,127]. Snakes responsible for biting three of the 82 cases at Wonju Union Christian Hospital were identified as being *A saxatilis*, but the clinical features were not identified in this account[127].

6. Shedao mamushi (A. shedaoensis)

No data are available.

7. Ussuri mamushi (A. ussuriensis)

In South Korea, 13 of 82 patients presenting to Wonju Union Christin Hospital in South Korea were thought to have been bitten by *A ussuriensis*[127]. In one case, identified as a bite by *A. caliginosus* (now included in *A ussuriensis*), there was marked oedema, ecchymoses and blistering. The majority of snakebite cases in a series of 126 reported from five hospitals in Seoul, Jeounju, Wonju, Gwangju and Incheon (1976-1977) were suspected to be due to *A. ussuriensis*[131]. There were no deaths. Three patients were bitten by this species in Japan[132]. One developed severe pain and swelling of the whole arm, which subsided in 72 hours, and blister formation. Three hours after the bite he had difficulty in walking and developed blurred vision which persisted for more than a week. One of the other two cases also had blurred vision. The venom of *A ussuriensis* is the most toxic, in mice, of all the Korean Agkistrodon species. It contains two thrombin-like enzymes, a capillary permeability increasing enzyme and a neurotoxin[133].

8. High mountain viper pit vipers (A. monticola and A. strauchi)

No clinical data are available.

b. Envenoming by the Malayan pit viper (Calloselasma rhodostoma)

In Thailand, this species is the commonest and most widespread venomous snake responsible for bites. Thirty-eight per cent of the dead snakes brought by the bitten patients were *C. rhodostoma*[8]. In a study of 46 cases of fatal snakebite in Thailand, *C. rhodostoma*, with *B. candidus*, was the commonest cause (13 cases)[76]. Malayan pit viper bite is mainly an occupational disease of rubber plantation and other plantation workers and is common in southwestern Vietnam (especially Songbe Province), Cambodia, Laos, Java and especially in northwestern Malaysia. Thirty-three per cent of snakebites in Indonesia are said to be caused by this species with 3.5% fatality rate[134]. Sixty-three per cent of identified snakebites in north Malaya were attributed to this species[135]. At Sungi Patani Hospital (1960-61), Reid and his colleagues studied 250 cases of proven bites by *C rhodostoma*[136]. Forty-four per cent were in rubber plantation workers. Local swelling started within minutes and reached its maximum after 24 to 72 hours, but about half the patients developed slight or no envenoming. Local necrosis developed in 11% of patients (Figure 54c). It was always preceded by blistering (Figure 54b) but not all patients with blistering developed necrosis.

The risk of necrosis was greatest when bites were on the digits (27%). Necrosis affected only superficial tissues (Figure 54d) but secondary bacterial infection could result in bone and joint involvement. In most cases necrosis ranged from 0.25 to 9.0 (mean 3.3) cm^2 and healed in 13-86 (mean 47) days. In the most severe case there was 300 cm^2 of skin loss which healed in 322 days. Bacterial infection was seen only in necrotic wounds. Systemic haemorrhage was seen in only 15% of cases. The earliest haemorrhagic manifestation was "haemoptysis" demonstrated by asking the patient to cough hard in order to produce sputum. This was seen as early as 20 minutes after the bite. Reid was convinced that the bloodstained spit was from the lungs and was not due to bleeding from the gums which was less common and followed later after the bite. Hess's (tourniquet) test was usually positive. Slightly raised "discoid ecchymoses" 3-15 mm in diameter were seen scattered over the body in severe cases (Figure 54e). No haemorrhages were seen in the optic fundi or on the eardrums. Shock developed in 22% of severe cases. It was manifested by apathy, thirst, a rapid thready pulse and fall in blood pressure. ECG T wave inversion and ST segment depression were seen in some of the cases.

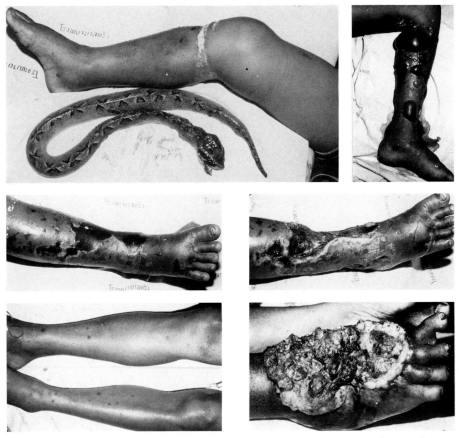

Figure 54. Envenoming by the Malayan pit viper (*Calloselasma rhodostoma*) in Thailand (photos © Dr. D.A. Warrell except as noted).
54a. (top left) Tense oedema of the whole limb (courtesy of Prof. Sornchai Looareesuwan, Bangkok).
54b. (top right) Tense oedema, bruising and blistering 48 hours after the bite.
54c. (middle left) Demarcated blackened areas of necrosis.
54d. (middle right) The same patient after surgical debridement.
54e. (bottom left) Discoid haemorrhages.
54f. (bottom right) Squamous cell carcinoma developing at the site of a chronic skin ulcer with osteomyelitis 8 years after the bite.

Blood became incoagulable in all the patients with systemic envenoming. This was seen as early as 30 minutes after the bite. In untreated patients this coagulopathy persisted for 1-26 days[137]. Profound thrombocytopenia was found in most of the patients with systemic envenoming; the platelet count returned to normal in 3-6 days. In patients with proven bites by *C rhodostoma* in eastern (Chantaburi) and southern Thailand (Trang), spontaneous systemic bleeding was seen in 24% of those with systemic envenoming[138]. Bleeding was usually from the gingival sulci and haemoptysis was seen in only one patient who had cavitating pulmonary tuberculosis. Peripheral leucocytosis was common[138]. Despite the rapid loss of platelets from the peripheral blood during defibrinogenation, there was little evidence of platelet activation and the rapid rise in platelet count after specific antivenom treatment suggested platelet sequestration (R.A. Hutton, unpublished). Mortality from *C. rhodostoma* bites, attributable to haemorrhage or secondary infection of necrotic wounds (including tetanus), is relatively low. In Malaya, Reid saw two fatalities, from tetanus and cerebral haemorrhage. In 23 fatal hospital cases of *C. rhodostoma* bite in north Malaya (1955-60) the interval between bite and death was 5-240 (mean 65, median 32) hours[136]. In Thailand, 13 deaths after proven *C. rhodostoma* bites were attributed to cerebral haemorrhage (6), shock (4), tetanus (2), septicaemia and anaphylaxis (1 each). The interval between bite and death was 5.5 to 576 (median 61) hours[76]. The locally necrotic effect of the venom is a frequent cause of morbidity. Gangrene may result in loss of a digit or limb, or in crippling deformity, while chronic infection such as osteomyelitis may lead to malignant change (Figure 54f). Clinical reports of proven or suspected *C. rhodostoma* bites have also been published from Java[93], Laos, Cambodia[138] and from other parts of Thailand and west Malaysia[39].

c. Envenoming by the sharp-nosed pit viper or "hundred pacer" (Deinagkistrodon acutus)

Six per cent of all the snakebite cases reviewed in Guangxi in 1990 were attributed to this species[36]. Of the 64 cases, seven had been bitten while handling captive snakes. This is one of the species which has high commercial value for food and medicinal purposes in China. All the bites occurred in Guilin, mostly in the fields and mountains. In two cases these snakes had struck the bars of their cages so forcibly that venom had been ejected into the eyes of onlookers who were standing too close. At Jianning Hospital, Fujian Province, 111 cases of *D. acutus* bite were treated, 72% inflicted on the feet[139]. Seventy-three per cent of the victims were peasants. In Taiwan from 1904 to 1971 there were 278 records of *D. acutus* bites, 2.4% of all snakebites, with 66 deaths (mortality 24%). Although Taiwan was separated from mainland China about a million years ago, the venoms of *D. acutus* in Taiwan and the mainland seem remarkably similar[140]. Clinical effects of envenoming resemble those in victims of *C. rhodostoma*, but tend to be more severe. In Taiwan, aborigines living in the San Di-Mon mountains seem to be particularly vulnerable to bites by this species[80]. Severe pain and bleeding from the fang marks begins almost immediately. Bleeding from the bite can persist for days in patients with untreated coagulopathy. The swelling may be very extensive, and blistering is common. In the Jianning series, swelling involved more than half the bitten limb in 55% of cases and more than the whole limb in 24% and may encroach on the abdomen or chest[139]. Necrosis is evident in 3-5 days in about 10% of patients. After necrosis, amputation of digits or limbs was required in 8% of cases. Swelling subsides in about 12 days, but necrosis may take months to heal[80]. Local bruising, initially around the site of the bite, may extend up the bitten limb in 60% of cases with development of large haematomas in severe cases. Spontaneous systemic bleeding is common, occurring in 41% of the Jianning series[139]. Sites of bleeding include nose, gums, urinary tract, old wounds and venepuncture sites. Petechiae have been described on the limbs, face and oral mucosa[141].

Blood usually becomes incoagulable within a few hours of the bite and there is thrombocytopenia. Peripheral leucocytosis is reported. Persistent bleeding has resulted in severe anaemia. Shock developed from seven hours to six days after the bite especially in children and elderly debilitated patients in 31% of the Jianning series[139]. Symptoms included syncope, dyspnoea, tachypnoea, dizziness, blurred vision, sweating and prostration. In Guangxi the case fatality was 4.7%,[36] in Jianning 5.4%[139].

d. Envenoming by hump-nosed vipers (genus Hypnale)

No bites by *H. hypnale* have been reported from India this century, but in Sri Lanka it accounts for 27% of all snakebites. This high incidence may be explained by the large populations of this species in rubber, tea, coffee, coconut, cocoa, herb and other plantations.

1. Merrem's hump-nosed viper (H hypnale)

Most bites result in local pain and swelling resolving in a few days without residual necrosis and with no systemic problems. However, since 1930, there has been increasing suspicion that bites by this small snake could occasionally give rise to severe envenoming[142]. In 1930 a collector for the Colombo Museum was bitten by an *H. hypnale*. Within 10 minutes he developed stinging pains all over the body and later felt faint. There was swelling of the wrist, a burning sensation in the stomach, thirst, smarting of the eyes and some delirium. He was treated by an ayurvedic physician. He twice vomited blood, swelling extended to the shoulder, he developed a high fever and became unconscious. Although "given up" by the physician, he began to improve on the fifth day after the bite and eventually recovered completely[143]. Cases of fatal bilateral renal cortical necrosis[144], coagulopathy and renal failure, which was fatal in two out of eight cases[145-147], and bleeding tendency and acute renal failure with recovery[148] were attributed to this species, but in all these cases there was some doubt about the identification of the snake, which had usually been based on patients' or their relatives' descriptions[142]. An immature Russell's viper, particularly one in which the characteristic spots were obscured by mud or imminent sloughing of the skin, might have been mistaken for *H. hypnale*. However, a five year old boy bitten by a 427 mm long *H hypnale*, developed local swelling, incoagulable blood, thrombocytopenia, bleeding into the gastrointestinal tract and acute renal failure which was successfully treated with peritoneal dialysis[142]. Laboratory studies demonstrated that the venom of *H. hypnale* was procoagulant, fibrinolytic and aggregated platelets. Nearly four months after the bite a Tc^{99} DTPA renogram showed evidence of a non-functioning left kidney. Recently, more cases of bleeding and clotting disorder with renal failure have been seen in patients with proven bites by *H hypnale*.

2. Millard's hump-nosed viper (H. nepa)

In four cases of proven bites by *H. nepa*, there was pain and swelling which subsided within 3-5 days[47].

e. Envenoming by Indo-Chinese mountain vipers (genus Ovophis)

1. Mount Kinabalu mountain viper (O. chaseni)

Near the Belalong River, a tributary of the Temburong River in eastern Brunei, at an altitude of about 700 metres, Dr Peter Ashton, a botanist, was bitten on the ankle by "the cryptically mottled dark olive-green and brown" *O. chaseni*, approximately 38 cm long[149]. There was severe pain within five minutes, considerable swelling in one hour and pain, swelling and bruising extending beyond the knee after 24 hours. The accompanying Ibans reassured him that the effects would wear off after several days, but he had to be carried back to Brunei State Hospital, a journey taking five days. During the journey he developed pain in the groin as swelling spread to involve the lower abdomen, ecchymoses in the bitten limb, fainted and was incontinent of faeces and had difficulty passing urine. On the sixth day after the bite he fainted, vomited profusely and became pale and shocked with abdominal distention, bruising around the umbilicus (signifying intraperitoneal bleeding), ecchymoses over both loins, a large scrotal haematoma and tenderness in both iliac fossae. His haemoglobin concentration had fallen to 4.4 g/dl, the urine contained a few erythrocytes and there was evidence of haemolysis (methaemoglobinuria), urobilinogen in the urine and a reticulocyte count of 5.7%. He recovered after blood transfusion and palliative treatment and was able to leave hospital 12 days after the bite[149].

2. Mountain pit viper (O. monticola)

A snake man was bitten on the finger by a 53 cm long specimen of *O monticola* at Shillong, Khasi Hills, Assam (1500 metres altitude). He developed swelling, severe bleeding at the site of incisions and his blood was incoagulable[92]. A man bitten on the hand in Hong Kong developed local swelling[150]. He became thrombocytopenic with a coagulopathy (greatly prolonged prothrombin time, activated partial thromboplastin time and thrombin time, elevated FDP, greatly reduced fibrinogen concentration and detectable soluble fibrin monomer complex) maximal on the day after the bite. Coagulation returned to normal in four days and he recovered with conservative treatment. In six cases at Shillong, Meghalaya, India, there were no signs of envenoming, but a fatal case was reported in an elderly woman[92]. In other envenomed patients there was local swelling involving half the bitten limb, transient shivering and sloughing of the wound.

3. Hime-habu (Ovophis okinavensis)

A bite on the thumb was followed by pain, swelling and redness extending up to the elbow, associated with axillary lymphadenopathy and subsiding in eight days[151].

f. Envenoming by Asian arboreal pit vipers (genus Trimeresurus)

1. White-lipped green pit viper (T. albolabris)

In a survey of venomous snakes and snakebite in Thailand, this species was the second most frequently brought by victims of snakebite (27% of all bites) and the most widely distributed (at 65% of participating hospitals nationwide). The length of the snakes ranged from 120-895 (mean 487) mm (n=307)[8]. Fifty per cent of snakebites in Indonesia are thought to be caused by this species with 2.4% fatality rate[134]. Twenty-nine patients with proven bites by *T albolabris* were studied in Bangkok, Trang and Kanchanaburi in Thailand[152]. Thirty-one per cent were bitten while cutting or collecting grass, flowers, trees, branches or other plants and in 54% bites were on the upper limb. Pain and swelling developed early after the bite and spread to involve more than half the bitten limb in 46% of cases (Figure 55a,b). Local bruising (58%) and tender enlargement of local lymph nodes (46%) were common, but local blisters were seen in only six cases and local necrosis in only two (both bites being on digits). More extensive necrosis has been seen in other patients (Figure 55c). In this series, systemic signs and symptoms were rare. Two patients were hypotensive and shocked on admission to hospital. Only one bled from the gums, two had petechial haemorrhages and one had menorrhagia. Six patients had incoagulable blood when they were first seen and another seven developed incoagulable blood while under observation in hospital 9-47 hours after admission. Half had a neutrophil leucocytosis and 38% were thrombocytopenic. All patients made a full recovery but complete restoration of function in the bitten limb took up to two months. Evidence of coagulopathy and fibrinolytic activity were found in 10 patients. Intense hypofibrinogenaemia was observed in all cases, but levels of other clotting factors and of the physiological coagulation inhibitors were within normal. FDP were predominantly uncrosslinked. There was little evidence of platelet activation and platelet aggregation was generally normal[152]. *T albolabris* is probably the most common venomous snake in urban Bangkok and bites by this species are a frequent cause of admission to Chulalongkorn and other hospitals in the city. In some parts of Vietnam (for example Lamdong Province) it is the commonest cause of snakebite. Bites among tea-pickers in Java were not uncommon and fatal cases are known[93]. It is responsible for 54% of identifiable cases of snakebite in the New Territories of Hong Kong. At Chulalongkorn Hospital, Bangkok, 72 children, aged between 1.5 months and 14 years, had been bitten by green pit vipers[153]. The precise species was not identified, but they were likely to have been either *T. albolabris* or *T. macrops*. Symptoms included pain, oozing from the site of the bite and swelling which appeared within 2-4 hours, reached a peak at 3-4 days and took a week to subside. Swelling involved more than half the bitten limb in 25% of patients, 85% had ecchymoses, 21% developed blistering and two developed necrosis. Thirty-five per cent of these children had systemic bleeding (from the gastrointestinal tract and gums, and as epistaxis and haematuria) and one became shocked. Other symptoms were nausea, vomiting, diarrhoea, abdominal discomfort, lethargy and mild fever. Seventy-five per cent had a peripheral leucocytosis of more than 10×10^9/litre[153]. Eighteen adult patients bitten by green pit vipers were also seen at Chulalongkorn Hospital and showed similar effects of envenoming[117]. One developed angio-oedema of the lips and tongue after sucking his wound. Local haemorrhagic blistering appeared in four cases. Two of the nine digital bites were complicated by gangrene requiring amputation. Two elderly patients died of intracranial haemorrhage[117]. Duodenal obstruction from a haematoma, systemic bleeding, defibrination, gastrointestinal symptoms, melaena, vomiting, haematemesis and acute renal failure have also been described[152]. In Hong Kong, among 152 cases of proven or suspected *T. albolabris* bite, local swelling (84%) usually subsided within 2-3 days, 9% of patients had regional lymphadenopathy and a few developed blistering and local necrosis[114]. There was a fatal intracranial bleed in an adult patient and fatal cases in children have also been described in Hong Kong.

2. Cantor's pit viper

Bites by this species are not regarded as fatal by the natives of the Andaman and Nicobar Islands[92].

3. Sakishima-habu (T. elegans)

In Okinawa, 30-60 bites by *T. elegans* are reported each year with a morbidity of 0.73 to 1.32 per 1000 population per year. In the whole of Japan about 100 cases are reported annually (morbidity 3.0 per 1000 population per year). Deaths and severe necrosis have not been reported. However, in Shika, Ishigaki Island, among 24 cases seen between 1950 and 1955, 22 developed local signs only, including swelling, tenderness and local necrosis requiring amputation or leading to permanent deformity[154]. Two patients developed systemic symptoms; one of them became tachypnoeic, shocked, peripherally cyanosed and comatose three hours after the bite but recovered apart from local necrosis and loss of his thumb. Only one death had been seen, in 1926; the patient had become dyspnoeic with pain in the chest, tachycardia, shock and peripheral cyanosis several hours after the bite and died 24 hours after the bite.

4. Red-tailed green pit viper (T. erythrurus)

Of 20 patients studied in Burma, 65% showed no evidence of envenoming and there were no deaths[155]. All envenomed patients had local swelling but no necrosis or ulceration developed. In severe cases, incoagulable blood and thrombocytopenia was observed; the coagulopathy could persist for up to 12 days. At Mandalay, a patient died with intra-abdominal haemorrhage after being massaged.

5. Yellow spotted pit viper (T. flavomaculatus)

Only one case of a bite has been reported, inflicted on Mr McGregor by the subspecies *T. f mcgregori* which he discovered[156]. On Batan Island he was scratched by the fangs on his thumb. There was very little pain and the swelling subsided within a couple of days.

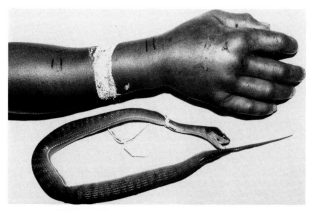

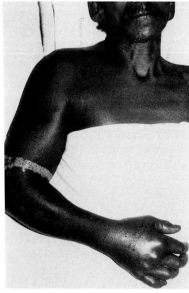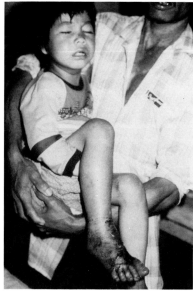

Figure 55. Envenoming by the white-lipped green pit viper (*Trimeresurus albolabris*) in Thailand (photos © Dr. D.A. Warrell).
55a. (top) Swelling of the hand and forearm.
55b. (bottom left) Swelling of the whole bitten limb and adjacent area of the trunk.
55c. (bottom right) Necrosis of the bitten foot in a Vietnamese child.

6. Japanese habu (T. flavoviridis)

The incidence of habu bites in the Amami Islands has averaged 176-206 per 100,000 per year, and in the Ryukyu Islands 15-19 per 100,000 per year. Before the introduction of antivenom in about 1905, the fatality rate was 11-15% in the Amami Islands and 18-24% in the Ryukyu Islands[21]. Forty-two per cent of bites were inflicted in the fields and 22% in the home, 54% to the lower and 41% to the upper limbs. There was intense pain, swelling, blistering and bruising of the bitten limb. Swelling frequently involves the whole limb and adjacent areas of the trunk. Patients bitten in the lower limb may develop anterior tibial compartment syndrome. Local necrosis developed in 6.8% and in 4.5% there was residual dysfunction resulting from amputation or ankylosis. Necrosis of digits is particularly common. Systemic symptoms develop in about 14% of patients. There is a fall in blood pressure and pulse volume, peripheral cyanosis, fever, vomiting, abdominal pain and impaired consciousness. Systemic symptoms may occur without local necrosis (about 10%) and necrosis without systemic symptoms (about 3%). Despite the discovery of several haemorrhagins in the venom of *T. flavoviridis*, spontaneous systemic haemorrhage has not been described and there is no mention in the reports of incoagulable blood. About 75% of deaths occurred within 24 hours, the earliest being only five hours after the bite. Fifteen per cent occurred within 48 hours and 10% within 3-9 days of the bite[157].

7. Indian green pit viper (.T gramineus)

Considering that this is the most abundant pit viper in the southern half of India, it is surprising that there is little reliable information about the effects of envenoming. In the past the name *T. gramineus* has been applied to many other green arboreal pit vipers of this genus, as far afield as in Taiwan (*T. stejnegeri*). Local pain and swelling are reported with nausea, vomiting and fever. There is no mention of bleeding, coagulopathy or local necrosis. According to Wall[92], "the bite is rarely, if ever, fatal, but severe local effects and constitutional disturbances are usually attendant".

8. Jerdon's pit viper (.T jerdonii)

"One bite by *T jerdonii* showing local signs of swelling and haemorrhage occurred in Guilin District."[36]

9. Kanchanaburi pit viper (T. kanburiensis)

A woman was bitten on the foot by a 50 cm long specimen of *T. kanburiensis* while searching for bamboo shoots on a hill near to where the type specimen was collected in 1927[22]. She developed severe pain and swelling which eventually involved the whole limb and the right flank (Figure 56), bruising of the calf, tender popliteal lymph nodes, recurrent shock probably attributable to hypovolaemia, peripheral leucocytosis, anaemia and a mild coagulopathy (hypofibrinogenaemia, elevated fibrin(ogen) degradation products and modest reduction in plasminogen and alpha-2 antiplasmin without thrombocytopenia). She was treated conservatively and was fit to leave hospital after four days. Such serious symptoms in a healthy young woman suggest that, in the absence of the specific antivenom, bites by this species could prove fatal in very young, very old or debilitated patients.

10. Large-scaled pit viper (T. macrolepis)

Tea-pickers in the Western Ghats of India, bitten on the hands or feet by this species, developed intense burning pain at the site of the bite with swelling extending to the shoulder or knee which persisted for three or four days[158]. Secondary infection was rare and there was no mortality or more serious symptoms caused by the bites.

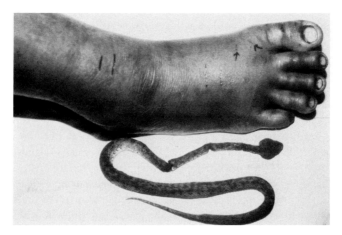

Figure 56. Envenoming by the Kanchanaburi pit viper (*Trimeresurus kanaburiensis*). 25 year old woman bitten on the dorsum of the foot (arrowed) showing swelling of the foot and ankle 1½ hours after the bite and the snake responsible. (British Museum of Natural History, London, Accession number 1988.383) (courtesy of Prof. Sornchai Looareesuwan, Bangkok).[22]

11. Dark green pit viper (T. macrops)

In a nationwide survey of venomous snakes responsible for bites in Thailand, this species was recorded in 10% of participating hospitals and constituted 1% of all snakes collected[8]. In Bangkok, it is second only to *T albolabris* as a cause of snakebite but, as with other species of this genus, it has been misidentified and misnamed (for example as *T. popeorum*) in many publications[8,23]. In a study of five proven cases in Bangkok, the patients were bitten while in their gardens picking flowers, cutting grass or collecting firewood. There was painful swelling involving less than half of the bitten limb but no local blistering or necrosis and no systemic symptoms. Three of the patients had a neutrophil leucocytosis; only one had thrombocytopenia and none had incoagulable blood. Studies in which the biting species was not definitely confirmed have suggested that more severe bleeding and clotting disturbances can occur after envenoming by this species[159].

12. Anamallay or Malabar rock pit viper (T. malabaracius)

Bites by this species have been reported but none had proved fatal. Pain, swelling and local bleeding occur[92].

13. Chinese habu (.T mucrosquamatus)

From 1904 to 1971, 30% of venomous snakebites in Taiwan were caused by this species with an 8% mortality. In Guangxi, China, 13.4% of bites were attributed to *T. mucrosquamatus*; 28.5% developed systemic envenoming and 94.3% local swelling with necrosis in 1.6%[36]. Bites have been described from Taiwan, China and the northeast frontier of India. There is severe local pain and swelling which may involve the entire bitten limb with tender enlargement of regional lymph nodes. Serosanguinous discharge from the fang marks, local blistering, bruising and the development of intracompartmental syndromes, especially anterior tibial compartment syndrome, are described. Systemic symptoms include nausea, vomiting, epigastric pain, fever and shock which may cause impaired consciousness or even generalised convulsions. Peripheral leucocytosis is common and there may be thrombocytopenia, evidence of coagulopathy (but this has not been investigated thoroughly) and spontaneous bleeding including an intracranial haemorrhage in one case[80]. Other severe complications include oliguric renal failure and ECG changes suggesting myocardial damage[80]. In Wujin County, Giangsu Province, China, *T. mucrosquamatus* is the only venomous species responsible for all the bites and a few deaths each year. This species is often found in and around human dwellings; 30% of the bites in Guangxi occurred in the patients' homes[36].

14. Pope's pit viper (T. popeiorum)

This species has never been proved to be responsible for a case of snakebite in any part of its range, but its name has been confused with other arboreal green pit vipers such as *T albolabris* and *T macrops*[23].

15. Flat-nosed pit viper (T. puniceus)

A bite on the foot that occurred near Kuala Lumpur, western Malaysia, resulted in immediate burning pain and swelling which extended up to the knee.

16. Mangrove pit viper (.T purpureomaculatus)

Bites by this species are said to be common in those who work in swamp and mangrove forests in western Malaysia. Tweedie[160] considered that bites by this species produced trivial envenoming in virtually every case. Three bites by *T. purpureomaculatus* were reported in southwest Thailand without evidence of envenoming[8]. However, envenoming may cause severe pain, local swelling which may involve the entire bitten limb, tender enlargement of local lymph nodes, local necrosis and incoagulable blood. In a series of 28 cases observed in western Malaysia, seven had incoagulable blood, 15 local swelling and two necrosis. A three year old child died 12 hours after the bite[74].

17. Chinese green pit viper (T. stejnegeri)

In areas where this species is sympatric with *T. albolabris* and *T. popeiorum*, bites by the three species are likely to be confused. However, in Taiwan, *T stejnegeri* is very common and responsible for 53% of bites but with less than 1% mortality[80]. In Guangxi, China, most patients were bitten on the lower limbs while in the fields or mountains; 91% developed local swelling, 23% systemic envenoming but there was only one case of necrosis and one fatality[36]. Another fatality has been reported following a bite on the head. Symptoms include severe local pain, oozing from the fang marks, extensive local swelling (which may involve the entire limb and adjacent trunk), bruising, nausea and vomiting. Peripheral leucocytosis and mild elevation of serum alkaline phosphatase and aminotransferases was common in Taiwan but in a study of 16 patients coagulopathy was rare[80]. A man bitten by a green pit viper (probably *T. stejnegeri*) in a mountainous area of Fukien Province in China, rapidly developed extensive swelling and bruising, became unconscious in 20 minutes and died in about three hours.

18. Horse-shoe pit viper (T. strigatus)

In one reported case there was no envenoming[92].

19. Sumatran pit viper (T. sumatranus)

T sumatranus is said to be "the most aggressive among the viper species". Bites by this snake in plantations in east Malaysia are quite common[40,161]. Envenoming is said to cause severe pain and swelling. No detailed reports are available. In Thailand and western Malaysia there have been no reported cases of bites by *T. hageni*.

20. Tokara-habu (T. tokarensis)

Only one or two bites are reported each year in the population of about 600 in the islands inhabited by this species. Neither death nor severe necrosis has been reported.

21. Sri Lankan green pit viper (T. trigonocephalus)

Bites by this species are uncommon. Immediate pain and swelling, involving almost the entire bitten limb, are described. There may be local blistering but local necrosis, bleeding and clotting disturbances and other systemic symptoms have not been observed. Swelling subsides in a few days. One case of "drooping of eyelids" has not been confirmed[162].

g. Envenoming by Wagler's pit viper (Tropidolaemus wagleri)

Twenty-four of 48 cases of proven *T. wagleri* bites in western Malaysia developed no envenoming. There was local swelling in the other 24 cases and in one necrosis ensued. Blood coagulation remained normal in the six cases in which it was assessed[74]. Three patients bitten on Negros in the Philippines suffered immediate bleeding, pain and swelling at the site of the bite with persistent numbness for a month or more. However, in some parts of its range, this species has a terrifying reputation. According to Beccari[163] the Malays believe that, if bitten by this species, they have no time even to take their jacket off before they die.

VI. PREVENTION OF SNAKEBITE

A better understanding of diurnal and seasonal patterns of snake activity and their preferred habitats, avoidance of unnecessarily high risk activities and the use of protective clothing, such as shoes or boots, would reduce the risk of bites. In the Philippines the provision of raised walkways through marshy areas reduced the incidence of cobra bites, and in Thailand the wearing of boots reduced the risk of bites by cobras in fish farmers. Educating the community in correct methods of first aid, dissuading them from wasting valuable time indulging in useless and potentially dangerous traditional treatments and improving the understanding and treatment of snakebite at primary health care posts, rural dispensaries and district hospitals in Asia could reduce the incidence of severe envenoming.

Amateur herpetologists and others should be dissuaded from picking up dangerous or potentially dangerous species as many bites result from this behaviour. Snakes should never be disturbed, attacked, cornered or handled even if they are thought to be harmless species or appear to be dead. Venomous species should never be kept as pets or as performing animals. In high risk areas, boots, socks and long trousers should be worn for walks in undergrowth or deep sand and a light should always be carried at night. Unfortunately, even such simple precautions may be impracticable in many rural areas, because of climate, poverty and local beliefs. For example, in some parts of the rice-growing area of central Burma, rice farmers are reluctant to wear shoes of any kind when they go into the paddy fields because they fear it will offend the Russell's vipers and make them more likely to bite. Collecting firewood, dislodging logs or boulders with bare hands, pushing sticks or fingers into burrows, holes and crevices, climbing rocks and trees covered with dense foliage and swimming in overgrown lakes and rivers are particularly hazardous activities. Unlit paths and gutters are particularly dangerous at night after heavy rains. It is difficult to exclude snakes from fields and gardens. It is futile and ecologically undesirable to attempt the extermination of venomous snakes and at present there is no "snake repellant" that is effective without poisoning the snake. These compounds include naphthalene, sulphur, nicotine sulphate, strichnine, insecticides (such as DDT and dieldrin), organophosphates and fumigants such as calcium cyanide, formaldehyde, tetrachloroethane and methyl bromide.

Prophylactic immunization against snake venom has been experimented with in several Asian countries and even taken as far as field trials in Japan,[164] but there are theoretical and practical problems which make it unlikely that this will provide the answer to rural snakebite in Asia.

VII. FIRST AID TREATMENT OF SNAKEBITE IN ASIA[165,166]

Patients bitten by snakes need urgent medical assessment, but rural health stations or district hospitals often serve large areas and many agricultural areas infested with snakes may be relatively inaccessible by road, especially during the rainy season. It may take a patient hours or even days to reach the nearest medical facility. Education of rural communities in good first aid practice may prevent time-wasting and dangerous customs and could prolong a patient's life until they reach medical care.

The principles of first aid are

1. The delivery of snakebite victims as quickly as possible to a place where they can be seen by medical staff.

2. The use of methods to delay the evolution of life-threatening envenoming at least until the patient reaches a place where they can receive medical care.

3. The alleviation of severe and possibly life-threatening early symptoms of envenoming.

Advice about first aid must take into account the fact that it can only be carried out by the snakebite victim or by those who are nearby or arrive quickly on the scene. In most cases, medically-trained people will not be available to give first aid. Only in zoos, snake farms, research stations and organised expeditions is it possible to provide equipment, even as simple as splints and crepe bandages, to be used soon after the accident has occurred. First aid treatment of snakebites is an important subject for health education in the community, especially among high risk groups such as agricultural workers and their families.

A. GENERAL RECOMMENDATIONS FOR FIRST AID

1. The bitten person should be reassured. Many will be terrified, fearing sudden death and, in this state of mind, they may behave irrationally or even hysterically. The basis for reassurance is the fact that many venomous bites do not result in envenoming, the relatively slow progression to severe envenoming (hours following elapid bites, days following viper bites) and the effectiveness of modern medical treatment.

2. The bite wound should not be tampered with in any way. Wiping it once with a damp cloth to remove surface venom is unlikely to do much harm (or good) but the wound must not be massaged.

3. The bitten limb should be immobilised as effectively as possible using a makeshift splint or sling; if available, crepe bandaging of the splinted limb is an effective form of immobilisation.

4. The snakebite victim should be transported as quickly and as passively as possible to the nearest place where they can be seen by a medically-trained person (health station, dispensary, clinic or hospital). The bitten limb must not be exercised as muscular contraction will promote systemic absorption of venom. If no motor vehicle, train or boat is available, the patient can be carried on a stretcher or hurdle, on the pillion or crossbar of a bicycle or on someone's back. Most traditional, and many of the more recently fashionable, first aid measures are useless and potentially dangerous. These include local cauterization, incision, excision, amputation, suction by mouth, vacuum pump or syringe, combined incision and suction ("venom-ex" apparatus), injection or instillation of compounds such as potassium permanganate, phenol (carbolic soap) and trypsin, application of electric shocks or ice (cryotherapy), use of traditional herbal, folk and other remedies including the ingestion of emetic plant products and parts of the snake, multiple incisions and tattooing (Burma) and ayurvedic treatments such as instillation of oil blown through a tube into the trachea ("nasna kireema") and heating over a fire ("vadu" or "dum ellima") (Sri Lanka)[51].

5. If the snake responsible for the bite has been killed, it should be taken along with the patient for identification, but it should not be touched with bare hands even if it appears dead and no attempt should be made to chase the snake into the undergrowth as this will risk further bites.

B. DANGERS OF TOURNIQUETS, LIGATURES AND COMPRESSION BANDS

Systemic envenoming by some elapid snakes (for example *O hannah* and Naja species) may develop so rapidly that fatal respiratory paralysis may ensue, exceptionally, within 30 minutes of the bite. In these cases there is a strong argument for attempting to impede the systemic uptake of venom to allow more time to transport the patient to hospital. Tourniquets of some sort are still the most popular first aid method in developing countries and most medical staff working in areas where snakebite is common will have been impressed by the damaging effects of this technique; ischaemia and gangrene, damage to superficial peripheral nerves, increased fibrinolytic activity and congestion and swelling in the occluded limb leading to increased bleeding, shock or acute development of systemic envenoming after release of the tourniquet and intensification of local effects of venom in the occluded limb. Studies in Thailand, Burma and the Philippines showed that the majority of tourniquets applied in rural areas were ineffective in preventing the systemic spread of venom.[165,166] *For all these reasons, the use of tourniquets, ligatures and pressure bands is not recommended.*

1. Sutherland's compression immobilisation method

In animals, arterial-occlusive ligatures or tourniquets have been shown to prevent the absorption of venom and to prolong survival after the injection of elapid and viper venoms. Immobilisation of the injected limb without occlusion was shown to delay the absorption of higher molecular weight toxins (eg in *Notechis scutatus* and *Daboia russelii* venoms) spread through the lymphatics, but not smaller molecular weight toxins (e.g. in cobra venom) absorbed directly into the bloodstream. Venom procoagulants in some venoms seem to be permanently localised (perhaps through local thrombosis) or inactivated in occluded limbs. Sutherland et al[167] found that in restrained monkeys compression and immobilisation of the injected limb in a pneumatic chamber at 55 mmHg and crepe bandaging and splinting judged to exert the same compressive effect delayed the movement of labelled venom from the injected limb without causing the ischaemia inevitable with conventional tourniquets. In monkeys, this method was effective with 13 Australasian elapid venoms, and the venoms of the Indian cobra (*N. naja*) and the eastern diamond back rattlesnake (*Crotalus adamanteus*). The method was formally endorsed by the Australian National Health and Medical Research Council in 1979 and has been enthusiastically promoted in Australasia, Southern Africa and elsewhere. However, even in Australia it is still used in only 18-45% of snakebite cases[168]. Unfortunately, there have been few clinical reports of the use of this method and no attempt at comparative or controlled studies. The rapid development of systemic envenoming with increasing systemic venous venom antigen concentration has been observed in several cases after the release of crepe or Biscard bandages. In Australia, the method has proved safe, but prolonged application of pressure immobilisation has produced evidence of intensification of local effects of neurotoxic and cytotoxic venom components in a few patients. Compared with the venoms of Asian vipers and cobras, Australasian elapid venoms produce little or no tissue damage at the site of the bite. Pressure immobilisation is likely to cause the intensification of locally necrotic effects of Asian snake venoms with secondary ischaemic effects resulting from increased pressure in tight fascial compartments, especially the anterior tibial compartment. *For this reason pressure immobilisation is not recommended in patients bitten by Asian vipers and cobras.*

For victims of snakebite in rural areas of Asia, the pressure immobilisation method raises difficult practical problems. Long stretchy bandages are unlikely to be available except to wealthy outsiders such as campers, hikers and expedition members. It is difficult to judge the pressure applied by a crepe bandage. If it is too loose it will be ineffective and if too tight it could produce the same risk of ischaemia and gangrene as an arterial tourniquet. Finally, the application of the bandage may prove difficult or impossible if the victim is on their own, especially if the bite is on the dominant arm.

However, Sutherland's pressure immobilisation method, when correctly applied, is undoubtedly far more tolerable and less dangerous than tight tourniquets or ligatures. *The method is recommended after bites by dangerous neurotoxic species such as kraits (Bungarus), cobras which cause little local envenoming (Naja philippinensis) and the king cobra (Ophiophagus hannah).*

2. Treatment of early symptoms of envenoming before the patient reaches hospital[166]

Anaphylaxis: as early as a few minutes and up to several hours after bites by some Vipera species and Russell's vipers, patients may develop symptoms of anaphylaxis and stimulation of the autonomic nervous system: hypotension, tachycardia, shock, impaired consciousness, angio-oedema of the tongue, mouth, gums, lips and face, urticaria, abdominal colic, nausea, retching, vomiting and diarrhoea (sometimes repeated and profuse), sweating and "gooseflesh" and in some cases breathlessness and bronchospasm. These features are attributable to autopharmacological effects of venom, releasing endogenous mediators or activating precursors such as bradykinin. On rare occasions, people (usually herpetologists or snake handlers) who have been bitten or exposed in other ways to a specific snake venom may become sensitized and develop true immediate-type I hypersensitivity after a bite or contact of mucosae such as the lips and mouth with venom when applying suction to a wound. *The treatment of all these anaphylactic syndromes is subcutaneous or intramuscular injection of 0.1% adrenaline, followed by an intravenous injection of an antihistamine H_1 antagonist* (see below). Hypotensive patients should be tipped head downwards and those with severe bronchospasm, dyspnoea or cyanosis should be given oxygen by any available means.

Pain in the bitten limb may be severe. Oral paracetamol is preferable to aspirin which commonly causes gastric erosions even in healthy people and could lead to persistent gastric bleeding in patients with incoagulable blood.

Vomiting is a common early symptom of severe systemic envenoming by any species of snake. Patients should lie on their side to prevent aspiration of vomit. Persistent vomiting can be treated with an injection[****] of chlorpromazine (25-50 mg for adults, 1 mg/kg for children).

Respiratory distress and cyanosis may indicate paralysis of the respiratory muscles or blockage of the airway in a patient with respiratory or circulatory failure. The patient should be laid on their side, the airway cleared by elevating the jaw, removing foreign bodies and inserting oral airway if available. If respiratory distress and cyanosis persist, oxygen should be given and, if there are still signs of respiratory failure, ventilation will have to be assisted. In the absence of any special equipment, mouth-to-mouth or mouth-to-nose ventilation can be life-saving. If the patient is unconscious and no femoral or carotid pulse can be felt, external cardiac massage and mouth-to-mouth ventilation should be started without delay.

Community first aid workers can be trained to place snakebite victims in the correct position, maintain the airway and even to do cardiopulmonary resuscitation. In some countries dispensers, nurses and ambulancemen can be trained to give adrenaline, antihistamines, chlorpromazine and other drugs, to insert oral airways, administer oxygen and carry out CPR.

VIII. MEDICAL TREATMENT IN HEALTH STATIONS, DISPENSARIES AND HOSPITALS[166]

Snakebite is a medical emergency. Ideally, all patients bitten by snakes should be assessed by medically trained staff. In most patients, uncertainties such as the species responsible, the amount of venom injected and the variable time course for development of signs require that patients should be kept under observation for at least 24 hours. Exceptions are those cases in which the bite was by an unequivocally non-venomous species such as legless lizards (Amphisbaenids or worm lizards - Amphisbaenia; legless skinks (Scincidae) - *Berkudia*, *Isopachys* and *Ophioscincus*) and other legless lizards such as Anguidae (*Ophisaurus* sp) and Dibamidae (*Dibamus* sp); legless amphibians (caecilians - Ichthyophiidae - *Gymnophiona*) and non-venomous snakes (blind snakes - Typhlopidae and

---

[****]*Patients with incoagulable blood may develop massive haematomas after intramuscular and subcutaneous injections. Except in the case of adrenaline, the intravenous route should be used whenever possible.*

Leptotyphlopidae; boas and pythons - Boidae; uropelts or shield tails - Uropeltidae; pipe snakes - Anilidae; and Xenopeltidae) and those colubrid snakes known to be non-venomous. Medical staff must decide quickly whether the patient has been bitten by a snake, whether there are signs of envenoming and whether antivenom or ancillary treatment is needed. Three important initial questions are:

1. On which part of your body were you bitten?
2. How long ago were you bitten?
3. Have you brought the snake and, if not, can anyone describe it?

Patients should be asked to describe their symptoms and then questioned directly about local pain, swelling, tenderness, regional lymph nodes, bleeding, motor and sensory symptoms, vomiting, fainting and abdominal pain. The time after the bite when these symptoms appeared and their progression should be noted. Details of pre-hospital treatment (tourniquets, herbal remedies etc) should also be recorded as these may, themselves, cause symptoms.

1. Examination

The absence of discernible fang marks does not exclude snakebite, but the discovery of two or more discrete puncture marks suggests a bite by a venomous snake. The pattern of fang punctures is rarely helpful as there may be marks by accessory fangs, other teeth and multiple bites. The distance between the fang marks is proportional to the size of the snake. Local swelling and enlargement and tenderness of regional lymph nodes are often the earliest signs of envenoming, but factitious swelling may be caused by a tourniquet. Most cases of significant envenoming by Asian vipers and cobras are associated with the development of local swelling within two hours of the bite but there have been exceptions to this rule. Systemic envenoming by most Asian species is associated with local swelling, although in the case of some bites by colubrids, kraits, Philippine cobra (*N. philippinensis*) and even Russell's vipers, this may be negligible. Persistent bleeding from the fang marks, other recent wounds and venepuncture sites suggest that the blood is incoagulable. The gums should be examined thoroughly as these are usually the first site of spontaneous systemic bleeding. The signs of shock are fall in blood pressure, collapse, cold cyanosed and sweaty skin and impaired consciousness. The foot of the bed should be raised and an intravenous infusion of isotonic saline or a plasma expander such as haemaccel, gelofuse, dextran or fresh frozen plasma should be started immediately. The earliest symptoms of neurotoxicity after elapid bites is often blurred vision, a feeling of heaviness of the eyelids and drowsiness. The frontalis muscle is contracted, raising the eyebrows and puckering the forehead, even before ptosis can be demonstrated. Respiratory muscle paralysis with imminent respiratory failure is suggested by dyspnoea, restlessness, sweating, exaggerated abdominal respiration, central cyanosis and coma. If there is any suggestion of respiratory muscle weakness, objective monitoring should be attempted by measuring peak expiratory flow, vital capacity or expiratory pressure using the mercury manometer of a sphygmomanometer. Coma is usually the result of respiratory or circulatory failure. Patients with widespread flaccid paralysis may seem deeply comatose because they are unresponsive and arreflexic but, provided they are adequately ventilated, they are likely to be fully conscious. Enough distal motor function may be retained to allow them to signal by flexing a finger or toe in response to questions.

2. Monitoring of snake-bitten patients

Patients bitten by snakes should, ideally, be observed in hospital for at least 24 hours after the bite. The following should be checked at least once an hour:

1. level of consciousness
2. presence or absence of ptosis

3. pulse rate and rhythm
4. blood pressure
5. respiratory rate
6. extent of local swelling
7. new symptoms or signs.

A. DIAGNOSIS

In most patients, the history of snakebite will be clear-cut and the clinician will have to decide which species was likely to be responsible and whether there are signs of envenoming. However, some patients may only suspect that they have been bitten by a snake because they experienced a sharp pricking pain while walking in the dark or in undergrowth, collecting firewood or even while asleep on the floor in their hut. Thorns, rodent bites and bites and stings by arthropods could produce immediate local pain and one or more puncture marks. Bites and stings by venomous Asian arthropods (for example, hymenoptera, scorpions, spiders, centipedes) can cause mild local swelling and severe systemic symptoms. Local swelling and inflammation, sometimes resulting in a hot, red, swollen limb with enlarged regional nodes, can result from secondary infection (cellulitis) following penetrating wounds from thorns or rodent bites. The interval between the accident and the development of inflammatory swelling is usually more than 24 hours, but in the case of *Pasteurella multocida* infection following mammal bites, this interval may be as short as 6-12 hours.

1. Species diagnosis

Descriptions of snakes by snakebite victims and onlookers, and the use of local names for snakes, are often misleading and so, unless the snake has been brought for identification, the clinician will have to rely on the clinical picture and the results of laboratory tests to make a species diagnosis. Unfortunately, clinical features are rarely diagnostic. The circumstances of the bite can be helpful. Kraits are most likely to be responsible for bites inflicted at night on people asleep on the floor of their huts. In and near rivers, lakes and marshy areas, cobras are most likely to be responsible.

In most parts of Asia there are four main clinical syndromes of envenoming:
1. Severe local swelling, blistering and necrosis with coagulable blood; cobras are usually responsible.
2. Severe local envenoming (as above) with incoagulable blood and spontaneous systemic bleeding - Viperidae (vipers or pit vipers) are usually responsible.
3. Mild or absent local swelling with neurotoxic symptoms - kraits (*Bungarus*) are usually responsible (or Philippine cobras - *N. philippinensis* in the appropriate geographical area).
4. Mild or negligible local envenoming with incoagulable blood and spontaneous systemic bleeding - Russell's vipers are usually responsible. Colubrids (*Rhabdophis*) are very rarely responsible.

2. The 20 minute whole blood clotting test (20WBCT)

This is a simple and rapid "bedside" test which must be carried out, on admission and repeated subsequently, in all patients with suspected snakebite. A few ml of venous blood are placed in a new, clean, dry, glass test tube and left upright and undisturbed at room temperature for 20 minutes. The tube is then tipped. If the blood is still liquid and runs out of the tube, the patient is defibrinogenated, suggesting systemic envenoming by a viper or, much more rarely, a colubrid (*Rhabdophis*).

3. Immunodiagnosis[30]

Specific snake venom antigens can be detected in wound aspirate, swabs or biopsies, serum urine, cerebrospinal fluid and other body fluids. Enzyme immunoassay has been the most widely used. For the Asian region, no commercial test is available, but immunoassay has proved a valuable tool in the clinical investigation of snakebite and the assessment of antivenom efficacy. Nonspecific ("heterophile") reactions are common with sera from rural populations. In the case of venom antigen detection, this problem can be partly overcome by technique and by using a large number of unenvenomed controls from the same population to establish the background absorbence[30]. Detection of venom antibodies in patients bitten by snakes in the past remains too unreliable to be useful for individual diagnosis or epidemiological studies.

C. ANTIVENOM TREATMENT

The most important and urgent decision to be made in any patient bitten by a snake is whether or not to give antivenom, the only specific antidote to venom. Antivenom is the hyperimmune serum or plasma of animals, usually horses or sheep, which have been immunized with snake venoms. Most commercial antivenoms consist largely of $F(ab)_2$ fragments of immunoglobulin obtained by pepsin digestion and ammonium sulphate precipitation. For the following reasons, antivenom should never be used routinely and indiscriminately, but only when indicated.

1. All commercial antivenoms carry a risk of potentially dangerous serum reactions.

2. Antivenom is not always necessary: some patients are bitten by non-venomous snakes and 10-50% of those bitten by venomous snakes are not envenomed.

3. Antivenoms have a range of specific and paraspecific neutralizing activity but are useless for venoms outside that range. Specific antivenoms are not available for treatment of envenoming by some species (eg elapid species which rarely bite - *Calliophis*, *Maticora*; Sri Lankan Russell's viper; several *Agkistrodon* and many *Trimeresurus* species).

4. Antivenom is very expensive, usually in short supply and has a limited shelf life. Scarce and valuable supplies must not be wasted.

1. Indications for antivenom

Antivenom is indicated in all cases of systemic and severe local envenoming (Table 5).

Table 5
Indications for antivenom treatment after bites by Asian snakes

A	**Systemic envenoming**
1.	Neurotoxicity
2.	Spontaneous systemic bleeding
3.	Incoagulable blood (20 minute whole blood clotting test)
4.	Cardiovascular abnormality: hypotension, shock, arrhythmia, abnormal electrocardiogram
5.	Impaired consciousness
B	**Local envenoming by species known to cause local necrosis***
1.	Swelling involving more than half the bitten limb
2.	Rapidly progressive swelling
3.	Bites on fingers and toes

*Cobras and Viperidae

2. Contraindications to antivenom

There is no absolute contraindication to antivenom when a patient has life-threatening systemic envenoming. However, patients with an atopic history (asthma, hay fever, eczema, drug and food allergies etc) and those with a history of reactions to equine antisera have an increased risk of severe reactions. In those cases, pretreatment with subcutaneous adrenaline and intravenous antihistamine and hydrocortisone may prevent or diminish the reaction. There is not time for desensitization.

3. Hypersensitivity testing

Intradermal, subcutaneous or intraconjunctival tests with diluted antivenom have no predictive value for early anaphylactic or late serum sickness type antivenom reactions and should no longer be used[169,170].

4. Timing of antivenom treatment

Antivenom should be given as soon as possible once signs of systemic or severe local envenoming are evident (Table 5). It is almost never too late to try antivenom treatment; it has proved effective in reversing coagulopathy several days after bites by Echis species and *Calloselasma rhodostoma*. When patients arrive in hospital with a tourniquet or other constricting band in place, antivenom treatment, if it is thought necessary, should be started before these are released or there is a risk of severe envenoming when the venom in the occluded limb is released into the general circulation.

5. Antivenom specificity

If the species responsible for the bite is known, monospecific antivenom is the optimal treatment. However, in areas where the venoms of a number of different species produce similar clinical effects, polyspecific antivenoms must be used in the majority of patients who do not bring the dead snake for identification. Polyspecific antivenoms are specific for the range of venoms which they cover, but a larger dose is required to provide the same specific neutralizing power as a monospecific antivenom.

6. Antivenom administration

Ideally, antivenom should be used before its expiry date, but these stated dates are usually very conservative, partly for commercial reasons. It has been found that most liquid antivenoms retain 90% of their activity for years even when stored at high ambient temperatures (25 or 30°C) and that lyophilized antisera are much more stable[171]. However, antivenom solutions which have become opaque should not be used as protein precipitation is associated with loss of activity and an increased risk of reactions. Antivenom is most effective when given intravenously. Freeze-dried (lyophilized) antivenom is dissolved in sterile water. Antivenom can be given by intravenous injection at a rate of about 5 ml per minute, or diluted in isotonic fluid and infused over 30-60 minutes. The incidence and severity of antivenom reactions was the same with these two methods[169]. The advantage of intravenous infusion is ease of control, but intravenous "push" injection requires less expensive equipment, is quicker to set up and ensures that someone remains at the patient's side during the crucial first 10-15 minutes after the start of treatment, when early reactions are most likely to occur.

When intravenous administration is impossible, antivenom can be given by deep intramuscular injection at multiple sites in the anterior and lateral aspects of the thighs, followed by massage to promote absorption. Absorption from intragluteal injection is unreliable. There is a limit to the volume of antivenom that can be given by this route and there is a risk of haematoma formation in patients with incoagulable blood.

Table 6

Guide to initial dosage of some important antivenoms for Asian snake bites

Scientific Name	English Name	T&W Number	Manufacturer / Antivenom	Approximate Initial Dose	Incidence of Antivenom Reaction*	Reference
Agkistrodon b blomhoffii	Japanese mamushi	110, 111, 113-115	Japanese manufacturers, monospecific	20 ml		124
A b brevicaudus	Chinese mamushi	105	Shanghai Vaccine & Serum Inst, monospecific	20 ml		125
Bungarus caeruleus	Common (Indian) krait	67,70,73,74,78	Indian manufacturers, polyspecific	100 ml	T&W no73-52% (63%)	51,71,72
Calloselasma rhodostoma	Malayan pit viper	93	TRCS monospecific	100 ml	87%	138
		94	Thai Government Pharmaceutical Organisation, monospecific	50 ml	40%	138
Daboia russelii India	Russell's viper	67,68,71,73,76,78, 79	Indian manufacturers, polyspecific	50 ml		51
Daboia russelii Sri Lanka	Russell's viper	73,78	Indian manufacturers, polyspecific	100 ml	T&W no 73-52% (63%)	50
Daboia russelii Burma	Russell's viper	87	Industry & Pharm Corp., Yangoon, monospecific	40 ml	13% (100%)	17
Daboia russelii Thailand	Russell's viper	92	TRCS, monospecific	50 ml		116,176
Echis carinatus	Saw scaled viper	67,72,73,77	Indian manufacturers, polyspecific	10-30 ml	T&W no 67-7.4%	176
		78,79		40 ml		99
Echis sochureki		100,102	Nat Inst Prev Med, Taiwan	100 ml		80
Naja atra	Chinese cobra	89	TRCS, monospecific	100 ml		29,89,172
Naja kaouthia	Monocellate Thai cobra	67,68,69,73,75,78	Indian manufacturers, polyspecific	100 ml	T&W no 73-52% (63%)	51
Naja naja	Indian cobra	131	Twyford Pharmaceuticals, monospecific	50 ml		
Naja sumatrana	Sumatran/Malay cobra	90	TRCS, monospecific	200 ml		94
Ophiophagus hannah	King cobra	112	Japan Snake Institute, anti-yamakagashi	20 ml		
Rhabdophis subminiatus	Red-necked keelback			20 ml		177-179
R. tigrinus	Yamakagashi	88	TRCS, monospecific	100 ml	45%	152,190
Trimeresurus albolabris	White-lipped green pit viper	109	Chemo-Sero-Therap Res Inst, Kumamoto, Japan	20 ml	15%	191
T. flavoviridis	Japanese habu					

TRCS = Thai Red Cross Society; T&W = Theakston & Warrell, 1991[176]; *antivenom reactions: % early anaphylactic (pyrogenic)

7. Dosage of antivenom

Guidelines for initial dosage based on clinical studies are available for some important antivenoms used in the Asian region (Table 6). In most cases, manufacturer's recommendations given in the "package insert" are based on mouse assays which may not correlate with clinical findings. The initial dose of antivenom, however large, may not completely neutralize the depot of venom at the site of injection. Patients should therefore be observed for several days even if they show a good clinical response to the initial dose of antivenom. Continuing absorption of venom may cause recurrent neurotoxicity or haemostatic problems after the serum antivenom concentration has declined[30].
Children must be given the same dose of antivenom as adults.

8. Response to antivenom treatment

Neurotoxic signs often respond slowly, after several hours, or unconvincingly but, in the case of envenoming by *N. kaouthia* in Thailand, improvement after 30 minutes has been observed[172]. Cardiovascular effects such as hypotension and sinus bradycardia (for example after bites by *Daboia* and *Vipera* species) may respond within 10-20 minutes. Spontaneous systemic bleeding usually stops within 15-30 minutes and blood coagulability is restored within about six hours if an adequate dose of antivenom has been given. The 20WBCT (see above) should be used to monitor the dose of antivenom in patients with coagulopathy. If the blood remains incoagulable six hours after the first dose, the dose should be repeated and so on, every six hours, until blood coagulability is restored. Antivenom treatment has undoubtedly reduced snakebite mortality: for example, in Japan, mortality from habu bites (*T. flavoviridis*) was reduced to one-third after the introduction of antivenom in 1904-5[157].

Some antivenoms are capable of rapidly eliminating venom antigenaemia and haemostatic and cardiovascular abnormalities. Efficacy against neurotoxicity, even against predominantly post-synaptic neurotoxins of Asian cobras, is less convincing. The efficacy of antivenoms against local necrosis is controversial. Laboratory studies have shown that the antivenom must be given very early after envenoming to prevent these changes.

9. Antivenom reactions

Early (anaphylactic), pyrogenic and late (serum sickness type) reactions may occur.

Early reactions begin 10-60 minutes after starting intravenous administration of antivenom. Cough, tachycardia, itching (especially of the scalp), urticaria, fever, nausea, vomiting and headache are common symptoms. More than 5% of patients with early reactions develop systemic anaphylaxis - hypotension, bronchospasm and angio-oedema; but there are few reports of deaths reliably attributed to these reactions. The incidence of these reactions varies from 3-54% depending on manufacturer, refinement, dose and route of administration. *The vast majority of early anaphylactic antivenom reactions are not immediate type I hypersensitivity reactions but result from complement activation by IgG aggregates present in the antivenom.* Adrenaline (epinephrine) 0.1% (1 in 1000) should be given subcutaneously or intramuscularly in a dose of 0.5-1.0 ml for adults, 0.01 mg/kg for children. This should be followed by an intravenous injection of an H_1 antagonist (antihistamine) such as chlorpheniramine maleate (10 mg for adults, 0.2 mg/kg for children).

Pyrogenic reactions, which result from pyrogen contamination of the antivenom during manufacture, begin 1-2 hours after treatment. There is an initial chill with cutaneous vasoconstriction, gooseflesh and shivering. Temperature rises sharply during the rigors and there is intense vasodilatation, widening of the pulse pressure and eventual fall in mean arterial pressure. In children, febrile convulsions may occur at the peak of the fever. Patients should be laid flat to prevent postural hypotension. Their temperature should be reduced by fanning, tepid sponging and antipyretic drugs such as paracetamol (15 mg/kg) given by mouth, suppository or via nasogastric tube.

Late (serum sickness type) reactions occur 5-24 (average 7) days after treatment. The higher the dose of antivenom, the higher the incidence, the greater the severity and the shorter the interval before symptoms appear. There is itching, urticaria, fever, arthralgia, proteinuria and sometimes neurological symptoms. Antihistamines are used for milder attacks, but in severe cases, including those with neurological symptoms, a short course of prednisolone should be given.

D. ANCILLARY TREATMENT
1. Treatment of local envenoming

Although most local effects of snakebite are attributable directly to cytolytic and other activities of the venom itself, the bite may introduce bacteria and the risk of local infections greatly increases if the wound has been incised with an unsterile instrument or tampered with in some other way. The pattern of bacterial flora may vary in different countries[173]. It is appropriate to give prophylactic antimicrobials and a booster dose of tetanus toxoid. The wound should be cleaned with antiseptic. Blisters and bullae should be aspirated to dryness with a fine sterile needle rather than allowing them to rupture. Snake bitten limbs should be nursed in the most comfortable position. The wound should be examined frequently for evidence of necrosis: blistering, blackening or depigmentation of the skin, loss of sensation and a characteristic smell of putrefaction. Necrotic tissue should not be left to slough spontaneously but should be debrided by a surgeon under general or local anaesthesia as soon as possible to reduce the risk of secondary infection and to promote eventual healing. Skin appearances may be deceptive, for necrosis can undermine apparently normal skin. Large areas may be denuded of skin; recovery can be accelerated by applying split skin grafts immediately after debridement provided that the wound is not infected. Debrided tissue, serosanguinous discharge and pus should be cultured and the patient treated with appropriate antimicrobials. Fluctuant areas, suggestive of an underlying abscess, should be aspirated and opened for drainage.

Severe pain, especially in the lower leg, may indicate an intracompartmental syndrome or thrombosis of a major artery. Fasciotomies are performed far too readily by many surgeons impressed by tensely swollen limbs, pale, tight, cool skin and difficulty in palpating peripheral arteries. These clinical signs may be misleading; the limb may be cool only because of the insulating layer of extravasated fluid; normal arterial flow may be detectable with a doppler ultrasound probe and measurement of intracompartmental pressure may reveal reassuringly normal pressures, well below the figure of 45 mmHg (60 cmH_2O) associated with a high risk of ischaemic necrosis. Fasciotomy may be disastrous if it is performed while the patient's blood is still incoagulable and there is severe thrombocytopenia. Animal studies showed that fasciotomy was not effective in saving envenomed muscles[86]. Provided that adequate antivenom treatment is given as soon as possible after the bite, fasciotomy is rarely if ever needed. However, bites involving the finger pulps are frequently complicated by necrosis. Expert surgical advice should be sought, especially if the thumb or index finger is involved.

Arterial thrombosis is a rare complication, of viper bites (eg *Daboia russelii*). It should be suspected in a patient who rapidly developed severe pain in a limb with a sharply demarcated cold distal area and arterial pulses that were undetectable by doppler. Cerebral artery thrombosis has also been described. Once any haemostatic abnormality had been corrected, this could be investigated by arteriography and the possibility of angioplasty, thrombectomy or reconstructive arterial surgery considered.

2. Haemostatic abnormalities

Once adequate doses of antivenom have been given to neutralize venom antihaemostatic factors, recovery of normal haemostatic function may be accelerated by giving fresh whole blood, fresh frozen plasma, cryoprecipitates or platelet concentrates. *Heparin and antifibrinolytic agents should not be used.*

3. Neurotoxic envenoming

The airway must be protected in patients developing bulbar and respiratory paralysis. Once secretions begin to pool in the pharynx, a cuffed endotracheal tube should be introduced. Mechanical ventilation is usually required for only a few days but patients have recovered after 10 weeks of mechanical ventilation and 30 days of manual ventilation by ambu bag or anaesthetic bag. Antivenoms cannot be relied upon to reverse neurotoxicity or prevent its progression to respiratory paralysis.

Anticholinesterases: Neuromuscular blockade by post-synaptic neurotoxins may be partly overcome by the use of anticholinesterase drugs. For example, in this region, these drugs have been used successfully to treat patients envenomed by cobras (*Naja naja*[48], *N. philippinensis*[174], *N. kaouthia*[89] and kraits *B. caeruleus*[175], *B. candidus*[75]).

All patients with neurotoxic symptoms should be given a "Tensilon" (edrophonium) test as in the case of patients with suspected myasthenia gravis. Atropine sulphate (0.6 mg for adults, 50 µg/kg for children) is given by intravenous injection to block the muscarinic effects of acetylcholine. This is followed by edrophonium chloride (10 mg in adults, 0.25 mg/kg in children) by slow intravenous injection. The response should be assessed objectively. Those who respond convincingly can be maintained on neostigmine, methyl sulphate and atropine sulphate.

4. Hypotension and shock

Specific antivenom can reverse the direct myocardial and vasodilating effects of some venoms, but in patients who have leaked large amounts of blood and plasma into the bitten limb and elsewhere, a plasma expander is needed to correct hypovolaemia. The foot of the bed should be raised in an attempt to improve cardiac filling while an intravenous infusion is set up. Central venous pressure should be monitored to prevent fluid overload. Other causes of hypotension, such as a massive concealed haemorrhage or an autopharmacological effect of the venom, should be considered. In victims of Russell's viper in Burma and India, acute pituitary/adrenal insufficiency may develop as a result of haemorrhagic infarction of the anterior pituitary as in Sheehan's syndrome. In these cases, hypoglycaemia should be corrected with intravenous 50% glucose and hydrocortisone should be given[50,87].

5. Renal failure

Acute renal failure may be caused by haemorrhage, ischaemia resulting from hypotension, disseminated intravascular coagulation and renal vasoconstriction, pigment nephropathy caused by haemoglobinuria, direct nephrotoxicity and immune complex glomerulonephritis caused by serum sickness reactions. Renal failure is a common feature of Russell's viper bites, but can occur in patients severely envenomed by any species. If the urine output falls below 400 ml in 24 hours, central venous pressure should be monitored and a urethral catheter inserted. Cautious rehydration with isotonic fluid (to increase the central venous pressure to +10 cmH$_2$O) can be followed by high dose frusemide (up to 100 mg intravenously) and finally dopamine (2.5 µg/kg/minute) by continuous infusion into a central vein. If these measures fail to increase urine output, patients should be managed conservatively until dialysis is indicated.

E. SNAKE VENOM OPHTHALMIA

The four species of cobra in this region which commonly "spit" their venom (*N. philippinensis, N. samarensis, N. sputatrix* and *N. sumatranus*) can cause intense conjunctivitis with a risk of corneal erosions, complicated by secondary infection, anterior uveitis and even permanent blindness. First aid treatment consists of irrigating the eye or other affected mucous membrane as soon as possible using large volumes of water or any other available bland fluid. Unless a corneal abrasion can be excluded by slit lamp examination or fluorescein staining, the patient should be treated as for a corneal injury with a topical antimicrobial agent (tetracycline and chloramphenicol). Topical or systemic antivenom treatment is not indicated. 0.5% adrenaline eye drops are said to relieve the burning sensation instantaneously.

F. TREATMENT OF BITES BY PARTICULAR SPECIES IN ASIA
1. Colubridae

Antivenom is available for the treatment of bites by only two species of Asian colubrid - *Rhabdophis tigrinus* and *R. subminiatus* ("anti-yamakagashi" made by the Japan Snake Institute ([176] no 112). Venom extracted from the Duvernoy's glands of *R. tigrinus* was toxoided with formalin and used to immunise rabbits. In three patients who developed spontaneous systemic bleeding from the gums, gastrointestinal and urinary tracts and subcutaneously with coagulopathy, there was a rapid resolution of these effects of envenoming after intravenous administration of 10-20 ml of anti-yamakagashi antivenom intravenously[177-179]. If this antivenom were not available, or if systemic symptoms developed after envenoming by other species of colubrid, conservative treatment should aim at the control of bleeding and prevention of renal failure. ***Heparin should not be used.*** Platelets and clotting factors can be replenished, but since the procoagulant venom factors from the venom may persist for days or even weeks, patients may continue to bleed. Exchange transfusion has been used in cases of *R. tigrinus* envenoming before the advent of antivenom, with some success[180].

2. Elapidae
a. Bungarus

Polyspecific antivenoms are available covering *B caeruleus, B ceylonicus* and *B fasciatus* ([176] no 78) and *B. caeruleus* and *B. fasciatus* ([176] nos 67 & 80) and there are monospecific antivenoms for *B. caeruleus* ([176] nos 70, 73 & 74) and *B fasciatus* ([176] nos 91, 97 & 103). Antivenoms for *B. multicinctus* are manufactured in Taiwan ([176] no 100) and Shanghai ([176] no 107). Mortality from *B. caeruleus* bites was 77% before the introduction of specific antivenom[69], but in a series of 17 cases of *B. caeruleus* envenoming in India, 90-430 ml of Haffkine polyspecific antivenom was found to be "very effective". Only two patients (12%) died but the speed of response in the remainder was not mentioned[71]. In another series from India, 20 patients who awoke in the morning with paralytic symptoms and were presumed to have been bitten by *B. caeruleus* were given doses of 100 ml of Haffkine antivenom on admission, after six hours and again within the first 24 hours[72]. There was "demonstrable recovery" within 3-8 hours and "full recovery" within 12-36 hours in 15 patients. The other five died within two hours of admission (apparently mechanical ventilation was not attempted). This more rapid response may be attributable to the adjunctive use of anticholinesterase, but the response to these drugs has been very variable in patients envenomed by *Bungarus* species. Patients envenomed by *B. caeruleus* in India[181] and Sri Lanka[51], by *B. candidus* in western Malaysia[75] and by *B. ceylonicus*[52] did not respond, but there was definite improvement in cases of neurotoxic envenoming by *B. candidus* in Thailand[75] and *B. caeruleus* in India[175]. These differences may be explicable by the relative proportion of pre- and post-synaptic neurotoxins injected in the particular case or to the timing of treatment in relation to the evolution or recovery from the effects of these two types of neurotoxins. In four cases of proven *B. caeruleus* neurotoxic envenoming in Sri Lanka, treatment with 100-340 ml of Haffkine polyvalent antivenom cleared venom antigenaemia within 15 minutes to one hour in all cases but the clinical response was not impressive[51]. Convincing improvement in the neurological signs was not seen until 24 hours after the start of antivenom treatment (Figures 45a & b). Another patient bitten in Sri Lanka showed no response to an initial dose of 50 ml of Haffkine antivenom and was ventilated for 18 hours, receiving a total dose of 100 ml of antivenom[182].

It is worth trying the "Tensilon" test in all patients with neurotoxic envenoming. Bulbar and respiratory function must be carefully monitored. Patients should be intubated once their secretions begin to pool in the pharynx, and ventilation should be assisted if respiratory failure develops. A mechanical ventilator is not essential; one patient with severe envenoming by *B. multicinctus* was cured after 30 days of manual ventilation[183].

b. Calliophis

CRI Kasauli "polyvalent snake venom antiserum" ([176] no 67) and "monovalent krait venom antiserum" ([176] no 70) are said to have "probable" activity against Indian *Calliophis* species. In the only reported case of fatal neurotoxic envenoming[9] the patient's life could almost certainly have been saved with assisted ventilation.

c. Maticora

No specific antivenom is available. The rare deaths could probably have been prevented by assisted ventilation.

d. Naja

For envenoming by the Chinese cobra (*N. atra*) the National Institute of Preventive Medicine in Taiwan manufactures a *Naja-Bungarus* bivalent and *Naja* monovalent antivenom ([176] nos 100 and 102). Two patients with severe systemic symptoms after *N atra* bites in Taiwan showed improvement 2-6 hours after treatment with 40 and 100 ml of antivenom[80]. Apparently, most patients in Taiwan do not visit hospitals after snakebites and so antivenom treatment has not been widely used[39]. It is interesting that, on the Chinese mainland, no antivenom is manufactured for the treatment of cobra envenoming. One hundred and twenty-six cases treated with local trypsin, with or without other drugs, but apparently not treated with antivenom, recovered with not more than two deaths[86].

For bites by the monocellate cobra (*N. kaouthia*) the Thai Red Cross Society manufactures a monospecific antivenom ([176] no 89), the Industry and Pharmaceutical Corporation Yangon, Burma, manufactures a monospecific and bispecific antivenom ([176] nos 86 & 85) and CRI Kasauli, India, manufactures a "monovalent cobra venom antiserum" ([176] no 69). In Reid's series of 47 patients with cobra bites in western Malaysia (mostly caused by *N. kaouthia*)[88], four patients were treated with Thai Red Cross *Naja* monospecific antivenom and six with Haffkine polyspecific in doses of 20-150 ml. "Neither antivenom appeared to prevent or ameliorate local necrosis. In systemic poisoning improvement followed, but it was not dramatic"[88]. Five patients bitten by *N. kaouthia* near Bangkok who developed neurotoxic symptoms were treated with 40-60 ml of (presumably) Thai Red Cross antivenom. All showed improvement in their neurotoxic symptoms within 30 minutes and complete recovery by two hours but three went on to develop local necrosis[172]. In Bangkok, 39 children, presumed to have been bitten by *N. kaouthia*, developed respiratory paralysis. Mechanical ventilation could be stopped 1-21 hours after starting antivenom and the patients appeared neurologically normal 2-23 hours after antivenom. The dose of Thai Red Cross antivenom ranged from 30-340 (average about 160) ml[89]. In Samut Prakan Province, Thailand, the large amounts of antivenom required (up to 600 ml) suggested that Thai Red Cross antivenom was not particularly effective in neutralizing the neurotoxic effects of *N. kaouthia* venom even when it was given by the intravenous route soon after the bite[29]. In the 1980s, a group of physicians at Chulalongkorn Hospital, Bangkok, believed that antivenom treatment was ineffective and possibly harmful, and chose to treat their patients conservatively with mechanical ventilation, forced diuresis and ancillary drugs. However, in a group of 37 patients treated in this way, 16 (46%) developed tissue necrosis requiring grafting in 14 cases, an incidence and severity far higher than in patients treated with antivenom[184].

Ptosis responded dramatically to edrophonium chloride treatment in two patients thought to have been envenomed by *N. kaouthia*[189].

Envenoming by Indian spectacled cobras (*N naja*)
A number of antivenoms are available ([176] nos 67-69, 73, 75, 78, 80, 81 & 120). There have been no critical studies of the efficacy of antivenom treatment in *N naja* envenoming. The much lower mortality of cobra bites (8.4%) than krait bites (78.1%) at a time when only specific cobra antivenom was available suggested marked efficacy[69] but, in the 1970s, continuing high mortalities from neuroparalytic envenoming encouraged the search for ancillary treatments[48]. Addition of neostigmine was claimed to reduce the mortality from 77.4 to 4.2% in patients with neurotoxic envenoming[48]. In Sri Lanka, 300 ml of Haffkine polyspecific antivenom eliminated venom antigenaemia, but there was no convincing response in neurotoxic signs[51].

Antivenoms for Oxus cobra (*N. oxiana*) envenoming are manufactured in Iran ([176] nos 60 & 61), Pakistan ([176] nos 80 & 81) and the Russian Federation ([176] nos 140, 142, 144, 146 & 147). Efficacy has not been tested clinically.

Antivenom for Philippine cobra (*N. philippinensis*) envenoming is manufactured in the Philippines ([176] no 99). In a study of eight patients with neurotoxic envenoming, 20, 50 or 100 ml of Philippine cobra antivenom failed to produce marked improvement within two hours. Edrophonium was significantly more effective than antivenom at increasing the duration of upward gaze and either completely reversed or markedly decreased paralysis in every patient[185].

No specific antivenom is produced for envenoming by the Thai spitting cobra (*N. siamensis*) although paraspecific activity is claimed for Thai Red Cross cobra antivenom ([176]no 89). For Javan and Sunda Island spitting cobra (*N sputatrix*) envenoming, a polyvalent and monospecific antivenom is produced by Perum Bio Farma, Bandung ([176] nos 95 & 98). Their clinical efficacy has not been tested.

For envenoming by the Sumatran/Malay spitting cobra (*N. sumatrana*) one monospecific antivenom is available ([176] no 131). This antivenom, raised against "Malayan *N. n. sputatrix*" (= *N. sumatrana*) venom was effective against *N sumatrana* venom from Malaysia but was ineffective against *N. kaouthia* venom from Thailand and *N. naja* venoms from India and Sri Lanka (RDG Theakston, unpublished observations). In one of Reid's patients envenomed by a yellow cobra (*N. sumatrana*), there was neurological improvement one hour after the infusion of 100 ml of Haffkine polyspecific antivenom had been completed[88].

a. Ophiophagus
Several polyspecific antivenoms are claimed to have paraspecific activity against the venom of the king cobra (*O. hannah*) ([176] nos 6, 67, 78 & 89), but only one antivenom is raised against the venom of this species (Thai Red Cross king cobra antivenin [176] no 90).

Several studies have shown a lack of cross-neutralization between antivenoms raised against venoms of *Naja* species and *O. hannah* but, in one study, mice were protected against 8-10 $LD_{50}s$ of *O. hannah* venom by Iranian *N oxiana*, Australian tiger snake and death adder antivenoms, Thai *N kaouthia* antivenom and Australian sea snake antivenoms[186]. The enormous volumes of specific antivenom (up to 1150 ml) used to treat several of the reported cases may be explained by the large amount of venom injected, by the low potency of the antivenom or by administration of excessive volumes of antivenom before a clinical response could reasonably be expected. Those faced with the rare problem of treating cases of envenoming by this species should be encouraged by the recovery of several reported patients with severe envenoming. Conservative treatment of respiratory and circulatory failure can be life-saving. If specific *O. hannah* antivenom is not available, cobra antivenom or preferably tiger snake or death adder antivenom would be worth giving in the hope of paraspecific activity[94].

b. Walterinnesia

Specific antivenom is available on request from the Department of Zoology, Tel Aviv University ([176] no 58) and paraspecific activity is claimed for South African Institute for Medical Research polyvalent antivenom ([176] no 6) (see chapter on African and Middle Eastern snakes).

4. Viperidae

a. Azemiops

No specific antivenom is available.

b. Cerastes

See chapter on African and Middle Eastern snakes.

c. Daboia

No specific antivenoms have been prepared against the venoms of *D. r. formosensis* (Taiwan), *D. r. limitis* (Indonesia) or *D. r. pulchella* (Sri Lanka).

For the treatment of Indian *D r russelii* envenoming, a variety of polyspecific, bispecific and monospecific antivenoms are available, manufactured by CRI, Kasauli ([176] nos 67, 68 & 71), Haffkine ([176] nos 73 & 76), SII Pune ([176] nos 78 & 79) and in Pakistan ([176] nos 80 & 83). No formal studies of the clinical efficacy of antivenom has been published but, in India, the high mortality of *Echis* bites (32.8%) compared to Russell's viper bites (11.3%), at a time when only antivenom specific for Russell's viper was available, has been cited as evidence of the efficacy of this treatment[69]. However, the high mortality (54.2%) of "hospitalised patients presenting haemorrhagic snake venom poisoning and treated by conventional methods of antivenin therapy with supportive whole blood transfusion" has been used as an argument for ancillary treatment with heparin[48].

In Sri Lanka, 21 patients with proven systemic envenoming by *D. r. pulchella* were treated with 50-200 ml of Haffkine polyspecific antivenom[50]. Mean venom antigenaemia fell from 375 to 104 ng/ml six hours after the first dose of antivenom but was permanently cleared in only one patient. In the remainder there was persistent or recurrent antigenaemia up to seven days after the bite[50]. There was no dramatic reversal of neurotoxic signs after antivenom treatment and blood coagulability was restored between one and 25 hours after the first dose of antivenom. This Haffkine antivenom, raised against the venom of Indian *D. r. russelii*, has a variable reputation in Sri Lanka but, although some have found it rapidly effective, doses of up to 530 ml have proved necessary and doses of 450 ml have failed to correct the haemostatic defect[50]. In the standard mouse assay, the ED_{50} of two batches of

Haffkine antivenom against Sri Lankan *D. .r pulchella* venom was 59.9 and 31.3 µl/mouse and for two batches of IPC Yangon Burma antivenom was 80.6 and 85.2 µl/mouse[50].

For *D. r. siamensis* envenoming in Burma, a highly effective antivenom is manufactured by Industry and Pharmaceutical Corporation, Yangon, Burma ([176] nos 85 & 87). In mouse assays, the IPC Yangon monospecific Russell's viper antivenom was very effective against venom from Burmese, Thai and Indian Russell's viper venoms (ED$_{50}$s 2.3, 2.0 and 1.1 µl/mouse)[50]. In Burma, this antivenom was effective clinically in restoring blood coagulability and stopping spontaneous bleeding[17]. However, it seemed relatively ineffective in preventing the development of renal failure even in cases where it was given 60 minutes after the bite[17,34].

The Thai Red Cross Society manufactures a monospecific *D. r. siamensis* antivenom ([176] no 92). In Prachinburi, Thailand, 41 patients who developed incoagulable blood 15 minutes to 10 hours after the bite were treated with 20-440 ml of this antivenom. The initial dose was 10-20 ml, repeated hourly until the blood became coagulable. This usually happened within 6-10 hours, and so a dose of 60-100 ml of antivenom was usually sufficient, but in an exceptional case whose blood remained incoagulable for 50 hours, 440 ml of antivenom were given[115]. At Manorom, Thailand, five patients who had an abnormal clot quality test and evidence of systemic bleeding were given 20-50 ml of Thai Red Cross antivenom intravenously at 3-8 hour intervals until normal clot quality had been restored and bleeding had stopped[116]. Forty to 80 ml were required over 9½-12 hours. This antivenom is currently in short supply. If it were not available, IPC Yangon antivenom would be a highly effective alternative treatment judging by the results of mouse assays[50].

No specific antivenom for Russell's viper envenoming is manufactured in China, but in Guangxi "antivenom (5000 units/ampoule) was injected intravenously into four patients"[36]. Efficacy is not mentioned and there are no published studies of antivenom treatment. Seventeen cases were treated by local injection of trypsin and ancillary drugs with not more than two fatalities[86].

Ancillary treatment is extremely important in patients with severe systemic envenoming by Russell's vipers. Relatively normal levels of antithrombin III in victims of envenoming provide a theoretical basis for ancillary treatment with heparin although this would be potentially dangerous by enhancing the bleeding tendency. Preliminary studies of early low dose heparin treatment have been carried out in Burma[187]. Shock should be treated by correcting hypovolaemia with a plasma expander. Intravenous dopamine (2-15 µg/kg/minute) was effective in some refractory cases in Burma, but naloxone and methylprednisolone were not effective[34]. Acute pituitary adrenal insufficiency should be suspected (especially in Burma and India) if shock is associated with severe headache, deterioration in consciousness and neurological signs of hypoglycaemia such as extensor posturing. In these cases glucose and hydrocortisone should be given intravenously[115]. Renal failure is the commonest severe manifestation and cause of death in Russell's viper victims throughout the geographical range. Less than one-third of patients who develop oliguria are likely to respond to conservative measures such as rehydration, diuretics and dopamine, but peritoneal dialysis, usually for only 72 hours, has been effective in reducing the mortality of acute renal failure from 80% to less than 20% in Rangoon and to 15% in Colombo[17]. In patients with haemoglobinuria or myoglobinuria, renal damage may be prevented by correcting hypovolaemia and acidosis and improving urine output with an intravenous infusion of mannitol and bicarbonate. Patients with neuromyotoxicity (Sri Lanka and possibly India) should be carefully observed in hospital in case they develop bulbar and respiratory paralysis requiring endotracheal intubation and mechanical ventilation. Anticholinesterases are not effective[50]. Patients with symptoms of chronic pituitary insufficiency after Russell's viper bite should be investigated and, if necessary, treated with hormone replacement[113].

d. Echis

The variability of composition and immunogenicity of *Echis* venoms throughout their geographical range has been increasingly recognised over the past 20 years. However, national antivenom manufacturers may not have taken account of this intra- and inter-species variability in choosing an appropriately pooled venom for immunization. In India, where two species (*E. carinatus* in the south and *E. sochureki* in the north) are now recognised, polyspecific and monospecific antivenoms are manufactured by CRI Kasauli, Haffkine and SII Pune ([176] nos 67, 72, 73, 77-79). No formal studies of antivenom efficacy have been published from the areas of India and Sri Lanka where *E. carinatus* occurs, but in the Deogad area of Ratnagiri District, Maharashtra State, India, Haffkine polyspecific antivenom in doses of 10-30 ml given by slow intravenous injection produces rapid cessation of pain and bleeding[121]. Among 300 cases, only three developed limited local necrosis and four died. Before the advent of antivenom treatment, the mortality from *Echis* bites in this area was very high[119].

E. sochureki occurs in Iraq, Iran, Afghanistan, Pakistan and northern India. Antivenoms which seem likely, geographically, to be raised against the venom of this species are manufactured in Iran ([176] nos 60 & 62), Pakistan ([176] nos 80 & 84) and possibly in India. However, in a salutary case of severe envenoming by a 74 cm long *E. sochureki* from Pakistan, 160 ml of Haffkine polyspecific antivenom had little or no effect on the coagulopathy[122]. In mouse assays, Behringwerke "Near and Middle East polyvalent" antivenom ([176] no 129), which is raised against *Echis* venom from East Africa and Pakistan, was as effective in neutralizing haemorrhage and prothrombin activation as Razi Institute, Iran polyvalent and Haffkine polyvalent antivenoms. However, in the patient, 100 ml of Behringwerke antivenom seemed to have little effect on the bleeding and clotting problems[122]. In Jammu, in the north of India, Bhat treated 293 patients with viperine envenoming (mostly attributable to *E. sochureki*) with CRI Kasauli polyvalent antisnake venom serum in an initial dose of 20 ml by slow intravenous injection, repeated every 4-6 hours until the blood coaglation time had returned to normal[99]. In 120 patients, the bleeding and clotting defect was corrected in 24 hours with 60-120 (average 80) ml of antivenom. In the remaining patients doses of 120-270 ml of antivenom, together with blood transfusion, were needed and correction of the bleeding and clotting defect took up to four days.

E. multisquamatus occurs in Uzbekistan, Turkmenistan, Iran, Tajikistan, Afghanistan and Pakistan. On geographical grounds, antivenoms manufactured in the Russian Federation ([176] nos 140, 143 146), Iran ([176] nos 60 & 62) and Pakistan ([176] nos 80 & 84) might be expected to have some specificity, but no studies have been reported.

e. Eristocophis

No specific antivenom is available.

f. Pseudocerastes

Mono- and poly-specific antivenoms are manufactured in Iran ([176] nos 60, 63 & 64) but no studies of clinical efficacy have been published.

g. Vipera

For envenoming by the Middle Eastern mountain vipers of the *Vipera xanthina* complex, specific antivenoms are manufactured for *V. latifii* in Iran ([176] nos 63 & 64) and *V. xanthina* in Iran ([176] no 60) and Europe ([176] nos 126, 129 & 134). No clinical studies have been reported. For *V. berus* envenoming, a number of polyspecific antivenoms are manufactured in Europe ([176] nos 117, 123-126, 132, 134-136, 139). Their efficacy against venoms of Asian *V. berus* is unknown. For *V. lebetina* envenoming, a number of mono- and poly-specific antivenoms are available. For the Asian area, polyspecific and monospecific antivenoms are manufactured in Iran ([176] nos 60, 63, 64), Pakistan ([176] nos 80 & 83), the Russian Federation ([176] nos 140, 141, 145, 147). Since geographical variation in the venom's antigenicity and composition can be expected, it would be wise to choose an antivenom raised against venoms from the appropriate country. The few case reports of bites by this species contain little information about the efficacy of antivenom. For *V. ursinii* envenoming, polyspecific antivenoms are manufactured in Europe ([176] nos 126, 132, 134). Their efficacy against the venom of Asian *V. ursinii* is unknown.

h. Agkistrodon

For envenoming by *A. b. blomhoffii* in Japan, a number of locally manufactured mono- and poly-specific antivenoms are available ([176] nos 109-111, 113-115). In Japan, there are now very few fatalities despite an estimated more than 1,000 bites per year. In mild or moderately envenomed cases, 20 ml of antivenom appears effective, although swelling may progress after treatment, pain and oedema subside in 7-10 days[124]. One patient died with haemorrhage and pulmonary oedema despite being given an initial dose of 20 ml of antivenom three hours after the bite and 120 ml altogether. In China, the Shanghai Vaccine and Serum Institute manufactures a monospecific antivenom for *A. blomhoffii brevicaudus* ([176] no 105). Five hundred and thirty patients were treated in Jiangsu and Zhejiang, with 5-20 (usually 10) ml of antivenom[125]. The mortality was 1.1%. Most physical signs disappeared or were relieved in 1-3 days and in some within 3-5 hours, but neurotoxic symptoms (blurred vision, dyplopia and ptosis) persisted in some patients. In most patients local swelling subsided within three days but in 45 it continued to extend after antivenom treatment. In Jiangsu, mortality from *A. blomhoffii brevicaudus* bites had fallen from 3-5% in the pre-antivenom era (1959-1971) to 0.62% in 1972-73, after introduction of antivenom treatment[125].

No specific antivenom is manufactured for the treatment of envenoming by the Central Asian pit viper (*A. halys*) or the Himalayan pit viper (*A. himalayanus*). In Iran, polyspecific and monospecific antivenom is manufactured against the venom of *A. intermedius* ([176] nos 60 & 66). Clinical efficacy has not been reported. For two of the three mamushis (*A. saxatilis* and *A. ussuriensis*) found in Korea (and elsewhere) no specific antivenoms are manufactured. In 14 patients treated with antivenin (Crotalidae) polyvalent from Wyeth Laboratories, U.S. "a more rapid cessation of systemic symptoms and a reduction in limb oedema was obvious". In Wonju, South Korea, 15 of 82 cases of mamushi bite were treated with Wyeth polyvalent antivenin given up to six days after the bite. There were four deaths and 14 cases of crippling deformity including nine amputations[127]. This Wyeth antivenom ([176] no 11) is raised against *Crotalus* and *Bothrops* venoms but is claimed to neutralize "other Agkistrodon species". Japanese *A b blomhoffii* antivenom ([176] no) is said to neutralise the venom of the Korean mamushis. No antivenoms are available for treatment of envenoming by *A. shedaoensis, A. monticola* or *A. strauchi*.

i. Calloselasma

Mono- and a poly-specific antivenom for treatment of *C. rhodostoma* envenoming are manufactured in Thailand and Bandung, Indonesia ([176] nos 93-96). The Thai Red Cross Society monospecific antivenom has been produced in Bangkok since 1939. It was evaluated clinically by Reid and his colleagues in western Malaysia[135,137]. Fifty to 100 ml of this antivenom restored blood coagulability permanently in all but one of the 23 patients treated, but smaller doses (10-20 ml) appeared to be ineffective. At Trang in southern Thailand, a randomized comparative trial of three monospecific antivenoms (Thai Red Cross Society (TCRS), Thai Government Pharmaceutical Organisation (TGPO) and Twyford Pharmaceutical). was carried out in 4-6 patients with proven bites by *C. rhodostoma* whose blood was incoagulable on admission to hospital[138]. TGPO and Twyford antivenoms rapidly and permanently restored blood coagulability, but TRCS antivenom failed to do so in two out of 15 cases. The greatest increase in plasma fibrinogen concentration during the first 24 hours after treatment was in the TGPO group. In parallel laboratory assays, TRCS antivenom was significantly inferior to the other two in anti-lethal potency, TGPO was superior in anti-haemorrhagic and anti-necrotic potency and Twyford antivenom was superior in anti-procoagulant and anti-defibrinogenating potency. Clinical efficacy of these antivenoms against local necrosis remains equivocal. An initial dose of 5 ampoules of TGPO or Twyford antivenoms was recommended for treatment of systemic envenoming by *C. rhodostoma*. The case fatality rate for *C rhodostoma* envenoming is low, but deaths have been attributed to cerebrovascular accidents, shock, tetanus, septicaemia and anaphylaxis[76]. The severe local envenoming typical of bites by this species can contribute to shock (through hypovolaemia) and tetanus and septicaemia from secondary infection of the necrotic wounds. Oropharyngeal swabs and venom samples from freshly captured specimens of *C. rhodostoma* in southern Thailand yielded a variety of bacteria including gram negative rods (eg Enterobacter and Pseudomonas species), Staphylococci and Clostridia[173]. Prophylaxis with a combination of gentamicin and benzylpenicillin was recommended for bites by this species. Ancillary treatment of severe envenoming by *C. rhodostoma* should include circulating volume repletion, assessment of intracompartmental pressure, especially if the bite is on the lower leg, and early debridement and grafting of necrotic areas of skin[166]. Prednisolone and epsilon aminocaproic acid were tested in western Malaysia and found to be ineffective[188,189].

j. Deinagkistrodon

Monospecific antivenoms for *D agkistrodon* envenoming are manufactured in Taiwan and Shanghai ([176] nos 104, 106 & 108). One hundred and eleven patients bitten by *D. acutus* were treated in Fujian Province using traditional remedies including "Wuyashan brand drug for curing snakebites" and "Fujian-made drug for curing snakebites"[139]. In a group of 95 patients "mainly treated" with these remedies, the cure rate was 94%, but 17-19% developed necrotic ulcers at the site of the bite. It is not clear how many of the patients received antivenom although this treatment was recommended for "emergency treatment in severe or lethal cases"[139]. In Guangxi, 29 patients, 11 with severe envenoming, were treated with 1-4 ampoules of antivenom[36]. The outcome is not mentioned. Three of the fatal cases had not received antivenom[36]. In another study, five patients were treated by local injection of trypsin, apparently with good results[86]. In Kaohsiung, Taiwan, two patients stopped bleeding and showed improvement in coagulopathy after being given 20 and 40 ml of monospecific antivenom but local necrosis of the wound was not prevented[80]. The clinical effects of envenoming are similar to those caused by *C. rhodostoma* and similar ancillary treatments are recommended.

k. Hypnale

No specific antivenom is available but paraspecific activity is claimed for SII, Pune polyvalent antisnake venom serum ([176] no 78 & 79). In Sri Lanka, where bites by *H. hypnale* are common, most patients seek traditional ayurvedic treatment. SII or Haffkine polyspecific antivenoms are used in some hospitals but there is no evidence of efficacy and it would be surprising if these antivenoms had any neutralizing activity against *H. hypnale* venom, for the venoms used in their production do not include any species of the subfamily Crotalinae[142]. In the absence of specific antivenom, ancillary treatment may be needed for the rare cases of bleeding coagulopathy and acute renal failure.

l. Ovophis

No specific antivenoms are available for the treatment of envenoming by *O. chaseni, O. monticola* or *O. okinavensis*. In Japan, some patients are treated with habu (*T. flavoviridis*) antivenom.

m. Trimeresurus

Three polyspecific antivenoms manufactured in the U.S. and India are claimed to have paraspecific activity against *Trimeresurus* species ([176] nos 11, 78 & 79), but the only available antivenom raised against (Thai) *T. albolabris* venom is the Thai Red Cross Society (TRCS) "green pit viper antivenin" ([176] no 88). In Thailand, an initial dose of 50 ml of this antivenom was given by intravenous infusion to 11 patients with incoagulable blood[152]. Venom antigen was no longer detectable in serum one hour after the start of treatment in nine of the patients and blood coagulability was restored after a median of five hours. In the two patients with the highest serum venom antigen levels on admission, antigenaemia was still detectable 48 and 72 hours after antivenom, but blood coagulability was restored after six and two hours. In three patients there was recurrent venom antigenaemia associated with a fall in fibrinogen concentration, increased FDP and deteriorating clot quality 1-12 hours after initial clearance of antigenaemia. Further doses of antivenom were required to a total of 100-150 ml[152]. In a group of 72 children with "viper bites" treated in Chulalongkorn Hospital, Bangkok, the snake responsible had been identified as a green pit viper (*T. albolabris* or *T. macrops*) in 29 cases[153]. The author concluded that TRCS monospecific green pit viper antivenom in doses of 10-70 (average 24) ml was ineffective[153]. In another study in Bangkok, 60 patients envenomed by "green pit vipers" were treated with 60, 80 or 160 ml of antivenom or no antivenom. Antivenom produced a significant increase in the speed of restoration of normal blood clotting and the authors recommended 40 ml as the minimal therapeutic dose[190]. Ancillary treatment with heparin is not recommended[152] and, in the absence of specific antivenom, the use of clotting factors is likely to result in only transient increase in plasma fibrinogen concentration. Local necrosis is an uncommon complication.

For patients envenomed by *T. elegans* in Japan, no specific antivenom is available. Habu (*T. flavoviridis*) antivenom is used, but has poor neutralising activity.

No antivenoms are available for the treatment of envenoming by *T. cantori*, *T. erythrurus* or *T. flavomaculatus*.

Japanese habu (*T flavoviridis*) antivenom is manufactured in Japan ([176] no 109). In rabbits, this antivenom prevented death and local necrosis when given intramuscularly one or three hours after venom injection[191]. Most of the bitten patients are able to receive 20-40 ml of this antivenom by intravenous infusion within one hour of the bite. Ancillary treatment consists of vasopressor drugs in patients with hypotension and consideration of fasciotomy in patients with bites on the fingers or with evidence of anterior tibial compartment and other compartmental syndromes. The introduction of antivenom treatment in Japan in 1904 and improvements in general medical care have resulted in a decline in case fatalities, from more than 11% (1898-1903) in the Amami Islands and more than 18% in the Ryukyu Islands, to current levels of less than 1%[21].

There are no specific antivenoms for Indian *T. gramineus, T. macrolepis* and *T. malabaricus* envenoming, but paraspecific activity is claimed for two SII polyspecific antivenoms ([176] nos 78 & 79). No antivenoms are manufactured for *T. jerdonii* or *T. kanburiensis* bites. Envenoming by *T. macrops* is usually mild, but some venom of this species may be used (inadvertently!) in the production of TRCS "green pit viper" antivenom ([176] no 88) which is claimed also to neutralize "*T. popeiorum*" (=*T. macrops*) venom. A specific antivenom for *T. mucrosquamatus* is produced in Taiwan ([176] no 101) but not on the Chinese mainland. There are no reports of clinical efficacy. As with Japanese habu (*T. flavoviridis*) bites, local envenoming may be severe resulting in intracompartmental syndromes and raising the question of fasciotomy.

No specific antivenoms are available for treating bites by *T. popeiorum, T. puniceus* and *T. purpureomaculatus*. Envenoming by *T. purpureomaculatus* may be severe and life-threatening with bleeding and coagulopathy. Conservative treatment with clotting factors and platelets might be necessary but heparin should not be used.

Bites by *T. stejnegeri* are common in Taiwan and parts of mainland China. Specific antivenom is manufactured in Taiwan ([176] no 101). Clinical efficacy has not been reported. No antivenoms are available for the treatment of bites by *T. trigonocephalus* or *T. tokarensis*.

n. Tropidolaemus
No antivenom is available.

IX. REFERENCES

1. **WÜSTER W, OTSUKA S, MALHOTRA A, THORPE RS.** Population systematics of Russell's viper: a multivariate study. *Biol J Linnean Soc* **47**:97-113, 1992.
2. **GLOYD HK, CONANT R.** *Snakes of the Agkistrodon complex: a monographic review.* Oxford, Ohio, USA: Society for the study of amphibians and reptiles, 1990.
3. **VOGEL JP.** Indian serpent-lore or the Nagas in Hindu legend and art. London: Arthur Probsthain, 1926:
4. **ZHAO E-M, ADLER K.** *Herpetology of China.* Oxford, Ohio: Society for the Study of Amphibians and Reptiles, 1993.
5. **KUNTZ RE.** Snakes of Taiwan. *Quart J Taiwan Mus*; XVI (122), 1963.
6. **URAGODA CG.** *A history of medicine in Sri Lanka - from the earliest times to 1948.* Sri Lanka Medical Association, 1987.
7. **TORIBA M, SAWAI Y.** Venomous snakes of medicinal importance in Japan. In: Gopalakrishnakone P, Chou LM, eds. *Snakes of Medical Importance (Asia-Pacific Region).* National University Singapore,:323-347, 1990.
8. **VIRAVAN C, LOOAREESUWAN S, KOSAKARN W, et al.** A national hospital-based survey of snakes responsible for bites in Thailand. *Trans R Soc Trop Med Hyg*; **86**:100-106, 1992.
9. **KRAMER E.** Zur Schlangen fauna von Nepal. *Rev Suisse Zool*; **84 (3)**:721-761, 1977.
10. **WARRELL DA.** Tropical snakebite: clinical studies in Southeast Asia. In: Harris JB, Ed. *Natural Toxins. Animal, plant and microbial.* Oxford: Clarendon Press,:25-45, 1986.
11. **WÜSTER W, THORPE RS.** Systematics and biography of the Asiatic cobra *Naja naja* species complex in the Philippine Islands. In: Peters G, Hutterer R, eds. *Vertebrates in the tropics.* Bonn: Museum Alexander Koenig,:333-344, 1990.
12. **WÜSTER W, THORPE RS.** Asiatic cobras: systematics and snakebite. *Experientia*; **47**:205-209, 1991.
13. **WÜSTER W, THORPE RS.** Asiatic cobras: population systematics of the *Naja naja* species complex (Serpentes: Elapidae) in India and Central Asia. *Herpetologica*; **48 (1)**:69-85, 1992.
14. **WÜSTER W, THORPE RS.** Dentitional phenomena in cobras revisited: spitting and fang structure in the Asiatic species of *Naja* (Serpentes: Elapidae). *Herpetologica*; **48 (4)**:424-434, 1992.
15. **WÜSTER W, THORPE RS.** *Naja siamensis,* a cryptic species of venomous snake revealed by mt DNA sequencing. *Experientia*; **50**:75-79, 1994.
16. **YOUNG BA.** Morphological basis of "growling" in the king cobra, *Ophiophagus hannah. J Exper Zool*; **260**:275-287, 1991.
17. **WARRELL DA.** Snake venoms in science and clinical medicine 1. Russell's viper: biology, venom and treatment of bites. *Trans R Soc Trop Med Hyg*; **83**:732-740, 1989.
18. **WALL F.** A popular treatise on the common Indian snakes. Part V The Russell's viper *Vipera russelii. J Bombay Nat Hist Soc*; **18 (1)**:1-17, 1907.
19. **AUFFENBERG W, REHMAN H.** Studies on Pakistan reptiles. Pt 1 The genus *Echis* (Viperidae*). Bull Florida Mus Nat Hist Biol Sci*; **35 (5)**:263-314, 1991.
20. **NILSON G, ANDRÉN C.** *The mountain vipers of the Middle East - the Vipera xanthina complex (Reptilia, Viperidae).* Bonner Zoologische Monographien; 20, 1986.
21. **SASA M, TERUYA K, UCHIYAMA H, IWAI S.** Epidemiology of the poisonous snakebite in the Amami and the Ryukyu Islands. *Jap J Exper Med*; **29**:417-444, 1959.
22. **WARRELL DA, LOOAREESUWAN S, STIMSON AF, HUTTON RA.** Rediscovery and redefinition of Malcolm Smith's *Trimeresurus kanburiensis* in Thailand, with a report of envenoming. *Trans R Soc Trop Med Hyg*; **86**:95-99, 1992.
23. **WARRELL DA.** Dark green pit viper bites (correspondence). *Am J Trop Med Hyg*; **42 (6)**:623-624, 1990.
24. **TUN-PE , BA-AYE , AYE-AYE-MYINT , TIN-NU-SWE , WARRELL DA.** Bites by Russell's vipers (*Daboia russelii siamensis* in Myanmar: effect of the snake's length and recent feeding on venom antigenaemia and severity of envenoming. *Trans R Soc Trop Med Hyg*; **85**:804-808, 1991.
25. **SWAROOP S, GRAB B.** Snakebite mortality in the world. *Bull WHO*; **10**:35-76, 1954.

26. **DE SILVA A.** The pattern of snake bite in Sri Lanka. *Snake*; **8**:43-51, 1976.

27. **BERNATZIK HA.** *The spirits of the yellow leaves*. London: Robert Hale, 1958.

28. **SAWAI Y, TORIBA M, ITOKAWA H, DE SILVA A, PERERA GLS, KOTTEGODA MB.** Study on deaths due to snakebite in Anuradhapura district, Sri Lanka. *The Snake*; **16**:7-15, 1984.

29. **VIRAVAN C, VEERAVAT U, WARRELL MJ, THEAKSTON RDG, WARRELL DA.** ELISA confirmation of acute and past envenoming by the monocellate Thai cobra (*Naja kaouthia*). *Am J Trop Med Hyg*; **35 (1)**:173-181, 1986.

30. **HO M, WARRELL MJ, WARRELL DA, BIDWELL D, VOLLER A.** Review. A crtical reappraisal of the use of enzyme-linked immunosorbent assays in the study of snake bite. *Toxicon*; **24 (3)**:211-221, 1986.

31. **REID HA, LIM KJ.** Sea-snakebite. A survey of fishing villages in north-west Malaya. *BMJ*; **2**:1266-1272, 1957.

32. **FAYRER J.** The venomous snakes of India and the mortality caused by them. *BMJ*; **2**:620, 1892.

33. **ALI Z, BEGUM M.** Snake bite - a medical and public health problem in Pakistan. In: Gopalakrishnakone P, Chou LM, eds. *Snakes of Medical Importance (Asia-Pacific region)*. National University Singapore,:447-461, 1990.

34. **MYINT-LWIN, WARRELL DA, PHILLIPS RE, TIN-NU-SWE, TUN-PE , MAUNG-MAUNG-LAY.** Bites by Russell's viper (*Vipera russelii siamensis*) in Burma: haemostatic, vascular and renal disturbances and response to treatment. *Lancet*; **ii**:1259-1264, 1985.

35. **ZHAO E.** Venomous snakes of China. In: Gopalakrishnakone P, Chou LM, eds. *Snakes of Medical Importance (Asia-Pacific Region)*. National University Singapore,243-268, 1990.

36. **SAWAI Y, KAWAMURA Y, TORIBA M, et al.** An epidemiological study on the snakebites in Guangxi Zhuang autonomous region, China in 1990. *Snake*; **24**:1-15, 1992.

37. **SAWAI Y, TSENG CS.** Snakebites in Taiwan Paper VI-2. In: de Vries , Kochva , eds. *Toxins of animal and plant origin.*:985-991, 1973.

38. **REID HA, THEAN PC, MARTIN WJ.** Epidemiology of snake bite in North Malaya. *BMJ*; **1**:992-997, 1963.

39. **SAWAI Y, KOBA K, OKONOGI T, et al.** An epidemiological study of snakebites in Southeast Asia. *Jap J Exper Med*; **42 (3)**:283-307, 1972.

40. **LIM B-L.** Venomous land snakes of Malaysia. In: Gopalakrishnakone P, Chou LM, eds. *Snakes of medical importance (Asia-Pacific region)*. National University Singapore:387-417, 1990.

41. **TORIBA M.** Venomous snakes of medical importance in Korea. In: Gopalakrishnakone P, Chou LM, eds. *Snakes of medical importance (Asia-Pacific region)*. National University Singapore,:377-386, 1990.

42. **KOPSTEIN F.** *Bungarus javanicus*, een nieuwe Javaansche giftslang. Mededeelling over een doodelijke Bungarus-beet. *Gneeskunde Tijdschrift Nederland-Indies*; **LXXII**:136-140, 1932.

43. **LATIFI M.** *The snakes of Iran*. Oxford, Ohio: Society for the Study of Amphibians and Reptiles, 1991:

44. **SMITH MA.** *The fauna of British India, Ceylon and Burma, including the whole of the Indo-Chinese sub-region. Reptilia and Amphibia Vol III - Serpentes*. London: Taylor & Francis, 1943:

45. **WHO .** Zoonotic Disease Control. Baseline epidemiological study on snake-bite treatment and management. *Wkly Epidem Rec*; **42**:319-320, 1987.

46. **TOMARI T.** An epidemiological study of the occurrence of Habu snake bite on the Amami Islands, Japan. *Int J Epidemiol*; **16 (3)**:451-461, 1987.

47. **DE SILVA A.** Venomous snakes, their bites and treatment in Sri Lanka. In: Gopalakrishnakone P, Chou LM, eds. *Snakes of medical importance*. National University Singapore:479-556, 1990.

48. **BANERJEE RN.** Poisonous snakes of India, their venoms, symptomatology and treatment of envenomation. In: Ahuja MMS, ed. *Progress in Clinical Medicine*. New Delhi: Arnold-Heinemann, 136-179, 1978.

49. **REID HA, THEAN PC, CHAN KE, BAHAROM AR.** Clinical effects of bites by Malayan viper *Ancistrodon rhodostoma*. *Lancet*; **1**:617-621, 1963.

50. **PHILLIPS RE, THEAKSTON RDG, WARRELL DA, et al.** Paralysis, rhabdomyolysis and haemolysis caused by bites of Russell's viper (*Vipera russelii pulchella*) in Sri Lanka: failure of Indian (Haffkine) antivenom. *QJM*; **68 (257)**:691-716, 1988.

51. **THEAKSTON RDG, PHILLIPS RE, WARRELL DA, ET AL.** Envenoming by the common krait (*Bungarus caeruleus*) and Sri Lankan cobra (*Naja naja naja*): efficacy and complications of therapy with Haffkine antivenom. *Trans R Soc Trop Med Hyg*; **84 (2)**:301-308, 1990.

52. **DE SILVA A, MENDIS S, WARRELL DA.** Neurotoxic envenoming by the Sri Lankan krait (*Bungarus ceylonicus*) complicated by traditional treatment and a reaction to antivenom. *Trans R Soc Trop Med Hyg*; **87**:682-684, 1993.

53. **MATHER HM, MAYNE S, McMONAGLE TM.** Severe envenomation from "harmless" pet snake. *BMJ*; **1**:1324-1325, 1978.

54. **ZOTZ RB, MEBS D, HIRCHE H, PAAR D.** Hemostatic changes due to the venom gland extract of the red-necked keelback snake (*Rhabdophis subminiatus*). *Toxicon*; **29 (12)**:1501-1508, 1991.

55. **CABLE D, McGEHEE W, WINGERT WA, RUSSELL FE.** Prolonged defibrination after a bite from a "non-venomous" snake. *JAMA*; **251 (7)**:925-926, 1984.

56.   **SMEETS REH, MELMAN PG, HOFFMANN JJML, MULDER AW.** Case report. Severe coagulopathy after a bite from a "harmless" snake (*Rhabdophis subminiatus*). *J Int Med*; **230**:351-354, 1991.

57.   **HOFFMANN JJML, VIJGEN M, SMEETS REH, MELMAN PG.** Haemostatic effects *in vivo* after snakebite by the red-necked keelback (*Rhabdophis subminiatus*). *Blood Coag & Fibrinolysis*; **3**:461-464, 1992.

58.   **MITTLEMAN MB, GORIS RC.** Envenomation from the bite of the Japanese colubrid snake *Rhabdophis tigrinus* (Boie). *Herpetologica*; **30** (2):113-119, 1974.

59.   **MANDELL F, BATES J, MITTLEMAN MB, LOY JW.** Major coagulopathy and "non-poisonous" snake bites. *Pediatrics*; **62** (2):314-317, 1980.

60.   **MITTLEMAN MB, GORIS RC.** Death caused by the bite of the Japanese Colubrid snake Rhabdophis tigrinus (Boie) (Reptilia, Serpentes, Colubridae). *J Herpetol*; **12 (1)**:109-111, 1978.

61.   **OGAWA H, SAWAI Y.** Fatal bite of the yamakagashi (*Rhabdophis tigrinus*). *The Snake*; **18**:53-54, 1986.

62.   **DE SILVA A, ALOYSIUS DJ.** Moderately and mildly venomous snakes of Sri Lanka. *Ceylon Med J*; **28 (3)**:118-127, 1983.

63.   **WHITAKER R.** Slight reaction from bites of the near-fanged snakes *Boiga ceylonensis* (Gunther) and *Dryophis nasutus* (Lacepede). *J Bombay Nat Hist Soc*; **67**:113, 1970.

64.   **BURGER WL.** A case of mild envenomation by the mangrove snake *Boiga dendrophila*. *The Snake*; **76**:99-100, 1974.

65.   **MAMONOV G.** Case report of envenomation by the mountain racer *Coluber ravergieri* in USSR. *The Snake*; **9**:27-28, 1977.

66.   **D'ABREU E.A.** . Effect of a bite from Schneider's water snake (*Hypsirhina enhydris*). *J Bombay Nat Hist Soc*; **xxii**:203, 1913.

67.   **PERRY G.** Mild toxic effects resulting from the bites of Jan's desert racer, *Coluber rhodorachis*, and Moila's snake, *Malpolon moilensis* (Ophidia: Colubridae). *Toxicon*; **26 (6)**:523-524, 1988.

68.   **WATT G, PADRE L, TUAZON ML, THEAKSTON RDG, LAUGHLIN L.** Bites by the Philippine cobra (*Naja naja philippinensis*): prominent neurotoxicity with minimal local signs. *Am J Trop Med Hyg*; **39 (3)**:306-311, 1988.

69.   **AHUJA ML, SINGH G.** Snake bite in India. *Indian J Med Res*; **42 (4)**:661-686, 1954.

70.   **DE SILVA A.** Snakebites in Anuradhapura District. *The Snake*; **13**:117-130, 1981.

71.   **HATI AK, SAHA SG, BANERJEE D, BANERJEE S, PANDA D.** Clinical features of poisoning by common kraits and treatment with polyvalent antivenin. *The Snake*; **20**:140-143, 1988.

72.   **SAINI RK, SINGH S, SHARMA S, RAMPAL V, MANHAS AS, GUPTA VK.** Snake bite poisoning presenting as early morning neuroparalytic syndrome in jhuggi dwellers. *J Assoc Physns India*; **34 (6)**:415-417, 1986.

73.   **FAYRER J.** Deaths from snakebites; a trial condensed from the sessions' report. *Indian Med Gaz*; **iv**:156-157, 1869.

74.   **REID HA.** Symptomatology, pathology and treatment of land snake bite in India and Southeast Asia. In: Bücherl W, Buckley EE, Deulofeu V, eds. *Venomous animals and their venoms.* New York: Academic Press,611-642, 1968.

75.   **WARRELL DA, LOOAREESUWAN S, WHITE NJ, et al.** Severe neurotoxic envenoming by the Malayan krait *Bungarus cnadidus* (Linnaeus): response to antivenom and anticholinesterase. *BMJ*; **286**:678-680, 1983.

76.   **LOOAREESUWAN S, VIRAVAN C, WARRELL DA.** Factors contributing to fatal snake bite in the rural tropics: analysis of 46 cases in Thailand. *Trans R Soc Trop Med Hyg*; **82**:930-934, 1988.

77.   **KARALLIEDDE LD, SANMUGANATHAN PS.** Respiratory failure following envenomation. *Anaesthesia*; **43**:753-754, 1988.

78.   **MAUNG-MAUNG-AYE** . Some experience in the management of snake-bite. *Burma Med J*; **20**:33-40, 1972.

79.   **BADER A.** *Bisse durch nicht einhermische Giftschlangen.* Inaugural Dissertation for the degree of Doctor of Medicine. Frankfurt am Main: Johann Wolfgang Goethe-Universität, 1976.

80.   **KUO T-P, WU C-S.** Clinicopathological studies on snake bites in Taiwan. *The Snake*; **4**:1-22, 1972.

81.   **HAILE NS.** The snakes of Borneo, with a key to the species. *Sarawak Mus J Kuching*; **8**:743-771, 1958.

82.   **HARRISON JL.** The bite of a blue Malaysian coral snake or ular matahari. *Malayan Nature Journal*; **11**:130-132, 1957.

83.   **LIM-LEONG-KENG F, LEE-TAT-MONG M.** *Fascinating snakes of Southeast Asia - an introduction.* Kuala Lumpur: Tropical Press,107, 1989.

84.   **JACOBSON E.** A case of snake-bite (*Maticora intestinalis*). *Bull Raffles Mus*; **13**:77-79, 1937.

85.   **WALL AJ.** *Indian snake poisons, their nature and effects.* London: WH Allen & Co, 1883.

86.   **XIONG YL, ZOU RJ, YE ZZ, CHEU XL.** Experimental studies on treatment of Viperidae snake bite with trypsin. *Yao Hsueh Hsueh Pao*; **14 (7)**:385-388, 1979.

87.   **MAUNG-MAUNG-AYE.** *Snakes of Burma with venomology and envenomation.* Rangoon: Arts & Science University, 1976.

88. **REID HA.** Cobra bites. *BMJ*; **2**:540-545, 1964.
89. **MITRAKUL C, DHAMKRONG AT, FUTRAKUL P, ET AL.** Clinical features of neurotoxic snake bite and response to antivenom in 47 children. *Am J Trop Med Hyg*; **33 (6)**:1258-1266, 1984.
90. **TRISHNANANDA M, OONSOMBAT P, DUMAVIBHAT B, YONGCHAIYUDHA S, BOONYAPISIT V.** Clinical manifestations of cobra bite in the Thai farmer. *Am J Trop Med Hyg*; **28 (1)**:165-166, 1979.
91. **SAWAI Y, HONMA M.** *Snake bites in India*.451-460, 1976.
92. **WALL F.** *The poisonous terrestrial snakes of our British Indian Dominians (including Ceylon) and how to recognize them with symptoms of snake poisoning and treatment.* 3rd ed. Bombay: Natural History Society, 1913.
93. **KOPSTEIN F.** *De Javaansche gifslangen en haar beteekenis voor den mensch.* Weltevreden: Visser, 1930:
94. **SHATTOCK FM.** Injuries caused by wild animals. *Lancet*; **1**:412-415, 1968.
95. **TIN-MYINT, RAI-MRA, MAUNG-CHIT, TUN-PE, WARRELL DA.** Bites by the king cobra (*Ophiophagus hannah*) in Myanmar: successful treatment of severe neurotoxic envenoming. *QJM*; **80 (293)**:751-762, 1991.
96. **CHEN H-C, LAI Y-H, TSAI J-H.** Acute renal failure following Russell's viper envenomation: a report of two cases. *Kaohsiung J Med Sci*; **4 (8)**:467-472, 1988.
97. **WANG Y-M, LU P-J, HO C-L, TSAI I-H.** Characterization and molecular cloning of neurotoxic phospholipases A2 from Taiwan viper (*Vipera russelii formosensis*). *Eur J Biochem*; **209**:635-641, 1992.
98. **AUFFENBERG W.** The herpetofauna of Komodo, with notes on adjacent areas. *Bull Florida State Mus Biol Sci*; **25 (2)**:1-156, 1980.
99. **BHAT RN.** Viperine snake bite poisoning in Jammu. *J Indian Med Ass*; **63**:383-392, 1974.
100. **EAPEN CK, CHANDY N, KOCHUVARKEY KL, ZACHARIA PK, THOMAS PJ, IPE TI.** Unusual complications of snake bite: hypopituitarism after viper bites. In: Ohsaka A, Hayashi K, Sawai Y, eds. *Animal, plant and microbial toxins.* New York: Plenum ,467-473, 1976.
101. **EAPEN CK, CHANDY N, JOSEPH JK.** A study of 1000 cases of snake envenomation. In*: XI International Congress of Tropical Medicine* & Malaria. Calgary: 1984.
102. **MATTHAI TP, DATE A.** Acute renal failure in children following snake bite. *Ann Trop Paediat*; **1**:73-76, 1981.
103. **BASU J, MAJUMDAR G, DUTTA A, ET AL.** Acute renal failure following snake bite (viper). *J Assoc Physns India*; **25 (12)**:883-890, 1977.
104. **CHUGH KS, AIKAT BK, SHARMA BK, DASH SC, MATHEW MT, DAS KC.** Acute renal failure following snake bite. *Am J Trop Med Hyg*; **24 (4)**:692-697, 1975.
105. **SHASTRY JCM, DATE A, CARMAN RH, JOHNY KV.** Renal failure following snake bite. A clinicopathological study of nineteen patients. *Am J Trop Med Hyg*; **26 (5)**:1032-1038, 1977.
106. **DATE A, SHASTRY JCM.** Renal ultrastructure in acute tubular necrosis following Russell's viper envenomation. *J Pathol*; **137**:225-241, 1982.
107. **DATE A, PULIMOOD R, JACOB CK, KIRUBAKARAN MG, SHASTRY JCM.** Haemolytic-uraemic syndrome complicating snake bite. *Nephron*; **42**:89-90, 1986.
108. **THEIN-THAN, TIN-TUN, HLA-PE, et al.** Development of renal function abnormalities following bites by Russell's vipers (*Daboia russelii siamensis*) in Myanmar. *Trans Roy Soc Trop Med Hyg*; **85**:404-409, 1991.
109. **TIN-NU-SWE, TIN-TUN, MYINT-LWIN, et al.** Renal ischaemia, transient glomerular leak and acute renal tubular damage in patients envenomed by Russell's vipers (*Daboia russelii siamensis*) in Myanmar. *Trans R Soc Trop Med Hyg*; **87**:678-681, 1993.
110. **THAN-THAN, HUTTON RA, MYINT-LWIN, et al.** Haemostatic disturbances in patients bitten by Russell's viper (*Vipera russelii siamensis*) in Burma. *Brit J Haematol*; **69**:513-520, 1988.
111. **THAN-THAN, KHIN-EI-HAN, HUTTON RA, et al.** Evolution of coagulation abnormalities following Russell's viper bite in Burma. *Brit J Haematol*; **65**:193-198, 1987.
112. **THAN-THAN, FRANCIS N, TIN-NU-SWE, et al.** Contribution of focal haemorrhage and microvascular fibrin deposition to fatal envenoming by Russell's viper (*Vipera russelii siamensis*) in Burma: clinicopathological studies. *Acta Tropica, Basel*; **46**:23-28, 1989.
113. **TUN-PE, PHILLIPS RE, WARRELL DA, et al.** Acute and chronic pituitary failure resembling Sheehan's syndrome following bites by Russell's viper in Burma. *Lancet*; **ii**:763-767, 1987.
114. **COCKRAM CS, CHAN JC, CHOW KY.** Bites by the white-lipped pit viper (*Trimeresurus albolabris*) and other species in Hong Kong. A survey of 4 years' experience at the Prince of Wales Hospital. *J Trop Med Hyg*; **93 (2)**:79-86, 1990.
115. **KANJANAJATANEE J, VISUTIPANT S.** Russell's viper bite: clinical manifestations and treatment. *Thai Med Council Bull*; **13 (1)**:25-38, 1984.
116. **MITRAKUL C, JUZI U, PONGRUJIKORN W.** Antivenom therapy in Russell's viper bite. *Am J Clin Pathol*; **95 (3)**:412-417, 1991.

117. **MAHASANDANA S, RUNGRUXSIRIVORN Y, CHANTARANGKUL V.** Clinical manifestations of bleeding following Russell's viper and green pit viper bites in adults. *SE Asian J Trop Med Pub Hlth*; **11** (2):285-293, 1980.

118. **SITPRIJA V, BOONPUCKNAVIG V.** Snake venoms and nephrotoxicity. In: Lee CY, ed. *Snake Venoms. Handbook of Experimental Pharmacology.* Berlin: Springer-Verlag,:997-1018, 1979.

119. **WARRELL DA, ARNETT C.** The importance of bites by the saw-scaled or carpet viper (*Echis carinatus*). Epidemiological studies in Nigeria and a review of the world literature. *Acta Tropica, Basel*; **33 (4)**:307-341, 1976.

120. **WHITAKER R.** Snake bite case histories. *J Bombay Nat Hist Soc*; **70 (2)**:382-387, 1974.

121. **WHITAKER R.** Miscellaneous notes. Notes on bites by the saw-scaled viper, *Echis carinatus* in the Deogad area of Ratnagiri district, Maharashtra. *J Bombay Nat Hist Soc*; **67 (2)**:335-337, 1970.

122. **WEIS JR, WHATLEY RE, GLENN JL, RODGERS GM.** Prolonged hypofibrinogenemia and protein C activation after envenoming by *Echis carinatus sochureki*. *Am J Trop Med Hyg*; **44 (4)**:452-460, 1991.

123. **SHAW CJ.** Notes on the effect of the bite of McMahon's viper (*E macmahonii*). *J Bombay Nat Hist Soc*; **30**:485-486, 1925.

124. **TATENO I, SAWAI Y, MAKINO M.** Current status of Mamushi snake (*Agkistrodon halys*) bite in Japan with special reference to severe and fatal cases. *Jap J Exper Med*; **33 (6)**:331-346, 1963.

125. **SHANGHAI VACCINE & SERUM INSTITUTE.** *Agkistrodon halys* bite treated with specific antivenin. Observation of 530 cases. *Chinese Med J*; **2 (1)**:59-62, 1976.

126. **MOORE TC.** Snakebite from the Korean pit viper. *Mil Med*; **142 (7)**:546-549, 1977.

127. **SAWAI Y, LAH K-Y.** Snakebites in South Korea. *Snake*; **9**:38-47, 1978.

128. **SUN-KINSHEN.** Successful treatment of 9 cases of respiratory paralysis caused by Pallas pit viper bite. *Chinese Med J*; **94 (9)**:624, 1981.

129. **MEISSNER A, HAUSMANN B, LINN C, ET AL.** Defibrierungssyndrom nach Schlangenbissverletzungen. *Deutsche med Wschr*; **114**:1484-1487, 1989.

130. **CHEN Y-C.** Venomous snake bites and snake venom research in China. In: Gopalakrishnakone P, Chou LM, eds. *Snakes of Medical Importance (Asia-Pacific Region).* National University Singapore,:269-279, 1990.

131. **SOH C-T, MIN H-K, BAE S-K, IM S-C, KIM S-K.** Current status of snakebite in Korea. *Yonsei Reports on Trop Med*; **9 (1)**:48-56, 1978.

132. **SAWAI Y.** Snakebites by Korean Mamushi in Japan. *Snake*; **7**:40-41, 1975.

133. **ZHAO E-M, WU G, YANG W.** Comparisons of toxicity and neutralization test among Pallas' viper, Snake-island pit viper and black eye-brow pit viper. *Acta Herpetologica Sinica*; **1 (3)**:1-6, 1979.

134. **KAWAMURA Y, SAWAI Y, JIANG K.** Comparative potency of antivenoms against Japanese and Chinese mamushi venoms. *Snake*; **17**:82-83, 1985.

135. **REID HA, THEAN PC, MARTIN WJ.** Epidemiology of snake bite in North Malaya. *BMJ*; **1**:992-997, 1963.

136. **REID HA, THEAN PC, CHAN KE, BAHAROM AR.** Clinical effects of bites by Malayan viper (*Ancistrodon rhodomstoma*). *Lancet*; **I**:617-621, 1963.

137. **REID HA, CHAN KE, THEAN PC.** Prolonged coagulation defect (defibrination syndrome) in Malayan viper bite. *Lancet*; **I**:621-626, 1963.

138. **WARRELL DA, LOOAREESUWAN S, THEAKSTON RDG, et al.** Randomized comparative trial of three monospecific antivenoms for bites by the Malayan pit viper (*Calloselasma rhodostoma*) in southern Thailand: clinical and laboratory correlations. *Am J Trop Med Hyg*; **35 (6)**:1235-1247, 1986.

139. **JINGCHENG Z, DASHAN R.** 111 cases of snake-bite (*Agkistrodon acutus* Gunther) treated by combined traditional Chinese and Western medicine. *J Trad Chinese Med*; **2 (2)**:119-123, 1982.

140. **KOMORI Y, NIKAI T, SUGIHARA H.** Comparative study of *Agkistrodon acutus* venoms from China and Taiwan. *Comp Biochem Physiol*; **79 (1)**:51-57, 1984.

141. **SHEN M-C.** Afibrinogenemia and thrombocytopenia following crotalid snake bites in Taiwan. *J Formosan Med Ass*; **82**:239-244, 1983.

142. **DE SILVA A, WIJEKOON ASB, JAYASENA L, et al.** Haemostatic dysfunction and acute renal failure following envenoming by Merrem's hump-nosed viper (*Hypnale hypnale*) in Sri Lanka: first authenticated case. *Trans R Soc Trop Med Hyg*; **88**:209-212, 1994.

143. **DERANIYAGALA PEP.** *A coloured atlas of some vertebrates from Ceylon. Vol 3 Serpentoid Reptilia.* Colombo: Government Press, 1955.

144. **VARAGUNAM T, PANABOKKE RG.** Bilateral cortical necrosis of the kidney following snakebite. *Postgrad Med J*; **46**:449-451, 1970.

145. **PERUMAINAR M.** Pathogenesis of microclots formation following viper bites. *Sri Lanka Assoc Adv Sci* 1975; (abstract).

146. **PERUMAINAR M.** Renal damage following hump-nosed viper bite. *Sri Lanka Assoc Adv Sci* 1975; (abstract).

147. **PERUMAINAR M.** Clinical manifestations following hump-nosed viper bites. In: *SLMA 90th Anniversary Sessions.* SLMA, 10, 1977.

148. **DHARMARATNE L, GUNAWARDENA U.** Generalised bleeding tendency and acute renal failure following Merrem's hump-nosed viper bite. *J Ceylon Coll Physns*; **21**:37-42, 1988.

149. **HAILE NS.** Snake bites man: two recent Borneo cases. *Sarawak Mus J*; **11 (21-22)**:291-298, 1963.

150. **KWONG YL, CHAN GTC.** Coagulation problems in pit viper bite. *J Hong Kong Med Assoc*; **40 (3)**:210-212, 1988.

151. **SUGANO H, SAWAI Y.** A case of mild envenomation by the Hime-habu, *Trimersurus okinavensis* Boulenger. *Snake*; **14**:143-144, 1982.

152. **HUTTON RA, LOOAREESUWAN S, HO M, et al.** Arboreal green pit vipers (genus Trimersurus) of Southeast Asia: bites by *T albolabris* and *T macrops* in Thailand and a review of the literature. *Trans R Soc Trop Med Hyg*; **84**:866-874, 1990.

153. **MITRAKUL C.** Clinical features of viper bites in 72 Thai children. *SE Asian J Trop Med Pub Hlth*; **13 (4)**:628-636, 1982.

154. **KEEGAN HL, YOSHINO K.** *Trimeresurus elegans* (Gray 1849), the Sakishima habu, a venomous pit viper from the Ryukyu Islands. *Am J Trop Med Hyg*; **8 (2)**:124-133, 1959.

155. **MAUNG-MAUNG-AYE.** Venomous snakes of medical importance in Burma. In: Gopalakrishnakone P, Chou LM, eds. *Snakes of medical importance (Asia-Pacific region)*. National University Singapore,:211-241, 1990.

156. **TAYLOR EH.** *The snakes of the Philippine Islands*. Manila: Monog Bureau Sci, 1922.

157. **SAWAI Y, KAWAMURA Y, EBIHARA I, OKONOGI T, HOKAMA Z, YAMAKAWA M.** Studies on the improvement of treatment of habu (*Trimeresurus flavoviridis*) bites: 6. Habu bites on the Amami and Ryukyu Islands in 1964. *Jap J Exper Med*; **37**:51-61, 1967.

158. **WHITAKER R.** Pit viper (*Trimeresurus macrolepis* Beddome) bites at a South Indian tea estate. *J Bombay Nat Hist Soc*; **70 (1)**:207-208, 1973.

159. **VISUDHIPHAN S, TONMUKAYAKUL A, TUMLIANG S, DUMAVIBHAT B, DIANKIJAGUM A.** Dark green pit viper (*Trimeresurus popeorum*) bite: clinical and serial coagulation profiles in 51 cases. *Am J Trop Med Hyg*; **41 (5)**:570-575, 1989.

160. **TWEEDIE MWF.** *The snakes of Malaya. 3rd ed*. Singapore National Printers, 1983.

161. **LIM B-L.** *Poisonous snakes of Peninsular Malaysia*. Malayan Nature Society & Institute for Medical Research, 1979.

162. **DE SILVA A.** *Trimeresurus trigonocephalus* bites. *The Snake*; **15**:91-94, 1983.

163. **BECCARI O.** *Wanderings in the great forests of Borneo*. London: Archibald & Constable, 1904.

164. **SAWAI Y.** Vaccination against snake bite poisoning. In: Lee C-Y, ed. *Snake Venoms*. Berlin: Springer-Verlag,881-897, 1979.

165. **WARRELL DA.** The global problem of snake bite: its prevention and treatment. In: Gopalakrishnakone P, Tan CK, eds. *Recent Advances in Toxinology Research Vol 1*. Venom & Toxin Research Group, National University of Singapore,121-153, 1992.

166. **WARRELL DA.** Treatment of snake bite in the Asia-Pacific region: a personal view. In: Gopalakrishnakone P, Chou LM, eds. *Snakes of medical importance (Asia-Pacific region)*. Singapore University Press,641-670, 1990.

167. **SUTHERLAND SK, COULTER AR, HARRIS RD.** Rationalisation of first-aid measures for elapid snakebite. *Lancet*; **I**:183-186, 1979.

168. **CURRIE B.** Pressure-immobilization first aid for snakebite - fact and fancy. XIII International Congress for Tropical Medicine and Malaria. Jomtien, Pattaya, Thailand 29 Nov-4 Dec 1992. *Toxicon*; **31 (8)**:931-932.(abstract), 1993.

169. **MALASIT P, WARRELL DA, CHANTHAVANICH P, et al.** Prediction, prevention and mechanism of early (anaphylactic) antivenom reactons in victims of snake bites. *BMJ*; **292**:17-20, 1986.

170. **CUPO P, AZEVEDO-MARQUES MM, DE MENEZES JP, HERING SE.** Reaçoes de hipersensitclidade imediats apó uso intravenoso de soros antivenenos: valor prognóstico dos testes de sensibilidade intradérmicos. *Rev Inst Med Trop Sao Paulo*; **33 (2)**:115-122, 1991.

171. **WHO.** *Progress in the characterization of venoms and standardization of antivenoms*. Geneva: WHO Offset Publications No 58, 1981.

172. **TRISHNANANDA M, YONGCHAIYUDHA S, CHAYODOM V.** Clinical observations on glucocorticoids in cobra envenomation. *SE Asian J Trop Med Pub Hlth*; **9 (1)**:71-73, 1978.

173. **THEAKSTON RDG, PHILLIPS RE, LOOAREESUWAN S, ECHEVERRIA P, MAKIN T, WARRELL DA.** Bacteriological studies of the venom and mouth cavities of wild Malayan pit vipers (*Calloselasma rhodostoma*) in southern Thailand. *Trans R Soc Trop Med Hyg*; **84**:875-879, 1990.

174. **WATT G, THEAKSTON RDG, HAYES CG, et al.** Positive response to edrophonium in patients with neurotoxic envenoming by cobras (*Naja naja philippinensis*). A placebo-controlled study. *NEJM*; **315**:1444-1448, 1986.

175. **RAMAKRISHNAN MR, SANKARAN K, GUPTA GD, CHANDRASEKAR S.** External ophthalmoplegia in Elapidae bites and its response to neostigmine. *Neurology India*; **23 (2)**:109-110, 1975.

176. **THEAKSTON RDG, WARRELL DA.** Antivenoms: a list of hyperimmune sera currently available for the treatment of envenoming by bites and stings. *Toxicon*; **29 (12)**:1419-1470, 1991.

177. **WAKAMATSU T, KAWAMURA Y, SAWAI Y.** A successful trial of yamakagashi antivenom. *Snake*; **18**:4-5, 1986.

178. **NOMURA T, NAGATA T, KAWAMURA Y, SAWAI Y.** A case of severe yamakagashi (*Rhabdophis tigrinus*) bite treated by antivenom. *Snake*; **21**:85-86, 1989.

179. **AKIMOTO R, WATANABE Y, SAKAI A, KAWAMURA Y, SAWAI Y.** A case of defibrination syndrome due to Japanese colubrid snake, yamakagashi (*Rhabdophis t tigrinus*) bite, treated with antivenom. *Snake*; **23 (1)**:36-39, 1991.

180. **MORI K, HISA S, SUZUKI S, et al.** A case of severe defibrination syndrome due to snake (*Rhabdophis tigrinus*) bite. *Japan J Clin Haematol*; **24 (3)**:256-262, 1983.

181. **SETHI PK, RASTOGI JK.** Neurological aspects of ophitoxemia (Indian krait) - a clinico-electromyographic study. *Ind J Med Res*; **73**:269-276, 1981.

182. **FERNANDO P, DIAS S.** A case report. Indian krait bite poisoning. *Ceylon Med J*; **27**:39-41, 1982.

183. **LIN-ZHEN-YAO, OU-MING.** The cure of a patient with respiratory paralysis for thirty days after *Bungarus multicinctus* bite. *New Traditional Chinese Medicine*; **4**:24 28, 1976.

184. **POCHANUGOOL C, LIMTHONGKUL S, MEEMANO K.** Clinical features of 37 non-antivenin treated neurotoxic snake bite patients. In: Gopalakrishnakone P, Tan CK, eds. *Progress in venom and toxin research*. Faculty of Medicine, National University Singapore,:46-51, 1987.

185. **WATT G, MEADE BD, THEAKSTON RDG, et al.** Comparison of Tensilon and antivenom for the treatment of cobra-bite paralysis. *Trans R Soc Trop Med Hyg*; **83**:570-573, 1989.

186. **MINTON SA.** Paraspecific protection by elapid and seasnake antivenins. *Toxicon*; **5 (1)**:47-55, 1967.

187. **MYINT-LWIN, TIN-NU-SWE, MYINT-AYE-MU, THAN-THAN, THEIN-THAN, TUN-PE.** Heparin therapy in Russell's viper bite victims with impending DIC (a controlled trial). *SE Asian J Trop Med Pub Hlth*; **20 (2)**:271-272, 1989.

188. **REID HA, THEAN PC, MARTIN WJ.** Specific antivenene and prednisone in viper-bite poisoning: controlled trial. *BMJ*; **2**:1378-1380, 1963.

189. **REID HA.** E-amino caproic acid and fibrinolysis in viper-bite defibrination. *Lancet*; **2**:5-7, 1965.

190. **MAHASANDANA S, RATANANDA S, KHUNPRAYOON S.** Antivenom treatment for green pit viper bite. In: *XI International Cognress for Tropical Medicine & Malaria*. Calgary, Canada. 1984.

191. **SAWAI Y, MAKINO M, MIYAZAKI S, et al.** Studies on the improvement of treatment of habu snake (*Trimersurus flavoviridis*) bites. 1. Studies on the improvement of habu snake antivenin. *Jap J Exper Med*; **31**:137-150, 1961.

Chapter 28

CLINICAL TOXICOLOGY OF SNAKEBITE IN AUSTRALIA AND NEW GUINEA

Julian White

TABLE OF CONTENTS

I. INTRODUCTION

Australia and New Guinea have developed a unique fauna as a result of prolonged isolation from other continents following the separation from Gondwanaland over 60 million years ago. Repeated glacial/ interglacial cycles during the Pleistocene have also exerted an effect on the evolution and distribution of fauna, both through climatic variation and changes in sea level, the latter also allowing successive waves of invaders via land bridges with adjacent Asia. These effects are most evident in the mammal fauna but Australia and New Guinea also have a very distinctive snake fauna, in part distinguished by a higher proportion of venomous species than any other continental region. In addition the significant venomous snakes are limited to the families Elapidae and Hydrophiidae, both closely related. There are no vipers native to this region. The Australian snakes and their cousins in New Guinea have evolved some of the most potent venoms and venom components of any snakes in the world and Australia is often characterized as home to the world's most dangerous snakes, particularly by Australians, many of whom are very aware of the hazards presented by this portion of their country's fauna. Yet despite the potency of these snake's venoms, snakebite is only an infrequent event in Australia, and death is rare. In New Guinea however snakebite is a significant medical problem.

II. EPIDEMIOLOGY OF SNAKEBITE IN AUSTRALIA AND NEW GUINEA

A. THE SNAKES: DISTRIBUTION, VENOMS, CHARACTERISTICS

Three families of venomous snakes are found in Australia and New Guinea: Colubridae, a few backfanged species only, none of which appear to cause significant envenoming in man (possible exception, the brown tree snake, *Boiga irregularis*); Hydrophiidae, the sea snakes, which are discussed in Chapter 13; Elapidae, the front fanged terrestrial snakes which dominate the Australian snake fauna, both in terms of numbers, and species. The rest of this Chapter will be limited to discussion of this group, with emphasis on those species known to cause dangerous envenoming in man.

Of the approximately 80 species of elapid snakes in Australia and New Guinea, at least 20 are large enough and have sufficiently potent venoms to severely envenom, or even kill man[1,2]. All have fangs at the front of the mouth, placed on maxillae with only limited rotation, thus limiting fang length[3]. In many the venom glands, situated in the upper jaw region posterior to the eye, are small and capable of producing only small quantities of venom. However this venom is often very potent and some Australian elapids produce the most toxic snake venoms known[4]. The toxicity and specific effects of the venom varies between species, but four principal effects are seen in human envenoming by these snakes, though not all are present in every venom[2,5]. These four toxin groups/ envenoming effects are: paralysis caused by neurotoxins (pre- and/or post-synaptic); coagulopathy caused mostly by potent procoagulants which induce defibrination, though in some species there are true anticoagulant toxins; muscle damage caused by myotoxins (phospholipases); renal damage/ failure the mechanisms for which are multifactorial, but may include direct nephrotoxins (not yet clearly demonstrated)[6].

The majority of the dangerous species are almost exclusively terrestrial and diurnal, although most will also be crepuscular, or even nocturnal, on hot summer nights[7,8]. The death adders (*Acanthophis* spp.) are unusual in several ways, and are the only dangerous snakes which are habitually active at night (also active during the day). Food items are quite variable, usually including a mix of both endo- and ecto-thermic prey. Habitats vary from the wet cool subtemperate regions of Tasmania in the south, through temperate woodland, semi-arid and arid scrub and desert, to tropical habitats in the north of Australia and in New

Guinea. Essentially no part of Australia is free of dangerous venomous snakes. Some species do not adjust well to habitat disturbance (eg death adders) while others have adapted to changing environments and are common in rural areas and even in metropolitan areas (eg brown snakes, *Pseudonaja* spp.). Recent changes in faunal structure may also affect snake populations as illustrated by the effect of the cane toad, *Bufo marinus*, an introduced species now expanding its range from Queensland, across the top of Australia and down the east coast. This toad has highly toxic skin secretions which kill most predators trying to eat the toad, including snakes. In addition the toad has a voracious appetite, eating many animals smaller than it, thus potentially decreasing the natural prey of venomous snakes. There is mounting opinion that in Queensland the effects of this toad have included a decline in the populations of most species of dangerous venomous snake, with the exception of the taipan, *Oxyuranus scutellatus*, a mammal feeder[9], with a consequent increase in the populations of this snake. As the taipan is the most dangerous snake in Australia such a change may affect the epidemiology of snakebite in coastal Queensland, with a possible increase in the proportion of bites developing severe envenoming.

The snakes considered dangerous to man are listed in Table 1, including scientific and common names, basic distribution, general habitat type, size, principle diagnostic features (scale counts), fang length, venom quantity (milking), venom toxicity, and principle venom effects in man. Several works are published on the biology, taxonomy and distribution of the venomous snakes of Australia and New Guinea and the reader is referred to these for further information[1,7,10,11,12]. Approximate distribution for some of the major species of Australian elapid snakes is shown in Figure 1, and representative species are shown in Figures 2 to 10.

B. SNAKEBITE IN AUSTRALIA

In common with most regions of the world, statistics on the incidence of snakebite in Australia are incomplete. Snakebite is not a notifiable disease and hospital records include cases listed as snakebite, yet without envenoming and probably due to some other cause/bite. Conversely, some cases of snakebite, especially fatal cases, may not be recognized as due to snakebite. Most authorities estimate that there are between 1,000 and 3,000 cases of snakebite in Australia annually, with an average of 2 fatalities[13,14,15]. Statistics on fatalities for each State are given in Table 2. Not surprisingly the most fatalities are recorded in the most populous states, particularly Queensland which has a large rural population in areas of relatively high snake density, including the taipan. Current evidence suggests that there has been a steady decline in the number of fatalities, both in absolute terms and relative to population increase[14]. The reasons for this include: (i) availability of high quality antivenoms; (ii) availability of intensive care units; (iii) sophisticated medical evacuation resources servicing even the most remote areas; (iv) incorporation of training on the management of snakebite in both medical and paramedical courses; (v) promotion of appropriate first aid techniques; (vi) a decrease in the number of individuals in high risk activities for snakebite due to declining rural populations and increasing mechanization.

Information on the epidemiology of snakebite related to particular species of snakes is not extensive.

It appears that brown snakes cause more bites and probably more deaths than any other species group, but this may just reflect the very wide distribution of these snakes and their ability to adapt to life in close association with man. The most common biting species will clearly vary from State to State and within each State, reflecting differences in local snake fauna. Information from South Australia is given in Table 3 while Table 4 lists the most likely species to cause snakebite in each State.

Table 1
Principal dangerous snakes of Australia and New Guinea

Scientific Name	Common Name	Distribution (1)	Habitat (2)	Size (3)	Scales (4)	Anals/subcaudals (4)
BROWN SNAKE GROUP						
Pseudonaja textilis	eastern brown snake	SA,QLD,NT,NSW,VIC,NG	A,SA,F,T,U	1.5m	17 rows	divided/45-75divided
Pseudonaja nuchalis	western brown snake, gwardar	SA,NT,WA,QLD,NSW	A,SA,F,T,U,	1.5m	17-19 rows	divided/50/70divided
Pseudonaja affinis	dugite	SA,WA	SA,F,U	1.5m	19 rows	divided/50-70divided
TIGER SNAKE GROUP						
Notechis scutatus	eastern tiger snake	SA,NSW,VIC,QLD	F,W,U	1.2m	17 rows	single/35-65single
Notechis ater	black tiger snake	SA,TAS,WA	SA,F,W,U	1.5m	17-19 rows	single/35-60single
Notechis a. occidentalis	western tiger snake	WA	F,W,U	1.2m	17-19 rows	single/35-50single
Tropidechis carinatus	rough scale snake	QLD,NSW	F,W,T	0.8m	23 rows	single/50-60single
Austrelaps superbus	common copperhead	SA,VIC,TAS	F,W,U	1.3m	15-17 rows	single/35-55single
Austrelaps labialis	Adelaide Hills copperhead	SA	F,W,U	0.7m	15-17 rows	single/35-55single
Austrelaps ramsayi	highlands copperhead	VIC,NSW	F,W	0.8m	15-17 rows	single/35-55single
BLACK SNAKE GROUP						
Pseudechis australis	mulga snake, king brown	WA,SA,QLD,NSW,NT,NG	A,SA,F,T	2m	17 rows	divided/50-75single>divided
Pseudechis porphyriacus	red bellied black snake	SA,VIC,NSW,QLD	F,W,T,U	1.5m	17 rows	divided/40-65single>divided
Pseudechis butleri	spotted mulga snake	WA	A,SA	1.6m	17 rows	divided/55-65single>divided
Pseudechis colletti	Colletts snake	QLD	A,SA	1.5m	19 rows	divided/50-70single>divided
Pseudechis guttatus	spotted black snake	QLD,NSW	F,W	1.5m	19 rows	divided/45-65single>divided
Pseudechis papuanus	Papuan black snake	NG	F,W,T	2.1m	19 rows	divided/45-75single>divided
DEATH ADDERS						
Acanthophis antarcticus	common death adder	WA,SA,VIC,NSW,QLD,NT,NG	A,SA,F,H,T	1m	21-23 rows	single/38-55single
Acanthophis pyrrhus	desert death adder	WA,SA,NT,QLD	A,SA	0.8m	21 rows	single/45-60single>divided
Acanthophis praelongus	northern death adder	WA,NT,QLD	SA,F	0.8m	19-23 rows	single/39-57single
TAIPANS						
Oxyuranus scutellatus	common taipan	QLD,NT,WA	F,W,T	2m	21-23 rows	single/45-80divided
Oxyuranus microlepidotus	inland taipan	SA,QLD,NT	A,SA	2m	23 rows	single/55-70divided
Oxyuranus S. canni	New Guinea taipan	NG	F,W,T	2m	21-23 rows	single/45-80divided
SMALL EYED SNAKE						
Micropechis ikaheka	small eyed snake	NG	F,W,T	2m		

KEY 1: SA=South Australia; QLD=Queensland; NT=Northern Territory; WA=Western Australia; NSW=New South Wales; VIC=Victoria; TAS=Tasmania; NG=New Guinea.
KEY 2: A=arid; SA=semi arid /bushland; F=forest; W=wetlands; T=tropical; H=New Guinea highlands; U=urban/semi urban areas.
KEY 3,4: Size=average adult length; Scales=mid body scale count; Anals=anal scale; Subcaudals=subcaudal scales number/if single or divided.

Table 1. (continued)
Principal dangerous snakes of Australia and New Guinea

Scientific Name	Fang Length (5)	Venom Quantity (6)	Mean Venom Injected (7)	Venom Toxicity LD$_{50}$ (8)	Principal Venom Actions (9)
BROWN SNAKE GROUP					
Pseudonaja textilis	2.8mm (2.0-4.0)	2-6mg(max 67mg)	4.5mg(0.03-9.10mg)	sc(mice) 0.053mg/kg	PC,PreN, ?K, ?C
Pseudonaja nuchalis	aprox. 2.5mm	aprox. 18mg	NA	sc(mice) 0.473mg/kg	PC, ?PreN, ?K, ?C
Pseudonaja affinis	aprox. 2.5mm	aprox. 18mg	NA	sc(mice) 0.660mg/kg	PC, ?PreN, ?k, ?C
TIGER SNAKE GROUP					
Notechis scutatus	3.5mm(2.0-5.5mm)	35mg(max 189mg)	12.7mg(1.1-31.9mg)	sc(mice) 0.118mg/kg	PreN, PostN, PC, M
Notechis ater	NA	23-75mg(max 388mg)	NA	sc(mice) 0.051-0.338mg/kg	PreN, PostN, PC, M
Notechis a. occidentalis	NA	35mg	NA	sc(mice) 0.194mg/kg	PreN, PostN, PC, M
Tropidechis carinatus	aprox. 2.5mm	6mg	6.0mg(0.23-22.57mg)	sc(mice) 1.36mg/kg	PreN, PostN, PC, M
Austrelaps superbus	3.3mm(3.0-4.5mm)	20mg(max 85mg)	NA	sc(mice) 0.560mg/kg	?PreN, ?PC, ?M
Austrelaps labialis	NA	NA	NA	NA	?PreN, ?PC, ?M
Austrelaps ramsayi	NA	NA	NA	NA	?PreN, ?PC, ?M
BLACK SNAKE GROUP					
Pseudechis australis	6.5mm	180mg(max 600mg)	61.6mg	sc(mice) 2.38mg/kg	M, AC, ?N
Pseudechis porphyriacus	4.0mm(3.5-5.0mm)	40mg(max 75mg)	1.3mg	sc(mice) 2.52mg/kg	M
Pseudechis butleri	NA	NA	NA	NA	? as for *P. australis*
Pseudechis colletti	NA	48mg	NA	sc(mice) 2.38mg/kg	M
Pseudechis guttatus	NA	32mg	NA	sc(mice) 2.13mg/kg	M
Pseudechis papuanus	NA	NA	NA	sc(mice) 1.09mg/kg	N, Bleeding (?PC, AC 0r H)
DEATH ADDERS					
Acanthophis antarcticus	6.2mm(5.0-8.3mm)	78mg(max 238mg)	36mg(3.4-99mg)	sc(mice) 0.400mg/kg	PostN
Acanthophis pyrrhus	NA	NA	NA	NA	?PostN
Acanthophis praelongus	NA	NA	NA	NA	?PostN
TAIPANS					
Oxyuranus scutellatus	7.9-12.1mm	120mg(max 400mg)	20.8mg(0.6-68.9mg)	sc(mice) 0.099mg/kg	PreN, PC, M
Oxyuranus microlepidotus	3.5-6.2mm	44mg(max 110mg)	17.3mg(0.7-45.6mg)	sc(mice) 0.025mg/kg	PreN, PC, ?M
Oxyuranus S. canni	NA	NA	NA	NA	PreN, PC, ?H, M
SMALL EYED SNAKE					
Micropechis ikaheka	NA	NA	NA	NA	?N, ?M

KEY 5: average adult fang length.
KEY 6: average dry weight of milked venom.
KEY 7: venom injected in experimental conditions.
KEY 8: toxicity of whole venom as LD$_{50}$ (sc=subcutaneous).
KEY 9: N=neurotoxin; PreN=presynaptic N; PostN=postsynaptic N; PC=procoagulant; AC=anticoagulant; H=haemorrhagin; M=myotoxin; K=nephrotoxin; C=cardiotoxin.

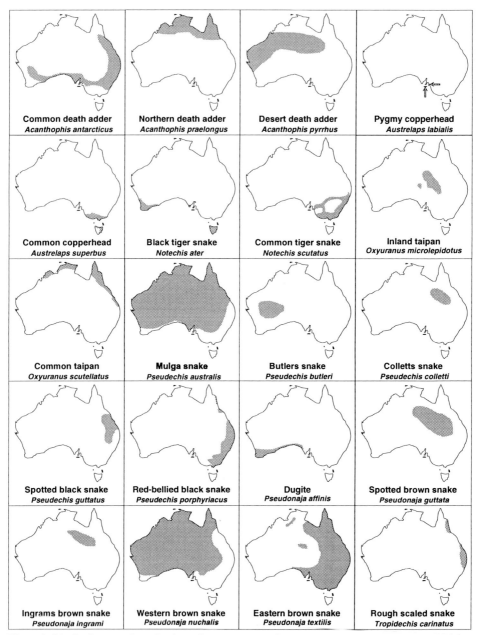

Figure 1: Distribution maps for major Australian venomous snakes.

C. SNAKEBITE IN NEW GUINEA

New Guinea, a large island immediately to the north of Australia, shares much of its fauna with Australia, including venomous snakes. Politically it is divided into two countries; the western half, West Irian, is politically part of Indonesia, while the eastern half is the principal component of the nation, Papua New Guinea (PNG). It is only for PNG that there is substantial published information on snakebite, and from both this database and comments of those who have worked in the PNG medical system, it is clear that snakebite is a frequent occurrence, and that through hospital time and antivenom purchases, it is a major component of the national medical budget[16,17].

601

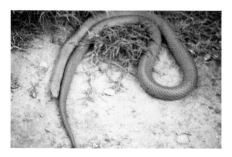

Figure 2. Common brown snake *Pseudonaja textilis* (photo © Dr. J. White).

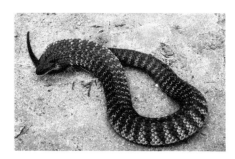

Figure 3. Tiger snake, *Notechis scutatus* (photo © Dr. J. White).

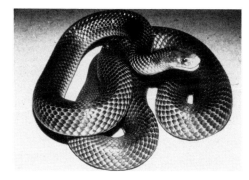

Figure 4. Mulga snake, *Pseudechis australis* (photo © Dr. J. White).

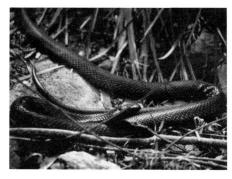

Figure 5: Red bellied black snake, *Pseudechis porphyriacus* (photo © Dr. J. White).

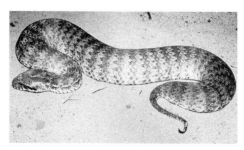

Figure 6. Death adder, *Acanthophis antarcticus* (photo © Dr. J. White).

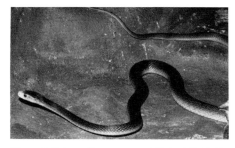

Figure 7. Taipan, *Oxyuranus scutellatus* (photo © Dr. J. White).

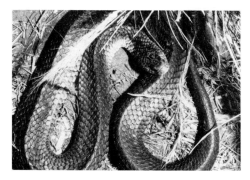

Figure 8. Copperhead, *Austrelaps superbus* (photo © Dr. J. White).

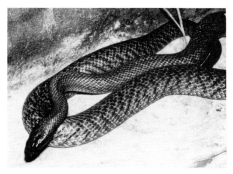

Figure 9. Inland taipan, *Oxyuranus microlepidotus* (photo © Dr. J. White).

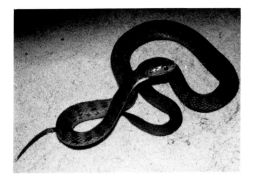

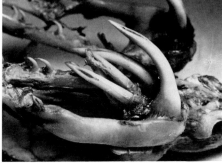

Figure 10. Rough scale snake, *Tropidechis carinatus* (photo © Dr. J. White).

Figure 11. Taipan skull showing fangs, other teeth (photo © Dr. J. White).

Table 2
Snakebite fatalities by region in Australia

State	Pre-Antivenom Era 1910-1926	1945-49	Antivenom Era 1952-61	1968-82
Queensland	74	18	18	15
New South Wales	57	6	9	9
Victoria	43	-	9	11
Western Australia	6	3	6	7
South Australia	8	-	1	2
Tasmania	8	1	-	3
Northern Territory	1	-	1	9
ACT	1	-	1	-
TOTAL	198	28	45	56
Fatality Rate Per Year	12.4	5.6	4.5	3.7

NOTE: Fatality rate per year is for the total population at that time. As the total population has been steadily rising, the rate per head of population would have fallen more dramatically than the above figures suggest.

Table 3
Epidemiology of snakebite in South Australia

Type of Snake	No. of Cases	Illegitimate	No. with envenoming	Coag.	Neuro.	Myo.	Renal
Brown S.	85	17	23	13	2	0	5
Tiger S.	20	8	17	10	7	2	1
Mulga S.	15	6	12	2	0	4	0
Black S.	15	7	13	2	0	0	0
Death Adder	12	12	6	0	2	0	0
Taipan	3	3	3	3	2	1	2
Other	14	3	9	0	0	0	0
Unknown	79	0	7	1	3	1	1
Total	243	56	90	31	16	8	9

KEY: No. of Cases=total number in survey; Illegitimate=people bitten while catching/handling/keeping snakes; No. with envenoming=all patients in group showing clear evidence of venom effects, from local to severe; Coag.=patients with coagulopathy*; Neuro.=patients with evidence of paralysis, minor to complete*; Myo.=patients with myolysis*; Renal=patients with evidence of renal function impairment or renal failure*. *=patients where this problem was checked for and documented, not necessarily all patients with this problem, as in some it was not checked for, may have been present but not documented.

Table 4
Snakes most likely to cause bites for each state

Snake		Qld.	NSW	ACT	Vic.	SA	NT	WA	Tas
Brown Snakes	U	H	H	M	M	H	H	H	-
	R	H	H	M	H	H	H	H	-
Tiger Snakes	U	L	L	L	H	L	-	L	H
	R	L	M	L	H	M	-	M	H
Copperhead	U	-	L	L	M	L	-	-	M
	R	L	L	L	M	L	-	-	M
Rough Scale S.	U	L	L	-	-	-	-	-	-
	R	L	L	-	-	-	-	-	-
Mulga Snake	U	L	L	-	-	L	M	L	-
	R	M	M	-	-	M	H	H	-
Black Snake	U	L	M	L	L	M	-	-	-
	R	L	M	L	M	M	-	-	-
Death Adders	U	L	L	-	-	L	L	L	-
	R	L	L	-	-	L	L	L	-
Taipans	U	M	-	-	-	-	M	-	-
	R	H	L	-	-	L	H	L	-

KEY: U=urban; R=rural; H=highly likely to be present and cause bites; M=moderately common only;
L=uncommon or rare, therefore unlikely to cause bites.

III. SYMPTOMS AND SIGNS

A. GENERAL CONCEPTS OF ENVENOMING

As with snakebite in other regions of the world, there is a misconception amongst many in the community that any bite by a dangerous snake will result in lethal envenoming with dire consequences unless urgent remedial action is taken. A corollary of this is that most people who think they have suffered a snakebite will be anxious, with attendant symptomatology which may confuse the diagnostic process.

The health professional managing a case of suspected snakebite should understand that venomous snakes may strike, and even bite, without injecting a dangerous quantity of venom. Thus a definite bite by even the most lethal species of snake, with clear bite marks and venom on the skin surface, will not necessarily develop evidence of envenoming. There are many and recent examples where failure to understand this basic point has led to misunderstandings about the diagnosis and treatment of snakebite.

Of all suspected snakebites presenting for treatment in Australia, probably less than 1 in 2 develop envenoming sufficient to warrant antivenom therapy. In some series in children the figure is as low as 1 in 20 cases[18], although this probably represents an overdiagnosis of snakebite in this special group. The likelihood of failure to significantly envenom is probably different for each species group of snakes. The most common culprit in snakebite in Australia is the brown snake group, *Pseudonaja* sp., with about 1 in 4 cases of definite bite actually developing significant envenoming[19]. However, this should not lead to complacency, for bites by these snakes can cause very severe envenoming and still are thought to cause more deaths than bites by any other species group. Tiger snakes, *Notechis* sp., cause significant envenoming in at least 1 in 2 cases[15,19]. Taipans, *Oxyuranus* spp., are most likely to cause significant envenoming, with about 3 out of 4 taipan bites being fatal unless adequately treated, making these snakes amongst the most lethal in the world[9,15]. Taipans also have the longest fangs of any Australian snake (Figure 11). About 1 in 2 death adder, *Acanthophis* sp., bites were lethal in the past in Australia, with similar experience in New Guinea, although in recent years in Australia bites by these snakes are rare except in reptile keepers[15,19,20]. In this latter group the incidence of envenoming by death adders is much lower, probably less than 1 in 5, which may reflect both the size of the snake and the mechanism of the bite, often a glancing blow only[19]. The mulga snake, *Pseudechis australis*, is a frequent cause of snakebite in arid and northern Australia, but case reports are few which limits prognostic data; however, it is likely that at least 1 in 3 bites are severe[15,19]. The red bellied black snake, *Pseudechis porphyriacus*, though common and a frequent cause of bites, is very unlikely to cause severe or lethal envenoming, but quite likely to cause mild symptomatic envenoming[15,19]. For all other species data are scant. The rough scale snake, *Tropidechis carinatus*, should be considered in the same group as the tiger snakes, as should the copperheads (or at least *Austrelaps superbus*), though neither are likely, on average, to be quite as severe as the tiger snake.

B. THE ONSET AND DEVELOPMENT OF ENVENOMING

Envenoming is not an inevitable consequence of a bite by a dangerous snake, but when it does occur it usually does so rapidly. However this is not always the case and there have been tragedies where a patient was discharged well after several hours of observation following a snakebite, only to develop severe, even fatal envenoming many hours later[21]. Except in extraordinary cases there will be some evidence of envenoming within 18 to 24 hours of the bite, although rarely the major complications of envenoming, notably myolysis, renal failure, and less likely neurotoxic paralysis, will first manifest more than 24 hours post bite[6,15,22].

The likelihood of developing envenoming depends on a number of factors: (i) the size and species of snake; (ii) the number of bites inflicted and the nature of the bites; (iii) the size and health of the victim. The rapidity of onset of envenoming similarly is governed by several variables: (i) the number of bites; (ii) the age, size and health of the victim; (iii) the activity of the victim following the bite; (iv) the effectiveness of first aid therapy. Small children are more likely to develop severe envenoming, and do so more rapidly than adults. This is not just due to small body mass in children. A young child is usually less coordinated when under stress, will more often sustain multiple bites, is usually very active after the bite and application of first aid will usually be delayed until after the child has been running, seeking comfort.

From the onset of first symptoms of envenoming to development of severe and life threatening envenoming may occasionally be a very short time span[23], but in most cases this progression will take many hours. Patients dying from snakebite in Australia in the early part of the 20th century, prior to the advent of either antivenoms or intensive therapy facilities, mostly died many hours after the bite[20]. In nearly half of these cases death occurred more than 24 hours post bite, and in only 16% did death occur in the first 6 hours. These figures may help to explain why death from snakebite is now rare in Australia, but also disguise the fact that in a significant number of those cases dying late, the severe effects of envenoming, which ultimately resulted in death, actually occurred in the first 12 hours. This is confirmed by more recent surveys of snakebite fatalities[15], where the complications that ultimately led to death, such as cerebral haemorrhage or severe renal damage, may have occurred many hours or days prior to death.

C. GENERAL SYMPTOMS AND SIGNS OF ENVENOMING

While there are some variations between species, in essence the general symptoms and signs of envenoming can be considered as common for all species, except for local effects at the bite site[2,15]. The bite site may be painless and hard to discern, or painful, swollen, bruised, and quite obvious, with clear fang marks. The characteristic appearances of the bite site and features of systemic envenoming for each major snake group are given in Table 5. A painless and trivial bite site does not imply a trivial bite. The corollary is also true, that an obvious and painful bite site does not imply significant systemic envenoming will ensue (e.g. bites by the red bellied black snake, *Pseudechis porphyriacus*). Multiple bites are almost invariably associated with severe envenoming. Bite marks may be indistinct, or 1 or

2 fang marks, or scratch marks, or a mixture of scratches and fang marks[15,24,25]. Typical cases are illustrated in Figures 12 to 15.

Table 5
Major features of envenoming for each snake group

Snake	Pain	Local Swelling	Necrosis	Systemic Paralysis	Coag.	Myolysis	Renal
Brown Snakes	U	R	-	U	C☆	-	C
Tiger Snakes	C	C	U	C☆	C	C	U
Mulga Snake	C	C☆	R	?R	-(AC)	C☆	U
Black Snakes	C	C	R	-	-	?R	-
Death Adders	C	U	-	C	-	-	-
Taipans	U	U	R	C☆	C☆	U	U

KEY: ☆=major feature of envenoming; C=common; U=uncommon; R=rare; (AC)=anticoagulant; Coag=defibrination type coagulopathy; Renal=evidence of renal function impairment.

Classic symptoms of systemic envenoming include headache, nausea, vomiting, abdominal pain, and dizziness. Blurred vision is also not uncommon, and may not indicate early paralysis. Collapse, unconsciousness, and even convulsions may occur within 60 mins. of the bite, particularly in the patient who remains active (walking, running), with convulsions more usually seen in small children, in which group they may be the presenting feature of envenoming in children too young to complain specifically of snakebite[15,26]. Early collapse is often accompanied by spontaneous recovery within 10 to 30 mins.[15]

Anxiety can also result in many of the above symptoms and signs, and it may be difficult in some cases to determine whether the patient is actually envenomed, or just very anxious. Tingling in the limbs associated with rapid respirations may suggest hyperventilation due to anxiety rather than envenoming.

D. SPECIFIC TOXIN EFFECTS AND COMPLICATIONS
1. Neurotoxic paralysis: symptoms and signs

Neurotoxic paralysis remains the most widely known and feared complication of snakebite, despite the fact that respiratory paralysis and its secondary complications are now a rare cause of snakebite fatality[15]. In the early part of this century respiratory paralysis was the most common cause of snakebite deaths, but the advent of antivenom, and more importantly, intensive therapy units with the capacity to ventilate patients, has greatly reduced the importance of this classic effect of envenoming. It remains, however, an important complication of envenoming, and produces classic symptoms and signs that unequivocally announce the development of systemic envenoming and the need for antivenom therapy.

Paralysis is due to either pre- or post-synaptic neurotoxins, or a mixture of the two[5,15]. Not all dangerous Australian snakes have either or both (see Tables 1, 5). The post-synaptic neurotoxins in general act more rapidly, but their effects are reversible with antivenom therapy, while the pre-synaptic neurotoxins take longer to manifest, but are often not reversible with antivenom therapy[15].

The first evidence of paralysis is usually ptosis (Figure 16), followed by blurred vision, diplopia on lateral gaze (Figure 17), then dysarthria, with progressive development of peripheral muscle weakness and respiratory muscle paralysis. The patient may first complain of "heavy" or "sleepy" eyes, then blurred or double vision. These first symptoms of paralysis usually occur more than one hour after the bite, often at 2 to 3 hours post bite, with progressive development of paralysis over the next 1 to 4 hours, by which time, in a severe case, there will be evidence of respiratory embarrassment. However, full paralysis of all the muscles of respiration including the diaphragm may take 20 or more hours, although the patient will probably have earnt intubation and ventilation well before this[15,27]. Occasionally the onset and progress of paralysis is far more rapid, with progression to severe paralysis within 2 to 3 hours post bite. At the other end of the spectrum, onset of paralysis may be delayed by many hours, and fail to manifest until 12 or more hours post bite.

2. Coagulopathy: symptoms and signs

Coagulopathy following Australian snakebite has often been underrated in the past, but current evidence suggests it is a major complication of envenoming by some species (see Tables 1, 5) and a leading cause of snakebite mortality[15,28,29]. Symptoms and signs specific for coagulopathy are few, and while the patient with coagulopathy will usually have other evidence of envenoming, this is not always the case. It is not rare for the patient to be essentially symptom free and apparently well while having a significant coagulopathy with unclottable blood. Persistent bleeding from the bite wound and venepuncture sites is very suggestive of coagulopathy. Major spontaneous haemorrhage in association with coagulopathy is mercifully uncommon, but when present may result in specific symptoms and signs. The most important and common site for spontaneous haemorrhage is in the brain, with consequent loss of consciousness and other neurological signs, the ultimate outcome usually being death.

The cause of the coagulopathy is mostly potent venom procoagulants, which convert prothrombin to either thrombin or meizothrombin, and clinically cause a defibrination type consumptive coagulopathy[5,15,30]. For a few species the altered clotting state is due to true anticoagulants, but the effects of these appears far less profound than the procoagulants.

3. Myotoxicity: symptoms and signs

Several Australian snakes contain potent myotoxins in their venom, often associated with neurotoxins (see Tables 1, 5)[5,15]. The widespread myolysis caused by these toxins results in the release of muscle breakdown products, notably creatine kinase and myoglobin. The former may rise to very high levels (inexcess of 100,000IU). The latter colours the urine red or muddy brown, a classic sign of myolysis (Figure 18). The muscle damage, if severe, will usually result in muscle pain, especially on contraction against resistance as in muscle power testing, and also muscle weakness which may be mistaken for true paralysis. The quantity of myoglobin passed through the kidneys is usually said to be a risk for renal failure; however, the author has treated a number of cases with very severe myolysis without evidence of renal damage[19]. In severe cases of myolysis muscle wasting may occur (Figure 19). There may be a severe hyperkalaemia in association with severe myolysis, which may prove very difficult to manage and result in cardiac problems which are likely to be symptomatic.

4. Renal Failure: symptoms and signs

It is not clear if Australian snake venoms contain primary nephrotoxins, or if the renal failure seen after severe envenomation is purely a secondary complication. There is one case of envenoming by a brown snake which is quite suggestive of a primary nephrotoxic effect[6], and certainly brown snake bites are the leading cause of snakebite renal failure, even though they do not cause myolysis[2,15,19].

The symptoms and signs of snakebite renal failure are the same as for any other cause of kidney damage. Urine output should be carefully monitored in all snakebite patients.

E. PROGNOSTIC INDICATORS

A patient with multiple bites, or intoxicated with alcohol, is more likely to develop severe envenoming. Early onset of symptoms and signs, particularly paralytic signs or coagulopathy, suggests severe envenoming. A patient who remains subjectively and objectively free of envenoming for 6 hours post bite in the absence of continued first aid is unlikely to develop severe envenoming, and in most cases will remain well. Beware the occasional case developing late envenoming however, and avoid the dangers of discharging an apparently well patient only 6 hours post bite. Early collapse, while indicative of envenoming, does not necessarily correspond with ultimately severe envenoming. Bites by the red bellied black snake are a good example of this, as envenoming by this species is very rarely life threatening, but early collapse is not uncommon.

IV. PROPHYLAXIS

A. AVOIDANCE OF BITES

The most important measure in preventing snakebite is avoidance of bites through eliminating inappropriate or risky behaviour and by minimizing the chances of human-snake encounters. Essentially this amounts to common sense. Walking through long grass, or barefoot, especially on warm nights, putting hands into hollows or other possible retreats where the occupant cannot be visualized are all activities associated with snakebite. Young children playing outdoors unsupervised are similarly at risk. Snake handlers are at special risk. Snakes will sometimes frequent areas close to human habitation, particularly if there is debris harbouring food items (eg. mice, lizards, frogs), potential shelter for the snake, or available water in hot dry areas. Houses raised above ground level offer good shelter for snakes beneath the house, and snakes quite frequently will enter houses if given access. There is a common misconception that snakebite only occurs outdoors; though not common, snakebite can and does occur inside dwellings, even hospitals, and fatalities have occurred, often because snakebite was not considered as a possible diagnosis.

B. PUBLIC EDUCATION ON SNAKEBITE

Public education about the causes and first aid treatment of snakebite is clearly of benefit in reducing the risk of bites and ensuring those bitten reach medical aid in as good a condition as possible. There are no government schemes to ensure such education, but most schools run programmes on bites and stings, there are a number of private "wildlife specialists" giving both school and public lectures on avoidance and treatment of bites and stings, and within Australia there are numerous publications on this subject for general sale. In recent years groups of snake enthusiasts have banded together to provide a public service collecting snakes found in gardens, houses etc. (eg.Adelaide Snake Catchers Inc.) and while reducing the number of snakes in proximity to man, they also distribute information on snakebite to a motivated audience. It is too soon to determine if such activities are resulting in a reduction in the incidence of snakebite.

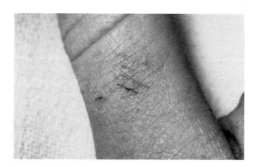

Figure 12. Bite site, brown snake bite (photo © Dr. J. White).

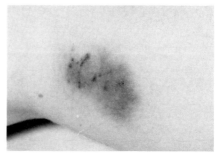

Figure 13. Bite site, tiger snake bite (photo © Dr. J. White).

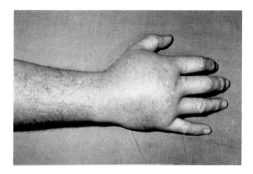

Figure 14. Mulga snake bite with local swelling (photo © Dr. J. White).

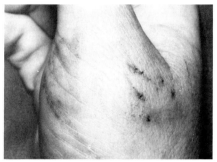

Figure 15. Taipan bite showing multiple teeth marks (photo © Dr. J. White).

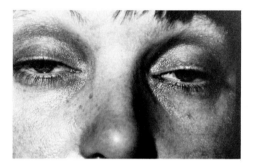

Figure 16. Ptosis following tiger snake bite (photo © Dr. J. White).

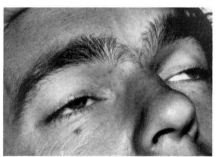

Figure 17. Sixth nerve palsy with diplopia and squint on lateral gaze, death adder bite (photo © Dr. J. White).

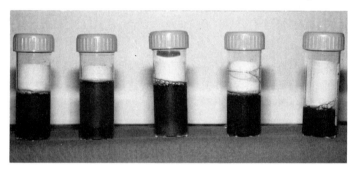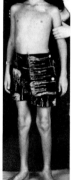

Figure 18: Myoglobinuria following tiger snake bite (photo © Dr. J. White).

Figure 19: Muscle wasting due to myolysis, tiger snake bite (photo © Dr. J. White).

C. IMMUNIZATION AGAINST SNAKE VENOMS

Snakebite is not nearly common enough in Australia to justify mass immunization programmes, even were such programmes shown to be effective. The situation in certain regions of New Guinea is less clear. For the present no proven immunization is available. Special cases have arisen in the past where immunization of an individual at high risk has been undertaken. The best known case was a reptile handler who milked snakes for antivenom production and who became allergic to antivenom after several bites requiring treatment[31]. This individual was progressively immunized against tiger snake venom and a subsequent bite was thought to have been milder than expected due to the immunization.

V. FIRST AID TREATMENT

A. PRINCIPLES AND THEORY OF FIRST AID

The key principle in first aid must be to do the patient no harm. Most past snakebite first aid treatments have violated this principle. The aim of first aid for snakebite is to maximize the chance of patient survival by: (i) reducing the rate of venom absorption; (ii) reducing the rate of venom movement from the bite site; (iii) ensuring continuance of vital functions.

Most research has indicated that the majority of venom is transported from the bite site by the lymphatic system; therefore, any muscle movement in the bitten limb/area will speed venom movement, as will general activity by the victim, such as running or even walking[32,33]. Immobilization of the bitten limb alone has been shown to retard venom movement[34]. When combined with a broad bandage compressing superficial lymph vessels, limb immobilization has been shown experimentally (in monkeys) to greatly retard venom movement[32]. It is effective as an arterial tourniquet, but can be left on for several hours and is clearly both safer and more practical than a tourniquet. This method of first aid for Australian snakebite is commonly referred to as the "pressure immobilization bandage" and has gained wide acceptance. There are several published case reports suggesting the clinical effectiveness of the method, though no controlled trials[35,36]. It is the only method of first aid for snakebite recommended in Australia and New Guinea. While it may be applicable to bites for some non-Australian snakes, it may cause problems if used for a bite which causes significant local tissue damage (e.g. many viper bites and some cobra bites) and so is not generally accepted outside of Australia.

B. RECOMMENDED FIRST AID

(a) If the patient develops evidence of respiratory or cardiac failure, use standard cardio-pulmonary resuscitation techniques to maintain life.

(b) The patient should be encouraged to lie still, and reassured, to avoid panic.

(c) A broad compression bandage should be applied over the bitten area, at about the same pressure as for a sprained ankle. A second bandage should then be applied distally, moving proximally, to cover as much of the bitten limb as possible. If bandage is not available then torn up strips of clothing, or even pantyhose, may be used.

(d) The bandaged limb should be firmly immobilised using a splint.

(e) The bite site wound should not be washed, cleaned, cut, sucked, or treated with any substance.

(f) Tourniquets should not be used.

(g) The patient should be transported to appropriate medical care.

(h) Nil orally unless the patient will not reach medical care for a prolonged period of time in which case only water should be given by mouth. No food should be consumed. Alcohol should not be used.

(i) If the offending snake has been killed it should be brought with the patient for identification.

(j) Remove any rings, bangles etc. from the bitten limb.

VI. CLINICAL MANAGEMENT

A. GENERAL CONSIDERATIONS

The patient presenting with possible snakebite should be considered as a medical emergency and managed expeditiously. Particularly in children, where a history may not be available or reliable, a high index of suspicion for snakebite is the wisest policy. As many Australian snakes may not leave very obvious bite marks, the diagnosis may not be obvious. In the patient who is clearly unwell it is important to coordinate diagnostic and management activities to speed the process of treatment. All patients with suspected snakebite should be admitted to hospital and closely monitored.

B. DIAGNOSIS

1. Approach to diagnosis

The key to effective treatment is rapid and accurate diagnosis. The patient presenting with a history of possible snakebite has already performed a crucial step in this process. However, also consider snakebite in the patient who might have been exposed to a bite, yet is unaware of a bite or unable to give any history. Young children severely bitten may present first with a convulsion, which may distract from considering snakebite as a diagnosis. The patient found unconscious in a bush area or where snakes are found may also prove a diagnostic difficulty. If the patient is unconscious or has significant respiratory impairment then attend to this as a priority.

Quickly ascertain if a snake was seen or if a bite was felt, and if symptoms of envenoming have subsequently occurred (see Section III). Initial examination can commence at the same time. While the patient gives the history observe if there is ptosis or dysarthria, then test for ophthalmoplegia or other muscle weakness. If there is appropriate first aid in place, consider that this may be delaying onset of envenoming if the patient is ostensibly well. Cut away the bandage over the bite site, check the wound for multiple bites while swabbing for venom detection (keep overlying bandage for latter venom assay if necessary). The key points in history, examination and laboratory investigations are listed in Table 6.

2. Role of venom detection

Venom detection has assumed an increasing role in the management of Australian snakebite, but its role in New Guinea is less certain. The Venom Detection Kit (VDK) is produced by the antivenom manufacturer for Australia (CSL Ltd., Melbourne; "CSL") and uses an ELISA principle to qualitatively detect nanogram quantities of venom from the wound site or urine[37,38,39]. It will determine if snake venom is present and which type, corresponding to the five major snake groups and equivalent monovalent antivenoms. Some less common species give positive reactions to more than one venom type. A result can be obtained in less than 20 mins. A positive result from a wound swab does not indicate systemic envenoming and is not an indication for antivenom therapy. A positive result from urine is only likely if there is systemic envenoming, and in the absence of this there is little point in testing urine. Blood has proved an unreliable test sample and is not recommended. The VDK has enabled monovalent antivenom to be used much more frequently, thus reducing the need for the more expensive and complication prone polyvalent antivenom. However in New Guinea, where the range of dangerous species in any given area is often less, and costs preclude the stocking of a wide range of monovalent antivenoms, polyvalent antivenom is often the first choice, hence the comparative unimportance of the VDK at this time. This situation may change in the future.

3. Role of laboratory investigations

Apart from venom detection, which does not need laboratory facilities, standard blood tests can be most helpful in assessing and treating snakebite. Principle tests are listed in Table 6. Three key complications are best demonstrated by lab tests: coagulopathy, myolysis and renal damage. Serial extended coagulation tests are very useful in treating snakebite coagulopathy of the defibrination type, titrating antivenom therapy against recovery in coagulation parameters[15,26,40,41]. In the absence of a laboratory this can be achieved using the bedside whole blood clotting time. Myolysis can be measured by serum/plasma creatine kinase and by urine myoglobin. In the absence of a laboratory check urine colour and test for haemoglobin (dipstick). Renal function can be followed with creatinine and urea levels, but urine output is also a valuable guide.

Table 6
History, examination and laboratory investigations

Problem	History	Examination	Investigation
Circumstances of the bite	Geographic area, Snake size, colour, ?multiple bites ?first aid activity after the bite	Cut bandage away over bite site to check for multiple bites, local redness, swelling	Venom detection from bite site
Local Effects	Pain, swelling	Redness, swelling, tender draining lymph nodes	
General Symptoms and Signs	Headache, nausea, vomiting, abdominal pain, collapse, dizziness.	Tachycardia, hypertension, conscious state (irritability)	?ECG
Paralysis	Sleepy eyes, heavy eyelids, speech difficulty, weakness, breathing problems.	Ptosis, lateral gaze paresis, fixed dilated pupils, dysarthria, peripheral muscle weakness, respiratory impairment.	Arterial Blood Gas FEV Pulse Oximetry
Coagulopathy	Persistent bleeding from bite site, other bleeding	Ooze from bite, or venepuncture sites	Whole blood clotting time CBP, INR, APTT, TCT, Fibrinogen titre, FDP/XDP.
Myolysis	Muscle pain or weakness or cramps, red or brown urine.	Pain on contracting muscles against resistance, muscle weakness.	Serum CK Urine myoglobin Serum K^+ Serum LDH
Renal	Poor urine output		Serum creatinine, urea, K^+
Background Information	Past snakebites, past exposure to antivenom, allergic history, past kidney problems		

4. Assessing extent of envenoming

As the key decision in treatment is whether or not to give antivenom therapy, any assessment of extent of envenoming must be directed towards this. A patient with a bite site and with general symptoms of envenoming (headache, vomiting etc.) may be developing early systemic envenoming, but beware of anxiety. If there is evidence of paralysis, coagulopathy or myolysis then there is significant systemic envenoming. If there has been a convulsion or collapse then there is significant envenoming. If there is progressive or extensive paralysis, full defibrination, or frank myoglobinuria, then there is severe envenoming[2,41,42].

A patient who presents symptom free with effective first aid in place, which was promptly applied, may develop envenoming rapidly after removal of the first aid, or may not develop envenoming for several hours. The initially well patient needs frequent reassessment.

C. TREATMENT

1. General approach to treatment

The aims of treatment are to minimize patient morbidity and mortality at the least cost. Quick assessment and institution of appropriate treatment will minimize the extent of any envenoming and so reduce the occurrence and severity of complications. On this basis it might be suggested that prompt use of antivenom to all patients with suspected snakebite would be beneficial. Indeed, this was a policy adopted by some hospitals in the past. Antivenom is both potentially hazardous and very expensive (see Table 7) and it is most inadvisable to use it unless there is a clear indication, that is there is evidence of significant envenoming by a snake capable of causing either major complications or death[41,42].

Table 7
Available snake antivenoms (from CSL Ltd., Melbourne)

Antivenom	Species Covered	Volume	Cost (Aust. $)	Minimum Dose
BROWN AV 1000units/amp.	*Pseudonaja textilis*	4ml	$129.60	1 amp.
	Pseudonaja nuchalis			1 amp.
	Pseudonaja affinis			1 amp.
	Pseudonaja guttata			1 amp.
	Pseudonaja ingrami			1 amp.
TIGER AV 3000units/amp.	*Notechis scutatus*	6.8ml	$190.10	1 amp.
	Notechis ater			2 amps.
	Notechis a. serventyi			4 amps.
	Austrelaps superbus			1 amp.
	Austrelaps labialis			1 amp.
	Austrelaps ramsayi			1 amp.
	Tropidechis carinatus			1 amp.
	Pseudechis porphyriacus			1 amp.
	Pseudechis colletti			1 amp.
	Pseudechis gutattus			1 amp.
	?Micropechis ikaheka			1 amp.
BLACK AV 18000units/amp.	*Pseudechis australis*	35ml	$840.25	1 amp.
	Pseudechis butleri			1 amp.
	Pseudechis papuanus			1 amp.
	(*Pseudechis porphyriacus*)			(½ amp.)
	(*Pseudechis colletti*)			(½ amp.)
	(*Pseudechis gutattus*)			(½ amp.)
DEATH ADDER AV 6000units/amp.	*Acanthophis antarcticus*	20ml	$661.00	1 amp.
	Acanthophis pyrrhus			1 amp.
	Acanthophis praelongus			1 amp.
TAIPAN AV 12000units/amp.	*Oxyuranus scutellatus*	40ml	$1,044.40	1 amp.
	Oxyuranus s. canni			1 amp.
	Oxyuranus microlepidotus			1 amp.
POLYVALENT	Covers all above	48ml	$1,131.85	1 amp.

The patient should have urgent matters dealt with first, such as maintenance of airway/respiration if this is imperiled, and an iv line inserted, taking blood for relevant investigations at that time. Lie the patient on his side if there is a degree of paralysis as the gag reflex may be impaired and inhalation of vomitus may occur. Once basic needs have been dealt with, then remove any first aid, except if the patient has severe envenoming, in which case remove the first aid only after initial antivenom therapy is complete. If the patient is initially well then remove first aid immediately after first assessment.

When taking blood or inserting iv lines, be aware of the possibility of coagulopathy and avoid vessels where application of local pressure may be difficult. In particular, avoid venepuncture of the femorals or in the neck, and avoid iv line/CVP line insertion in the femoral, neck, or subclavian vessels.

Ensure the patient is adequately monitored, particularly noting fluid balance and urine output (plus colour). Arrhythmias are infrequent in Australian snakebite patients, and no cardiac toxins have been described, although there is a suspicion that some venoms, notably brown snake venom, may interfere with cardiac function at high concentrations[43]. Continuous cardiac monitoring is therefore advisable but not mandatory. If the patient is initially well, make sure that ward staff are aware of the signs of paralysis and regularly check for them in addition to standard observations.

2. Antivenom therapy and its complications

The cornerstone of snakebite treatment is antivenom therapy[13,41]. There are monovalent antivenoms for each major group of Australian venomous snakes, and for New Guinea snakes, with the exception of the small eyed snake, *Micropechis* spp. There is also a polyvalent antivenom covering all species, except *Micropechis*. The antivenoms, the species they cover, average volume, current cost, and recommended minimum dose are listed in Table 7.

Antivenom is indicated if there is significant envenoming, as discussed earlier. It is the definitive treatment of coagulopathy (see below), but may not reverse paralysis, myolysis, or renal damage[41]. It should be given as soon as safely possible once indicated. Because it is essentially refined horse serum it is allergenic and may stimulate both early and late reactions[44,45]. Anaphylactic type early reactions may occur, both in the patient who has received antivenom previously, and also *de novo* in a patient never previously exposed. For this reason some experts recommend using prophylactic medications prior to commencing antivenom therapy[13]. These include sc adrenaline, iv antihistamine and iv hydrocortisone. The value of these premedications is not proven, and their use is controversial. It has been theorized that sc adrenaline, by increasing blood pressure, may put the patient with coagulopathy at greater risk of severe haemorrhage[41]. This has not been proven although there is some evidence implicating adrenaline in lethal intracerebral haemorrhage in this situation[27,28]. Pre-therapy sensitivity testing is of no value and not recommended[13,41].

If the patient does exhibit a severe early reaction to antivenom, but has severe envenoming, especially if there is a coagulopathy, then after initial stabilization by stopping the antivenom infusion and giving adrenaline, it will be necessary to restart the antivenom infusion, possibly under cover of continuous adrenaline infusion (if indicated)[9,41,42]. In this setting the dose of antivenom may need to be increased substantially. Antivenom may also cause late reactions, particularly serum sickness, the frequency of which increases with total volume of antivenom given. Less than 50 ml of antivenom rarely results in serum sickness, but above this it is far more common (one ampoule of polyvalent antivenom is about 50 mls). If more than 50 mls of antivenom is given then consider prescribing prophylactic oral steroids. All patients given antivenom therapy should be told of the symptoms of serum sickness before leaving hospital and asked to report back if they develop.

Antivenom should be given iv, preferably diluted about 1:10 to 1:5 (depending on the total volume and size of patient, ie less dilution may be needed in children to avoid fluid overload), and given through an iv line, commencing very slowly and increasing the rate if no reactions occur, aiming to give the whole dose over 15 to 20 mins.[41] Before commencing the infusion, have adrenaline ready to give (diluted and ready to run piggyback using a pump is preferred) to treat severe early reactions, together with standard resuscitation equipment[42]. Stay with the patient during and for at least 30 mins. after the infusion. The initial and subsequent doses will depend on the clinical situation, but if there is severe envenoming or multiple bites, commence with at least twice the minimum dosage (see Table 7). Monovalent antivenom specific for the snake involved is always preferable to polyvalent antivenom. If the snake cannot be identified prior to commencing therapy, consider mixing 2 monovalent antivenoms rather than using polyvalent, providing that the mixture will cover all likely culprit species. The commonest such mixture is brown snake and tiger snake antivenoms.

3. Neurotoxicity and its treatment

The symptoms and signs of neurotoxic paralysis have already been discussed, as have the time frame of onset. Full paralysis may take days or even weeks to reverse if caused by pre-synaptic neurotoxins (particularly bites by tiger snakes and taipans). As there is a delay between binding to the terminal axon and onset of paralysis there is a latent period when damage is occurring without clinical manifestation. The sooner antivenom is given after onset of first signs of paralysis, the more effective it will be in preventing progression. If the neurotoxins are purely post-synaptic (eg death adders) then there is a possibility of reversal of paralysis. Experience outside Australia has suggested that anticholinesterase therapy may also reverse some post-synaptic paralysis, but this has only been tried with a few cases of death adder bite and its place is uncertain[46,47]. If proven reliable, given the cost of death adder antivenom, it may well become the primary treatment in some areas, especially in New Guinea.

The patient with severe paralysis will require ventilation, usually using endotracheal intubation in the first instance. Tracheostomy should be avoided, at least in the early stages, due to bleeding problems if there is an associated coagulopathy.

4. Coagulopathy and its treatment

On present evidence it appears that only the defibrination type coagulopathy is associated with the likelihood of major haemorrhage, and even then major bleeding is uncommon[40]. It is a consumptive coagulopathy, unresponsive to inhibitors (eg heparin) and use of factor replacement such as Fresh Frozen Plasma while there is still circulating venom and consumption is not advisable as it adds more substrate for the venom and will increase levels of degradation products, which are also anticoagulant. The best therapy is to expeditiously neutralize all circulating venom using antivenom. Once this is achieved normal homeostatic mechanisms quickly return clotting function to safe, if not normal, levels, obviating the need for any replacement therapy in most cases. It is possible to titrate antivenom against clotting results. Clinical experience suggests that fibrinogen will reach protective levels in much less than 6 hours[15,24,26,39,47].

The classic defibrination coagulopathy, as seen after bites by brown snakes, tiger snakes and taipans (and some other species), may develop very rapidly after the bite (within 15 mins. in active children) and is typified by unclottable blood (whole blood clotting time > 15 mins.), grossly prolonged intrinsic and extrinsic clotting times (APTT > 150 secs.; INR > 12), undetectable fibrinogen level and grossly elevated degradation products, both FDP and cross linked (D-Dimer) FDP, and a normal or near normal platelet count[39]. Thrombin clotting time is also grossly prolonged, but is a sensitive measure of fibrinogen concentration, and may show improvement before any other parameter, once sufficient antivenom has been given.

5. Myotoxicity and its treatment

Myotoxicity is best measured by serum/plasma creatine kinase levels and presence of myoglobin in the urine. Quantitative measurement of urinary myoglobin, while interesting, is expensive and usually not justified. Muscle biopsy will not change therapy and so is hard to justify, though of considerable interest. It is unknown if antivenom therapy can reverse myolysis, but it seems unlikely; thus once detected, myolysis is probably not affected by antivenom. Early antivenom therapy for other reasons (eg coagulopathy) may reduce the extent of myolysis. Once established, renal function and throughput should be monitored, giving a fluid load and possibly alkalinization of the urine. Regular physiotherapy and possibly a high protein diet are useful in the recovery phase of severe cases, where a high proportion of total voluntary muscle mass may be lost, with marked wasting and contractures. Experimental evidence suggests that the regrown muscle may be deficient in fast fibres.

6. Renal failure and its treatment

It is uncertain why some snakebite victims develop renal failure, but it is not uncommon in adult patients, and may be seen following even quite mild envenoming, particularly by brown snakes. At least in adults, careful monitoring of urine output (if necessary, using catheterization) and renal function is warranted. Many patients may be slightly dry on arrival at hospital and an iv fluid load initially is often advisable. The management of renal failure is beyond the scope of this publication.

7. Other issues in treatment

Local tissue injury at the bite site is either mild or not present in all but an exceptional few cases of Australian snakebite[15,24]. Should marked local swelling develop with evidence of pressure induced pathology such as compartment syndrome, then management should be as for other causes of this problem. Surgical intervention should be very rare in Australian snakebite.

As with any bite, there is a chance of local infection, but this is not common, and most often seen with bites by red bellied black snakes and their generic relatives. Tetanus prophylaxis should always be considered. Routine prophylactic antibiotics are not indicated. Analgesia is rarely a major problem, but narcotic analgesics should be avoided in the early stages if possible, as should platelet active drugs (eg aspirin).

VII. REFERENCES

1. **COGGER, H.G.** *Reptiles and Amphibians of Australia.* Sydney, A.H. & A.W. Reed, 1975.
2. **WHITE, J.** Snakebite;an Australian perspective. *J. Wilderness Med.*, **2**: 219-244, 1991
3. **WHITE, J.** Elapid snakes: venom production and bite mechanism. In COVACEVICH, J., DAVIE, P. and PEARN, J. Eds. *Toxic Plants and Animals: a guide for Australia*, Queensland Museum, 504 pp, 1987.
4. **BROAD, A.J., SUTHERLAND, S.K. and COULTER, A.R.** The lethality in mice of dangerous Australian and other snake venoms. *Toxicon*, **17**: 661-664, 1979.
5. **WHITE, J.** Elapid snakes: venom toxicity and actions. In COVACEVICH, J., DAVIE, P. and PEARN, J. Eds. *Toxic Plants and Animals: a guide for Australia*, Queensland Museum, 504 pp, 1987.
6. **ACOTT, C.J** Acute renal failure after envenomation by the common brown snake. *Med. J. Aust.*, **149**: 709-710, 1988.
7. **WILSON, S.K. and KNOWLES, D.G.** *Australia's Reptiles.* Sydney, Collins, 447pp, 1988.
8. **SHINE, R.** *Australian Snakes: A Natural History.* Sydney: Reed Books 1991.
9. **COVACEVICH, J., PEARN, J. and WHITE, J.** The world's most venomous snake. In PEARN, J. and COVACEVICH, J. Eds. *Venoms and Victims*, The Queensland Museum and Amphion Press, pp 111-120, 1988.
10. **MIRTSCHIN, P.J., CROWE, G.R. and DAVIS, R.** Dangerous snakes of Australia. In GOPALAKRISHNAKONE, P. and CHOU, L.M. *Snakes of Medical Importance (Asia Pacific Region).* National University of Singapore, Singapore. pp 1-174, 1990.
11. **EHMANN, H.** *Australias Reptiles, Australian Natural History Series.* Australian Museum, Sydney, 1992.
12. **COGGER, H.G.** The venomous snakes of Australia and Melanesia. In BUCHERL, W. and BUCKLEY, E.E. Eds. *Venomous Animals And Their Venoms* (Vol 2). Academic Press, London, pp. 35-77, 1971.
13. **SUTHERLAND, S.K.** *Australian Animal Toxins.* Melbourne, Oxford University Press, 1983.
14. **WHITE, J., POUNDER, D., PEARN, J.H. and MORRISON, J.J.** A perspective on the problems of snakebite in Australia. In GRIGG, G., SHINE, R. and EHMANN, H. Eds. *Biology of Australasian Frogs and Reptiles*, Royal Zoological Society of New South Wales, 1985.

15. **WHITE, J.** Elapid snakes: aspects of envenomation. In COVACEVICH, J., DAVIE, P. and PEARN, J. Eds. *Toxic Plants and Animals: a guide for Australia,* Queensland Museum, 504 pp, 1987.

16. **CURRIE, B.J., SUTHERLAND, S.K., HUDSON, B.J. and SMITH, A.M.A.** An epidemiological study of snake bite envenomation in Papua New Guinea. *Med. J. Aust.,* **154:** 266-268, 1991.

17. **CURRIE, B., NARAQUI, S., and KEVAU, I.** Snakebite in Papua New Guinea; rising costs and unanswered questions. *Abstracts of the 23rd Annual Medical Symposium of the Medical Society of Papua New Guinea.* September 4-5, 1987.

18. **JAMIESON, R. and PEARN, J.** An epidemiological and clinical study of snake-bites in childhood. *Med. J. Aust.,* **150:** 698-702, 1989.

19. **WHITE, J.** A review of snakebites and suspected snakebites treated in South Australia with particular reference to reptile handlers. *Proceedings 10th World Cong. Animal, Plant and Microbial Toxins.* National University of Singapore, 1991.

20. **FAIRLEY, N.H.** The present position of snakebite and the snake bitten in Australia. *Med. J. Aust.,* **1:** 296-313, 1929.

21. **WHITE, J., WILLIAMS, V.** Severe envenomation with convulsion following multiple bites by a common brown snake, *Pseudonaja textilis; Aust. Paediatr. J.,* **25:**109-111, 1989.

22. **FURTADO, M.A., and LESTER, I.A.** Myoglobinuria following snake bite. *Med. J. Aust.,* **1:** 674-6, 1968.

23. **SUTHERLAND, S.K., COULTER, A.R. and HARRIS, R.D.** Rapid death of a child after a taipan bite. *Med. J. Aust.,* **1:** 136, 1980.

24. **WHITE, J.** Ophidian envenomation; a South Australian perspective. *Records of the Adelaide Children's Hospital,* **2(3):** 311-421, 1981.

25. **PEARN, J. and COVACEVICH, J.** An atlas of the skin lesions in snakebite. *Med. J. Aust.,* **2:** 568, 1981.

26. **CAMPBELL, C.H.** Snake bite and snake venoms: their effects on the nervous system. In: VINKEN, P.J. and BRUYN, G.W. Eds. *Handbook of Clinical Neurology, Vol. 37, Intoxications of the Nervous System,* North Holland Publishing Co, 1979.

27. **TIBBALLS, J., HENNING, R.D., SUTHERLAND, S.K. and KERR, A.R.** Fatal cerebral haemorrhage after tiger snake (*Notechis scutatus*) envenomation. *Med. J. Aust.,* **154,** 275-276, 1991.

28. **McGARITY, B.H., MARSHALL, G.P., LOADSMAN, J.A., CARR, S.J. and HARPER, C.G.** Fatal cerebral haemorrhage after tiger snake bite. *Med. J. Aust.,* **155,** 61-62, 1991.

29. **MARSHALL, L.R. and HERRMANN, R.P.** Coagulant and anticoagulant actions of Australian snake venoms. *Thrombosis and Haemostasis Research (Stuttgart),* **50(3):** 707-711, 1983.

30. **WIENER, S.** Snakebite in a subject actively immunized against snake venom. *Med. J. Aust.,* **1:** 658-661, 1961.

31. **SUTHERLAND, S.K., COULTER, A.R. and HARRIS, R.D.** Rationalisation of first-aid measures for elapid snakebite. *Lancet,* 183-186, 1979.

32. **SUTHERLAND, S.K., COULTER, A.R., HARRIS, R.D., LOVERING, K.E. and ROBERTS, I.D.** A study of the major Australian snake venoms in the monkey *(Macaca fascicularis);* in the movement of injected venom; methods which retard this movement, and the response to antivenoms. *Pathology,* **13:** 13-27, 1981.

33. **BARNES, J.M. and TRUETA, J.** Absorption of bacteria toxins and snake venoms from the tissues: importance of the lymphatic circulation. *Lancet,* **1:** 623-626, 1941.

34. **MURRELL, G.** The effectiveness of the pressure/immobilization first aid technique in the case of a tiger snake bite. *Med. J. Aust.,* **2:** 295, 1981.

35. **PEARN, J.H., MORRISON, J.J., CHARLES, N. and MURI, V.** First aid for snakebite. *Med. J. Aust.,* **2:** 293-4, 1981.

36. **SUTHERLAND, S.K. and COULTER, A.R.** Snake bite: detection of venom by radioimmunoassay. *Med. J. Aust.,* **2:** 683-684, 1977.

37. **HURRELL, J.G.R. and CHANDLER, H.W.** Capillary enzyme immunoassay field kits for the detection of snake venom in clinical specimens: a review of two years' use. *Med. J. Aust.,* **2:** 236-237, 1982.

38. **COULTER, A.R., COX, J.C., SUTHERLAND, S.K. and WADDELL, C.J.** A new solid phase sandwich radioimmunoassay and its application to the detection of snake venom. *Journal of Immunological Methods,* **23:**241-252, 1978.

39. **WHITE, J., DUNCAN, B., WILSON, C., WILLIAMS, V. and LLOYD, J.** Coagulopathy following Australian elapid snakebite; a review of 20 cases. *Proceedings 10th World Cong. Animal, Plant and Microbial Toxins.* National University of Singapore, 1991.

40. **WHITE, J.** Elapid snakes: management of bites. In COVACEVICH, J., DAVIE, P. and PEARN, J. Eds. *Toxic Plants and Animals: a guide for Australia,* Queensland Museum, 504 pp, 1987.

41. **WHITE, J.** *Management of snakebite in South Australia; a management plan.* South Australian Health Commission, 36 pp.. 1991

42. **SUTHERLAND, S.K.** pers com 1992.

43. **SUTHERLAND, S.K. and LOVERING, K.E.** Antivenoms: use and adverse reactions over a 12 month period in Australia and Papua New Guinea. *Med. J. Aust.,* **2:** 671-674, 1979.

44. **SUTHERLAND, S.K.** Serum reactions: an analysis of commercial antivenoms and the possible role of anticomplementary activity in de-novo reactions to antivenoms and antitoxins. *Med. J. Aust.,* **1:** 613-615, 1977.

45. **WATT, G., THEAKSTON, R.D.G, HAYES, C.G.** *et al* Positive response to edrophonium in patients with neurotoxic envenoming by cobras (*Naja naja philippinensis*). *New Engl. J. Med.,* **315:** 1444-8, 1986.

46. **CURRIE, B., FITZMAURICE, M. and OAKLEY, J.** Resolution of neurotoxicity with anticholinesterase therapy in death adder envenomation. *Med. J. Aust.,* **148:** 522-5251988, .

47. **WHITE, J., TOMKINS, D., STEVEN, I. and WILLIAMS, V.** Tiger Snake bite. *Records of the Adelaide Children's Hospital,* **3(2):** 169-173, 1984.

Chapter 29

CLINICAL TOXICOLOGY OF SNAKEBITE IN NORTH AMERICA

Hernan F. Gomez and Richard C. Dart

TABLE OF CONTENTS

I. INTRODUCTION

The history of snakebite treatment has been characterized by the bizarre and unusual. Whether it be the snake sideshows common 50 years ago or the rattlesnake roundups and electric shock cures of today, it is clear that snakebite has captured the imagination and interest of us all.

Our fear and fascination were well founded in the past. Before modern medical care, the available treatments were as dangerous as the disease; many died of either the snakebite or the cure. Mortality in the 1800 's and early 1900 's was estimated at 5% to 25%[1-3]. Today the incidence is certainly below one-half percent[1,4].

Sadly, the advances that improved the outcome of snakebite have generally been unappreciated. Perhaps the most important is the advent of rapid prehospital transportation. Antivenom or other hospital based treatments have little effect if the victim must travel hours to receive care. Another important development has been the evolution of intensive care medicine and critical care units. Finally, the introduction of specific antivenoms provided an effective method to reduce venom injury. All of these components are needed to manage a snakebite case adequately.

II. EPIDEMIOLOGY OF SNAKEBITE IN NORTH AMERICA

A. SNAKE DISTRIBUTION IN THE UNITED STATES

There are approximately 115 species of snakes in the United States, 19 of which are considered venomous[5]. Approximately 45,000 snakebites occur each year. 8,000 of these are inflicted by venomous snakes[6], resulting in 9 - 14 deaths. Most bites occur between March and October, when snakes and victims are most active. See Table 1 for a list of major venomous snakes found in the United States. Distribution maps for major venomous snakes found in the U.S. are shown in Figure 1.

Table 1
Principal venomous snakes of the United States[53]

Scientific Name	Common Name	Original Describer/Year
Crotalus	**Rattlesnake**	**Linnaeus,1758**
C. adamanteus	Eastern Diamondback Rattlesnake	Palisot de Beauvois,1799
C.atrox	Western Diamondback Rattlesnake	Baird & Girard,1853
C.cerastes	Sidewinder	Hallowell,1854
C.c.cerastes	Mojave Desert Sidewinder	Hallowell,1854
C.c.cercobombus	Sonoran Sidewinder	Savage & Cliff,1953
C.c.laterorepens	Colorado Desert Sidewinder	Klauber,1944
C.horridus	Timber Rattlesnake	Linnaeus,1758
C.lepidus	Rock Rattlesnake	Kennicott,1861
C. l . klauberi	Banded Rock Rattlesnake	Gloyd,1936
C.l.lepidus	Mottled Rock Rattlesnake	Kennicott,1861
C.mitchellii	Speckled Rattlesnake	Cope,1861
C.m.pyrrhus	Southwestern Speckled Rattlesnake	Cope,1866
C.m.stenhensi	Panamint Rattlesnake	Klauber,1930
C. molossus	Blacktail Rattlesnake	Baird & Girard,1853
C.m.molossus	Blacktail Rattlesnake	Baird & Girard,1853
C.pricei	Twin-spotted Rattlesnake	Van Denburgh,1895
C.p.pricei	Twin-spotted Rattlesnake	Van Denburgh,1895
C. ruber	Red Diamond Rattlesnake	Cope,1892
C.r.ruber	Red Diamond Rattlesnake	Cope,1892
C.scutulatus	Mojave Rattlesnake	Kennicott,1861
C.s.scutulatus	Mojave Rattlesnake	Kennicott,1861
C. tigris	Tiger Rattlesnake	Kennicott,1861
C.viridis	Western Rattlesnake	Rafinesque,1818
C.v.abyssus	Grand Canyon Rattlesnake	Klauber,1930
C.v.cerberus	Arizona Black Rattlesnake	Coues,1875
C.v.concolor	Midget Faded Rattlesnake	Woodbury,1929
C.v.helleri	Southern Pacific Rattlesnake	Meek,1905
C.v.lutosus	Great Basin Rattlesnake	Klauber,1930
C.v.nuntius	Hopi Rattlesnake	Holbrook,1840
C.v.viridis	Prairie Rattlesnake	Rafinesque,1818
C.willardi	Ridgenose Rattlesnake	Meek,1905
C.w.obscurus	New Mexico Ridgenose Rattlesnake	Harris,1974
C.w.willardi	Arizona Ridgenose Rattlesnake	Meek,1905
Sistrurus	**Pigmy Rattlesnakes & Massasauga**	**Garman,1883**
S.catenatus	Massasauga	Rafinesque,1818
S.c.catenatus	Eastern Massasauga	Rafinesque,1818
S.c.ewardsii	Desert Massauga	Baird & Girard,1853
S.c.tergeminus	Western Massauga	Say,1823

Scientific Name	Common Name	Original Describer/Year
S.miliarius	Pigmy Rattlesnake	Linnaeus,1766
S.m.barbouri	Dusky Pigmy Rattlesnake	Gloyd,1935
S.m.miliarius	Carolina Pigmy Rattlesnake	Linnaeus,1966
S.m. steckeri	Western Pigmy Rattlesnake	Gloyd,1935
Micruroides	**Western Coral Snake**	**Schmidt,1928**
M.euryxanthus	Western Coral Snake	Kennicot,1860
M.e.euryxanthus	Arizona Coral Snake	Kennicot,1860
Micrurus	**Eastern Coral Snake**	**Wagler,1824**
M.fulvius	Eastern Coral Snake	Linnaeus,1766
M.f.fulvius	Eastern Coral Snake	Linnaeus,1766
M.f.tenere	Texas Coral Snake	Baird & Girard,1853
Agkistrodon	**Copperhead & Cottonmouth**	**Palisot de Beauvois,1799**
A.contortrix	Copperhead	Linnaeus,1766
A.c.contortrix	Southern Copperhead	Linnaeus,1766
A.c.laticinctus	Broad-banded Copperhead	Gloyd & Conant,1934
A.c.mokasen	Northern Copperhead	Palisot de Beauvois,1799
A.c.phaeogaster	Osage Copperhead	Gloyd,1969
A.c.pictigaster	Trans-pecos Copperhead	Gloyd & Conant,1943
A.piscivorus	Cottonmouth	Lacepede,1789
A.p.conanti	Florida Cottonmouth	Gloyd,1969
A.p.leucostoma	Western Cottonmouth	Troost,1836
A.p.piscivorus	Eastern cottonmouth	Lacepede,1789

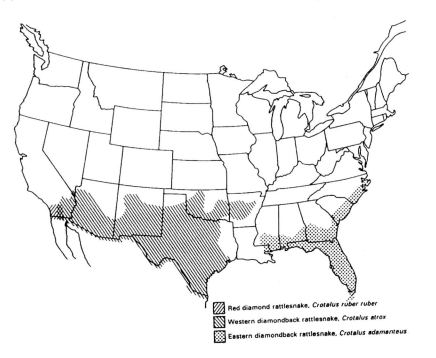

Figure 1. Distribution maps for major United States venomous snakes (Courtesy F.E. Russell).

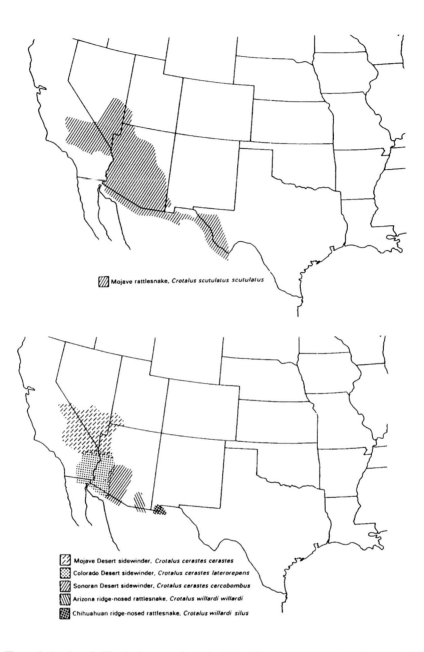

Figure 1. (continued): Distribution maps for major United States venomous snakes (Courtesy F.E. Russell).

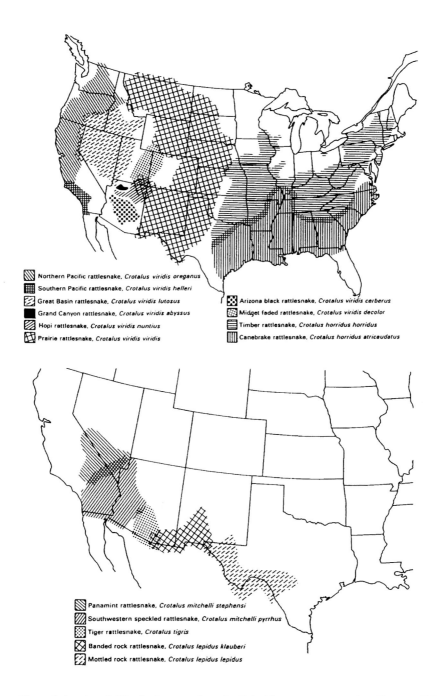

Figure 1. (continued): Distribution maps for major United States venomous snakes (Courtesy F.E. Russell).

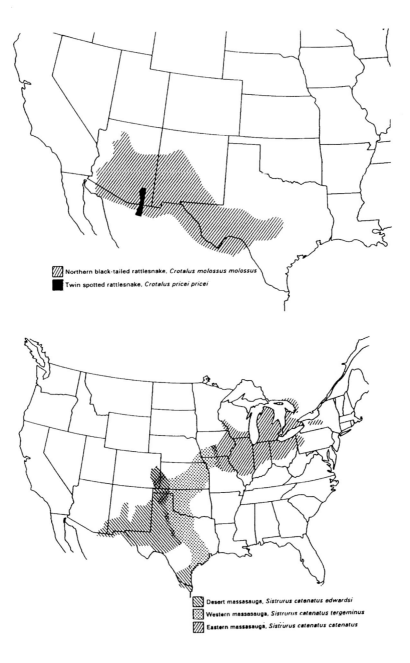

Figure 1. (continued): Distribution maps for major United States venomous snakes (Courtesy F.E. Russell).

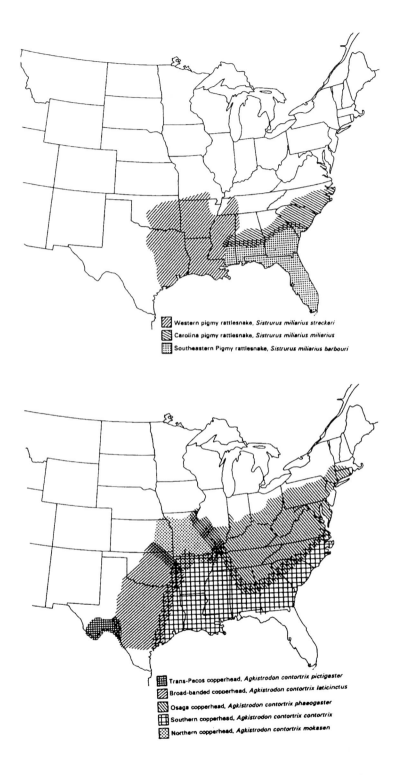

Figure 1. (continued): Distribution maps for major United States venomous snakes (Courtesy F.E. Russell).

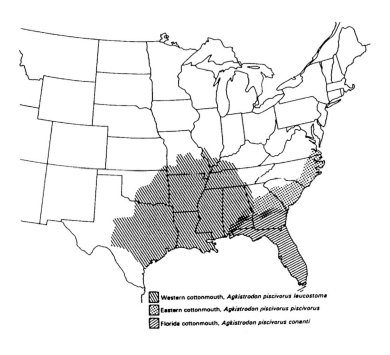

Western cottonmouth, *Agkistrodon piscivorus leucostoma*
Eastern cottonmouth, *Agkistrodon piscivorus piscivorus*
Florida cottonmouth, *Agkistrodon piscivorus conanti*

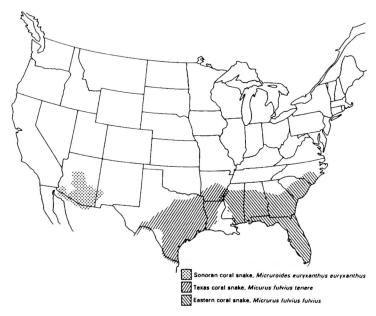

Sonoran coral snake, *Micruroides euryxanthus euryxanthus*
Texas coral snake, *Micurus fulvius tenere*
Eastern coral snake, *Micrurus fulvius fulvius*

Figure 1. (continued): Distribution maps for major United States venomous snakes (Courtesy F.E. Russell).

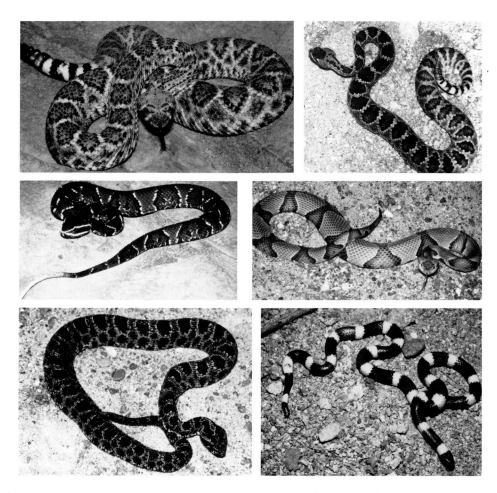

Figure 2. Some major venomous snakes of North America (photos © Dr. J. White). From top left clockwise: *Crotalus atrox, C. scutelatus, Agkistrodon contortrix, Micruroides euryxanthus, Sistrurus miliaris, A. bilineatus.*

Poisonous snakebites in the United States involve members of the family Crotalidae (pit vipers), and the family Elapidae. Three genera from the family Crotalidae inhabit the United States: *Crotalus* (rattlesnakes), *Sistrurus* (pygmy rattlesnake and massasauga), and *Agkistrodon* (copperheads and water moccasins).

Coral snakes are representatives of the Elapidae family in North America. These include the eastern coral snake *(Micrurus fulvius fulvius)*, and the Texas coral snake *(Micrurus fulvius tenere)*, and the Arizona (Sonoran) coral snake *(Micruroides euryxanthus)*. The Texas and Arizona coral snakes are found primarily in the states that bear their names, and the eastern coral snake is found primarily in the extreme southeast United States[1]. Overall, coral snakes account for only 20 to 25 bites a year[7].

Envenomations also occur by exotic species: species not indigenous to the United States. Although the incidence of poisonous snake bites from exotic species is low, medically important snakebites by exotic species not indigenous to the United States may occur in zoo personnel as well as in amateur herpetologists[8].

B. SNAKE DISTRIBUTION IN MEXICO

Mexico possesses a larger number of dangerously venomous snakes (59 species) than any other country in the New World[9]. Included in its fauna are practically every species of venomous snake occurring in the United States and Belize[9]. See Table 2 for a list of major venomous snakes found in Mexico. Distribution maps for major venomous snakes found in Mexico are shown in Figure 3. As in the continental United States, the most important snake family in terms of the abundance of species and subspecies, as well as the incidence of morbidity and mortality, is the Crotalidae family[10].

Table 2
Principal venomous snake species of Mexico[9,11,53]

Scientific Name	Common Name	Original Describer/Year
Bothrops	**Lancehead**	**Wagler,1824**
Bothrops asper	Vibora Sorda, ahueyactli, Barba Amarilla, Cuatro Narices	Garman,1884
Crotalus	**Rattlesnake**	**Linnaeus,1758**
Crotalus atrox	Vipora Serrana	Baird & Girard,1953
C.basiliscus	Saye (Cora Indians)	Cope,1864
C.catalinensis	Vibora de Cascabel	Cliff,1954
C.cerastes	Vibora Cornuda	Hallowell,1854
C.durissus	Cascabel Tropical	Linnaeus,1758
C.enyo	Vipora de Cascabel	Cope,1861
C.exsul	Vipora de Cascabel	Garman,1884
C.intermedius	Colcoatl,V lbora Sorda	Troschel,1866
C.lannomi	Vibora de cascabel	Tanner,1966
C.mitchellii	Vibora Blanca	Cope,1861
C. molossus	Vibora de Cascabel de Cola Negra	Baird & Girard,1953
C. polystictus	Chiauhcoatl, Tlehua (Nahuatl)	Cope,1865
C. pricei	Vibora de Cascabel	Van Denburgh,1895
C. pusillus	Vibora de Cascabel	Klauber,1952
C.ruber	Vibora de Cascabel	Cope,1861
C.scutulatus	Chiauhcoatl (Nahuatl)	Kennicott,1861
C.stejnegeri	Vibora de Cascabel	Dunn,1919
C.tigris	Vibora de Cascabel	Kennicott,1861
C.tortugensis	Vibora de Cascabel	V.Denburgh & Slevin,1921
C.transversus	Vibora de Cascabel	Taylor,1944
C.triseriatus	Hocico de Puerco	Wagler,1830
C.viridis	Vibora de Cascabel	Rafinesque,1818
C.willardi	Vibora de Cascabel	Meek,1906
Sistrurus	**Pigmy Rattlesnakes & Massasauga**	**Garman,1883**
Sistrurus catenatus	Vibora de Cascabel	Rafinesque,1818
S. ravus	Cascabel Enana,Colcoatl, Rotalo Pigmeo	Cope,1865
Micruroides	**Western Coral Snake**	**Schmidt,1928**
M.euryxanthus	Coralillo de Sonora	Kennicot,1860
Micrurus	**Eastern Coral Snake**	**Wagler,1824**
Micrurus bernadi	Coral, Coralillo	Cope,1887
M.bogerti	Coral, Coralillo	Roze,1967
M.browni	Coral de Canutos (Chiapas)	Schmidt & Smith, 1943
M.diastema	Coral Anillado	Dumeril, Bibron
M.distans	Coral, Coralillo	Kennicott,1860
M.elegans	Coral Punteado (Chiapas)	Jan,1858
M.ephippifer	Coral, Coralillo	Cope,1865
M.fulvius	Coral, Coralillo	Linnaeus
M.laticollaris	Coral, Coralillo	Peters,1869
M.latifasciatus	Coral, Coralillo	Schmidt,1933
M.limbatus	Coral, Coralillo	Fraser,1964
M.proximans	Coral, Coralillo	Smith & Chrapliwy,1966

0

0

0

0

0

629

Scientific Name	Common Name	Original Describer/Year
M.nigrocinctus	Coral, Coralillo, Gargantilla	Girard
Agkistrodon	**Cottonmouth & Copperhead**	**Palisot de Beauvois,1799**
A.bilineatus	Cantil de agua	Gunther,1863
A.contortrix	Local name unknown (Copperhead)	Linnaeus,1776

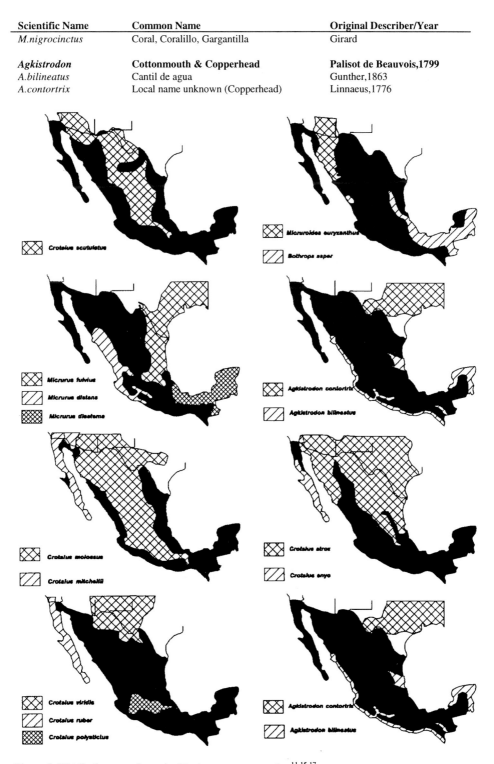

Figure 3. Distribution maps for major Mexican venomous snakes[11,15,17].

Much of Mexico and Central America has been cleared for agriculture. This has resulted in areas of secondary growth which provides a suitable habitat for numerous venomous snake species such as *Bothrops asper*[9]. The genus *Bothrops* is distributed primarily in South America, with the exception of "cuatro narices" *Bothrops asper*, which extends through Central America into northern Mexico along the Atlantic versant[11,12]. This snake is responsible for the majority of snakebites in Mexico and is found in a variety of habitats in its range[11]. In general, however, *B. asper* is found principally in tropical rainforest and tropical evergreen forest[12]. *Bothrops asper* is primarily a lowland form, with its distribution ranging from sea level up to a maximum of 1,200-1,300 meters[13]. The snake is considered to be particularly large and aggressive, and may grow up to 2.5 meters in length[11].

The rattlesnakes (genera *Crotalus* and *Sistrurus*) undergo their maximum radiation in Mexico with the Mexican Plateau and its fringing mountains possessing the greatest diversity of rattlesnakes[9]. Mainland Mexico is the approximate center of rattlesnake geographic distribution, and also has the greatest variety of rattlesnakes[14]. The United States follows Mexico in rattlesnake diversity[14]. There are 26 species[9] and 54 subspecies[14] that inhabit the Mexican mainland, Baja peninsula, and the islands of the Pacific and Gulf of California[14].

The genus *Sistrurus* is represented in Mexico by 2 species, *S. ravus* and *S. catenatus*. *Sistrurus ravus*, known locally as the cascabel enana or colcoatl (Mexican pygmy rattlesnake), is distributed in the highlands of central and southern Mexico[15]. The distribution of *S. catenatus* (massasauga) is mainly restricted to the continental United States; however, this species has been identified in north-central and north-eastern Mexico[15].

The Crotalidae family in Mexico is also represented by 2 *Agkistrodon* species[11,16]. *Agkistrodon contortrix* (copperhead) barely ranges into north central Mexico. Its range in Mexico extends along the banks of the Rio Grande and in canyons from northeastern Chihuahua through northern Coahuila, and from the Sierra del Camden to Piedra Negroes[16]. The range of *A. balanites* is much more extensive and includes northern Mexico from Tamaulipas and Sonora, Mexico, southward to northwestern Costa Rica[16]. Throughout its range the species is distributed in seasonally dry forest habitats[16].

The Elapidae family in Mexico, as in the United States, is made up of different species of coral snake. They include at least 14 different species consisting of 1 from the genus *Micruroides* and 13 from the genus *Micrurus*[17]. The genus *Micrurus* is thought to contain 53 species in the western hemisphere. Mexico is represented by at least 13 species distributed in a variety of habitats, ranging from desert to cloud forest[17].

C. CHARACTERISTICS OF SNAKES AND VENOMS IN NORTH AMERICA

Members of the Crotalidae family are called pit vipers because of bilateral depressions or pits located midway between and below the level of the eye and the nostril (Figure 4). The pit is a heat-receptor organ[18] which senses the presence and location of warm-blooded prey or predators[5]. The pit also guides the direction of a strike. The maximal range of effectiveness of this organ is approximately 14 inches[19]. The Crotalid snakes are also distinguished by two fangs (elongated, upper maxillary teeth) which can be folded against the roof of the mouth (Figures 5 and 6). This is in contrast to the Elapids (coral snakes) which have shorter fangs that are fixed in an erect position[6]. The presence of a rattle distinguishes the rattlesnake from all other Crotalids. Neonate rattlesnakes may lack functional rattle segments and are often practically soundless. An indestructible myth that rattlesnakes always rattle before striking has persisted for 250 years[19]. In truth, many strikes occur without a warning rattle.

The venom gland in all crotalids is located in the upper jaw area posterior to the eye. This gland is surrounded by striated muscle which enables the snake to inject large doses of venom[1]. Crotalid venom is a complex mixture of proteins which have enzymatic activities that can cause local tissue injury, systemic vascular damage, hemolysis, fibrinolysis, and neuromuscular dysfunction, resulting in a combination of local and systemic effects. These proteins include: transaminase, hyaluronidase, phospholipase, phosphodiesterase, cholinesterase, and endonucleases (Table 3). Venom proteins range in molecular weight from less than 6,000 to over 100,000[20]. The peptides in snake venom appear to bind to multiple receptor sites in their prey[21]. Because there are multiple sites of action, it is prudent not to label or treat a poisoning as a "neurotoxin", "hemotoxin" or "cardiotoxin".[1] Collectively, crotalid snake venom components affect almost every organ system. In crotalid envenomations, the most deleterious effects are seen in the cardiovascular, hematologic, respiratory and nervous systems.

Coral snakes are representatives of the Elapidae family in North America. They are all brightly colored snakes with black, red, and yellow rings that entirely encircle their bodies. The red and yellow rings touch in coral snakes, but are separated by black rings in nonpoisonous snakes. This has given rise to the well known rhyme: "red on yellow, kill a fellow; red on black, venom lack." This rule is not true for countries other than the United States.

Elapids lack the heat-sensing facial pits found in Crotalids and have nearly round pupils. Coral snakes are smaller and more docile than crotalids. The fangs on the coral snake are small and fixed, making it necessary for coral snakes to hold onto their prey for significant envenomation to take place[1]. Coral snake venom is primarily composed of neurotoxic components that do not cause marked local injury. The incidence of serious human envenomations by coral snakes is much lower than that for Crotalids, but serious envenomations still occur[22,23].

D. SNAKEBITE IN NORTH AMERICA

Statistics on the incidence of snakebites in North America should be viewed with caution. They most likely underestimate the true incidence overall since health care facilities in Mexico[24] and in the United States[25] are not required to report snakebites. Bearing that in mind, it has been estimated that 45,000 bites by all snakes in the United States occur each year, with about 6,680 persons treated for snake venom poisoning[6]. Fatalities from snakebite have ranged from 9 -14 deaths per year with most deaths attributed to rattlesnakes[6]. Out of 76,941 animal bites in the United States reported voluntarily to the American Association of Poison Control Centers during 1991, 4,408 were due to snakebites. Rattlesnakes accounted for 13.7%, copperheads 8.8%, cottonmouths 1.5%, unknown crotalids 0.2%, coral snakes 0.6%, poisonous exotic snakes 19.5%, nonpoisonous snakes 23.6%, and the remainder were unknown snakes[26]. Bites by poisonous snakes occur only occasionally during the colder months of the year (November - March). This is because humans generally spend less time out of doors and snakes are generally inactive during the winter months. Parrish et al. found that during a ten year period (1950 -1959) 95% of snakebite incidents happened from April through October[27]. Table 4 lists the estimated incidence of poisonous snakebite in the United States by region and state.

It is estimated that approximately 27,480 snakebites occur in Mexico per year[28,29]. During the years 1960 to 1974 there were 291 reported deaths from snakebites in Mexico[11]. This would be an annual incidence of 20.8 snakebite fatalities per year during this 14 year time period. The highest percentage of deaths were reported from the states of Oaxaca (21.6%) and Veracruz (15.8%)[11]. Table 5 summarizes the snakebite fatality rate by region and state.

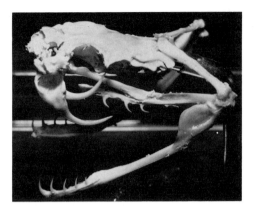

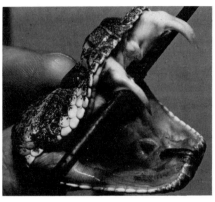

Figures 4. Skull of *C. atrox* showing fangs and non fang teeth (photo © Dr. J. White).

Figure 5. Live specimen of *C. atrox*, showing erect fangs (photo © Dr. J. White).

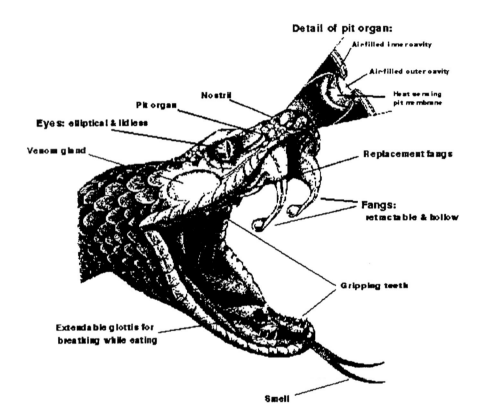

Figure 6. Crotalidae envenomation and heat sensing structures (with permission from the New York Times).

Table 3
Enzymes in North American snake venoms[1] (courtesy F.E. Russell)

	Crotalus	*Sistrurus*	*Agkistrodon*	*Micrurus*
Proteolytic enzymes	+	+	+	+
Arginine ester ester hydrolase	+	NK*	+	NK
Thrombin -like enzyme	+	NK	+	NK
Collagenase	+	NK	+	NK
Hyaluronidase	+	NK	+	NK
Phospholipase A_2(A)	+	N K	+	+
Phospholipase B	?	NK	NK	NK
Phosphomonoesterase	+	NK	+	NK
Acetylcholinesterase	0	0	0	NK
RNase	+	NK	NK	NK
DNase	+	NK	NK	NK
5'-Nucleotidase	+	NK	+	NK
NAD-Nucleotidase	0	0	+	NK
L-Amino acid oxidase	+	+	+	NK
Lactate dehydrogenase	NK	NK	NK	NK

*NK= Not Known

Table 4
Estimated incidence of poisonous snakebite by region and state[4]

Region and State	Inpatient	Outpatient	Total Bites	Per 100,000 /Year
New England	**7.6**	**0.0**	**7.6**	**0.07**
Maine	0.0	0.0	0.0	0.0
New Hampshire	1.0	0.0	1.0	0.16
Vermont	0.3	0.0	0.0	0.08
Massachusetts	2.0	0.0	2.0	0.04
Rhode Island	0.3	0.0	0.3	0.04
Connecticut	4.0	0.0	4.0	0.16
Middle Atlantic	**57.0**	**79.0**	**136.0**	**0.40**
New York	12.0	25.0	37.0	0.22
New Jersey	15.0	10.0	25.0	0.41
Pennsylvania	30.0	44.0	74.0	0.65
East North Central	**88.0**	**110.0**	**19 8.0**	**0. 55**
Ohio	24.0	21.0	45.0	0.46
Indiana	20.0	25.0	45.0	0.97
Illinois	11.0	24.0	35.0	0.35
Michigan	26.0	32.0	58.0	0.74
West North Central	**215.0**	**228.0**	**443.0**	**2.88**
Minnesota	3.0	0.0	3.0	0.09
Iowa	6.0	3.0	9.0	0.33
Missouri	111.0	123.0	234.0	5.42
North Dakota	5.0	0.0	5.0	0.79
South Dakota	22.0	9.0	31.0	4.56
Nebraska	20.0	26.0	46.0	3.26
Kansas	48.0	67.0	115.0	5.28
South Atlantic	**1,255.0**	**1,147.0**	**2,402.0**	**9.25**
Florida	209.0	141.0	350.0	7.07
Georgia	304.0	226.0	530.0	13.44
South Carolina	104.0	80.0	184.0	7.72
North Carolina	392.0	464.0	856.0	18.79
Virginia	112.0	105.0	217.0	5.47
West Virginia	111.0	99.0	210.0	11.29
Maryland	18.0	24.0	42.0	1.35
Delaware	2.0	6.0	8.0	1.79
District of Columbia	3.0	2.0	5.0	0.65
East South Central	**356.0**	**310.0**	**666.0**	**5.53**
Tennessee	43.0	36.0	79.0	2.21
Kentucky	92.0	51.0	143.0	4.71
Alabama	108.0	100.0	208.0	6.37
Mississippi	113.0	123.0	236.0	10.83

Region and State	Inpatient	Outpatient	Total Bites	Per 100,000 /Year
West South Central	**1,251.0**	**1,004.0**	**2,255.0**	**13.30**
Arkansas	152.0	155.0	307.0	17.19
Louisiana	195.0	139.0	334.0	10.25
Oklahoma	120.0	86.0	206.0	8.85
Texas	784.0	624.0	1,408.0	14.70
Mountain	**210.0**	**100.0**	**310.0**	**4.52**
Montana	18.0	20.0	38.0	5.63
Idaho	6.0	4.0	10.0	1.50
Wyoming	12.0	9.0	21.0	6.36
Colorado	30.0	11.0	41.0	2.34
New Mexico	59. 0	12.0	71.0	7.47
Arizona	72. 0	30.0	102.0	7.83
Utah	9. 0	11.0	20.0	2.25
Nevada	4. 0	3.0	7.0	2.45
Pacific	**163. 0**	**97.0**	**260.0**	**1.28**
Washington	20. 0	5.0	25.0	0.88
Oregon	5. 0	9.0	14.0	0.79
California	138. 0	83.0	221.0	1.41

Table 5
Annual fatality rate in 10 states* of Mexico 1960 -1974[11]

State*	Fatalities per year	Percent of total (%)
Oaxaca	32.7	22.0
Veracruz	22.7	15.2
Puebla	12.7	8.5
Chiapas	11.7	7.8
Hidalgo	10.5	7.1
San Luis Potosi	8.3	5.6
Tabasco	7.7	5.2
Michoacan	5.0	3.4
Yucatan	5.0	3.4
Jalisco	4.0	2.7
Total	**120.3**	**80.9**
All of Mexico	*148.7*	*100.0*

* 10 States with the highest snakebite fatality rate

The large pitviper *Bothrops asper* is abundant in Mexico and is considered the principle cause of snakebite envenomation throughout its range[9,11], although one study conducted in Merida, Yucatan, revealed an equal number of hospital admissions for *B. asper* and *C. terrificus*[30]. As one might imagine from the great diversity of rattlesnake species in Mexico, the overall incidence of rattlesnake bite is second only to bites from *Bothrops* species[9]. Avila (1980) reported that the highest incidence of rattlesnake bites resulting in hospital admissions occurred between the months of March and November in data collected over 4 years (1975 -1978)[24]. The peak month for admissions was September, which the authors attributed to climatic factors (e.g. peak seasonal humidity)[24].

III. SYMPTOMS AND SIGNS

A. GENERAL CONCEPTS OF ENVENOMATION
Many frightened patients have been bitten by nonvenomous snakes, and not all victims of poisonous snakebite are envenomed. Since snakebite treatment itself may cause medical complications, it is important to recognize the signs and symptoms of envenomation. Up to 25% of crotalid snakebites do not result in envenomation[6]. The severity of poisoning following a crotalid bite is therefore variable. Crotalid bites are generally classified as *minimal, moderate,* or *severe* depending on the degree of local and

systemic injury (Table 6)[31]. The gravity of envenomation is dependent on several factors including: location, depth, and number of bites; the amount of venom injected, the species and size of the snake involved, the age and size of the victim, and the time post snakebite of definitive therapy[6].

B. GENERAL SYMPTOMS AND SIGNS OF ENVENOMATION

Crotalid envenomation is characterized by the presence of one or more fang marks, burning pain[5], and early progressive local edema around the area of the bite site[6]. Common symptoms and signs of rattlesnake bite are listed in Table 7. In general, when envenomation has occurred, some swelling becomes apparent within 10 -20 minutes following the bite[25] secondary to small vessel and capillary injury[31]. Crotalid venom quickly alters blood vessel permeability, leading to loss of plasma and blood into the surrounding tissue. In severe Crotalidae envenomations the progressive edema may involve an entire limb within one to two hours. In contrast, the edema may slowly progress over a one to two day period in less severe envenomations[5]. Edema in a particular area, such as the face or a muscle compartment, may threaten life or limb without the presence of apparent systemic effects[31].

Table 6
Procedure for assessment of crotalid bite severity[31] (30 min-4hr)

The grading of a bite should be based on the physician's assessment of local injury, systemic signs and symptoms, and the results of laboratory tests. The grading of the bite should be determined by the most severe symptom or sign (e.g., a patient with no swelling but having a systolic blood pressure of 70 mm/hg should be considered a severe envenomation).

Minimal Envenomation
Swelling, erythema, or ecchymosis limited to immediate area of the bite site
Systemic signs and symptoms not present or minimal
Coagulation parameters all normal. No other significant laboratory abnormalities.

Moderate Envenomation
Swelling, erythema or ecchymosis present, may involve most of an extremity, and may be spreading slowly.
Systemic signs and symptoms present, but not life-threatening. These may include nausea, vomiting, oral paresthesias or unusual tastes, mild hypotension (SBP > 80 mm/hg), mild tachycardia, and tachypnea.
Coagulation parameters may be abnormal, but no clinically significant bleeding is present. Severe abnormalities of other laboratory tests are not present.

Severe Envenomation
Swelling or ecchymosis involve the entire extremity and are spreading rapidly.
Systemic signs and symptoms are markedly abnormal, including severe alteration of mental status, nausea and vomiting, hypotension (SBP < 80), severe tachycardia, tachypnea, or other respiratory compromise.
Coagulation parameters abnormal with serious bleeding present or threat of spontaneous bleeding, including PT unmeasurable, PTT unmeasurable, platelets <20,000/μL, or fibrinogen undetectable. Severe abnormalities of other laboratory values should also be considered severe envenomations.

Swelling is especially prominent in bites by the eastern diamondback and may be less marked in bites by the Mojave, prairie, timber, red, Pacific, black-tailed rattlesnakes[6], copperhead, pygmy rattler, and massasauga snakes[5]. Lymphangitis and regional lymph nodes tenderness often occur[25]. Progressive ecchymosis is also seen because of leakage of red blood cells into subcutaneous tissue[25]. Ecchymosis and discoloration of the skin may appear within minutes or hours in the area of the snakebite[6]. Hemorrhagic blebs may also occur within several hours for similar reasons. Of interest, hemoconcentration may initially be present as a result of the leakage of fluid into subcutaneous tissue, followed by a decrease in hemoglobin over several days from blood loss secondary to coagulopathy[5].

Table 7
Incidence of symptoms of rattlesnake venom poisoning[25] (courtesy F.E. Russell)

Symptom or Sign	Incidence	Symptom or Sign	Incidence
Fang marks	100%	Increased blood clotting time	37%
Swelling and edema	74%	Decreased hemoglobin	37%
Weakness	70%	Thirst	34%
Pain	65%	Necrosis	27%
Numbness of tingling of tongue and mouth, or scalp or feet	63%	Abnormal electrocardiogram	26%
Changes in pulse rate	60%	Glycosuria	20%
Tingling or numbness of affected part	57%	Increased salivation	20%
Faintness or dizziness	57%	Sphering of red blood cells	18%
Blood pressure changes	54%	Proteinuria	16%
Ecchymosis	51%	Cyanosis	16%
Sweating and/or chills	43%	Increased blood platelets	16%
Nausea, vomiting, or both	42%	Hematemesis, hematuria, or melena	15%
Change in body temperature	42%	Unconsciousness	12%
Decreased blood platelets	42%	Blurring of vision	12%
Fasciculations	41%	Swollen eyelids	7%
Swelling regional lymph nodes	40%	Muscle contractions	6%
Vesiculations	40%	Retinal hemorrhage	5%
Respiratory rate changes	40%	Convulsions	1%

Other systemic symptoms include generalized weakness, diaphoresis, nausea and vomiting, hyperthermia, paresthesias, altered level of consciousness (including syncope), perioral and periorbital muscular fasciculations[25]. Muscle fasciculations may also be seen in the area of the bite site. Victims may note a metallic, minty, or rubbery taste in their mouths[25]. Paresthesias or numbness is frequently noted in the face, scalp, around the lips, and at the tips of fingers and toes, particularly following bites by the Mojave and eastern diamondback rattlesnakes[5,25].

Coral snake venom is primarily composed of neurotoxic components. Unlike pit viper venoms, coral snake venom lacks significant proteolytic enzymatic function, which explains paucity of local signs and symptoms following envenomation[32]. Elapid bites may result in tremors, marked salivation, and mental status changes - including drowsiness and euphoria. Signs and symptoms may be delayed[33] up to 12 hours post envenomation[22]. The neurological signs including dysarthria and diplopia, may herald the onset of cranial nerve palsies and bulbar paralysis with ptosis, fixed and contracted pupils, dysphagia, dyspnea, and seizures. The immediate cause of death is paralysis of muscles of respiration[5,22,33].

IV. FIRST AID TREATMENT

A. PRINCIPLES AND THEORY OF FIRST AID

First aid measures should never be regarded as a substitute for definitive medical care, nor should they be instituted at the expense of delaying the administration of antivenom[6]. Since the benefit of first aid has not been proven, but has on occasion produced morbidity, controversy continues as to appropriate early treatment following a snakebite[34]. The standard of practice recommended by a national symposium in 1960 included incision, suction, and application of a constriction band. These recommendations are potentially harmful and have given way to more conservative, less invasive first aid procedures (described below)[1,34].

B. RECOMMENDED FIRST AID

- The victim should retreat beyond striking range[5]. Some patients have been bitten more than once by the same snake[35], usually by persons who persist in handling the snake in spite of the first bite[5].
- Victims and helpers should remain calm. Even experienced snake handlers may panic and use inappropriate measures.
- The extremity should be immobilized in a neutral position below the level of the heart.
- The victim's physical activity should be kept minimal.
- Because antivenom cannot be administered if the patient is not in a medical facility, the victim should be promptly transported regardless of whether they have overt signs of envenomation. Since the signs and symptoms of snakebites may be delayed, it is prudent for clinical effects to develop under the watchful eye of trained medical personnel. Further aid by laypersons other than the 5 measures listed above is of questionable value[6].

Prehospital personnel should be directed to establish intravenous access, administer oxygen, and transport victims to a medical facility. Previously placed tourniquets and constriction bands should not be removed until intravenous access has been established.

C. FIRST AID KITS AND ELECTRIC SHOCK THERAPY

Several commercially available first aid products deserve comment. The well known Cutter Snakebite Kit® contains suction cups that produce little suction, and often produce an ineffective seal on digits. The scalpel blade in the kit can injure digital nerves, arteries, and tendons[34] and is not recommended. Another product, the Sawyer Extractor Vacuum Pump®, can produce up to 750 mm/hg of negative pressure over the puncture site without incision. Although this device has been shown to remove some snake venom in one animal study[36], the clinical efficacy of this device is unproven.

Electric shock treatment of snakebite has garnered much publicity since being reported in a letter to *The Lancet* describing dramatic improvement of pain and swelling in snakebite victims in a remote region of Ecuador[37]. Efficacy of this dangerous procedure has never been proven in animal[38] or human studies and has resulted in serious electrical injuries[39-41]. We strongly advise against the use of any form of this potentially harmful technique.

Current medical opinion on the use of constriction bands is divided. In theory, the use of a constriction band retards venom absorption, which should increase local tissue injury while reducing the incidence and severity of systemic manifestations. An animal study (porcine model) using constriction bands designed to restrict only superficial venous and lymphatic flow while allowing arterial and deep venous flow found that constriction band use delayed venom absorption without causing increased swelling[42]. Although constriction band use may prove to be a useful first aid measure in humans, additional controlled studies are needed to better define the clinical indications for the use of this technique.

V. LABORATORY TESTS

Evaluation in a health care facility includes obtaining blood and urine for laboratory testing. The choice of the test will depend on the family of snakes involved[25], and the presentation of physical and systemic findings. For example, a coagulation abnormality resembling disseminated intravascular coagulation is a common laboratory finding in rattlesnake bites[31]. Although evidence of intravascular hemolysis on the peripheral blood smear is unusual, decreased fibrinogen, increased prothrombin time (PT) and activated partial thromboplastin time (PTT), and thrombocytopenia are common[31]. Urinalysis may occasionally reveal hematuria, glycosuria, and proteinuria. Bleeding and clotting times are usually prolonged[6].

Laboratory evaluation in rattlesnake envenomations include complete blood count and platelet counts, coagulation parameters (including prothrombin and partial thromboplastin times, fibrinogen level), renal function tests, urinalysis, and electrolytes. In severe poisonings it is advisable to type and cross-match[6], and obtain an arterial blood gas as well as an electrocardiogram[25]. In severe envenomations by rattlesnakes, complete blood and platelet counts, and coagulation parameters should be determined serially.

Since signs and symptoms of coral snake bite are neurological in nature, the emphasis on blood screens is not warranted[25]. However, since respiratory failure may result from clinical effects of the neurotoxin, baseline and serial pulmonary function parameters (such as inspiratory pressure and vital capacity) in addition to ICU observation may be useful.

VI. CLINICAL MANAGEMENT

A. GENERAL CONSIDERATIONS

Initial management in the treatment of snakebite, as in any emergency, should include advanced cardiac life support as necessary with appropriate attention to Airway, Breathing and Circulation. Prehospital personnel should be directed to establish intravenous access, administer oxygen, and transport victims to a medical facility. The initial management of hypotension should be rapid intravenous isotonic fluid infusion. Tourniquets and constriction bands should not be removed until intravenous access is established. Other recommended supportive care measures include immobilization of the limb in a functional position until swelling is clearly receding and coagulation tests are normal. During recovery, the bitten part (particularly the hand) should be regularly exercised in order to preserve as much function and strength as possible[31]. The wound area should be cleaned and the need for tetanus booster should be determined[25]. Cultures and antibiotic therapy should be initiated only if clinical signs of infection develop. Blebs, bloody vesicles, or superficial necrosis can be debrided several days after the injury. The area may then be treated as a second-degree burn[31].

Physicians who are not familiar with the management of snake envenomation or who encounter problematical clinical issues should contact a toxicologist or a regional certified Poison Center with experience in the management of such cases. Hospital pharmacies in those regions of the United States where poisonous snakes are prevalent should maintain adequate stocks of antivenom[35]. Unfortunately, many hospitals stock insufficient amounts of antivenom, even in endemic areas[43].

B. ANTIVENOM (GENERAL): CROTALIDAE AND ELAPIDAE

One commercial pit viper antivenom is available in the United States: Antivenin (Crotalidae) Polyvalent, produced by Wyeth-Ayerst Laboratories. Since the venoms of all pit vipers, including rattlesnakes, copperheads, and moccasins share some common antigens, Wyeth has manufactured an antivenom produced from hyperimmune serum. The venoms used in eliciting an immune response are: *Crotalus atrox, C. adamanteus, C. terrificus, and Bothrops atrox*[1]. Wyeth-Ayerst Laboratories also manufactures a commercial antivenom against the venom of the eastern coral snake *(Micrurus fulvius)*. This antivenom is probably effective against venom of other *Micrurus* species[44]; however, it is not effective for bites of the Arizona coral snake *(Micruroides euryxanthus)*[5]. Both antisera are prepared by immunization of horses (e.g. equine derived antivenom).

C. EVALUATION FOR POTENTIAL IMMUNE REACTIONS

Since Antivenin (Crotalidae) Polyvalent is derived from horse serum, it is common for patients to develop an allergic reaction during antivenom infusion. These are classified as acute and delayed serum reactions. Early reactions are type I hypersensitivity reactions mediated by histamine. Delayed serum reactions (serum sickness) are type III reactions.

An intradermal skin test should be applied before antivenom is given but only when a definite decision to administer the antivenom has been made. A true positive test (weal or erythema >10 mm in diameter appearing within 30 min) suggests that the patient may develop an allergic reaction to antivenom infusion, whereas a negative result usually indicates that the patient will tolerate the infusion[31,45]. However, some patients with negative skin tests will develop acute allergic reactions; likewise, some patients with positive skin tests tolerate antivenom infusion without difficulty. The skin test is a guide and antivenom decisions should be based on a risk-benefit analysis of the patient's condition. In addition to skin testing, a history of allergy to horse serum or previous reactions to antivenom should be obtained[35]. To prevent a delay while waiting for the skin test results, mixing of the initial dose of antivenom should be performed simultaneously with placement of the skin test. Since the antivenom takes about 30 minutes to go into solution, it will be ready when the skin test is interpreted[31].

D. ADMINISTRATION OF ANTIVENOM

All Crotalidae bites that show evidence of progressive signs and symptoms of envenomation should immediately receive the Antivenin (Crotalidae) Polyvalent. Progression is defined as worsening of local injury (e.g., pain, ecchymosis and swelling); laboratory abnormalities (e.g., worsening hemoglobin, platelet count, clotting times or other tests); or systemic manifestations (e.g., unstable vital signs or abnormal mental status)[31]. The recommended dose of antivenom has increased over the years. Originally, only 2-4 vials were recommended. Today 10 vials are recommended as the initial dose in rattlesnake bites. In rapidly progressive envenomations or cases developing hemodynamic instability, an initial dose of at least 20 vials of antivenom is recommended in addition to aggressive supportive care. Overall, poisoning by water moccasins usually requires lesser doses and in copperhead bites, antivenom is rarely required, except for in children and the elderly[6].

Under no circumstances should antivenom be injected directly into finger or toes[6]. Intramuscular injection is also not recommended as venom induced hypovolemia may retard absorption of antivenom.

It is recommended that the package insert may be used as a guide for preparation of the antivenom. In general, once mixed, the antivenom should be diluted in 250 to 500 cc of crystalloid and slowly infused, until it is evident that anaphylaxis will not occur. If a reaction does not develop, the rate should be increased in a stepwise manner until the rate will complete the antivenom infusion within one hour[31]. Infusion of antivenom should be done under the supervision of a physician until it has become clear that anaphylaxis will not take place[5].

Most patients will show arrest or reversal of their symptoms and signs during the first antivenom infusion; however, it is extremely important that observation for progression of edema and systemic symptoms of envenomation be continued even after antivenom has been infused. Limb circumference should be measured at several sites above and below the bite, and the advancing border of edema should be outlined with a pen every 15 -30 minutes. This serves as an index of the progression, as well as a guide for antivenom administration[25]. Laboratory determinations are repeated every 4 hours or after each course of antivenom therapy, whichever is more frequent. If any of the parameters worsen, additional antivenom therapy may be warranted.

It should be emphasized that one can easily be deceived by a bite that appears innocuous at first. An unremarkable physical and laboratory exam at presentation does not reliably indicate an insignificant envenomation. We recommended that physicians observe patients with a history of snakebite at least 8 hours[42]. Patients with dry bites may be discharged after 8 to 12 hours of observation. Patients with severe or life-threatening bites and patients receiving antivenom should be admitted to an intensive care unit. The general ward is appropriate for patients with mild or moderate envenomations who have completed or do not require further antivenom therapy.

Patients are ready for discharge when swelling begins to resolve, the coagulopathy has been reversed, and the patient is ambulatory. Outpatient follow-up is necessary to monitor for infection and serum sickness.

The value of aggressive supportive care cannot be overemphasized. Isotonic fluid resuscitation followed by pressor agents is appropriate for hypotension. Antivenom is the best treatment for coagulopathy, but if active bleeding has already started, blood component replacement such as fresh frozen plasma, platelets, and packed red blood cells may be necessary.

E. TREATMENT OF IMMUNE REACTIONS

If a reaction develops, the antivenom infusion should be immediately discontinued. Isotonic fluids, epinephrine and H_1- and H_2-receptor blocking drugs should be given to control the acute reaction. The severity of the envenomation must then be compared to the risks of restarting the antivenom infusion. In general, the antivenom can be restarted after dilution and slowing of the infusion. Positive skin tests may be handled in a similar manner: reassessment of the need for antivenom, pretreatment with histamine blockers, and dilution and slowing of the infusion. Since negative skin tests do not absolutely guarantee that a reaction will not take place during antivenom infusion, equipment for endotracheal intubation, cricothyrotomy[6], and medications for advanced cardiac life support should be immediately available. Delayed serum reactions (serum sickness) are type III hypersensitivity reactions. Type III reactions will usually occur 1-2 weeks after antivenom administration. Symptoms include malaise, fever, arthralgia, proteinuria, swollen joints, urticaria, lymphadenopathy, and occasionally peripheral neuritis manifested by pain and weakness of the extremities. The incidence of type III hypersensitivity increases with the number of vials used to treat the envenomation. McCollough[46] has reported an incidence of serum sickness of up to 75%[47]. Signs and symptoms of serum sickness may be treated with antihistamines and corticosteroids. Symptoms of serum sickness range from a mild viral-type illness to severe urticaria, rash, arthralgias, and other complications. Most patients who receive more than 5 vials develop serum sickness. Appropriate therapy includes anti-inflammatory analgesics, antihistamines, and corticosteroids.

F. ALTERNATIVE THERAPIES

The effectiveness of antivenom has been well established[11]. Fasciotomy and supportive care alone has been advocated by some, but evidence does not support this approach[25]. If a compartment syndrome is suspected, the compartment pressure should be documented before fasciotomy is performed. Fasciotomy should not be done unless the arterial blood supply has clearly been impaired[31]. This procedure may be considered in patients with elevated compartment pressure (>30 mm/hg) that is unresponsive to limb elevation, mannitol (1 to 2 grams per kg), and antivenom (an additional 10 vials). Insufficient venom neutralization has been more common than overneutralization. Our approach to potential compartment syndrome is shown in Table 8[31]. Morbidity and mortality from snakebite appears to be related to lack of treatment or undertreatment of the envenomation syndrome[48].

Table 8
Management of possible compartment syndrome after Crotalid envenomation[31]

1. Determine intracompartmental pressure.
2. If not elevated, continue standard management.
3. If signs of compartment syndrome are present and compartment pressure is > 30 mm/hg:
   a. Elevate limb.
   b. Administer mannitol 1 to 2 g/kg IV over 30 minutes.
   c. Simultaneously administer additional Antivenin (Crotalidae) Polyvalent, 10 to 15 vials IV over 60 minutes.
   d. If elevated compartment pressure persists another 60 minutes, consider fasciotomy.

Notes: 1. Elevated compartment pressure is caused by the action of the venom on the tissues, and thus, the most effective treatment is to neutralize the venom, which in many cases will reduce the compartment pressure.

2. This protocol delivers a high osmotic load and should not be used when contraindicated. The protocol must be completed promptly so that, if ever needed, fasciotomy may be performed as early as possible.

Although recommended by some authors, there is no objective evidence to support the use of prophylactic antibiotics. Wound infections are surprisingly rare after crotalid snake bites. As noted for other uses of prophylactic antibiotic treatment, infection may occur despite prophylactic antibiotic administration. Therefore, antibiotics are warranted only when evidence of infection is present.

The use of corticosteroids for the treatment of venom injury has been controversial for many years. To date, no convincing evidence of efficacy has been published, but several studies indicating lack of efficacy have been published[49-51]. Steroids should be reserved for the treatment of allergic reactions or as an adjunct in the treatment of serum sickness.

G. CORAL SNAKEBITE TREATMENT

Bites by coral snakes should be handled in a manner different from bites from Crotalidae species. Although the same general considerations for pit viper snakebites should be applied, the potential coral snake victim should be admitted to the hospital for

24-48 hours of observation if it is impossible to recover the snake[35]. Coral snake venom effects may develop hours after envenomation and are not easily reversed. It is suggested that 3 vials of the antivenom (*Micrurus fulvius*) be administered to all patients who have definitely been bitten by *M. fulvius* [25,31], since experience has shown that once symptoms and signs appear, it may not be possible to prevent further effects or reverse those changes that have already occurred[25]. Additional coral snake antivenom is reserved for the appearance of symptoms or signs of coral snake envenomation[35]. Ventilatory support may be required, and the patient must be observed closely for signs of respiratory muscle weakness and hypoventilation.[6] Since observation for mental status changes and other neurological signs is fundamental in the assessment of coral snake envenomations, it is best to avoid the use of sedatives[25].

H. SEQUELAE OF NORTH AMERICAN SNAKE POISONING

Although envenomation by coral snakes may certainly result in mortality[22], little or no data has been reported concerning permanent sequelae in coral snake bite survivors. Kitchens[22] and Parrish[33] reported no permanent sequelae in their respective case series. In contrast, permanent sequelae of pit viper envenomation are common. These may be divided into local or systemic manifestations, as summarized in Table 9. Overall, the reported outcomes are generally limited to amputation and obvious dysfunction of an area, usually an extremity. Local sequelae from scar formation may occur from local necrosis and stricture as a result of the venom itself [1], or secondary to treatment. Although disfiguring scars may develop following tissue excision or fasciotomy, they are generally not reported in the literature. Overall the reported incidence of permanent local sequelae is below 10% of all bites, excluding sequelae due to the surgery itself[1,53].

Table 9
Potential sequelae of pitviper poisoning[48]

Injury	Example
LOCAL	
Necrosis	Loss of all or part of fingers, hands, toes, feet, skin, lip etc.
Loss of function	Contractures, joint stiffness
Discomfort	Pain or numbness of bite site or in involved joints, recurrent swelling, numbness
Abnormal appearance	Discoloration of bite site or areas involved in swelling, scarring at bite site.
SYSTEMIC	
Soft tissue	Diffuse soft tissue swelling
Kidney injury	Renal failure
Hypersensitivity	Snake venom allergy
Multiple organ failure	Death

Systemic sequelae include renal failure, persistent neurological syndromes, tetanus and persistent neuromuscular syndromes. The incidence of death, the ultimate form of systemic sequelae, is fortunately a rare occurrence. Mortality has been estimated at 5-25% before antivenom and intensive care units were available[1-3]. However, since the introduction of antivenom and modern intensive care technology, the incidence of death has decreased to 0 to 1.5%[1,4,48]. When death occurs, it is usually related to improper handling of pit viper envenomation or insufficient medical attention. In order to reduce the possibility of a fatal outcome, the individual choosing to handle a pit viper should do so in close proximity to a medical facility, preferably with a companion who can notify emergency medical services in the area, or who can transport the potential victim to a medical facility. In addition, if the treating physician has had little or no experience in the management of snakebite victims, he or she would be wise to contact an experienced consultant.

VII. REFERENCES

1. **RUSSELL,F.E.** *Snake Venom Poisoning.* 3rd ed. Great Neck, New York, Scholium International, Inc., pp 60 -234, 1983.
2. **WILLSON,P** Snake poisoning in the United States: a study based on analysis of 740 cases. *Arch Int Med,* **1:**516 -570, 1908.
3. **BARRINGER, P.B.** The venomous reptiles of the United States, with the treatment of wounds inflicted by them. *S Ned Surg Gyne Assoc,* **4:**283 -300, 1892.
4. **PARRISH, H.M.** Incidence of treated snakebites in the United States. *Public Health Reports,* **81:**269-276, 1966.
5. **WINGERT,W.A. AND WAINSCHEL,J.** Diagnosis and management of envenomation by poisonous snakes. *Southern Med Journal,* **68:** 1015 -1026, 1975.
6. **RUSSELL,F.E., CARLSON R.W., WAINSCHEL J. AND OSBORNE A.H.** Snake venom poisoning in the United States. *JAMA,* 233: 341 -344, . 1975
7. **RUSSELL,F.E., AND DART R.C.** Toxic effects of animal toxins. In AMDUR, M.O., DOULL, J., KLAASSEN, C.D. Eds. *CASARETT & DOULL'S Toxicology:The Basic Science of Poisons.* 4th ed. New York, Macmillan Publishing pp 104 -136, 1990.
8. **TRESTRAIL, J.H.** The "underground zoo"-the problem of exotic venomous snakes in private possession in the United States. Vet *Hum Toxicol,* (suppl): 144 -149, 1982.
9. **CAMPBELL, J.A. AND LAMAR, W.W.** Regional accounts and keys to venomous snakes-Mexico and Central America. In CAMPBELL, J.A. & LAMAR, W.W. Eds. *The Venomous Reptiles of Latin America,*Cornell University Press,Ithaca,pp24-33, 1989.
10. **ZAVALA, J.T., ALARCON, L.C. AND CABELLO, R.R.** Tratamiento de las mordeduras por serpientes ponzo f iosas. Sal P , *Qbl M 6x,***23:**457-472, 1981.
11. **JULIA ZERTUCHE, J.** Reptiles mexicanos de importancia para la salud publica y su distribucion geographica. *Salud Publica* Mex, **23(4):**329-343, 1981.
12. **CAMPBELL, J.A. AND LAMAR, W.W.** Regional accounts and keys to venomous snakes-Mexico and Central America. In CAMPBELL, J.A. & LAMAR, W.W. Eds. *The Venomous Reptiles of Latin America,*Cornell University Press,Ithaca,pp 180 -192, 1989.
13. **CAMPBELL, J.A. AND LAMAR, W .W .** Regional accounts and keys to venomous snakes-Mexico and Central America. In CAMPBELL, J.A. & LAMAR, W.W. Eds. *The Venomous Reptiles* of *Latin America,*Cornell University Press,Ithaca,pp 189 -192 , 1989.
14. **GLENN, J.L. AND STRAIGHT, R.C.** The rattlesnakes and their venom yield and lethal toxicity. In TU A.T. Ed. *Rattlesnake Venoms: Their Actions and Treatment.* New York, Marcel Dekker, Inc., pp 3-56, 1982.
15. **CAMPBELL, J.A. AND LAMAR, W.W.** Regional accouts and keys to venomous snakes-Mexico and Central America. In CAMPBELL, J.A. & LAMAR, W.W. Eds. *The Venomous Reptiles of Latin America,*Cornell University Press,Ithaca,pp 374-376, 1989.
16. **CAMPBELL, J.A. AND LAMAR, W.W.** Regional accounts and keys to venomous snakes-Mexico and Central America. In CAMPBELL, J.A. & LAMAR, W.W. Eds. *The Venomous Reptiles of Latin America,*Cornell University Press,Ithaca,pp 158 -161, 1989.
17. **CAMPBELL, J.A. AND LAMAR, W.W.** Regional accouts and keys to venomous snakes-Mexico and Central America. In CAMPBELL, J.A. & LAMAR, W.W. Eds. *The Venomous Reptiles of Latin America,*Cornell University Press,Ithaca,pp 150-155, 1989.
18. **BLOCK,M.D.** Function and operation of the facial pit of the pit vipers. *Nature [New Biol],* **165:** 284-285, 1950.
19. **KLAUBER, L.M.** *Rattlesnakes: Their habits, life, histories and influence on mankind.* 2nd ed.Vol 2, University of California Press, Zoological Society of San Diego, 1972.
20. **STOCKER, K.F.** Composition of snake venoms. In Stocker K.W. ed. *Medical Use of Snake Venom Proteins.* CRC Press, Boca Raton , Florida,pp 33-56, 1990.
21. **RUSSELL,F.E.** *Snake Venom Poisoning.* 3rd ed. Great Neck, New York, Scholium International, Inc., 163 pp, 1983.
22. **KITCHENS, C.S. AND VAN MIEROP, L.H.S.** Envenomation by the Eastern Coral Snake *(Micrurus fulvius fulvius)* a study of 39 victims. *JAMA,* **258:**1615 -1618, 1987.
23. **MOSELY, T.** Coral snake bite: Recovery following symptoms of respiratory paralysis. *Ann Surg,* **163:**943, 1966.
24. **AVILA, G.C., ESTRADA, J., AND GARCIA, J.P.** Picados de vibora de cascabel. *Plana Medica,* **27:**35-46, 1980.
25. **RUSSELL, F.E.** Snake venom poisoning in the United States. *Ann Rev Med,* **31:**247-259, 1980.
26. **LITOVITZ, T.L., HOLM, K.C., BAILEY, K.M. AND SCHMITZ B.F.** 1991 annual report of the American Association of Poison Control Centers National Data Collection System. *Am. J. Emerg Med,* **10:**452 -505, 1992.

27. **PARRISH, H.M., GOLDNER, J.C. AND SILBERG S.L.** Comparison between snakebites in children and adults. *Pediatrics,* **36:**251 -256, 1965.
28. **TAY, Z.J., CASTILLO, A.L., JULIA Z.J., ROMERO C.R. AND VELASCO, C.O.** Accidentes por mordedura de animales ponzonosos. *Revista de la Facultad de Medicina, U.N.A.M. (Mexico),* **23** (7): 4 - 17, 1980.
29. **TAY, Z.J., CASTILLO, A.L., JULIA Z.J., ROMERO C.R. Y VELASCO, C.O.** Accidentes por mordedura de animales ponzonosos. *Revista de la Facultad* de Medicina, *U.N.A.M.* (Mexico), **23** (8): 6 - 19, 1980.
30. **ROSADO-LOPEZ, L. AND LAVIADA-ARRIGUNAGA, F.A.** Accidente ofidico communicaion de 38 casos. *Investigación Clinica,***62:**409 -412, 1977.
31. **DART, R.C. AND RUSSELL F.E.** Animal Poisoning. In Hall, Schmidt & Wood Eds.*P rinciples of Critical Care. ist* ed. New York, New York, McGraw-Hill, Inc, pp 2163 -2171, 1992.
32. **NORRIS, R.L. AND DART, R.C.** Apparent Coral snake envenomation in a patient without visible fang marks. *Am J Emerg Med,* **7:**402 -405, 1989.
33. **PARRISH, H.M. AND KHAN, M.S.** Bites by Coral snakes: report of 11 representative cases. *Am J Med Sci,* May: 561 -568, 1967.
34. **HARDY SR., D.L.** A review of first aid measures for pitviper bite in North America with an appraisal of extractor suction and stun gun electroshock. In CAMPBELL & BRODIES *Eds.Biology of the Pitvipers.* 1st ed.Arlington, Texas, Selva Publishing, pp 405 -414, 1992.
35. **WATT, C.H.** Poisonous snakebite treatment in the United States. *JAMA,* **240:**654-656, 1978.
36 **BRONSTEIN, A.C., RUSSELL F.E. AND SULLIVAN J.B.** Negative pressure suction in the field treatment of rattlesnake bite victims (abstract) *Vet Hum Toxicol,* **28:**485, 1985.
37. **GUDERIAN, R.H., MACKENZIE, C.D. AND WILLIAMS, J.F.** High voltage shock treatment for snake bite. (letter) *Lancet* **2:**229, 1986.
38. **HOWE, N.R. AND MEISENHEIMER, J.L.** Electric shock does not save snakebitten rats. *Ann Emerg Med* **17:**254-256, 1988.
39. **DART, R.C. AND GUSTAFSON, R.A.** Failure of electric shock treatment for rattlesnake envenomation. *Ann Emerg Med,* **20:**659-661, 1991.
40. **RUSSELL F.E.** A letter on electroshock for snakebite. (letter) *Vet Hum Toxicol,* **29:**320 -321, 1987.
41. **RYAN, A.J.** Don't use electric shock for snakebite. (letter) *Postgrad Med* **83:**52-75, 1987.
42. **HURLBUT K.M., DART R.C., SPAITE D. AND MCNALLY J.** Reliability of clinical presentation for predicting significant pit viper envenomation. *Ann Emerg Med,* **17:**438, 1988.
43. **DART, R.C., DUNCAN, C. AND MCNALLY, J.** Effect of inadequate antivenin stores on the medical treatment of crotalid envenomation. *Vet Hum Toxicol* **33:**267-269, 1991.
44. **DART R.C., O'BRIEN P.C., GARCIA R.A., JARCHOW J.C. AND MCNALLY J.** Neutralization of *Micrurus distans distans* venom by antivenin *(Micrurus fulvius). J Wild Med,* **3:**377-381, 1992.
45. **SPAITE, D.W., DART, R.C., HURLBUT K. AND MCNALLY J.T.** Skin testing: implications in the management of pit viper envenomation. *Ann Emerg Med,* (abstract) **17:**389, 1988.
46. **MCCOLLOUGH N.C. AND GENNARO J.F.** Treatment of venomous snakebites. *Snake Venoms and Envenomation,* New York, Marcel Dekker, Inc., pp 80 -101, 1971.
47. **CORRIGAN, P. AND RUSSELL, F.E.** Clinical reactions to antivenom. In ROSENBERG, P ed. *Toxins: Animal, Plant, and Microbial,* Pergamon Press, Oxford, pp 457-465, . 1976
48. **DART, R.C., MCNALLY D.W., SPAITE D.W. AND GUSTAFSON R.** The sequelae of pitviper poisoning in the United States. In CAMPBELL & BRODIES *Eds.Biology of the Pitvipers.* 1st ed.Arlington, Texas, Selva Publishing, pp 395 -403, 1992.
49. **REID, H.A., THEAN, P.C. AND MARTIN, W.J.** Specific antivenene and prednisone in viper bite poisoning-controlled trial. *B M J,* **2:**1378, 1963.
50. **RUSSELL, F.E., AND EMORY, J.A.** Effects of corticosteroids on lethality of *Ancistrodon contortix* venom. *Am J Med Sci,* **241:**507, 1961.
51. **SCHOTTLER, W.H.A.** Antihistamine, ACTH, cortisone, hydrocortisone and anesthetics in snake bite. *Am J Trop Med Hyg,* **3:**1083, 1954.
52. **RUSSELL F.E.** Clinical aspects of snake venom poisoning in North America. *Toxicon,* **7:**33-37, 1969.
53. **COLLINS, J.T.** Standard Common and Current Scientific Names for North American Amphibians and Reptiles 3rd ed. *SSAR Herp Circ,* **19:**26-33, 1990.

Chapter 30

CLINICAL TOXICOLOGY OF SNAKEBITE IN CENTRAL AMERICA

José María Gutiérrez

TABLE OF CONTENTS

I. INTRODUCTION

A large variety of snakes are found in Central America. In Costa Rica, for instance, there are about 123 species, distributed in many habitats, particularly in the tropical rain forests[1]. The majority of snakes belong to the family Colubridae, although the most important species from a medical point of view are classified within the family Viperidae (subfamily Crotalinae), commonly known as pit vipers or "tobobas"[1,2]. In addition, the family Elapidae, which in Central America includes coral snakes (subfamily Elapinae) and the sea snake (subfamily Hydrophiinae), have species which, despite the fact that they cause relatively few accidents, can induce potentially fatal envenomings[2,3]. Snakebite envenomings constitute a significant public health problem in this area of the world, mainly affecting the rural population[2,3]. In some regions of Central America the problem is aggravated by inadequate medical facilities and training to deal with these envenomings.

II. EPIDEMIOLOGY OF SNAKEBITE IN CENTRAL AMERICA

A. THE SNAKES: DISTRIBUTION, VENOM AND CHARACTERISTICS

Species classified in three families produce toxic secretions and possess a delivery system that allows them to inject their venom:

1. Family Colubridae

Within this family there are several rear-fanged snakes which could inject their venom into humans. However, even in cases where venom has been inoculated, most of these species do not cause relevant envenomings in humans. There are reports of bites by *Conophis lineatus* (locally known as "guarda camino") in which some degree of envenoming was described[4].

2. Family Elapidae

Subfamily Hydrophiinae: There is only one species of sea snake in Central America, the yellow bellied sea snake, *Pelamis platurus*, locally known as "serpiente de mar". This pelagic sea snake is found only in the Pacific Ocean, where it dwells in large numbers in offshore waters[5,6]. It has a pair of frontally-located fixed fangs and a highly neurotoxic venom containing post-synaptic type neurotoxins[7]. The venom yield is very low and the snake is not aggressive, unless it is caught; moreover, due to the small size of its mouth it is very difficult for this snake to bite a human being. Thus, very few cases of bites by *Pelamis platurus* are described in the literature[7].

Subfamily Elapinae: In Central America there are 14 species of coral snakes (*Micrurus* sp)[5], *M. nigrocinctus* being the most abundant species and accountable for the majority of the accidents. Coral snakes can be found in a variety of habitats[5]. Some species are present not only in the forests, but also in urban areas. Coral snakes in Central America have a color pattern characterized by the following sequence of rings: red-yellow-black-yellow-red. In addition, rings are "complete", i.e., present not only dorsally but also ventrally. There are two exceptions in Central America to this general pattern: *M. mipartitus* ("gargantilla") which has complete rings of only two colors, orange and black, although sometimes orange rings are replaced by white rings; and *M. dissoleucus*, which has the triad pattern typical of many South American coral snakes[5]. By using these morphological criteria, poisonous coral snakes can be distinguished from non-venomous colubrid snakes that have colored rings. Although the natural history of these reptiles is poorly studied, it is known that coral snakes are fossorial[5] and that some species feed on eels, lizards, caecilians, amphisbaenians and colubrid snakes[8]. They have a highly potent neurotoxic venom synthesized in a gland located in the upper jaw region. Venom is injected through fixed frontally-located grooved fangs. Due to the small size of their mouth, coral snakes bite humans usually on the fingers[2,3].

Table 1
Poisonous snakes of Central America

Scientific Name	Common Name	Distribution
Family VIPERIDAE		
Bothrops asper	Terciopelo, Barba amarilla	G,B,H,N,CR,P
Bothrops (Porthidium) nummifer	Mano de piedra, timbo	G,B,H,S,N,CR,P
Bothrops (Porthidium) picadoi	Mano de piedra	CR, P
Bothrops (Porthidium) nasutus	Tamagá	G,B,H,N,CR,P
Bothrops (Porthidium) godmani	Toboba de altura	G,N,CR,P
Bothrops (Porthidium) ophryomegas	Toboba chinga	G,H,S,N,CR,P
Bothrops (Porthidium) lansbergii	Tamagá, patoco	P
Bothrops (Bothriechis) aurifer	Cantil loro, cantil verde	G
Bothrops (Bothriechis) bicolor	Víbora verde	G,H
Bothrops (Bothriechis) schlegelii	Bocaracá, toboba de pestaña	G,H,N,CR,P
Bothrops (Bothriechis) lateralis	Lora	CR,P
Bothrops (Bothriechis) nigroviridis	Toboba de árbol	CR,P
Bothrops (Bothriechis) marchi	Lora, tamagá verde	H,N
Agkistrodon bilineatus	Cantil, mocasina, castellana	G,B,H,S,N,CR
Crotalus durissus	Cascabel, chischil	G,B,H,S,N,CR
Lachesis muta	Cascabela muda, Matabuey, verrugosa	N,CR,P
Family ELAPIDAE		
Pelamis platurus	Serpiente de mar	G,H,S,N,CR,P
Micrurus nigrocinctus	Coral, coralillo	G,B,H,S,N,CR,P
Micrurus browni	Coral, coralillo	G
Micrurus diastema	Coral, coralillo	G,B,H
Micrurus elegans	Coral, coralillo	G
Micrurus hippocrepis	Coral, coralillo	G,B
Micrurus latifasciatus	Coral, coralillo	G
Micrurus stuarti	Coral, coralillo	G
Micrurus ruatanus	Coral, coralillo	H
Micrurus alleni	Coral, coralilla	N,CR,P
Micrurus clarki	Coral, coralilla	CR, P
Micrurus ancoralis	Coral, coralilla	P
Micrurus dissoleucus	Coral, coralilla	P
Micrurus mipartitus	Coral, gargantilla	N,CR,P
Micrurus stewarti	Coral, gargantilla	P

G = Guatemala; B = Belize; H = Honduras; S = El Salvador; N = Nicaragua; CR = Costa Rica; P = Panamá.

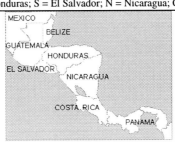

Figure 1a. Countries of Central America.

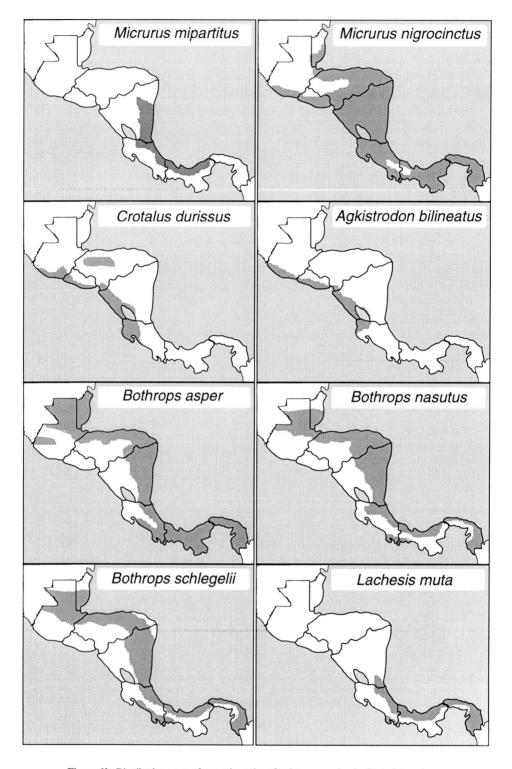

Figure 1b. Distribution maps of several species of poisonous snakes in Central America.

3. Family Viperidae (subfamily Crotalinae)

There are 16 species of pit vipers in Central America, found in a variety of ecological conditions[5]. Crotaline snakes are characterized by the presence of a loreal pit located between the nostril and the eye; this morphological feature allows a rapid differential diagnosis between pit vipers and other snakes. Pit vipers in Central America are classified in the genera *Bothrops, Crotalus, Lachesis* and *Agkistrodon*, although recent herpetological studies have split the species formerly classified as *Bothrops* into the genera *Bothrops, Bothriechis* and *Porthidium*[5]. Pit vipers have a diverse diet; some species like *Bothrops asper* (adult specimens), *Crotalus durissus* and *Lachesis muta* feed mainly on small mammals, particularly rodents[9], whereas *Bothrops (Porthidium) godmani* has a diet that includes invertebrates, amphibians, reptiles, birds and mammals[10]. The reproductive cycles of several species of Central American pit vipers have been studied[11-13].

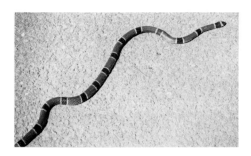

Figure 2. *Micrurus nigrocinctus* (coral, coralillo).

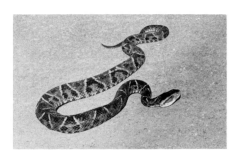

e 3. *Bothrops asper* (terciopelo, barba amarilla).

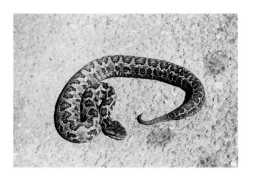

Figure 4. *Bothrops (Porthidium) godmani* (toboba de altura).

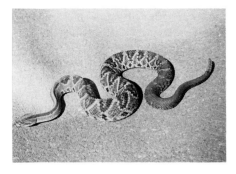

Figure 5. *Crotalus durissus durissus* (cascabel, chischil).

This group of snakes has a highly developed and efficient venom-delivery system in which the venom is conducted from the gland, through a duct, to a large pair of frontally-located fangs with an enclosed venom channel. The fangs are folded back when the mouth is closed and protrude when it opens. In addition, these snakes can open their mouth widely, allowing them to bite in various anatomical locations.

Pit viper venoms comprise a complex mixture of toxins, enzymes, peptides, nucleotides, biogenic amines, carbohydrates, salts and organic acids[14]. Of particular relevance is the presence of many proteases, esterases and phospholipases A_2, responsible for a variety of pharmacological effects. In addition, other components such as lectins and nerve growth factor have been described in these venoms, although their role in envenoming has not been studied. The reader is referred to Chapter 24 of this volume (by Meier and Stocker) for a description of the various toxins and enzymes present in snake venoms. The pathophysiology of pit viper envoming in Central America is characterized by local tissue damage (myonecrosis, hemorrhage and edema) and systemic alterations such as hemorrhage, coagulopathy, renal failure and cardiovascular shock[2,3]. No neurotoxic signs and symptoms have been described in crotaline envenomings in Central America. Table 1 summarizes some features of the poisonous snakes distributed in the area and Figure 1 depicts the distribution of some of these species in the various countries of the region. Some of the poisonous snakes of this region are shown in Figures 2 to 6. A comprehensive review of the biology of Latin American poisonous snakes has been published[5].

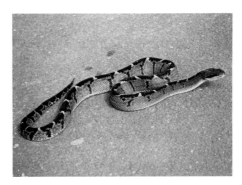

Figure 6. *Lachesis muta stenophrys* (cascabela muda, matabuey, verrugosa).

B. SNAKEBITE IN CENTRAL AMERICA

There is not a systematic collection of epidemiological data related to snakebites in Central America. In Costa Rica, an estimated number of about 600 patients attend health centers each year as a consequence of snakebites, giving a morbidity rate of approximately 20 per 100,000 per year[2,15]. This is most likely an underestimation, since an unknown number of cases do not seek medical treatment for various reasons. Probably a similar incidence occurs in other Central American countries, with the exception of El Salvador, where snakebites are less common. In Costa Rica, where antivenom is widely distributed, about 1-2% of snakebitten patients die (Table 2). It has been assumed that lethality is higher in other Central American countries, since antivenom is not readily available, particularly in rural areas.

Most snakebites happen to agricultural workers while laboring in the field[2,3]. The majority of accidents take place in lowland agricultural regions where snakes are abundant and young males 5 to 25 years old constitute the age group with the highest incidence (Figure 7). The vast majority of bites are inflicted by pit vipers, among which *Bothrops asper* ("terciopelo" or "barba amarilla") is responsible for almost half of the cases; only about 2% of bites are due to coral snakes[3]. In El Salvador, however, the rattlesnake *Crotalus durissus durissus* is responsible for many accidents. Data collected in Costa Rica indicate that approximately 10% of the bites are caused by non-venomous colubrid species[3].

Regarding the anatomical location of the bites, approximately 50% of bites are on the feet, 18% involve the rest of the lower limb, and the other 32% occur in the upper extremity, predominantly in the hands[3]. This distribution emphasizes the relevance of the fact that many workers perform their duties with inadequate or no footwear, thereby increasing the possibilities of being bitten.

Table 2
Snakebite fatalities in Costa Rica

Year	Number of Fatalities	Mortality Rate (per Million inhabitants)
1980	9	4.0
1981	5	2.2
1982	7	2.9
1983	8	3.3
1984	6	2.3
1985	5	1.9
1986	11	4.1
1987	11	3.9
1988	5	1.7
1989	9	3.1

Source: Dirección General de Estadística y Censos, Ministerio de Economía y Comercio and Caja Costarricense del Seguro Social, Costa Rica.

III. SYMPTOMS AND SIGNS

A. GENERAL CONCEPTS OF ENVENOMING

When treating a snakebite, it is important to keep in mind that many bites do not end in severe envenoming because: (i) non-venomous snakes often bite people without causing any harm; (ii) a number of bites by poisonous snakes do not result in venom injection; and (iii) even bites where venom is delivered might cause only mild envenoming if the amount of venom injected is low. Thus, only a fraction of snakebites result in serious envenoming. This is important, since treatment with specific antivenom is indicated only when objective signs of envenoming are observed. Table 3 summarizes the most relevant pathophysiological alterations induced by the venoms of Central American snakes.

Table 3
Pathophysiology of snakebite envenoming in Central America

Family	Genus	Venom Effects
Elapidae	*Pelamis, Micrurus*	Neurotoxic paralysis
Viperidae	*Agkistrodon, Bothrops*[a], *Crotalus, Lachesis*	*Local effects*: Edema, hemorrhage, necrosis. *Systemic effects*: Hemorrhage, coagulopathy[b], cardiovascular, shock, renal failure

[a]Several species formerly classified within the genus *Bothrops* have been recently classified in the genera *Bothriechis* and *Porthidium*.

[b]Venoms of several species of *Bothrops* do not induce coagulopathy (see text).

Studies on the ontogenetic variation in biochemical composition and pharmacological activities of the venoms show the existence of major qualitative and quantitative changes that develop as snakes age. For instance, experimental studies indicate that venoms from newborn specimens of *Bothrops asper* and *Crotalus durissus durissus* are more toxic than those of adults[16-18], whereas the venom of newborn specimens of *Lachesis muta* is almost devoid of toxicity[19]. However, since the absolute amount of venom injected is less in the case of newborn and juvenile specimens than in bites inflicted by adults, the overall envenoming is usually not as severe. Thus, despite a qualitatively common pathophysiology in pit viper envenomings, there are variations not only from species to species, but also within a single species, due to geographic[16,20] and ontogenetic factors.

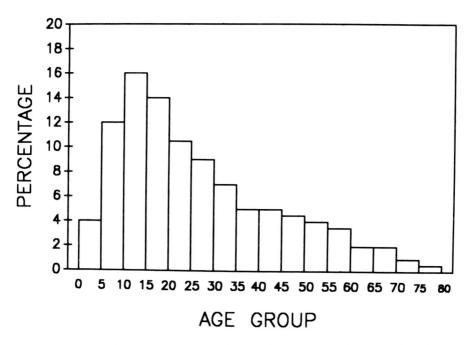

Figure 7. Distribution of snakebite cases in Costa Rica according to age groups (in years). Information was obtained from Bolaños[2] and from unpublished data collected by Instituto Clodomiro Picado.

B. THE ONSET AND DEVELOPMENT OF ENVENOMING

In pit viper bites where venom has been injected, the onset of envenoming is very rapid, as local effects (edema, pain and bleeding at the site of venom inoculation) start within the first few minutes after the bite[3,21,22]. In these cases, local tissue damage spreads rapidly whereas systemic envenoming appears later on, usually between 1 to 6 hours depending on the circumstances of the accident. In contrast, coral snake bites are not characterized by prominent local effects, with the exception of local pain and edema. Instead, in these cases the onset of envenoming usually occurs after 2 or more hours and is characterized by the appearance of neurotoxic signs and symptoms[3,22]. In some patients, the onset of envenoming might be delayed for several hours, making the observation of the bitten patient necessary for at least six hours.

Several factors determine the severity of envenoming as well as the time of its onset: (i) the amount of venom injected; for instance, *Bothrops asper* delivers a much larger amount of venom than other Central American snakes[23]; as a consequence its bites are usually more severe. (ii) The number of bites inflicted and the route of venom injection; most accidents by pit vipers are due to a single bite and venom is injected intramuscularly or subcutaneously. In these cases the severity of envenoming is not as drastic as when several bites occur or when venom is injected directly into a vein. (iii) The condition of the victim, not only in terms of size and weight, but also in terms of the overall physiological status. Usually children develop more serious envenomings than adults and the onset of systemic alterations appears earlier.

After initial pain, swelling and bleeding, the progression of symptoms and signs in pit viper envenoming consists of the spreading of local tissue damage and, in moderate and severe cases, the appearance of systemic alterations such as hemorrhage, coagulopathy, hypotension and renal failure[3,21,22]. The time-course of these systemic alterations depends on factors like amount of venom injected, anatomic region where the bite occurs and the species responsible for the accident. Bites by the bushmaster, *Lachesis muta*, locally known as "mata buey" or "verrugosa", often result in severe envenoming, with a rapid development of systemic alterations[24]. Similarly, bites by "terciopelo" (*Bothrops asper*) usually result in the appearance of coagulopathy, hemorrhage and hypotension[3,22]. In contrast, accidents due to species that deliver relatively low amounts of venom, such as "lora" (*Bothrops lateralis*), "toboba de árbol" (*Bothrops nigroviridis*) and "bocaracá" (*Bothrops schlegelii*), are usually characterized by local effects with no significant systemic alterations, with the exception of a moderate coagulopathy in some cases. In the case of "cascabel" (*Crotalus durissus durissus*), most accidents in Central America are graded as mild[25], in contrast to the South American subspecies which induces rather severe envenomings[26,27]. On the other hand, in coral snake bites envenoming develops rapidly once neurotoxic signs appear, with paralysis of various muscles, including respiratory muscles[3,28].

C. GENERAL SIGNS AND SYMPTOMS OF ENVENOMING

Local signs and symptoms in pit viper bites appear rapidly after venom injection and, depending upon the severity of the case, may include swelling, pain, bleeding, ecchymosis and necrosis[2,3,22]. Mild cases develop only swelling, pain and sometimes bleeding through the fang marks. Patients bitten by coral snakes, even in severe cases, do not develop conspicuous local signs and symptoms, except for pain and mild edema[2,3,28].

Systemic envenoming in pit viper bites is characterized by nausea, dizziness, fever, vomiting, hypotension, gingival bleeding, hemoptysis, hematuria and oliguria[2,3,22]. The proper evaluation of these signs and symptoms can be obscured by the anxiety of snakebitten patients; thus, a meticulous and objective clinical assessment is needed. Cases of systemic coral snake envenomings are characterized by ptosis, generalized muscle weakness and respiratory problems, together with dizziness, dysarthria, dysphagia, ophthalmoplegia, blurred vision and, sometimes, muscle fasciculations[2,3,28].

D. SPECIFIC TOXIN EFFECTS AND COMPLICATIONS
1. Pit viper envenoming
a. Hemorrhage

Both local and systemic bleeding typically occur in pit viper envenoming. Local bleeding takes place both through the fang marks and around the site of venom injection, as ecchymosis and blisters may develop. As systemic envenoming ensues, hemorrhage also develops in organs such as lungs, kidneys, stomach and, in severe cases, brain. Hemoptysis often occurs and gingival bleeding is not uncommon. The main consequence of such extensive bleeding is hypovolemia and cardiovascular shock, a typical complication in severe pit viper envenomings in Central America. Hemorrhage is caused by the action of hemorrhagic toxins, zinc-dependent metalloproteinases that degrade the components of the basal lamina located in the periphery of capillary vessels and venules[29,30]. The action of hemorrhagic toxins results in the collapse of the microvessel wall with blood escaping into the interstitial space[30,31]. Blood incoagulability (see below) may enhance the bleeding in pit viper envenomings, but coagulopathy per se is not the leading cause of hemorrhage induced by these venoms[32].

b. Edema

Local edema is one of the most common consequences of pit viper envenoming in Central America. Its pathogenesis is multifactorial, as venoms exert a variety of actions which result in the imbalance between interstitial and intravascular fluids, causing edema. Some of these actions are: (i) venoms directly affect endothelial cells, promoting the escape of plasma to the interstitium[29,30]; (ii) venoms induce the release of histamine, bradykinin, prostaglandins and complement anaphylatoxins by the action of components such as kallikrein-like proteases and phospholipases A_2[33]. Besides its effects on interstitial fluid imbalance, edema may also contribute to tissue damage by causing an increment in the interstitial pressure in muscle compartments[2,21]; in some cases, when interstitial pressure rises above 30 mm Hg, a compartmental syndrome develops, drastically impairing the blood supply to distal areas of the extremities. In addition to local edema, pulmonary edema is often observed in severe pit viper envenomings, probably resulting from both direct and indirect effects of venom components on lung vasculature.

c. Myotoxicity

Together with hemorrhage and edema, myonecrosis is a common local effect in pit viper bites. If extensive, myonecrosis results in pain which, however, cannot be distinguished from the pain associated with the acute inflammatory reaction induced by the venom. In the case of Central American pit viper venoms, myonecrosis is mainly due to the action of myotoxins having phospholipase A_2 structure[34,35]. These toxins induce acute muscle cell damage by directly disrupting the integrity of the plasma membrane of skeletal muscle cells[34-36]. In addition, muscle cells are probably affected by the ischemia that results from hemorrhage and swelling and from the direct effect of the venom on larger vessels, since angionecrosis and thrombosis have been described[37,38]. There is no evidence of systemic myotoxicity even in severe cases and usually no myoglobinuria is observed in these patients.

d. Coagulopathy

Blood incoagulability is one of the most typical findings in pit viper envenomings in Central America. Laboratory tests such as prothrombin time and whole blood clotting time are widely used to monitor the development of envenoming[3,22,39]. Incoagulability results mainly from defibrination, due to the action of thrombin-like proteases present in the venoms[3,22,40,41]. In addition, some *Bothrops* venoms contain factor X-activators[42] and prothrombin activators that cause a complex derangement of hemostatic mechanisms (see Chapter 24 by Meier and Stocker in this volume). Thus, disseminated intravascular coagulation is often a consequence of pit viper envenomings. Incoagulability is associated with a drop in the concentration of fibrinogen and other coagulation factors. Concomitantly, the fibrinolytic system is activated and, consequently, fibrin-degradation products appear[43]. It is important to note that defibrination per se does not necessarily lead to bleeding, although the concomitant action of hemorrhagic metalloproteinases and thrombin-like enzymes may enhance the hemorrhagic condition.

Not all Central American pit viper venoms induce defibrination. It was reported that the venoms of *Bothrops lateralis*, *B. nasutus*, *B. ophryomegas* and *B. picadoi* are devoid of blood clotting activity on human plasma and do not induce defibrination in experimental animals[44]. Thus, it is very likely that coagulopathy does not develop in patients bitten by any of these species. Besides their effects on plasma clotting factors, pit viper envenomings are sometimes associated with thrombocytopenia[22].

e. Renal failure

Severe envenomings by pit vipers may result in acute renal failure[3,21,45]. In these cases, oliguria or anuria appear usually six or more hours after the bite; therefore, urine output should be carefully monitored, together with serum levels of creatinine and urea. The pathogenesis of renal alterations in pit viper envenomings has not been fully understood, although it probably results from the combination of several factors, such as tubular necrosis as a consequence of ischemia and direct action of venom components on the kidney. It is likely that hypovolemia and inadequate renal perfusion are the most important causes of kidney damage in pit viper bites. Pathological studies in humans have demonstrated the presence of distal nephron nephrosis, acute tubular necrosis and cortical necrosis[46,47]. In contrast to South American rattlesnake venom, which induces myoglobinuria and acute renal failure[48], envenomings by the Central American rattlesnake *Crotalus durissus durissus* are not characterized by renal alterations, since this venom does not cause rhabdomyolysis and renal function is not significantly impaired[25].

2. Coral snake envenoming
a. Neurotoxic paralysis

When a significant amount of venom is injected in a coral snake bite, ptosis is usually the first sign of neurotoxicity, appearing 2 to 6 hours after the accident, although there are reports of cases where the onset of envenoming was delayed more than 6 hours[28]. Afterwards, the patient develops blurred vision, ophthalmoplegia, dysarthria and a generalized and progressive muscle weakness which includes respiratory muscles, thereby causing respiratory paralysis[3,28]. Coral snake venoms have been poorly studied, but it is known that neurotoxicity is primarily due to a post-synaptic blockade of neuromuscular transmission by typical alpha neurotoxins[49] (see Chapter 24 by Meier and Stocker in this volume). Nevertheless, in the case of *Micrurus nigrocinctus*, the most abundant coral snake in Central America, experimental studies have demonstrated a presynaptic effect as well[50]. On the other hand, although there are no descriptions of human envenomings in Central America by the yellow bellied sea snake, *Pelamis platurus*, it can be assumed that signs and symptoms of such an envenoming would resemble those described for coral snakes, as alpha neurotoxins have been purified from this venom[51].

E. PROGNOSTIC INDICATORS
1. Pit viper envenoming

Rapid development of severe local effects is suggestive of a severe envenoming, although all envenomings, even the ones that do not result in systemic poisoning, usually include local edema and pain[3,21,22]. If no local effects develop in the first hour after the bite, this strongly suggests that envenoming is not going to develop or will be mild. To monitor systemic poisoning, defibrination is a useful parameter; thus, laboratory tests such as whole blood clotting and prothrombin times are useful tools to follow the course of envenoming and the success of antivenom therapy[39,43]. However, it must be kept in mind that some crotaline venoms do not induce defibrination.

2. Coral snake envenoming

In coral snake bites local effects are not relevant and should not be used as criteria to judge the severity of envenoming. In contrast, an early onset of paralytic signs is the most clear evidence that a severe envenoming is likely to occur. Nevertheless, due to variations in the absorption of the venom from the site of the bite, the onset of neurotoxic paralytic effects might be delayed several hours, even in severe cases.

IV. PROPHYLAXIS

The avoidance of bites constitute the most important factor in the prevention of snakebite envenomings. People, especially residents of rural areas and agricultural workers, must be aware of some basic precautions which reduce the probability of a bite:

- Always wear leather shoes or, preferably, boots. Since about 50% of bites occur in the feet[3], this will greatly reduce the number of envenomings.
- Do not place hands directly on the ground, inside hollow pieces of wood, small caves or under logs or rocks, as snakes frequently hide in these locations. It is useful to carry a stick that aids in the inspection of the ground before stepping on it.
- Exercise care not only in the woods, but also around human settlements, where snakes can also be found.
- Since some pit vipers live in trees and bushes, be cautious when collecting crops.
- Instruct children about venomous snakes and their bites, since they often play with snakes, increasing the risk of being bitten.
- Do not try to handle a poisonous snake, no matter how expert the person thinks he/she is. If a snake is observed in the field, just avoid it instead of trying to kill it.

There are many misconceptions concerning snakes and snakebites in Central America. Therefore, it is very important to promote extensive public educational programs in order to provide the general population with basic knowledge on the identification of poisonous snakes and prevention of bites. In Costa Rica, the Instituto Clodomiro Picado has a permanent extension program which benefits communities, students, local leaders, medical and paramedical personnel, farmers and tourists. This program, which has been active for several years, has increased the general knowledge on the subject[52].

V. FIRST AID TREATMENT

A. PRINCIPLES OF FIRST AID

The aim of first aid treatment in snakebite envenomings is to reduce the rate of venom absorption and, consequently, to delay the onset of envenoming, in such a way that no additional harm is inflicted on the patient[53]. The immobilization of the bitten part, together with rapid transportation of the patient to the nearest health center, are the two key elements in an efficient first aid treatment. Despite the fact that many people suggest the use of suction devices that would remove part of the inoculated venom, there is no clear evidence that such measures indeed result in significant venom elimination. Suction procedures performed without making incisions are not apparently harmful, although their effectiveness is dubious.

The use of pressure immobilization bandages has gained wide acceptance as a means of retarding venom absorption in other regions of the world[54]. However, in the case of pit viper venoms, which cause prominent swelling and vascular damage, this method is not recommended as it may complicate the local tissue damage induced by these venoms. The use of stun gun electroshock treatment has been promoted by some people[55]; however, neither clinical nor experimental evidence support the value of this procedure and, therefore, it is not recommended[53,56].

B. FIRST AID TREATMENT

- Both the bitten person and other people around should remain calm after the accident.
- If the snake has been killed, take it to the health center for identification.
- Immobilize the bitten body part in order to retard venom absorption.
- Decrease general physical activity as much as possible.
- Do not make incisions, since profuse bleeding may occur in patients with coagulopathy.
- Do not use tourniquets, nor pressure immobilization bandages, since they worsen the already impaired perfusion to affected tissue. If a tourniquet has been already applied, caution should be exercised when releasing as rapid systemic envenoming may ensue.

- Do not apply ice bags to affected tissue. Avoid administration of food or alcohol; only water can be given if hospitalization is going to be delayed.
- Transport the patient as soon as possible to the nearest health center where antivenom is available.

VI. CLINICAL MANAGEMENT

A. GENERAL CONSIDERATIONS

Any patient with evidence of envenoming or of having being bitten by a snake should be regarded as a medical emergency and must be treated accordingly. All snakebite cases must be admitted to health centers and observed meticulously. In pit viper bites, fang marks are usually present, although their absence does not preclude envenoming. Even in patients that claim not to have been envenomed, a close monitoring of local and systemic signs and symptoms is strongly recommended.

B. DIAGNOSIS

1. Approach to diagnosis

A key initial goal in a diagnostic protocol is to find if the bite was caused by a pit viper, a coral snake or a non-poisonous snake. In the latter case, no local signs and symptoms develop, with the exception of mild pain and swelling. Pit viper envenomings typically cause early development of local effects, whereas in coral snake bites there is only mild pain and swelling at the bite site. Therefore, in Central America, evidence of local tissue damage implies that the patient was bitten by a pit viper. Since coral snake bites are not characterized by local effects, and since neurotoxic effects appear later on, diagnosis of these bites must rely on the patient's description of the snake and on the fact that coral snakes frequently remain attached to the bitten part after they bite.

If the patient brings the offending snake, some key morphological features are helpful to differentiate between poisonous and non-poisonous species: (i) Pit vipers have two orifices at each side of the head; one of them is the nostril and the other, located between the nostril and the eye, is the loreal pit, a thermoreceptor organ that helps pit vipers in defensive as well as in feeding behaviour. Thus, the presence of two orifices on each side of the head indicates, without exception, that the snake is a pit viper. In contrast, coral snakes and non-poisonous snakes have the nostril, but lack the loreal pit, therefore having only one orifice at each side of the head. (ii) To distinguish coral snakes from non-poisonous colubrid species having colored rings, the key features are the sequence of the colors and the completeness of the rings. In the case of true coral snakes, the rings are placed in the sequence red-yellow-black-yellow-red. In addition, rings are complete, i.e., present both dorsally and ventrally in a continuous fashion. The only exceptions to this scheme in Central America is *Micrurus mipartitus* and *M. dissoleucus*. The former is distributed in Costa Rica and Panamá and has rings of only two colors, black and orange, whereas the latter has the triad pattern of rings that typifies many South American *Micrurus*. Quite often, however, the patient does not bring the offending snake and is too confused to give a reliable description of it. In these cases the diagnosis must be based on clinical and laboratory findings but, again, the distinction that has to be made in order to select the proper antivenom is between pit viper, coral snake or non-poisonous snake.

2. Role of laboratory investigations

Pit viper envenomings: Coagulation tests are widely used and recommended in pit viper envenomings in order to demonstrate defibrination and to evaluate the success of antivenom therapy[39,43]. Prothrombin time and partial thromboplastin time are prolonged in these cases, although a simple whole-blood clotting time can be easily carried out wherever laboratory facilities are not available. In addition, quantification of fibrinogen and fibrin-degradation products are often performed[43] (Table 4). It must be kept in mind that several pit viper venoms in Central America do not induce defibrination; however, usually these envenomings are not characterized by severe systemic poisoning and other laboratory tests can be used to monitor the severity of the case. In addition to clotting tests, a platelet count is recommended, as thrombocytopenia has been described in systemic envenomings. Since renal damage is often present, serum levels of urea and creatinine must be determined, together with urianalysis and estimation of urine volume output.

Table 4
Basic laboratory tests recommended in pit viper envenomings

Prothrombin time (or whole blood clotting time)

Fibrinogen concentration

Fibrin(ogen) degradation products

Platelet count

Serum urea and creatinine concentration

Urianalysis

The use of serum levels of various enzymes (creatine kinase, lactate dehydrogenase) might be useful to monitor tissue damage[57]. However, caution must be kept in interpreting these results, as the levels of some enzymes drop rapidly after they peak; consequently, adequate serial sampling must be done. Other haematologic alterations in pit viper envenomings include moderate leucocytosis and neutrophilia, together with a reduction in hemoglobin concentration[22,45].

Coral snake envenoming: In general, no laboratory tests are necessary in coral snake bites. In severe envenomings, colored urine may appear, since these venoms have been shown to be myotoxic in experimental animals[58,59]. If this happens, myoglobin levels in urine and creatine kinase levels in serum must be determined.

3. Assessing the extent of envenoming

Pit viper envenomings: An integral approach using both clinical and laboratory criteria is strongly recommended. Meticulous clinical observations must be done to follow changes in blood pressure, body temperature, urine output, local swelling, increments in intracompartmental pressure and bleeding. Together with clinical appraisal, laboratory tests such as prothrombin time or whole blood clotting time, as well as serum urea and creatinine determinations, must be carried out. The simplistic view that coagulation tests are the only parameter to evaluate the extent of envenoming is misleading, as some pit viper venoms do not affect coagulation tests[44]. If only local alterations are present, i.e. if there is local swelling, bleeding and pain, but no evidence of coagulopathy nor of systemic bleeding, the case can be considered as a mild envenoming. In contrast, if systemic manifestations of poisoning develop besides local effects, then the envenoming must be considered as either moderate or severe, depending upon how drastic these systemic disturbances are. This broad gradation of the severity of the envenomings is relevant in order to determine the volume of antivenom that needs to be administered. Table 5 classifies envenomings on the basis of their severity.

Coral snake envenomings: An early development of neurotoxic paralysis is a clear indication of a severe envenoming and should be handled accordingly. Moderate envenomings usually develop only limited muscle paralysis without extensive involvement of respiratory muscles. The intensity of local effects should not be used as a criterion to assess the severity of envenoming in coral snakebites.

Table 5
Classification of pit viper envenomings in Central America according to severity

Severity	Local Effects	Systemic Effects	Initial Antivenom Dose[a]
Mild	Mild edema	-	4 vials
Moderate	Moderate edema	Coagulopathy,	6 vials
	Mild bleeding	Minor cardiovascular	
		disturbances	
Severe	Pronounced edema	Coagulopathy	10 vials
	Profuse bleeding	Extensive bleeding	
	Necrosis	Hypovolemic shock	
		Renal failure	

[a]Antivenom dose refers to the polyvalent antivenom produced by Instituto Clodomiro Picado, Costa Rica. Each vial of this antivenom neutralizes at least 30 mg of *Bothrops asper* venom, 20 mg of *Lachesis muta stenophrys* venom and 20 mg of *Crotalus durissus durissus* venom.

C. TREATMENT
1. General approach to treatment

A rapid identification of the offending snake as a pit viper, coral snake or non-poisonous snake, together with a careful early monitoring of the severity of envenoming, are cornerstone elements in a successful treatment of a snakebite case. As soon as the patient arrives at the health center, medical and paramedical personnel must be aware of the clinical and laboratory features that need to be monitored. Tourniquets or any other type of ligature have to be removed once antivenom infusion has started. It is recommended that an i.v. line is inserted immediately upon admission, although antivenom must be administered only if there is evidence of envenoming. An indiscriminate administration of antivenom is discouraged since this heterologous antiserum may induce harmful secondary reactions. Even when signs of envenoming are not present, the patient must remain in the health center for observation for at least 6 hours, as it has been demonstrated that the onset of envenoming is delayed several hours in some cases. A key element in a successful treatment is the periodic clinical monitoring of the patient, together with laboratory determinations, in order to objectively determine progress of both envenoming and the effects of treatment.

Infections often develop in pit viper bites, due in part to the presence of abundant bacteria in the venoms, and also to the severe tissue necrosis which contributes to the colonization by microorganisms[60,61]. Awareness of this possibility is necessary in order to determine if antibiotics have to be administered. Surgical measures are not recommended, except when a compartmental syndrome develops. Any early surgical procedure in the bitten region is strongly discouraged since it may result in extensive bleeding due to the coagulopathy present in these patients.

2. Antivenom therapy

Antivenom administration is indicated when there is evidence of envenoming. The two most important antivenoms produced in Central America by the Instituto Clodomiro Picado (University of Costa Rica, Costa Rica) are polyvalent antivenom and anti-coral antivenom[62]. The former is effective against the venoms of all the pit vipers in the region, including *Crotalus durissus durissus* and *Lachesis muta*, whereas anti-coral antivenom neutralizes the venoms of the most abundant species of *Micrurus*. However, it must be kept in mind that this antivenom is not effective against the venom of coral "gargantilla" (*Micrurus mipartitus*). Fortunately, bites by this species are very rare and a specific antivenom produced in small amounts and kept at Instituto Clodomiro Picado has to be used[63]. In addition, a multivalent coral snake antivenom was produced in the late seventies, being effective in the neutralization of several Central and South American coral snake venoms[64]. Besides their well demonstrated clinical efficacy, experimental studies have corroborated the ability of these antivenoms in the neutralization of the most relevant toxic effects induced by Central American snake venoms[62,65-68]. The recommended doses of polyvalent antivenom to be administered in pit viper envenomings are indicated in Table 5. Besides these products made and distributed by Instituto Clodomiro Picado, there are other sources of polyvalent antivenom available in the region[69]; however, there are no published studies on the efficacy of these products in the neutralization of Central American pit viper venoms.

If a patient shows signs of envenoming, an initial dose of antivenom must be administered as soon as possible (Table 5). In health centers, antivenom should be given only i.v. and diluted in isotonic solutions, as other routes are by far less effective. However, if access to a health center is many hours away, and if there is conclusive evidence that the patient is severely envenomed, administration of antivenom in the field can be considered. In these cases, antivenom is injected undiluted, by the intramuscular route, although it should be kept in mind that there is always a risk of life-threatening allergic reactions. Even if antivenom is given in the field, the patient must be transported to a medical facility in order to assure a comprehensive treatment.

The personnel administering antivenom must be aware that acute allergic reactions may occur within the first 30 minutes of infusion, including true anaphylactic as well as anaphylactoid reactions[70,71]. These may develop even when there is not a history of previous heterologous equine serum administration. The performance of skin tests to predict the occurrence of allergic reactions is not recommended in hospitals, since it is highly unreliable[70,71]. Thus, in order to deal with a potential early reaction, some physicians recommend a prophylactic i.v. administration of antihistamine drugs and hydrocortisone[71]. However, this is a controversial issue since it has not been conclusively demonstrated that this procedure reduces the incidence of immediate reactions to antivenom administration. In any case, the initial infusion of antivenom has to be made slowly and, if there is evidence of reaction, it must be stopped and both anti-histamines (e.g. diphenhydramine) and hydrocortisone have to be injected i.v. In addition, adrenaline must be available for the treatment of severe reactions, together with standard resuscitation equipment. Once these drugs have been administered, antivenom administration must be restarted, albeit with caution. Besides the horse-derived antivenom, Instituto Clodomiro Picado also manufactures a sheep-derived polyvalent antivenom for people known to be allergic to horse serum.

In adults, antivenom must be diluted with physiologic solutions for its administration in a total volume of 500 ml[72]. If early reactions do not occur, the infusion flow rate must be increased so that the total volume is given in 2-3 hours. In children, the same number of antivenom vials have to be administered, but the total volume of diluted solution must be reduced in order to avoid fluid overload. If the patient has a tourniquet and there is evidence of significant envenoming, antivenom therapy must start before releasing the tourniquet.

In some cases it may be necessary to give additional doses of antivenom, depending upon the evolution of local and systemic signs and symptoms. If there is evidence that envenoming has not been controlled, then an additional volume of antivenom is required. Again, the careful monitoring of each case is the only acceptable method of determining the precise dose to be given. Thus, in pit viper envenomings in Central America, the required number of antivenom vials for a single treatment may go from 4 in mild cases, to as many as 20 in very severe cases. The few well demonstrated cases of envenomings by *Lachesis muta* in Costa Rica have been extremely severe, with a rapid onset of systemic effects[24]. Thus, until a more comprehensive clinical appraisal of this problem is performed, envenomings by this pit viper have to be treated with an initial dose of 10-15 vials of polyvalent antivenom.

Besides the early reactions described, patients may also develop a delayed reaction (serum sickness) 8 to 15 days after antivenom injection[73]; this is characterized by urticaria, pruritus, edema, arthralgia and fever[21,74]. Patients must know about this possibility and they should be asked to return to the health center if such reaction takes place in order to receive a treatment based on steroids.

3. Pit viper bites
a. Local tissue damage and its treatment

Local tissue effects constitute a serious challenge for those managing pit viper envenomings. On one hand, these effects develop very rapidly; thus, a delay in antivenom administration greatly reduces the success of therapy. Although various drugs have been tried, both experimentally and clinically, in an attempt to reduce local tissue damage, there is no consistent evidence of efficacy with any of them. In the case of edema and other vascular alterations, it is necessary to monitor the perfusion to distal parts of the bitten extremity, by the use of doppler or similar techniques, as well as to detect changes in the subfascial pressure. If there is evidence that a compartmental syndrome has developed, i.e., if interstitial fluid pressure in a given muscle compartment rises above 30 mm Hg, fasciotomy might be indicated[2,21,76]. However, this judgement should be made with extreme caution, as this procedure introduces potentially serious complications. Fasciotomy should be performed only after coagulation disorders have been controlled by antivenom infusion, in order to avoid extensive bleeding. On the other hand, surgical debridement is indicated in order to remove necrotic tissue.

b. Infection and its treatment

Local infection develops in a number of pit viper envenomings, mainly due to the presence of large amounts of bacteria in the venoms[2,22,60]. This may cause local abscesses and sepsis; thus, when evidence of infection appears, antibiotics are indicated. Despite the recommendation by some clinicians for prophylactic antibiotic administration, this is not encouraged until there is objective evidence of infection. The bacteria that have been isolated from the venoms of Central American pit vipers require the use of a combination of penicillin and a broad spectrum antibiotic[2,72]. However, caution must be exercised when using antibiotics that may affect renal function, as in many cases of pit viper envenomings the kidney is already impaired. In addition, surgical drainage of abscesses might be necessary.

c. Coagulopathy and its treatment

Defibrination is a consequence of the direct action of venom components on clotting factors, especially on fibrinogen. This activity is not inhibited by heparin, making this drug useless in handling the coagulopathy characteristic of these envenomings[2]. On the other hand, administration of plasma to replace clotting factors is not recommended until the venom has been neutralized by antivenom. Therefore, coagulopathy must be treated with a dose of antivenom large enough to neutralize circulating venom factors. Afterwards, levels of clotting factors increase and functional tests of coagulation return to normal values within 6 to 12 hours after an adequate dose of antivenom has been administered.

d. Renal failure and its treatment

A meticulous record of urine output, as well as of serum urea and creatinine levels, is very important to detect the onset of acute renal failure. The maintenance of an adequate fluid load is crucial in preventing renal damage and the induction of osmotic diuresis, by administration of mannitol, has been successful in preventing renal failure[2,76]. If acute renal failure develops, it needs to be treated accordingly, a subject that goes beyond the scope of this chapter.

e. Cardiovascular shock and its treatment

The cardiovascular status of patients envenomed by pit vipers has to be monitored carefully in order to detect hypotension and the onset of shock. Venom-induced bleeding causes hypovolemia that may eventually lead to cardiovascular shock[3,21,74]. Administration of whole fresh blood or plasma expanders needs to be considered in these circumstances[3,72,74,76]. The use of steroids in the treatment of pit viper venom-induced shock is not supported by any conclusive evidence and therefore is not recommended.

f. Other issues in treatment of pit viper envenomings

Tetanus prophylaxis (tetanus toxoid) is advisable as a routine procedure[2,72]. Analgesics can be administered. In addition, it is important to monitor serum electrolyte and blood pH alterations since they may develop in severe cases and need to be dealt with.

4. Coral snake bites
a. Neurotoxicity and its treatment

Careful attention must be paid to patients bitten by coral snakes to detect the first signs of neurotoxicity which may take several hours to appear and usually progress very rapidly after their onset. Any evidence of neurotoxicity must be followed by a rapid administration of anti-coral antivenom. The time interval between onset of envenoming and initiation of antivenom infusion is a critical factor in the prognosis of these cases. Antivenom is indicated even when envenoming is well advanced, as there are clinical reports showing the reversal of neurotoxic effects. The risk of aspiration pneumonia has to be considered and caution should be taken to avoid it. Endotracheal intubation is urged in patients with evidence of envenoming, in order to be prepared for artificial ventilation. This is recommended also because some Central American coral snake venoms might not be neutralized by the commercially-available anti-coral antivenom. In Brazil, the use of anticholinesterase drugs, in combination with atropine, has been effective in the treatment of envenomings by coral snakes which induce only postsynaptic effects[49,75]. However, preliminary studies carried out with the venom of *Micrurus nigrocinctus* in Central America strongly indicate that anticholinesterase drugs are ineffective in patients bitten by this species, probably because this venom also induces presynaptic effects at the neuromuscular junction[50]. The usefulness of these drugs in envenomings induced by other coral snake species needs to be studied.

ACKNOWLEDGEMENTS: The author thanks Javier Núñez, Abel Robles, Irma Arguedas, Rocío Monge, Gustavo Rojas and Danilo Chacón for their collaboration in the preparation of the manuscript.

VII. REFERENCES

1. **SAVAGE, J. M.**, *A Preliminary Handlist of the Herpetofauna of Costa Rica*, Universidad de Costa Rica, San José, 1976,
2. **BOLAÑOS, R.**, *Serpientes, Venenos y Ofidismo en Centroamérica*, Editorial Universidad de Costa Rica, San José, 136 p, 1984.
3. **BOLAÑOS, R.**, Las serpientes venenosas de Centroamérica y el problema del ofidismo. Primera parte. Aspectos zoológicos, epidemiológicos y biomédicos, *Revista Costarricense de Ciencias Médicas*, 3, 165, 1982.
4. **JOHANBOCKE, M. M.**, Effects of a bite by *Conophis lineatus* (Squamata, Colubridae), *Bull. Phil. Herp. Soc.*, 22, 39, 1974.
5. **CAMPBELL, J. A., AND LAMAR, W. W.**, *The Venomous Reptiles of Latin America*, Cornell University Press, Ithaca, 425 p, 1989.
6. **VORIS, H. K.**, *Pelamis platurus* (Culebra de mar, pelagic sea snake), in *Costa Rican Natural History*, Janzen, D., Ed., The University of Chicago Press, Chicago, 411, 1983.
7. **TU, T., TU, A. T., AND LIN, T. S.**, Some pharmacological properties of the venom, venom fractions and pure toxin of the yellow-bellied sea snake *Pelamis platurus*, *J. Pharm. Pharmac.*, 28, 139, 1976.
8. **GREENE, H., AND SEIB, R. L.**, *Micrurus nigrocinctus* (Corál, coral snake, coralillo), in *Costa Rican Natural History*, Janzen, D., Ed., The University of Chicago Press, Chicago, 406, 1983.
9. **GREENE, H. W.**, The ecological and behavioral context for pitviper evolution, in *Biology of the Pitvipers*, Campbell, J. A. and Brodie, E. D., Eds., Selva, Texas, 107, 1992.
10. **CAMPBELL, J. A., AND SOLÓRZANO, A.**, The distribution, variation, and natural history of the Middle American montane pitviper, *Porthidium godmani*, in *Biology of the Pitvipers*, Campbell, J. A., and Brodie, E. D., Eds., Selva, Texas, 223, 1992.
11. **SOLÓRZANO, A., AND CERDAS, L.**, Biología reproductiva de la cascabel centroamericana *Crotalus durissus durissus* (Serpentes: Viperidae) en Costa Rica, *Rev. Biol. Trop.*, 36, 221, 1988.
12. **SOLÓRZANO, A., AND CERDAS, L.**, Reproductive biology and distribution of the terciopelo, *Bothrops asper* Garman (Serpentes: Viperidae), in Costa Rica, *Herpetologica*, 45, 444, 1989.
13. **SOLÓRZANO, A.**, Distribución y aspectos reproductivos de la mano de piedra, *Bothrops nummifer* (Serpentes: Viperidae), en Costa Rica, *Rev. Biol. Trop.*, 37, 133, 1989.
14. **TU, A. T.**, *Venoms: Chemistry and Molecular Biology*, John Wiley & Sons, New York, 1977, 560 p.
15. **ROJAS, G.**, Unpublished data, 1992.
16. **GUTIÉRREZ, J. M., CHAVES, F., AND BOLAÑOS, R.**, Estudio comparativo de venenos de ejemplares recién nacidos y adultos de *Bothrops asper*, *Rev. Biol. Trop.*, 28, 341, 1980.
17. **LOMONTE, B., GENÉ, J. A., GUTIÉRREZ, J. M., AND CERDAS, L.**, Estudio comparativo de los venenos de serpiente cascabel (*Crotalus durissus durissus*) de ejemplares adultos y recién nacidos, *Toxicon*, 21, 379, 1983.
18. **GUTIÉRREZ, J. M., DOS SANTOS, M. C., FURTADO, M. F., AND ROJAS, G.**, Biochemical and pharmacological similarities between the venoms of newborn *Crotalus durissus durissus* and adult *Crotalus durissus terrificus* rattlesnakes, *Toxicon*, 29, 1273, 1991.
19. **GUTIÉRREZ, J. M., AVILA, C., CAMACHO, Z., AND LOMONTE, B.**, Ontogenetic changes in the venom of the snake *Lachesis muta stenophrys* (bushmaster) from Costa Rica, *Toxicon*, 28, 419, 1990.
20. **JIMÉNEZ-PORRAS, J. M.**, Venom proteins of the fer-de-lance, *Bothrops atrox*, from Costa Rica, *Toxicon*, 2, 115, 1964.
21. **WINGERT, W. A.**, Management of crotalid envenomations, in *Handbook of Natural Toxins*, Vol 5, *Reptile Venoms and Toxins*, Tu, A. T., Ed., Marcel Dekker, New York, Chap. 20, 1991.
22. **DE FRANCO, D., ALVAREZ, I., AND MORA, L. A.**, Mordedura de ofidios venenosos en niños en la región Pacífico Sur. Análisis de ciento sesenta casos, *Acta Médica Costarricense*, 26, 61, 1983.
23. **BOLAÑOS, R.**, Toxicity of Costa Rican snake venoms for the white mouse, *Am. J. Trop. Med. Hyg.*, 21, 360, 1972.
24. **BOLAÑOS, R., ROJAS, O., AND ULLOA, C. E.**, Aspectos biomédicos de cuatro casos de mordeduras de serpiente por *Lachesis muta* (Ophidia: Viperidae) en Costa Rica, *Rev. Biol. Trop.*, 30, 53, 1982.
25. **BOLAÑOS, R., MARÍN, O., MORA, E., AND ALFARO, E.**, El accidente ofídico por cascabela (*Crotalus durissus durissus*) en Costa Rica, *Acta Médica Costarricense*, 24, 211, 1981.
26. **ROSENFELD, G.**, Symptomatology, pathology and treatment of snake bites in South America, in *Venomous Animals and Their Venoms, Vol II, Venomous Vertebrates*, Bucherl, W., and Buckley, E., Eds, Academic Press, New York, 345, 1971.
27. **CUPO, P., AZEVEDO-MARQUES, M. M., AND HERING, S. E.**, Acidente crotálico na infancia: aspectos clínicos, laboratoriais, epidemiológicos e abordagem terapeutica, *Revista da Sociedade Brasileira de Medicina Tropical*, 24, 87, 1991.
28. **KITCHENS, C. S., AND VAN MIEROP, L. H. S.**, Envenomation by the eastern coral snake (*Micrurus fulvius fulvius*). A study of 39 victims, *J.A.M.A.*, 258, 1615, 1987.

29. **OHSAKA, A.**, Hemorrhagic, necrotizing and edema-forming effects of snake venoms, in *Snake Venoms*, Lee, C. Y., Ed., Springer-Verlag, Berlin, 480, 1979.
30. **OWNBY, C. L.**, Pathology of rattlesnake envenomation, in *Rattlesnake Venoms, Their Actions and Treatment*, Tu, A. T., Ed., Marcel Dekker, New York, 163, 1982.
31. **MOREIRA, L., GUTIÉRREZ, J. M., BORKOW, G., AND OVADIA, M.**, Ultrastructural alterations in mouse capillary blood vessels after experimental injection of venom from the snake *Bothrops asper* (terciopelo), *Exp. Mol. Pathol.*, 57, 124, 1992.
32. **KAMIGUTI, A. S., CARDOSO, J. L. C., THEAKSTON, R. D. G., SANO-MARTINS, I. S., HUTTON, R. A., RUGMAN, F. P., WARRELL, D. A., AND HAY, C. R. M.**, Coagulopathy and hemorrhage in human victims of *Bothrops jararaca* envenoming in Brazil, *Toxicon*, 29, 961, 1991.
33. **HAWGOOD, B. J.**, Physiological and pharmacological effects of rattlesnake venoms, in *Rattlesnake Venoms, Their Actions and Treatment*, Tu, A. T., Ed., Marcel Dekker, New York, 121, 1982.
34. **GUTIÉRREZ, J. M.**, Mechanism of action of myotoxins isolated from crotaline snake venoms, in *Proceedings of the First Brazilian Congress on Proteins*, Oliveira, B., and Sgarbieri, V., Eds., Editora da UNICAMP, Campinas, 336, 1991.
35. **GUTIÉRREZ, J. M., AND LOMONTE, B.**, Local tissue damage induced by *Bothrops* snake venoms. A review, *Memorias Instituto Butantan*, 51, 211, 1989.
36. **GUTIÉRREZ, J. M., OWNBY, C. L., AND ODELL, G. V.**, Pathogenesis of myonecrosis induced by crude venom and a myotoxin of *Bothrops asper*, *Exp. Mol. Pathol.*, 40, 367, 1984.
37. **HOMMA, M., AND TU, A. T.**, Morphology of local tissue damage in experimental snake envenomation, *Br. J. Exp. Path.*, 52, 538, 1971.
38. **ARCE, V., BRENES, F., AND GUTIÉRREZ, J. M.**, Degenerative and regenerative changes in murine skeletal muscle after injection of venom from the snake *Bothrops asper*: a histochemical and immunocytochemical study, *Int. J. Exp. Path.*, 72, 211, 1991.
39. **PEÑA-CHAVARRÍA, A., VILLAREJOS, V. M., AND ZOMER, M.**, Clinical importance of prothrombin time determination in snake venom poisoning, *Am. J. Trop. Med. Hyg.*, 19, 342, 1970.
40. **ARAGÓN-ORTIZ, F., AND GUBENSEK, F.**, Characterization of thrombin-like proteinase from *Bothrops asper* venom, in *Toxins: Animal, Plant and Microbial*, Rosenberg, P., Ed., Pergamon Press, Oxford, 107, 1978.
41. **ARAGÓN-ORTIZ, F.**, Isolation and partial characterization of *Lachesis muta melanocephala* coagulant proteinase: biochemical parameters of the venom, *Rev. Biol. Trop.*, 36, 387, 1988.
42. **HOFMANN, H., AND BON, C.**, Blood coagulation induced by the venom of *Bothrops atrox*. 2. Identification, purification and properties of two factor X activators, *Biochemistry*, 26, 780, 1987.
43. **BARRANTES, A., SOLÍS, V., AND BOLAÑOS, R.**, Alteración en los mecanismos de la coagulación en el envenenamiento por *Bothrops asper* (terciopelo), *Toxicon*, 23, 399, 1985.
44. **GENÉ, J. A., ROY, A., ROJAS, G., GUTIÉRREZ, J. M., AND CERDAS, L.**, Comparative study on coagulant, defibrinating, fibrinolytic and fibrinogenolytic activities of Costa Rican crotaline snake venoms and their neutralization by a polyvalent antivenom, *Toxicon*, 27, 841, 1989.
45. **OTERO, R., TOBÓN, G. S., GÓMEZ, L. F., OSORIO, R., VALDERRAMA, R., HOYOS, D., URRETA, J. E., MOLINA, S., AND ARBOLEDA, J. J.**, Accidente ofídico en Antioquia y Chocó. Aspectos clínicos y epidemiológicos (marzo de 1989-febrero de 1990), *Acta Médica Colombiana*, 17, 229, 1992.
46. **MEKBEL, S. T., AND CÉSPEDES, R.**, Las lesiones renales en el ofidismo, *Acta Médica Costarricense*, 6, 111, 1963.
47. **VARGAS-BALDARES, M.**, Renal lesions in snake bite in Costa Rica, in *Toxins: Animal, Plant and Microbial*, Rosenberg, P., Ed., Pergamon Press, Oxford, 497, 1978.
48. **AZEVEDO-MARQUES, M. M., CUPO, P., COIMBRA, T. M., HERING, S. E., ROSSI, M. A., AND LAURE, C. J.**, Myonecrosis, myoglobinuria and acute renal failure induced by South American rattlesnake (*Crotalus durissus terrificus*) envenomation in Brazil, *Toxicon*, 23, 631, 1985.
49. **VITAL-BRAZIL, O.**, Coral snake venoms: mode of action and pathophysiology of experimental envenomation, *Rev. Inst. Med. Trop. Sao Paulo*, 29, 119, 1987.
50. **RODRIGUES-SIMIONI, L., COGO, J C., GUTIÉRREZ, J. M., AND PRADO-FRANCESCHI, J.**, *Micrurus nigrocinctus* venom induced effects on isolated mouse phrenic-nerve diaphragm and chick biventer cervicis preparations, in *I Symposio da Sociedade Brasileira de Toxicología*, Instituto Butantan, Sao Paulo, 7, 1990.
51. **TU, A. T., LIN, T. S., AND BIEBER, A. L.**, Purification and chemical characterization of the major neurotoxin from the venom of *Pelamis platurus*, *Biochemistry*, 14, 3408, 1975.
52. **GUTIÉRREZ, J.M., SEGURA, M., AND AYMERICH, R.**, Historia del Instituto Clodomiro Picado, in *Ciencia y Tecnología en la Construcción del Futuro*, Ruiz, A., Ed., Asociación Costarricense de Historia y Filosofía de la Ciencia, San José, 203, 1991.
53. **HARDY, D. L.**, A review of first aid measures for pit viper bite in North America with an appraisal of extractor[tm] suction and stun gun electroshock, in *Biology of the Pitvipers*, Campbell, J. A., and Brodie, E. D., Eds., Selva, Texas, 405, 1992.

54. **SUTHERLAND, S. K., COULTER, A. R., AND HARRIS, R. D.**, Rationalisation of first-aid measures for elapid snakebite, *Lancet*, 1, 183, 1979.

55. **GUDERIAN, R. H., MACKENZIE, C. D., AND WILLIAMS, J. F.**, High voltage shock treatment for snake bite (letter), *Lancet*, 2, 229, 1986.

56. **HOWE, N. R., AND MEISENHEIMER, J. L.**, Electric shock does not save snakebitten rats, *Ann. Emerg. Med.*, 17, 254, 1988.

57. **GUTIÉRREZ, J. M., ARROYO, O., AND BOLAÑOS, R.**, Mionecrosis, hemorragia y edema inducidos por el veneno de *Bothrops asper* en ratón blanco, *Toxicon*, 18, 603, 1980.

58. **GUTIÉRREZ, J. M., LOMONTE, B., PORTILLA, E., CERDAS, L., AND ROJAS, E.**, Local effects induced by coral snake venoms: evidence of myonecrosis after experimental inoculations of venoms from five species, *Toxicon*, 21, 77, 1983.

59. **GUTIÉRREZ, J. M., ARROYO, O., CHAVES, F., LOMONTE, B., AND CERDAS, L.**, Pathogenesis of myonecrosis induced by coral snake (*Micrurus nigrocinctus*) venom in mice, *Br. J. Exp. Path.*, 67, 1, 1986.

60. **ARROYO, O., BOLAÑOS, R., AND MUÑOZ, G.**, The bacterial flora of venom and mouth cavities of Costa Rican snakes, *Bull. Pan Am. Hlth. Org.*, 14, 280, 1980.

61. **BOLAÑOS, R., AND BRUNKER, T.**, Bacteriología del veneno y de las glándulas veneníferas de *Bothrops asper* y *Crotalus durissus durissus* de Costa Rica, *Revista Costarricense de Ciencias Médicas*, 4, 27, 1983.

62. **BOLAÑOS, R., AND CERDAS, L.**, La producción y control de sueros antiofídicos en Costa Rica, *Bol. Of. Sanit. Panam.*, 88, 189, 1980

63. **BOLAÑOS, R., CERDAS, L., AND TAYLOR, R.**, The production and characteristics of a coral snake (*Micrurus mipartitus hertwigi*) antivenin, *Toxicon*, 13, 139, 1975.

64. **BOLAÑOS, R., CERDAS, L., AND ABALOS, J. W.**, Venenos de serpientes coral (*Micrurus* spp): informe sobre un antiveneno polivalente para las Américas, *Bol. Of. Sanit. Panam.*, 84, 128, 1978.

65. **GUTIÉRREZ, J. M., GENÉ, J. A., ROJAS, G., AND CERDAS, L.**, Neutralization of proteolytic and hemorrhagic activities of Costa Rican snake venoms by a polyvalent antivenom, *Toxicon*, 23, 887, 1985.

66. **ROJAS, G., GUTIÉRREZ, J. M., GENÉ, J. A., GÓMEZ, M., AND CERDAS, L.**, Neutralización de las actividades tóxicas y enzimáticas de cuatro venenos de serpientes de Guatemala y Honduras por el antiveneno polivalente producido en Costa Rica, *Rev. Biol. Trop.*, 35, 59, 1987.

67. **GUTIÉRREZ, J. M., ROJAS, G., AND CERDAS, L.**, Ability of a polyvalent antivenom to neutralize the venom of *Lachesis muta melanocephala*, a new Costa Rican subspecies of the bushmaster, *Toxicon*, 25, 713, 1987.

68. **GUTIÉRREZ, J. M., ROJAS, G., PÉREZ, A., ARGUELLO, I., AND LOMONTE, B.**, Neutralization of coral snake *Micrurus nigrocinctus* venom by a monovalent antivenom, *Brazilian J. Med. Biol. Res.*, 24, 701, 1991.

69. **THEAKSTON, R. D. G., AND WARRELL, D. A.**, Antivenoms: a list of hyperimmune sera currently available for the treatment of envenomings by bites and stings, *Toxicon*, 29, 1419, 1991.

70. **MALASIT, P., WARRELL, D. A., CHANTHAVANICH, P., VIRAVAN, C., MONGKOLSAPAYA, J., SINGHTHONG, B., AND SUPICH, C.**, Prediction, prevention and mechanism of early (anaphylactic) antivenom reactions in victims of snake bites, *Br. Med. J.*, 292, 17, 1986.

71. **CUPO, P., AZEVEDO-MARQUES, M. M., MENEZES, J. B., AND HERING, S. E.**, Reacoes de hipersensibilidade imediatas apos uso intravenoso de soros antivenenos: valor diagnóstico dos testes de sensibilidade intradérmicos, *Rev. Inst. Med. Trop. Sao Paulo*, 33, 115, 1991.

72. **MOYA, J., AND GUTIÉRREZ, J. M.**, Mordedura de serpiente, in *Emergencias Médicas*, Quesada, O., Ed., Pfizer, San José, 253, 1987.

73. **CORRIGAN, P., RUSSELL, F. E., AND WAINSCHEL, J.**, Clinical reactions to antivenin, in *Toxins: Animal, Plant and Microbial*, Rosenberg, P., Ed., Pergamon Press, Oxford, 437, 1978.

74. **WATT, G.**, Snakebite treatment and first aid, in *The Venomous Reptiles of Latin America*, Campbell, J. A., and Lamar, W. W., Eds., Cornell University Press, Ithaca, New York, 6, 1989.

75. **VITAL-BRAZIL, O., PELLEGRINI, A., AND DIAS-FONTANA, M.**, Antagonism of *Micrurus frontalis* venom by neostigmine. Treatment of experimental envenomation, in *Toxins: Animal, Plant and Microbial*, Rosenberg, P., Ed., Pergamon Press, Oxford, 437, 1978.

76. **DE FRANCO, D., ALVAREZ, I., AND MORA, L. A.**, Terapia de la mordedura de ofidios venenosos en niños en la región Pacífico Sur. Análisis en ciento sesenta casos, *Acta Médica Costarricense*, 26, 76, 1983.

Chapter 31

CLINICAL TOXICOLOGY OF SNAKE BITES IN SOUTH AMERICA

Hui Wen Fan and J.L. Cardoso

TABLE OF CONTENTS

I. INTRODUCTION

Snake envenoming represents a significant public health problem in tropical countries. Data from South America are fragmentary although snake bites in the sub-continent are not uncommon and the policy of collection of data has been neglected.

Immunisation of pigeons against the lethal effects of snake venom was first demonstrated by Sewall[1]. Simultaneously in 1894, Phisalix & Bertrand[2] and Calmette[3] established the basis for serumtherapy in the treatment of snakebite. Vital Brazil was a pioneer who, in 1901, prepared the first antivenom against South American venomous snakes. His great contribution to snake bite serumtherapy literature was the demonstration of antivenom specificity[4].

The first studies on snakebites in Brazil, including aetiological, clinical and epidemiological figures, were performed by the same auhtor in the classical "La defense contre l'ophidisme"[5]. Other authors of importance include Houssay[6] who started the production of antivenom in Argentina and Posados Arango[7] who proposed the utilization of antivenom in Colombia.

Much of the information referred to in this chapter is based on the experience of the authors at Hospital Vital Brazil (HVB) - Instituto Butantan (Sao Paulo, Brazil) and a review of the literature.

II. EPIDEMIOLOGY

A. VENOMOUS SNAKES OF INTEREST IN SOUTH AMERICA

Until the recent taxonomic review of Campbell and Lamar[8], who proposed three new genera created from genus *Bothrops*: *Bothriechis* (Palm-pitvipers); *Bothriopsis* (Forest-pitvipers) and *Porthridium* (Hognosed and montane pitvipers), only four genera of snakes were responsible for human envenoming in South America. Because few human cases are described and the venoms' activities are poorly studied for many species of the former genus *Bothrops*, from the medical point of view these snakebites have still been considered as bothropic envenoming.

- Snakes of the genus *Bothrops* (lance-headed vipers) are responsible for about 90% of snake bites in almost all of South America[7];
- Snakes of the genus *Lachesis* (bushmaster) in Amazonia are of particular interest due to the similarities with *Bothrops* envenoming;
- *Crotalus* snakebites are related to neurotoxic and myotoxic effects of *C.d.terrificus* (South-American rattlesnake) venom;
- Snakes of the genus *Micrurus* are not frequent causes of envenoming and data about human snakebites are scarce.

The most important species known in South America are listed in Table 1[8].

B. SNAKE BITE IN SOUTH AMERICA

Human snakebites occur more frequently in rural areas, affecting mainly agricultural workers deprived of basic protection equipment. In rain forest snake bite injuries assume a particular importance because adequate medical facilities and personnel needed to provide specific treatment are often lacking.

669

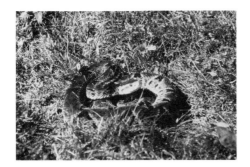

Figure 1. *Bothrops atrox* (courtesy Dr. J. Meier, Basel).

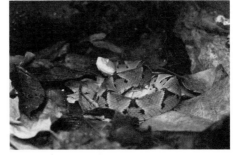

Figure 2. *Bothrops brazili* (courtesy Dr. G. Puorto, Sao Paulo, Brazil).

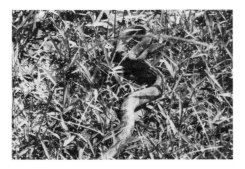

Figure 3. *Bothrops jararaca* (courtesy Dr. J. Meier)

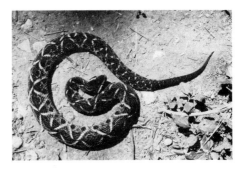

Figure 4. *Bothrops jararacussu* (courtesy Dr. G. Puorto, Sao Paulo, Brazil).

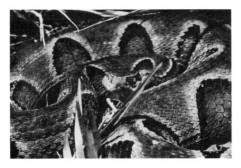

Figure 5. *Bothrops moojeni* (courtesy Dr. J. Meier).

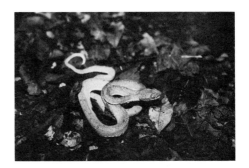

Figure 6. *Bothriopsis bilineata* (courtesy Dr. G. Puorto, Sao Paulo, Brazil).

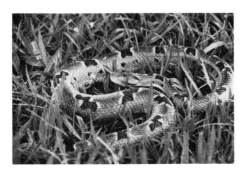

Figure 7. *Bothrops neuwiedi* (courtesy Dr. J. Meier).

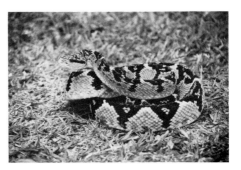

Figure 8. *Lachesis muta* (courtesy Dr. G. Puorto, Sao Paulo, Brazil).

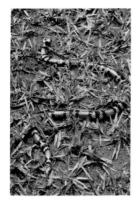

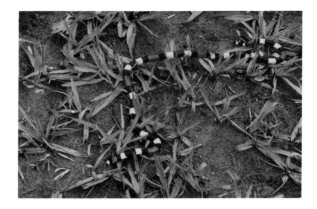

Figure 9. *Micrurus frontalis* (courtesy Dr. J. Meier).

Figure 10. *Micrurus ibibaboca* (courtesy Dr. J. Meier).

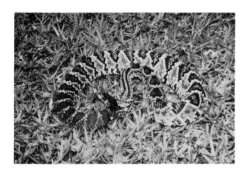

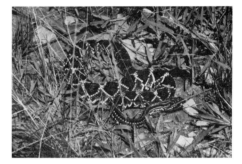

Figure 11. *Crotalus durissus durissus* (courtesy Dr. J. Meier).

Figure 12. *Crotalus durissus terrificus* (courtesy Dr. J. Meier).

1. Incidence of snakebites according to the type of snake

Information from the WHO[7] for South America reveals that about 90% of venomous snake bites are caused by *Bothrops* of several species. The genera *Crotalus*, *Lachesis* and *Micrurus* are responsible for the remaining 10%. Data from Hospital Vital Brazil (HVB) reveal that about 50% of snakebite cases had no signs/symptoms of envenoming. This emphasises that snake bite is not always synonymous with envenoming. This occurs because most snakes are non-venomous or even those with a venom apparatus can fail to envenom human beings[10,11](Table 2).

A morbidity rate of 54.5 per 100,000 population was estimated in 1972 using partial data from southeast region of Brazil[12]. In 1986, a National Program on Snakebite ("Programa Nacional de Ofidismo"-PNO.) was started in Brazil sponsored by the Ministry of Health. Since then more accurate data have been available for the country as a whole[13]. For other countries, data are fragmentary and based on surveys and case reports. Those records reveal 20,000 snakebites occur per year in Brazil (13-15 snakebites/100,000 population). It is known that many cases are not notified, mainly in rural areas, leading to underestimation of the number of cases.

In Argentina, the estimated number of cases reaches 1,500 snakebites per year (5/100,000 population per year)[14]. Most snakebites take place in the north of the country.

In Colombia about 2,000 new cases are referred each year, 90% caused by *Bothrops*, mainly *B. atrox*[15,16]. The snakebites caused by *Crotalus*, *Lachesis* and *Micrurus* are rare. Cases of envenoming by *Palamis platurus*, the sea snake from the Pacific Ocean, are exceptionally uncommon[17]. Data about mortality are fragmentary but it seems to be decreasing[16].

Table 1
Venomous snakes in South America[6]

Snake	Country											
	FG	S	G	V	BR	C	E	PE	BO	PA	A	U
Bothrops												
atrox	X	X	X	X	X	X	X	X	X			
brazili	X	X	X	X	X	X	X	X	X			
neuwiedi					X				X	X	X	X
jararacussu					X				X	X	X	
jararaca					X					X	X	
alternatus					X					X	X	X
moojeni					X						X	
erithromelas					X							
Bothriopsis												
bilineata	X	X	X	X	X	X	X	X	X			
taeniata	X	X	X	X	X	X	X	X	X			
Lachesis muta	X	X	X	X	X	X	X	X	X			
Crotalus durissus												
durissus												
dryinas	X	X	X		X							
ruruima				X	X							
cumanensis			?	X		X						
terrificus					X		X		X	X	X	X
collilineatus					X				?			
cascavella					X							
Micrurus												
hemprichi	X	X	X	X	X	X	X	X				
surinamensis	X	X	X	X	X	X	X	X	X			
leminiscatus	X	X	X	X	X	X	X	X	X			
spixii				X	X	X	X	X	X			
frontalis					X				X	X	X	X
corallinus					X					X	X	?
ibibboca	?	?			X							

X = present; ? = dubious identification; FG = French Guiana; S = Suriname: G = Guiana; V = Venezuela; BR = Brazil; C = Colombia; E = Ecuador; PE = Peru; BO = Bolivia; PA = Paraguay; A = Argentina; U = Uruguay.

Venomous snake bites are important among the population of Ecuador's eastern jungle (Oriente) due to *Bothrops* and *Lachesis*. The morbidity rate of 25% is the result of delays in initiation of appropriate treatment[18].

The risk of envenoming by snake bite in French Guiana varies from 45/100,000 inhabitants in the cities up to 590/100,000 population living within the primary forests[19]. Snakebites are caused by *Bothrops* (*B.atrox, B.brazili, B.bilineatus*); *Crotalus durissus;*

Lachesis muta and *Micrurus* sp, but *B.atrox* and *Crotalus durissus* are the most medically important species.

In Uruguay data on snakebites by *B. alternatus* and *B. neuwiedii* are obtained from Centro de Información y Asesoramiento Toxicológico de Montevidéu, a national reference center[20].

The morbidity rate in Venezuela reported from 1978 to 1982 was 7.7 snakebites/100,000 population with 4.97% mortality. *Bothrops atrox* was the species that caused most snakebites while *Crotalus* and *Micrurus* represented less than 10% of snake bites[21].

Table 2

Snakebites in Brazil: number of cases according to type of snake in three different periods of time

Genus	1902-45*		1966-77**		1986-1990***	
	Number	%	Number	%	Number	%
Bothrops	4906	73.67	2709	49.31	60647	66.96
Crotalus	738	11.08	183	3.33	6204	6.85
Micrurus	15	0.23	14	0.25	415	0.45
Lachesis	16	0.24	2	0.03	1529	1.68
Non venomous	58	0.87	2585	47.05	1577	1.74
Unknown	926	13.91	-	-	20190	22.29
TOTAL	6659	100.00	5493	100.00	90562	100.00

Sources: *Fonseca, F. (1949); **Nahas (1978) unpublished; ***Brasil (1993)

2. Identification of snake

The identification of the snake responsible for the snakebite has a great value in epidemiological studies, both for an understanding of medically important snakes in different areas and the clinical picture caused by different species. For documentation it is important to define by an appropriate terminology the criterion used for the diagnosis of the snakebite. At HVB it is classed a "PROBABLE" snakebite by a particular snake species/group if the snake was not brought in for identification but the diagnosis was based on the clinical picture. At HVB, 61.9% (1803/2908) of the patients fulfilled clinical criteria for diagnosis of snakebite, while in about 40% (1105/2908) diagnosis was made by identification of the offending snake (Table 3).

3. Age and Sex

The highest incidence (64%) is observed in patients between 15-49 years old representing the active work group (Figure 13). About 70% of the cases are male. In Brazil, as in many other tropical countries, snake bites are predominantly in rural workers.

4. Seasonal and diurnal variation

Most snakebites occur during hot and rainy months, corresponding to the period between September to March in the Brazilian Southeast region (Figure 14) and Argentina, February through May in Ecuador[18] and June to November in Venezuela[21]. This coincides with information on the seasonality of snakebites in Southeast Asia[22] and in South Africa[23].

With respect to diurnal variation, the majority of snakebites occurs between 5 a.m. and 5 p.m. (76.4%) which corresponds to the period of most agricultural activities.

Table 3
iological and clinical classification of snakes responsible for snakebites at HVB, 1966-77

Classification	Number of cases
Bothrops jararaca	958
Bothrops sp*	48
B. neuwiedi	16
B. moojeni	6
B. alternatus	4
B. jararacussu	3
Crotalus durissus terrificus	53
C.d. sp*	6
C.d. collilineatus	1
C.d. cascavella	1
Micrurus corallinus	5
M. lemniscatus	2
M. frontalis	1
Lachesis muta	1
SUBTOTAL	1105
Bothrops probable	1674
Crotalus probable	122
Micrurus probable	6
Lachesis probable	1
SUBTOTAL	1803
TOTAL	2908

* Species not determined

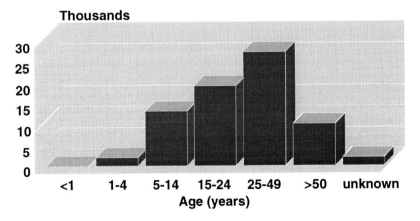

Figure 13: Age of patients bitten by snakes, Brazil, 1986-1989.

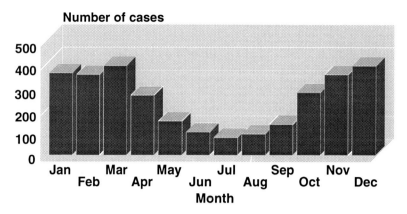

Figure 14. Seasonality of the snakebites(*Bothrops* HVB, 1966-1977).

5. Site of bite

About 75% of the bites are located on the foot and legs; about 20% on hands. This observation resulted in the prophylactic recommendation to use boots and to avoid handling objects in places where snakes are possibly living.

6. Lethality

The first data from Vital Brazil (1914)[24] referred to about 4,800 deaths per year in Brazil. The subsequent rates showed a reduction in the various periods of study. In 1949 there was a mortality rate of 2.43 %[25] whereas in 1972 it was 1.75%[26]. The most recent data are provided by the Ministry of Health where a mortality rate of 0.59% was found in 90,562 cases (Table 4).

Table 4
Deaths in snakebite patients: lethality due to various genera, Brazil, 1986-1990

Genus	Number of Cases	Number of Deaths	Coefficient of Lethality
Bothrops	60,647	234	0.39
Crotalus	6,204	157	2.53
Lachesis	1,529	19	1.24
Micrurus	415	03	0.73
Not informed	20,190	117	0.58
Non venomous	1,577	-	-
TOTAL	90,562	530	0.59

Source: Brazil, Ministério da Saúde (1993). Unpublished data.

The mortality in Argentina in 1979 was 5.5% (6/109)[27], similar to Ecuador where 5.4% (16/294) of patients died following venomous snakebites[18]. These rates are extremely high and may not be representative since deaths were registered in referral health care hospitals. Data from French Guiana show that the mortality rate reaches 2% of the total number of snakebites.

It is believed that the best prognosis is reserved for patients seen and treated in the first 3 hours after the snakebite. In Brazil most deaths occur in patients with a delay of 6 hours or more before being treated with antivenom (Figure 15). At HVB, 47.3% of the patients are treated in the first 3hrs after the bite and 75.8% in the first 6 hours. In Ecuador only 47% arrive within 6 hours of the bite, probably because most of these snakebites occur in jungle areas[18].

Number of deaths

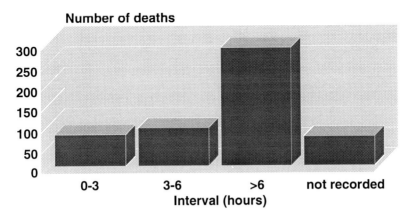

Figure 15: Interval between snakebite /serum therapy in fatal cases, Brazil, 1986-1990.

III. MECHANISMS OF ACTION OF BRAZILIAN SNAKE VENOMS

A. PROTEOLYTIC ACTIVITY

Present in *Bothrops* and *Lachesis* venom, this activity is attributed to a complex mixture of proteolytic enzymes known to produce local tissue damage. The venom factors responsible include proteases, phospholipases, membrane damaging polypeptide toxins, etc. The mode of action can be direct by cellular destruction or by secondary activation of inflammatory mediators, such as leucotriens, prostaglandins, and other substances[28]. Edema and necrosis are the most important clinical features observed in human envenoming. Besides these local effects, proteolytic venoms can produce systemic effects like shock, changes in the coagulation system, platelet aggregation and liberation of endogenous autocoids, such as histamine, serotonin and bradykinin[29].

B. COAGULANT ACTIVITY

Defibrination syndrome has been observed in *Bothrops, Lachesis* and *Crotalus* envenomation[30]. The coagulation activators of the South-American vipers act at three different points of the coagulation cascade: Factor I (thrombin-like activity), prothrombin and Factor X (pro-coagulant activity)[31]. As a consequence, patients may have incoagulable blood with reduced fibrinogen levels[32].

C. HEMORRHAGIC ACTIVITY

Metalloproteins, called hemorrhagins, have been isolated from *Bothrops* and *Lachesis* venoms[33]. Increased permeability of the capillary endothelium is observed in experimental models[34]. Hemorrhagin levels in serum have been correlated with occurrence of bleeding phenomena in human envenoming[35].

D. MYOTOXIC ACTIVITY

Muscle necrosis caused by *Crotalus* venom is attributed to crotoxin, compounded by crotapotin (without enzymatic activity) and phospholipase A_2. The myotoxicity in human envenoming by *Crotalus* was first described in 1985[36], demonstrating lack of haemolysis in patients bitten by South American rattlesnakes[37]. Degenerative/necrotic changes and regeneration signs in striated muscle fibers type I or IIa are observed[38]. Experimentally many species of *Micrurus* from Brazil and Colombia induce myotoxicity[39]. The correlation of this finding with clinical envenoming needs further studies

Table 5
Classification of the venoms of South American snakes, according to their physiopathological activities

Snake	Activity
Bothrops	Proteolytic
	Coagulant
	Haemorrhagic
Lachesis	Proteolytic
	Coagulant
	Haemorrhagic
	"Neurotoxic"
Crotalus	Neurotoxic
	Myotoxic
	Coagulant
Micrurus	Neurotoxic

E. NEUROTOXIC ACTIVITY

The Brazilian snake neurotoxins can be divided into two groups:

- pre-synaptic neurotoxins: are one of the most potent components in snake venom. They act at the motor end-plates, impairing acetylcholine (Ach) liberation[40-42]. This kind of neuromuscular blockade is documented in *C. d. terrificus*, *C. d. cascavella*, and *Micrurus corallinus* venoms[41].

- post-synaptic neurotoxins: the blockade of nervous impulse is due to a binding between neurotoxin and cholinergic receptors at the post-junctional membrane of myoneural end-plates. It causes a syndrome similar to myasthenia gravis. Post-synaptic neurotoxins are found in *Micrurus frontalis* and *M. lemniscatus* venoms[41].

In Brazil, correlation between the fundamental pathophysiological effects of the venoms and clinical aspects of the envenomation are due to Rosenfeld[12,26,43], leading to simplified and rational diagnosis criteria. (Table 5).

IV. *BOTHROPS* SNAKEBITES

Many species of *Bothrops* snakes cause snakebites in South America; however, a common clinical picture, with some regional particularities, has been reported by the different authors. Local and systemic envenoming are attributed to proteolytic, haemorrhagic and coagulant activities of *Bothrops* venom.

A. LOCAL ENVENOMING

The inflammatory local picture of *Bothrops* envenoming can be explained by the interaction of several factors, including proteolytic enzymes (proteases, phospholipase, hyaluronidase, etc), secondary activation of inflammation mediators (bradykinin, serotonin, leucotriens), ischemia provoked by microthrombi or by massive edema, and muscular necrosis due to haemorrhagic action.

Bleeding from the site of bite is relatively common although fang marks are not always visible. **Solid edema** is the most frequent of the signs of envenoming (Figure 16). Swelling appears in minutes and is accompanied by **local pain**. Swelling may be massive, involving the whole limb. The venom components are taken up by lymphatics so local lymph nodes draining the bitten area may become enlarged and tender. Bruising may be seen at the site of bite and along the line of superficial lymphatics and **painful enlargement of regional**

ganglia is seen. In about 12 hours, **blisters** can be present with haemorrhagic or necrotic contents. The local effects tend to progress in the first 24 hours after the bite.

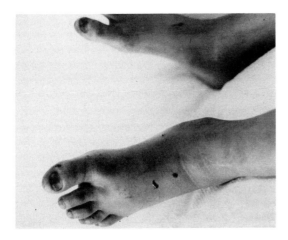

Figure 16. Bleeding from the bite site, with obvious fang marks, ecchymosis and edema following envenoming by *Bothrops* sp.

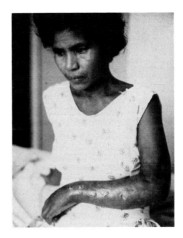

Figure 17. Residual tissue damage following snakebite.

Necrosis is an important local complication occurring in about 10% of *Bothrops* snakebites seen at HVB where *B. jararaca* is the predominant species. The intensity and extent are generally correlated with the length of the snake, bites on digits, use of tourniquet and other first aid procedures, and time elapsed between bite and antivenom therapy. It is limited to subcutaneous tissue in most of the cases, but deeper structures like muscle, tendon and bone can also be compromised (Figure 17) leading to prolonged or permanent disability[7]. Fortunately **amputation** is rare (less than 1% in HVB cases).

Secondary infection observed with necrosis is related to bacteria of the buccal flora of the snake. The most frequent agents isolated from abscesses are Gram negative aerobics, *Staphylococcus aureus* and anaerobic microorganisms[44]. Microbiological studies performed in Brazil reveal that *Morganella morganii, E. coli,* and *Providencia* sp were the most common agents isolated from abscesses by *Bothrops* snakebites caused by *B. jararaca* and *B. moojeni* bites[45,46]. The frequency of local necrosis/abscesses in Brazil depends on the prevalent species of *Bothrops*, which varies from region to region. The incidence differs from 16-18%[47], 15.7%[45] in *B. moojeni* distribution areas, and 12.8% of patients bitten predominantly by *B. jararaca* (HVB data, unpublished). In the area of *B. erithromelas* (Northeast) figures are not available.

Extensive swelling can lead to **compartmental syndrome** which requires surgical intervention. Data from HVB showed that 1.23% of patients bitten by *Bothrops* were submitted to fasciotomy.

B. SYSTEMIC ENVENOMING

Hypotension and peripheral shock (Figure 18) are described early in severe envenoming and are due to massive release of vasoactive substances such as bradykinin[12]. Hypovolaemia may be caused by massive sequestration of plasma volume into the bitten limb, increase in capillary permeability or massive haemorrhage[48].

Consumption coagulopathy is the clinical result of coagulant activity. Defibrination syndrome can be easily detected by the Clotting Time test in remote areas without laboratory facilities. The reversal of coagulation disturbances occurs, in general, in 6 to 12 hours. After antivenom administration, the fibrinogen curve shows a tendency to increase at the same time as decrease of fibrin/fibrinogen degradation products[49]. As a rule unclottable blood doesn't represent a risk factor in the prognosis. Young *Bothrops* snakes cause milder edema than adults and, in some cases, only coagulation disturbances may be detectable as a sign of envenoming[50].

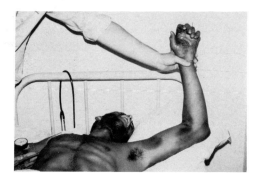

Figure 18. Extensive bruising and shock.

Hemorrhagic phenomena are relatively common but are of little clinical importance in most cases. Bleeding from the gums, bleeding from recent wounds, purpura and haematuria are the most frequent manifestations of hemorrhagic venom. These haematological abnormalities increase the patients risk severity since incoagulability of blood facilitates bleeding from different sites. Shock and death may occur due to massive loss of blood or intracranial hemorrhage[18,51].

The commonest cause of deaths in *Bothrops* snakebites is **acute renal failure** (ARF). The etiology is multifactorial involving hypovolaemia (caused by shock, systemic bleeding and/or sequestration of fluids in the bitten limb), disseminated intravascular coagulation with intraglomerular deposits of fibrin, and a possible direct nephrotoxic activity. Histopathological examination reveals acute tubular necrosis in most cases, while cortical necrosis is less frequent[52].

C. TREATMENT

Many of the traditional first aid treatments recommended for snakebite are harmful and without benefit. The use of tourniquets or local incisions is responsible for aggravation of local effects of envenoming caused by proteolytic snake venoms[9,23,53,54]. The recommended measures are reassurance of the patient, immobilization of the bitten limb, moving the patient to hospital as quickly as possible and avoiding unhelpful or damaging first aid procedures (constricting bands, incisions, instillation of chemicals, etc).

Table 6
Classification and dose of *Bothrops* antivenom therapy in Brazil

Clinical Picture	Severity		
	Mild	Moderate	Severe
Local manifestation (mainly oedema)	absent or mild	present	present
Intense bleeding	absent	absent	present
Hypotension/shock	absent	absent	present
Oliguria or anuria	absent	absent	present
Dose of Antivenom (in no. of ampoules)	4	8	12 or more

After treatment patients bitten by venomous snakes should be observed in hospital for at least 24 hours. Specific antivenom should be given if there are signs of envenoming. The amount of antivenom to be administered depends on the severity of envenoming. The Brazilian Ministry of Health uses three grades of severity according to the clinical picture. The classification and schedule for antivenom therapy is described in Table 6[55].

V. *LACHESIS* SNAKEBITES

The surucucu represents the largest venomous snake found in Latin America, reaching almost 4m length. Its habitat is the rain forest of several countries located in the Amazon region.

Human snakebites caused by *Lachesis* are rare and few cases have been reported in the literature. Cases reported in Costa Rica[56], and in Colombia[57], showed that the clinical picture produced by *Lachesis* envenoming was similar to that caused by *Bothrops* in many aspects.

Human envenomings by *Lachesis muta* have been described where the clinical picture was compatible with "neurotoxic" activity[58]. Disturbance of the autonomic nervous system, leading to vagal stimulation, could be responsible for early hypotension, drowsiness, abdominal pain, vomiting and diarrhoea. In severe cases bradycardia, cardiac arrhythmia and shock are a cause of death. In Brazil, a human envenoming by *Lachesis muta muta* was reported in which systemic symptoms (nausea, vomiting, diarrhoea, abdominal pain) corresponded with those reported elsewhere[59].

A. TREATMENT

The doses of *Lachesis* antivenom recommended by the Brazilian Ministry of Health are 10 to 20 ampoules given by the intravenous route. In the Amazon region it's important to have *Bothrops-Lachesis* antivenom available to be used when it's not possible to identify the snake responsible for the snakebite or if the clinical picture is not clear enough for diagnosis of the type of snake.

VI. *CROTALUS* SNAKEBITES

The South American rattlesnake is irregularly distributed along the continent, mainly in dry areas, and it is not found in the Amazon nor on the sea-board.

Crotalus snakebites are less common than *Bothrops* envenoming. They are responsible for about 7.5% of snake bites in Brazil, but some regional variances occur[13]. The majority of cases are described in areas of distribution of *C.d.terrificus* and *C.d.collilineatus*, while human cases of envenoming by other subspecies are poorly documented.

A. SITE OF BITE

Local signs of envenoming are not significant. When present they are characterized by mild edema and hyperemia restricted to the site of the bite. Pain is not common but parestheseae may persist for weeks. Fang marks are not always evident.

B. NEUROTOXIC MANIFESTATIONS

Rosenfeld[12] first described the typical "neurotoxic" facies in *Crotalus* envenoming. In the first six hours, most cases develop uni- or bilateral ptosis and paralysis of facial muscles. Other ocular signs and symptoms include ophthalmoplegia, midriasis, blindness and diplopia. Less frequent are difficulty in swallowing and alteration in taste and smell due to involvement of cranial nerves.

C. MYOTOXIC MANIFESTATIONS

The first clinical evidence of *Crotalus* myotoxicity was reported in 1985 when "intravascular hemolysis" *in vivo* was noted[36,37]. Patients usually complain of generalized muscle pain which appears early and it is more intense in severe cases. Red or dark urine reflects myoglobin elimination and it is proportional to rhabdomyolysis (Figure 19). Laboratory data reveal an early increase of serum creatine kinase (CK), especially of two isoenzymes: CK_3 (MM) and CK_2 (MB), whereas elevation of LDH is slower and more gradual[60]. These fractions can achieve levels comparable with myocardial infarction[61]. Histological studies reveal selective damage by the venom to type I and/or IIa striated muscle, rich in MB-CK[38].

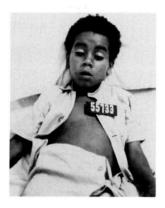

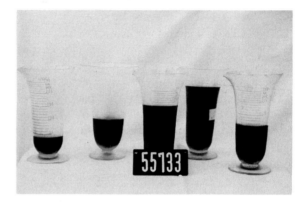

Figure 19. Paralysis after *Crotalus* envenoming.

Figure 20. Myoglobinuria following *Crotalus* envenoming.

D. HAEMATOLOGICAL MANIFESTATIONS

The thrombin-like activity was first described in 1964[62]. Afibrinogenemia and unclottable blood were reported in 1980[63]. Almost half of patients bitten by *C. d. terrificus* have a coagulation disturbance with consumption of fibrinogen[30]. Few cases develop bleeding phenomena.

Human envenoming can be complicated by acute respiratory failure. Neurotoxic and myotoxic activities of venom have been reported as the mechanism of ventilatory disorders leading to impairment of respiratory muscle function. However, significant respiratory failure is only occasionally reported in victims of South American rattlesnake bite; it generally occurs in the first 24 hours after the bite and is transitory.

Myoglobinuric acute renal failure is the commonest cause of deaths in *Crotalus* snakebites. It is attributed to myotoxic effects (with myoglobin liberation and excretion in the urine) and a possible nephrotoxic effect of the venom. Its occurrence is related to severity of envenoming and time elapsed between snakebite and antivenom therapy[64]. Acute tubular necrosis (ATN) with oliguria or anuria generally occurs in the first 48 hours and requires early dialysis[52].

E. TREATMENT

The severity of cases and schedules of *Crotalus* antivenom recommended in Brazil are given in Table 7[55].

Table 7
Crotalus snakebite severity classification and dose of antivenom therapy in Brazil

Clinical Picture	Severity	
	Moderate	Severe
Neurotoxic facies blurred vision	mild or evident	evident
Myalgia	mild or absent	present
Dark urine	not evident or absent	present
Oliguria/anuria	absent	present or absent
Blood	generally clottable	clottable or unclottable
Dose of antivenom (no. of ampoules)	10	20 or more

VII. *MICRURUS* SNAKEBITES

Elapidae are represented in South America by the genus *Micrurus*. Human snakebites by *Micrurus* species are relatively rare in Brazil, representing less than 1% of venomous snake bites.

Elapid neurotoxins are responsible for the clinical picture observed in patients bitten by coral snakes. These low molecular weight toxins have no significant enzymatic activity and are rapidly absorbed. The mechanism of action of *Micrurus* venom is predominantly a post-synaptic blockade of the neuromuscular junction.

Like *Crotalus* local signs of envenoming are restricted to mild edema, pain or parestheseae at the site of bite. In most cases fang marks are not obvious or characteristic.

Neurotoxic manifestations of *Micrurus* envenoming appear in minutes to hours after the bite. The clinical picture is characterized by ptosis and facial muscle paralysis ("neurotoxic" or "myasthenic" facies of Rosenfeld); involvement of intrinsic ocular muscles with blurred vision, diplopia; ophthalmoplegia; anisocoria; disphagia; drooling of saliva due to paralysis of deglutition; and respiratory difficulties due to paralysis of thoracic and diaphragmatic muscles. Death occurs as a consequence of acute respiratory failure (Figure 21).

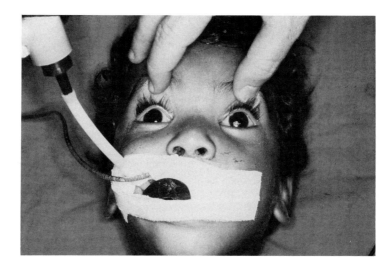

Figure 21. Paralysis with respiratory failure following *Micrurus* envenoming.

A. TREATMENT

For all patients envenomed by coral snakes in Brazil the dose of *Micrurus* antivenom recommended is 10 ampoules given by the intravenous route.

As a complementary treatment, anticholinesterase drugs have been recommended in elapid snakebites[65]. In Brazil, reversion of clinical signs in *Micrurus* envenoming has been reported with neostigmine, without use of specific antivenom[66]. The schedule, according to the Brazilian Ministry of Health, consists of 5 intravenous injections of 0.5mg of neostigmine at intervals of 30 minutes, followed by longer intervals according to the rate of improvement of respiratory function. Each administration should be preceded by 0.6mg of atropine sulphate 15 minutes before, in order to neutralize the muscarinic effects.

VIII. COLUBRIDAE SNAKEBITES

About 40% of patients complaining of snakebite don't develop evidence of envenoming. In some cases this may be due to snakebites by non-venomous snakes, mainly members of *Colubridae* family, although some are undoubtedly due to "dry bites" by otherwise dangerously venomous species. At HVB, in 5,493 snake bites, 2,585 (47.6%) were diagnosed as "non venomous snake bite" or "non envenoming" snakebite. Few snakes were brought for identification and most of these were Colubridae (see Table 8).

Table 8
Non-venomous snake /non envenoming snakebites, HVB, 1966-77

Snake	Number	%
Heliocops modesta	106	4.10
Philodryas patagoniensis	81	3.13
Oxyrhopus trigeminus	49	1.89
Thamnodynastes strigatus	41	1.58
Philodryas olfersii	36	1.39
Xenodon merremii	26	1.00
"Probable" diagnosis	2074	80.23
Other *Colubridae* and *Boidae*	172	6.65
TOTAL	2585	100.00

Colubrid snakes are found on all continents except Antarctica and they are especially numerous in tropical and subtropical regions. The scarcity of human envenoming by colubrid snakes may be due to their non-aggressive behavior and the fangs situated towards the back of the mouth ("back fanged"). Nevertheless some species have reportedly caused severe reactions with local and systemic envenoming[67,68].

In Brazil, there are a few case reports of envenoming by *Philodryas olfersii* and *Clelia clelia pumblea* where patients developed local swelling and ecchymosis without coagulation disturbances[11,69-71]. The treatment in all cases was symptomatic. Reversion of the clinical picture occurred without complications.

Few Colubrid venoms are studied because the snakes are primarily considered "non-venomous". Haemorrhagic, oedematogenic, and fibrinolytic activities have been shown in *P. olfersii* venom, which was devoid of procoagulant action[72]. It appears that the venom shares some common antigen with *Bothrops* species since the haemorrhagic activity was neutralized by *Bothrops* antivenom.

IX. DIAGNOSIS

Snakebites by venomous animals can be diagnosed by the identification of the offending animal - ETIOLOGIC DIAGNOSIS, by the symptoms and clinical signs of envenomation - CLINICAL DIAGNOSIS or by detection of venom in immunoassays- IMMUNOLOGICAL DIAGNOSIS.

Diagnosis based on clinical figures is more familiar for health staff and must be emphasised. In this respect Rosenfeld[12] observed: "There was need for establishing a symptomatologic clinical criterion that would permit a diagnosis of the snakebites and consequent therapeutic handling and prognosis WITHOUT identification of the snake. This was proposed because most physicians are unable to classify venomous snakes and it is rare for the patients, or his family, to bring the animal that caused the snakebite".

Immunodiagnostic methods, such as enzyme-linked immunosorbent assay (ELISA) and radioimmunoassay (RIA), have been available for clinical studies in many countries. In Brazil, immunoassays have been utilized in studies about kinetics of venom/heterologous antivenom in patients' sera. A correlation has been established between the severity of *Bothrops* envenoming and levels of circulating venom in human snakebites[73]. Theakston[74] demonstrated in human snakebites by *Bothrops* that circulating venom is quickly eliminated (3-4 days), while serum antivenom concentration is detectable for up to 40 days.

To evaluate efficacy of antivenom, Cardoso[49] performed a clinical trial to compare the three antivenoms produced in Brazil in the treatment of envenoming by lanced-head vipers. All Brazilian *Bothrops* antivenoms effectively eliminated venom antigenemia.

An immunoassay was proposed in order to discriminate between *Bothrops atrox* and *Lachesis muta muta* venoms, as these species are assumed to be responsible for most snakebites in Amazonia and cause similar clinical symptoms[75].

Detection of IgM and IgG antibodies against *Bothrops* venom was developed as part of epidemological studies of snakebites[76,77].

X. ANTIVENOM THERAPY

The first steps in the history of serumtherapy against snakebites in South America started with Vital Brazil[4]. In 1898, working with Calmette's antivenom, he observed that it was not effective against the venom of some Brazilian snakes. This observation led to the discovery of the antivenom's specificity: "Having immunized some dogs against (Brazilian) rattlesnake venom and others against (*Bothrops*) jararaca venom, I obtained quite active sera, and I realized that sera from animals immunized against jararaca venom did not neutralize that of rattlesnake."[4].

The first guidelines for serumtherapy in Brazil were based on two factors: 1.) severity of envenoming, defined by clinical parameters, and 2.) average amount of venom each species of snake was able to produce when milked. Vital Brazil[4] proposed the following schedule for *Bothrops* envenoming:

Table 9
Antivenom therapy in *Bothrops* envenoming proposed by Vital Brazil (1901)

SEVERITY	VIALS	ROUTE
MILD	2	SC
MODERATE	4	SC
SEVERE	1 + 5	SC/IV

Rosenfeld[78] maintained the same schedules of dosage for antivenom and established the following principles of serumtherapy: 1.) specificity of antivenom; 2.) early administration; 3.) sufficient dose; 4.) whole dose at once; 5.) proper injection route. Following these criteria, the author reported a reduction of mortality of 7 to 10 times in patients submitted to serumtherapy when compared to cases which didn't receive antivenom[12].

In the last 20 years there has been a tendency towards increasing doses for antivenom therapy. However, these changes were established based only on clinical impressions without controlled studies. Nowadays a critical reappraisal of *Bothrops* envenoming suggests that patients may be being treated with excessive amounts of antivenom in Brazil[74].

Snakebite antivenom produced in Brazil is basically composed of horse immunoglobulins digested with pepsin. Potency of the antivenom is assessed by the ED_{50} test by intraperitoneal injection in mice[79].

The main producers of antivenoms in South America are listed in Table 10.

The routine schedule for antivenom therapy in Brazil includes:
- prior parenteral administration of anti-histamine to prevent or reduce early reactions,
- diluted solution of antivenom given by intravenous route,
- vigilant monitoring of patient during infusion and in the first 24 hours after antivenom.

The skin/conjunctival test has been abolished in practice since it is shown to be ineffective in predicting immediate-type hypersensitivity reactions in patients given heterologous antivenom[81,82].

A. UNTOWARD REACTIONS

Early and late reactions may occur with variable frequency but severe or lethal complications have not been reported.

1. Early reactions

Incidence rates of early reactions to Brazilian antivenoms vary depending on the authors, from 25.6 to 87%[49,81]. Anaphylactic and/or anaphylactoid type reactions are clinically undistinguishable. The commonest manifestations include: chills, nausea, vomiting and generalized urticaria. The treatment is based on stopping antivenom administration and giving 0.1% adrenaline subcutaneously. After the symptoms of reactions subside antivenom administration should be resumed cautiously.

2. Late reactions

Serum sickness occurred in 5 to 9% of patients followed up to four weeks after antivenom therapy at HBV. The symptomatology included fever, lymphadenopathy, urticaria, local pruritis and oedema. All were treated with corticosteroids, anti-histamine and aspirin with good prognosis.

Table 10
Main producers of hyperimmune equine antisera (antivenom) in South America

Country	Producer	Antidote
Argentina	Instituto Nacional de Microbiologia "Dr.Carlos G. Malbran" av.Velez Sarsfield 563 Buenos Aires	Antibothrops bivalente Antibothrops tetravalente Anticrotalus Antimicrurus Tropical trivalente
	Ejercito Argentino* Campo de Mayo Batallon 601, Pcia de Buenos Aires	Antibothrops bivalente Antimicrurus
Brazil	Instituto Butantan av.Vital Brazil, 1500 Caixa Postal 65 Sao Paulo-SP	Antibotrópico Antilaquético Antibotrópico-laquético Anticrotálico Antiophidico polyvalente Antielapídico
	Instituto Vital Brazil Caixa Postal 28 Niterói-RJ	Antibotrópico Anticrotálico Antiophidico polyvalente
	FundaçÆo Ezequiel Dias r.Conde Pereira Carneiro, 80 30.500-000 Belo Horizonte-MG	Antibotrópico Anticrotálico Antibotrópico-crotálico Antibotrópico-laquético
Colombia	Instituto Nacional de Salud av.Eldorado con Carrera, Zona G, Bogota	Antiophidico polylavente
Ecuador	Instituto Nacional de Higiene y Medicina Tropical "Leopoldo Izquieta Perez" Casilla Postal 3961, Guayaquil	Anti-Bothrops
Peru	Institutos Nacionales Salud Depart. Animales Venenosos* Calle Capac Yupanqui no 1400 Apartade n° 451 Lima	Suero antibotropico polyvalente Suero antilachesico Suero anticrotalico
	Instituto Nacional de Higiene, Lima	Bothrops polyvalent Anti-coral polyvalent Suero antilachesico Suero anticrotalico
Venezuela	Universidad Cental de Venezuela Caracas	Suero antiofidico polyvalente UCV

* Lyophilized final product   Source: Theakston and Warrell, 1991[80].

XI. REFERENCES

1. **SEWALL, H.** Experiments on the preventive inoculation of rattlesnake venom. *J Phisiol* **8**: 203-210, 1887.
2. **PHISALIX, C., BERTRAND, G.** Sur la propriete antitoxique du sang des animaux vaccines contre le venin de vipere. *C. R. Soc. Biol.*, **46**:111-114, 1894.
3. **CALMETTE A.** L'immunisation artificielle des animaux contre le venin des serpents et la therapeutic experimentale de morsure venimeuses. *C. R. Soc. Biol.*, **46**: 120-124, 1894.
4. **BRAZIL, V.** Contribuicao ao estudo de veneno ophidico III. Tratamentos das mordeduras das cobras. *Rev. med. Sao Paulo*, **4**:375-380, 1901.

5. **VITAL BRAZIL, O.** *A defesa contra o Ophidismo.* SÆo Paulo, Pocai & Weiss, 1911.
6. **HOUSSAY, B.A., SORDELLI, A., NEGRETE.** Estudios sobre venenos de serpientes. *R. Inst. Bact. C. Malbran,* **1:**341, 1915.
7. **POSADAS ARANGO, A.** Estudios cientificos. In MOLINA, C.A. ed. *Las Serpientes.* Mellin, Columbia: Imprensa Oficial, pp 253-283, 1909.
8. **CAMPBELL, J.A. & LAMAR, W.W.** *The Venomous Reptiles in Latin America.* New York: Cornell University Press, 1989.
9. **WORLD HEALTH ORGANIZATION** *Progress in the Characterization of Venoms and Standardization of Antivenoms.* WHO Offset Publication n° 58. Geneva, 44 pgs, 1981.
10. **WARRELL, D.A.** Snake bites in five continents. In: BUNCH, C. ed. *Horizons in Medicine* no 1. Baillière Tindall, London, p.106-114, 1989.
11. **PINTO, R.N.L.; da SILVA Jr, N.J.& AIRD, S.D.** Human envenomation by the South American opisthoglyph *Clelia clelia plumbea. Toxicon* **29 (12):** 1512-1516, 1991.
12. **ROSENFELD, G.** Symptomatology, Pathology and Treatment of Snake Bites in South America. In: BUCHERL,W. & BUCKLEY,E.E. eds *Venomous Animal and Their Venoms* vol.2. Academic Press, New York, Cap. 34, p.345-384, 1971.
13. **BRAZIL, MINISTERIO DA SAUDE,** *Ofidismo: Analise Epidemiologica.* Brasilia-DF, pps 49, 1991.
14. **ESTESO, S.C.** *Ofidismo en la republica Argentina.* Editorial Arpon, Córdoba- Argentina, 166 pgs, 1985.
15. **OTERO, R.; VALDERRAMA, R.; OSORIO, R.G. & POSADA, L.E.** Programa de atencíon primaria del snakebitee ofídico. *Iatréia* 5 (2): 96-102, 1992.
16. **SILVA, J.J.** Las serpientes del género Bothrops en la amazonia colombiana. *Acta Medica Colombiana* **14 (3):** 148-165, 1989.
17. **ANGEL MEJIA, R.** *Serpientes de Colombia: su relacion con el hombre.* Secretaría de Educacíon y Cultura de Antioquia. Medellin, 229 pgs, 1987.
18. **KERRIGAN, K.R.** Venomous snakebite in Eastern Ecuador. *Am J Trop Med Hyg* **44 (1):** 93-99, 1991.
19. **CHIPPAUX, J.P.** Les serpents de la Guyane française. *Collection Faune Tropicale XXVII,* 165 pgs, 1986.
20. **PURTSCHER, H.; BURGER, M.; SAVIO, E.; JUANIC, L.R.; DOMINGUEZ, B.V.; CAORSI, E.; TAMBLER, M. & LABORDE, A.** Ofidismo y Aracnidismo en el Uruguay. *Rev Med Uruguay* **7 (1):** 1-37, 1983.
21. **PARRA, M.A.A.; LA ROSA, G.C.; CASTILLO F., E.; ALBERT, S. & CORDERO, O.** *Ofidismo en Venezuela.* Alpha Impressores, Valencia- Venezuela, 104 pg, 1987.
22. **SAWAI, Y.; KOBA, K.; OKONOGI, T.; MISHIMA, S.; KAWAMURA, Y.; CHINZEI, H.; ABU BAKAR, BIN I.; DEVARAJ, T.; PHONG-AKSARA, S.; PURANANANDA, C.; SALAFRANCA, E.S.; SUMPAICO, J.S.; TSENG, C.S.; TAYLOR, J.F.; WU, C.S. & KUO, T.P.** An epidemiological study of snakebites in the Southeast Asia. *Japan J Exp Med* **42 (3):** 283-307, 1972.
23. **CHAPMAN, D.D.** The symptomatology, pathology and treatment of the bites of venomous snakes of Central and Southern Africa. In: BÜCHERL, W.; BUCKELEY, E.E. & DEULOFEU, V. eds *Venomous Animals and their Venoms* vol.1, 463-527. New York, Academic Press, 1968.
24. **VITAL BRAZIL,** *La defense contre l'ophidisme.* 2nd edn., Sao Paulo: Pocai & Weiss, p 319, 1914.
25. **FONSECA, F.** *Animais Peçonhentos.* SÆo Paulo, Instituto Butantan, 1949.
26. **ROSENFELD,G.** Animais peçonhentos e tóxicos do Brasil. In LACAZ, C.S.; BARUZZI, R.G. & SIQUEIRA Jr, W. *IntroduçÆo à Geografia Médica do Brasil* Chapter 19: 430-475. SÆo Paulo, EDUSP, 1a ediçÆo, 1972.
27. **MARTINO, O.A.; MATHET, H.; MASINI, R.D.; IBARRA-GRASSO, A.; THOMPSON, R.; GONDELL, C. & BOSCH, J.E.** *Emponzoñamiento humano provocado por venenos de origen animal.* Ministerio de Bienestar Social, Buenos Aires, 240 pgs, 1979.
28. **VARGAFTIG, B.B.; BHARGAVA, N. & BONTA, I.L.** Haemorrhagic and permeability increasing effects of *Bothrops jararaca* and other *Crotalidae* venoms as related to anime or kinin release. *Agents and Actions* **4:** 163-168, 1974.
29. **VITAL BRAZIL, O.** Peçonhas. In CORBETT, C.E. ed. *Farmacodinâmica* pp.1044-1074. Rio de Janeiro: Guanabara Koogan, 1982.
30. **KAMIGUTI, A.S. & CARDOSO, J.L.C.** Haemostatic changes caused by the venoms of South American snakes. *Toxicon* **27:** 955-963, 1989.
31. **NAHAS, L.; KAMIGUTI, A.S. & BARROS, A.R.** Thrombin - like and factor X - activator components of *Bothrops* snake venoms. *Thromb Haemostasis* **41:** 314-328, 1979.
32. **MARUYAMA, M.; KAMIGUTI, A.S.; CARDOSO, J.L.C.; SANO-MARTINS, I.; CHUDZINSKY, A.M.; SANTORO, M.L.; MORENA, P.; TOMY, S.C.; ANTONIO, L.C.; MIHARA, H. & KELEN, E.M.A.** Studies on blood coagulation and fibrinolysis in patients bitten by *Bothrops jararaca. Thromb Haemost* **63:** 449-453, 1990.
33. **MANDELBAUM, F.R.; ASSAKURA, M.T.; REICHL, A.P.** Characterization of two hemorrhagic factors isolated from the venom of *Bothrops neuwiedi* (jararaca pintada). *Toxicon* **22:** 193-206, 1984.

34. **QUEIROZ, L.S.; SANTO NETO, H.; ASSAKURA, M.T.; REICHL, A.P. & MANDELBAUM, F.R.** Pathological changes in muscle caused by haemorrhagic and proteolytic factors from *Bothrops jararaca* snake venom. *Toxicon 23*: 341-345, 1984.

35. **KAMIGUTI, A.S.; RUGMAN, F.P.; THEAKSTON, R.D.G.; FRANÇA, F.O.S.; ISHII, H.; HAY, C.R.M. & BIAS, G.** The role of venom haemorrhagin in spontaneous bleeding in *Bothrops jararaca* envenoming. *Thromb and Haemostasis 67*(4): 484-488, 1992.

36. **AZEVEDO-MARQUES, M.M.; CUPO, P.; COIMBRA, T.M.; HERING, S.E.; ROSSI, M.A. & LAURE, C.J.** Myonecrosis, myoglobinuria and acute renal failure induced by South American rattlesnake (*Crotalus durissus terrificus*) envenomation in Brazil. *Toxicon 23*: 631-636, 1985.

37. **AZEVEDO-MARQUES, M.M.; CUPO, P. & HERING, S.E.** Evidence that *Crotalus durissus terrificus* (South American rattlesnake) envenomation in humans causes myolysis rather than hemolysis. *Toxicon 11*: 1163-1168, 1987.

38. **CUPO, P.; MELLO DE OLIVEIRA, J.A.; HERING, S.E. & AZEVEDO-MARQUES, M.M.** Myopathology in human striated muscle in *Crotalus* envenomation: a clinical and histoenzymological study. In: (WEGMANN, RJ. & WEGMANN, M.A. eds) *Recent Advances in Cellular and Molecular Biology vol.5*, p. 45-50. Peeters Press, Leuven, Belgium, 1992.

39. **GUTIÉRREZ, J.M.; ROJAS, G.; DA SILVA Jr, J.N. & NUNES, J.** Experimental myonecrosis induced by the venoms of South American *Micrurus* (coral snakes). *Toxicon 30* (10): 1299-1302, 1992.

40. **VITAL BRAZIL, O. & EXCELL, B.J.** Action of crotoxin and crotactin from the venom of *Crotalus durissus terrificus* (South American rattlesnake) on the frog neuromuscular junction. *J Physiol 212*: 34-35, 1970.

41. **VITAL BRAZIL, O.** Coral snake venoms: mode of action and pathophysiology of experimental envenomation. *Rev Inst Med trop SÆo Paulo 29* (3): 119-126, 1987.

42. **VITAL BRAZIL, O.** Mecanismos de açÆo das toxinas peptídicas em nervos, músculos e sinapses. *Anais do XII simpósio anual da ACIESP sobre toxinas proteicas vol.II.* Campinas, PublicaçÆo ACIESP n⁰ 57-II, 1988.

43. **ROSENFELD, G.** Molestias por venenos animais. *Pinheiros Terapeutico*, 17:3-15, 1965.

44. **GOLDSTEIN, J.C.; CITRON, D.M.; GONZALEZ, H.; RUSSELL, F. & FINEGOLD, S.M.** Bacteriology of rattlesnake venom and implications for therapy. *J Infect Dis 140* (5): 818-821, 1979.

45. **PINTO, R.N.L.** Snakebite accidents in Goias. *Mem. Inst. Butantan*, 52(suppl.):47-48, 1990.

46. **JORGE, M.T. & RIBEIRO, L.A.R.** Acidentes por Serpentes Peçonhentas do Brasil. *Rev Assoc Med Bras 36* (2): 66-77, 1990.

47. **NISHIOKA, S.A., SILVERA, P.V.P.** A clinical and epidemiologic study of 292 cases of lance-headed viper bite in a Brazilian teaching hospital. *Am. J. Trop. Med. Hyg.*, 47(6):805-810, 1992.

48. **RUSSELL. F.E.; CARLSON, R.W.; WAINSCHEL, J. & OSBORNE, A.H.** Snake venom poisoning in the United States. Experience with 550 cases. *JAMA 233*; 341-4, 1975.

49. **CARDOSO, J.L.C.; FAN, H.W.; FRANÇA, F.O.S.; JORGE, M.T.; LEITE, R.P.; NISHIOKA, S.A.; AVILA, A.; SANO-MARTINS, I.S.; TOMY, S.C.; SANTORO, M.L.; CHUDZINSKI, A.M.; CASTRO, S.B.; KAMIGUTI, A.S.; KELEN, E.M.A.; HIRATA, M.H.; MIRANDOLA, R.M.S.; THEAKSTON, R.D.G. & WARRELL, D.A.** Randomized comparative trial of three antivenoms in the treatment of envenoming by lance-headed vipers (*Bothrops jararaca*) in SÆo Paulo, Brazil. *Q J Med 86*: 315-325, 1993.

50. **RIBEIRO, L.A. & JORGE, M.T.** Epidemiologia e quadro clínico dos acidentes por serpentess *Bothrops jararaca* adultas e filhores. *Rev Inst Med trop SÆo Paulo 32* (6): 436-442, 1990.

51. **KOUYOUMDIJAN, J.A.; POLIZELLI, C.; LOBO, S.M.A.; GUIMARÇES, S.M.** Fatal extradural haematoma after snake bite (*Bothrops moojeni*). *Trans R Soc Trop Med Hyg 85*: 552, 1991.

52. **AMARAL, C.F.S.; REZENDE, N.A.; DA SILVA, O.A.; RIBEIRO, M.M.F.; MAGALHÇES, R.A.; DOS REIS, R.J.; CARNEIRO, J.G. & CASTRO, J.R.S.** Insuficiência renal aguda secundária a acidentes ofídicos botrópico e crotálico. Análise de 63 casos. *Rev Inst Med trop SÆo Paulo 28*(4): 220-227, 1986.

53. **ARNOLD, R.E.** Treatment of rattlesnake bites. In: TU, A.T. ed *Rattlesnake venoms, their actions and treatment*, p. 324. New York: Marcel Dekker, 1982.

54. **TUN-PE, TIN-NU-SWE, MYINT-LWIN, WARRELL, D.A. & THAN WIN** The efficacy of tourniquets as a first-aid measure for Russell's viper bites in Burma. *Trans R Soc Trop Med Hyg 81*: 403-405, 1987.

55. **BRASIL, MINISTÉRIO DA SAØDE** (1987) *Manual de Diagnóstico e Tratamento dos Acidentes Ofídicos.* Brasília, 53 pgs.

56. **BOLAÑOS, R. ROJAS, O., ULLOA FLORES, C.E.** Aspectos biomedicos de cuatro caso de mordedura de serpiente por *Lachesis muta* (Ophidia: Viperidae) en Costa Rica. *Rev. Biol. Trop.* 30:53-58, 1982.

57. **OTERO, P.R., TOBON, J.G.S., GOMEZ, G.L.F., OSORIO, G.R.G., VALDERAMA, H.R.** Bites from the bushmaster (*Lachesis muta*) in Antioquia and Choco, Columbia, report of five accidents. *Toxicon* 31(2):158, 1993.

58. **HAAD, J.L.** Accidentes humanos por las serpientes de los generos *Bothrops* y *Lachesis. Mem. Inst. Butantan* 44/45:403-423, 1980/1981.

59. **JORGE, M.T., SANO-MARTINS, I.S., FERRARI, R.S., RIBEIRO, L.A., TOMY, S.C., CASTRO, S.C.B.** Envenoming by *Lachesis muta* in Brazil. *Toxicon* 31(2):140-141, 1993.

60. **CUPO, P.; AVEZEDO-MARQUES, M.M. & HERING, S.E.** Clinical and laboratory features of South American rattlesnake (*Crotalus durissus terrificus*) in children. *Trans R Soc trop Med Hyg 82*: 924-929, 1988.

61. **CUPO, P.; AVEZEDO-MARQUES, M.M. & HERING, S.E.** Acute myocardial infarction-like enzyme profile in human victims of *C. durissus terrificus* envenoming. *Trans R Soc trop Med Hyg 84*: 447-451, 1990.

62. **NAHAS, L.; DENSON, K.W.E. & MACFARLAINE, R.G.** A study of the coagulant action of eight snake venoms. *Thrombosis et Diathesis Haemorrhagica (Stuttg) 12*: 355-367, 1964.

63. **AMARAL, C.F.S.; DA SILVA, O.A.; LOPES, M. & PEDROSO, E.R.P.** Afibrinogenemia following snake bite (*Crotalus durissus terrificus*). *Am J Trop Med Hyg 29*: 1453, 1980.

64. **SILVEIRA, P.V.P. & NISHIOKA, S.A.** South American rattlesnake bite in a Brazilian teaching hospital. Clinical and epidemiological study of 87 cases, with analysis of factors predictive of renal failure. *Trans R Soc trop Med Hyg 86*: 562-564, 1992.

65. **BANERJEE, R.N.; SAIINI, A.L. & CHACKO, K.A.** Neostigmine in the treatment of Elapidae bites. In OHSAKA, A.; HAYASHI, K. & SAWAI, Y. eds *Animal, Plant,and Microbial Toxins* v.2: 475-481. Plenum Press, New York, 1974.

66. **COELHO, L.K.; SILVA, E.; ESPOSITTO, C. & ZANIN, M.** Clinical features and treatment of Elapidea bites: report of three cases. *Human Exp Toxicol 11*: 135-137, 1992.

67. **MINTON, S.A.** Venomous bites by nonvenomous snakes: an annoted bibliography of colubrid envenomation. *J Wild Med 1*: 119-127, 1990.

68. **DATTA, G. & TU, A.** Toxicology and Biochemistry of *Colubridae* venom. *J Toxicol-Toxins Reviews 12* (1): 63-89, 1993.

65. **NICKERSON, M.A., HENDERSON, R.W.** A case of envenomation by the South American Colubrid, *Phulodryas olfersii* (green snake). *Herpetologica, 32*:197-198, 1976.

70. **SILVA, M.V. & BUONONATO, M.A.** Relato clínico de envenenamento humano por *Philodryas olfersii*. *Mem I Butantan 47/48*: 121-126, 1984.

71. **SILVEIRA, P.V.P. & NISHIOKA, S.A.** Non-venomous snake bite and snake bite without envenoming in a Brazilian teaching hospital. Analysis of 91 cases. *Rev Inst Med trop SÆo Paulo 34* (6): 499-503, 1992.

72. **ASSAKURA, M.T., SALOMAO, M.G., PUORTO, G., MANDELBAUM, F.R.** Haemorrhagic, fibrinogenolytic and edema forming activities of the venom of the Colubrid snake *Philodryas olfersii* (green snake). *Toxicon 30*(4):427-438, 1992.

73. **BARRAL-NETTO, M.; SCHRIEFER, A.; BARRAL, A.; ALMEIDA, A.R.P. & MANGABEIRA, A.** Serum levels of bothropic venom in patients without antivenom intervention. *Am. J.Trop. Med. Hyg. 45*(6): 751-754, 1991.

74. **THEAKSTON, R.D.G.; FAN, H.W.; WARRELL, D.A.; DIAS DA SILVA, W.D.; WARD, S.A.; HIGASHI, H.G. & THE BUTANTAN INSTITUTE ANTIVENOM STUDY GROUP-BIASG** Use of enzyme immnoassays to compare the effect and assess the dosage regimens of three Brazilian *Bothrops* antivenoms. *Am J Trop Med Hyg 47*(5): 593-604, 1992.

75. **CHAVEZ-OLORTEGUI, C.; LOPES, C.S.; CORDEIRO, F.D. ;GRANIER, C. & DINIZ, C.S.** An enzyme linked immunoabsorbent assay (ELISA) that discriminates between *Bothorps atrox* and *Lachesis muta muta* venoms. *Toxicon 31* (4): 417-425, 1993.

76. **THEAKSTON, R.D.G.; REID, H.A.; LARRICK, J.W.; KAPLAN, J. & YOST, J.A.** Snake venom antibodies in Ecuadorian indians.*J Trop Med Hyg 84*: 203-208, 1981.

77. **DOMINGOS, M.O.; CARDOSO, J.L.C.; MOURA DA SILVA, A.M. & MOTA, I.** The humoral immune responses of patients bitten by snake *Bothrops jararaca* (jararaca). *Toxicon 28*: 723-726, 1990.

78. **ROSENFELD, G.; NAHAS, L.; DE CILLO, D.M. & FLEURY, C.T.** Envenenamentos por serpentes, aranhas e escorpiones. In: PRADO, F.C.; RAMOS, J.A. & VALLE, J.R. eds *AtualizaçÆo Terapêutica*: 931-944. Livraria Luso-Espanhola e Brasileira Ltda., Rio de Janeiro, 1957.

79. **RAW, I.; GUIDOLIN, R.; HIGASHI, H.G. & KELEN, E.M.A.** Antivenoms in Brazil: preparation. In TU, A.T.T. ed *Handbook of natural toxins*, vol.5 chapter 18, pp.557-581. Marcel Dekker Inc., New York, 1991.

80. **THEAKSTON, R.D.G. & WARRELL, D.A.** Antivenoms: a list of hyperimmune sera currently available for the treatment of envenoming by bites and stings. *Toxicon 29*(12): 1419-1470, 1991.

81. **MALASIT, P.; WARRELL, D.A.; CHANTHAVANICH, P.; VIRAVAN, C.; MONGKOLSAPAYA, J.; SINGHTOHONG, B.; SUPICH, C.** Prediction, prevention, and mechanism of early (anaphylactic) antivenom reactions in victims of snake bites. *B Med J 292*: 17-20, 1986.

82. **CUPO, P.; AZEVEDO-MARQUES, M.M.; MENEZES, J.B. & HERING, S.E.** Reaçes de Hipersensibilidade imediatas após uso intravenoso de soros antivenenos: Valor Prognóstico dos testes de sensibilidade intradérmicos. *Rev Inst Med trop SÆo Paulo 33* (2): 115-122, 1991.

Chapter 32

COMMERCIALLY AVAILABLE ANTIVENOMS ("HYPERIMMUNE SERA", "ANTIVENINS", "ANTISERA") FOR ANTIVENOM THERAPY

Jürg Meier

TABLE OF CONTENTS

I. INTRODUCTION

In 1971, the WHO Expert Committee on Biological Standardization proposed the international name for antivenoms produced for the treatment of envenomation caused by venomous animals being *antivenenum*, followed by the zoological species name(s) of the animal(s), the venom of which was used as antigen(s) and the name of the animal species in which the hyperimmune serum was produced[1]. However, this proposal did not find consequent application. Therefore, the terms *antivenom* and *antivenin,* respectively*,* are used synonymously throughout the literature.

Today, serotherapy is the only method of choice for the specific treatment of envenomation caused by venomous animals. Notes on the principles of antivenom therapy, where applicable, are found in the respective clinical chapters of this handbook. Several registers of commercially available antivenoms against bites and stings of venomous animals, as well as notes on the production of such sera, have been published in recent years[2-8]. This chapter summarizes the actual situation and provides data for an easy access to antivenoms against animal envenomations. No details on manufacturing procedures and product specifications are included in this chapter, since these products are subject to drug registration procedures in their respective countries of origin and the manufacturers therefore are inspected by the respective public health authorities to guarantee the quality of these medical products.

The selection of the adequate hyperimmune serum has to meet the following requirements:

1) Specificity: The hyperimmune serum used should be able to effectively neutralize the venom of the venomous animal involved in a given case of envenomation. Since geographical variability in animal venoms may be pronounced, the hyperimmune serum produced with the venom of a population of the respective venomous animal species, which occurs in the region of origin of the animal specimen that envenomed the patient to be cured, may be the preferable choice for use.

2) Availability: While the different products are usually easily available in the countries of origin, import into other countries may often be timeconsuming, if ever possible. However, local poison control centers may inform about the nearest place, where the respective antivenom is on stock.

Travellers often wonder whether or not they should take an antivenom along with them, while travelling through tropical countries, where encounters with venomous animals might be expected. Since due to the risk of anaphylactic complications, an antivenin therapy should only be performed by experienced medical doctors on one hand, and since on the other hand a five to ten ampoule package of a hyperimmune serum necessary for such a treatment is quite expensive, such prerequisites make sense only under certain circumstances. Instead, to follow the prophylactic measures to decrease the risk usually prevents any injury and envenomation by venomous animals.

Unfortunately, in those countries where envenomations caused by venomous animals form a considerable public health problem for the population, antivenom is often not available or if so, often too expensive in relation to the general way of life.

The present list was prepared by a thorough evaluation of our files of correspondence with the different institutions manufacturing antivenoms and the recently published lists available[2,3,8]. The updated files then were sent to the different institutions for "proof reading" and as an invitation to change whatever should be changed in the eyes of the institutions. While some institutions, like the Lister Institute in UK[10] and FitzSimmons in Africa[11], informed that they ceased production of their antivenoms already years ago, the majority of the institutions kindly provided updated data to the authors. Some of the institutions, which can however be found in antivenom lists published earlier, did not respond to multiple inquiries from our side. Since it is of no use to include doubtful sources, it was decided to include into this list only those manufacturers of antivenoms who clearly stated that they produce the respective antivenoms to date.

The antivenoms listed throughout Tables 1 to 13 have a code number, which is formed as shown in Figure 1. This code consisting of three letters followed by a number includes as abbreviation the animal group against the envenomations of which the antivenom is active as well as the continent, where the respective venomous animals occur.

Figure 2 provides the algorithm of the whole key structure. It is possible *1)* to start a search with the institution which manufactures antivenoms, *2)* to start with the scientific name of a venomous animal species, *3)* to start with the animal group and *4)* to start with the geographic region.

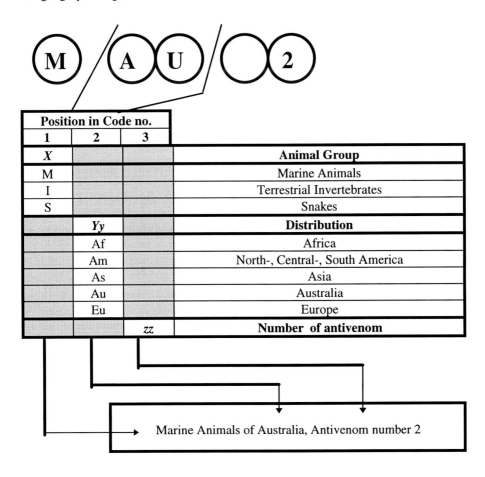

Figure 1. Code number used in Tables 1 to 13.

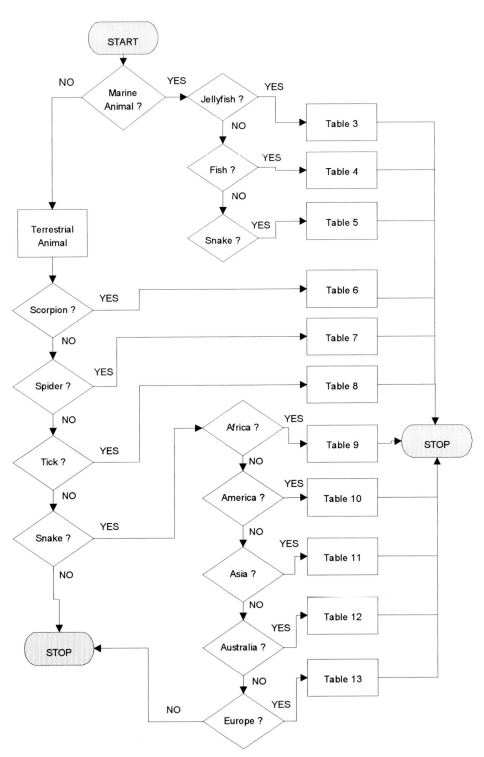

Figure2. Algorithm for an easy access to the tables of this antivenom list.

II. KEY TO HYPERIMMUNESERA ACCORDING TO MANUFACTURERS

Table 1
Manufacturers of antivenoms

Address of Manufacturer	Code No. of Antivenoms (Table No.)
Behringwerke AG Postfach 1140 35001 Marburg/Lahn Federal Republic of Germany Phone: ++49-6421-390 Fax: ++49-6421-31388 Telex: 0482320	SAF 8,9(9) / SAS 52(11) / SEU 3(13)
Biologials Production Service Alabang, 1702 Muntinlupa Metro Manila, Philippines Phone: ++1-632-8421333 Fax: ++1-632-8421285	SAS 38(11)
Central Research Institute 173 204 (H.P.) Kasauli, India Phone: ++91-1793-2060 Fax: ++91-1793-2049	IAS 3(6) / SAS 12,13,14,15,16,17(11)
Centro de Biotecnologia Facultad de Farmacia, Universida Central Av. de Los Llustres Los Chaguaramos Caracas, Venezuela Phone: ++58-2 -693-1026/-6615102	SAM 30(10)
Chemapol, Co. Ltd. Kodanska 46 100 10 Prague 10, The Czech Republic Phone: ++42-2-734737 Fax: ++42-2-734576	SEU 7(13)
Commonwealth Serum Laboratories 45 Poplar Road Parkville, Victoria 3052 Australia Phone: ++61-3-3891911 Fax: ++61-3-3891434 Telex: AA 32789	MAU 1(3) / MAU,2(4) ,3(5) / IAU 1,2(7) / IAU 3(8) / SAU 1,2,3,4,5,6(12)
Fundaçao Ezequiel Dias Rua Conde Pereira Carneiro 80 30500 Belo Horizonte, M.G., Brazil Phone: ++55-31-332-2077/-7222 Fax: ++55-31-332-2534 Telex: 392417 FEDS BR	SAM 22,23,24,25(10)

Table 1, continued

Address of Manufacturer	Code No. of Antivenoms (Table No.)
Gerencia General de Biologicos y Reactivos, Minidterio de Salud, M. Escobado 20, C.P. 11400 Mexico, D.F., Mexico Phone: ++52-527-6127/-7368 Fax: ++52-527-6693	IAM 1(6) / SAM 7,8,9(10)
Haffkine Biopharmaceutical Co. Ltd. Acharya Donde Marg, Parel, Bombay 400012, India Phone: ++91-22-4129320-23/-4129224 Telex: 11-71427 HBPC IN	SAS 18,19,20,21,22(11)
Institut d'Etat des Sérums et Vaccine Razi Hessarek B.P. 656 Teheran, Iran Phone: ++98-21-2005	IAS 2(6) / SAS 5,6,7,8,9,10,11(11)
Institute of Immunology Rockefellerova 2, P.O.Box 266 41000 Zagreb, Croatia Phone: ++38-41-430333 Fax: ++38-41-277278	IEU 3(7) / SEU 5(13)
Institut Pasteur Rue du Docteur Laveran Algiers, Algeria Phone: ++21-32-672511 Fax: ++21-32-672503	IAF 1(6) / SAF 1(9)
Institut Pasteur Place Charles-Nicolle Casablanca, Morocco Phone: ++21-22-275778 Fax: ++21-22-260957	IAF 2(6) / SAF 2(9)
Institut Pasteur, 13 Place Pasteur, Tunis, Tunisia Phone: ++21-61-283022 Fax: ++21-61-791833	IAF 3(6) / SAF 3(9)
Instituto Butantan Av. Vital Brazil 1500 Caixa Postal 65 05504 Sao Paulo, S.P. Brazil Phone: ++55-11-8137222 Fax: ++55-11-8151505 Telex: 83325 BUTA BR	IAM 3,4(6) / IAM 6,7(7) / SAM 13,14,15,16,17,18(10)

Table 1, continued

Address of Manufacturer	Code No. of Antivenoms (Table No.)
Instituto Clodomiro Picado Universidade de Costa Rica Ciudad Universitaria Rodrigo Facio, San José Costa Rica Phone: ++506-290344 Fax: ++506-249367 Telex: UNICORI 2544	SAM 10,11,12(10)
Instituto Sieroterapico Vaccinogeno Toscana SCLAVO Via Fiorentina 1 53100 Siena, Italy Phone: ++39-577-293111 Fax: ++39-577-293493	SEU 4(13)
Instituto Vital Brazil Rua Vital Brasil Filho 64, Santa Rosa 24230-340 Niteroi, R.J., Brazil Phone: ++55-21-711-0012 Fax: ++55-21-714-3198	SAM 19,20,21(10)
Kitasato Institute Minato-ku, Tokyo, Japan Phone: ++81-3-4446161	SAS 50(11)
Laboratorios BIOCLON Calzada de Tlalpan 4687 C.P. 14050 Mexico, D.F., Mexico Phone: ++52-665-4111/-4317/-4309 Fax: ++52-666-1036	IAM 2(6) / SAM 3,4,5,6(10)
Laboratorios Vencofarma do Brasil Ltda. Traves Rua de Oliveira 237 Parque das Indûstrias 86030-380 Londrina, Paranà Brasil Phone: ++55-43-339-1350 Fax: ++55-43-235-4073	SAM 26,27,28,29(10)
Merck, Sharp and Dohme International P.O.Box 2000 Rahway, N.J. 07065, U.S. Phone: ++1-215-661 5477 Fax: ++1-215-661 5319	IAM 5(7)
Ministry of Health, Central Laboratories P.O.Box 6115 Jerusalem 91060 Israel Phone: ++97-22-381631 Fax: ++97-22-781456	IAS 1(6) / SAS 1,2,3,4(11)

Table 1, continued

Address of Manufacturer	Code No. of Antivenoms (Table No.)
National Center of Infectious and Parasitic Diseases 26, Y Sakasov Blvd., 1504 Sofia, Bulgaria Phone: ++35-92-43471 Fax: ++35-92-442260	SEU 6(13)
National Institute of Health Biological Production Division Islamabad, Pakistan Phone: ++92-51-240946/-240973 ++92-51-240544-548 ++92-51-241720 Telex: 5811-NAIB-PK Fax: ++92-51-20797	SAS 26,27,28,29,30(11)
National Instit. of Preventive Medicine 161 Kun Yang Street, Nan-Kang, Taipei, Taiwan 115 Phone: ++88-62-7857559 Fax: ++88-62-7853944	SAS 39,40,41(11)
Pasteur-Mérieux Sérum et Vaccins Avenue Général Leclerc 69007 Lyon Phone: ++33-72-737707 Fax: ++33-72-737737	IEU 2(6) / SAF 7(9) / SAS 51(11) / SEU 1,2(13)
Perum Bio Farma (Pasteur Institute) Jl. Pasteur 28, Post Box 1136 Bandung 40161, Indonesia Phone: ++62-22-83755 Fax: ++62-22-210299 Telex: 28432 biofar ia	SAS 37(11)
Res. Foundation for Microbial Diseases Osaka University Osaka, Japan Phone: ++81-6-8775121 Fax: ++81-6-8761984	SAS 49(11)
Serum Institute of India Ltd. 212/2 Hadapsar Pune - 411 028, India Phone: ++91-212-672016 Fax: ++91-212-672040 Telex: 145-7317 SERA IN 145-7216 SEAL IN	SAS 23,24,25(11)
SEVAC Institute for Sera and Vaccines Korunni 108 101 03 Prague, Czech Republic Phone: ++42-2-734751 Telex: 121852; Fax: ++42-2-737183	SEU 8(13)

Table 1, continued

Address of Manufacturer	Code No. of Antivenoms (Table No.)
Shanghai Inst. of Biological Products Ministry of Health 1262 Yan An Road Shanghai, People's Republic China Phone: ++86-21-2513189 Fax: ++86-21-2511807	SAS 42,43,44(11)
South African Institute for Medical Research Serum and Vaccine Department P.O.Box 28999 Sandringham 2131 South Africa Phone: ++27-11-8829940 Fax: ++27-11-8820812	IAF 5(7) / SAF 4,5,6(9)
Takeda Chemical Industries Ltd. Osaka, Japan Phone: ++81-6-2042111 Fax: ++81-6-2042880	SAS 47(11)
The Chemo-Serotherap. Res. Institute 668 Okubo, Shimizu Kumamoto 860, Japan Phone: ++81-96-3441211 Fax: ++81-96-3449269	SAS 45,46(11)
Thai Red Cross Society Queen Saovabha Memorial Institute Bangkok, Thailand Phone: ++66-2-2520161-4 Fax: ++66-2-2540212 Telex: 82535 THRESCO TH	SAS 31,32,33,34,35,36(11)
The Japan Snake Institute Yabuzuka-honmachi Nittagun, Gunma Prefecture 379-23 Japan Phone: ++81-277-785193 Fax: ++81-277-785520	SAS 48(11)
Twyford Pharmaceuticals GmbH Postfach 210805 67008 Ludwigshafen Fed. Republic of Germany Phone: ++49-621-5892688 Fax: ++49-621-5891530 Telex: 464823	IEU 1(6)
Wyeth - Ayerst Laboratories P.O. Box 8299 Philadelphia, PA 19101-1245 U.S. Phone: ++1-215-688-4400 Fax: ++1-215-9649743 Telex: 0236851323	SAM 1,2(10)

III. KEY TO ANTIVENOMS ACCORDING TO SPECIES NAMES

Table 2
Key according to scientific species names

Scientific Species Name	Antivenom Code No. (Table No.)
MARINE ANIMALS	
Chironex fleckeri	MAU 1(3)
Chiropsalmus quadrigatus	MAU 1(3)
Synanceja trachynis	MAU 2(4)
Synanceja sp.	MAU 2(4)
SNAKES	
Acanthophis antarcticus	SAU 1,6(12)
Acanthophis pyrrhus	SAU 1(12)
Acanthophis praelongus	SAU 1(12)
Agkistrodon acutus	SAS 46,48(11)
Agkistrodon bilineatus	SAM 3, 8(10)
Agkistrodon blomhoffi	SAS 51,52(11)
Agkistrodon b. brevicaudatus	SAS 47(11)
Agkistrodon halys	SAS 6, 12,54,55,56(11)
Agkistrodon rhodostoma	SAS 40, 41,42(11)
Agkistrodon sp.	SAM 1(10)
Aipysurus laevis	MAU 3(5)
Astrotia stokesii	MAU 3(5)
Austrelaps superba	SAU 4,6(12)
Austrelaps ramsayi	SAU 4,6(12)
Bitis arietans	SAF 9,10,11(9)
Bitis gabonica	SAF 9,10,11(9)
Bitis gabonica rhinoceros	SAS 26(11)
Bitis nasicornis	SAF 10(9)
Bitis sp.	SAF 6(9)
Bothriopsis bilineata smaragdina	SAM 32(10)
Bothrops alternatus	SAM 15,18,19,21,23,24,26,27,28,29,35,39,40,43(10)
Bothrops ammodytoides	SAM 39(10)
Bothrops (atrox) asper	SAM 3, 4, 6, 8,11,13,14, 32(10)
Bothrops (atrox) atrox	SAM 1, 9, 26, 27(10)
Bothrops bilineatus smaragdinus	SAM 32(10)
Bothrops brazili	SAM 32(10)
Bothrops castelnaudi	SAM 32(10)
Bothrops colombiensis	SAM 46(10)
Bothrops cotiara	SAM 15, 18, 19, 21, 23, 28, 29(10)
Bothrops jararaca	SAM 15, 18, 19, 21, 23, 24, 26, 27, 28,29,40(10)
Bothrops jararacussu	SAM 15, 18, 19, 21, 23, 24, 26, 27, 28, 29,40(10)
Bothrops (atrox) moojeni	SAM 15, 18, 19, 21, 23, 24, 26, 27, 28, 29(10)
Bothrops neuwiedi	SAM 15, 18, 19, 21, 23, 24, 26, 27, 28, 29,40,43(10)
Bothrops neuwiedi diporus	SAM 39(10)
Bothrops nummifer	SAM 3(10)
Bothrops pictus	SAM 32(10)
Bothrops pradoi	SAM 15, 18, 19, 21, 23, 28, 29(10)

Scientific Species Name	Antivenom Code No. (Table No.)
Bothrops sp.	SAM 44(10)
Bungarus caeruleus	SAS 13,16,19,20,24,27,29(11)
Bungarus fasciatus	SAS 6,27,29,38,42(11)
Bungarus multicinctus	SAS 44,49(11)
Calloselasma rhodostoma	SAM 1(10) / SAS 36,37(11)
Cerastes cerastes	SAF 1,2,3,5,9,11(9) / SAS 5,51,52(11)
Cerastes vipera	SAF 1,2,3,5,9,11(9) / SAS 51,52(11)
Crotalus adamanteus	SAM 1(10)
Crotalus atrox	SAM 1, 3, 5, 6, 7(10)
Crotalus basiliscus	SAM 7(10)
Crotalus durrissus	SAM 3, 7(10)
Crotalus durrissus cumanensis	SAM 30(10)
Crotalus durrissus durrissus	SAM 11(10)
Crotalus durrissus terrificus	SAM 1,5,6,9,14,17,20,21,23,24,26,28(10)
Crotalus mollosus	SAM 7(10)
Crotalus nigrescens	SAM 3(10)
Crotalus sp	SAM 1(10)
Crotalus tigris	SAM 3, 5, 6(10)
Deinagkistrodon acutus	SAS 41,43(11)
Deinagkistrodon sp.	SAM 1(10)
Dendroaspis jamesoni	SAF 7(9)
Dendroaspis polylepis	SAF 7,8(9) / SAS 25(11)
Dendroaspis sp.	SAF 4(9)
Dendroaspis viridis	SAF 7,8(9)
Dispholidus typus	SAF 6(9)
Echis carinatus	SAF 5,9(9)/SAS 5,7,12,17,18,20,23,24,25,26,30,51,52(11)
Echis coloratus	SAF 9,10(9) / SAS 1, 3,52(11)
Echis multisquamatus	SAS 7(11)
Enhydrina schistosa	MAU 3(5)
Haemachatus haemachatus	SAF 4,8(9)
Hydrophis sp.	MAU 3(5)
Lachesis muta	SAM 1,11,13,15,25(10)
Lachesis muta stenophrys	SAM 11(10)
Lapemis hardwickii	MAU 3(5)
Laticauda laticauda	MAU 3(5)
Laticauda semifasciata	MAU 3(5)
Microencephalophis gracilis	MAU 3(5)
Micrurus carinicauda	SAM 10(10)
Micrurus corallinus	SAM 18,29(10)
Micrurus frontalis	SAM 18,29(10)
Micrurus fulvius fulvius	SAM 2, 10(10)
Micrurus mipartitus	SAM 12(10)
Micrurus nigrocinctus	SAM 10(10)
Naja haje	SAF 4,7,8,9(9) / SAS 51,52(11)
Naja melanoleuca	SAF 4,7,8,9(9)
Naja mossambica	SAF 4(9)
Naja naja	SAS 12,13,18,21,23,26,27(11)
Naja naja atra	SAS 39(11)
Naja naja caeca	SAS 14(11)

Scientific Species Name	Antivenom Code No. (Table No.)
Naja naja kaouthia	SAS 14,32(11)
Naja naja naja	SAS 14(11)
Naja naja oxiana	SAS 5,6(11)
Naja naja philippinensis	SAS 38(11)
Naja naja sputatrix	SAS 37(11)
Naja nigricollis	SAF 7,8,9(9)
Naja nivea	SAF 4,8,9(9)
Naja sp.	SAS 6,32(11)
Notechis ater	SAU 4(12)
Notechis scutatus	SAU 4,6(12)
Ophiophagus hannah	SAS 33(11)
Oxyuranus microlepidotus	SAU 2,6(12)
Oxyuranus scutellatus	SAU 2,6(12)
Pelamis platurus	MAU 3(5)
Porthidium nummifer	SAM 3(10)
Praescutata viperina	MAU 3(5)
Pseudechis australis	SAU 3,6(12)
Tropidechis carinatus	SAU 4(12)
Pseudechis colletti	SAU 3,4(12)
Pseudechis guttatus	SAU 3,4(12)
Pseudechis papuanus	SAU 6(12)
Pseudechis porphyriacus	SAU 3,4(12)
Pseudocerastes persicus	SAS 5,10(11)
Pseudonaja affinis	SAU 5,6(12)
Pseudonaja nuchalis	SAU 5,6(12)
Pseudonaja textilis	SAU 5,6(12)
Rhabdophis tigrinus	SAS 48(11)
Rhabdophis sp.	SAS 48(11)
Sistrurus sp.	SAM 1(10)
Trimeresurus albolabris	SAS 31(11)
Trimeresurus flavoviridis	SAS 45(11)
Trimeresurus macrops	SAS 31(11)
Trimeresurus mucrosquamatus	SAS 40(11)
Trimeresurus sp.	SAM 1(10) / SAS 31(11)
Trimeresurus stejnegeri	SAS 40(11)
Vipera ammodytes	SAS 51,52(11) / SEU 1,3,4,6,8(13)
Vipera ammodytes ammodytes	SEU 5,7(13)
Vipera ammodytes meridionalis	SEU 5(13)
Vipera aspis	SEU 1,2,3,4,5,6(13)
Vipera berus	SEU 1,2,3,4,5,6,8(13)
Vipera kaznakovi	SEU 3(13)
Vipera latasti	SEU 3(13)
Vipera latifi	SAS 8(11)
Vipera lebetina	SAF 1,2,3,9(9) / SAS 51,52(11) / SEU 5(13)
Vipera lebetina obtusa	SAS 51(11)
Vipera mesocoronis	SEU 6(13)
Vipera (xanthina) palaestinae	SAF 10(9) / SAS 2,51,52(11) / SEU 3(13)
Vipera russelli	SAS 5,12,13,16,18,22,23,24,25,26,29(11)
Vipera russelli siamensis	SAS 35(11)
Vipera ursinii	SEU 3,4,5(13)

Scientific Species Name	Antivenom Code No. (Table No.)
Vipera xanthina	SAS 5,51,52(11)
Walterinnesia aegyptia	SAS 4(11)
TERRESTRIAL INVERTEBRATES	
Androctonus aeneas	IAF 3(6)
Androctonus australis	IAF 3(6) / IEU 1(6)
Androctonus australis hector	IAF 1(6)
Androctonus crassicauda	IAS 2(6)
Androctonus mauretanicus	IAF 2(6)
Androctonus sp.	IEU 2(6)
Atrax robustus	IAU 1(7)
Atrax sp.	IAU 1(7)
Buthotus salcyi	IAS 2(6)
Buthotus tamulus	IAS 3(6)
Buthus occitanus	IAF 3(6) / IEU 1(6)
Buthus sp.	IEU 2(6)
Centruroides limpidus limpidus	IAM 1(6),2(6)
Centruroides limpidus tecomanas	IAM 1(6),2(6)
Centruroides noxius	IAM 1(6),2(6)
Centruroides suffusus suffusus	IAM 1(6),2(6)
Centruroides sp.	IAM 1(6),2(6)
Hadronyche sp.	IAU 1(7)
Ixodes holocyclus	IAU 3(8)
Latrodectus hasselti	IEU 4(7) / IAU 2(7)
Latrodectus indistinctus	IAF 5(7) / IEU 4(7)
Latrodectus mactans	IAM 5(7)
Latrodectus m. tredecimguttatus	IEU 4(7)
Latrodectus sp.	IAF 5(7)
Leiurus quinquestriatus	IAF 3(6) / IEU 1,2(6) / IAS 1(6)
Loxosceles reclusa	IAM 7(7)
Loxosceles sp.	IAM 3(6),6(7)
Mesobuthus eupeus	IAS 2(6)
Odonthobuthus doriae	IAS 2(6)
Parabuthus transvaalicus	IAF 4(6)
Phoneutria sp.	IAM 3(6),6(7)
Tityus bahiensis	IAM 3,4(6),6(7)
Tityus serrulatus	IAM 3,4(6),6(7)

IV. LIST OF ANTIVENOMS FOR THE TREATMENT OF ENVENOMATIONS CAUSED BY VENOMOUS MARINE ANIMALS

A. ANTIVENOMS FOR THE TREATMENT OF ENVENOMATIONS CAUSED BY COELENTERATES

There is only one antivenin available for the highly toxic sea wasps *Chironex fleckeri* and *Chiropsalmus quadrigatus*, both species present in the coastal regions of Australia, and belonging to the coelenterate class Cubozoa (Box Jellyfish).

Table 3
Antivenoms available for the treatment of envenomations caused by marine invertebrates

Code No.	Product Name	Manufacturer	Venoms Covered
MAU 1	Box jellyfish antivenom	Commonwealth Serum Laboratories Parkville, Victoria 3052 Australia Phone: ++61-3-3891911 Fax: ++61-3-3891434 Telex: AA 32789	*Chironex fleckeri Chiropsalmus quadrigatus*

B. ANTIVENOMS FOR THE TREATMENT OF ENVENOMATIONS CAUSED BY VENOMOUS FISHES

There existed monovalent antivenins for the Mediterranean fish species of the genus Trachinus and Scorpaena, respectively and a polyvalent antivenin which is said to neutralize also envenomations caused by *Uranoscopus scaber*. This species, however, seems to have no venomous glands at all, although spines on the operculum are present. Furhermore, it has been shown that *Uranoscopus* scaber stings as well as extracts of the tissue surrounding the spines are not able to envenomate experimental animals[9]. In a recent letter (to J.M., dated September 6, 1994) the Institute of Immunology of Zagreb, Croatia, informed us that they ceased production of their antivenoms against the above-mentioned venomous fishes. In Australia, stonefish stings form to some extent a public health problem. Therefore, a stonefish antivenin is available, which most probably neutralizes also the venoms of other *Synanceja* species.

Table 4
Antivenoms available for the treatment of envenomations caused by venomous fishes

Code No.	Product Name	Manufacturer	Venoms Covered
MAU 2	Stonefish antivenom	Commonwealth Serum Laboratories Parkville, Victoria 3052 Australia Phone: ++61-3-3891911 Fax: ++61-3-3891434 Telex: AA 32789	*Synanceja trachynis Synanceja* sp.

C. ANTIVENOMS FOR THE TREATMENT OF ENVENOMATION CAUSED BY SEA SNAKE BITE

Only one antivenin is available to date against sea snake bite envenomation. However, although extremely toxic, sea snakes use their venom in defence only on rare occasions (see Chapter 13).

Table 5
Antivenoms for the treatment of envenomations caused by sea snakes

Code No.	Product Name	Manufacturer	Venoms Covered
MAU 3	Sea snake antivenom	Commonwealth Serum Laboratories 45 Poplar Road Parkville, Victoria 3052, Australia Phone: ++61-3-3891911 Fax: ++61-3-3891434 Telex: AA 32789	*Notechis scutatus* *Enhydrina schistosa* *Aipysurus laevis* *Astrotia stokesii* *Hydrophis* sp. *Laticauda laticauda* *Laticauda semifasciata* *Lapemis hardwickii* *Microencephalophis gracilis* *Pelamis platurus* *Praescutata viperina*

V. LIST OF ANTIVENOMS FOR THE TREATMENT OF ENVENOMATIONS CAUSED BY VENOMOUS TERRESTRIAL INVERTEBRATES

A. ANTIVENOMS FOR THE TREATMENT OF ENVENOMATION CAUSED BY SCORPION STINGS

Table 6
Antivenoms for the treatment of envenomation caused by scorpion stings

Code No.	Product Name	Manufacturer	Venoms Covered
IAF 1	Scorpion antivenom	Institut Pasteur Rue du Docteur Laveran Algiers, Algeria Phone: ++21-32-672511 Fax: ++21-32-672503	*Androctonus australis hector*
IAF 2	Scorpion antivenom	Institut Pasteur Place Charles-Nicolle Casablanca, Morocco Phone: ++21-22-275778 Fax: ++21-22-260957	*Androctonus mauretanicus*

Code No.	Product Name	Manufacturer	Venoms Covered
IAF 3	Anti-scorpionic sera	Institut Pasteur 13, Place Pasteur Tunis, Tunisia Tel. ++21-61-283022 Fax: ++21-61-791833	*Androctonus aeneas* *Androctonus australis* *Buthus occitanus* *Leiurus* *quinquestriatus* Iranian scorpions
IAF 4	Scorpion antivenom	The South African Institute for Medical Research P.O.Box 1038 Johannesburg 2000 South Africa Phone: ++27-11-7250511 Telex: 4-22211	*Parabuthus* *transvaalicus*
IAM 1	Suero Antialacran	Gerencia General de Biologicos y Reactivos, Health Ministry M. Escobedo 20 C.P. 11400 Mexico D.F. Mexico	*Centruroides* *l.limpidus* *Centruroides l.* *tecomanas* *Centruroides noxius* *Centruroides s.* *suffusus* *Centruroides* sp.
IAM 2	Suero Antialacran Alacramyn®	Laboratorios BIOCLON Calzada de Tlalpan 4687 C.P. 14050 Mexico D.F. Mexico Phone: ++52-665-4111/- 4317/-4309 Fax: ++52-666-1036	*Centruroides l.* *limpidus* *Centruroides l.* *tecomanus* *Centruroides s.* *suffusus* *Centruroides noxius* *Centruroides* sp.
IAM 3	Soro-antiarachnidico	Instituto Butantan Av. Vital Brazil 1500 Caixa Postal 65 05504 Sao Paulo, S.P. Brazil Phone: ++55-11-8137222 Fax: ++55-11-8151505 Telex: 83325 BUTA BR	*Loxosceles* sp. *Phoneutria* sp. *Tityus bahiensis* *Tityus serrulatus*
IAM 4	Soro-antiscorpionico genus Tityus	Instituto Butantan 05504 Sao Paulo, S.P. (Details, see above)	*Tityus bahiensis* *Tityus serrulatus*
IEU 1	Scorpion antivenom Twyford (North Africa)	Twyford Pharmaceuticals GmbH Postfach 210805 67008 Ludwigshafen Fed. Republic of Germany Phone: ++49-621-5892688 Fax: ++49-621-5891530 Telex: 464823	*Androctonus australis* *Buthus occitanus* *Leiurus* *quinquestriatus*

Code No.	Product Name	Manufacturer	Venoms Covered
IEU 2	LABS 50	Pasteur-Mérieux Sérum et Vaccins Avenue Général Leclerc 69007 Lyon Phone: ++33-72-737707 Fax: ++33-72-737737	*Androctonus* sp. *Buthus* sp. *Leiurus* sp.
IAS 1	Scorpion Antivenom	Israel Association for Venom Research, Jerusalem, and Ministry of Health, Central Laboratories, P.O. Box 6115, Jerusalem, 91060 Phone: ++972-2-314819	*Leiurus quinquestriatus*
IAS 2	Polyvalent scorpion antivenom	Institut d'Etat des Sérums et Vaccine Razi Hessarek B.P. 656 Teheran, Iran Phone: ++98-21-2005	*Androctonus crassicauda* *Buthotus salcyi* *Mesobuthus eupeus* *Odonthobuthus doriae*
IAS 3	Monovalent scorpion anti-venom	Central Research Institute 173 204 (H.P.) Kasauli, India Phone: ++91-1793-2060 Fax: ++91-1793-2049	*Buthotus tamulus*

B. ANTIVENOMS FOR THE TREATMENT OF ENVENOMATION CAUSED BY SPIDER BITES

One antivenin is available against envenomation caused by the Australian mygalomorph Sidney Funnel-web spider (*Atrax robustus*) and a number of antivenins are available for the specific treatment of araneomorph spiders of the genera *Latrodectus*, *Loxosceles* and *Phoneutria*, respectively.

Table 7
Antivenoms for the treatment of spider bites

Code No.	Product Name	Manufacturer	Venoms Covered
IAF 5	Spider antivenom	The South African Institute for Medical Research P.O.Box 1038 Johannesburg 2000 South Africa Phone: ++27-11-7250511 Telex: 4-22211	*Latrodectus mactans (indistinctus)* *Latrodectus* sp.
IAU 1	Funnel-web spider antivenom	Commonwealth Serum Laboratories (Details, see IAU 2 below)	*Atrax robustus* *Atrax* sp. *Hadronyche* sp.

Code No.	Product Name	Manufacturer	Venoms Covered
IAM 5	Antivenin (Latrodectus mactans) MSD	Merck, Sharp and Dohme International P.O.Box 2000 Rahway, N.J. 07065, USA Phone: ++1-215-6615477 Fax: ++1-215-6615319	*Latrodectus mactans*
IAM 6	Soro-antiarachnidico polyvalente	Instituto Butantan Av. Vital Brazil 1500 Caixa Postal 65 05504 Sao Paulo, S.P. Brazil Phone: ++55-11-8137222 Fax: ++55-11-8151505 Telex: 83325 BUTA BR	*Loxosceles* sp. *Phoneutria* sp. *Tityus bahiensis* *Tityus serrulatus*
IAM 7	Soro-antiloxoscelico	Instituto Butantan Sao Paulo, Brasil (Details, see above)	*Loxosceles reclusa*
IEU 3	Anti-Latrodectus mactans tredecimguttatus serum	Institute of Immunology Rockefellerova 2, P.O.Box 266 41000 Zagreb, Croatia Phone: ++385-41-430333 Fax: ++385-41-277278	*Latrodectus mactans tredecimguttatus Latrodectus hasselti Latrodectus indistinctus*
IAU 2	Red-backed spider antivenom	Commonwealth Serum Laboratories 45 Poplar Road Parkville, Victoria 3052, Australia Phone: ++61-3-3891911 Fax: ++61-3-3891434 Telex: AA 32789	*Latrodectus hasselti*

C. ANTIVENOMS FOR THE TREATMENT OF ENVENOMATION CAUSED BY TICK BITES

Tick paralysis is a public health problem in some parts of the world (see Chapters 15 and 16). Therefore, an antivenin against tick venom has been prepared by the Commonwealth Serum Laboratories in Parkville, Australia.

Table 8
Antivenoms for the treatment of tick bites

Code No.	Product Name	Manufacturer	Venoms Covered
IAU 3	Tick antivenom	Commonwealth Serum Laboratories 45 Poplar Road Parkville, Victoria 3052, Australia Phone: ++61-3-3891911 Fax: ++61-3-3891434 Telex: AA 32789	*Ixodes holocyclus*

VI. LIST OF ANTIVENOMS FOR THE TREATMENT OF ENVENOMATIONS CAUSED BY VENOMOUS TERRESTRIAL SNAKES

The following paragraphs include one geographical map of each respective continent with the code numbers of antivenoms available, as shown in the respective table. Only product names, manufacturer addresses and the venoms to be covered by the respective products are given. No details about neutralization capacities and further product details are included to increase the lucidity of the tables. Wherever possible, fax and telex numbers were included to increase the speed in the context with orders and informational requests.

A. ANTIVENOMS FOR THE TREATMENT OF ENVENOMATIONS CAUSED BY VENOMOUS SNAKES IN AFRICA

These antivenoms are listed in Table 9.

Table 9
Antivenoms for the treatment of envenomations caused by venomous snakes in Africa

Code No.	Product Name	Manufacturer	Venoms Covered
SAF 1	Antiviperin	Institut Pasteur d'Algérie, Rue du Docteur Laveran, Algiers, Algeria Phone: ++21-32-672511 Fax: ++21-32-672503	*Cerastes cerastes* *Cerastes vipera* *Vipera lebetina*
SAF 2	Antiviperin Sera	Institut Pasteur, Place Charles-Nicolle, Casablanca, Marocco Phone: ++21-22-275778 Fax: ++21-22-260957	*Cerastes cerastes* *Cerastes vipera* *Vipera lebetina*
SAF 3	Antiviperin Sera	Institut Pasteur, 13 Place Pasteur, Tunis, Tunisia Phone: ++21-61-283022 Fax: ++21-61-791833	*Cerastes cerastes* *Cerastes vipera* *Vipera lebetina*
SAF 4	Polyvalent Antivenom	South African Institute for Medical Research - Serum and Vaccine Dept. P.O. Box 2899 Sandringham 2131 South Africa Phone: ++27-11-8829940 Fax: ++27-11-8820812	*Bitis* sp. *Dendroaspis* sp. *Haemachatus* sp. *Naja haje* *Naja melanoleuca* *Naja mossambica* *Naja nivea*
SAF 5	*Echis* - Antivenom	South African Institute for Medical Research Sandringham, South Africa (Details, see above)	*Echis carinatus* (Kenya) *Echis coloratus* *Cerastes cerastes* *Cerastes vipera*

Code No.	Product Name	Manufacturer	Venoms Covered
SAF 6	Boomslang Antivenom	South African Institute for Medical Research - Serum and Vaccine Dept. P.O. Box 2899 Sandringham 2131 South Africa Phone: ++27-11-8829940 Fax: ++27-11-8820812	*Dispholidus typus*
SAF 7	Ipser Afrique	Pasteur-Mérieux Sérum et Vaccins Avenue Général Leclerc 69007 Lyon Phone: ++33-72-737707 Fax: ++33-72-737737	*Bitis arietans* *Bitis gabonica* *Dendroaspis jamesoni* *Dendroaspis polylepis* *Dendroaspis viridis* *Naja haje* *Naja melanoleuca* *Naja nigricollis*
SAF 8	Zentralafrika-Serum	Behringwerke AG Postfach 1140 35001 Marburg/Lahn Federal Republic of Germany Phone: ++49-6421-390 Fax: ++49-6421-31388 Telex: 0482320	*Bitis arietans* *Bitis gabonica* *Bitis nasicornis* *Dendroaspis polylepis* *Dendroaspis viridis* *Haemachatus haemachatus* *Naja haje* *Naja melanoleuca* *Naja nigricollis* *Naja nivea*
SAF 9	Nord- und Westafrika-Serum	Behringwerke AG 35001 Marburg/Lahn (Details, see above)	*Bitis arietans* *Bitis gabonica* *Cerastes cerastes* *Cerastes vipera* *Echis carinatus* *Echis coloratus* *Naja haje* *Naja melanoleuca* *Naja nigricollis* *Naja nivea* *Vipera palaestinae* *Vipera lebetina*

B. ANTIVENOMS FOR THE TREATMENT OF ENVENOMATIONS CAUSED BY VENOMOUS SNAKES IN NORTH, CENTRAL AND SOUTH AMERICA

Table 10
Antivenoms for the treatment of envenomations caused by venomous snakes in North, Central and South America

Code No.	Product Name	Manufacturer	Venoms Covered
SAM 1	Wyeth Antivenin (Crotalidae) Polyvalent	Wyeth - Ayerst Laboratories P.O. Box 8299 Philadelphia, PA 19101-1245 U.S. Phone: ++1-215-688-4400 Fax: ++1-215-9649743 Telex: 0236851323	*Agkistrodon* sp. *Bothrops atrox* *Calloselasma* sp. *Crotalus* sp. *Deinagkistrodon* sp. *Crotalus adamanteus* *Crotalus atrox* *Crotalus durrissus terrificus* *Lachesis muta* *Sistrurus* sp. *Trimeresurus* sp.
SAM 2	Antivenin (*Micrurus fulvius*)	Wyeth - Ayerst Laboratories Philadelphia, U.S. (Details, see above)	*Micrurus fulvius fulvius*
SAM 3	Snake Antivenin	Laboratorios BIOCLON Calzada de Tlalpan 4687 C.P. 14050 Mexico, D.F., Mexico Phone: ++52-665-4111/-4317/-4309 Fax: ++52-666-1036	*Agkistrodon bilineatus* *Bothrops asper* *Porthidium nummifer* *Crotalus atrox* *Crotalus durrissus* *Crotalus nigrescens* *Crotalus tigris*
SAM 4	Monovalent Bothrops	Laboratorios BIOCLON 14050 Mexico, D.F., Mexico (Details, see above)	*Bothrops (atrox) asper*
SAM 5	Polyvalent Crotalus	Laboratorios BIOCLON 14050 Mexico, D.F., Mexico (Details, see above)	*Crotalus atrox* *Crotalus d. terrificus* *Crotalus tigris*
SAM 6	Polyvalent Mexico	Laboratorios BIOCLON 14050 Mexico, D.F., Mexico (Details, see above)	*Bothrops (atrox) asper* *Crotalus atrox* *Crotalus d. terrificus* *Crotalus tigris*

Code No.	Product Name	Manufacturer	Venoms Covered
SAM 7	Anti-Crotalus	Gerencia General de Biologicos y Reactivos, Minidterio de Salud, M. Escobado 20, C.P. 11400 Mexico, D.F., Mexico Phone: ++52-527-6127/-7368 Fax: ++52-527-6693	*Crotalus basiliscus Crotalus atrox Crotalus durrissus Crotalus mollosus*
SAM 8	Anti-Bothrops	Gerencia General de Biologicos y Reactivos, Minidterio de Salud, M. Escobado 20, C.P. 11400 Mexico, D.F., Mexico Phone: ++52-527-6127/-7368 Fax: ++52-527-6693	*Agkistrodon bilineatus Bothrops (atrox) asper*
SAM 9	Suero antiofidico export lyophilized	Gerencia General de Biologicos y Reactivos Mexico 03100 D.F., Mexico (Details, see above)	*Bothrops atrox Crotalus d. terrificus* Mexican and South American *Bothrops* and *Crotalus* sp.
SAM 10	Anticoral	Instituto Clodomiro Picado Universidade de Costa Rica Ciudad Universitaria Rodrigo Facio, San José Costa Rica Phone: ++506-290344 Fax: ++506-249367 Telex: UNICORI 2544	*Micrurus carinicauda Micrurus fulvius fulvius Micrurus nigrocinctus*
SAM 11	Polyvalent Antivenom	Instituto Clodomiro Picado San José, Costa Rica (Details, see above)	*Bothrops (atrox) asper Crotalus d. durrissus Lachesis muta stenophrys* Central and South American *Bothrops* sp.
SAM 12	Anti-mipartitus	Instituto Clodomiro Picado San José, Costa Rica (Details, see above)	*Micrurus mipartitus*
SAM 13	Antibotropico laquetico	Instituto Butantan Av. Vital Brazil 1500 Caixa Postal 65 05504 Sao Paulo, S.P., Brazil Phone: ++55-11-8137222 Fax: ++55-11-8151505 Telex: 83325 BUTA BR	*Bothrops alternatus Bothrops cotiara Bothrops jararaca Bothrops jararacussu Bothrops (atrox) moojeni Bothrops neuwiedi Bothrops pradoi Lachesis muta*

Code No.	Product Name	Manufacturer	Venoms Covered
SAM 14	Anticrotalico	Instituto Butantan 05504 Sao Paulo, S.P., Brazil (Details, see above)	*Crotalus d. terrificus*
SAM 15	Antilaquetico	Instituto Butantan 05504 Sao Paulo, S.P., Brazil (Details, see above)	*Lachesis muta*
SAM 16	Antibotropico	Instituto Butantan Av. Vital Brazil 1500 Caixa Postal 65 05504 Sao Paulo, S.P., Brazil Phone: ++55-11-8137222 Fax: ++55-11-8151505 Telex: 83325 BUTA BR	*Bothrops alternatus* *Bothrops cotiara* *Bothrops jararaca* *Bothrops jararacussu* *Bothrops (atrox) moojeni* *Bothrops neuwiedi* *Bothrops pradoi*
SAM 17	Antiophidico polyvalente	Instituto Butantan 05504 Sao Paulo, S.P., Brazil (Details, see above)	*Bothrops alternatus* *Bothrops cotiara* *Bothrops jararaca* *Bothrops jararacussu* *Bothrops (atrox) moojeni* *Bothrops neuwiedi* *Bothrops pradoi* *Crotalus d. terrificus*
SAM 18	Antielapidico	Instituto Butantan 05504 Sao Paulo, S.P., Brazil (Details, see above)	*Micrurus corallinus* *Micrurus frontalis*
SAM 19	Soro Antibotropico	Instituto Vital Brazil Rua Vital Brasil Filho 64, Santa Rosa 24230-340 Niteroi, R.J., Brazil Phone: ++55-21-711-0012 Fax: ++55-21-714-3198	*Bothrops alternatus* *Bothrops cotiara* *Bothrops jararaca* *Bothrops jararacussu* *Bothrops (atrox) moojeni* *Bothrops pradoi*
SAM 20	Soro Anticrotalico	Instituto Vital Brazil Niteroi, Rio de Janeiro, Brazil (Details, see above)	*Crotalus d. terrificus*

Code No.	Product Name	Manufacturer	Venoms Covered
SAM 21	Soro Antiofidico polyvalente	Instituto Vital Brazil Niteroi, Rio de Janeiro, Brazil (Details, see above)	*Bothrops alternatus* *Bothrops cotiara* *Bothrops jararaca* *Bothrops jararacussu* *Bothrops (atrox) moojeni* *Bothrops pradoi* *Crotalus d. terrificus*
SAM 22	Antibotropico	Fundaçao Ezequiel Dias Rua Conde Pereira Carneiro 80 30500 Belo Horizonte, M.G., Brazil Phone: ++55-31-332-2077/-7222 Fax: ++55-31-332-2534 Telex: 392417 FEDS BR	*Bothrops alternatus* *Bothrops jararaca* *Bothrops jararacussu* *Bothrops (atrox) moojeni* *Bothrops neuwiedi*
SAM 23	Antibotropico crotalico	Fundaçao Ezequiel Dias Rua Conde Pereira Carneiro 80 30500 Belo Horizonte, M.G., Brazil Phone: ++55-31-332-2077/-7222 Fax: ++55-31-332-2534 Telex: 392417 FEDS BR	*Bothrops alternatus* *Bothrops jararaca* *Bothrops jararacussu* *Bothrops (atrox) atrox* *Bothrops (atrox) moojeni* *Bothrops neuwiedi* *Crotalus d. terrificus*
SAM 24	Anticrotalico	Fundaçao Ezequiel Dias (Details, see above)	*Crotalus d. terrificus*
SAM 25	Antibotropico laquetico	Fundaçao Ezequiel Dias (Details, see above)	*Bothrops alternatus* *Bothrops jararaca* *Bothrops jararacussu* *Bothrops (atrox) atrox* *Bothrops (atrox) moojeni* *Bothrops neuwiedi* *Lachesis muta*

Code No.	Product Name	Manufacturer	Venoms Covered
SAM 26	Antiophidico polyvalente	Lab. Vencofarma do Brasil Ltda. Traves Rua de Oliveira 237 Parque das Indùstrias 86030-380 Londrinas, Paranà Brasil Phone: ++55-43-339-1350 Fax: ++55-43-235-4073	*Bothrops alternatus Bothrops cotiara Bothrops jararaca Bothrops jararacussu Bothrops (atrox) moojeni Bothrops neuwiedi Bothrops pradoi Crotalus d. terrificus*
SAM 27	Antibotropico	Lab. Vencofarma do Brasil Ltda. Londrinas, Paranà, Brasil (Details, see above)	*Bothrops alternatus Bothrops cotiara Bothrops jararaca Bothrops jararacussu Bothrops (atrox) moojeni Bothrops neuwiedi Bothrops pradoi*
SAM 28	Anticrotalico	Lab. Vencofarma do Brasil Ltda. Londrinas, Paranà, Brasil (Details, see above)	*Crotalus d. terrificus*
SAM 29	Antielapidico	Lab. Vencofarma do Brasil Ltda. Londrinas, Paranà, Brasil (Details, see above)	*Micrurus corallinus Micrurus frontalis*
SAM 30	Suero Antiofidico polyvalente	Centro de Biotecnologia Facultad de Farmacia, Universida Central, Av. de Los Llustres, Los Chaguaramos Caracas, Venezuela Phone: ++58-2 -693-1026/- 6615102	*Bothrops colombiensis Crotalus durrissus cumanensis*

C. ANTIVENOMS FOR THE TREATMENT OF ENVENOMATIONS CAUSED BY VENOMOUS SNAKES IN ASIA, INCLUDING NEAR AND MIDDLE EAST

Table 11
Antivenoms for the treatment of envenomations caused by venomous snakes in Asia, including Near and Middle East

Code No.	Product Name	Manufacturer	Venoms Covered
SAS 1	Anti-*Echis coloratus*	Ministry of Health, Central Laboratories P.O.Box 6115 Jerusalem 91060 Israel Phone: ++97-22-381631 Fax: ++97-22-781456	*Echis coloratus*
SAS 2	Anti-*Vipera palaestinae*	Ministry of Health, Israel (details, see above)	*Vipera palaestinae*
SAS 3	Arabian *Echis* Snake Antivenom	Ministry of Health, Israel (details, see above)	*Echis coloratus*
SAS 4	Anti-*Walterinnesia* Snake Antivenom	Ministry of Health, Israel (details, see above)	*Walterinnesia aegyptia*
SAS 5	Polyvalent Antivenom	Institut d'Etat des Serums et vaccins Razi Hessarek B.P. 656 Teheran, Iran Phone: ++98-21-2005	*Agkistrodon halys* *Bungarus fasciatus* *Cerastes cerastes* *Echis carinatus* *Pseudocerastes persicus* *Naja naja oxiana* *Vipera lebetina* *Vipera russelli* *Vipera xanthina*
SAS 6	Naja Antivenom	Institut d'Etat des serums et vaccins Teheran, Iran (details see above)	*Naja naja oxiana* *Naja* sp.
SAS 7	Echis Antivenom	Institut d'Etat des serums et vaccins Teheran, Iran (details see above)	*Echis carinatus* *Echis multisquamatus*
SAS 8	Latifi Antivenom	Institut d'Etat des serums et vaccins Teheran, Iran (details see above)	*Vipera latifi*
SAS 9	Lebetina Antivenom	Institut d'Etat des serums et vaccins Teheran, Iran (details see above)	*Vipera lebetina*
SAS 10	Persica Antivenom	Institut d'Etat des serums et vaccins Teheran, Iran (details see above)	*Pseudocerastes persicus*
SAS 11	Agkistrodon Antivenom	Institut d'Etat des serums et vaccins Teheran, Iran (details see above)	*Agkistrodon halys*

Code No.	Product Name	Manufacturer	Venoms Covered
SAS 12	Polyvalent Snake Venom Antiserum	Central Research Institute 173 204 (H.P.) Kasauli, India Phone: ++91-1793-2060 Fax: ++91-1793-2049	*Bungarus caeruleus* *Echis carinatus* *Naja naja* *Vipera russelli*
SAS 13	Bivalent Antiserum	Central Research Institute Kasauli (details, see above)	*Naja naja* *Vipera russelli*
SAS 14	Monovalent Cobra Venom Antiserum	Central Research Institute Kasauli (details, see above)	*Naja naja caeca* *Naja naja naja* *Naja naja kaouthia*
SAS 15	Monovalent Krait Venom Antiserum	Central Research Institute Kasauli (details, see above)	*Bungarus caeruleus*
SAS 16	Monovalent Russell's Viper Venom Antiserum	Central Research Institute Kasauli (details, see above)	*Vipera russelli*
SAS 17	Monovalent Echis Venom Antiserum	Central Research Institute Kasauli (details, see above)	*Echis carinatus*
SAS 18	Polyvalent Antisnake Venom Serum	Haffkine Biopharmaceutical Co. Ltd. Acharya Donde Marg, Parel, Bombay 400012, India Phone: ++91-22-4129320-23/-4129224 Telex: 11-71427 HBPC IN	*Bungarus caeruleus* *Echis carinatus* *Naja naja* *Vipera russelli*
SAS 19	Bungarus	Haffkine Biopharmaceutical Co. Ltd. Bombay, India (details, see above)	*Bungarus caeruleus*
SAS 20	Echis	Haffkine Biopharmaceutical Co. Ltd. Bombay, India (details, see above)	*Echis carinatus*
SAS 21	Naja	Haffkine Biopharmaceutical Co. Ltd. Bombay, India (details, see above)	*Naja naja*
SAS 22	Vipera	Haffkine Biopharmaceutical Co. Ltd. Bombay, India (details, see above)	*Vipera russelli*

Code No.	Product Name	Manufacturer	Venoms Covered
SAS 23	SII Polyvalent Antisnake Venom Serum (lyophilized)	Serum Institute of India Ltd. 212/2 Hadapsar Pune - 411 028, India Phone: ++91-212-672016 Fax: ++91-212-672040 Telex: 145-7317 SERA IN 145-7216 SEAL IN	*Bungarus caeruleus Echis carinatus Naja naja Vipera russelli*
SAS 24	SII Bivalent Antisnake Venom Serum (lyophilized)	Serum Institute of India Ltd. (details, see above)	*Echis carinatus Vipera russelli*
SAS 25	SII Polyvalent Antisnake Venom Serum (lyophilized) (Central Africa)	Serum Institute of India Ltd. (details, see above)	*Dendroaspis polylepis Bitis gabonica rhinoceros Echis carinatus Vipera russelli*
SAS 26	Polyvalent Antisnake Venom Serum	National Institute of Health Biological Production Division Islamabad, Pakistan Phone: ++92-51-240946/-240973 ++92-51-240544-548 ++92-51-241720 Telex: 5811-NAIB-PK Fax: ++92-51-20797	*Bungarus caeruleus Bungarus fasciatus Echis carinatus Naja naja Vipera lebetina Vipera russelli*
SAS 27	Monovalent (Naja naja)	National Institute of Health Pakistan (details, see above)	*Naja naja*
SAS 28	Monovalent (Krait)	National Institute of Health Pakistan (details, see above)	*Bungarus caeruleus Bungarus fasciatus*
SAS 29	Monovalent (Vipera russelli)	National Institute of Health Pakistan (details, see above)	*Vipera russelli Vipera lebetina*
SAS 30	Monovalent (Echis carinatus)	National Institute of Health Islamabad, Pakistan (details, see above)	*Echis carinatus*
SAS 31	Green Pit Viper Antivenin	Thai Red Cross Society Queen Saovabha Memorial Institute Bangkok, Thailand Phone: ++66-2-2520161-4 Fax: ++66-2-2540212 Telex: 82535 THRESCO TH	*Trimeresurus albolabris Trimeresurus macrops.* Other *Trimeresurus* sp. from Thailand
SAS 32	Cobra Antivenin	Thai Red Cross Society Queen Saovabha Memorial Institute Bangkok, Thailand Phone: ++66-2-2520161-4 Fax: ++66-2-2540212 Telex: 82535 THRESCO TH	*Naja naja kaouthia Naja* sp.

Code No.	Product Name	Manufacturer	Venoms Covered
SAS 33	King Cobra Antivenin	Thai Red Cross Society Bangkok, Thailand (details, see above)	*Ophiophagus hannah*
SAS 34	Banded Krait Antivenin	Thai Red Cross Society Bangkok, Thailand (details, see above)	*Bungarus fasciatus*
SAS 35	Russell's Viper Antivenin	Thai Red Cross Society Bangkok, Thailand (details, see above)	*Vipera russelli siamensis*
SAS 36	Malayan Pit Viper Antivenin	Thai Red Cross Society Bangkok, Thailand (details, see above)	*Calloselasma rhodostoma*
SAS 37	Polyvalent anti-venom serum	Perum Bio Farma (Pasteur Institute) Jl. Pasteur 28, Post Box 1136 Bandung 40161, Indonesia Phone: ++62-22-83755 Fax: ++62-22-210299 Telex: 28432 biofar ia	*Bungarus fasciatus Calloselasma rhodo-stoma Naja naja sputatrix*
SAS 38	Cobra Antivenin	Biologials Production Service Alabang, 1702 Muntinlupa Metro Manila, Philippines Phone: ++1-632-8421333 Fax: ++1-632-8421285	*Naja naja philippinensis*
SAS 39	Naja-Bungarus antivenin	National Inst. of Preventive Medicine 161 Kun Yang Street, Nan-Kang, Taipei, Taiwan 115 Phone: ++88-62-7857559 Fax: ++88-62-7853944	*Bungarus multicinctus Naja naja atra*
SAS 40	Trimeresurus antivenin	National Inst. of Preventive Medicine Taipei, Taiwan (Details, see above)	*Trimeresurus mucrosquamatus Trimeresurus stejnegeri*
SAS 41	Agkistrodon antivenin	National Inst. of Preventive Medicine Taipei, Taiwan (Details, see above)	*Agkistrodon acutus*
SAS 42	Mamushi	Shanghai Inst. of Biological Products Ministry of Health 1262 Yan An Road Shanghai, People's Republic China Phone: ++86-21-2513189 Fax: ++86-21-2511807	*Agkistrodon blomhoffi brevicaudatus*
SAS 43	D. acutus Antivenom	Shanghai Inst. of Biological Products (Details, see above)	*Deinagkistrodon acutus*

Code No.	Product Name	Manufacturer	Venoms Covered
SAS 44	B. multicinctus Antivenom	Shanghai Inst. of Biological Products (Details, see above)	*Bungarus multicinctus*
SAS 45	Habu antivenom	The Chemo-Serotherap. Res. Institute 668 Okubo, Shimizu Kumamoto 860, Japan Phone: ++81-96-3441211 Fax: ++81-96-3449269	*Trimeresurus flavoviridis*
SAS 46	Mamushi antivenom	The Chemo-Serotherap. Res. Institute Kumamoto, Japan (Details, see above)	*Agkistrodon blomhoffi*
SAS 47	Mamushi antivenom	Takeda Chemical Industries Ltd. Osaka, Japan Phone: ++81-6-2042111 Fax: ++81-6-2042880	*Agkistrodon blomhoffi*
SAS 48	Anti-Yamakagashi Antivenom	The Japan Snake Institute Yabuzuka-honmachi Nittagun, Gunma Prefecture 379-23 Japan Phone: ++81-277-785193 Fax: ++81-277-785520	*Rhabdophis tigrinus Rhabdophis* sp.
SAS 49	Dried Mamushi antivenom	Res. Foundation for Microbial Diseases Osaka University Osaka, Japan Phone: ++81-6-8775121 Fax: ++81-6-8761984	*Agkistrodon halys*
SAS 50	Mamushi antivenom	Kitasato Institute Minato-ku, Tokyo, Japan Phone: ++81-3-4446161	*Agkistrodon halys*
SAS 51	Antirept (African and Middle East Snakes)	Pasteur-Mérieux Sérum et Vaccins Avenue Général Leclerc 69007 Lyon Phone: ++33-72-737707 Fax: ++33-72-737737	*Cerastes cerastes Cerastes vipera Echis carinatus Naja haje Naja naja Naja naja kaouthia Vipera ammodytes Vipera lebetina obtusa Vipera palaestinae*

Code No.	Product Name	Manufacturer	Venoms Covered
SAS 52	Near and Middle East	Behringwerke AG Postfach 1140 35001 Marburg/Lahn 1 Federal Republic of Germany Phone: ++49-6421-390 Fax: ++49-6421-31388 Telex: 0482320	*Cerastes cerastes* *Cerastes vipera* *Echis carinatus* *Echis coloratus* *Naja haje* *Vipera ammodytes* *Vipera lebetina* *Vipera xanthina* *Vipera palaestinae*

D. ANTIVENOMS FOR THE TREATMENT OF ENVENOMATIONS CAUSED BY VENOMOUS SNAKES IN AUSTRALIA AND OCEANIA

Table 12
Antivenoms for the treatment of envenomations caused by venomous snakes in Australia and Oceania

Code No.	Product Name	Manufacturer	Venoms Covered
SAU 1	Death Adder Antivenom	Commonwealth Serum Laboratories 45 Poplar Road Parkville, Victoria 3052 Australia Phone: ++61-3-3891911 Fax: ++61-3-3891434 Telex: AA 32789	*Acanthophis antarcticus* *Acanthophis pyrrhus* *Acanthophis praelongus*
SAU 2	Taipan Antivenom	Commonwealth Serum Laboratories Parkville, Victoria, Australia (Details, see above)	*Oxyuranus microlepidotus* *Oxyuranus scutellatus*
SAU 3	Black Snake Antivenom	Commonwealth Serum Laboratories 45 Poplar Road Parkville, Victoria 3052 Australia (Details, see above)	*Pseudechis australis* *Pseudechis colletti* *Pseudechis guttatus* *Pseudechis porphyriacus*
SAU 4	Tiger Snake	Commonwealth Serum Laboratories Parkville, Victoria, Australia (Details, see above)	*Austrelaps superba* *Austrelaps ramsayi* *Notechis ater* *Notechis scutatus* *Pseudechis colletti* *Pseudechis guttatus* *Pseudechis porphyriacus* *Tropidechis carinatus*
SAU 5	Brown Snake	Commonwealth Serum Laboratories, Parkville, Victoria, Australia (Details, see above)	*Pseudonaja affinis* *Pseudonaja nuchalis* *Pseudonaja textilis*

Code No.	Product Name	Manufacturer	Venoms Covered
SAU 6	Polyvalent Snake Antivenom (Australia - New Guinea)	Commonwealth Serum Laboratories Parkville, Victoria, Australia (Details, see above)	*Acanthophis antarcticus* *Austrelaps superba* *Notechis scutatus* *Oxyuranus microlepida* *Oxyuranus scutellatus* *Pseudechis australis* *Pseudechis papuanus* *Pseudonaja affinis* *Pseudonaja nuchalis* *Pseudonaja textilis*

E. ANTIVENOMS FOR THE TREATMENT OF ENVENOMATIONS CAUSED BY VENOMOUS SNAKES IN EUROPE

After completion of this list, a new ovine antivenom against European vipers, initially based on *Vipera berus,* was released by Therapeutic Antibodies Inc. ("Beritab"), after successful clinical trials in Sweden. This is now the antivenom of choice for European *Vipera* bites.

Table 13
Antivenoms for the treatment of envenomations caused by venomous snakes in Europe

Code No.	Product Name	Manufacturer	Venoms Covered
SEU 1	Ipser Europe	Pasteur-Mérieux Sérum et Vaccins Avenue Général Leclerc 69007 Lyon Phone: ++33-72-737707 Fax: ++33-72-737737	*Vipera ammodytes* *Vipera aspis* *Vipera berus*
SEU 2	Sérum antivenimeux purifié Mérieux	Pasteur Mérieux Lyon, France (Details, see above)	*Vipera aspis* *Vipera berus*
SEU 3	Europe	Behringwerke AG Postfach 1140 35001 Marburg/Lahn Federal Republic of Germany Phone: ++49-6421-390 Fax: ++49-6421-31388 Telex: 042320	*Vipera ammodytes* *Vipera aspis* *Vipera berus* *Vipera kaznakovi* *Vipera latasti* *Vipera palaestinae* *Vipera ursinii* *Vipera xanthina*
SEU 4	Serum antiviperin	Instituto Sieroterapico Vaccinogeno Toscana SCLAVO Via Fiorentina 1 53100Siena, Italy Phone: ++39-577-293111 Fax: ++39-577-293493	*Vipera ammodytes* *Vipera aspis* *Vipera berus* *Vipera ursinii*

Code No.	Product Name	Manufacturer	Venoms Covered
SEU 5	Antiviperinum	Institute of Immunology Rockefellerova 2 Zagreb, Croatia Phone: ++38-41-430333 Fax: ++38-41-277278	*Vipera a. ammodytes Vipera a. meridionalis Vipera aspis Vipera berus Vipera lebetina Vipera mesocoronis Vipera ursinii Vipera xanthina*
SEU 6	Monovalent	National Center of Infectious and Parasitic Diseases 26, Y Sakasov Blvd., 1504 Sofia, Bulgaria Phone: ++35-92-43471 Fax: ++35-92-442260	*Vipera ammodytes Vipera aspis Vipera berus*
SEU 7	Anti-Vipera	Chemapol, Co. Ltd. Kodanska 46 100 10 Prague 10, The Czech Republic Phone: ++42-2-734737 Fax: ++42-2-734576	*Vipera a.ammodytes*
SEU 8	Venise	SEVAC Institute for Sera and Vaccines Korunni 108 101 03 Prague, Czech Republic Phone: ++42-2-734751 Telex: 121852 Fax: ++42-2-737183	*Vipera ammodytes Vipera berus*

VII. REFERENCES

1. **WHO EXPERT COMMITTEE ON BIOLOGICAL STANDARDIZATION**, *Requirements for snake antivenins* (Requirements for biological substances No.21), *World Health Org. techn.Rep.Series*, No.463, 27, 1971.
2. **CHIPPAUX, J.P. AND GOYFFON, M.,** Producers of antivenomous sera, *Toxicon*, 21, 739, 1983.
3. **CHIPPAUX, J.P. AND GOYFFON, M.,** Production and use of snake antivenin, in *Handbook of Natural Toxins*, A.T.Tu, Ed., Dekker, New York, 1991, 529.
4. **DETRAIT, J.,** Repertoire des instituts et laboratoires producteurs de sérums antivenimeux, *Bull.Soc.herpet.France*, 21, 44, 1982.
5. **RUSSELL, F.,** *Snake Venom Poisoning*, 562 pp., Lippincott, Philadelphia, 1980.
6. **RUSSELL, F.E. AND LAURITZEN, L.,** Antivenins, *Trans.Royal Soc.trop.Med.Hyg.*,60, 797,1966.
7. **WORLD HEALTH ORGANIZATION**, Progress in the characterization of venoms and standardization of antivenoms, *WHO Offset Publ.* 58, 1981.
8. **THEAKSTON R.D.G. AND WARRELL, D.A.,** Antivenoms: a list of hyperimmune sera currently available for the treatment of envenoming by bites and stings, *Toxicon*, 29, 1419, 1991.
9. **MARETIC, Z.,** Fish venoms, in *Handbook of natural toxins*, Vol. 3, A.T.Tu, Ed., Dekker, New York, 1988, 445.
10. Personal communication, from The Lister Institute of Preventive Medicine, Brockley Hill, Stanmore, Middlesex HA7 4JD, U.K. stating that they "ceased production 1978 and sale of antivenom in 1984".
11. Personal communication, fax from S.A.I.M.R., Sandringham, South Africa, stating that "FitzSimmons do not manufacture antivenoms and ceased to distribute SAIMR antivenoms years ago".